STANDARDS OF PSYCHIATRIC AND MENTAL HEALTH NURSING PRACTICE

STANDARD I. ASSESSMENT

The Psychiatric–Mental Health Nurse Collects Client Health Data.

Rationale: The assessment interview—which requires linguistically and culturally effective communication skills, interviewing, behavioral observation, database record review, and comprehensive assessment of the client and relevant systems—enables the psychiatric–mental health nurse to make sound clinical judgments and plan appropriate interventions with the client.

STANDARD II. DIAGNOSIS

The Psychiatric–Mental Health Nurse Analyzes the Assessment Data in Determining Diagnoses.

Rationale: The basis for providing psychiatric–mental health nursing care is the recognition and identification of patterns of response to actual or potential psychiatric illnesses and mental health problems.

STANDARD III. OUTCOME IDENTIFICATION

The Psychiatric–Mental Health Nurse Identifies Expected Outcomes Individualized to the Client.

Rationale: Within the context of providing nursing care, the ultimate goal is to influence health outcomes and improve the client's health status.

STANDARD IV. PLANNING

The Psychiatric–Mental Health Nurse Develops a Plan of Care that Prescribes Interventions to Attain Expected Outcomes.

Rationale: A plan of care is used to guide therapeutic intervention systematically and achieve the expected client outcomes.

STANDARD V. IMPLEMENTATION

The Psychiatric–Mental Health Nurse Implements the Interventions Identified in the Plan of Care.

Rationale: **At the basic level,** the nurse may select counseling, milieu therapy, self-care activities, psychobiological interventions, health teaching, case management, health promotion and health maintenance, and a variety of other approaches to meet the mental health needs of clients. In addition to the intervention options available to the basic-level psychiatric–mental health nurse, **at the advanced level,** the certified specialist may provide consultation, engage in psychotherapy, and prescribe pharmacological agents where permitted by state statutes or regulations.

STANDARD Va. COUNSELING
STANDARD Vb. MILIEU THERAPY
STANDARD Vc. SELF-CARE ACTIVITIES
STANDARD Vd. PSYCHOBIOLOGICAL INTERVENTIONS
STANDARD Ve. HEALTH TEACHING
STANDARD Vf. CASE MANAGEMENT
STANDARD Vg. HEALTH PROMOTION AND HEALTH MAINTENANCE

Advanced Practice Interventions Vh–Vj

The following interventions (Vh–Vj) may be performed only by the certified specialist in psychiatric–mental health nursing.

STANDARD Vh. PSYCHOTHERAPY
STANDARD Vi. PRESCRIPTION OF PHARMACOLOGICAL AGENTS
STANDARD Vj. CONSULTATION

STANDARD VI. EVALUATION

The Psychiatric–Mental Health Nurse Evaluates the Client's Progress in Attaining Expected Outcomes.

Rationale: Nursing care is a dynamic process involving change in the client's health status over time, giving rise to the need for new data, different diagnoses, and modifications in the plan of care. Therefore, evaluation is a continuous process of appraising the effect of nursing interventions and the treatment regimen on the client's health status and expected health outcomes.

Foundations of
Psychiatric –
Mental Health Nursing

Elizabeth M. Varcarolis, RN, MA
Professor
Deputy Chairperson
School of Nursing
Borough of Manhattan Community College
City University of New York
New York, New York

Foundations of Psychiatric–Mental Health Nursing

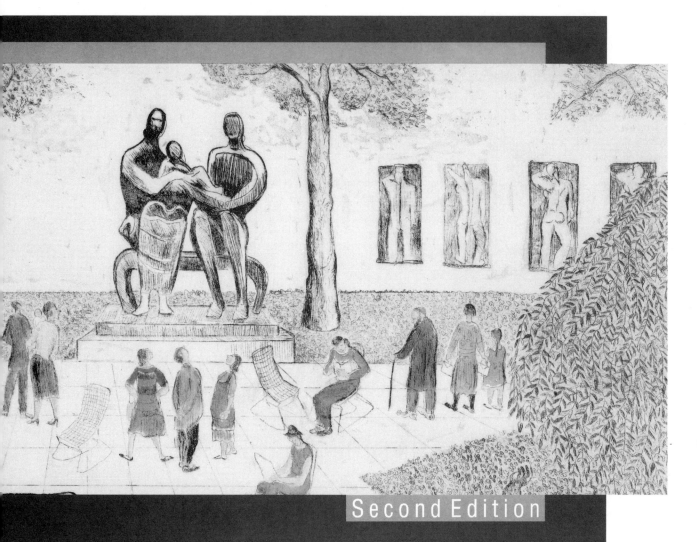

Second Edition

W.B. SAUNDERS COMPANY
A Division of Harcourt Brace & Company
Philadelphia London Toronto Montreal Sydney Tokyo

W.B. Saunders Company
A *Division of Harcourt Brace & Company*

The Curtis Center
Independence Square West
Philadelphia, Pennsylvania 19106

Cover by Aida Anthony Whedon

Library of Congress Cataloging-in-Publication Data

Varcarolis, Elizabeth M.
    Foundations of psychiatric–mental health nursing / Elizabeth M.
Varcarolis.—2nd ed.
      p.   cm.
    Includes bibliographical references and index.
    ISBN 0-7216-3765-5
    1. Psychiatric nursing. I. Title.
    [DNLM: 1. Mental Disorders—nursing. 2. Psychiatric Nursing.   WY
160 V278f 1944]
    RC440.V37 1994
    610.73'68—dc20
    DNLM/DLC   93-4467

Foundations of Psychiatric–Mental Health Nursing, 2nd ed.   ISBN 0-7216-3765-5

Printed in the United States of America.

Last digit is the print number: 9   8   7   6   5   4

To the memory of my father Josiah Merrill, who I
miss every day
and
To my mother Ruth Merrill

With love to my husband, Paul
Who gladdens my heart and centers my life

To the memory of friends who were nurses and who
left behind memories of laughter and warmth,
and unfilled voids

Ruth Ann Geise Pettengill
Cindy Swoards
Aubrey Robinson
Sylvia Vincent Corliss

Contributors

Barbara B. Bauer, RN, MSN
Adult Continuing Education Faculty, Northeast Wisconsin Technical College, Green Bay, Wisconsin; Senior VIP Educator, St. Mary's Hospital Medical Center, Green Bay, Wisconsin; Board Member, Bellin Psychiatric Center, Green Bay, Wisconsin
People Who Defend Against Anxiety Through Aggression Toward Others

Beth Bonham, RN, MSN, CS
Family Support Services Coordinator, Indiana Juvenile Justice Task Force; Formerly Assistant Professor of Nursing, Marian College, Indianapolis, Indiana
Infants, Children, and Adolescents

Penny S. Brooke, RN, MS, JD
Assistant Dean for Student Affairs and Associate Professor, University of Utah College of Nursing, Salt Lake City, Utah; Boards of Trustees, Intermountain Health Care and the Valley Hospitals (LDS, Alta View, and Cottonwood); Nursing Collaborative Council, University of Utah Health Sciences Center, Salt Lake City, Utah
Legal and Ethical Issues

Ann Marie Brown, RNCS, MSN
Director, Mobile Crisis Service, Columbia Presbyterian Medical Center, New York, New York; Private Practice, Individual and Group Psychotherapy
Selected vignettes for defense mechanisms in Anxiety Disorders

Helene S. Charron, RN, MS
Professor and Chairperson, Department of Nursing, Monroe Community College, Rochester, New York
Anxiety Disorders; Somatoform and Dissociative Disorders

Brenda Lewis Cleary, RN, PhD, CS
Regional Dean and Professor, Texas Tech Health Sciences Center School of Nursing, Permian Basin, Odessa, Texas; Gerontological Clinical Nurse Specialist, Seabury Nursing Center, Odessa, Texas
Cognitive Impairment Disorders

Mattie Collins, RN, EdD
Adjunct Nursing Professor, Borough of Manhattan Community College, City University of New York, New York, New York
Communication: The Clinical Interview and the Nurse-Client Relationship

Michelle J. Conant, RN, MSN, CS
Former Adjunct Professor, Nursing Faculty Department of Nursing, Borough of Manhattan Community College, New York, New York; Lehman College, New York, New York; Fairleigh Dickinson University, Madison, New Jersey; Private Practice, Livingston, New Jersey and New York, New York
People Who Defend Against Anxiety Through Eating Disorders

Mary Jane Herron, PhD
Private Practice, Woodcliff Lake, New Jersey
Adult Relationships and Sexuality

William G. Herron, PhD
Private Practice, Woodcliff Lake, New Jersey; Professor, Psychology Department, St. John's University, Jamaica, New York; Faculty Senior Supervisor and Training Analyst, Center for Advanced Psychoanalytic Studies, Teaneck, NJ
Adult Relationships and Sexuality

Anne Cowley Herzog, RN, MSN
Instructor, Department of Nursing, Cypress College, Cypress, California; Educator, University of California Irvine Medical Center, Orange, California
Chronic Mental Illness and the Mentally Ill Who Are Homeless; A Nurse Speaks, Unit V

Signe S. Hill, RN, BSN, MA
Former Instructor, Northeast Wisconsin Technical College, Green Bay, Wisconsin
People Who Defend Against Anxiety Through Aggression Toward Others

Sally Kennedy Holzapfel, RN, MSN, CS, CETN, CGNP
Clinical Nurse Specialist in Gerontology, Department of Veterans Affairs Medical Center, Lyons, New Jersey; Clinical Assistant Professor, University of Medicine and Dentistry of New Jersey, School of Nursing, Newark, New Jersey
Families in Crisis: Family Violence; The Elderly

Catherine M. Lala, RNC, MSN, CNS
Psychiatric–Mental Health Clinical Nurse Specialist, Albany Medical Center, Albany New York
Communication Within Groups

Suzanne Lego, RN, PhD, CS, FAAN
Director, Advanced Certificate Program in Psychoanalytic Training, Columbia University School of Nursing, New York, New York; Private Practice, New York, New York, Pittsburgh, Pennsylvania, and Kent, Ohio
Evolution of Nursing in Psychiatric Settings; Personality Disorders: Antisocial, Paranoid, and Borderline

Kem B. Louie, RN, PhD, CS, FAAN
Associate Professor and Chairperson, Graduate Nursing Program, College of Mount Saint Vincent, Bronx, New York; Adjunct Visiting Assistant Professor, Bronx Municipal Hospital Center, Department of Psychiatry, Bronx, New York

Margie Lovett-Scott, RN, MSN, EdD
Associate Professor, Nursing, State University of New York College at Brockport, Brockport, New York
Cultural Diversity in Mental Health Nursing

Mary McAndrew, RN, MS
Hospital Administrator, Mount Carmel Guild Hospital, Newark, New Jersey
People Who Depend on Substances Other Than Alcohol

Peggy Miller, RN, BSN, MSN Candidate
Associate Professor, Health Science Division, Cypress College, Cypress, California
Chronic Mental Illness and the Mentally Ill Who Are Homeless

Jane Bryant Neese, RN, MS, CS, PhD Candidate
Fellow, WK Kellogg Foundation and Fellow, Center on Aging and Health, University of Virginia, Charlottesville, Virginia; Fellow, National Center for Nursing Research, National Institutes of Health, Bethesda, Maryland
The Hospitalized Person

John A. Payne, RN, MA
Assistant Professor, Borough of Manhattan Community College, City University of New York, New York, New York
A Nurse Speaks, Unit II

Hildegard E. Peplau, RN, EdD, FAAN
Professor Emerita, Rutgers, The State University of New Jersey, New Brunswick, New Jersey
Evolution of Nursing in Psychiatric Settings

Carla E. Randall, RN, MSN
Second Year Coordinator, Salish Kootenai College, Pablo, Montana
A Nurse Speaks, Unit VII

John Raynor, PhD
Professor, Department of Science, Borough of Manhattan Community College, City University of New York, New York, New York

Arnette D. Robinson, RN MSN, DSW
Assistant Professor, Nursing, Borough of Manhattan Community College, City University of New York, New York, New York; Clinical Instructor, Lenox Hill and VA Hospital, New York, New York

L. Sharon Shisler, RN, MA, CS
Psychiatric Clinical Nurse Specialist and Psychiatric Liaison Coordinator, Greenwich Hospital, Greenwich, Connecticut; Group Facilitator for Parent Partnering Program, White Plains Child Care Program, White Plains, New York; Group Facilitator for Women with HIV and AIDS, Greenwich AIDS Alliance Group, Greenwich, Connecticut
A Nurse Speaks, Unit III

Kathleen Smith-DiJulio, RN, MA
Psychosocial Clinical Nurse Specialist, Group Health Cooperative, Seattle, Washington
Families in Crisis: Family Violence; Evidence of Maladaptive Responses to Crisis: Rape; People Who Depend on Alcohol

Judith Sutherland, RN, PhD
Associate Professor, Abilene Intercollegiate School of Nursing, Abilene, Texas
Contributions to Communication: The Client Interview and the Nurse–Client Relationship, text on empathy

Margaret R. Swisher, RN, MSN
Psychiatric Instructor, Brandywine School of Nursing, Coatesville, Pennsylvania
A Nurse Speaks, Unit IV

Julius Trubowitz, EdD
Assistant Professor, Queens College, City University of New York, New York, New York; Private Practice, New York, New York
Historical Overview, Personality Theories, and Classification of Mental Illness; Predominant Therapies and Contemporary Issues

Marcia A. Ullman, RN, MSC
Assistant Professor, Department of Nursing, State University of New York College at Brockport, Brockport, New York
Cultural Diversity in Mental Health Nursing

Elizabeth M. Varcarolis, RN, MA
Professor and Deputy Chairperson, School of Nursing, Borough of Manhattan Community College, City University of New York, New York, New York
Communication: The Clinical Interview and the Nurse–Client Relationship; The Nursing Process in Psychiatric Settings; Anxiety; Crisis and Crisis Intervention; Alterations in Mood: Grief and Depression; Alterations in Mood: Elation in Bipolar Disorder; Schizophrenic Disorders; People Who Contemplate Suicide: Aggression Toward Self

Thomas Wenzka, RN, MSN
Assistant Professor, Department of Nursing, Brunswick College, Brunswick, Georgia; Intake and Group Therapist, Charter By-the-Sea Hospital, St. Simons Island, Georgia
Anxiety and the Mental Health Continuum as a Conceptual Framework

Preface

The 1990s are decidedly complex times. Daily advances in the fields of neurobiology, pharmacology, and immunology need to be integrated within a health care system that is now in transition and within a society that is still evolving and reverberating with change.

There are many social issues that have an impact on the mental and physical health of our children, adults, and the elderly. AIDS, addiction, domestic violence, homelessness and impaired colleagues are some of the phenomena nurses deal with all the time. Concurrently, we are flooded with neurobiological findings that reveal possible causes of some mental health disorders and that point the way to new medications promising the potential to alleviate mental anguish.

It is hoped that the second edition of *Foundations of Psychiatric—Mental Health Nursing* will provide the student with the tools to assess, plan for, and intervene with a diverse client population stricken with multiple common mental health problems and disorders.

FAMILIAR FEATURES RETAINED IN THIS EDITION

The second edition retains the basic nursing process format and uses anxiety and the mental health continuum as the organizing framework, while updating clinical treatments, drug therapies, and social issues.

The clinical chapters (Chapters 11 to 25) continue to use the following format: Theory, Nursing Process, Case Study, and Nursing Care Plan.

- The "assessment" provides standard tools.
- "Planning" includes goals as well as identifying and planning for possible personal thoughts and feelings health care workers often experience.
- "Interventions" include psychotherapeutic intervention, health teaching, somatic therapies, and psychotherapy that is applicable for each group of disorders.
- A case study is presented at the end, followed by a nursing care plan that helps the student translate the theoretical material into a clinical situation.

Self-study exercises and perforated drug cards remain. A new expanded **instructor's manual** provides learning activities, creative games, teaching ideas, up-to-date audio/visual information, as well as new updated multiple choice questions. A **computerized ExaMaster** provides fast and flexible testing options to the instructor. Qualified instructors who have adopted the text for classroom use can request the testbank by contacting their local W. B. Saunders textbook representative or by writing to the Textbook Department, W. B. Saunders Company, The Curtis Center, Independence Square West, Philadelphia, PA 19106-3399.

NEW TO THE SECOND EDITION

- Careful integration of latest findings on biological bases of mental illness has been incorporated into every clinical chapter.
- New chapters include Communications within Groups and Dealing with People with Aggressive Behaviors.

- A separate chapter on the Anxiety Disorders and a second that combines the Somatoform and Dissociative Disorders.
- The topics *child abuse, spouse abuse,* and *elder abuse* are combined in one chapter that highlights the similarities but continues to present the differences in intervention for these situations.
- Psychophysiological disorders have been placed in Chapter 26, The Hospitalized Person, along with updated psychosocial interventions for the person with AIDS, the person who is dying, and a person in chronic pain.
- The chapters on cultural diversity and the chronic mentally ill/homeless client are totally new.
- All chapters have been updated and have undergone significant revisions. The chapters on infants, children, and adolescents and legal and ethical issues have new authors who have made substantial updates.
- Highlights from the DSM-1V *Options* book have been included in the clinical chapters, where appropriate.
- A glossary has been added.

I am heartened and grateful for the support and comments of so many faculty throughout the country. The additions and changes reflect your suggestions offered through the mail survey, those of the reviewers, and through personal correspondence. I welcome your comments and hope you find in this edition the easy reading style, clarity of presenting concepts, and relevance to today's nursing practice that many of you valued in the first edition.

ELIZABETH M. VARCAROLIS

Acknowledgments

I wish to thank all the chapter authors who helped reshape and redefine the second edition of *Foundations of Psychiatric—Mental Health Nursing*. These chapters represent an enormous amount of work and thought, and the book attests to the expertise of these authors. Special thanks to the new authors, some of whom submitted numerous drafts with grace and enthusiasm.

I also wish to thank past contributors whose diligence and knowledge helped make the first edition a success: Juliet L. Tien-Hyatt, Lorenzo M. Valvo, Mary Ursula Guthormsen, Ardis R. Swanson, Margaret H. Pipchick, and Jeffrey S. Grunberg.

Thanks go to Mattie Collins and Judith Sutherland for their contributions to the Communications chapter. Acknowledgment goes to Jeanne Underwood for her review of and suggestions for the group chapter, and to Ann Marie Brown for short clinical vignettes demonstrating defense mechanisms in the Anxiety Disorders chapter.

A special thanks to Kay Charron, who developed a marvelously innovative and refreshing instructor's manual to accompany this edition. It is full of games, crossword puzzles, questions, information on the latest audio/visual materials, and so much more. I thank you, Kay.

Gratitude and appreciation go to colleagues at the Borough of Manhattan Community College who extended themselves on my behalf. Everett Flannery, Chairperson of Allied Health, for his generosity in facilitating my research through computer searches. John Raynor, Department of Sciences, who wrote the "How Does It Work?" pieces on the psychotropic drugs. To my chairperson, Veronica Coleman, whose obvious pleasure in having this text come from our nursing department, always makes my day.

So many creative minds have added to the personality of this second edition. Aida Wheadon, artist and lifelong friend, graciously agreed to provide the cover for this edition. James Varcarolis, my nephew, stole time from his three lives to submit new photographs. The contributors to "A Nurse Speaks" continue to add humanness and warmth in the telling of their stories, and I thank them for what is for me a special part of this text.

As always, thanks to Ilze S. Rader, my editor, whose humor, interest, and creativity continue to keep my enthusiasm high. Thanks to Marie Thomas, editorial assistant, whose gracious manner and efficient style keep things moving along smoothly. I offer sincere thanks to Dave Prout, my developmental editor. We talked, fought, discussed, and disagreed, and consequently, made an excellent team. His ideas and input were invaluable in putting this all together. And to my copy editor, Liz Gauger, whose smooth style and clarifications make us all look good.

I must state emphatically, that what has made working on the revisions exciting and come alive is the dialogue with my talented and knowledgeable reviewers. Teachers from all over the country have shared their opinions, expertise, experience, suggestions, and their warm support for this text. So much of the credit for the positive changes, additions, clarifications, and rethinking goes to them. I truly enjoyed working with you all.

Barbara Aldinger, RN, MSN
Episcopal Hospital
Philadelphia, Pennsylvania

Tracey A. Bergeron, RN, MS, C
Portsmouth Hospital
Portsmouth, New Hampshire

Florence P. Best, RN, MS, BSN
Providence Hospital
Sandusky, Ohio

Elizabeth Bonham, RN, MSN, CS
Marian College
Indianapolis, Indiana

Lorraine M. Clarke, RN, EdM
University of Vermont
Burlington, Vermont

Joyce A. Edwards, PhD
Psychologist, Private Practice
Graduate Faculty, St. Michael's College
Winooski, Vermont

Karen S. Gingrow, RN, PhD
Valdosta State College
Valdosta, Georgia

Helen E. Lowe, RN, MEd, BA
Amarillo College
Amarillo, Texas

Truda Jane McGrew, RN, MSN, BSN
Southwest Mississippi Community
College
Summit, Mississippi

Cleo Newtown-Watkins, RN, MSN
Millard Fillmore Hospital
Buffalo, New York

Almetria Anne Poole, RN, MSN
Itawamba Community College
Fulton, Mississippi

Carla E. Randall, RN, MSN, BSN
Salish Kootenai College
Pablo, Montana

Deborah Ann Rorick, RN, MSN, BSN
Lakeland Community College
Mentor, Ohio

Cynthia Ann Schaeffer, RN, BSN
Pottsville Hospital
Pottsville, Pennsylvania

Rebecca A. Sherwood, RN, DNSc, CS
DeAnza College
Cupertino California

Joanne W. Springer, RN, MSN, CS
Boise State University
Boise Idaho

Judith A. Sutherland, RN, PhD
University of Texas
Tyler, Texas

Joann E. Bohm, RN, MS
Grayson County College
Denison, Texas

Mary Ann Camann, RN, MN, CS
Kennesaw State College
Marietta, Georgia

Anita Deitrick, RN, BSN
Des Moines Area Community College
Ankeny, Iowa

Marsha Garfinkel, RN, MSN
Greater Hartford Community College
Hartford, Connecticut

Alice B. Jehle, RN, MS
Berkshire Community College
Pittsfield, Massachusetts

Christine W. Massey, RN, C
Barton College
Wilson, North Carolina

Marilyn Meder, RN, MSN, CS
Grandview Hospital
Sellersville, Pennsylvania

Joyce Ott, RN, MSN, CS
Community College of Beaver County
Monaca, Pennsylvania

Patricia A. Rahe, RN, BSN, C
Indiana Vocational Technical College
Madison, Indiana

Sandra Roberson, RN, MSN, BSN
Amarillo College
Amarillo, Texas

Elizabeth Savaria-Porter, RN, MS, BS
St. Joseph Hospital
North Providence, Rhode Island

Sandra Schuler, RN, MSN
Montgomery College
Takoma Park, Maryland

Rosanne C. Shinkle, RN, MN
University of North Dakota
Grand Forks, North Dakota

Judy Stovall Leggett, RN, MSN
Itawamba Community College
Fulton, Mississippi

Margaret R. Swisher, RN, MSN, BSN, BA
Brandywine School of Nursing
Caln Township, Pennsylvania

Cheryl Ann Thornburg, RN, MSN
Florence-Darlington Technical College
Florence, South Carolina

Sylvia A. Whiting, RN, PhD, CS
South Carolina State University
Orangeburg, South Carolina

Betty L. Whigham, ARNP, BSN, MEd
Hillsborough Community College
Tampa, Florida

And still through it all, with humor and grace, my husband Paul stands as a constant reminder of what is, after all, the most essential ingredient for growth. Love.

Brief Contents

Contents

Key to Special Features

PART ONE

FOUNDATIONS IN THEORY

BASIC
PSYCHIATRIC CONCEPTS

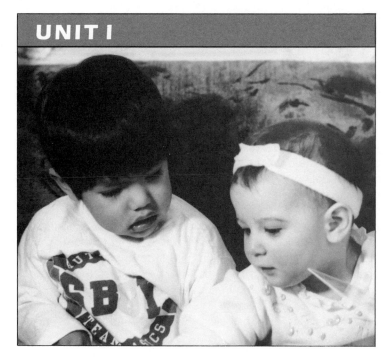

UNIT I

The reward of friendship is itself. The man who hopes for anything else does not understand what true friendship is.

SAINT AILRED OF RIEVAULX

A Nurse Speaks

by Kem Louie

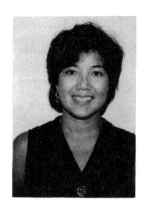

My interest in drug prevention began in the fall of 1987, when I was working as an assistant professor at Lehman College, the Bronx, New York. For decades, this community has existed in the midst of a drug epidemic. Perhaps the most heartbreaking of the innocent victims are the babies born to crack- and substance-abusing mothers. Of these, many are born to AIDS-infected mothers. Nurses are on the front lines in caring for these mothers and babies. Young children are used to sell drugs and as lookouts for law enforcement officers while dealers sell drugs in the streets.

The solution to the drug epidemic is a complex one that involves the commitment of the community. The dean of nursing of the college and the district attorney of Bronx County met to develop a community-based drug prevention program. The idea of nurses and district attorneys educating children about drugs seemed innovative. This is the story of PLAN (Pupils, Lawyers, and Nurses) Against Drugs.

Criminal justice and health care professionals fight drug use in different ways. District attorneys seek to bring those who violate narcotics laws to justice while protecting the rights of both society and the accused. Nurses, on the other hand, educate, counsel, and care for drug-addicted adults and infants. The program emphasizes how each of these professions can combat the effects of drug use in the community.

PLAN Against Drugs consists of four three-hour weekly sessions with a class of 30 10-year-old children, predominantly African Americans and Latino Americans. This age group was chosen for the drug prevention education program because this is the age when children are believed to begin thinking about drug use.

At the first session, a team consisting of a nurse and an assistant district attorney introduces the program and reviews how each professional works to combat drug use in the community. Nurses view drug addiction as a disease and addicts as people who need treatment. I reviewed in simple terms the effects of illicit drugs on body systems. The potential for contracting AIDS through intravenous drug use and transnatal routes is discussed. The children seem to know as much as the professionals in many instances. Many of these young children tell stories of people they know who are addicted to drugs or who have AIDS. Some mention family members. The assistant district attorney discusses undercover police "buy and bust" operations to catch drug dealers and the role of the assistant district attorney in prosecuting defendants. Many of the children also can identify or know drug dealers in their neighborhoods. Incredibly enough, one elementary school was located next door to a crack house.

In the second session, the children go on a field trip to a local hospital to see various settings in which nurses and other health professionals work. The tours are led by nurses in the hospitals. Especially powerful for the children is the tour of the neonatal intensive care unit, where many infants are born drug addicted or HIV infected. During the tour, many of the children express concern for these youngest victims. Many ask if they can touch or hold these babies in their arms. Comments range from "How could these mothers do this to them?" to "Will they live?" I usually responded to their concerns, and sometimes the only answer I could give was "I really don't know."

In the third session, the children are sent to the county courthouse, where they see part of an undercover police officer's testimony on the "buy and bust" operation. The undercover officer testifies about what took place before the arrest of the accused. The defendant is in the courtroom and is sometimes seen in handcuffs. The assistant district attorney in the case generally describes his or her role in the courtroom. Before the court session begins, the judge speaks to the children about being a judge and the judge's role during the court proceedings. The children are usually impressed with the judge's authority and caring concern.

In the fourth and last session, the children go back to the county courthouse, where they conduct their own mock narcotics trial. The script is given to the teacher at the first session. In the script, a 10-year-old is mistakenly accused of selling crack in the school playground. All of the children in the class take part in the trial as judge, defendant, defense lawyers, assistant district attorneys, jury members, and witnesses. The script calls for the school nurse to be a witness and to testify for the "accused" 10-year-old child. This reinforces the nurse's role in educating children about drug prevention. At the conclusion of the mock trial, the 12-member jury deliberates the defendant's guilt or innocence. The trial is videotaped by court technicians, and the tape is given to the teacher on return to the school. One poignant response by a young child will always be remembered: As we left the courthouse, she asked "Why are all the defendants minorities, are we all bad?" This astute observation reveals the complex connections among poverty, high unemployment, and drug use in many urban communities.

This drug prevention program in part addresses the child's self-esteem and self-image in a somewhat powerless society. At the end of four weeks, the children and I were on a first-name basis and generally felt good. The children experienced firsthand the devastating results of drug use, and we were able to share with them our adult world and our concerns for their future.

CHAPTER 1

Historical Overview, Personality Theories, and Classification of Mental Illness

Julius Trubowitz

OUTLINE •

KEY TERMS AND CONCEPTS • • • • • • • • • • • • • • •

The key terms and concepts listed here also appear in bold where they are defined or discussed in this chapter.

ACCOMMODATION

ADAPTIVE-MALADAPTIVE CONTINUUM

ASSIMILATION

CONSCIOUS

CONSTRUCTIVE-DESTRUCTIVE
    CONTINUUM

DEFENSE MECHANISM

DIAGNOSTIC AND STATISTICAL
    MANUAL OF MENTAL DISORDERS
    (DSM)

DISSOCIATION

DSM-III-R

EGO

ID

PLEASURE PRINCIPLE

PRECONSCIOUS

PRIMARY PROCESS

PSYCHIATRY

PSYCHOSEXUAL STAGES OF
  DEVELOPMENT
Anal
Genital
Latency
Oral
Phallic
REALITY PRINCIPLE

SECONDARY PROCESS
SELECTIVE INATTENTION
SELF-SYSTEM
SUBLIMATION
SUPEREGO
UNCONSCIOUS

OBJECTIVES ■

After studying this chapter, the student will be able to

1. Assess his or her own mental health using five important signs of mental health and mental illness identified in this chapter.
2. Name one contribution of each of the following figures: Hippocrates, Plato, Aristotle, Asclepiades, Johann Weyer, Phillippe Pinel, and Benjamin Rush.
3. Identify Freud's basic assumptions of personality development and discuss his theory of development of personality as it relates to:
   A. Levels of awareness
   B. Agencies of the mind (id, ego, superego)
   C. Defenses against anxiety
4. Compare and contrast the developmental stages of Freud, Erikson, and Piaget.
5. Relate Sullivan's security operations to a personal experience.
6. Examine the basic assumptions of cognitive therapy.
7. Identify the strengths and weaknesses of the DSM-III-R classification of mental disorders.

Mental Health and Mental Illness

CONCEPTS OF MENTAL HEALTH AND MENTAL ILLNESS

Mental health professionals are faced with the problem of defining mental illness and mental health. Agreement on the definition of mental illness and mental health has been elusive throughout history. In the past, definitions have used statistical measures. The term *mental illness* was applied to behaviors, described as strange and different, that deviated from an established norm. However, such criteria are inadequate because they may suggest that mental health is based on conformity. If such definitions were used, nonconformists and independent thinkers, such as Abraham Lincoln, Mahatma Gandhi, Socrates, and Martin Luther King, Jr., would be judged mentally ill.

The field of mental illness is plagued by a host of myths and misconceptions. One myth is that to be mentally ill is to be different and odd. Another misconception is that to be healthy, one must be logical and rational. But many of those suffering from mental illness are not different and odd, and no "healthy" human is fully logical and rational. There are people who show extremely abnormal behavior and are characterized as mentally ill who are far more like the rest of us than different from us. There is no obvious and consistent line between mental illness and mental health. *In fact, all human behavior lies somewhere along a continuum of mental health and mental illness.*

A helpful approach in defining mental illness and mental health is based on evaluating individual behavior in two dimensions:

1. On a continuum from *adaptive* to *maladaptive.*
2. On a continuum from *constructive* to *destructive.*

Along the **adaptive-maladaptive continuum,** behaviors are assessed to the degree that they contribute to or are detrimental to the individual's psychological well-being. For example, does the behavior widen or restrict the range of possible responses to a problem of living? Does it raise or lower self-esteem? Does it create situations in which the individual or others are more likely to experience relief of tension or stress?

Maladaptive behavior allows a problem to continue and often generates new problems, interfering significantly —often over an extended period of time—with an individual's ability to function in such important areas

Table 1-1 ■ MENTAL HEALTH VERSUS MENTAL ILLNESS	
SIGNS OF MENTAL HEALTH	**SIGNS OF MENTAL ILLNESS**
Happiness A. Finds life enjoyable. B. Can see in objects, people, and activities their possibilities for meeting one's needs.	**Major Depressive Episode** A. Loss of interest or pleasure in all or almost all usual activities and pastimes. B. Mood as described by person is depressed, sad, hopeless, discouraged, "down in the dumps."
Control Over Behavior A. Can recognize and act on cues to existing limits. B. Can respond to the rules, routines, and customs of any group to which one belongs.	**Control Disorder, Undersocialized, Aggressive** A. A repetitive and persistent pattern of aggressive conduct in which the basic rights of others are violated.
Appraisal of Reality A. Accurate picture of what is happening around one. B. Good sense of the consequences, both good and bad, that will follow one's acts. C. Can see the difference between the "as if" and "for real" in situations.	**Schizophrenic Disorder** A. Bizarre delusions, such as delusions of being controlled. B. Auditory hallucinations. C. Delusions with persecutory or jealous content.
Effectiveness in Work A. Within limits set by abilities, can do well in tasks attempted. B. When meeting mild failure, persists until determines whether or not one can do the job.	**Adjustment Disorder with Work (or Academic) Inhibition** A. Inhibition in work or academic functioning where previously there was adequate performance.
A Healthy Self-concept A. Sees self as approaching one's ideals, as capable of meeting demands. B. Reasonable degree of self-confidence helps in being resourceful under stress.	**Dependent Personality Disorder** A. Passively allows others to assume responsibility for major areas of life because of inability to function independently. B. Lacks self-confidence, e.g., sees self as helpless, stupid.

Data from Redl F, Wattenberg W. Mental Hygiene in Teaching. New York: Harcourt, Brace & World, 1959, pp 198–201; American Psychiatric Association. Diagnostic and Statistical Manual of Mental Disorders, 3rd ed, revised (DSM-III-R). Washington, DC: American Psychiatric Association, 1987.

of life as health, work, love, and interpersonal relationships. On the other hand, *adaptive behavior* solves problems in living and enhances an individual's life.

Table 1-1 identifies important aspects of mental health on a continuum. These aspects include degree of (1) happiness, (2) control over behavior, (3) appraisal of reality, (4) effectiveness in work, and (5) health of self-concept.

Regarding the second dimension, behavior along the **constructive-destructive continuum** often affects others as much as the individual. *Destructive behavior* not only results in failure to deal with a problem — and thus is maladaptive — but also undermines or destroys the psychological and often biological well-being of the individual and others. Such behavior — whether it occurs once or repeatedly — may seriously undermine health, significantly increase chances of (or actually bring about) death, or drastically affect psychological functioning in the individual or others. On the other hand, *constructive behavior* contributes to psy-

chological growth and biological well-being. It improves the health and positively influences the psychological functioning of the individual and others.

Historical Overview

Psychiatry can trace its origins to the beginning of the history of humanity. Its earliest roots are found in primitive peoples' conception of illness and treatment. In the prescientific era of primitive humanity, the approach to illness and treatment was based on magic and superstition (as were all life's phenomena). It was only with the development of scientific medicine during the Greek era that psychiatry moved out of the realm of the supernatural and established a true scientific beginning. The Greeks perceived disease as a natural development, and mental illness was observed and studied as a disease phenomenon. It was the great scholars of ancient Greece—Hippocrates, Plato, and Aristotle—who influenced the development of psychiatry through the modern era.

The value of clinical observation, the beginning of personality theory, the relationship between mental health and mental illness, and the first steps in the humane treatment of the mentally ill client were all contributions of Greek thinking.

Psychiatry is the science of curing or healing disorders of the psyche. It is the medical specialty that is derived from the study, diagnosis, treatment, and pre-

vention of mental disorders. The following section traces the development of psychiatry from primitive cultures through the development of dynamic psychiatry. Follow the narrative by using Table 1–2 as a guide.

PRIMITIVE CULTURES

The field of psychiatry evolved from our first primitive attempts to understand and treat our own illnesses and abnormal behaviors. All physical or mental disorders had superstitious or supernatural explanations.

Table 1–2 ■ HISTORICAL OVERVIEW—MENTAL HEALTH DEVELOPMENT

	CONCEPTIONS OF ABNORMAL BEHAVIOR		CONTRIBUTIONS	
Culture	**Principal Theories of Causation**	**Characteristic Methods of Helping**	**Positive**	**Negative**
Primitive cultures	Possession by evil spirits, sorcerers, ghosts	Magic, exorcism		
Ancient Greece	Supernatural forces and divine intervention; beginning of naturalistic explanation of sickness	Observation replaces superstition; still mainly primitive physical methods; start of humane treatment approaches	Beginning of concern with humanity of individual	Continuation of confinement; little recognition of psychological or social factors
Medieval period	Possession by devils and sorcerers	Harsh, primitive methods; banishment; first hospitals established	Establishment of first hospitals	Movement back to irrational explanation and harsh treatment of mentally ill
Renaissance	Sorcery, witchcraft, and naturalistic explanation of sickness	Harsh physical punishment; death; rebirth of humane attitude; clinical observation and description	Forerunner of modern clinical description	Ruthless persecution of the mentally ill
17th and 18th centuries	Irrationality and social deviance	Isolation and inhumane physical treatment		Isolation and harsh physical treatment
Mid-18th and early 19th centuries	Sickness; mental illness	Humane treatment; discovery of animal magnetism and hypnosis impetus for psychotherapy	Pinel—"breaking the chains," changes in mental hospitals, less barbaric treatment	
Late 19th and early 20th centuries	Intrapsychic, usually unconscious conflict	Emergence of psychotherapy; analysis and interpretation of free associations, dreams, and other behaviors	Recognition of importance of motivation and early childhood development	Overemphasis on past and unconscious factors as compared with interpersonal and social factors
Mid-20th century	Conflicts between individuals; family, community, and social forces	Marital, family, and community interventions designed to deal with problems of interaction between and among people	Recognition of importance of interaction among individual, family, and society	Interpersonal-social approach can ignore biological and other individual factors
1970–1990s	Neurobiochemical abnormalities in combination with psychological factors	Chemical therapies	Discovery of neurobiological factors influencing mental disease; proliferation of newer biochemical therapies effective in treating mental disorders	Overemphasis on view that "it all comes down to chemistry"

Adapted from Altrocchi J. Abnormal Behavior. New York: Harcourt Brace Jovanovich, 1980, p 30.

Whether a person suffered from headaches and fever or displayed aberrant, bizarre thinking and behavior, primitive humanity attributed it all to the intervention of supernatural forces, such as evil spirits, gods, witches, and magicians. Primitive humanity believed that illness resulted from violations of the group's laws and taboos.

Treatment methods and techniques of primitive medicine belong in the realm of the magical. The role of treating illness was vested in the medicine man or woman, the shaman, or the healer.

GREEK AND ROMAN BELIEFS

The true history of psychiatry, like that of scientific medicine, begins with the Greeks. The Greeks are generally credited with providing the first scientific view of mental disorders.

Hippocrates (460–377 B.C.) epitomized the movement away from the supernatural and toward the natural explanation of mental illness. Called the **Father of Medicine,** Hippocrates, who devised an oath of ethical behavior that has guided physicians for centuries, advocated the separation of medicine from philosophy and theology. He vehemently attacked magical and religious explanations of illness.

Plato (427?–347 B.C.) believed that an individual's entire life merited study. His *Republic* mentions that one could write a psychological biography of a man from his earliest years, when "the soul is easily molded," through his relationship with other members of his family and his educational process. There are striking parallels between Plato's three-part division of the human soul and Freud's theories. Plato's three-part division and the Freudian model of id, ego, and superego (to be discussed more fully later) are strikingly similar.

Aristotle, Plato's pupil (384–322 B.C.), made a significant contribution to the use of clinical observation. Although he is thought of as a great philosopher, Aristotle was a physician who observed a continuum in psychological reactions from normal to pathological behavior. Aristotle viewed psychological reactions as expressions of the total person rather than manifestations of a specific diseased part (Zilboorg and Henry 1941). This point has contemporary relevance in light of the current emphasis on holistic medicine.

Clinical observation was further developed and emphasized by Asclepiades (around 100 B.C.), whom some have called the Father of Psychiatry (Lewis 1942). As a pioneer in the application of humane treatment methods, Asclepiades opposed the use of mechanical restraints, an issue that recurs in the history of the treatment of the mentally ill. Asclepiades prescribed occupational therapy to increase attention span and memory and introduced music therapy for calming agitated clients (Major 1954).

MEDIEVAL PERIOD

Although Western culture attempted to preserve the Greek traditions of psychiatry, there were few positive developments during the Middle Ages, a period of about 1000 years from the fifth century to the fifteenth century. In Europe, this period was characterized by a breakdown of social conditions, with wars, plagues, and migrations. Life was unpredictable and precarious. Surgery was taken up by barbers and their assistants, obstetrics was handled by midwives, and psychiatry was practiced by exorcising priests and witch-hunting clerics. Clerics gradually assumed an important role in medical writing and practice, and pertinent clinical observation on mental illness began to dwindle. The mentally ill inspired great fear and were regarded as being possessed by the devil and by evil spirits. Harsh physical treatment and severe punishments were used to purge the mentally ill of their evil spirits. The severely mentally ill were often turned out of their houses and left to fend for themselves. In central Europe, they were placed on boats, "ships of fools," to wander along the rivers of that region. The boat became a symbol of the wandering mind deprived of guidance.

However, in the fourth century, general hospitals were established, and a few possessed separate sections for the mentally ill. According to Lewis (1942), a hospital specifically for clients with mental disease opened in Jerusalem in 490 A.D.

THE RENAISSANCE

Three major conflicting trends regarding the care of the mentally ill developed during the Renaissance. They were (1) the increase in witch hunting, (2) the rebirth of humane attitudes toward the mentally ill, and (3) greater progress toward a scientific explanation of mental illness.

This period was one of profound contradictions. On one hand, there was the ruthless persecution of the mentally ill as witches. Those who showed the slightest psychological deviation or peculiarity were suspected of being witches or sorcerers. All of life's misfortunes (e.g., a poor harvest, death, or a broken marriage) were seen as the work of the devil.

A textbook, *The Witch Hammer*, was published in 1489 by two German theologians. Fanatical in their approach, these theologians had as their goal the extermination of witches. With political, religious, and scientific support and the authority of Pope Innocent VIII in 1484 (Zilboorg and Henry 1941), they set out on a witch hunt. Thousands of mentally ill people were put to death, along with those who were political and religious dissenters (who were then deemed witches) (Bromberg 1954).

In sharp contrast to this callous, cruel persecution, the Renaissance later brought the rebirth of a humane attitude toward the mentally ill. A deep sympathy for the unfortunate sick was nurtured.

Johann Weyer (1515–1588), a major figure identified with humane treatment of the mentally ill, is regarded as having made the greatest contribution to psychiatry during the Renaissance (Zilboorg and Henry 1941). Weyer, considered today to be the Father of Modern Psychiatry (Mora 1967), recognized that "witches" and those "possessed" were mentally ill and demanded that they be treated by doctors rather than by priests.

Another contribution to psychiatry at this time was made by Paracelsus (1493–1541). He is credited with having made the first reference to unconscious motivation in metal illness (Zilboorg and Henry 1941).

THE 17TH AND 18TH CENTURIES

During the seventeenth and eighteenth centuries, two historic developments changed the way the mentally ill were perceived and treated. *First*, beginning in the seventeenth century, reason came to prevail in science, philosophy, and religion. Reason took the place of God. The attitude toward mental illness in seventeenth- and eighteenth-century western Europe was one of shame, because mental illness did not fit the scheme of reason.

Second, as the mentally ill populations became less identified with the devil and witchcraft, they, along with the poor, were viewed as a social problem. The governments decided to resolve their social crisis by putting all these unfortunates in prison. This type of prison was called a "hôpital général" in France, a "Zuchthaus" in Germany, and a "workhouse" in Great Britain. Four years after its opening, the general hospital in Paris housed 6000 people, including beggars, vagrants, prostitutes, criminals, cripples, old people, orphans, those suffering from venereal disease, homosexuals, "unbelievers," and the mentally ill. This became the rule under governments of the mid-seventeenth century.

In these institutions, the mentally ill were chained, and doctors were practically never consulted. During this period, physical treatment methods designed to serve as shock therapy for the mentally ill were actively developed. One such treatment was "ducking." The client was plunged again and again into water as a shock measure.

THE MID-18TH AND EARLY 19TH CENTURIES

Phillippe Pinel (1745–1826) is credited with the beginning of humane treatment of the mentally ill. In 1793, Pinel was put in charge of the Bicêtre asylum and, in 1795, of the Salpêtrière, both in Paris. He was a reformer and humanitarian who opposed the traditional view of punishment for the mentally ill. He objected to bloodletting; he opposed indiscriminate prescription of drugs; and he rejected beatings. Pinel described ducking as a "medical delirium, more serious than the delirium of patients" (Ackerknecht 1968). He directed restraints to be removed and chains to be broken.

Pinel was also a gifted therapist. He sought to make contact with, and understand the inner experiences of, his mentally ill clients. His concerned attitude and his emphasis on establishing a trusting relationship with his clients have led some historians to consider Pinel a pioneer in the use of psychotherapy for the severely mentally ill (Reik 1956).

Pinel made daily rounds, examining clients, observing their behavior, and taking notes on their conversations. Historians trace the development of psychiatric case reports and case histories to Pinel's observational methods (Zilboorg and Henry 1941).

Under Pinel's leadership, the hospital became the main tool in treating the mentally ill client. Psychotherapeutic measures were to be based strictly on the authority and expert knowledge of the physician. More humane treatment methods were introduced, appropriate segregation of types of mental clients was instituted, and occupational and recreational therapeutic programs were established in the hospital regimen.

Benjamin Rush, another leader, called the Father of American Psychiatry, wrote the first American textbook of psychiatry in 1812.

THE EMERGENCE OF DYNAMIC PSYCHIATRY

Psychiatry had made great strides since the era of primitive medicine. However, the way the mind functioned remained largely an uncharted, undiscovered world.

Franz Anton Mesmer (1734–1815), a controversial Austrian physician, presented a theory of mental operations that, although flawed, led toward the understanding of the workings of the mind. He claimed that through his mysterious powers, called animal magnetism, he could cure a whole range of physical and mental disorders. He was able to provoke the appearance of symptoms in clients by his physical presence or by his gestures.

It was a disciple of Mesmer, Marquis de Puysegur (1751–1825), who made the discovery that provided the impetus for the development of the movement called dynamic psychiatry. Puysegur "magnetized" a young peasant named Victor Race, who fell into a strange sleep in which he seemed to be more awake and aware than in his normal waking state. Victor retained no memory of that state once it had passed.

Puysegur's discovery provided a new understanding of what would later be called the unconscious. Mental life began to be seen as a dynamic energy system of forces. The therapeutic implications of the psychological tie between the client and magnetizer (later the hypnotist and then the psychotherapist) came into the mainstream of psychiatry a century later in the work of Jean-Martin Charcot (1835–1893) and his contemporaries. Charcot, a leading neurologist, conferred a scientific dignity on hypnosis when he read his famous paper on hypnosis at the Academie des Sciences in Paris in 1882.

It was Pierre Janet (1859–1947) who advanced the knowledge of the functioning of the mind and whose contributions brought a rich harvest of ideas to dynamic psychiatry. Mainly using hypnosis, Janet was the first to demonstrate that many symptoms of hysteria and other "neuroses" lay in what he called "subconscious fixed ideas" (Ellenberger 1970). In the development of dynamic psychiatry from Charcot and Janet, the path leads to Sigmund Freud.

Major Theories of Personality

All people go through a series of stages in their development from infancy through old age. Each stage has its own character and offers its own unique opportunities for growth. The meaning of particular events and relationships is deeply influenced by the stage in the life cycle in which they occur. Although each of us is unique, we all go through the same basic stages of growth. Each has its own special contribution to the individual as a whole. Hebrew, Chinese, and Greek writings dating back over 2000 years attest to our interest in and observation of the "stages of man." Each ancient writing has identified similar stages in the human life cycle (Levison and Gooden 1985).

Nurses draw on relevant theories of personality and human development as a basis for assessment, nursing diagnosis, planning, intervention, and evaluation. Different theorists view the life cycle through their own disciplines and individual theories of personality development.

The contributions of Freud, Erikson, Sullivan, Piaget, and the cognitive theorists form important theoretical foundations used in all medical and nursing practices, not just in the specialties of psychiatry or psychiatric nursing.

FREUD

Sigmund Freud (1856–1939), an Austrian psychiatrist and the founder of psychoanalysis, developed a complex theoretical formulation of the nature of the human personality. The following major components of his theory are discussed in the following sections: (1) levels of awareness, (2) personality structure, (3) the concept of anxiety and defense mechanisms, and (4) psychosexual stages of development.

Levels of Awareness

Essentially, Freud's levels of awareness provide a mental typography that is divided into three parts: (1) the conscious, (2) the preconscious, and (3) the unconscious.

CONSCIOUS. The **conscious** includes all experiences that are within a person's awareness at any given time. For example, all intellectual, emotional, and interpersonal aspects of a person's behavior that *a person is aware of and is able to control* are within conscious awareness. All information that is easily remembered and immediately available to an individual is in the conscious mind. The conscious mind is logical and, according to Freud, regulated by the reality principle.

PRECONSCIOUS. The **preconscious** includes experiences, thoughts, feelings, or desires that might not be in immediate awareness but can be recalled to consciousness. The preconscious (sometimes called subconscious) can help screen out extraneous information and can enhance concentration. The preconscious can censor certain wishes and thinking and helps repress unpleasant thoughts or feelings.

UNCONSCIOUS. Although Freud cannot be credited with discovering the unconscious, it was Freud who developed the concept of the unconscious in clear, rich, and original terms. Freud described the mind as an iceberg to convey the relationship between the conscious and the unconscious. The water's surface represents the boundary between conscious and unconscious, with nine tenths of the mind submerged under water (Fig. 1–1).

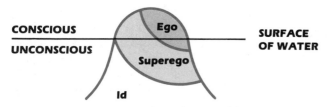

Figure 1–1. *The mind as an iceberg.*

The **unconscious** refers to all memories, feelings, thoughts, or wishes that are not available to the conscious mind. Often these repressed memories, thoughts, feelings, or wishes could, if made prematurely conscious, trigger enormous anxiety. However, unconscious material often does become manifest in dreams, slips of the tongue, or jokes, or through the use of hypnosis, therapy, or certain drugs (e.g., sodium pentothal and hallucinogens).

The unconscious exists comfortably with extreme contradictions and ambivalence (love and hate toward the same object), intense emotions, and strong sexual urges. The unconscious is not logical, has no conception of time, and is governed by what Freud calls the pleasure principle.

Conscious, preconscious, and *unconscious* are not mental processes or systems. They are adjectives that describe the quality of psychological activity.

Personality Structure

Freud sought to describe what he called the "anatomy of the mental personality." He isolated three categories of experience—the id, the ego, and the superego—which represent a method of looking at the way an individual functions. They are not separate entities or sections of the mind. Very roughly, they may be identified as biologically driven energy (id), ways of coping with reality (ego), and finally, conscience (superego). The way the three interact, the conflicts they produce, and their blendings provide a comprehensive picture of the behavior of the individual.

THE ID. The **id** is the "core of our being." It is the source of all drives and the reservoir of instincts. The id is the oldest and the first original function of the personality, and it is the basis out of which the ego and the superego develop. The id includes all of our genetic inheritance, our reflexes, and our capacities to respond, including our instincts, basic drives, needs, and wishes that motivate us. It is the reservoir of psychic energy and furnishes all of the power for the operation of the other two systems. It is with us at birth.

The id operates according to the **pleasure principle** and uses primary processes. The pleasure principle

refers to seeking immediate tension reduction. The id cannot tolerate increases in libido, or tension, which are experienced as uncomfortable states. Therefore, the id seeks to discharge the tension and return to a more comfortable, constant level of energy. To avoid painful tension and obtain pleasure, the id acts immediately in an impulsive, irrational way. It pays no attention to the consequences of actions and therefore often behaves in ways harmful to self and others.

Freud makes a distinction between primary process thinking and secondary process thinking. **Primary process** is a psychological activity in which the id attempts to reduce tension by hallucinating or forming an image of the object that will satisfy its needs and remove the tension. For example, the primary process provides the hungry individual with a mental picture of food. Picturing a hamburger momentarily reduces hunger pangs. This hallucinatory experience in which the desired object is present in the form of a memory image is called wish fulfillment. This activity is present in the mental functioning of newborns, in nocturnal dreams, and in the hallucinations of psychotics. Picturing a bottle or the breast partially pacifies the hungry infant, but it does not satisfy his or her need. The primary process by itself is not capable of reducing tension. The hungry infant cannot eat mental images of food. A new or secondary psychological process must develop if the individual is to survive. When this occurs, the structure of the second system of the personality, the ego, begins to take form.

THE EGO. The **ego** emerges because the needs, wishes, and demands of the id require appropriate exchanges with the outside world of reality. The hungry person has to be able to seek, find, and eat food in order to meet his or her needs and survive. The ego emerges out of the id and acts as an intermediary between the id and the external world. The ego is said to begin its development during the fourth or fifth month of life. The ego distinguishes between things in the mind and things in the external world, whereas the id knows only the subjective reality of the mind. *Reality testing is one function of the ego.*

The ego follows the reality principle and operates by means of the **secondary process,** i.e., realistic thinking. The aim of the reality principle is to satisfy the id's impulses in the external world with an object that is suitable. The **reality principle** determines whether an experience is true or false and whether it has external existence or not. Whereas the id employs fantasies and wishes of the primary process to satisfy a need, the ego uses the realistic thinking characteristic of the secondary process. Using the secondary process, the ego devises a plan and then tests the plan, usually by some kind of action, to see whether it will work. *Problem solving, then, is another function of the ego.* For example, the hungry person figures out where to find food and then proceeds to look for it in that place.

The ego has been called the executive of the personality. The ego becomes the mediator between the organism and the outer world. Through the use of mental functions of judgment and intelligence, the ego selects the parts of the environment to which it will respond and decides what instincts will be satisfied, and in what fashion. Carrying out its executive function is not an easy task for the ego. The ego has to try to integrate the often conflicting demands of its "three harsh masters"—external reality, the id, and the superego.

THE SUPEREGO. The third and last system of personality to be developed is the **superego.** It is the internal representative of the values, ideals, and moral standards of society. It comes from the interactions with one's parents during the extended period of childhood dependency. From a system of rewards and punishments originally imposed on the child from without, the child internalizes the moral standards of parents and society. The superego is the moral arm of personality. It strives for perfection rather than pleasure and represents the ideal rather than the real.

The superego consists of two subsystems: the conscience and the ego-ideal. What parents view as improper and what they punish the child for doing become incorporated into the child's conscience. The conscience refers to the capacity for self-evaluation and criticism. When moral codes are violated, the conscience punishes the person by instilling guilt. A maladaptive example of this behavior is seen in the extreme condition of depression, in which people berate themselves cruelly for minor actions and trivial shortcomings.

What parents approve of and what they reward the child for doing become incorporated as the ego-ideal. The mechanism by which this incorporation takes place is called introjection. Living up to one's ego-ideal results in the person's feeling proud and increases self-esteem.

The development of the superego is a necessary part of socialization because young children's egos are too weak to control their impulses. Parental "thou shalt nots" are needed for a period of time. But a harsh superego can be uncompromising and may lead to blocking necessary and reasonable satisfactions. Furthermore, a rigid superego can create feelings of inferiority, expressed as "I'm a bad person," when the individual fails to meet parental dictates. The superego is said to have its development during the phallic stage (3–5 years).

The three systems of the personality, the id, the ego, and the superego, are names for the psychological processes that follow different operating principles. In a mature and well-adjusted personality, they work together as a team under the administrative leadership of the ego. However, development does not always proceed smoothly. Too powerful an id or a superego may gain control, and imbalance and maladjustment may be the result. Let's take a look at a hypothetical situation and consider the roles of the id, ego, and superego. In the case of a young man or woman out on a date with an attractive member of the opposite sex with whom he or she might wish to have a sexual relationship, the id would declare, "I want, I want!" while the superego might assert, "Thou shalt not!" The ego would be faced with the problem of meeting the id's demands within the limitations and standards of society. A solution might involve the young person's waiting until he or she becomes better acquainted with the other individual or some other social norm is met.

Defense Mechanisms

Freud believed that anxiety was an inevitable part of living. The environment, physical and social, presents dangers and insecurities, threats and satisfactions. It can produce pain and increases in tension as well as pleasure and reductions in tension. Everyone must cope with anxiety. The ego develops defenses, or **defense mechanisms,** to ward off anxiety by preventing conscious awareness of threatening feelings. Without defense mechanisms, anxiety might overwhelm and paralyze us and interfere with daily living.

Defense mechanisms share two common features: (1) they operate on an unconscious level (except suppression), so that we are not aware of their operation, and (2) they deny, falsify, or distort reality to make it less threatening. We cannot survive without defense mechanisms. However, if they become too extreme in distorting reality, interference with healthy adjustment and personal growth may occur. A fuller discussion of defense mechanisms is found in Chapter 9. Table 1–3 includes an overview of some common defense mechanisms and a brief description of their characteristics, with examples from daily living.

Psychosexual Stages of Development

Freud believed that human development proceeds through a series of stages, from infancy to adulthood. Each stage is characterized by the inborn tendency of

Table 1–3 ■ COMMON DEFENSE MECHANISMS

DEFENSE MECHANISM	CHARACTERISTICS	EXAMPLE
Repression	Blocking a wish or desire from conscious expression	You forget the name of someone for whom you have intense negative feelings
Projection	Attributing an unconscious impulse, attitude, or behavior to someone else (blaming or scapegoating behavior)	A man who is attracted to his friend's wife on an unconscious level accuses his wife of flirting with his friend
Reaction-formation	An intense feeling regarding an object, person, or feeling is beyond awareness and acted out consciously in an opposite manner	You treat someone whom you unconsciously dislike intensely in an overly friendly manner
Regression	Returning to an earlier form of expressing an impulse	A child resumes bed-wetting after having long since stopped (after the birth of a child, a baby brother)
Rationalization	Unconsciously falsifying an experience by giving a "rational" explanation	A student who did not study for an exam blames his failure on the teacher's poor lecture material and the unfairness of the exam
Identification	Modeling behavior after someone else	A six-year-old girl dresses up in her mother's dress and high-heeled shoes
Displacement	Discharging intense feelings for one person onto another object or person who is less threatening, thereby satisfying an impulse with a substitute object	A child who has been scolded by her mother hits her doll with a hairbrush
Sublimation	Rechanneling an impulse into a more socially desirable outlet	A student satisfies sexual curiosity by conducting sophisticated research into sexual behaviors

all individuals to reduce tension and seek pleasure. Each stage of development during the first five years is defined and named for those parts of the body (erogenous zones) that produce the main source of gratification during that stage. Each stage is associated with a particular conflict that must be resolved before the child can move successfully to the next stage. Freud believed that the experiences during the early stages determine an individual's adjustment patterns and the personality traits that person has as an adult. In fact, Freud thought that the personality was rather well formed by the time the child entered school and that subsequent growth consisted of elaborating this basic structure.

The three early stages, collectively called the pregenital stage, are the oral, anal, and phallic stages. The child then enters a prolonged latency period, the quiet years in which the dynamics become more or less stabilized. With the arrival of adolescence, there is a burst of libidinal forces, primitive impulses from the id, which upsets the stabilization of the latency period and gradually comes under control as the adolescent moves into adulthood. The final developmental stage of adolescence and adulthood is the genital stage. Table 1–4 summarizes Freud's **psychosexual stages of development** and can be used to follow the narrative.

ORAL STAGE (0–1 year). The first stage is the **oral stage,** which lasts from birth to age one year. The baby is "all mouth," getting most of his or her gratification from sucking. The erogenous zones are the lips and mouth, through which the infant receives nourishment, has the closest contact with the mother (in breast-feeding), and discovers information about the world.

During this stage, which Freud called "primary narcissism," the infant is concerned only with his or her own gratification. The infant is all id, operating on the pleasure principle and striving for immediate gratification of needs. The ego begins to emerge during this time (fourth or fifth month of life), as the infant begins to see him- or herself as separate from the mothering one. This is the beginning of the development of a "sense of self." When the infant experiences gratification of basic needs, a sense of trust and security begins.

ANAL STAGE (1–3 years). Freud's second psychosexual stage is the **anal stage,** which is experienced in the second year of life. Generally, toilet training occurs during this period. According to Freud, the child gains pleasure both from the elimination of the feces and from their retention. Toilet training involves converting an involuntary activity, the elimination of bodily wastes, into a voluntary one. Until this time,

Table 1–4 ■ FREUD'S PSYCHOSEXUAL STAGES OF DEVELOPMENT

STAGE (AGE)	SOURCE OF SATISFACTION	PRIMARY CONFLICT	TASKS	DESIRED OUTCOME	OTHER POSSIBLE PERSONALITY TRAITS
Oral (0–1 year)	Mouth (sucking, biting, chewing)	Weaning	Mastery of gratification of oral needs; **beginning of ego development (4–5 months)**	Trust in the environment develops with the realization that needs can be met	Fixation at the oral stage is associated with passivity, gullibility and dependence, the use of sarcasm, and the development of orally focused habits (e.g., smoking, nail-biting)
Anal (1–3 years)	Anal region (expulsion and retention of feces)	Toilet training	Beginning to gain a sense of control over instinctual drives; learns to delay immediate gratification to gain a future goal	Control over impulses	Fixation associated with anal retentiveness (stinginess, rigid thought patterns, obsessive-compulsive disorder) or anal expulsive character (messiness, destructiveness, cruelty)
Phallic (Oedipal) (3–6 years)	Genitals (masturbation)	Oedipus and Electra complexes	Sexual identity with parent of same sex; **beginning of superego development**	Identification with parent of same sex	Unresolved outcomes may result in difficulties with sexual identity and difficulties with authority figures
Latency (6–12 years)	—	—	Growth of ego functions (social, intellectual, mechanical) and the ability to care about and relate to others outside the home (peers of the same sex)	The development of skills needed to cope with the environment	Fixations can result in difficulty in identifying with others and in developing social skills, resulting in a sense of inadequacy and inferiority
Genital (13 years and beyond)	**Genitals** (sexual intercourse)	—	Developing satisfying sexual and emotional relationships with members of the opposite sex; emancipation from parents—planning life goals and gaining a strong sense of personal identity	The ability to be creative and find pleasure in "love and work"	Inability to negotiate this stage could result in difficulties in becoming emotionally and financially independent, lack of strong personal identity and future goals, and inability to form satisfying intimate relationships

Data from Gleitman H. Psychology. New York: WW Norton, 1981.

the infant has experienced few demands from others, but now there appear to be direct attempts by the parents to interfere with the pleasure obtained from the excretory functions. Thus, the conflict of this stage is between those demands from society in the persons of the parents and the sensations of pleasure associated with the anus.

According to Freud, parents' reactions during this stage may have far-reaching effects on the formation of specific traits and values. If the mother is very strict and repressive in her methods, the child may hold back the feces in defiance and become constipated. If this mode of reaction generalizes to other forms of behavior, the child will develop a retentive character: that is, the child will become stubborn and stingy, unwilling to give. Or, under the pressure of coercive

measures in toilet training, the child may vent rage by expelling the feces at the most inappropriate times. This can become the original model for all kinds of expulsive traits—cruelty, malicious destructiveness, temper tantrums, and messy disorderliness. On the other hand, if the mother is warm and sensitive in her urging and extravagantly praises the child in toilet activity, the child will acquire the notion that the whole activity of producing feces is extremely important. This idea may be the basis for creativity and productivity. The child learns to delay immediate gratification (expelling feces) to obtain a future goal (parental approval).

PHALLIC STAGE (3–6 years). The **phallic stage** of development occurs between the ages of three and six years. The child experiences both pleasurable and conflicting feelings associated with the genital organs. At this time, children devote much energy to examining their genitalia, masturbating, and expressing interest in sexual matters. Children are curious about everything, including anatomical differences between the sexes and the origin of babies. They create unconscious fantasies about the sexual act itself and the birth process. Their ideas are frequently inaccurate and unrealistic, such as believing that a pregnant woman has eaten her baby and that a baby is expelled through the mouth or anus.

The pleasures of masturbation and the fantasy life of children set the stage for the Oedipus complex, which Freud considered to be one of his greatest contributions to the study of personality development. Freud's concept of the Oedipus complex was suggested by the Greek tragedy of Sophocles in which King Oedipus unwittingly murdered his father and married his mother. To Freud, the Greek myth symbolized the unconscious psychological conflict that each child faces: the child's unconscious sexual attraction to, and wish to possess, the parent of the opposite sex, and the hostility and desire to remove the parent of the same sex, as well as subsequent guilt for these wishes. The conflict is resolved when the child identifies with the parent of the same sex.

According to Freud, the emergence of the superego is both the solution to, and the result of, these intense forbidden impulses. Because these intense erotic and murderous impulses have no prospect of succeeding, children channel this emotional energy through the defense mechanisms of identification and introjection. As a result, children not only identify with the parent of the same sex but also incorporate into their own belief system the values and social standards of their parents and those of their culture and subculture.

LATENCY PERIOD (6–12 years). After the phallic stage, the child enters elementary school and begins what Freud termed the **latency stage.** This period, encompassing approximately six years between the phallic and genital stages, is marked by a tapering off of conscious biological and sexual urges. The sexual impulses, which are unacceptable in their direct expression, are channeled and elevated into more culturally accepted levels of activity, such as sports, intellectual interests, and peer relations. Freud was relatively silent about the latency period. He did not consider it a genuine psychosexual stage, but rather a period of transition and comparative sexual quiescence.

Today, Freud's view of latency has been questioned by most critics. They believe that it is more accurate to observe that during this period children learn to hide their sexuality from disapproving adults.

GENITAL STAGE (13–20 years). Freud's final stage is termed the **genital stage**. It emerges at adolescence with the onset of puberty, when the genital organs mature. The impulses of the pregenital period are narcissistic in character: that is, the individual gains gratification from his or her own body. The child values other people because they satisfy his or her narcissistic pleasures. During adolescence, some of this self-love or narcissism becomes redirected toward gratification involving genuine interaction with other people. Sexual attraction, socialization, group activities, vocational planning, and preparation for marrying and raising a family begin to manifest themselves. By the end of adolescence, the person becomes transformed from what was originally a pleasure-seeking individual to a more reality-oriented, socialized adult.

A mature individual is one who has reached conventional genital sexuality; one who satisfies his or her needs in socially approved ways; and one who is able, in Freud's words, "to love and to work."

Although Freud differentiated five stages of personality growth, he did not assume that there were any sharp breaks or abrupt transitions in proceeding from one stage into another. The final organization of personality represents contributions from all stages.

Long Term Effects of Freud's Psychosexual Stages

Some theorists contend that the effects of Freud's psychosexual stages can be seen in various adult character types or traits. They believe that if a child has been either unduly frustrated or overindulged, the child may become fixated on a particular stage. Fixation refers to growth arrestment in which excessive needs, characteristic of an earlier stage, are recreated.

For example, a child who persists in thumb-sucking well beyond the preschool years may be showing evidence of being fixated at the oral stage. These theorists believe that the child has an inability to satisfy oral needs in an age-appropriate manner. The example of a chain-smoking adult who persists in smoking despite of all health warnings also suggests a fixation on oral needs. Character traits of an orally fixated person include being dependent on and easily influenced by others.

Likewise, adults who experienced frustration or overindulgence at the anal stage, according to Freudian thought, may be described as having anal personalities. They may be orderly, parsimonious, and stubborn, or the opposite—disorganized, explosive, and uncontrolled. Most of us do not reflect a pure type, but these personality types and their opposites are

Table 1-5 ■ FREUD'S PSYCHOSEXUAL TRAITS AS BIPOLAR DIMENSIONS

ORAL TRAITS

Optimism	Pessimism
Gullibility	Suspiciousness
Manipulativeness	Passivity
Admiration	Envy
Cockiness	Self-belittlement

ANAL TRAITS

Stinginess	Overgenerosity
Constrictedness	Expansiveness
Stubborness	Acquiescence
Orderliness	Messiness
Rigid punctuality	Tardiness
Meticulousness	Dirtiness
Precision	Vagueness

PHALLIC TRAITS

Vanity	Self-hatred
Pride	Humility
Blind courage	Timidity
Brashness	Bashfulness
Gregariousness	Isolation
Stylishness	Plainness
Flirtatiousness	Avoidance of heterosexuality
Chastity	Promiscuity
Gaiety	Sadness

From Engler BO. Personality Theories: An Introduction. Boston: Houghton Mifflin, 1979, p 55; adapted from Maddi SR. Personality Theories: A Comparative Analysis. Holmwood, Ill: Dorsey Press, 1972, pp 271–276.

thought to have their origin in the various psychosexual stages.

Freud viewed "neurosis" as the product of an inadequate emotional development. In cases of neurosis, the individual continues to mature physically, passing from stage to subsequent stage, but with heavy residues of negative attitudes and emotions that prevent the individual from functioning optimally and dealing adequately with stress and anxiety. Such individuals are bound to their unhappy past and respond emotionally in immature ways. These unrealistic responses are not helpful in the everyday world.

Maddi (1972) summarized the various character traits described by Freud as bipolar dimensions. These traits may be seen as attitudes that develop initially during the various psychosexual stages. Consider each of the traits in Table 1-5. See if you recognize them as characteristics of yourself or someone you know.

ERIKSON'S PSYCHOSOCIAL STAGES OF DEVELOPMENT

Erik Erikson, an American psychoanalyst and initially a close follower of Freud, broadened Freud's theory of human development. First, Erikson stressed the role of the ego, or the rational part of the personality, whereas Freud concentrated largely on the nonrational, instinctual parts of the personality (the id). Second, Erikson viewed the growing individual within the larger social setting of the family and its cultural heritage rather than in the more restricted triangle of mother-child-father. Third, Erikson's stages span the full life cycle, in contrast to Freudian theory, which views basic personality as established by age five years. Fourth, Erikson differed from Freud in that he studied healthy personalities to arrive at his theory, rather than analyzing neurotic clients, as Freud had done.

In summary, Erikson remolded Freud's psychosexual stages of development into psychosocial stages, emphasizing the growth of individuals as they establish new ways of understanding and relating to themselves and to their changing social world throughout the whole life cycle.

Erikson's recognition that humans continue to develop throughout their life span resulted in a developmental scheme of eight stages, extending from infancy to old age. Erikson states that at each stage individuals are faced with a particular crisis or conflict, which can have a positive or a negative outcome.

The stages listed in Table 1-6 are the major stages in the life cycle as described by Erikson. They clearly build on Freud's psychosexual stages, but they emphasize the social determinants of personality development. The conflicts are not simply caused by frustration of instinctual drives early in one's life; they take into account the roles that society and the individual play throughout life in the formation of the personality. Furthermore, Erikson's view of the individual is an optimistic one in that he demonstrates that each phase of growth has its strengths as well as its weaknesses and that failures at one stage of development can be rectified by successes at later stages.

SULLIVAN'S INTERPERSONAL THEORY

Harry Stack Sullivan (1892–1949), an American-born theorist in interpersonal psychiatry, used the Freudian framework early in his career. Later he developed a new concept of personality. Sullivan stopped trying to deal with what he considered unseen and private mental processes within the individual (Freud's intrapsychic processes) and began to focus on interpersonal processes that could be observed in a social framework. The basis of his theory was the contention that personality can be observed and studied only when a person is actually behaving in relation to one

Table 1–6 ■ ERIKSON'S EIGHT STAGES OF DEVELOPMENT

APPROXIMATE AGE	DEVELOPMENTAL TASK	PSYCHOSOCIAL CRISIS	SUCCESSFUL RESOLUTION OF CRISIS	UNSUCCESSFUL RESOLUTION OF CRISIS
Infancy (0–1½ years)	Attachment to mother, which lays foundations for later trust in others	Trust versus mistrust	Sound basis for relating to other people; trust in people; faith and hope about the environment and the future	General difficulties relating to people effectively; suspicion; trust-fear conflict; fear of the future
Early childhood (1½–3 years)	Gaining some basic control of self and environment (e.g., toilet training, exploration)	Autonomy versus shame and doubt	Sense of self-control and adequacy; willpower	Independence-fear conflict; severe feelings of self-doubt
Late childhood (3–6 years)	Becoming purposeful and directive	Initiative versus guilt	Ability to initiate one's own activities; sense of purpose	Aggression-fear conflict; sense of inadequacy or guilt
School age 6–12 years	Developing social, physical, and school skills	Industry versus inferiority	Competence; ability to learn and work	Sense of inferiority; difficulty learning and working
Adolescence 12–20 years	Making transition from childhood to adulthood; developing a sense of identity	Identity versus role confusion	Sense of personal identity; fidelity	Confusion about who one is; identity submerged in relationships or group memberships
Early adulthood 20–35 years	Establishing intimate bonds of love and friendship	Intimacy versus isolation	Ability to love deeply and commit oneself	Emotional isolation; egocentricity
Middle adulthood 35–65 years	Fulfilling life goals that involve family, career, and society; developing concerns that embrace future generations	Generativity versus self-absorption	Ability to give and care for others	Self-absorption; inability to grow as a person
Later years 65 years to death	Looking back over one's life and accepting its meaning	Integrity versus despair	Sense of integrity and fulfillment; willingness to face death; wisdom	Dissatisfaction with life; denial of or despair over prospect of death

Data from Erikson EH. Childhood and Society. New York: WW Norton, 1963; Altrocchi J. Abnormal Psychology. New York: Harcourt Brace Jovanovich, 1980, p 196.

or more other individuals. Thus, Sullivan defines personality as "the group of characteristic ways in which an individual relates to others" (Sullivan 1953). According to Sullivan, personality consists of behavior that can be observed.

Sullivan believes that individuals are motivated by two sets of purposes or goals: (1) the pursuit of satisfactions and (2) the pursuit of security. *Satisfactions* refer to biological needs, including sleep and rest, sexual fulfillment, food and drink, and physical closeness to other humans. *Security* was used by Sullivan to refer to a state of well-being, of belonging, and of

being accepted. Sullivan used the term *dynamism* to describe those characteristic patterns of interpersonal behavior that the individual develops in the pursuit of the two goals of satisfaction and security.

Anxiety and the Self or Self-system

Anxiety is a key concept in Sullivan's interpersonal psychiatry. It refers to any painful feeling or emotion. It comes from tension that arises from social insecurity or blocks to satisfaction (organic needs). According to Sullivan, there are a number of characteristics of anxiety. First, it is interpersonal in origin. For example, a mother's anxious feelings can be transmitted to a child. Second, anxiety can be described, and behaviors stemming from anxiety can be observed. The anxious person can tell how he or she feels, and behavior resulting from anxiety can be observed and studied. Third, individuals strive to reduce anxiety. For example, children learn that they can avoid anxiety that comes from punishment and the threat to their security by conforming to their parents' wishes.

Sullivan used the term *security operations* to describe those measures that the individual employs to reduce anxiety and enhance security. Collectively, all of the security operations an individual uses to defend him- or herself against anxiety and ensure self-esteem make up the **self-system.**

Sullivan identified three components of the self-system, which is based on the child's experiences with others early in life. These three components are

- The *good-me.* The good-me represents that part of the personality that develops in response to rewarding appraisals from others.
- The *bad-me.* The bad-me develops in response to anxiety-producing appraisals from others. The child learns to avoid these feelings of discomfort and distress by altering certain behaviors.
- The *not-me.* The not-me develops in response to overwhelming feelings of horror, dread, and loathing. In an effort to relieve anxiety, the child represses or dissociates these intense feelings. These feelings, now gone from awareness, become the not-me.

There are many parallels between Sullivan's notion of security operations and Freud's concept of defense mechanisms. Both are processes of which we are unaware, and both are ways in which we reduce anxiety. Although at times the concepts overlap, the major difference between security operations and defense mechanisms is Sullivan's emphasis on what is observable. For example, Freud's defense mechanism of repression is an *intrapsychic* activity, whereas Sullivan's security operations are *interpersonal* relationship activities that can be observed. Some examples of the observable manifestations of security operations are sublimation, selective inattention, and dissociation.

SUBLIMATION. When a child's behavior brings disapproval, the child experiences anxiety and threats to self-esteem. The child learns to reduce the anxiety by behaving in a more acceptable manner. For example, the child learns to express anger verbally instead of biting, hitting, or kicking the person with whom he or she is angry. This expression of unacceptable drives as more acceptable behaviors is called **sublimation.**

SELECTIVE INATTENTION. Sullivan states that **selective inattention** refers to an individual who "doesn't happen to notice an almost infinite series of more-or-less meaningful details of one's living" that might cause anxiety (1953). For example, a husband may not notice his wife's seductive behavior toward other men because it threatens his own self-esteem.

DISSOCIATION. Some things are so threatening to the security of the self that they cannot be faced by the individual. For example, the abused child, needy, helpless, and dependent on the abusing parent, blocks out or dissociates the experience of hate or anger toward his or her parent or parents. Such feelings are excluded from conscious awareness before they are able to trigger overwhelming and intolerable anxiety. Thus, **dissociation** is similar to the defense Freud referred to as repression.

Sullivan's interpersonal theory has had a great impact on the direction of nursing practice. Hildegard Peplau, influenced by the work of Sullivan and learning theory, developed the first systematic theoretical framework in psychiatric nursing. In her book *Interpersonal Relationships in Nursing* (1952), Peplau laid the foundation for the professional practice of psychiatric nursing and has continued to enrich psychiatric nursing theory and the advancement of nursing practice. The discussions of the one-to-one nurse-client relationship and the clinical interview (Chapter 6) illustrate how Peplau's theoretical framework has become a cornerstone for the practice of psychiatric nursing and consequently all nursing practice.

PIAGET

Jean Piaget (1896–1980), after earning a doctorate in zoology in his home town in Switzerland, went on to explore the field of psychology. Piaget believed that just as other living organisms *adapt* to their environment biologically, so, too, do humans adapt to their environment psychologically. He considered cognitive acts as ways in which the mind organizes and adapts to its environment. Piaget used the word *schema* to refer to the child's cognitive structure or framework of thought. Schemata are categories that people form in their minds to organize and understand the world. At the beginning, the young child has only a few schemata with which to understand the world. Gradually these are increased. Adults use a wide variety of schemata to comprehend the world.

Two complementary processes of adaptation help in the development of schemata: assimilation and accommodation. **Assimilation** refers to the ability to incorporate new ideas, objects, and experiences into the framework of one's thoughts. Through assimilation, the growing child will perceive and give meaning to new information according to what he or she already knows and understands. Assimilation is conservative in that its main function is to make the unfamiliar familiar, to reduce the new to the old. In contrast, **accommodation** refers to the ability to change one's schema in order to introduce new ideas, objects, or experiences. Whereas the process of assimilation molds the object or event to fit the child's existing frame of reference, accommodation changes the mental structure in order that new experiences may be added. These two processes are constantly working together to produce changes in the growing child's understanding of the world.

The acquisition of knowledge is an active process that depends on interaction between the child and his or her environment. Children do not passively receive stimulation from the environment. They learn about the world through active encounters with it. The development of the child's thinking relies on changes made in the mental structure of the child as he or she interacts with the environment. The true measure of a child's intellectual growth depends on the ability to change old ways of thinking to solve new problems.

Piaget's Stages of Cognitive Development

The development of children's thinking progresses through a sequence of four major stages, each of which is very different from the others. They are the (1) sensorimotor period (0–2 years), (2) preoperational period (2–7 years), (3) period of concrete operations (7–11 years), and (4) period of formal operations (age 11 years through adulthood) (Table 1–7).

The sequence of these four stages and of the substages they comprise never varies; no stage is ever skipped, because each one further develops the preceding stage and lays the groundwork for the next. The stages are somewhat related to chronological age. As with all development, however, each individual reaches each stage according to his or her own timetable. For this reason—and also because there is considerable overlapping between the stages of retention, and some characteristics from preceding stages occur in those that follow—all age norms must be considered approximate.

Table 1–7 ■ PIAGET'S STAGES OF COGNITIVE DEVELOPMENT

PERIOD	CHARACTERISTICS OF THE PERIOD	MAJOR CHANGE OF THE PERIOD
Sensorimotor (0–2 years)	—	
Stage 1 (0–1 month)	Reflex activity only; no differentiation	Development proceeds from reflex activity to representation and sensorimotor solutions to problems
Stage 2 (1–4 months)	Hand-mouth coordination; differentiation via sucking reflex	
Stage 3 (4–8 months)	Hand-eye coordination; repeats unusual events	
Stage 4 (8–12 months)	Coordination of two schemata; object permanence attained	
Stage 5 (12–18 months)	New means through experimentation— follows sequential displacements	
Stage 6 (18–24 months)	Internal representation; new means through mental combinations	
Preoperational (2–7 years)	Problems solved through representation; language development (2–4 years); thought and language both egocentric; cannot solve conservation problems	Development proceeds from sensorimotor representation to prelogical thought and solutions to problems
Concrete operational (7–11 years)	Reversibility attained; can solve conservation problems—logical operations developed and applied to concrete problems; cannot solve complex verbal problems	Development proceeds from prelogical thought to logical solutions to concrete problems
Formal operational (11 years to adulthood)	Logically solves all types of problems— thinks scientifically; solves complex verbal problems; cognitive structures mature	Development proceeds from logical solutions to concrete problems to logical solutions to all classes of problems

KOHLBERG'S THEORY OF MORAL DEVELOPMENT

Lawrence Kohlberg's theory of moral development is deeply rooted in Piaget's work. Kohlberg's unique contribution was to apply to the study of moral development the concept of a progression of stages that Piaget worked out in relation to cognitive development. Kohlberg's research in psychology demonstrated that our conception of justice (what is right?) changes and develops over time as we interact with our environment. Building on the work of Piaget, Kohlberg described a series of six stages of moral development, with each subsequent stage providing a more complex system of moral reasoning and hence a more adequate conception of what is just and right.

COGNITIVE THEORISTS

A more recent approach to understanding personality development and mental illness, called cognitive psychology, has shifted attention away from the individual's biology and the dynamic mind. It focuses on the individual's thought processes. The aim of cognitive theorists is to understand the individual through an examination of his or her cognition (thought processes) and cognitive development. In growing up, individuals learn certain thoughts about themselves and their world. These learned thoughts become the basis for emotions and behavior. This approach assumes that it is the individual's faulty thought processes that are at the basis of his or her mental disorder. For example, Albert Ellis (1957) states that an individual may learn that "it is a dire necessity . . . to be approved or loved by almost everyone for almost everything he does" or that "it is terrible, horrible, and catastrophic when things are not the way one would like them to be." With these thoughts, individuals may feel excessively anxious and dependent. They may look to others for approval and feel unworthy when they do not get it. In addition, such thoughts may lead to frustration and an inability to deal with thwarting and unexpected events.

Aaron Beck, one of the major proponents of the cognitive approach, maintains that the individual's fallacious thinking, due to faulty learning during development, is at the root of mental disorders. Beck (1976) states that individuals with faulty thoughts use the following thinking processes: (1) they are likely to distort reality, (2) they have unreasonable attitudes, (3) they make incorrect inferences on the basis of inadequate and incorrect information, (4) they have trouble distinguishing between imagination and reality, and (5) they use incorrect premises and assumptions in making judgments and decisions.

Cognitive theorists affirm that this new approach to mental disorders changes our perspectives of ourselves and our problems. Instead of viewing ourselves as helpless in the face of our biological reactions or as swayed by unconscious drives and impulses, we can regard ourselves as products of faulty learning and self-defeating ideas who are thus capable of unlearning and correcting faulty thinking. Changing self-defeating ideas can open the way to more adaptive and self-rewarding behaviors.

Toward *DSM-IV*

To carry out their professional responsibilities, clinicians and researchers need accurate and clear-cut guidelines for identifying and categorizing mental illness. Such guidelines help clinicians plan and evaluate the success or failure of a treatment plan for their clients. Several elements are necessary to identify and clearly categorize types of mental illness. There must be agreement as to what specific behaviors—along the adaptive-maladaptive and constructive-destructive lines—constitute mental illness. A common language has to be agreed on so that behaviors can be properly identified and organized into acceptable diagnostic categories.

In 1952, the American Psychiatric Association set out to classify abnormal behavior and provide an official manual of mental disorders, including descriptions of diagnostic categories. It is called the **Diagnostic and Statistical Manual of Mental Disorders (DSM)** and is now the most widely accepted system of classifying abnormal behavior in the United States today, consistent in many respects with the World Health Organization's International Classification of Diseases. The manual is the system used by trained professionals in most US hospitals and other clinical settings.

There have been revisions to the original 1952 manual: the DSM-II in 1968, the DSM-III in 1980, and the **DSM-III-R** (third edition, revised) in 1987. The changes that have been made include moving away from any particular theoretical framework for understanding mental disorders and establishing more specific criteria to identify disorders.

In the DSM-III (1980) and the DSM-III-R (1987), for the first time, the criteria for classification of mental disorders were sufficiently detailed for clinical, teaching, and research purposes. For example, the DSM-III-R provides the following specific criteria for the diagnosis of generalized anxiety disorder:

Generalized Anxiety Disorder

A. Generalized, persistent anxiety is manifested by symptoms from *three of the following four categories*: (a) *motor tension*: shakiness, jitteriness, jumpiness, trembling, tension, muscle aches, fatigability, inability to relax, eyelid twitch, furrowed brow, strained face, fidgeting, restlessness, easy startle; (b) *autonomic hyperactivity*: sweating, heart pounding or racing, cold, clammy hands, dry mouth, dizziness, light-headedness, paresthesia (tingling in hands or feet), upset stomach, hot or cold spells, frequent urination, diarrhea, discomfort in the pit of the stomach, lump in the throat, flushing, pallor, high resting pulse and respiration rate; (c) *apprehensive expectation*: anxiety, worry, fear, rumination, anticipation of misfortune to self or others; (d) *vigilance and scanning*: hyperattentiveness resulting in distractibility, difficulty in concentration, insomnia, feeling "on edge," irritability, impatience.

B. The anxious mood has been continuous for at least one month.

C. Not due to another mental disorder, such as Depressive Disorder or Schizophrenia.

D. At least 18 years of age.

The DSM-III and DSM-III-R introduced a new multiaxial system of classification to allow for multiple complexities of people's lives. DSM-IV continues individual evaluation on five dimensions (Table 1–8) as well as addressing ethnic and cultural considerations.

The term clinical disorder on axis I refers to the collection of signs and symptoms that together constitute a particular disorder. Axis II refers to long-term patterns of behavior and mental retardation. Axis III notes medical conditions potentially relevant to understanding and helping the person. Axis IV is for reporting psychosocial and environmental problems that may affect the diagnosis, treatment, and prognosis of a mental disorder. Axis V, called global assessment of functioning (GAF), gives an indication of the person's best level of psychological, social, and occupational functioning during the preceding year, rated on a scale of one to 100 (from persistent danger of severely hurting one's self or others to superior functioning in a variety of activities) at the time of the

---

Table 1–8 ■ DSM-IV MULTIAXIAL SYSTEM OF EVALUATION	
Axis I	Clinical disorders
	Other conditions that may be a focus of clinical attention
Axis II	Personality disorders
	Mental retardation
Axis III	General medical conditions
Axis IV	Psychosocial and environmental problems
Axis V	Global assessment of functioning

Reprinted with permission from the Diagnostic and Statistical Manual of Mental Disorders, fourth edition (DSM-IV). Washington, DC: American Psychiatric Association, 1994.

---

evaluation, as well as the highest level of functioning for at least a few months during the past year. For children and adolescents, this should include at least one month during the school year. Ratings of current functioning generally reflect the current need for treatment or care. Ratings of the highest level of functioning during the past year frequently have prognostic significance because often the goal of treatment is to return the person to his or her previous level of functioning after an episode of illness. Table 1–9 illustrates how the multiaxial system of classification might be applied to a hypothetical case.

According to the American Psychiatric Association's Task Force on Nomenclature and Statistics, axes I, II, and III constitute the official DSM-IV diagnosis; axes IV and V provide additional information that may be useful in decisions about the therapeutic intervention and in the prediction of likely outcome.

Evaluation and revision are ongoing processes, and the DSM-IV revisions were published in 1994. The DSM-IV will maintain more consistency with the International Classification of Diseases, which is compiled by the World Health Organization. One aim of the DSM-IV is to increase the validity and reliability for each diagnostic category through extensive review of research results, clinical data, and field trials (APA 1994).

However, caution needs to be exercised in diagnosing or labeling, whether a medical diagnosis or a nursing diagnosis is being formulated. The premise that every society has its own view of health and illness and its own classification of diseases has long been observed by anthropologists, historians, and students of cross-cultural society (Klerman 1986).

The DSM-III and DSM-III-R have been criticized for their lack of emphasis on the individual within his or her cultural context (Rothblum et al. 1986). Although the authors of the DSM-III state that abnormality is on a continuum with wellness, the medical perspective reflected in the DSM-III-R can lead to a search for pathological characteristics in those who might otherwise be considered healthy individuals. DSM-IV encourages cultural and ethnic awareness.

The process of psychiatric labeling can have harmful effects on an individual and his or her family, especially if the diagnosis was made on insufficient evidence and proves faulty. A cross-national study of the diagnosis of mental disorders demonstrates, for example, a dramatic difference between British and American psychiatrists. The study revealed that London psychiatrists tend to "diagnose" people more frequently as manic or having character disorders, whereas New York psychiatrists use the diagnosis of schizophrenia much more readily (Rothblum et al. 1986). Psychiatric classifications are at present based

Table 1–9 ■ CLINICAL EXAMPLE DEMONSTRATING DSM-III-AXES

EVALUATION	DATA
Axis I	
Schizophrenic disorder, paranoid	For the past nine months, Michael, a 33-year-old sales representative, has suffered delusions of grandeur and persecution. Believing himself to be a genius, he became convinced that another salesman in his firm was trying to kill him because the other man could not tolerate Michael's superiority. In the past two weeks, Michael has become certain that this other man has had a pale green gas pumped into his office through the air-conditioning ducts, but there is no objective evidence of such gas or any other malfunctioning of the air-conditioning system.
Axis II	
Paranoid traits, no personality disorder	Michael has always tended to be suspicious and distrustful of people. He looks constantly for evidence that others are trying to get the better of him or to harm him, and his manner is guarded. He has trouble relaxing, and others see him as cold and unemotional. He has no close friends and is considered a "loner." He was extremely jealous of his wife, from whom he is now separated, and often accused her, falsely, of having affairs with other men.
Axis III	
Colitis	Michael sees a flare-up of his colitis (inflammation of the colon) as evidence that the salesman is poisoning him, even though Michael has had the same symptoms many times before.
Axis IV	
Psychosocial and environmental problems: a. Marital separation b. Loss of work responsibility Rated severe	Michael left his wife 10 months ago. Two months ago, the president of Michael's firm reassigned one of Michael's most important accounts to the salesman Michael now suspects of hostile intent. Michael thinks this was maneuvered by the other salesman, but in fact, the president acted because the quality of Michael's work was deteriorating. His work had slowed visibly, and coworkers complained that they could not perform their own work properly when he was present.
Axis V	
Highest level of adaptive functioning in past year (GAF) Rated fair	Michael's functioning was adequate until he separated from his wife. At that point, he began to withdraw further from friends and acquaintances. He appeared to concentrate more on his job but actually spent his time checking and rechecking his work. When the firm's president reassigned his major account, Michael's work deteriorated further, and Michael began to air some of his suspicions about the partner who took over the account. When his colitis flared up two weeks ago, he requested an appointment with the president and accused the partner openly. Michael was fired.

Adapted from Altrocchi J. Abnormal Behavior. New York: Harcourt Brace Jovanovich, 1980.

mostly on clinical observations, to some degree on theoretical viewpoints, and least of all on empirical studies (Boxer 1987).

An example of cultural and social bias influencing psychiatric diagnosis is the fact that homosexuality was labeled a psychiatric disease in the DSM-I and DSM-II. All research consistently failed to demonstrate that people with a homosexual orientation were any more maladjusted than heterosexuals. Despite the research data, change occurred in the medical community only when gay rights activists advocated an end to discrimination against lesbians and gay men. No longer is homosexuality classified as a mental disorder.

Bias in a social system extends to many minority groups. Some examples include blacks, elderly persons, children, women, and those with homosexual orientation. These biases are often reflected in our power structures and political systems.

A proposed category thought by many to reflect social bias was *self-defeating personality disorder*, found in the appendix to the DSM-III-R (APA 1987). Most people who would come under this category are women. The American Psychological Association has declared this new diagnosis potentially dangerous to women and without scientific basis (Boxer 1987). This category was not adopted for the DSM-IV.

A syndrome often takes different superficial forms in different cultures. Also, people from minority or migrant populations may have good reason to be distrustful, and it should not be assumed that these clients are suffering from paranoia or paranoid schizophrenia (Westmeyer 1986). Refer to Chapter 4 for further discussions on culture and inherent pitfalls in formulating a DSM diagnosis.

Awareness of the cultural bias and dangers inherent in labeling has enormous implications for nursing practice, especially in the field of mental health, because nurses often take their cues from the medical structure. Doctors diagnose "diseases." Nurses diagnose "a perceived difficulty or need" (ANA 1980). The more objectively we as nurses observe, assess, and diagnose the individuals under our care, the more effectively we will administer our skills.

Summary

Defining mental illness or recognizing mental health may change with the culture, the time in history, the political system and power, and the person or group doing the defining. There is no question that mental health and mental illness do exist on a continuum. One continuum is called adaptive-maladaptive; another is termed constructive-destructive. General indications of a mentally healthy person can be assessed by the degree of (1) happiness, (2) control over behavior, (3) appraisal of reality, (4) effectiveness in work, and (5) self-concept (see Table 1–1).

The history of psychiatry dates back to primitive cultures. Progress in the understanding of mental illness and the treatment of the mentally ill was made in ancient Greece.

Subsequently, the development of psychiatry has been influenced by many factors. Religious fanaticism resulted in many mentally ill persons' being condemned as witches. Later, the mentally ill were viewed as social problems to be kept in places of confinement. Changes in the treatment of the mentally ill and a more humane attitude were advanced by Phillippe Pinel in the late eighteenth and early nineteenth centuries.

Sigmund Freud advanced the first theory of personality development, which in part still influences the thinking of mental health workers today. He articulated levels of awareness (unconscious, preconscious, conscious) and demonstrated the influence of one's unconscious on behavior in everyday life, as evidenced by the use of defense mechanisms. Freud identified three psychological processes of personality (id, ego, and superego) and described how they operate and develop. He proposed one of the first modern developmental theories of personality based on five psychosexual stages of human growth from infancy to adulthood.

Erik Erikson viewed the growth of the individual in terms of the social setting (family, community, and culture). Erikson expanded on Freud's developmental stages to include middle age through old age. Erikson called his stages psychosocial and emphasized the social aspect of personality development.

Harry Stack Sullivan proposed the interpersonal theory of personality development, which focuses on interpersonal processes that can be observed in a social framework. Anxiety is a key concept in Sullivan's theory, and he described certain "security operations" people use to decrease anxiety, such as sublimation, selective inattention, and dissociation. Hildegard Peplau was influenced by Sullivan's interpersonal theory. Peplau's theoretical framework in psychiatric nursing has become the foundation of psychiatric nursing practice.

Jean Piaget added to the understanding of personality development by identifying four cognitive stages in an individual's development. These are the (1) sensorimotor period, (2) preoperational period, (3) period of concrete operations, and (4) period of formal operations. All stages follow this sequence, and each stage lays the groundwork for the next stage. Lawrence Kohlberg applied Piaget's concept of stage development to the study of moral development.

Cognitive theorists focus on an individual's thoughts, with the premise that thoughts become the basis for emotions and behaviors. Cognitive therapy is based on the assumption that if one changes patterns of thinking, changes in behavior will follow.

The DSM-III and DSM-III-R provide specific behavioral criteria for each diagnostic category of mental disorder and include axes to incorporate other data relevant in best diagnosing and planning appropriate care. The DSM-IV increases the validity and reliability of each diagnostic category through the extensive use of research results and addresses cultural influences.

However, caution in adopting labels is advised, and some problems in applying information from the DSM-III-R and DSM-IV were identified, such as the diagnostician's potential or actual bias toward specific minority groups and the need to incorporate cultural norms when making a diagnosis. Awareness of these biases and caution in adopting and promoting labeling have enormous implications for nurses.

References

Ackerknecht EH. A Short History of Psychiatry, 2nd ed, revised (Wolff S, trans). New York: Hafner Publishing Company, 1968. (Original work published 1959).

Altrocchi J. Abnormal Behavior. New York: Harcourt Brace Jovanovich, 1980.

American Nurses' Association. Nursing: A Social Policy Statement. Kansas City, MO: American Nurses' Association, 1980.

American Psychiatric Association. Diagnostic and Statistical Manual of Mental Disorders, 3rd ed, revised (DSM-III-R). Washington, DC: American Psychiatric Association, 1987.

American Psychiatric Association, DSM-IV Options Book: Work in Progress. Washington, DC: American Psychiatric Association, 1991.

American Psychiatric Association. Diagnostic and Statistical Manual of Mental Disorders, 4th ed (DSM-IV). Washington, DC: American Psychiatric Association, 1994.

Beck AJ. Cognitive Therapy and the Emotional Disorders. New York: The New American Library, 1976.

Boxer S. The parable of the check turners and the check-smiters. Discover, 8(6):80, 1987.

Bromberg W. Man Above Humanity. Philadelphia: JB Lippincott, 1954.

Ellenberger HF. The Discovery of the Unconscious: The History and Evolution of Dynamic Psychiatry. New York: Basic Books, 1970.

Ellis A. How to Live With a Neurotic. New York: Crown, 1957,

Gleitman H. Psychology. New York: WW Norton, 1981.

Klerman GL. Historical perspectives on contemporary schools of psychotherapy. In Millon T, Klerman GL (eds). Contemporary Directions in Psychopathology Towards the DSM-IV. New York: The Guilford Press, 1986.

Levison DJ, Gooden WE. Theoretical trends in psychiatry. In Kaplan HI, Sadock BJ (eds). Comprehensive Textbook of Psychiatry, 4th ed. Baltimore: Williams & Wilkins, 1985.

Lewis NDC. A Short History of Psychiatric Achievement. London: Chapman & Hall, 1942.

Maddi SR. Personality Theories: A Comparative Analysis, revised. Homewood, IL: Dorsey Press, 1972.

Major RH. A History of Medicine. Springfield, IL: Charles C Thomas, 1954.

Mora G. From demonology to the Narrenturm. In Gladstone I (ed). Historic Derivations of Modern Psychiatry. New York: McGraw-Hill, 1967, pp 41–73.

Peplau HE. Interpersonal Relations in Nursing. New York, GP Putnam's Sons, 1952.

Reik LE. The historical foundations of psychotherapy in schizophrenias. American Journal of Psychology, 10:241, 1956.

Rothblum ED, Solomon LJ, Albee GW. A sociological perspective of the DSM-III. In Millon T, Klerman GL (eds). Contemporary Directions in Psychopathology Towards the DSM-IV. New York: The Guilford Press, 1986.

Sullivan HS. The Interpersonal Theory of Psychiatry. New York: WW Norton, 1953.

Westmeyer J. Cross cultural diagnosis. The Harvard Medical School Mental Health Letter, 2(12):4, 1986.

Zilboorg G, Henry GW. A History of Medical Psychology. New York: WW Norton, 1941.

FURTHER READING

Chapman AN. Harry Stack Sullivan: His Life and Work. New York: Putnam, 1976.

Cornford FM. The Republic of Plato. Oxford, MA: Oxford University Press, 1970.

Engler B. Personality Theories: An Introduction. Boston: Houghton Mifflin, 1979.

Erikson EH. Studies in the interpretation of play. Part I: Clinical observations of play disruption in young children. Genetic Psychology Monograph, 22:557, 1940.

Erikson EH. Ego development and historical change. In Greenacre P, et al (eds). The Psychoanalytic Study of the Child, vol II. New York: International Universities Press, 1946, pp 350–396.

Erikson EH. Sex differences in the play configurations of pre-adolescents. American Journal of Orthopsychiatry, 21(4):667, 1951.

Erikson EH. Childhood and Society, 2nd ed. New York: WW Norton, 1963.

Groddeck G. The Book of the Id (English trans). New York: Funk & Wagnalls, 1950. (Original work published 1923.)

Hinsie LE, Campbell RJ. Psychiatric Dictionary, 4th ed. New York: Oxford University Press, 1973.

Kohlberg L. Stages of moral development as a basis for moral education. In Beck CM, Crittender BS, Sullivan EV (eds). Moral Education. New York: Newman Press, 1971.

Piaget J. The Construction of Reality in the Child. New York: Basic Books, 1954.

Piaget J. The Psychology of Intelligence. Paterson, NJ: Littlefield Adama, 1963.

Piaget J. Six Psychological Studies. New York: Random House, 1967.

Strachey J (ed and trans). The Standard Edition of the Complete Psychological Works of Sigmund Freud. London: The Hogarth Press, 1961. (Original work published 1923.)

Wadsworth BJ. Piaget's Theory of Cognitive Development: An Introduction for Students of Psychology and Education. New York: David McKay, 1971.

Self-study Exercises

True or false. Correct the false statements.

1. _____ Happiness, control of behavior, sound reality testing, ability to work effectively, and good self-concept are measures of mental health.

2. _____ Behaviors that allow problems to continue and that interfere with an individual's health and ability to function in work, love, or interpersonal relationships are deemed maladaptive behaviors.

3. _____ Destructive behaviors undermine or destroy the psychological or physical well-being of a person or others around the person.

4. _____ The DSM-IV provides specific diagnostic criteria as guides for diagnosis of mental disorders.

5. _____ The DSM-III-R is free of cultural, social, and political bias and always provides accurate labels.

Match the major contribution to mental health development with the correct time or person.

6. _____ Called the Father of Medicine. Encouraged the thinking that mental illness had a natural explanation and was not caused by evil spirits.

7. _____ Called the Father of Psychiatry. Placed emphasis on clinical observation. First to prescribe music and occupational therapy.

8. _____ Although a barbaric time dominated by superstition, wars, and plagues, this period saw the establishment of the first hospitals.

9. _____ Time when the mentally ill were isolated and banished to prisons and workhouses and treated atrociously.

10. _____ A reformer and humanitarian. A gifted therapist. First to keep case records. Treated the mentally ill with respect and compassion.

11. _____ Introduced hypnosis to psychiatry as a useful tool.

12. _____ A humanitarian called the Father of American Psychiatry.

13. _____ Known for humane treatment of the mentally ill. Called father of modern psychiatry.

A. Asclepiades

B. Phillippe Pinel

C. Hippocrates

D. Benjamin Rush

E. Medieval period

F. Pierre Janet

G. Johann Weyer

H. 17th and 18th centuries

I. Harry Stack Sullivan

Choose the answer that most accurately completes the statement.

14. The psychoanalytical theory of Freud placed major emphasis on

   A. Sex instincts
   B. Unconscious motivation
   C. Fixation in psychosexual stages
   D. All of the above

15. Freud called the structure of personality that represents our basic drives, needs, and wishes the

   A. Id
   B. Ego
   C. Superego
   D. Unconscious

16. According to Freud, the ego

   A. Is totally conscious
   B. Obeys the pleasure principle
   C. Follows the reality principle
   D. Is in control of the personality

17. The order in which Freud's three personality components appear as a result of the division of psychic energy is

   A. Ego, id, superego
   B. Superego, ego, id
   C. Id, ego, superego
   D. Ego, superego, id

18. Defense mechanisms

    A. Ward off anxiety
    B. Occur on an unconscious level
    C. Deny or distort reality
    D. All of the above

19. According to Freud, anxiety

    A. Is an inevitable aspect of the human condition
    B. Is a cultural and social product
    C. Has its source in the birth trauma
    D. Invariably leads to severe neurosis

20. A child identifies with the parent of the same sex and starts to take in the values and standards of his or parents (superego) during the

    A. Oral stage
    B. Anal stage
    C. Phallic (oedipal) stage
    D. Genital stage

Match the stage of psychosocial development (Erikson) with the correct age group.

21. _____ Initiative versus guilt
22. _____ Identity versus role confusion
23. _____ Generativity versus stagnation
24. _____ Integrity versus despair
25. _____ Autonomy versus shame
26. _____ Intimacy versus isolation
27. _____ Trust versus mistrust
28. _____ Industry versus inferiority

A. Infancy (birth to 12–18 months)

B. Eighteen months to three years

C. Third to sixth years

D. School age (sixth year to puberty)

E. Adolescence (12–20 years)

F. Early adulthood (20–35 years)

G. Middle adulthood (35–65 years)

H. Later years (65 to death)

Choose the answer that most accurately completes the statement.

29. The stage that is NOT one of the four major stages of cognitive development according to Piaget is

   A. Sensorimotor period (0–2 years)
   B. Preoperational period (2–7 years)
   C. Period of concrete operations (7–11 years)
   D. Period of adolescence (11–21 years)

30. According to Piaget's theory, children progress from one stage to another

   A. In an orderly and invariant sequence
   B. Totally on the basis of chronological age
   C. And occasionally may skip a stage
   D. Only when their behavior is consistent with the final stage

31. Sullivan believed that anxiety

   A. Usually leads to ineffective relationships
   B. Results from failure to satisfy physiological needs
   C. Is interpersonal in origin
   D. Enhances an individual's self-esteem

32. The security operation in which one fails to observe some factor in interpersonal relations that might cause anxiety is termed

   A. Sublimation
   B. Selective inattention
   C. "As if"
   D. Suppression

33. Cognitive theories of personality emphasize

   A. Unconscious modes of perception and awareness
   B. Motivational factors in personality development
   C. Behavioral responses to the environment
   D. Processes of knowing and understanding the world

CHAPTER 2

Predominant Therapies and Contemporary Issues

Julius Trubowitz

OUTLINE •

MAJOR SOMATIC TREATMENTS AND PSYCHOTHERAPEUTIC APPROACHES
Somatic Therapy
    Psychopharmacological Therapy
    Electroconvulsive Therapy
Psychotherapy
    Individual Psychotherapy
    Group Psychotherapy
    Other Therapeutic Approaches

ISSUES IN MENTAL HEALTH NURSING FOR THE 1990s
Community Mental Health Programs
Deinstitutionalization
Self-help Groups
The Homeless
Acquired Immunodeficiency Syndrome
Biological Revolution
Neglected Populations

SUMMARY

KEY TERMS AND CONCEPTS • • • • • • • • • • • • • •

The key terms and concepts listed here also appear in bold where they are defined or discussed in this chapter.

ANTIANXIETY DRUGS
Anxiolytics

ANTIDEPRESSANT DRUGS

ANTIMANIC DRUGS

ANTIPSYCHOTIC DRUGS
Neuroleptics

FREE ASSOCIATION

GROUP PSYCHOTHERAPY
Family Therapy
Psychoanalytically Oriented Group
   Therapy
Psychodrama

INDIVIDUAL PSYCHOTHERAPY
Behavioral Therapy
Classical Psychoanalysis

Cognitive Psychotherapy
Gestalt Therapy
Psychoanalytical Psychotherapy
Short Term Dynamic Psychotherapy
Transactional Analysis

OTHER THERAPEUTIC APPROACHES
Crisis Therapy
Hypnotherapy
Milieu Therapy
Sex Therapy

PSYCHOTHERAPY

PSYCHOTROPIC DRUGS

SOMATIC THERAPY

TRANSFERENCE FEELING

OBJECTIVES ■

After studying this chapter, the student will be able to

1. Compare and contrast the four major groups of psychotropic drugs used today.
2. Describe the treatment style of each of the seven subtypes of individual therapy discussed in this chapter.
3. Discuss three group modalities in terms of their indications and methods of effecting change.
4. Identify specific indications for sex therapy, hypnotherapy, crisis intervention, and milieu therapy.
5. Discuss three issues in the mental health field today that are identified in this chapter.

Major Somatic Treatments and Psychotherapeutic Approaches

Like all diseases, diseases of the mind (mental disorders) necessitate a variety of treatment approaches. This chapter provides an overview of some of the more prevalent treatments. Within individual chapters covering specific mental disorders, these approaches are discussed in more detail, involving the relevance for nursing practice and outlining the nurse's responsibilities. Therapies to be covered are outlined in Table 2–1.

Two broad approaches to the treatment of mental disorders are practiced today: *somatic therapy* and *psychotherapy*.

Somatic therapy involves various manipulations of the body. It constitutes medicine's classic attack on mental disease through the use of medications and electroconvulsive therapy.

Psychotherapy can be defined as "a process by which one or more mental health professionals help,

through psychological methods, one or more other people who have significant psychological difficulties in living" (Altrocchi 1980). Psychotherapy continues the analytical tradition in helping people resolve areas of conflict, diminish psychic pain, and develop more effective ways of getting their needs met.

SOMATIC THERAPY

Two major areas of treatment involving the body are discussed: (1) psychopharmacological therapy and (2) electroconvulsive therapy.

Psychopharmacological Therapy

Since 1955, psychopharmacology has become an important scientific discipline in its own right. In addition, through the development of new chemical agents, psychopharmacological therapy has become a major treatment method for a variety of mental disor-

Table 2–1 ■ SUMMARY OF CURRENT THERAPIES

SOMATIC THERAPY	INDIVIDUAL PSYCHOTHERAPY	GROUP PSYCHOTHERAPY	OTHER THERAPIES
Psychopharmacological therapy	Classical psychoanalysis	Psychoanalytically oriented group therapy	Sex therapy
• Antianxiety	Psychoanalytically oriented psychotherapy	Psychodrama	Hypnotherapy
• Antipsychotic	Short term dynamic psychotherapy	Family therapy	Crisis therapy
• Antidepressant	Transactional analysis		Milieu therapy
• Antimanic	Cognitive psychotherapy		
Electroconvulsive therapy	Behavioral therapy		
	Gestalt therapy		

ders. The use of psychopharmaceuticals has radically improved the treatment of the mentally ill, both within and outside the hospital. With the use of these agents, it has become possible for some families to hold together and for some individuals to hold jobs, make use of psychotherapy, or both.

Drugs that have an effect on brain function, behavior, or experience are called **psychotropic drugs.** Most of the prescribed medications for people with some form of mental disorder come under the category of psychotropic drugs.

Since the advent of psychotropic drugs in psychiatry, nurses have had to accept the responsibility of evaluating therapeutic effects, observing for and teaching clients about potential harmful effects, and administering these drugs. An overview of the four categories of psychotropic drugs—antipsychotic, antianxiety, antidepressant, and antimanic (lithium carbonate)—is provided in this chapter. These drugs are discussed in detail in the clinical chapters addressing the disorders for which they are indicated. Psychotropic drugs are discussed under the heading Somatic Therapies in each of the clinical chapters.

ANTIPSYCHOTIC DRUGS. The antipsychotic drugs, often called **neuroleptics,** have the ability to

1. Decrease psychotic, paranoid, and disorganized thinking
2. Alter bizarre behavior
3. Decrease dangerous levels of hyperactivity
4. Increase the activity level of severely withdrawn individuals
5. Help clients become more amenable to psychotherapy

Standard neuroleptic therapy involves the phenothiazine-like drugs. These drugs are believed to be effective because of their action in reducing the effect of the neurotransmitter dopamine by blocking the dopamine receptors. This has the effect of reducing distorted perceptions and misinterpretations of reality. These drugs are useful in acute psychotic episodes (e.g., schizophrenia, manic phase of bipolar disorder, agitated psychotic depressions, and organic brain syndromes). Examples of these drugs include the phenothiazines (e.g., chlorpromazine [Thorazine]), the thioxanthenes, and the butyrophenones. The antipsychotic (neuroleptic) drugs and specific side effects, nursing implications, and responsibilities are discussed at length in Chapter 19.

More recently, another group of drugs have been released that target a larger number of the debilitating symptoms of schizophrenia (both the negative and positive symptoms of schizophrenia) and have fewer side effects. Two of these drugs are clozapine (Clozaril) and risperidone (Risperdal). Clozaril is given to treatment-resistant schizophrenics, and for many, it has brought relief of symptoms when other neuroleptics have failed. However, Clozaril causes 1–2% of patients to develop agranulocytosis when taking this drug. Risperdal, however, is safer and often used as a first choice to improve both the positive (delusions and hallucinations) and the negative symptoms of schizophrenia, such as lack of motivation, difficulty initiating contacts with others, and apathy (see Chapter 19).

Antiparkinsonian drugs are often given to prevent or minimize the extrapyramidal side effects of standard neuroleptic therapy. They are assumed to work by their anticholinergic effects. Antiparkinsonian drugs are not helpful in the prevention or treatment of tardive dyskinesia (see Chapter 19). Popular examples include benztropine mesylate (Cogentin), biperiden (Akineton), and trihexyphenidyl (Artane).

ANTIANXIETY DRUGS. The antianxiety drugs are also referred to as **anxiolytics.** Essentially, these drugs are used for

1. Management of anxiety disorders
2. Short term relief of acute anxiety
3. Reduction of anxiety associated with depression
4. Preoperative procedures

The most widely prescribed antianxiety or anxiolytic drugs used today are the benzodiazepines. These drugs are central nervous system depressants. The calming effect appears to be related to their effect on the limbic system and reticular formation. Common drugs in this group include chlordiazepoxide hydrochloride (Librium), diazepam (Valium), lorazepam (Ativan), and oxazepam (Serax). Many of these drugs are used as muscle relaxants or anticonvulsants, and in acute alcohol withdrawal. Tolerance to these drugs develops, and withdrawal should be gradual (see Chapter 14 for a fuller discussion).

Several antidepressants, such as trazodone (Desyrel), doxepin (Sinequan), imipramine (Tofranil), and phenelzine (Nardil), also appear to have antianxiety effects and are effective in the treatment of both generalized anxiety disorder and panic disorder. Clomipramine (Anafranil) is effective in selected people with obsessive-compulsive disorder.

ANTIDEPRESSANT DRUGS. Essentially, the antidepressant drugs are used for the treatment of depression. Some desired effects of the drugs include

1. Elevated mood
2. Increased concentration
3. Increased socialization
4. Increased energy levels

There are three major categories of antidepressants: (1) the tricyclic antidepressants, (2) the monoamine oxidase inhibitors, and (3) the selective serotonin reuptake inhibitors (SSRIs). In special instances, the tricyclic antidepressants are used in the treatment of phobias and childhood enuresis. Popular tricyclics include amitriptyline hydrochloride (Elavil), imipramine hydrochloride, and doxepin hydrochloride. Of the monoamine oxidase inhibitors, isocarboxazid (Marplan), phenelzine sulfate, and tranylcypromine sulfate (Parnate) are used. SSRIs include fluoxetine (Prozac), sertraline (Zoloft), and paroxetine HCL (Paxil). At present, these drugs boast the lowest side effect profile of the antidepressants, although other antidepressants continue to be studied.

Several other drugs used as antidepressants have been approved for the treatment of depression in the United States. Alprazolam (Xanax), an antianxiety medication, also works as a mild antidepressant. Other antidepressants include amoxapine (Asendin), maprotiline (Ludiomil), and trazodone. The side effects, actions, and nursing responsibilities regarding antidepressant drugs are covered in Chapter 17.

ANTIMANIC DRUGS. Lithium carbonate is the drug of choice for treating individuals with acute manic behavior and for preventing the recurrence of manic-depressive episodes. Essentially, lithium helps normalize some of the following behaviors in a client with bipolar disorder

1. An elevated, unstable mood
2. Grandiosity and aggressiveness
3. Psychomotor agitation
4. Extreme talkativeness (logorrhea)
5. Extreme irritability

It is thought that lithium acts by altering the sodium transport in the nerve and muscle cells, causing a shift toward intraneural metabolism of catecholamines. The contraindications for the drug, along with its actions and side effects, are covered at length in Chapter 18.

Increasing attention has been given to the use of anticonvulsant medications to promote mood stabilization in people with a bipolar disorder. Carbamazepine (Tegretol) and valproic acid (Depakene) are examples of anticonvulsants that have proved successful in the treatment of manic episodes in bipolar disorders.

Electroconvulsive Therapy

Electroconvulsive therapy (ECT) is an effective therapy for treating some people with severe depression, especially those who are acutely suicidal, are unwilling to eat, do not respond to tricyclic antidepressants and monoamine oxidase inhibitors (antidepressants), and are unable to tolerate medication.

Since the introduction of ECT in 1938, its popularity has waxed and waned, but today ECT is becoming more widely and successfully used in many parts of the United States. Essentially, while the client is under the effects of anesthesia and muscle relaxants, an electrical stimulus is passed through the temporal lobes, causing seizure activity in the brain. Short term memory loss is experienced with bilateral treatment. Nursing responsibilities and implications in relation to ECT are discussed in Chapter 17.

Insulin shock or coma therapy, popular in the 1930s, has been replaced by the use of psychotropic drugs and ECT. Psychosurgery is another procedure that was used before the advent of psychotropic drugs. Psychosurgery was dramatized to the lay public in *One Flew Over the Cuckoo's Nest*. Prefrontal lobotomies are rarely used today. These procedures have potential complications and negative side effects, and they are thought by many to be unethical and unacceptable. Their use is indicated for clients who have chronic conditions and intractable assaultiveness, when all other approaches have failed.

PSYCHOTHERAPY

There are many different schools of psychotherapy. According to one author, there were 36 different systems in 1959 (Harper 1974). This number has substantially increased since then. Different systems of psychotherapy vary in goals and techniques. The following discussion separates major psychotherapies practiced today into three categories: (1) individual psychotherapy, (2) group psychotherapy, and (3) other therapeutic approaches. Refer to Table 2–1 for an overview of the therapies to be discussed.

Individual Psychotherapy

Seven subtypes of psychotherapy conducted with individual clients are discussed in the following section: classical psychoanalysis, psychoanalytically oriented psychotherapy, short term dynamic psychotherapy, transactional analysis, cognitive psychotherapy, behavioral therapy, and gestalt therapy.

CLASSICAL PSYCHOANALYSIS. The term *psychoanalysis* describes the school and the system of therapy based on Freud's theory of personality and developed from Freud's treatment methods with neurotic clients in Vienna at the beginning of the twentieth century.

A number of techniques are employed by the analyst to uncover unconscious feelings and thoughts that interfere with the client's living a fuller life. One such technique is called **free association.** When a client free-associates, he or she is encouraged to say anything that comes to mind, without censoring thoughts or feelings. Another method of uncovering unconscious material is through dream analysis. During sleep, one's defenses are weakened, and unconscious material often becomes conscious, although in symbolic forms.

During treatment, the client traditionally lies on a couch, in a relaxed posture, which helps bring unconscious processes to the surface. The client faces away from the analyst and is encouraged to project his or her fantasies onto the unseen, relatively neutral analyst. Through development of transference, the client experiences the therapist as if he or she were a significant person in the client's life and transfers feelings for that person or persons onto the analyst. The client re-experiences childhood conflicts that are inappropriate to his or her adult life. The analyst facilitates awareness of these **transference feelings** and fantasies. The process of repeated interpretation to the person of his or her unconscious processes has the effect of bringing about change and is called "working through."

PSYCHOANALYTICAL PSYCHOTHERAPY. The psychoanalytical model of psychotherapy uses many of the tools of psychoanalysis, such as free association, dream analysis, and transference, but the therapist is much more involved and interacts with the client more freely. Clinical nurse specialists with special training at the master's level may do psychotherapy with clients in private practice. Lego (1984) states that the nurse/therapist works with the client to uncover unconscious material that appears in the form of symptoms or unsatisfactory life patterns. This is done through an intimate professional relationship between the nurse/therapist and the client over a period of time. The process proceeds through stages—the introductory, working, and termination stages. These stages are described with examples in Chapter 6.

SHORT TERM DYNAMIC PSYCHOTHERAPY. Short term dynamic psychotherapy is usually indicated when a person has a specific symptom or interpersonal problem he or she wants to work on. The therapist participates actively and influences the direction of the content more than in either of the models discussed previously.

Although many of the tools employed in traditional psychotherapy are used, such as uncovering unconscious processes through transference and dream interpretations, other methods such as free association are discouraged. Sessions are held weekly, and the total number of sessions to be held (anywhere from 12 to 30) is determined at the outset of therapy. This type of intervention is successful for highly motivated individuals who have insight and who indicate a positive relationship with the therapist from the beginning.

TRANSACTIONAL ANALYSIS. Transactional analysis is both a theory and a therapeutic approach developed by Eric Berne in the early 1960s. As a personality theory, transactional analysis incorporates concepts from orthodox Freudian psychoanalysis and ego psychology. Berne states that each person has three ego states or personality parts. People respond to others from these ego states and change from one to another frequently (Aldinger 1992). All people do this.

1. Parent—concepts of standards of behavior and how things should be done
2. Adult—rational-thinking and data-analyzing part of the personality.
3. Child—feelings associated with persons, things, or incidents represent the need-gratifying aspects of the personality

The ego state a person is using can be identified from the type of words used, the voice tone, gestures, and so forth. Berne states that problems arise when there is an incongruity between the ego states of people interacting with each other. For example:

WIFE (adult):	Would you please take out the garbage?
HUSBAND (child):	Is that why you married me? To be your garbage man?
WIFE (child):	Well, you're not good for much else!

As a therapeutic approach, transactional analysis can be used with groups and families, as well as in individual therapy. The client is taught to be able to identify his or her ego states, evaluate which ego states (child, adult, or parent) are operating in a given situation, and identify the pattern of his or her communication with others. Maladaptive patterns, which Berne calls games, interfere with relationships and effective functioning.

The continuation of maladaptive communication patterns is often rewarded positively or negatively with "strokes," and the client is taught how to identify these reinforcers and initiate alternate methods of getting the needed reinforcement. In effect, the therapist works with the client using here-and-now experiences.

COGNITIVE (INSIGHT) PSYCHOTHERAPY. Cognitive psychotherapists emphasize the importance of restructuring, or changing the ways in which people think about themselves, and thus changing the ways they behave in the world. Aaron Beck's approach to therapy with people suffering from depression illustrates the major components of cognitive therapy. Early in therapy, the client's life history is reviewed. The client's patterns of response to certain types of experiences are identified. For example, a person may come to recognize that he generally thinks of himself as worthless whenever he is not getting "enough" attention from others. This faulty thinking is what the therapist would target. Much of the work in cognitive therapy for depressed individuals consists of focusing on the client's specific depression-generating thoughts.

Albert Ellis (1962) refers to these thoughts as "self-statements" or "internalized verbalizations," "things the patient tells himself." These self-statements or thoughts reflect the distortions that occur in people's feelings and consequent behavior. Cognitive therapists help people identify distorted thoughts, acquire objectivity toward them, correct them, and consequently neutralize their power.

BEHAVIORAL THERAPY. Behavioral therapists work on the assumption that changes in maladapted behavior can occur without insight into the underlying cause. Behavioral therapy is based on learning theory. This therapy works best when it is directed at specific problems and the goals are well defined. Behavioral therapy is effective in people with agoraphobia (graded exposure and flooding) and other phobias (desensitization), alcoholism (aversion therapy), schizophrenia (token economy), and many other conditions.

The many types of behavioral therapy can be grouped into five categories: (1) modeling, (2) operant conditioning, (3) self-control therapy, (4) systematic desensitization, and (5) aversion therapy.

Modeling. In modeling, the therapist provides a role model for specific identified behaviors, and the client learns through imitation. The therapist may do the modeling, provide another person to model the behaviors, or present a video for the purpose. Modeling is frequently used in conjunction with other behavioral therapy, as well as with other therapeutic approaches.

Operant Conditioning. Operant conditioning entails rewarding a person for desired behaviors. Called positive reinforcement, it is thought to be one of the best ways to increase desired behaviors. For example, when desired goals are achieved or behaviors are performed, clients are rewarded with "tokens." These tokens can be exchanged for food, small luxuries, or privileges. This reward system is known as "token economy."

Operant conditioning has been useful in improving verbal behaviors of mute, autistic, and developmentally disabled children. In hospitalized clients with chronic mental illness, behavioral therapy has been useful in increasing levels of self-care, social behavior, attendance in group activities, and more.

We use positive reinforcement in everyday life all of the time, whether we know it or not. Reinforcers can increase, decrease, or maintain a behavior. Here is an example of three ways in which behavior can be reinforced (Aldinger 1992). A mother takes her son to the market. The child starts acting out, wanting this and that, nagging, crying, and yelling.

Action	Result
1. The mother gives the child what he wants.	The child continues to use this behavior. This is positive reinforcement of negative behavior.
2. The mother scolds the child.	Acting out may continue because the child gets what he really wants—attention. This positively rewards negative behavior.
3. The mother ignores the acting out but gives attention to the child when he is acting appropriately.	The child gets positive rewards for appropriate behaviors.

Self-control Therapy. Self-control therapy is a combination of cognitive and behavioral approaches. A basic theme is that the "talking to ourselves" that we all do can be altered to help us direct and control our actions more effectively. Stress is one area in which self-control therapy can be useful. For example, the therapist would teach clients to say to themselves when they feel stress affecting their bodies, "All right . . . my chest is starting to feel tight. Take it easy. Sit down, and breathe deeply. There, I'm feeling calmer." One advantage of this technique is that change is likely to last in many cases, and it is easily applied to new situations in the future.

Systematic Desensitization. Systematic desensitization is another form of behavioral modification therapy. For example, a client who has a fear, or phobia, of a particular situation or object will be introduced to short periods of exposure to the phobic object or situation while in a relaxed state. Gradually, over a period of time, exposure is increased, until the anxiety or fear of the object or situation has ceased. This is a common treatment for a variety of phobias (e.g., school phobia, fear of flying, and fear of closed spaces). Refer to Chapter 14 for the application of systematic desensitization.

Aversion Therapy. Aversive "conditioning," or negative reinforcement, is another technique used to change behavior. One example of the use of aversion therapy is with people who have drinking problems. Each time the person takes a drink, he or she is given mild electric shock or an emetic. Over time, it is hoped that the taking of a drink will be associated with an unpleasant experience, which will eventually override the desire for a drink. Disulfiram (Antabuse), a medication, works on the same principle (see Chapter 23). Aversion therapy has also been used with people who have paraphilias. For example, an electric shock or other noxious stimulus is applied at the time of the paraphilic impulse.

GESTALT THERAPY. The evolution of gestalt therapy is closely related to the work of Fritz Perls (1893–1970). Although Perls was trained in the psychoanalytical tradition, he turned away from many of the basic proponents of psychoanalytical training. For example, gestalt therapy emphasizes the creative and expressive aspects of people, rather than the negative and distorted features. Another example is that the emphasis of living is on the "here and now," not the "then and there." Intellectual understanding of dysfunctional behavior is considered useless, because the gestaltists state that only present behavior can be changed, not history.

Gestalt therapy is noted for a variety of techniques that are geared toward uncovering repressed feelings and needs. For example, clients might be asked to carry out a dialogue between different parts of their personality. Another technique is to have a person behave the opposite of the way he or she feels, presuming that a person can then come into contact with a submerged part of the self. When dealing with dreams, a gestalt therapist might ask the client to play the part of various persons or objects in the dream in order to get in touch with a variety of repressed feelings.

Group Psychotherapy

Therapeutic work in groups provides an individual with opportunities not often possible in individual therapy. For example, distortions in interpersonal relationships revealed by peers may arouse less resistance than those revealed by an authority figure (therapist). The group provides validation from a variety of sources for erroneous thinking or distortions. A person may share with peers, perhaps for the first time, disturbing thoughts or feelings, thereby decreasing feelings of isolation. A group also provides the opportunity for participants to try out new ways of relating in a "safe environment."

Group therapy has the benefit of the therapist working with more than one client at a time. Therefore, group therapy is often less costly for individuals.

Three major group approaches are presented in this chapter: psychoanalytically oriented group therapy, psychodrama, and family therapy. Chapter 7 discusses group processes, members, and types of groups in more detail.

PSYCHOANALYTICALLY ORIENTED GROUP THERAPY. Problems of individuals in groups seem to parallel interpersonal problems and distortions in thinking that individuals first experienced in their family of origin. Psychoanalytically oriented group therapists use the phenomena of transference, resistance, interpretation, and working through as critical tools in group therapy. The goal is for people to work out unconscious conflicts within the group setting, in which the group members take an active role. Although called a leader, the therapist acts more as a facilitator of the group process.

Psychoanalytically oriented group therapy provides an atmosphere in which clients (usually seven or eight) gain reassurance in the knowledge that they are not alone or that their feelings, thoughts, and problems are not unique. The variety of group members enables an individual to form multiple transferences, which highlight unresolved emotional conflicts from childhood. The group provides a forum for recognizing and changing outmoded behaviors and adopting alternate and more satisfying styles of relating. Over time, group members are able to identify change and growth in themselves and others, reinforcing group cohesiveness and commitment toward growth.

PSYCHODRAMA. J. L. Moreno (1946) thought that emotional difficulties and maladaptive patterns could be seen and treated more readily in situations that involve action rather than just conversation. Using a play-like format, group members use dramatic techniques such as role-playing, role reversal, and soliloquies to portray intrapsychic and interpersonal conflicts and to play out pent-up feelings. Other members of the group serve as actors in each person's psychodrama. Role-switching within each psychodrama attempts to increase empathy and heighten the emotional reality of the scene. The therapist (called director) then works with group members to fantasize and play out more satisfying and constructive ways of dealing with their problems. Psychodrama is used effectively in prisons and addiction treatment settings.

FAMILY THERAPY. Family therapy is based on a systems theory in which a change in any part affects the entire system. The premise of family therapy is that the transactions within the family system determine the stability and later social adaptations of its members. It is within the family structure that people learn to trust, love, communicate, and function positively. If the family structure is faulty, then each member suffers. Dysfunctional patterns of one individual —say, a child—are thought to be the result of a dysfunctional family. Therefore, the dysfunctional member is said to be the "identified patient," or the one who acts out the pain in the family.

A family therapist might ask the family members about members of their extended family and about problems, such as personality traits and relationships. The therapist can then construct a chart visualizing generational relationships. This chart is called a genogram (see Chapter 27). Dysfunctional relationship problems are often handed down from one generation to another, and an understanding of complex relationships can help the therapist and the family better identify the process of faulty communication and erroneous beliefs. There are a variety of approaches therapists use in order to improve faulty communication, help families change dysfunctional behaviors, and develop support and satisfaction within the family unit. Refer to Chapter 7 for more on family therapy.

For many of the disorders discussed in this text, family therapy is one of a variety of appropriate treatment approaches.

Other Therapeutic Approaches

Four major treatment approaches that meet special needs or unique situations are sex therapy, hypnotherapy, crisis therapy, and milieu therapy.

SEX THERAPY. Sex therapy is essentially limited to the relief of an individual's or a couple's sexual symptoms and is geared toward improvement of sexual functioning. Sex therapy employs a combination of prescribed sexual experiences and psychotherapy sessions. Sex therapy is considered completed when a couple's or an individual's sexual difficulty is relieved.

Sex therapy aims to remove immediate obstacles to sexual functioning without seeking change in either the overall personality structure of the individuals or the fundamental nature of the marital relationship. It deals specifically with the present sexual aspects of the relationship that directly interfere with sexual functioning. Its goal is to improve a partner's or a couple's ability to communicate sexual feelings and sensations, wishes and fears to each other.

Treatment includes therapy sessions and prescribed experiences, to be conducted by the couple when they are alone together. The psychotherapeutic sessions and prescribed experiences help both to reveal and to resolve the sexual blocks, thereby allowing a more satisfying sexual relationship. At times hidden marital difficulties are revealed, and referrals for an appropriate therapeutic modality (e.g., individual, family, or couples) are made.

The Masters and Johnson (1966, 1970) treatment program has served as a model for sex therapy treatment formats. Generally, only couples are accepted for treatment. Masters and Johnson advocate a treatment program of a limited period, usually two weeks, conducted by cotherapists of both genders. During the treatment period, the couple reside away from their home, near the treatment center. Masters and Johnson believe that effective sex therapy requires clients to be free of the usual pressures of home and business, which necessitates a change of environment. Other treatment programs do not require change of residence, use a single therapist of either gender, and do not place a time limit on length of treatment (see Chapter 28).

HYPNOTHERAPY. Hypnosis has been successfully used by therapists to relieve specific target symptoms in their clients. Some therapeutic uses of hypnosis are (Kennedy 1984)

- Pain relief—may be used for some types of surgical anesthesia
- Anxiety and stress reduction
- Removal of undesirable habits (smoking, overeating, phobias)
- In conjunction with some therapies in unusual circumstances (age regression, multiple personality)
- Change in physiological mechanisms (blood pressure, heart rate)

Some disadvantages of hypnosis are

- Not all people can be hypnotized
- Suggestions may lose their effect over time
- Clients may become dependent on hypnosis instead of developing their own problem-solving skills

Hypnosis should be used only by trained individuals and is often used in conjunction with reconstructive forms of psychotherapy.

CRISIS THERAPY. Crisis therapy is covered in depth in Chapter 11. Essentially, crisis therapy is indicated for "normal" people whose usual coping patterns are not adequate when they are faced with a change they perceive as overwhelming. Crises can include maturational crises (e.g., midlife or adolescence), situational crises (e.g., death or loss of a job), or adventitious crises (e.g., flood or tornado). Crisis therapy is short term (usually 4–6 weeks), and the goal is to return people to their precrisis level of functioning. During a crisis, some people learn more mature adaptive patterns of functioning, whereas others (usually those lacking support from others) may come out at a lower level of functioning.

MILIEU THERAPY. Bruno Bettelheim coined the term *milieu therapy* in 1948 to describe his use of the total environment to treat disturbed children. Bettelheim created a comfortable, secure environment (or milieu) in which psychotic children were helped to form a new world. Staff members were trained to provide 24-hour support and understanding for each child on an individual basis. It was Bettelheim's goal "to create for (each child) a world that is totally different from the one he abandoned in despair, and moreover a world he can enter right now" (Bettelheim 1967).

There are certain basic characteristics of milieu therapy, whether the setting involves psychotic children, clients in a psychiatric hospital, drug abusers in a residential treatment center, or psychiatric clients in a day hospital. **Milieu therapy,** or therapeutic community, has as its locus a living, learning, or working environment. Milieu therapy may be based on any number of therapeutic modalities, from structured behavioral therapy to spontaneous, humanistically oriented approaches. However, most programs encompass the following (Liberman and Mueser 1989):

1. An emphasis on group and social interaction
2. Rules and expectations mediated by peer pressure
3. Blurring of the patient's role through viewing of patients as responsible human beings
4. An emphasis on patient's rights for involvement in setting goals
5. Freedom of movement and informality of relationships with staff

6. An emphasis on interdisciplinary participation
7. Goal-oriented, clear communication

Community meetings, activity groups, social skills groups, and physical exercise programs are some of the ways that milieu management is achieved.

Treatment units that set clearly defined and time-limited goals with patients and units that organize and schedule prosocial activities for most waking hours are thought to be the most effective.

Milieu therapy consists of the establishment of an environment that is adapted to the individual client's needs but that also provides greater comfort and freedom of expression than he or she has experienced in the past. The environment is staffed by persons who are trained to provide support and understanding and give individual attention. All members of the environment contribute to the planning and functioning of the setting. The power hierarchy is diminished, as all members are viewed as significant and valuable members of the community.

An overview of the major theoretical schools of thought, some major theorists, research emphases, and therapeutic approaches is given in Table 2–2.

Table 2–2 ■ SUMMARY OF SCHOOLS OF THOUGHT, THEORISTS, AND THERAPIES

SCHOOL	SOME AMERICAN THEORISTS	THEORETICAL INFLUENCES	RESEARCH EMPHASIS	THERAPEUTIC APPROACHES
Biological	Torry, Andreason	NIMH	Genetic studies; central nervous system research	Pharmacotherapy
Psychoanalytical	Erikson, Mahler, Kernberg	Freudian concepts and modifications, e.g., ego psychology	Personality disorders	Intensive insight psychotherapy and psychoanalysis
Interpersonal	Fromm-Reichmann, Ariete, Peplau, Rogers	Sullivan	Adult relations, e.g., marriage, work, and community	Broadened psychotherapeutic frameworks, e.g., families and groups; psychotherapy expanded for use with schizophrenia, depression, and other disorders
Social	Lindemann, Caplan, Meyer	Derived from sociology, anthropology, and other social sciences	Epidemiological studies and large-scale social analysis	Community mental health centers, e.g., crisis therapies
Behavioral-cognitive	Wolpe, Ellis, Beck	Based on pavlovian and skinnerian theories	Behavioral analysis of symptoms; learning theory	Behavioral therapies and learning theories, e.g., positive reinforcement, operant conditioning, systematic desensitization, aversion conditioning

Adapted from Klerman G. Historical perspectives on contemporary schools of psychopathology. *In* Millon T, Klerman G (eds). Contemporary Directions in Psychopathology Towards the DSM IV. New York: The Guilford Press, 1986, p 8.

Issues in Mental Health Nursing for the 1990s

COMMUNITY MENTAL HEALTH PROGRAMS

Mental health advocates support community mental health treatment programs to help people with mental illness cope more effectively with problems and achieve a better quality of life. Community-based programs for the mentally ill are set up to provide systems that can enable individuals to cope with daily life outside of institutions through rehabilitation and supportive therapy.

The Community Mental Health Centers Act of 1963 laid the basis for the delivery of services in the areas of mental health and mental illness. By the 1980s, this government-funded program had resulted in the establishment of about 800 community mental health centers. Because of significant financial constraints, the community mental health center function is severely limited, and this program is considered by many to be an ineffective one (Kaplan and Sadock 1991).

A disturbing trend within the community-based mental health programs of today is that the paraprofessional has moved into what is called the "new" professional status and has taken over more and more aspects of the care and treatment of the mentally ill. There has been a huge increase in the number of nontraditionally trained (and sometimes untrained) personnel in the human services fields. At the same time, PhD-level psychologists and psychiatrists are less and less involved in the care and treatment of the severely mentally ill, and professionally trained personnel constitute a decreasing percentage of community mental health workers in some areas of the country. Currently in the United States, large numbers of mental health staff service the least needy. Many psychiatrists, psychologists, social workers, and psychiatric nurses avoid working with the chronically ill psychotic population, preferring to practice psychodynamic psychotherapy privately (Test and Marks 1990). This lack of involvement by trained professionals has led to a crisis in patient care.

DEINSTITUTIONALIZATION

A controversial social and mental health issue of the 1980s and 1990s has been the process of deinstitutionalization, in which vast numbers of chronically mental ill patients have been discharged from mental hospitals and returned to the community. For example, in 1955 an estimated 560,000 people resided in psychiatric institutions, compared with 130,000 today (Kaplan and Sadock 1991). However, comprehensive community-based psychiatric and medical care is often not available for most discharged mentally ill patients. Of the 2000 community mental health centers originally proposed, only 800 were ever funded, often without providing the full range of clinical services required of them by law (Goldman et al. 1983). Consequently, discharge from the institution has in many cases resulted in increased exposure to a hostile environment and a lack of health care. Because the illness of many patients with chronic conditions interferes with their coping skills, there is a drift downward to even more stressful impoverished environments. The end result is homelessness in urban areas (Kaplan and Sadock 1991). Returning mental patients to the community has highlighted the crucial need for treatment resources and social support services, family involvement, and the provision of suitable living conditions to maintain the chronically ill in the community.

SELF-HELP GROUPS

A major community development in the mental health field in the 1980s was the rise of self-help groups throughout the United States, and these groups continue to proliferate in the 1990s. These programs are made up of persons experiencing similar circumstances or misfortunes either directly or indirectly concerned with mental health, such as Mothers Against Drunk Driving (MADD), Overeaters Anonymous (OA), and Gamblers Anonymous (GA). Most of these support groups incorporate the principles of Alcoholics Anonymous (AA), which was founded in 1935. The self-help groups function as a source of information as well as psychological support.

With dramatic increases in their membership, a number of these self-help groups have begun to emerge as constituencies in the mental health field. For example, the National Alliance of the Mentally Ill (NAMI) has become a powerful political force at the state and federal levels, advocating for the seriously mentally ill, particularly schizophrenics, and more recently for those suffering from depression and bipolar disorders. The alcoholism field is noted for the power of its constituency groups, notably the alliance between Alcoholics Anonymous and the National Council on Alcoholism. With these burgeoning groups, the mental health field can be compared to the general health field, in which constituency groups for cancer, heart disease, and arthritis have been important forces for the expansion of services and the support of research and innovation in treatment. There are, however, relatively few powerful advocacy groups for children and adolescents with mental illness.

THE HOMELESS

It has been estimated that providers of health care to the homeless may expect 40% of their clients to have mental illness, and many more will have emotional problems of some sort consequent to their homelessness (Breakey et al. 1989). In the 1980s, managers of shelters and meal sites started to experience increasing behavioral problems and untreated psychiatric illness among clients. Observers of areas where the homeless congregate noted that mentally ill men were starting to outnumber alcoholics (Blackwell et al. 1990). It has been increasingly recognized that a major issue facing community care in the 1990s, with the growing number of homeless persons who are mentally ill, is the need to successfully fulfill the necessary functions previously provided by mental hospitals, such as crisis intervention, daily social and recreational activities, housing, and medical and mental health care (Scott and Marks 1990).

ACQUIRED IMMUNODEFICIENCY SYNDROME

A major medical and mental health crisis facing the 1990s is the spread of acquired immunodeficiency syndrome (AIDS) throughout the world. It is believed that 1.5 million Americans are now infected with the human immunodeficiency virus. AIDS is now the most common cause of death in the United States.

AIDS has taken a heavy toll on the poor, urban, and minority populations in the United States. Moreover, AIDS has become the leading cause of death for 30- to 50-year-old men and 20- to 40-year-old women in New York City. There has been a sharp increase among people with AIDS in our teenage populations.

People with AIDS can show a full range of psychiatric symptoms—depression, mania, psychosis, general anxiety symptoms, and obsessive-compulsive symptoms, among others (Kaplan and Sadock 1991). Suicide is not uncommon among persons with AIDS or AIDS-related complex. Therefore, there is a large and vital role for mental health professionals to fill.

Another major challenge for the mental health community is meeting the mental health needs of health care workers and others who are directly involved in caring for persons with AIDS. Fear regarding

the transmission of AIDS may place stress on those who deal directly with individuals who have AIDs.

The day-to-day care of terminally ill AIDS clients carries with it a significant element of stress. If physicians, nurses, and others see their role primarily as one of saving lives, they may suffer because of their ineffectiveness. However, if they can view their role in the broader sense of ministering to the ill or dying, they may be better able to cope with their expectations and offer more comprehensive care.

BIOLOGICAL REVOLUTION

There is a biological revolution in psychiatry causing a move away from a psychological approach toward a more biological stance. Knowledge in the field of psychopharmacology has undergone unprecedented growth over the past quarter of a century. New developments are being announced monthly. New drug compounds have provided effective treatments for many psychiatric disorders, and new uses have been found for old medications. With the rapid expansion of biological and psychopharmacological information, the task of integrating biological and psychotherapeutic approaches to treatment has become more difficult. Some mental health professionals maintain that psychopharmacological approaches have become the essence of psychiatry, whereas others insist that these drugs merely mask the underlying psychological issues, work against conflict resolution, and interfere with therapy. However, the trend in treatment is to incorporate aspects of psychosocial, psychobiological, and psychopharmacological theories to form a new psychiatry (Schatzberg and Cole 1991). A major reason for this point of view is that although psychotropic drugs have profound and beneficial effects on cognition, mood, and behavior, they often do not change the underlying process, which is frequently highly sensitive to intrapsychic and psychosocial stressors. Beneficial outcomes can be best achieved by simultaneously reducing symptoms and promoting the capacity of the individual to adapt to the pressures and demands of his or her life.

NEGLECTED POPULATIONS

Finally, mental health care in the 1990s is confronted with the issue of caring for populations that have been traditionally underserved and unserved, such as women, children, the elderly, and those in rural populations. It has been calculated that 10% of the population at any time is in need of mental health services and that only about one third of this group comes to the attention of any sort of mental health treatment facility. The fate (good or bad) of the rest of this population is as yet undetermined. Women are still underserved or even harmed, particularly when their problems run counter to societal stereotypes, as is the case with female alcoholics. Two of three seriously disturbed children in the United States are not receiving the mental health services they need. Generally, there are few mental health services in rural areas.

By the year 2000, one of every six Americans will be over the age of 65. There has been no historical precedent for the aging of the population that will occur as we enter the twenty-first century. Never before have there been so many older people relative to the number of younger people, a situation presenting greater demands for mental health services. There is considerable evidence that older adults do not receive as much mental health care as would be desirable, and ethnic minority elders are even less well served (Roybal 1988; Fellin and Powell 1988). A number of reasons account for this inadequate level of mental health services: elders are reluctant to seek aid for emotional problems, funding to community mental health centers does not provide effective outreach to older adults, programs in some mental health professions (such as psychology) do not emphasize geriatric specialization, and there are few financial incentives for many private practitioners to seek out older patients who are provided with limited Medicare coverage. Attention needs to be given to the mental health needs of specific segments of the elderly population, including the frail and those living in poverty. Nursing home residents, older persons living alone, older women, older minorities, the elderly in rural areas, and the very old are especially vulnerable. Indeed, the current challenge to the mental health community and to society is to meet the needs of the vast numbers of underserved and unserved populations by the end of the twentieth century.

Summary

The four major categories of psychotropic drugs for treating mental disorders are (1) antipsychotics (neuroleptics), (2) antianxiety agents (anxiolytics), (3) antidepressants, and (4) antimanic drugs (for manic episodes in bipolar disorders). These are all discussed in detail in later chapters in this text.

Electroconvulsive therapy is extremely effective in major depressive disorders, in acutely suicidal clients, in clients who are not eating, and in those for whom medication is not effective.

This chapter provides an overview of some individual, group, and other psychotherapies. Many of these psychotherapies are explained in more detail within the chapters that deal with specific mental disorders. The individual therapies introduced were (1) classical psychoanalysis, (2) psychoanalytically oriented psychotherapy, (3) short term dynamic psychotherapy, (4) transactional analysis, (5) cognitive (insight) therapy, (6) the behavioral therapies, and (7) gestalt therapy.

The group therapies covered were (1) psychoanalytically oriented therapy, (2) psychodrama, and (3) family therapy. For each, the method of approach, the role of the participants, and the role of the therapist were discussed.

Other therapies useful in certain situations are (1) sex therapy, (2) hypnotherapy, (3) crisis therapy, and (4) milieu therapy. Conditions, indications, and contraindications for some were mentioned.

With regard to major issues in mental health care, there are a great many deficiencies in the number, type, and quality of services available to people needing mental health care. Political reasons, along with the existing dire economic conditions, have further served to highlight some of the deficits. Some trends seen during the 1980s were efforts to fill this need (increased use of paraprofessionals, the emergence of self-help groups, and the inclusion of mental health centers within existing health care centers). The 1980s saw the reverberations of deinstitutionalization, the increased incidence of the homeless who are mentally ill, the crisis of the AIDS epidemic, and the biological revolution in psychiatry with the availability of new drugs. The fact that a great majority of our population (women, children, the aged, refugees, those living in rural areas, and minorities) is still grossly underserved is of great concern to those working in the field of mental health. The challenge of the 1990s is to address deficiencies in the mental health needs of these populations.

References

Aldinger B. Personal communication, 1992.

Altrocchi J. Abnormal Psychology. New York: Harcourt Brace Jovanovich, 1980.

Beck AJ. Cognitive Therapy and the Emotional Disorders. New York: The New American Library, 1976.

Berne E. Games People Play. New York: Grove Press, 1964.

Bettleheim B. The Empty Fortress. New York: Free Press, 1967.

Bettleheim B. A Home for the Heart. New York: Knopf, 1974.

Blackwell B, et al. Psychiatric and mental health services. In Brickner P, et al (eds). Under the Safety Net. New York: WW Norton, 1990.

Breakey WR, et al. Health and mental health problems of homeless men and women in Baltimore. Journal of the American Medical Association, 262:1352, 1989.

Ellis A. Reason and Emotion in Psychotherapy. New York: Lyle Stuart, 1962.

Fellin PA, Powell TJ. Mental health services and older adult minorities: An assessment. The Gerontologist, 28:442, 1988.

Goldman HH, et al. Deinstitutionalization: The data demythologized. Hospital and Community Psychiatry, 34:129, 1983.

Harper RA. Psychoanalysis and Psychotherapy—36 Systems. New York: Jason Aronson, 1974.

Kaplan HI, Sadock BJ (eds). Synopis of Psychiatry, 6th ed. Baltimore: Williams & Wilkins, 1991.

Kennedy MS. Hypnosis. In Lego S (ed). The American Handbook of Psychiatric Nursing. Philadelphia: JB Lippincott, 1984.

Lego S. Individual therapy. In Lego S (ed). The American Handbook of Psychiatric Nursing. Philadelphia: JB Lippincott, 1984.

Liberman RP, Mueser KT. Schizophrenia: Psychosocial treatment. In Kaplan HI, Sadock BJ (eds). Comprehensive Textbook of Psychiatry (4th ed.). Baltimore, MD: Williams & Wilkins, 1989.

Masters WH, Johnson VE. Human Sexual Response. Boston: Little, Brown & Company, 1966.

Masters WH, Johnson VE. Human Sexual Inadequacy. Boston: Little, Brown & Company, 1970.

Moreno JL. Psychodrama. New York: Beacon, 1946.

Roybal ER. Mental health and aging: The need for an expanded federal response. American Psychologist, 43:189, 1988.

Schatzberg AF, Cole JO. Manual of Clinical Psychopharmacology, 2nd ed. Washington, DC: American Psychiatric Press, 1991.

Scott RA, Marks IM. Implementation and review. In Scott RA, Marks IM (eds). Mental Health Care Delivery: Innovations, Impediments, and Implementation. Cambridge: Cambridge University Press, 1990.

Test MA, Marks IM. Commentary. In Scott RA, Marks IM (eds). Mental Health Care Delivery: Innovations, Impediments, and Implementation. Cambridge: Cambridge University Press, 1990.

FURTHER READING

Andrulis DP, Mazade NA. American mental health policy: Changing directions in the 80s. Hospital and Community Psychiatry, 34:601, 1983.

Berlin RM, Kales JD, Humphrey FJ II, et al. The patient care crisis in community mental health centers: A need for more psychiatric involvement. American Journal of Psychiatry, 138:450, 1981.

Davison GC, Neale JM. Abnormal Psychology: An Experimental Clinical Approach. New York: John Wiley & Sons, 1982.

Fink P, Weinstein S. Whatever happened to psychiatry? The deprofessionalism of community mental health centers. American Journal of Psychiatry, 136:406, 1979.

Goldenberg I, Goldenberg H. Family Therapy: An Overview. Monterey, CA: Brooks/Cole, 1980.

Gruenberg EM, Archer J. Abandonment of responsibility for the seriously mentally ill. Milbank Memorial Fund Quarterly; Health and Society, 57:485, 1979.

Gutheil TG. The therapeutic milieu: Changing themes and theories. Hospital and Community Psychiatry, 36(12):1279, 1985.

Holzman D. New AIDS victim: Hospital budgets. Insight, 25:84, 1986.

Iscoe I, Harris LC. Social and community interventions. Annual Review of Psychology, 35:333, 1984.

Katz AH. Self-help and mutual aid: An emerging social movement. Annual Review of Psychology, 7:129, 1981.

Klerman GL. Report of the Administrator: Alcohol and Drug Abuse and Mental Health Administration, 1980. Washington, DC. DHHS Publications no. 81–1165, Washington, DC 1981.

Kolb LC, Brodie HK. Modern Clinical Psychiatry, 10th ed. Philadelphia: WB Saunders, 1982.

Lamb HR. What did we really expect from deinstitutionalization? Hospital and Community Psychiatry, 32:105, 1981.

Langsley DG. The community mental health center. Does it treat patients? Hospital and Community Psychiatry, 31:815, 1980.

Lipman RS. Pharmacotherapy of the anxiety disorders. In Fisher S. Greenberg RP (eds). The Limits of Biological Treatments for Psychological Distress. Hillsdale, NJ: Erlbaum Associates, 1989.

Mahoney MJ, Arnkoff DB. Congenitive and self-control therapies. In Garfield SI, Bergin AE (eds). Handbook of Psychotherapy and Behavior Change: An Empirical Analysis, 2nd ed. New York: John Wiley & Sons, 1978.

Mahoney MJ, Thoresen CE. Self-control: Power to the Person. Monterey, CA: Brooks/Cole, 1974.

Michenbaum D. Cognitive Behavior Modification. New York: Plenum, 1977.

Miller GE. Barriers to serving the chronically mentally ill. Psychiatric Quarterly, 53:118, 1981.

Redick RW, Witkin MJ. State and County Mental Hospitals, United States, 1979–1980 and 1980–1981. Rockville, MD: National Institute of Mental Health, 1983. Mental Health Statistical Note no. 165.

Riessman F. The role of the paraprofessional in the mental health crisis. Paraprofessional Journal, 1:1, 1980.

Rose SM. Deciphering and deinstitutionalization: Complexities in policy and program analysis. Milbank Memorial Fund Quarterly; Health and Society, 57:429, 1979.

Skinner BF. Science and Human Behavior. New York: MacMillan, 1953.

Sorensen JL, et al. Preventing AIDS in Drug Users and Their Sexual Partners. New York: The Guilford Press, 1991.

Thoresen CE, Coates TJ. Behavioral self-control: Some concerns. In Herson M. Eisler RM, Miller PM (eds). Progress in Behavior Modification, vol 2. New York: Academic Press, 1976.

Winslow WW. Changing trends in CMHCs: Keys to survival in the eighties. Hospital and Community Psychiatry, 3:273, 1982.

Self-study Exercises

Match the following.

1. _____ Are useful for short term relief of anxiety, management of anxiety disorders, and alcohol withdrawal

2. _____ Help normalize behaviors (e.g., grandiosity, psychomotor agitation, elevated unstable mood) in people in the manic state of bipolar illness

3. _____ Are used primarily for treating depressive disorders

4. _____ Can decrease bizarre behaviors and disorganized thinking and increase activity in severely withdrawn clients

A. Antimanic drugs (lithium)

B. Antipsychotics (neuroleptics)

C. Antianxiety drugs (anxiolytics)

D. Tricyclics, monoamine oxidase inhibitors, and serotonin reuptake inhibitors

Complete the statements by filling in the appropriate missing information.

5. Receiving a reward for a desired behavior is a form of _____ therapy.

6. Techniques used to get people in touch with different aspects of themselves, with emphasis on the "here and now" rather than the "then and there," are part of _____ therapy.

7. Lying on a couch, free-associating to a neutral analyst on whom transference feelings are directed, is part of _____ .

8. Identification of specific personality parts (child, parent, and adult) and the types of interactions (games) and recognition of maladaptive parental influences (scripts) are integral to _____ .

9. Therapy is limited in time, and although certain tools (e.g., transference and dream interpretation) are used, the therapist often influences the direction of the content. That is called _____ .

10. The therapist interacts actively with the client within the context of an intimate professional relationship to change symptoms or uncover unsatisfactory life patterns. This is called _____ .

Write a short answer to the questions that follow.

11. Indicate the advantage of each of the following:

    A. Group therapy: _____

    _____

    B. Family therapy: _____

    _____

    C. Psychodrama: _____

    _____

12. For each of the following therapeutic modalities, identify a circumstance that would indicate its use:

    A. Sex therapy: _____

    B. Hypnotherapy: _____

    C. Crisis therapy: _____

    D. Milieu therapy: _____

CHAPTER 3

Legal and Ethical Issues

Penny S. Brooke

OUTLINE ●

KEY TERMS AND CONCEPTS ● ● ● ● ● ● ● ● ● ● ● ● ● ● ● ● ●

The key terms and concepts listed here also appear in bold where they are defined or discussed in this chapter.

The author wishes to recognize and thank Lorenza M. Valvo and Mary Ursula Guthormsen for their contribution to the first edition.

INFORMED CONSENT

INTENTIONAL TORT

INVOLUNTARY ADMISSION

LEAST RESTRICTIVE ALTERNATIVE

NEGLIGENCE

PUNITIVE DAMAGES

RIGHT TO REFUSE TREATMENT

RIGHT TO TREATMENT

TARASOFF RULING: DUTY TO WARN
   THIRD PARTIES

TORTS

VOLUNTARY ADMISSION

OBJECTIVES ■

After studying this chapter, the student will be able to

1. Define the following terms:
   A. Ethics and bioethics
   B. Torts
   C. Battery
   D. Assault
   E. False imprisonment
   F. Negligence
2. Summarize the relationships between social norms, ethics, and mental deviation.
3. Compare (a) voluntary admission with two types of involuntary admission and (b) conditional release with discharge.
4. Discuss and give examples of what is meant by a client's civil rights, especially as they pertain to restraint and seclusion.
5. Discuss the standards of care for psychiatric nursing practice.
6. Describe the balance between patients' rights and the rights of society with respect to these legal concepts relevant in nursing and psychiatric nursing:
   A. Duty to intervene
   B. Documentation and charting
   C. Confidentiality
   D. Right to treatment
   E. Right to refuse treatment
   F. Informed consent

Through licensure, a state confers on the registered nurse the privilege of practicing the profession of nursing in that state. Implicit in this right to practice nursing is the responsibility to practice safely and competently and in a manner consistent with state laws and regulations. Nursing practice is regulated through licensure. Each state has a licensing agency, a state board of nursing that is charged with the implementation of the nurse practice act in that state. The state law sets forth the legal parameters of the practice of nursing, minimum qualifications for practicing nursing, and actionable offenses for disciplinary purposes. The state board of nursing is composed of experts in the field of nursing. The authority of the board varies according to the legislation of the state that creates and delegates responsibilities to the board. The board promulgates rules and regulations

that more specifically define the nurse practice act of its state. It also serves as the hearing panel in disciplinary matters.

The underlying premise of this chapter is that the patient's rights and the nurse's responsibilities are necessarily intertwined. Knowledge of the nurse practice act is merely a starting point because numerous statutes, regulations, and court decisions may affect the way a nurse practices. This is particularly true in the area of psychiatric nursing because every state has enacted mental health laws regarding the care and treatment of the mentally ill.

Nurses who work for the federal government in facilities such as Veterans Administration hospitals must also be aware of the policies and procedures of these institutions, as well as of the federal statutes that apply to these settings.

This chapter introduces the student to current legal and ethical issues that may be encountered in the practice of psychiatric nursing. Because the law is dynamic and evolving, it does not always lend itself to clear answers. Accordingly, in situations in which the law is not clearly stated by statute, regulation, or court decision, the nurse often encounters an ethical dilemma (i.e., a situation that requires a choice between morally conflicting alternatives).

The fundamental concept in any legal or ethical issue confronting the nurse in a psychiatric setting is striking the balance between the rights of the individual patient and the rights of society at large. This chapter is designed to assist the student in identifying competing ethical or legal interests involved in various nursing interventions and to help the student consider their impact on decision making.

Although the New York and California statutes and cases cited in the chapter might differ from those of the student's state, these statutes are representative of modern mental hygiene law in the United States. Different state cases are cited to demonstrate different principles of law. *The student is encouraged to be aware of the mental health statutes in his or her own state.*

Ethical Concepts

Ethics is the study of philosophical beliefs of what is considered right or wrong in a society. Discussions of ethical practice in nursing involve the topics of morals and values. Whenever morals and values are being debated, there is no right or wrong answer. Ethical beliefs are generally very personal beliefs that arise from one's experiences in society. Judgments made about the ethical beliefs of another are often unfounded. It is important for psychiatric nurses to be consciously aware of their own ethical beliefs. Nurses who are not aware of how they feel about ethical dilemmas are more likely to impose their beliefs on patients instead of being open to allowing patients to act autonomously according to their own beliefs. The term *bioethics* is used in relation to ethical dilemmas surrounding patient care. **Bioethics** in psychiatric nursing is the application of ethical principles within the scope of the psychiatric nursing practice setting.

The four principles of bioethics are (1) beneficience, (2) autonomy, (3) justice, and (4) fidelity. Beneficence is the doing of good; autonomy is the respect for others' rights to make decisions; justice is the treating of others fairly and equally; and fidelity is the strictest observance of loyalty and commitment to the patient.

An example of *beneficence* is the decision to remain by the bedside of an extremely anxious patient to be supportive, even if the shift has ended. Respecting others' rights to make treatment decisions that do not conform with the recommendation of the staff is an example of *autonomy*. Ensuring that equal staff attention is given to the depressed, disgruntled, disagreeable patient is an example of *justice*. An example of *fidelity* is demonstrated by the nurse's commitment to clinical expertise through participation in continuing education.

Everyone has an inner set of standards that results from the influences of family and teachers, as well as from life's experiences. The development of a value system is a dynamic process, and exposure to different values provides an opportunity for reordering and incorporating new values. Self-exploration to identify one's belief system through reading, questioning, and discussing ethical issues (i.e., clarifying one's own value system) is an essential element in the process of becoming a professional. Knowledge of one's value system helps in formulating a sturdy foundation for professional development. Without this knowledge, the nurse may feel vulnerable and become confused when confronted with work situations that present a different set of values. However, flexibility to allow one's values to grow, change, and evolve is necessary to professional development.

When the psychiatric nurse is presented with an ethical dilemma, it is often helpful to discuss possible solutions to the issues with others. Through small-group discussions, the nurse is able to clarify the facts of the situation and the real ethical decisions to be made. Input from several persons, including members of the health care team and the patient's family, may be most productive in clarifying these issues and in protecting the patient's autonomy and right to decide for him- or herself. There are no easy answers to ethical dilemmas, but having input from several persons helps to arrive at a reasonable solution. Ethical dilemmas typically result in final decisions that do not please everyone.

Because ethical decisions involve morals and values that may differ widely among decision makers, it is important to respect and protect the patient's autonomy and the patient's right to be the ultimate decision maker about decisions that affect the patient's life. The nurse must avoid trying to impose his or her personal morals and values on the patient. The nurse's life experiences may be dramatically different from those of the patient, and part of becoming a professional is developing the ability to recognize and accept the patient's right to have an opinion that differs from one's own.

The nurse's values may also conflict with the prevailing institutional value system. This situation further complicates the decision-making process and necessitates careful consideration of the patient's desires. For example, the nurse may experience a conflict in a setting in which there is abundant use of tranquilizers for the treatment of an elderly or a depressed patient. Whenever one's value system is compromised, increased stress results.

Ethical standards, although lacking the clarity and power of law, do serve as a field guide for decision making. As each generation advances in both knowledge and technology, society inherits increased options. Choices exist today that were nonexistent just 10 years ago. Such dynamic progress promotes more questions than answers. In such a society, the most limited, and thus the most dangerous, way of proceeding is to assume with moral certitude that there is only one "right" or "correct" thing to do. The nurse's role as a patient advocate is a prime example of the need to be able to view a situation from another vantage point: that is, through the eyes of the patient. The autonomy of psychiatric patients who have been judicially found to be incompetent is influenced by the court's appointment of a competent person to serve as the surrogate decision maker. The surrogate decision maker is chosen because of an ability to place him- or herself in the shoes of the patient. Clearly, this is not always a simple exercise; rather, it is one that demands empathy and understanding of all the critical elements of the situation.

The distinction between legal and ethical issues is often vague. However, there is an important distinction when the nurse relies on ethical guiding principles instead of on the guiding principles of law. The nurse is bound to comply with the laws, and even though the nurse may feel morally obligated to follow ethical guidelines, these guiding principles should not override laws. For example, if the nurse is aware of a statute, or of a specific rule or regulation created by the state board of nursing that prohibits certain behavior, such as restraining patients against their will, but the nurse feels an ethical obligation to protect the patient by using restraints, the nurse would be wise to follow the law. Laws override ethical principles, which do not have the same legal strength. Ethical issues are moral dilemmas that become laws if society is concerned enough to take the issues to the courts or to the legislature. Ethical issues become legal issues through court case decisions or when the legislature has heard from many people that a law is needed to protect certain rights. Laws are specific, and they address only what is wrong in a particular society. It is not always possible or desirable to translate an ethical principle into law. Laws protect people's rights and freedoms, but they also infringe on other rights and freedoms. Laws are fluid: they change from time

to time and from place to place. Laws reflect a community's standards, which is the reason nurses must become aware of the specific laws of the community in which they are practicing. The law is narrow and deals with a system of compliance in a given society. Laws are developed to protect the population as a whole, or at least a segment of the population. Specific laws are written to protect psychiatric patients and persons who are not competent to protect their own rights. Ethical principles are much broader and express more universal concepts than do laws. Ethical values address what is wrong or right or what the nurse's duties and obligations to the patient are. Ethical choices are based on the individual's attitudes, values, and beliefs. Although one's ethical beliefs are important to follow, they cannot be relied on as guiding principles when they contradict a stated law.

MENTAL ILLNESS AND THE SOCIAL NORM

Social norms are known to every society, and most members of society conform to these norms. However, some members of society do not conform. What happens to them? Must all people conform?

Thomas Szasz, a psychiatrist, questioned the basic concepts of mental illness (Szasz 1961, 1970; cited in Fenner 1980). He suggested that committing people to institutions for treatment was a mechanism used by society to come to terms with those who did not conform to society's mores. Thus, commitment to an institution was society's way of "dealing with" rather than "caring for" the deviants.

Does society need the nonconformist, the artist, the scientist, and the inventor? Does the majority have the right to impose its will on the individual?

What about the freedom of the individual to do what he or she wants to do when he or she wants to do it? When is the right of the individual curtailed for the benefit of society? Take, for example, the street lady who for years has been unobtrusively pilfering from trash containers every evening. This behavior, although not desirable, is acceptable. Eventually, she starts rummaging after midnight, and as the noise level escalates, the community responds by notifying authorities of the violation of the peace. What was once tolerable behavior becomes unacceptable. Davis and Aroskar (1978), when discussing mental illness, state that deviance is not the quality of the act the person commits but is a consequence of the application by others of rules or sanctions to the offender.

Therapy is always directed at restoring some functions and repressing others. According to Haring (1975), almost every therapeutic act contains some elements of manipulating or restructuring some biological or psychological functions. The objective of psychotherapy is to modify undesirable behavior and to increase the person's repertoire of more socially acceptable behavior. What constitutes desirable or acceptable behavior of the individual is decided on by the group that establishes the norms.

Methods of changing human behavior include behavior modification techniques and psychotherapy. Psychotropic drugs can also dramatically alter behavior and must therefore be prescribed carefully. All brain activity has a chemical component that affects behavior. A wide range of medications to alter behavior is now available, including psychotherapeutic drugs, tranquilizers, energizers, and hypnotics. Other methods of modifying behavior include psychosurgery, and electroshock therapy—all tremendously powerful means to treat the brain, the essence of the human. Freedom of expression is a fundamental value of our society, a right embodied in the Constitution. Some hold the view that many psychiatric treatment modalities alter the individual's thought processes and thus challenge our fundamental societal values.

Psychotherapy may consist of contrasting theoretical and methodological approaches to understanding human behavior. The therapeutic setting, the symbolism of how we behave and how we think, the process of developing a therapeutic relationship with a therapist, the resistance to treatment, the transference of feelings, and the termination of the therapeutic relationship are all important aspects of psychotherapy. Developmental theory, evaluation, and research are used in psychotherapy. The psychotherapeutic relationship is very crucial to the improvement of the patient's condition. The therapists using psychotherapy must be well trained in understanding human behavior. Many approaches and theories are available to assist the psychotherapist. This process does not necessarily have to be a lifelong one. Early intervention can help the patient avoid extended therapy by enabling the patient to understand the meaning of his or her behavior. Personal insight is an important aspect of the psychotherapeutic relationship. Children are especially responsive to psychotherapy because their defense mechanisms are not as complex as those of adults. The psychotherapeutic relationship carries with it serious ethical and legal obligations to the patient. The psychotherapist becomes extremely important to the patient and must assume this role conscientiously. Termination of the psychotherapeutic relationship can be traumatic to the patient if the break is not handled skillfully. The psychotherapist also has a legal and ethical obligation to the patient

and to society not to abuse the power that can exist when a patient relies on a therapist.

Protection of the patient when he or she is in a vulnerable state of mind must be considered. Sadly, many therapeutic relationships are in the news because of sexual abuse of clients by therapists. This type of misuse of the therapeutic relationship is grounds for losing one's license. Protection of the confidentiality and privacy of the patient's disclosures during therapeutic communication is also extremely important. Because of the complexity of human behavior, therapeutic relationships may be long-lasting and very complicated. Skilled psychotherapists must also have great insight into their own behavior.

In summary, essential to an understanding of ethical questions and issues is a knowledge of one's personal value system, the professional code of ethics, and societal values. Laws reflect society's values. In the area of mental health and psychiatric nursing, it is further necessary to understand the mental health laws at both the state and federal levels.

Mental Health Laws

A fundamental component of psychiatric nursing care is understanding the legal framework for the delivery and provision of mental health services in the particular state in which the nurse practices.

Laws have been enacted in each state to regulate the care and treatment of the mentally ill. Many of these laws have undergone major revision in the past 25 years, reflecting a shift in emphasis from state institutional care of the mentally ill to community-based care, heralded by the enactment of the Community Mental Health Center Act of 1963 under President John Kennedy. Along with this shift in emphasis has come the more widespread use of psychotropic drugs in the treatment of mental illness—enabling many people to integrate more readily into the larger community—and an increasing awareness of the need to provide the mentally ill with humane care that respects their civil rights.

Included in a patient's right to remain protected are the issues of inappropriate and indefinite involuntary commitment of mentally disordered persons, developmentally disordered persons, and persons with chronic alcoholism. The timeliness and appropriateness of evaluation and treatment of persons with serious mental disorders or chronic alcoholism are also issues of concern. An emphasis is now placed not only on protecting public safety but also on safeguarding the individual rights of persons through judicial review. Conservatorships for gravely disabled persons and better use of public funds for social service agencies that provide these services are being established by legislation at the state and federal levels. There can be competing interests between protection of the individual patient's rights and protection of the public safety. Public safety and health issues are generally legislated at the state level.

State laws are extensive, with a range in topics including types of admissions; appointments of conservators and guardians; treatment of minors; informed consent for electroconvulsive therapy, psychosurgery, and medication administration; civil rights; and treatment of disordered sex offenders.

The following section of this chapter provides an overview of the types of hospital admissions and discharges. **All students are encouraged to become familiar with the important provisions of the laws in their own states regarding admissions, discharges, patient rights, and informed consent** because a state-by-state review of the law is beyond the scope of this chapter.

ADMISSIONS TO THE HOSPITAL

Admissions to mental institutions are governed by statutes that vary from state to state. Admissions are either voluntary or involuntary, and this categorization affects a patient's rights with regard to release, notice of rights, and treatment.

VOLUNTARY HOSPITALIZATION. Generally, **voluntary admission** is sought by the patient or the patient's guardian through a written application to the facility. Voluntary patients have the right to demand and obtain release. If the patient is a minor, the release may be contingent on the consent of the parents or guardian. However, few states require voluntary patients to be notified of the rights associated with their status. Additionally, many states require that a patient submit a written release notice to the facility staff, who re-evaluate the patient's condition for possible conversion to involuntary status according to criteria established by the state law.

A minority of state statutes provide for a less restricted form of voluntary admission called informal admission. Informal admission permits a patient to make a verbal application for admission, similar to that made for hospital admission for medical treatment.

INVOLUNTARY HOSPITALIZATION. Involuntary admission presupposes the patient's lack of consent. Although criteria vary from state to state, there are two common threads found in state law that justify involuntary commitment. Involuntary admission is necessary when a person is a danger to him- or herself or others as a result of a mental disorder or when a person is in need of psychiatric treatment or care. Three different procedures are commonly available: judicial determination, administrative or agency determination, and certification by a specified number of physicians that a person's mental health justifies detention and treatment.

Involuntary hospitalization can be further categorized by the nature and the purpose of the involuntary admission. It may be emergency, observational or temporary, or indeterminate or extended.

Emergency Involuntary Hospitalization. Most states provide for emergency involuntary hospitalization for a specified period (3–10 days on the average) to prevent dangerous behavior likely to cause harm to self or others. Police officers, physicians, and mental health professionals may be designated by statute to authorize the detention of mentally ill persons who are dangers to themselves or others.

Observational or Temporary Involuntary Hospitalization. Observational or temporary involuntary hospitalization is of longer duration than emergency hospitalization. The primary purpose of this type of hospitalization is observation, diagnosis, and treatment of persons who suffer from mental illness or pose a danger to themselves or others. The length of time is specified by statute and varies markedly from state to state. Application for this type of admission can be made by a guardian, family member, physician, or other public health officer. Some states permit any citizen to make an application for aid to another. States vary as to their procedural requirements for this type of involuntary admission. Medical certification by two or more physicians that a person is mentally ill and in need of treatment or a judicial or administrative review and order are often required for involuntary admission.

Indeterminate or Extended Involuntary Hospitalization. Indeterminate or extended involuntary hospitalization has as its primary purpose extended care and treatment of the mentally ill. Like patients who undergo observational involuntary hospitalization, those who undergo extended involuntary hospitalization are committed solely through judicial or administrative action or medical certification. States that do not require a judicial hearing before commitment often provide the patient with an opportunity for a judicial review after commitment procedures. This type of involuntary hospitalization generally lasts from 60–180 days, but it may be for an indeterminate length of time.

Patients who are involuntarily committed do not lose their right of informed consent. Patients must be considered legally competent until they have been declared incompetent through a legal proceeding. Competency is related to the capacity to understand the consequences of one's decisions. If the psychiatric nurse believes a patient lacks this ability, action should be initiated to have a legal guardian appointed by the court.

RELEASE FROM THE HOSPITAL

Release from hospitalization depends on the patient's admission status. Patients who sought informal or voluntary admission, as previously discussed, have the right to demand and receive release. Some states, however, do provide for conditional release of voluntary patients, which enables the treating physician or administrator to order continued treatment on an outpatient basis if the clinical needs of the client warrant further care.

CONDITIONAL RELEASE. Conditional release usually requires outpatient treatment for a specified period to determine the client's compliance with medication protocols, ability to meet his or her basic needs, and ability to reintegrate into the community. Generally, a voluntary patient who is conditionally released cannot be reinstitutionalized without consent unless the institution complies with the procedures for involuntary hospitalization. However, an involuntary patient who is conditionally released may be reinstitutionalized at any time without recommencement of formal admission procedures.

DISCHARGE. Discharge, or unconditional release, is the termination of a patient-institution relationship. This release may be court ordered or administratively ordered by the institution's officials. Generally, the administrative officer of an institution has the discretion to discharge patients. In a majority of states, a patient can institute a court proceeding to seek a judicial discharge. Follow-up care is critical to these patients. Discharge planning is important for the continued well-being of the psychiatric patient. Aftercare case managers are needed to facilitate the patient's adaptation back into the community and to provide early referral if the treatment plan is not being followed.

CIVIL RIGHTS AND OTHER PATIENTS' RIGHTS

Most states specifically prohibit any person from depriving a recipient of mental health services of his or her civil rights, including the right to vote; the right to civil service ranking; rights related to granting, forfeit, or denial of license; and the right to make purchases and to enter contractual relationships, unless the patient has lost his or her legal capacity by being adjudicated incompetent. The psychiatric patient's rights include the right to humane care and treatment. The medical, dental, and psychiatric needs of the patient must be met in accordance with the prevailing standards accepted in these professions.

Proper orders for specific therapies and treatments are required and must be documented in the patients' charts. Consent for surgery, shock treatment, or the use of experimental drugs or procedures must be obtained. Patients have the right to communicate fully and privately with those outside of the facility. Patients have a right to have visitors, have reasonable access to phones and mail, and receive unopened correspondence.

Persons with mental illness are guaranteed the same rights under the federal and state laws as any other citizen. Included are the right to treatment provided by the least restrictive means, the right to prompt medical care and treatment, the right to be free from hazardous procedures, and the right to dignity, privacy, and humane care.

Most state laws also provide for the right to be free from harm, which includes freedom from unnecessary or excessive physical restraint, isolation, medication, abuse, or neglect. Use of medications for staff convenience, as a punishment, or as a substitute for treatment programs is explicitly prohibited. The right to religious freedom and practice, the right to social interaction, and the right to exercise and recreational opportunities are also protected.

Additionally, patients in psychiatric hospitals have the right to be treated with dignity and respect. These rights are not only ethically important but also legally protected. Patients have the right to be free from discrimination on the basis of ethnic origin, gender, age, handicap, or religion.

Confidentiality of care and treatment is also an important right for all psychiatric patients. The patient's records must be treated as confidential by the staff. Photographs may not be taken without the patient's consent. The patient's privacy is protected along with the confidentiality of the treatment. Any discussion or consultation involving a patient should be conducted discreetly and only with individuals who have a need and a right to know this privileged information. Discussions about a patient in public places such as elevators and the cafeteria, even when the patient's name is not mentioned, can lead to disclosures of confidential information and liabilities for the nurse and the hospital. The patient's permission must be given to share information with persons who are not directly involved in the patient's care. These protections also apply to the patient's medical record, which should be read only by individuals directly involved in the patient's treatment or in monitoring the quality of care given. The patient must issue a written authorization to allow others to read his or her medical record. The patient has a right to expect that all communications and other records relating to treatment are treated as confidential.

Additional rights the psychiatric patient enjoys include a written individualized treatment plan that is reviewed regularly and that involves the patient in the plan decisions. The treatment plan needs to include the least restrictive treatment environment that is appropriate. Reasonable safety is an expectation of this environment. If the patient is unable to make these decisions, the person legally authorized to act in the patient's behalf must be consulted.

Patients have the right to be informed by their physician of the benefits, risks, and side effects of all medications and treatment procedures used. Patients cannot be subjected to any procedure or treatment without their consent, or a battery will have occurred. (Assault is the threat of harm or putting a person in a state of apprehension; battery is the actual contact with the person. These principles are discussed in greater detail later in this chapter.)

Patients have the right to refuse participation in experimental treatments or research and the right to voice grievances and recommend changes in policies and services offered by the facility without fear of punishment or reprisal. Patients may seek, at their own expense, consultation with other mental health professionals or attorneys. Patients may not be forced to work for the hospital, with the exception of being assigned routine duties that are developed to enhance their living abilities outside of the agency. The rules and regulations of the hospital need to be explained to the patient, and the patient needs to have reasonable access for communicating with persons outside the hospital. Patients also have the right to receive an itemized, detailed explanation of their bill for services rendered while they were hospitalized. A discharge plan that includes follow-up care or continuing care requirements should also be explained to the patient.

RESTRAINT AND SECLUSION. Behavioral restraint and seclusion are authorized as an intervention (1) when behavior is physically harmful to the patient or a third party, (2) when the disruptive behavior presents a danger to the facility, (3) when alternative or less restrictive measures are insufficient in protecting the patient or others from harm, and (4) when the patient anticipates that a controlled environment would be helpful and requests seclusion.

As previously indicated, most state laws prohibit the use of unnecessary physical restraint or isolation.

The use of seclusion and restraint is permitted only on the written order of a physician, which must be reviewed and renewed every 24 hours and which also must specify the type of restraint to be used. "As necessary" orders are prohibited.

Only in an emergency may the charge nurse place a patient in seclusion or restraint and obtain a written or verbal order as soon as possible thereafter. Consent of the patient is also needed unless an emergency situation exists in which an immediate risk of harm to the patient or others can be documented. The patient must be removed from restraints when safer and quieter behavior is observed. While in restraints, the patient must be protected from all sources of harm. The nurse documents the behavior leading to restraint or seclusion and the time the patient is placed in and released from restraint. The patient in restraint must be assessed at regular and frequent intervals (e.g., every 15–30 minutes) for physical needs, safety, and comfort, and these observations are also documented.

Restraint and seclusion should never be used as punishment or for the convenience of the staff. For example, if the unit is short staffed, restraining a patient to protect the patient while the nurse passes medications is an inappropriate use of restraints. The least restrictive means of restraint for the shortest duration is always the general rule. Restraints are used only to prevent harm or to provide benefit to the patient. Chemical restraints are more subtle than physical restraints but can have a greater impact on the patient's ability to relate to the environment. The psychiatric nurse must be aware of the severe and powerful impact of chemical restraints on psychiatric patients. The patient's personality and ability to relate to others is greatly controlled by chemical restraints. The practice of secluding a patient is comparable to the practice of sedating a patient until the patient is secluded within him- or herself. An example of the misuse of chemical restraints is the case in which a verbally abusive or pacing patient is settled in his or her room through sedation in order to control the unit's environment. The nurse must always be able to document professional judgment for the use of physical or chemical restraint, as well as for the use of seclusion. With recent changes in the law regarding the use of restraint and seclusion that requires a patient's consent to be restrained, agencies have revised their policies and procedures, greatly limiting these practices of the past. Most agencies have found no negative impact associated with the reduced use of restraint and seclusion. Alternative methods of therapy and cooperation with the patient have been successful.

Patients' Rights

Nowhere is the conflict between the patient's expressed interests and the nurse's judgment of the patient's best interest more apparent than in the psychiatric setting. The nurse's role of patient advocate can be difficult to exercise in the psychiatric setting, given this inherent conflict. Questioning one's ability to be an effective advocate and separating one's clinical judgment from the patient's expressed desires are essential.

Some facilities may employ a designated institution-based patient advocate to mediate such conflicts. As Davis and Aroskar (1978) point out, the effectiveness of an institution-based patient advocate depends on access to hospital records, ability to call on qualified consultants, active participation in patient care conferences and quality-of-care committees, and direct access to the hospital administrator. This is an attempt to equalize the power of the individual and that of the institution.

Some states, recognizing the inability of mentally ill patients to assert their own rights effectively in the psychiatric setting, have developed ombudsmen programs for these patients. State law in California mandates an independent patient advocate, and New York provides for mental health legal services. Both programs ensure that patients' constitutional rights are protected and that their expressed interests are represented.

The single most important action a nurse can take to protect patients' rights is to be familiar with state laws regarding the care and treatment of mentally ill patients and any rights specified by the state. If state law mandates legal services for mental patients or a patients' rights advocate program, patient concerns regarding confinement, treatment, change in status, release, medication, and any other treatment modality can be referred to the appropriate offices.

Additionally, nurses need to be familiar with their own hospitals' policies regarding admission, change in status, release, medications, informed consent, and use of restraints. The next section discusses patients' rights in depth.

DUE PROCESS RIGHTS IN CIVIL COMMITMENT

The courts have recognized that involuntary civil commitment to a mental hospital is a "massive curtailment of liberty" (*Humphrey v. Cady* 1972, p. 509) requiring due process protections in the civil commit-

ment procedure. This right derives from the Fifth Amendment of the US Constitution, which states that "no person shall . . . be deprived of life, liberty or property without due process of law." The Fourteenth Amendment explicitly prohibits states from depriving citizens of life, liberty, and property without due process of law. State civil commitment statutes, if challenged in the courts on constitutional grounds, will have to afford minimal due process protections to pass the court's scrutiny.

A state's power in enacting civil commitment procedure is based either on the *parens patriae* power or on state police power. *Parens patriae* is the power of the state to act for the care, treatment, or protection of an individual or class of individuals who are unable to act on their own behalf in their own best interests.

For example, in an 1845 Massachusetts case, *In re Oakes*, the court found justification for depriving a person of liberty for his own safety and that of others when such restraint might be beneficial to him. Mr. Oakes, an elderly widower, was confined when he became engaged to a woman of questionable character and involved in speculative financial ventures after the death of his wife. This case is an example of early judicial application of the *parens patriae* doctrine to civil commitment of the mentally ill.

In contrast, a state's police power is a plenary power to make laws and regulations to protect the public health, safety, and welfare. Civil commitment statutes are enacted to protect societal interests and have their basis in the police power.

The privilege of the writ of habeas corpus and the least-restrictive-alternative doctrine are two other important concepts applicable to civil commitment cases. A writ of habeas corpus is the procedural mechanism, guaranteed by article I, section 9 of the US Constitution, used to challenge unlawful detention by the government. The doctrine of the **least restrictive alternative** mandates that the least drastic means be taken for achieving a specific purpose.

THE RIGHT TO TREATMENT

With enactment of the Hospitalization of Mentally Ill Act in 1964, the federal statutory **right to psychiatric treatment** in public hospitals was created. The statute requires that "a person hospitalized in a public hospital for a mental illness shall, during his hospitalization, be entitled to medical and psychiatric care and treatment."

Although state courts and lower federal courts have opined that there may be a federal constitutional right to treatment, the US Supreme Court has never firmly grounded the right to treatment in a constitutional principle. The evolution of these cases in the courts provides an interesting history of the development and shortcomings of our mental health delivery system.

The initial cases presenting the psychiatric patient's right to treatment arose in the criminal justice system. In *Rouse v. Cameron* (1966), the petitioner filed a writ of habeas corpus alleging that he was unlawfully detained and without psychiatric treatment after four years in a maximum security pavilion of St. Elizabeth Hospital. Mr. Rouse had pleaded not guilty by reason of insanity to a misdemeanor charge of having a dangerous weapon in his possession, which carried a one-year maximum sentence.

The court ruled that without treatment the petitioner would be deprived of liberty and, reaching its conclusion based on state law and citing a federal statutory right, indicated that there might also be a constitutional basis for the right to treatment.

The next significant right-to-treatment case served as a sorry indictment of mental health hospitals in Alabama. The central issue in *Wyatt v. Stickney* (1971) was the absence of adequate treatment for the involuntarily committed patients. Five thousand patients were cared for by a professional staff of 17 doctors, 21 registered nurses, 12 psychologists, and 13 social workers and a nonprofessional staff of 12 activity workers and 850 psychiatric aides.

The court found that the state hospitals lacked individualized patient treatment plans, adequate qualified professional staff to administer treatment, and a humane physical and psychological environment. In fashioning a remedy, the court issued several standards, including minimum staffing requirements, treatment in the least restrictive setting required by the individual, and development of a human rights committee in each institution. The court stated that "when patients are so committed for treatment purposes, they unquestionably have a right to receive such individualized treatment as will give each of them a realistic opportunity to be cured or improve his or her mental condition" (*Wyatt v. Stickney* 1971, p. 784).

The US Supreme Court first considered the right-to-treatment issue in *O'Connor v. Donaldson* (1975).

In 1957, Mr. Donaldson was involuntarily committed, on his father's initiation, to a Florida state hospital for care, treatment, and maintenance. For 14 years before his commitment, he was gainfully employed. Despite the fact that Mr. Donaldson posed no danger to himself or others, his requests for ground privileges, occupational training, and an opportunity to discuss his

case with the superintendent, Dr. O'Connor, or others were denied. During his 15 years of confinement, he was not provided with any treatment.

Mr. Donaldson frequently requested his release, which the superintendent was authorized to grant even though Mr. Donaldson was lawfully confined, because even if he continued to be mentally ill, he posed no danger to himself or others. Between 1964 and 1968, Mr. Donaldson's friend requested on four separate occasions that he be released into his custody. These requests, and requests made by a halfway house on Mr. Donaldson's behalf, were all denied by Dr. O'Connor, who believed that Mr. Donaldson should be released into his parents' custody. Dr. O'Connor further believed that Mr. Donaldson's parents were too old and infirm to care for him adequately.

The court found that Mr. Donaldson's care was merely custodial because he received no treatment. He was not dangerous, community alternatives were available for him, and the doctor's refusal to release him was "malicious." The Federal Court of Appeals ruled that Mr. Donaldson had a constitutional right to treatment and awarded him $38,000 in damages.

The US Supreme Court, in declining to affirm the lower court's finding of damages and a broad constitutional right to treatment, narrowly defined the issue for consideration: whether a finding of mental illness alone can justify the state's indefinite custodial confinement of a mentally ill person against his or her will. The Supreme Court held that a "state cannot constitutionally confine a nondangerous individual who is capable of surviving safely in freedom by himself or with the help of willing and responsible family members or friends" (*O'Connor v. Donaldson* 1975, p. 576).

In 1982, the US Supreme Court again considered an aspect of the right-to-treatment issue in *Youngberg v. Romeo*. The issue before the Supreme Court was whether involuntarily committed mentally retarded patients have a constitutionally protected interest in safety, freedom from undue restraint, and minimally adequate or reasonable training. Although the court affirmed these rights, it further noted that the substantive liberty interests established in the case were not absolute and that the patient's interests in liberty must be balanced against the state's reasons for restraint.

Although not specifically dealing with the rights of psychiatric patients, *Youngberg v. Romeo* has had an impact on cases regarding the psychiatric patient's right to refuse treatment. Recently enacted federal regulations on the use of restraints would override these case precedents.

INFORMED CONSENT

The principle of **informed consent** is based on a person's right to self-determination, as enunciated in the landmark case *Canterbury v. Spence* (1972, p. 780):

> The root premise is the concept, fundamental in American jurisprudence, that every human being of adult years and sound mind has a right to determine what shall be done with his own body . . . true consent to what happens to one's self is the informed exercise of choice, and that entails an opportunity to evaluate knowedgeably the options available and the risks attendant on each.

For consent to be effective legally, it must be informed. Generally, the informed consent of the patient or client must be obtained by the physician or other health professional to perform the treatment or procedure. Patients must be informed of the nature of their problem or condition, the nature and purpose of a proposed treatment, the risks and benefits of that treatment, alternative treatment options, the probability that the proposed treatment will be successful, and the risks of not consenting to treatment.

Because psychiatric nursing procedures are generally noninvasive and are commonly understood by the patient, the need for the nurse to obtain informed consent does not occur as frequently as in medical treatment. Many procedures that nurses perform have an element of implied consent attached. For example, if the nurse approaches the patient with a medication in hand and the patient indicates a willingness to receive the medication, implied consent has occurred. A general rule for the nurse to follow is that the more intrusive or risky the procedure, the higher the likelihood that informed consent must be obtained. The fact that the nurse may not have a legal duty to be the person to inform the patient of associated risks and benefits of a particular medical procedure does not excuse the nurse from explaining the procedure to the patient and obtaining the patient's expressed or implied consent. *Patient teaching is a recognized legal duty of nurses.*

THE RIGHT TO REFUSE TREATMENT

A corollary to the right to consent to treatment is the right to withhold consent. A patient may also withdraw consent at any time. Retraction of consent previously given must be honored, whether it is a verbal or written retraction. However, the mentally ill patient's **right to refuse treatment** with psychotropic drugs have been debated in the courts, turning in part on the issue of mental patients' competency to give consent or withhold consent to treatment and their status under the civil commitment statutes. These cases, initiated by state hospital patients, consider principles of constitutional law, balancing competing state interests and societal interests against the patient's interest in autonomy and self-determination in the face of the often permanent and disfiguring side effects of psychotropic drugs. The analyses in these cases included medical, legal, and ethical considerations, such as pragmatic treatment problems, the doctrine of informed consent, and the bioethical principle of autonomy.

The US Supreme Court, in two separate cases, *Mills v. Rogers* (1982) and *Rennie v. Klein* (1982), declined to rule on the issue of the right of the involuntarily committed mental patient to refuse treatment with antipsychotic drugs. Even without the enunciation of a federal constitutional right by the Supreme Court, these cases have had a significant, if not uniform, impact on the evolution of mental patients' rights.

In *Rogers v. Okin* (1979), the district court ruled that patients involuntarily committed are not incompetent and have constitutionally protected liberty and privacy interests in making treatment decisions for themselves. Without consent by the patient or the patient's guardian, this right could not be overridden except in an emergency. Forcible administration of medication is justified when the "need to prevent violence outweighs the possibility of harm to the medicated individual" and when reasonable alternatives to medication have been ruled out (*Rogers v. Okin* 1979, p. 1365).

The court of appeals (*Rogers v. Okin* 1980) affirmed the lower court's ruling that mental patients have the constitutionally protected right to make treatment decisions and refuse treatment. However, they differed with respect to the circumstances under which the state's police power interests in preventing violence and maintaining order in the institution and the state's *parens patriae* interest in alleviating the suffering of the mentally ill and providing effective treatment override the patient's liberty interests.

The court of appeals ruled that the police power provides the hospital staff with substantial discretion in an emergency and that the *parens patriae* doctrine justifies forcible administration of psychotropic medication to competent patients only when necessary to prevent further deterioration of a patient's mental health. The court of appeals reversed the lower court's conclusion that a guardian may make psychotropic drug treatment decisions for incompetent patients in nonemergency situations; instead, it decided that the patient's rights must be protected by a judicial determination of incompetency and application of the "substituted judgment rule." With a competent patient, then, treatment with antipsychotic medication is justified only if the patient has voluntarily accepted treatment.

Shortly after the US Supreme Court accepted the case of *Mills v. Rogers* to determine whether involuntarily committed mental patients have a constitutionally protected right to refuse forcible medication, the Supreme Judicial Court of Massachusetts decided, based on state law, that noninstitutionalized mentally ill patients have the right to refuse antipsychotic drugs. After noting that procedural and substantive issues were entwined with issues of state law, and consistent with their policy of avoiding unnecessary decisions of constitutional law, the Supreme Court sent the case back to the court of appeals to determine the effect of the Massachusetts case on its previous decision. The court of appeals then certified nine questions to the Massachusetts Supreme Judicial Court, focusing on the right of the involuntarily committed patient to refuse treatment and on standards and procedures that must be followed by institutions treating these patients.

Currently, Massachusetts prohibits nonconsensual, nonemergency forcible psychotropic drug treatment of involuntarily committed mental patients. The Supreme Judicial Court, in *Rogers v. Commissioner of the Department of Mental Health* (1983), ruled the following:

1. Involuntarily committed mental patients are competent and have the right to make treatment decisions until adjudicated incompetent by a judge.
2. If such patients are adjudicated incompetent, a judge, using the "substituted judgment" standard, will decide whether the patient would have consented to the administration of antipsychotic drugs.
3. Forcible administration of psychotropic drugs is justified without patient consent or court approval only when necessary to prevent "immediate, substantial and irreversible deterioration of a serious mental illness."

In upholding the institutionalized mental patient's right to bodily integrity, the Massachusetts court rejected physicians' assertions that they should have unqualified discretion in making treatment decisions. It further noted that informed consent and the right to privacy, which are the basis of the substituted judgment rule, outweigh institutional interests in forcible medication of patients to facilitate hospital administration, to reduce staff turnover, or to increase the number of patients treated and decrease each patient's length of stay. Additionally, the court rejected the argument that physicians are the appropriate party to make substituted judgment because the court deemed forcible administration of antipsychotic drugs to be an extraordinary treatment.

The precedent for the *Rogers* decision was set in the case *In re guardianship of Roe* (1981), which held that noninstitutionalized mental patients who are adjudicated incompetent have a right to refuse treatment with antipsychotic drugs by the use of a substituted judgment rule. The court enunciated general standards for courts to use in applying substituted judgment.

The factors underlying the court's decision that guardians do not have inherent authority to consent to antipsychotic drug treatment for their wards are (1) the intrusiveness of the treatment, (2) the potential for side effects, (3) the absence of an emergency, (4) the nature and extent of poor judicial involvement, and (5) the likelihood of conflicting interests.

In discussing the intrusiveness of the treatment and the possibility of adverse side effects, the court stated that there are "few . . . medical procedures which are more intrusive than forcible injection of antipsychotic medication" because it affects the person's thought processes and personality. It further noted that the very significant side effects "are frequently devastating and often irreversible" (*In re guardianship of Roe* 1981, p. 52).

After concluding that prior court approval was necessary in a substituted judgment, the court identified six relevant factors in applying this standard:

1. The person's expressed preferences regarding treatment when competent
2. The person's religious belief
3. The effect of treatment, or lack of it, on the person's family
4. The probability of an adverse side effect
5. The risks involved in the refusal of the treatment
6. The prognosis with treatment

In instances in which forcible medication is sought to prevent violence to third persons, to prevent suicide, or to preserve security, the court noted that the medication is being used as a "chemical restraint," and the justification for medication thus changes from individual treatment to public protection. Accordingly, the infringement on a person's liberty is at least equal to that with involuntary commitment. In this circumstance, the noninstitutionalized incompetent mentally ill patient has the right, through substituted judgment, to determine whether to be involuntarily committed or to be medicated.

In New Jersey, involuntarily committed psychiatric patients also brought a suit in federal court alleging violation of their constitutional rights through forcible administration of antipsychotic drugs. The district court in *Rennie v. Klein* (1979) recognized a qualified constitutional right (a limited right) based on four factors: (1) the physical danger posed by the patient to other patients and staff, (2) the patient's mental capacity to decide a course of treatment, (3) the availability of a less restrictive treatment, and (4) risk of permanent side effects.

Additionally, the court extended the right to refuse medication to voluntarily committed patients. On appeal, the right was reaffirmed, but it was limited by the state's ability to forcibly medicate when the patient is a danger to self or others, with the caveat that in nonemergency situations the patient must first be provided with procedural due process (*Rennie v. Klein* 1981). The US Supreme Court again declined to decide whether mental patients have a right to refuse treatment with psychotropic drugs, but this time it set aside the judgment of the Third Circuit Court of Appeals with instructions to reconsider the case in light of the Supreme Court ruling in *Youngberg v. Romeo* (*Rennie v. Klein* 1982).

In applying the "accepted professional judgment standard" of the *Youngberg* ruling, the Third Circuit Court of Appeals narrowed its previous ruling. The court ruled that involuntarily committed patients have the right to refuse administration of antipsychotic drugs, and the decision to administer such drugs against the patient's will must be based on an accepted professional judgment and be consistent with the procedures delineated in the New Jersey regulations, which satisfy due process requirements (*Rennie v. Klein* 1983).

In the court's analysis, the patient's right to refuse medications is weighed against whether the patient presents a danger to him- or herself or others. This evaluation is the product of a professional medical judgment. The decision of the medical staff would be presumed to be valid unless shown to be a "substantial departure from accepted practice." The factor to be considered is whether, and to what extent, the patient will suffer harmful side effects.

The contrast between the analyses in *Rogers* and *Rennie* is substantial. Whereas in *Rogers* the court recognized the individual's autonomy and right to self-determination, and even gave greater weight to the incompetent patient's previously expressed preference through substituted judgment, in *Rennie* the court of appeals substituted the physician's professional judgment for that of the patient's expressed preference. Tables 3–1 and 3–2 summarize the Massachusetts and New Jersey right-to-refuse-treatment cases.

Cases involving the right to refuse psychotropic drug treatment are still evolving. Without clear direction from the US Supreme Court, there will be different case outcomes in different jurisdictions. In the 1989 case of *State of Washington v. Harper*, the Supreme Court addressed whether mentally ill prisoners' refusal of medication can be overridden by administrative procedures or whether a full judicial hearing is required. The court held that the State of Washington Department of Corrections policy provided adequate due process protections and that prisoners were not entitled to a separate judicial hearing on the right to refuse medication. The court did not address the rights of involuntarily committed mentally ill patients.

Table 3–1 ■ RIGHT TO REFUSE TREATMENT: EVOLUTION OF MASSACHUSETTS CASE LAW TO PRESENT LAW

CASE	COURT	DECISION
Rogers v. Okin, 478 F Supp 1342 (D Mass 1979)	Federal District Court	Involuntary mental patients are competent and have the right to make treatment decisions Forcible administration of medication is justified in an emergency if needed to prevent violence and if other alternatives have been ruled out A guardian may make treatment decisions for an incompetent patient
Rogers v. Okin, 634 F2d 650 (1st Cir 1980)	Federal Court of Appeals	Affirmed that involuntary mental patients are competent and have the right to make treatment decisions The staff has substantial discretion in an emergency Forcible medication is also justified to prevent the patient's deterioration A patient's rights must be protected by judicial determination of incompetency
Mills v. Rogers, 457 US 291 (1982)	US Supreme Court	Set aside the judgment of the court of appeals with instructions to consider the effect of an intervening state court case
Rogers v. Commissioner of the Department of Mental Health, 458 NE2d 308 (Mass 1983)	Massachusetts Supreme Judicial Court answering questions certified by the Federal Court of Appeals	Involuntary patients are competent and have the right to make treatment decisions unless they are judicially determined to be incompetent

Table 3–2 ■ RIGHT TO REFUSE TREATMENT: EVOLUTION OF NEW JERSEY CASE LAW TO PRESENT LAW		
CASE	**COURT**	**DECISION**
Rennie v. Klein, 476 F Supp 1294 (D NJ 1979)	Federal District Court	Involuntary mental patients have a qualified constitutional right to refuse treatment with antipsychotic drugs Voluntary patients have an absolute right to refuse treatment with antipsychotic drugs under New Jersey law
Rennie v. Klein, 653 F2d 836 (3rd Cir 1981)	Federal Court of Appeals	Involuntary mental patients have a constitutional right to refuse antipsychotic drug treatment The state may override a patient's right when the patient poses a danger to self or others Due process protections are required before forcible medication of patients in nonemergency situations
Rennie v. Klein, 454 US 1078 (1982)	US Supreme Court	Set aside judgment of the court of appeals with instructions to consider the case in light of the US Supreme Court decision in *Youngberg v. Romeo*
Rennie v. Klein, 720 F2d 266 (3rd Cir 1983)	Federal Court of Appeals	Involuntary mental patients have the right to refuse treatment with antipsychotic medication Decisions to forcibly medicate must be based on "accepted professional judgment" and must comply with due process requirements of the New Jersey regulations

The policy of Washington's Corrections Department was similar to the process outlined in *Rennie v. Klein.*

The relationship between these cases on the right to refuse psychotropic drug treatment and cases on the right to terminate life support presents compelling ethical, legal, and philosophical questions. The Massachusetts courts, using a substituted judgment rule, and the New York courts, basing their rulings on common law, have honored incompetent medical patients' previously expressed desires, made while they were competent, to terminate life support. Other states, such as California, have enacted statutes that permit a person to designate a health care representative to consent to treatment should he or she become incompetent, with instructions delineating the patient's treatment desires.

These court cases and statutes are based on the individual's right to self-determination. The fundamental issue is whether there is a difference between medical and mental illness that justifies a distinction between the rights afforded to persons in making treatment decisions. The cases on the right to refuse medication have illustrated the complex and difficult task of translating social policy concerns into a clearly articulated legal standard.

On December 1, 1991, a federal law entitled the Patient Self-Determination Act became effective. This advance-directive law requires that all persons older than 18 years of age who are admitted to a hospital or to a Medicare and Medicaid–participating organization (e.g., home health agencies, prepaid health maintenance organizations, hospice programs, or skilled nursing facilities) be asked if they have an advance directive to clarify their wishes and philosophy regarding life, death, and medical care. The act does not require every person to have prepared a living will or special directive, but it is hoped that the inquiry will encourage patients to record their wishes. The act also requires that the agency provide written information regarding patients' rights under state law to accept or reject medical treatment and that the agency inform patients about durable powers of attorney (i.e., appointing a surrogate decision maker if the patient is unable to make decisions). The agency must document in the patient's record whether the patient has completed a directive. Agencies that do not comply with this law will lose their eligibility for federal funding reimbursement.

General Principles of Tort Law Applied to Psychiatric Settings

Although the statutes governing the delivery of mental health services clearly affect the rights of mental patients and the responsibilities of caregivers, the law that has evolved through court decisions plays an equally important role in defining rights and responsibilities generally.

Torts are civil wrongs for which money damages are collected by the injured party (the plaintiff) from the wrongdoer (the defendant). The injury can be to persons, property, or reputations. Because tort law has general applicability to nursing practice, this section may contain a review of material previously covered elsewhere in the student's nursing curriculum.

In a psychiatric setting, nurses are more likely to encounter provocative, threatening, or violent behavior. Such behavior might require the use of restraint or seclusion until a patient demonstrates quieter and safer behavior. Accordingly, the nurse in the psychiatric setting should understand the intentional torts of battery, assault, and false imprisonment.

INTENTIONAL TORTS

An **intentional tort** requires a voluntary act and an intent to bring about a physical consequence. In the most basic terms, a voluntary act is a voluntary movement of the body. The requirement for intent is met when the defendant acts purposefully to achieve a result or is substantially certain that the result will occur. If the injured party consents to participate in an act, there can be no intentional tort. Likewise, self-defense and defense of others are privileges that can be used to defend successfully against a court action for intentional torts. Reckless behavior may be classified as intentional or negligent. The forseeability that a suicidal patient will harm him- or herself if left alone with sharp objects or an open window to jump from is great enough that negligence would be found on the part of the nurse, who has a duty to protect the patient. If the nurse left the patient alone knowing that the patient would be likely to harm him- or herself, an intentional decision could be argued. It would not be a wise nursing judgment to test the suicidal patient's ability to be left alone with dangers in the immediate environment.

ASSAULT AND BATTERY. An **assault** is an act resulting in the plaintiff's apprehension of an immediate harmful or offensive touching (battery). In an assault, there is no actual contact. The defendant's act must amount to a threat to use force, although threatening words alone are not enough. The defendant must also have the opportunity and the ability to carry out the threatened act immediately. A **battery** is a harmful or offensive touching of another's person. For example, the nurse approaches the patient with a restraint in hand. The patient fearfully pleads not to be restrained. If the nurse proceeds to apply the restraints, both an assault and a battery may be charged against the nurse.

FALSE IMPRISONMENT. False imprisonment is an act with the intent to confine a person to a specific area. The use of seclusion or restraint that is not defensible as being necessary and in the patient's best interest may result in false imprisonment of the patient and liability for the nurse. As another example, if a psychiatric patient wants to leave the hospital and the nurse prohibits the patient from leaving, the nurse may have falsely imprisoned the patient if the patient was voluntarily admitted and if there are no agency or legal policies for detaining the patient. On the other hand, if the patient was involuntarily admitted or had agreed to an evaluation before discharge, the nurse's actions would be reasonable.

PUNITIVE DAMAGES. Punitive damages may be recoverable by an injured party in an intentional tort action. Because these damages are designed to punish and make an example, punitive damage awards can be very large. Often, the plaintiff's actual damages are insignificant, and nominal damages may be awarded in the sum of $1. However, intentional acts are not covered by malpractice insurance, making intentional torts a less attractive theory of liability for injured patients to pursue against health professionals and hospitals. The following case, *Plumadore v. State of New York* (1980), is illustrative of the use of intentional tort theory in the psychiatric setting.

Mrs. Plumadore was admitted to Saranac Lake General Hospital for a gallbladder condition. Her medical work-up revealed emotional problems stemming from marital difficulties, which had resulted in suicide attempts several years before her admission. After a series of consultations and tests, she was advised by the attending surgeon that she was scheduled to have gallbladder surgery later that day. After the surgeon's visit, a consulting psychiatrist who examined her directed her to dress and pack her belongings because he had arranged to have her admitted to a state hospital at Ogdensburg.

Subsequently, two uniformed state troopers handcuffed her and strapped her into the back seat of a patrol car. She was also accompanied by a female hospital employee and was transported to the state hospital. On arrival, the admitting psychiatrist recognized that the referring psychiatrist lacked the requisite authority to order her involuntary commitment. He therefore requested that she sign a voluntary admission form, which she refused to do. Despite Mrs. Plumadore's protests regarding her admission to the state hospital, the psychiatrist assigned her to a ward without physical or psychiatric examination and without the opportunity to contact her family or her medical doctor. The record of her admission to the state hospital noted an "informed admission," which is the patient-initiated voluntary admission in New York.

The court awarded $40,000 to Mrs. Plumadore for false imprisonment, negligence, and malpractice.

NEGLIGENCE

Negligence is an act or an omission to act that breaches the duty of due care and results in or is responsible for a person's injuries. The five elements required to prove negligence are (1) duty, (2) breach of duty, (3) cause in fact, (4) proximate cause, and (5) damages. Forseeability of harm is also evaluated.

Duty is measured by a standard of care. When a nurse represents him- or herself as being capable of caring for psychiatric patients and accepts employment, a duty of care has been assumed. The duty is owed to psychiatric patients to understand the theory and medications used in the specialty care of these patients. Persons who represent themselves as possessing superior knowledge and skill, such as psychiatric nurse specialists in nursing, are held to a higher standard of care in the practice of their profession. The staff nurse who is assigned to a psychiatric unit must be knowledgeable enough to assume a reasonable duty of care to the patients.

If the nurse is not capable of providing the standard of care that other nurses would be expected to supply under similar circumstances, the nurse has breached the duty of care. Breach of duty is the conduct that exposes the patient to an unreasonable risk of harm, through either commission or omission of acts on the part of the nurse. If a nurse does not have the required education and experience to know enough to provide certain interventions, the nurse has breached the duty by neglecting or omitting to provide necessary care. The nurse can also act in such a way that the patient is harmed and can thus be guilty of negligence through acts of commission.

Cause in fact may be evaluated by questioning: but for what the nurse did, would this injury have occurred? Proximate cause, or legal cause, may be evaluated by determining if there have been any intervening actions or persons that were, in fact, the causes of harm to the patient. Damages include actual damages (e.g., loss of earnings, medical expenses, and property damage) as well as pain and suffering.

Determining a Standard of Care for Psychiatric Nursing Practice

Professional standards of practice determined by professional associations differ from the minimum qualifications set forth by state licensure for entry into the profession of nursing. The American Nurses' Association (ANA) has established standards for psychiatric nursing practice and credentialing of clinical psychiatric nurse specialists (ANA 1982).

Standards for psychiatric nursing practice differ markedly from minimum state requirements because the primary purposes for setting these two types of qualifications are different. The state's qualifications for practice provide consumer protection by ensuring that all practicing nurses have successfully completed an approved nursing program and passed the national licensing examination. The professional association's primary focus is to elevate the practice of its members by setting standards of excellence. The ANA Standards of Psychiatric and Mental Health Nursing Practice are provided inside the front cover of this book.

Nurses are held to the standard of care exercised by other nurses possessing the same degree of skill or knowledge in the same or similar circumstances. In the past, community standards existed for urban and rural agencies. However, with greater mobility and expanded means of communication, national standards have evolved. Psychiatric patients have the right to receive the standard of care recognized by professional bodies governing nursing, whether they are in a large or a small, a rural or an urban facility. Nurses must participate in continuing education courses to stay current with existing standards of care.

The most common method of establishing a standard of care in a court case is through the use of an expert witness. Expert witnesses testify about their opinions and conclusions, usually based on a hypothetical fact pattern that is presented by counsel and that resembles the fact pattern of the actual case. The testimony of expert witnesses differs from that of other witnesses. Other witnesses can testify as to facts only. The expert's testimony carries no greater weight, except for credibility, than the testimony of any other witness.

In a professional negligence case or a disciplinary action, the expert witness testifying should not only be a member of the profession about which he or she is testifying but should also practice in the specialty area concerned in the case. The witness is qualified as an expert by reason of education, clinical practice, and research. An expert's opinion should not be bought: the integrity of the expert's opinion must be protected by the nurse acting as an expert.

Professional standards of practice for nursing promulgated by the ANA and other specialty nursing organizations are being advocated as a means of establishing a standard of care (Eccard 1977). This method, coupled with the use of a nurse expert, most accurately reflects nursing's view of appropriate intervention based on the use of the nursing process.

Hospital policies and procedures set up institutional criteria for care, and these criteria, such as the frequency of rounds on patients in seclusion, may be introduced to prove a standard that the nurse met or failed to meet. The shortcoming of this method is that the hospital's policy may be substandard. For example, the state licensing laws for institutions might set a minimum requirement for staffing or frequency of rounds on certain patients, and the hospital policy might fall below that minimum. Substandard institutional policies do not absolve the individual nurse of responsibility to practice based on professional standards of nursing care.

Like hospital policy and procedures, custom can be used as evidence of a standard of care. For example, in the absence of a written policy on the use of restraint, testimony might be offered regarding the customary use of restraint in emergency situations in which the combative, violent, or confused patient poses a threat of harm to self or others. Using custom to establish a standard of care may result in the same defect as using hospital policies and procedures: custom may not comply with the laws, accrediting body recommendations, or other recognized standards of care. Custom must be carefully and regularly evaluated to ensure that substandard routines have not developed. Substandard customs will not protect the nurse when a psychiatric patient charges that a right has been violated or that harm has been caused by the staff's common practices.

GUIDELINES FOR STUDENTS WHO SUSPECT NEGLIGENCE

It is not unusual for a student or practicing nurse to suspect negligence on the part of a peer. In most states, nurses have a legal duty to report such risks of harm to the patient. It is also very important that the nurse document clear and accurate evidence before making serious accusations against a peer. If the nurse questions a physician's orders or actions, or those of a fellow nurse, it is wise to communicate these concerns directly to the person involved. If the risky behavior continues, the nurse has an obligation to communicate these concerns to a supervisor, who should then intervene to ensure that the patient's rights and well-being are protected. If a nurse suspects a peer of being chemically impaired or practicing irresponsibly, the nurse has an obligation to protect not only the rights of the peer but also the rights of all patients who could be harmed by this impaired peer. If, after the nurse has reported suspected behavior of concern to a supervisor, the danger persists, the nurse has a duty to report the concern to someone at the next level of authority. It is important to follow the channels of communication in an organization, but it is also important to protect the safety of the patients. If the supervisor's actions or inactions do not rectify the dangerous situation, the nurse has a continuing duty to report the behavior of concern to the appropriate authority, such as the state board of nursing.

QUESTIONS FOR DISCUSSION

The distinction between minimum entry practice standards and professional practice standards is important in a discussion of standards of care for psychiatric nurses. Consider the legal and ethical issues posed by the following situations.

Nurse A has worked in a psychiatric setting for five years, since she was licensed by the state. She arrives at work on her unit and is informed that the nursing office has requested a nurse from the psychiatric unit to assist the intensive care unit staff in caring for an agitated car accident victim with a history of schizophrenia. Nurse A works with nurse B in caring for the patient. While the patient is sleeping, nurse B leaves the unit for a coffee break. Nurse A, unfamiliar with the telemetry equipment, fails to recognize an arrhythmia, and the patient has a cardiopulmonary arrest. The patient is successfully resuscitated after six minutes but suffers permanent brain damage.

- *Can nurse A legally practice? (That is, does her license permit her to practice in an intensive care unit?)*
- *Does the ability to practice legally in an area differ from the ability to practice competently in that area?*
- *Did nurse A have any legal or ethical grounds to refuse the assignment to the intensive care unit?*
- *What are the risks in accepting an assignment to an area of specialty practice in which you are professionally unprepared to practice?*
- *What are the risks in refusing an assignment to an area of specialty practice in which you are professionally unprepared to practice?*
- *Would there have been any way for nurse A to minimize the risk of an action for insubordination by the employer had she refused the assignment?*
- *What action could nurse A have taken to protect the patient and herself when nurse B left the unit for a coffee break?*
- *If nurse A is negligent, is the hospital liable for any harm to the patient caused by nurse A?*

A 40-year-old man who is admitted to the emergency room for a severe nosebleed has both nares packed. Because of his history of alcoholism and the probability of ensuing delirium tremens, the patient is transferred to the psychiatric unit. He is admitted to a private room, placed in restraints, and checked by a nurse every hour per physician order. While unattended, the patient suffocates, apparently by inhaling the nasal packing, which had become dislodged from the nares. On the next one-hour check, the nurse finds the patient without pulse or respirations.

A state statute requires that a restrained patient on a psychiatric unit be assessed by a nurse every hour for safety, comfort, and physical needs.

- *If standards are not otherwise specified, do statutory requirements set forth minimum or maximum standards?*
- *Does the nurse's compliance with the state statute relieve her of liability in the patient's death?*
- *Does the nurse's compliance with the physician's order relieve her of liability in the patient's death?*
- *Was the order for the restraint appropriate for this type of patient?*
- *What factors did you consider in making your determination?*
- *Was the frequency of rounds for assessment of patient needs appropriate in this situation?*
- *Did the nurse's conduct meet the standard of care for psychiatric nurses? Why or why not?*
- *What nursing action should the nurse have taken to protect the patient from harm?*

The Duty to Intervene

The psychiatric nurse has a duty to intervene when the safety or well-being of the patient or another person is obviously at risk. A nurse who follows an order that is known to be incorrect or that the nurse believes will harm the patient is responsible for the harm that results to the patient. If the nurse has information that leads him or her to believe that the doctor's orders need to be clarified or changed, it is the nurse's duty to intervene and protect the patient. It is important that the nurse communicate with the physician who has ordered the treatment to explain the concern. If the treating physician does not appear willing to consider the nurse's concerns, the nurse carries out the duty to intervene through other appropriate channels. It is important for the nurse to communicate concerns to his or her supervisor in order to allow the supervisor to communicate with the appropriate medical staff persons who can intervene in the

physician's treatment plan. The nurse, as the patient's advocate, has a duty to intervene to protect the patient; at the same time, however, the nurse does not have the right to interfere with the physician-patient relationship. It is very important to follow agency policies and procedures for communicating differences of opinion. If the nurse fails to intervene and the patient is injured, the nurse may be partially liable for the injuries that result because of the nurse's failure to use safe nursing practice and the nurse's own professional judgment. The legal concept of abandonment may also arise when a nurse does not leave a patient safely back in the hands of another health professional before discontinuing treatment. Abandonment issues arise when accurate, timely, and thorough reporting has not occurred or when follow-through of patient care, on which the patient is relying, has not occurred.

The duty to intervene on the patient's behalf poses many legal and ethical dilemmas for the nurse in the workplace. Institutions that have a chain-of-command policy or other reporting mechanisms offer some assurance that the proper authorities in the administration are notified. Most patient care issues regarding physician's orders or treatments usually can be settled fairly early in the process, with the nurse discussing his or her concerns with the physician. If further intervention by the nurse is required to protect the patient, the next step in the chain of command can be initiated. Generally, the nurse then notifies the immediate nursing supervisor; the supervisor discusses the problem with the physician and then with the chief of staff of a particular service until a resolution is reached. If there is no time to resolve the issue through the normal process because of the life-threatening nature of the situation, the nurse must act to protect the patient's life.

The issues become more complex when a professional colleague's conduct, including a student nurse's, is criminally unlawful, for example involving the diversion of drugs from the hospital or sexual misconduct with patients. Increasing media attention and the recognition of substance abuse as an occupational hazard for health professionals has led to substance abuse programs in many states. These programs provide appropriate treatment of impaired professionals in order to protect the public from harm and to rehabilitate the professional.

The problem previously discussed, of reporting impaired colleagues, becomes a very difficult one, particularly when no direct patient harm has occurred. Concern for professional reputations, damaged careers, and personal privacy rather than public protection has generated a code of silence regarding substance abuse among health professionals. Several states now require reporting of impaired or incompetent colleagues to the professional licensing boards. Without this legal mandate, the questions of whether to report and to whom to report become ethical ones.

QUESTIONS FOR DISCUSSION

Assume that there are no mandatory reporting laws for impaired or incompetent colleagues in the following clinical situations.

Jane Smith, 45 years of age, is admitted to the surgical unit for a biopsy of the thyroid gland. Her admitting physician has recommended a psychiatric consultation because Mrs. Smith has had a history of pronounced mood swings for the past three months, following the breakup of her marriage of 20 years. The nurse introduces the patient to the psychiatrist and is called away because of a new admission. Within the hour, the nurse is summoned to Mrs. Smith's room and finds the patient alone, agitated, and crying. The nurse encourages Mrs. Smith to share her concerns, and the patient then states that the doctor touched her "private areas" while talking with her and exposed himself to her. She states that she pushed him away as he advanced toward her. She tells the nurse that she feels violated and humiliated. What action, if any, can the nurse take?

- *Should the nurse chart the incident?*
- *Should the nurse inform the admitting physician?*
- *Should the nurse inform the nursing supervisor?*
- *Should the nurse talk with the consulting psychiatrist about the patient's allegations?*
- *Should the nurse inform the chief of staff of psychiatry of the patient's reported incident?*
- *Should the nurse report the incident to the chairperson of the peer review committee of the hospital?*
- *If the nurse initiates the reporting mechanism in her facility, must she take any further action?*
- *Should the nurse report the psychiatrist to the medical board?*
- *Should the nurse notify the police?*

Two nurses, Joe and Beth, have worked on the psychiatric unit for two years. During the past six months, Beth has confided to Joe that she has been going through a particularly difficult marital situation. Joe has noticed that for six months Beth has become increasingly irritable and difficult to work with. Joe notices that minor tranquilizers are frequently missing from the unit dose cart on the evening shift. Joe complains to the pharmacy and is informed that the drugs were stocked as ordered. Several patients state that they have not been receiving their usual drugs. Joe finds that Beth has recorded that the drugs have been given as ordered. Joe also notices that the patients appear more agitated. Joe suspects that Beth is diverting the drugs. What action, if any, should Joe take?

- *Should Joe confront Beth with his suspicion?*
- *If Beth admits that she has been diverting drugs, should Joe's next step be to report Beth to the supervisor or to the board of nursing?*
- *Should Joe make his concern known to the nursing supervisor directly by identifying Beth or should he state his concerns in general terms?*
- *Legally, must Joe report his suspicions to the board of nursing?*
- *Does the fact that harm to the patients is limited to increased agitation affect your responses?*

Documentation of Care

PURPOSE

The purpose of the medical record is to provide accurate and complete information about the care and treatment of patients and to give health care personnel responsible for that care a means of communicating with each other. The medical record allows for continuity of care. A record's usefulness is determined by evaluating, when the record is read at a later date, how accurately and completely the record portrays the patient's status at the time it was written.

Timeliness in recording nursing actions and observations is as important as the accuracy of the information shared. Miscommunications and delays in sharing pertinent information are major causes of legal liability. If a member of the health care team relies on old information because the nurse has not recently charted new data, and the patient is harmed, the nurse shares the responsibility for the resulting injury. For example, if a psychiatric patient describes to a nurse a plan to harm him- or herself or another, and the nurse fails to document the information, including the need to protect the patient or the identified victim, the information will be lost when the nurse leaves work and the patient's plan may be carried out. The harm caused could be linked directly to the nurse's failure to communicate this important information. Many nurses have the habit of carrying their nursing notes in a notebook in their pocket. This practice should be discouraged. Even though documentation takes time away from the patient, the importance of communicating and preserving the nurse's memory through the medical record cannot be overemphasized.

Accrediting agencies, such as the Joint Commission on Accreditation of Healthcare Organizations (JCAHO) and state regulatory agencies, require health care facilities to maintain records on patients' care and treatment. Noncompliance with record-keeping responsibilities may result in fines, loss of accreditation, or both.

FACILITY USE OF MEDICAL RECORDS

The medical record has many uses other than providing information on the course of the patient's care and treatment to health care professionals. Retrospective chart review can provide valuable information to the facility on the quality of care provided and on improving that care. Accordingly, the chart may be used to evaluate care for quality assurance or peer review. Utilization review analysts review the chart to determine appropriate use of hospital and staff resources consistent with reimbursement schedules. Insurance companies and other reimbursement agencies rely on the medical record in determining payments they will make on the patient's behalf.

Retrospective chart review can be performed for educational research and investigative purposes. Additionally, a facility may conduct reviews for risk management purposes, to determine areas of potential liability for the facility, and to evaluate methods used to reduce the facility's exposure to liability. These are just a few of many examples of the internal uses of the medical record.

THE MEDICAL RECORD AS EVIDENCE

From a legal perspective, the chart is a recording of data and opinions made in the normal course of the patient's hospital care. It is deemed to be good evidence because it is presumed to be true, honest, and untainted by memory lapses. Accordingly, the medical record finds its way into a variety of legal cases for a variety of reasons. Some examples of its use include to determine the extent of the patient's damages and pain and suffering in personal injury cases, such as when a psychiatric patient attempts suicide while under the protective care of a hospital; to determine the nature and extent of injuries in child abuse or elder abuse cases; to determine the nature and extent

of physical or mental disability in disability cases; and to determine the nature and extent of injury and rehabilitative potential in workers' compensation cases.

Medical records may also be used in police investigations, civil conservatorship proceedings, competency hearings, and commitment procedures. In states that mandate a mental health legal services or patients' rights advocacy program, audits may be performed to determine the facility's compliance with state laws or violation of patients' rights. Finally, medical records may be used in professional and hospital negligence cases.

During the discovery phase of litigation, the medical record is a pivotal source of information for attorneys in determining whether a cause of action exists in a professional negligence or hospital negligence case. Evidence of the nursing care rendered will be reflected in what the nurse charted at the time. Incomplete or poor notes will raise suspicion about the quality of care delivered.

NURSING GUIDELINES FOR CHARTING

Accurate, descriptive, and legible nursing notes serve the best interests of the patient, nurse, and institution. Integrated charting systems encourage all members of the health team to read each other's documentation of care. Any charting method that improves communication between care providers should be encouraged. Courts assume that nurses and physicians read each other's notes on patient progress. Many courts reflect the attitude that if care is not documented, it did not occur. The nurse's charting also serves as a valuable memory refresher if the patient sues years after the care is provided. In providing complete and timely information on the care and treatment of patients, the medical record enhances communication among health professionals. Internal, institutional audits of the record can improve the quality of care rendered. Following the guidelines in Box 3–1 will improve the nurse's charting.

QUESTIONS FOR DISCUSSION

A 23-year-old woman in an agitated state is admitted to a psychiatric unit and placed in a seclusion room without furniture, per physician order. Four days after her admission, a bed frame inexplicably arrives in the room. On the ninth day of hospitalization, her psychosis becomes more acute, and the staff intensify their care. The following day, the patient reports to the staff that she heard voices telling her to hurt herself. The

---

Box 3–1. DO'S AND DONT'S OF CHARTING

DO

- Chart in a timely manner all pertinent and factual information.
- Be familiar with the nursing documentation policy in your facility and make your charting conform to this standard. The policy will generally state the method of charting (e.g., SOAP, systems review, chronological block), the frequency, pertinent assessments, interventions, and outcomes. If your agency's policies and procedures do not encourage or allow for quality documentation, bring the need for change to the administration's attention.
- Chart legibly in ink.
- Chart facts fully, descriptively, and accurately.
- Chart what you see, hear, feel, and smell.
- Chart a total patient assessment on each shift and on admission, discharge, and transfer.
- Chart pertinent observations: psychosocial observations, physical symptoms pertinent to the medical diagnosis, and behaviors pertinent to the nursing diagnosis.
- Chart follow-up care provided when a problem has been identified in earlier documentation. For example, if a patient falls and injures a leg, describe how the wound is healing.
- Chart fully the facts surrounding unusual occurrences and incidents, but do not note in the chart that an incident report was filed. This form is generally a privileged communication between the hospital and the hospital's attorney. Charting it may destroy the privileged nature of the communication.
- Chart *all* nursing interventions, treatments, and outcomes, including teaching efforts and patient responses, and safety and patient protection interventions.
- Chart the patient's expressed subjective feelings.
- Chart each time you notify a physician, the reason for notification, what was communicated, the accurate time, the physician's instructions or orders, and the follow-up activity.
- Chart doctor visits and treatments.
- Chart discharge medications and instructions given for use, as well as all discharge teaching performed and what family members were included in the process.

DO NOT

- Do not chart opinions that are not supported by the facts.
- Do not defame patients by calling them names or by making derogatory statements about the patient (e.g., "an unlikable patient/person who is demanding unnecessary attention").
- Do not chart before an event occurs.
- Do not chart generalizations, suppositions, or "pat phrases" (e.g., "patient in good spirits").
- Do not obliterate, erase, alter, or destroy a record. If an error is made, draw one line through the error, write "mistaken entry" or "error," and initial. Follow your agency's guidelines closely.
- Do not leave blank spaces for chronological notes. If you must chart out of sequence, chart "late entry." Identify the time and date of the entry and the time and date of the occurrence.

SOAP = subjective data, objective data, assessment, and plan.

---

patient is sedated and locked in her room. Four hours later, the room is unlocked and the patient is found unconscious, with her head wedged between the bed frame and the side rails. She suffers neurological damage. The following day, the director of the nurses orders the staff to remove the original charting, rewrite their notes, and place the falsified notes in the chart.

- *Which acts or omissions by the staff breach the staff's duty to provide the patient with a safe environment?*

- *What nursing action should the staff have taken after sedating the patient to protect her from harm?*
- *Discuss the legal and ethical ramifications of the staff's falsification of the patient's record on the order of the director of nurses.*

This clinical situation was taken from the facts in a Connecticut case. In *Pisel v. Stamford Hospital* (1980), the falsification of the record was not disclosed until after a lawsuit had been filed. The Connecticut Supreme Court, in upholding a $3.6 million award for the patient, decided that the jury was entitled to consider the falsified record as evidence that the hospital was conscious of its negligence.

Maintaining Patient Confidentiality

ETHICAL CONSIDERATIONS: AMERICAN NURSES' ASSOCIATION CODE FOR NURSES

The ANA Code for Nurses states that "the nurse safeguards the client's right to privacy by judiciously protecting information of a confidential nature" (1985). The applicable interpretive statement provides further explanation for maintaining patient confidentiality and recognizes the distinction between legal and ethical obligations. The interpretive statement follows:

> The right of privacy is an inalienable right of all persons, and the nurse has a clear obligation to safeguard any confidential information about the client acquired from any source. The nurse-client relationship is built on trust. This relationship could be destroyed and the client's welfare and reputation jeopardized by injudicious disclosing of information provided in confidence. Since the concept of confidentiality has legal as well as ethical implications, an inappropriate breach of confidentiality may also expose the nurse to liability.

LEGAL CONSIDERATIONS

As previously stated, the patient's right to have his or her treatment and medical records kept confidential is legally protected. The fundamental principle underlying the ANA code on **confidentiality** is a person's constitutional **right to privacy.** Generally, the nurse's legal duty to maintain confidentiality is to act to protect the patient's right to privacy. Therefore, the nurse may not, without the patient's consent, disclose information obtained from the patient or information in the medical record to anyone except those necessary to carry out a patient's treatment plan.

For example, the nurse's release of information to the patient's employer about the patient's condition, without the patient's consent, is a breach of confidentiality that subjects the nurse to liability for the tort of invasion of privacy. On the other hand, discussion of patient's history with other staff members to ascertain a consistent treatment approach is not a breach of confidentiality.

Many states have enacted privileged communication statutes that prohibit specified health professionals from disclosing patient information unless the patient has either consented to the disclosure or waived the privilege of consent. These state statutes differ markedly.

Generally, to create a situation in which information is privileged, a patient–health professional relationship must exist, and the information must relate to the care and treatment of the patient. The health professional may refuse to disclose information in order to protect the patient's privacy. However, the right to privacy is the patient's right, and health professionals cannot involve confidentiality for their own defense or benefit.

A legal privilege of confidentiality is enacted legislatively, and exists to protect the confidentiality of professional communications (e.g., nurse-patient and attorney-client). The theory behind such privileged communications is that patients will not be comfortable or willing to disclose personal information about themselves if they fear that the nurse will repeat their confidential conversations. In some states in which the legal privilege of confidentiality has not been legislated for nurses, the nurse must respond to a court's inquiries regarding the patient's disclosures. In these states, the confidentiality of communications cannot be guaranteed.

EXCEPTIONS TO THE RULE

Duty to Warn Third Parties

The California Supreme Court, in its 1976 landmark decision ***Tarasoff*** v. *Regents of University of California,* ruled that a psychotherapist has the **duty to warn** his or her client's potential victim of potential harm. This decision created much controversy and confusion in the psychiatric and medical communities over breach of patient confidentiality and its impact on the therapeutic relationship in psychiatric care and on the psychotherapist's ability to predict patient dangerousness. This trend continues as other jurisdictions have adopted or modified the California rule despite the psychiatric community's objections. These jurisdictions view public safety to be more important than privacy in narrowly defined circumstances.

The *Tarasoff* case acknowledged that generally there is no common-law duty to aid third persons. An exception is when special relationships exist, and the court found the patient-therapist relationship sufficient to create a duty of the therapist to aid Ms. Tarasoff, the victim. The duty to protect the intended victim from danger arises when the therapist determines—or, pursuant to professional standards, should have determined—that the patient presents a serious danger to another. Any action reasonably necessary under the circumstances, including notification of the potential victim, the victim's family, and the police, discharges the therapist's duty to the potential victim.

Arguing that predictions of future violence are inaccurate at best and speculative at worst, the psychiatric community raised concerns over the use of a professional standard to determine when a therapist should have known of the client's future violence toward another, as required by *Tarasoff.* The courts and other legal commentators have recognized the therapist's difficulty in forecasting violence but have also noted that the therapist's prediction of violence is used in civil commitment procedures to determine whether a client or patient poses a threat to others.

The psychologist's diagnostic function, a professional service rendered within the legal scope of practice, was central to the California Supreme Court's ruling in *Hedlum v. Superior Court of Orange County* (1983). The court stated that the duty to warn was composed of two elements: (1) the duty to diagnose and predict the client's danger of violence and (2) the duty to take appropriate action to protect the identified victim. The court stated that "a negligent failure to diagnose dangerousness in a *Tarasoff* action is as much a basis for liability as is a negligent failure to warn a known victim once such a diagnosis has been made."

A limited duty to investigate the patient's history was enunciated in *Jablonski v. United States* (1983). Mr. Jablonski had attempted to rape his girlfriend's mother. He agreed to undergo psychiatric treatment. The police notified the chief psychiatrist that Mr. Jablonski had a criminal record that included threatening others and recommended that he be treated on an inpatient basis. The chief psychiatrist failed to communicate this information to the treating psychiatrist. The treating physician noted the patient's potential violence, learned of his criminal rape record, and noted his past psychiatric treatment during the initial interview. However, the treating psychiatrist did not attempt to locate the previous medical records and did not believe that the patient met the civil commitment criteria. While being treated on an outpatient basis, Mr. Jablonski killed his girlfriend.

The court found that the psychiatrist's failure to obtain the patient's records and the failure to record and communicate the telephone contact by the police were negligent acts. Although no specific threats were made toward the girlfriend, Mr. Jablonski's previous history indicated his violence would probably be directed toward her.

In *Thomas v. County of Alameda* (1980), a juvenile with dangerous and violent propensities toward young children was released from the custody of the county to the custody of his mother for a home visit. While home, he killed a neighborhood child, and the deceased child's parents sued the county for wrongful death, alleging that the county had a duty to warn the police, the juvenile's mother, and other local parents. The court held that there was no duty to warn because the victim was a "member of a large amorphous public group of potential targets and not a known, identifiable victim." This is distinguishable from the *Jablonski* case, in which sufficient information existed to identify the victim.

NURSING CONSIDERATIONS
As this trend to make it the therapist's duty to warn third persons of potential harm continues to gain wider acceptance, it is important for students and nurses to understand its implications for nursing practice. Although none of these cases to date has dealt with nurses, it is fair to assume that in jurisdictions that have adopted the *Tarasoff* doctrine, the duty to warn third persons will be applied to clinical psychiatric nurse specialists in private practice who engage in individual therapy.

It is unlikely that a duty to warn potential victims will be extended to staff psychiatric nurses working in the institutional setting because nurses do not have primary case management responsibilities. However, if a staff psychiatric nurse who is a member of a team of psychiatrists, psychologists, psychiatric social workers, and other psychiatric nurses does not report patient threats of harm against specified victims or classes of victims to the team of the patient's management psychotherapist for assessment and evaluation, this failure is likely to be considered substandard nursing care.

So, too, the failure to communicate and record relevant information from police, relatives, or the patient's old records might also be deemed negligent. Breach of patient-nurse confidentiality should not pose ethical or legal dilemmas for nurses in these situations because a team approach to the delivery of psychiatric care presumes communication of pertinent information to other staff members to develop a treatment plan in the patient's best interest.

Child and Elder Abuse Reporting Statutes

Because of their interest in protecting children, all 50 states, and the District of Columbia, have enacted **child abuse reporting statutes.** Although these statutes differ from state to state, they generally include a definition of child abuse, a list of persons required or encouraged to report, and the governmental agency designated to receive and investigate the reports. Most statutes include civil penalties for failure to report. Many states specifically require nurses to report cases of suspected abuse.

There is a conflict between federal and state laws with respect to child abuse reporting when the health care professional discovers child abuse or neglect during the suspected abuser's alcohol or drug treatment. Federal laws and regulations governing confidentiality of patient records, which apply to almost all drug abuse and alcohol treatment providers, prohibit any disclosure without a court order. In this case, federal law supersedes state reporting laws, although compliance with the state law may be maintained if a court order is obtained, pursuant to the regulations, if a report can be made without identifying the abuser as a patient in an alcohol or drug treatment program, or if the report is made anonymously. Some states do not allow anonymous reporting, in order to protect the rights of the accused.

As reported incidents of abuse to other persons in society surface, states may require health professionals to report other kinds of abuse. A growing number of states are enacting **elder abuse reporting laws,** which require registered nurses and others to report cases of abuse of the elderly. The elderly are defined as adults who are 65 years of age and older. These laws also apply to dependent adults—that is, adults between 18 and 64 years of age whose physical or mental limitations restrict their ability to carry out normal activities or protect themselves—when the registered nurse has actual knowledge that the person has been the victim of physical abuse. Additionally, the nurse may report knowledge of, or "reasonable suspicion" of, mental abuse or suffering. Both dependent adults and elders are protected by the law from purposeful physical or fiduciary neglect or abandonment. Because state laws vary, *students are encouraged to become conversant with the requirements of their state.*

QUESTIONS FOR DISCUSSION
In a private psychiatric unit in California, a 15-year-old boy is admitted voluntarily at the request of his parents because of violent, explosive behavior that seems to stem from his father's recent remarriage after his parents' divorce. A few days after admission, while in group therapy, he has an explosive reaction to a discussion about weekend passes for Mother's Day. He screams that he has been abandoned and that nobody cares about him. Several weeks later, on the day before his discharge, he elicits from the nurse a promise to keep his plan to kill his mother confidential.

Consider the ANA code of ethics on patient confidentiality, the principles of psychiatric nursing, and the duty to warn third parties in answering the following questions:

- *Did the nurse use appropriate nursing judgment in promising confidentiality?*
- *Discuss the bioethical principles of beneficence, justice, autonomy, and fidelity as they relate to the situation described.*
- *Does the nurse have a legal duty to warn the patient's mother of her son's threat?*
- *Is the duty owed to the patient's father and stepmother?*
- *Would a change in the admission status from voluntary to involuntary protect the patient's mother without violating the patient's confidentiality?*
- *Would your response be different depending on the state where the incident occurred? Why or why not?*
- *What nursing action, if any, should the nurse take after the disclosure by the patient?*

How would your responses to the concepts in the previous questions differ in relation to the changes in the following clinical situation?

A 25-year-old woman is attending a federally funded outpatient rehabilitative center for alcoholism after successfully completing the inpatient program. The patient's husband comments to the nurse that he believes his wife is showing improvement because she no longer beats their three-year-old son. A few weeks later, the son is admitted to the hospital with a fractured arm and several bruises and contusions over his body.

Summary

The states' power to enact laws for public health and safety and for the care of those unable to care for themselves often pits the rights of society against the rights of the individual. The complexities of these relationships can manifest as legal and ethical dilemmas in the psychiatric setting. More frequently, the nurse encounters problems requiring ethical choices. The nurse's privilege to practice nursing carries with it responsibility to practice safely, competently, and consistent with state and federal laws. Knowledge of the law, the ANA Code for Nurses, and the Standards of Psychiatric and Mental Health Nursing Practice will enhance the nurse's ability to provide safe, effective psychiatric nursing care and will serve as a framework for decision making when the nurse is presented with complex problems involving competing interests.

References

American Nurses' Association. Standards of Psychiatric and Mental Health Nursing Practice. Kansas City, MO: American Nurses' Association, 1982.

American Nurses' Association. Code for Nurses. Kansas City, MO: American Nurses' Association, 1985.

Canterbury v. Spence, 464 F2d 722 (DC Cir 1972), quoting Schloendorf v. Society of NY Hosp, 211 NY 125 105 NE2d 92, 93 (1914).

Davis A, Aroskar M. Ethical Dilemmas and Nursing Practice. New York: Appleton-Century-Crofts, 1978.

Eccard W. A revolution in white: New approaches to treating nurses as professionals. Vanderbilt Law Review, 30:839, 1977.

Fenner KM. Ethics and Law in Nursing. New York: Van Nostrand Reinhold, 1980.

Haring B. Ethics of Manipulation. New York: The Seabury Press, 1975.

Hedlum v. Superior Court of Orange County, 34 C3d 695 (1983).

Humphrey v. Cady, 405 US 504 (1972).

In re guardianship of Roe, 421 NE2d 40 (Mass 1981).

In re Oakes, 8 Law Rep 122 (Mass 1845).

Jablonski v. United States, 712 F2d 391 (9th Cir 1983).

Mills v. Rogers, 457 US 291 (1982).

O'Connor v. Donaldson, 422 US 563 (1975).

Pisel v. Stamford Hospital, 430 A2d 1 (Conn 1980).

Plumadore v. State of New York, 427 NYS2d 90 (1980).

Rennie v. Klein, 476 F Supp 1294 (DNJ 1979).

Rennie v. Klein, 653 F2d 836 (3rd Cir 1981).

Rennie v. Klein, 454 US 1078 (1982).

Rennie v. Klein, 720 F2d 266 (3rd Cir 1983).

Rogers v. Commissioner of the Department of Mental Health, 458 NE2d 308 (Mass 1983).

Rogers v. Okin, 478 F Supp 1342 (D Mass 1979).

Rogers v. Okin, 634 F2d 650 (1st Cir 1980).

Rouse v. Cameron, 373 F2d 451 (DC Cir 1966).

State of Washington v. Harper, 489 US 1064 (1989).

Tarasoff v. Regents of University of California, 17 C3d 425 (1976).

Thomas v. County of Alameda, 27 C3d 741 (1980).

Wyatt v. Stickney, 325 F Supp 781 (MD Ala 1971).

Youngberg v. Romeo, 457 US 307 (1982).

FURTHER READING

Bellah v. Greenson, 81 CA 3d 614 (1978).

Brennan J. Ethics and Morals. New York: Harper and Row, 1973.

California Department of Mental Health. Patients' Rights Advocacy Manual, 1985.

Chalmers-Frances v. Nelson, 6 C2d 402 (1936).

Cole R. Patients' rights to refuse antipsychotic drugs. Law, Medicine and Health Care, 9(4):19, 1981.

Darling v. Charleston Community Memorial Hospital, 211 NE2d 253 (Ill 1965).

Davis A. Ethical issues in nursing practice. Western Journal of Nursing Research, 2(3):135, 1980.

Davis A. Ethical issues in nursing research. Western Journal of Nursing Research, 2(4):760, 1980.

Davis A. Ethical issues in nursing research. Western Journal of Nursing Research, 5(1):97, 1983.

Development in the law: Civil commitment of the mentally ill. Harvard Law Review, 87:1193, 1974.

Fama AJ. Reporting incompetent physicians: A comparison of requirements in three states. Law, Medicine and Health Care, 11:111, 1983.

Furrow BR. Will psychotherapy be transformed in the 1980's? Law, Medicine and Health Care, 11:96, 1983.

Furrow BR. Public psychiatry and the right to refuse treatment: Toward an effective damage remedy. Harvard Civil Rights Civil Liberties Law Review, 19(1):20, 1984.

Gottlieb NR. Vitek v. Jones: Transfer of prisoner to mental institutions. American Journal of Law and Medicine, 8:175, 1982.

Greenlaw J. Documentation of patient care: An often underestimated responsibility. Law, Medicine and Health Care, 10:172, 1982.

Hawaii v. Standard Oil Company, 405 US 251 (1972), quoting 3 W Blackstone Commentaries, no. 47.

Health Law Center. Nursing and the Law, 2nd ed. Rockville, MD: Aspen Publications, 1975.

Helling v. Carey, 93 Wash2d 514 (1974).

In re detention of Harris, 654 P2d 109 (Wash 1982).

Keeton WP, Dobbs DB, Keeton RE, et al. Prosser and Keeton on Torts, 5th ed. St. Paul, MN: West Publishing Company, 1984.

Kjervik DK. The psychiatric nurse's duty to warn potential victims of homicidal psychotherapy outpatients. Law, Medicine and Health Care, 9(6):11, 1981.

Kravitz M. Informed consent: Must ethical responsibility conflict with professional conduct? Nursing Management, 16(11):34 A–H, 1985.

Lake v. Cameron, 364 F2d 657 (DC Cir 1966).

Litman J. Note, a common law remedy for forcible medication for the institutionalized mentally ill. Columbia Law Review, 82:1720, 1982.

Mavroudis v. Superior court of San Mateo, 102 CA3d 594 (1980).

Monius E. Introduction to bioethics. Center Nurse, The Washington Hospital Center, 2(1):4, 1986.

Nasbitt J. Megatrends. New York: Warner Books, 1982.

Project Release v. Prevost, 722 F2d 960 (2nd Cir 1983).

Rockford SH. More on the right to refuse treatment: Brother Fox and the mentally ill in New York. Law, Medicine and Health Care, 11(1):19, 1983.

Rosoff AJ. Informed Consent: A Guide for Health Care Providers. Rockville, MD: Aspen Publications, 1981.

Roth MD, Levin LJ. Dilemma of Tarasoff: Must physicians protect the public or their patients? Law, Medicine and Health Care, 11:104, 1983.

Selected recent court decisions, involuntary treatment with antipsychotic drugs—Mills v. Rogers. American Journal of Law and Medicine, 8:216, 1982.

Selected recent court decisions, mental patients—involuntary treatment—Rogers v. Commissioner of Department of Mental Health. American Journal of Law and Medicine, 9:522, 1984.

Southwick AF. The Law of Hospital and Health Care Administration. Ann Arbor, MI: Health Administration Press, 1978.

Taub J. Psychiatric malpractice in the 1980's: A look at some areas of concerns. Law, Medicine and Health Care, 11:97, 1983.

Winslade W. Choosing Life or Death: A Guide for Patients, Families and Professionals. New York: Macmillan, 1986.

Vitek v. Jones, 445 US 480 (1980).

Wyatt v. Aderholt, 503 F2d 1305 (5th Cir 1974).

Self-study Exercises

Match the word with the correct definition.

1. _____ Civil wrongs for which money damages are collected by the injured party.

2. _____ Harmful or offensive touching of another's person.

3. _____ The act or omission to act that breaches the duty or care and is the actual or proximate cause of a person's injuries.

4. _____ Based on the principle of a person's right to self-determination.

5. _____ Verbal or written retraction of consent previously given must be honored.

A. Negligence

B. Assault

C. Battery

D. Torts

E. Bioethics

F. Right to refuse treatment

G. Informed consent

True or false

6. _____ Voluntarily admitted patients have the right to demand and obtain release.

7. _____ In many states, common criteria for involuntary admission to mental health facilities include need for psychiatric treatment and danger to self and others.

For discussion

8. Discuss what is meant by *client's civil rights*, and give examples.

9. Discuss some of the legal responsibilities of the nurse in the care and discharge of a client in seclusion or restraints, as identified in this chapter.

10. Name at least four standards of care for psychiatric nursing practice.

11. Discuss guidelines for nurses who suspect negligence.

12. Define what is meant by confidentiality and right to privacy. Discuss two exceptions to the rule (see pages 64 to 66).

CHAPTER 4

Cultural Diversity in Mental Health Nursing

Margie Lovett-Scott
Marcia A. Ullman

OUTLINE

KEY TERMS AND CONCEPTS

The key terms and concepts listed here also appear in bold where they are defined or discussed in this chapter.

ACCULTURATION

ASSIMILATION

CULTURAL SHOCK

CULTURE

ENCULTURATION

ETHNICITY

ETHNOCENTRISM

FOLK BELIEFS

FOLK HEALERS

HERITAGE

RACE

SUBCULTURE

OBJECTIVES

After studying this chapter, the student will be able to

1. Explain the difference among race, ethnicity, and culture.
2. Discuss some folk beliefs about mental health and illness.

3. Identify strategies to improve communication across cultures.
4. Use part II of Leininger's acculturation tool with clients and discuss with them how this affects their approach to the health care professional.
5. Compare and contrast some cultural beliefs and values among African Americans, Asian Americans, Latino Americans, and Native Americans.
6. Identify two ways in which cultural beliefs can have an impact on the way each of the following cultures might use the health care system:
   A. African Americans
   B. Asian Americans
   C. Latino Americans
   D. Native Americans
7. Identify cultural values held by some practitioners that can impede their ability to work with culturally diverse clients or their families.

"The primary objective of the nursing curriculum is to prepare competent professional practitioners. Competency includes the ability to identify and use a variety of strategies to reach a given goal, the ability to use the resources of a variety of social systems (which include ethnic and racial subsystems within the society), the ability to engage in effective reality testing which includes a sophisticated understanding of the world, and the ability to learn from and respond to changing situations" (Osborne et al. 1983).

Few nursing curricula adequately address the issue of cultural congruency in treatment and practice. Consequently, nurses in general have, for too long, treated health matters as if racial, ethnic, and socio-cultural differences either did not exist or did not matter. Teaching students to respond to the cultural needs of clients must be a practice that is evident throughout the nursing curriculum. Students learning to perform physical assessments, for example, should be taught how to assess client and family needs within the appropriate cultural framework and how to plan nursing care interventions that use transcultural nursing concepts. A nurse who is unaware that Puerto Ricans believe that manipulating their female organs is wrong will be unprepared to teach breast self-examination to a Puerto Rican client. In addition, it is equally important to teach nursing students about racial variations in clinical findings; otherwise, important information about body functioning might not be revealed. For example, pallor and cyanosis appear differently in dark-skinned clients than in lighter-skinned ones.

Meeting the needs of a culturally diverse population requires self-awareness, sensitivity, and skill on the part of the nurse. According to Sands and Hale (1987), dehumanized care or conflict is likely to occur when nurses have not examined their knowledge of and attitudes toward different cultural groups. If unre- solved conflict exists between the nurse and the client, the relationship becomes nontherapeutic.

This chapter covers material that can heighten the nurse's awareness of, and appreciation for, the uniqueness of clients from culturally diverse back-grounds. Nurses who are culturally informed (i.e., are cognizant of the client's values, beliefs, lifeways, and cultural heritage) are much more likely to provide culturally congruent care and to veiw interactions with clients most unlike themselves as an exciting, enriching, reciprocally rewarding opportunity.

Scope and Significance of Cultural Diversity

By the year 2010, white Americans will be a minority, making up only 40% of the US population. Already several major cities have more minorities than whites (Fig. 4–1). For example, 70% of New York City residents are foreign born, 70% of the population of Washington, DC is African American, two thirds of the residents of Miami are Latino, one third of the population of San Francisco is Asian, and more than 8000 residents of St. Paul, Minnesota are Laotian (Copeland Griggs Productions 1987). Ideally, health care providers should be representative of the diverse clientele they serve.

In 1988, the American Nurses' Association (ANA) reported that of the 1,627,000 professional nurses practicing in the United States, 92.4% were white and 7.6% were nurses of color (Table 4–1). Although this figure represents an increase over the percentage of nurses of color practicing in 1979 (6.2% of the 1.5 million registered professional nurses) (ANA 1979), more significant strides must be made to diversify the

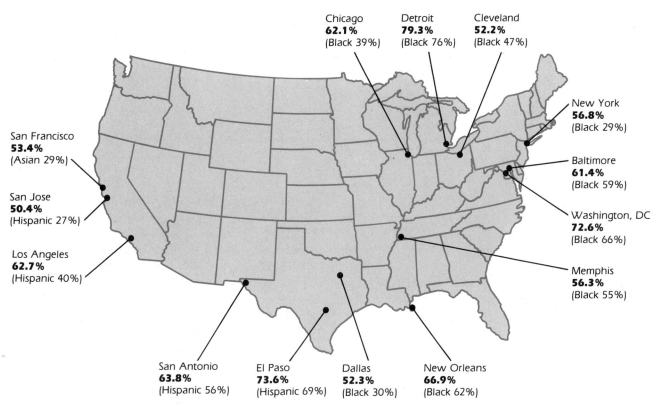

Figure 4–1. *Where minorities are the majority. In many of the largest US cities, minority groups make up more than half the population, as shown by the percentages. (The largest minority group is in parentheses.) (From Democrat and Chronicle, Rochester, NY. September 17, 1991.)*

nursing profession. Schools of nursing need to increase their efforts to recruit and retain more minorities, both as students and as faculty members.

Although it is not our intent to imply that membership in a particular race or cultural group automatically qualifies individuals to counsel or treat people within their own culture, it is our experience that minority clients respond more positively when people of color or other minorities are on the staff of the health agencies they use, even if their primary caregiver is white.

General Definitions and Concepts

Culture is a configuration of learned behaviors that are shared and transmitted in a society and by a particular group of people (Smith 1989). Persons born into a particular society are quickly socialized about what expectations the society has for them, as well as about the ones they have of others. These behaviors connote a particular way of life and enable the members in that society to survive and behave properly.

When anthropologists refer to culture in the broadest sense, they mean a way of life or belonging to a designated group of people. Culture is dynamic, changing, and diversified. Culture can be a major factor influencing how an individual perceives illness, nursing care, treatment, compliance, and recovery (Leininger 1990). Culture is a major determining factor in the use of mental health services (Wenger 1992).

Cultural shock is the mental or emotional confusion and distress that results from the interaction of two conflicting cultures. This is particularly significant if individuals bring into a situation various stereotypical beliefs that they consider to be factual. When their actual experiences prove their beliefs to be false, conflict results. Two-way culture shock is always a possibility when individuals who are culturally and ethnically different come together for the first time and have inaccurate information about each other's culture or ethnic group. For example, statements white individuals make to individuals of color once they get to know them, such as "You're not like the others" or "You're not what I expected," can sometimes be most confusing for those with a different stereotypical view of that cultural group.

Subculture refers to a smaller group within a larger cultural group that has its own particular set of cul-

Table 4–1 ■ PROFESSIONAL NURSES PRACTICING IN THE UNITED STATES	
African American	3.6%
Hispanic	1.3%
Native American	0.4%
Asian/Pacific Islander	2.3%
White	92.4%
	100.0%

Data from 1988 National Sample Survey. Bethesda, MD: US Department of Health and Human Services, 1988.

tural values, beliefs, and practices. Although it may be an integral member of a larger cultural group, it is somewhat different (Leininger 1990). A family member who practices a different religious faith than others in the family (e.g., one who practices Islam or is a Jehovah's Witness in a Roman Catholic family) may be as uniquely different from other family members as she or he is like them.

Black Muslims, more commonly referred to as members of the Nation of Islam, have religious beliefs that are an important part of their lifestyle, and health care providers should be familiar with them. For example, a newly admitted client who refuses to eat may be afraid of being served something with pork products or shellfish—foods that are prohibited. Muslims consider such foods filthy, and they are taught that a person is what he or she eats (Spector 1985).

Race, according to Johnson (1990, p. 41), "has typically represented an assumption of shared genetic heritage among groups of humans based on physical characteristics," such as skin and hair color or the shape of one's eyes, nose, and lips.

Ethnicity is a sense of belonging to a group with which one shares a unique cultural, social, and language identity. The group has in common distinctive identifying characteristics originating from a common national linguistic or racial orientation. Ethnicity iden-

tifies a person by his or her language, dialect, migratory status, race, religion, and sometimes food preferences.

Leininger (1989) defines **ethnocentrism** as the opinion that one's own beliefs, values, and lifeways are superior to or more desirable than another's. Table 4–2 defines terms that help clarify, at least in part, the influence that culture and beliefs exert on a person's attitudes and beliefs toward health care.

Folk Beliefs and Folk Healers

Folk beliefs are a group's health and illness belief systems. They may entail the practice of cultural medicine. For example, *asafetida*, a plant substance with a strong smell of garlic that looks like a dried-out sponge, is worn around the necks of some African Americans to prevent colds. Copper or silver bracelets worn around the wrists from birth to adulthood serve to protect the individual from illness and danger. If for any reason these bracelets are removed, it is believed that harm will befall the owner (Spector 1985).

Some individuals hold an almost fatalistic attitude about illness. They often believe that a situation or illness was "destined to happen" or that "God is pun-

Table 4–2 ■ CULTURAL CONCEPTS IMPORTANT IN HEALTH CARE	
TERM	**DEFINITION**
Enculturation	Learning about one's own culture and how outsiders see it. This information has of late been stressed as critical for all to know. A popular phrase today that exemplifies the importance of enculturation is, How can you know where you're going if you don't know where you've been?
Acculturation	A process that results when two autonomous cultures interact side by side for a period of time. Extensive changes in cultural patterns, beliefs, values, and behavior will occur in one or both cultures (Bullough and Bullough 1982, p. 105).
Assimilation	The process by which an individual belonging to a minority culture takes on behaviors of the majority culture. The members of the minority must often adopt the values and behaviors of the majority in order to succeed.
Heritage	Values and traditions passed from one generation to another. Each culture in our society has a health value system that affects members' beliefs about the health care services they receive. Knowing a client's heritage and how it relates to the majority culture helps the nurse anticipate how a client might perceive or interpret treatment interventions.

ishing me for some wrongdoing." These individuals experience denial, avoid treatment and care, and do not ascribe to prevention. The extreme of this is belief in witchcraft. Snow (1978) found this belief to be widespread among Puerto Ricans, Haitians, and African Americans. She estimated that one third of the African American clients treated at a southern United States psychiatric center believed they were victims of witchcraft.

Folk healers are individuals who are respected in their cultural communities as competent medical practitioners. Care should be used by health care professionals to avoid passing judgment on folk healers' competence as practitioners. Folk healers are widely used, especially by Native Americans, Puerto Ricans, and African Americans. Faith healers in Latino cultures, according to Wenger (1992), include

1. *Curanderos*, indigenous healers who use rituals, herbs, prayer, and massage in curing and caring practices
2. *Espiritualistas*, people born with a special talent for analyzing dreams or foretelling the future
3. *Verberos*, individuals who are knowledgeable in growing and prescribing herbs and in preventing and curing a variety of illnesses

Health care professionals generally do not know about the services of these healers because Latinos assume they would not want to know.

Root men and old ladies are folk healers who are respected by Africans and African Americans for their knowledge in curing disease and warding off evil harm. The spiritualist, an individual called by God to help with personal, financial, spiritual, emotional, or physical problems, is also revered by the African and African American communities. Herbalists are widely used by the Asian community for diagnostic and therapeutic interventions. Native Americans value the services of medicine men and witch doctors. Careless comments that devalue the services of folk healers that are made in the presence of members of these groups can lead to mistrust of the modern medical system.

Communicating Across Cultures

To be effective, health professionals must have the ability to communicate across cultures. Health care professionals need to learn to take into consideration an individual's communication pattern and the relationship of this pattern to a person's behavior, feelings, and attitudes. This requires a thorough initial

assessment of an individual's verbal and nonverbal communication patterns, including language style, dialect, use of touch, and kinesics. For example, some cultural groups such as Latinos use touch as an important means of communicating, whereas others interpret touch as intrusive and a violation of their personal space (Giger and Davidhizar 1990).

Persons in certain cultural groups amplify the volume of their voices when they are talking, whereas others lower their voices. A nurse who correlates loudness with anger may misinterpret what should be perceived as a normal communication pattern. The use of loud verbalization has long been misunderstood in Latinos and African Americans: it is often mislabeled as threatening.

Vignette

Two young Latino men visit their dad, who has been recently admitted to the hospital with a troubling hematological problem. In an attempt to cheer him up, they become loud and stay well beyond visiting hours. Anticipating resistance to her request for them to leave, a white nurse expresses concern and calls security to have them escorted out. However, her co-worker, an African American nurse, overhears the conversation and questions the need for security. The African American nurse politely explains to the family that visiting hours are over, and the family leaves.

Persons socialized to the Euro-American culture use eye contact when communicating with others. However, in some Asian cultures, looking a person of the opposite gender directly in the eyes suggests a sexual interest. Conversely, failure to look directly at African American clients is considered disrespectful.

Communication misunderstandings between the nurse and client can result in the client's withdrawing from treatment. This may occur without the nurse's ever knowing a misunderstanding existed. If good basic communication techniques are combined with cultural sensitivity, such misunderstandings can be kept to a minimum.

Assessing a Client's Cultural Needs

"If nursing is to promote and utilize the value of cultural diversity in health care and move beyond mere sensitivity to cultural difference to competence in the use of cultural knowledge then culture must be incorporated as a normal component of client assessment, as are physical and psychosocial dimensions" (DeSantiss 1988, p. 3).

Table 4–3 ▪ ACCULTURATION PROFILE FROM ASSESSMENT FACTORS

DIRECTIONS: Plot an **X** with the value numbers rated on this profile to discover the orientation or acculturation gradient of the informant. The clustering of numbers will give information about traditional or nontraditional patterns with respect to the criteria assessed*

CRITERIA	1 MAINLY TRADITIONAL	2 MODERATELY TRADITIONAL	3 AVERAGE	4 MODERATELY NONTRADITIONAL	5 MAINLY NONTRADITIONAL
1. Language and communication modes					
2. Physical environment					
3. Physical apparel and appearance					
4. Technology					
5. World view					
6. Family lifeways					
7. Social interaction and kinship					
8. Daily lifeways					
9. Religious orientation					
10. Economic factors					
11. Educational factors					
12. Political and legal factors					
13. Food uses					
14. Folk (generic) care-cure					
15. Professional care-cure expressions					
16. Caring patterns					
17. Curing patterns					
18. Prevention/maintenance factors					
19. Other indicators					

* The assessor will total numbers to get a summary orientation profile. Use of these ratings with written notations provides a holistic qualitative profile. Detailed notations are important to substantiate the ratings.

From Leininger M. Leininger's Acculturation Health Care Assessment Tool for Cultural Patterns in Traditional or Non-Traditional Lifeways. Journal of Transcultural Nursing, 2(2):40, 1991.

A client's cultural assessment is as important as the client's health history. A number of instruments have been developed to assist the practitioner in completing a cultural assessment of the client. We have chosen Leininger's widely used acculturation instrument. Part II of Leininger's assessment tool illustrates various areas health care workers may need to assess (Table 4–3). Once this assessment is completed, the nurse will be able to identify whether the client holds primarily traditional or nontraditional lifeways and will thus have the necessary information for planning care.

When performing a cultural assessment of a client, the nurse must remember that the client is part of a multifaceted system made up of the client; his or her nuclear and extended families; the ethnic community, including the church; and the traditional community. Each facet of this system is assessed to evaluate its relevance to the client. The nurse can then identify which areas are a source of support and which are a source of stress. For example, most members of a particular cultural group may view the church as a source of support and strength and may attend services regularly. For some members, however, the church may be a source of stress and they may rarely attend.

Although it is sometimes helpful to make generalizations about a particular culture's behaviors and beliefs, it is imperative that the nurse keep in mind the uniqueness of the person with whom she or he is working. "Generalizations are necessary for us to use; without them we would become inefficient creatures. However, they are guidelines for our behaviors, to be tentatively applied in new situations, and they should be open to change and challenge" (Sue and Sue 1990, p. 47).

Novice practitioners who work with clients who are culturally different from themselves often wish that they had a detailed guidebook that would tell them how to respond to a person from a particular cultural group. They quickly learn, however, that there is no expedient way to acquire knowledge about another person's culture. According to Sue and Sue (1990, p. 208), the complexity of human behavior makes it futile "to attempt an understanding of ethnic minorities without an adequate exploration of their historical background, subcultural values, and unique conflicts." Jones (1985) devised a model (Fig. 4–2) that incorporates these variables and provides a guide for conceptualizing psychological functioning in various cultural groups. The original model addresses only the African American client. However, Jones states that "while this framework was developed as a way of conceptualizing mental health problems in black therapy patients, the general approach might well be employed as a way of viewing psychological functioning in other ethnic minority patients as well" (p. 368). In Jones's model, four classes of variables comprise the structure of the

model: (1) reactions to racial oppression, (2) influence of the majority culture, (3) influence of the traditional culture, and (4) individual and family experiences and endowments (p. 364). Jones depicts these four classes of variables as overlapping circles. "The overlapping circles reflect the fact that each set of factors may be viewed as having both a separate influence on psychological functioning and an influence on the operation of the other factors. The specific content of each set of factors is derived from a clinical assessment of the individual patient" (p. 367). All four classes interacting together have an impact on the presenting problem. One of the major advantages of Jones's model is that it compels the mental health care provider to recognize that each client is an individual who has been influenced by a distinctive set of experiences and that even the interplay of each of these classes of variables is unique to the individual.

Andrews (1991), a noted transcultural nurse, suggests several guiding principles to be used in completing a cultural assessment of a client (Table 4–4).

Cultural Groups and Mental Health Concerns

Culture plays an important role in the diagnosis of mental disorders. Pitfalls can occur if statistical criteria are used that equate normalcy with those behaviors that occur most often in the general population. When deviations from the behaviors of the majority are considered abnormal, the conditions of many ethnic and racial minorities that exhibit strong subcul-

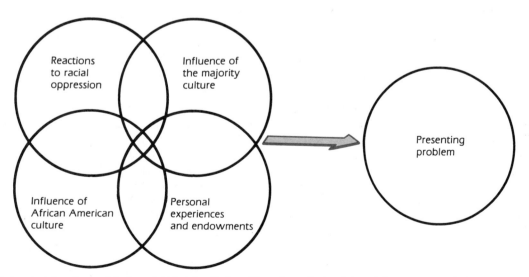

Figure 4–2. *Jones's interactive model of psychological functioning. (From Jones A. Psychological functioning in Black Americans: A conceptual guide for use in psychotherapy. Psychotherapy, 22(25):367, 1985.)*

Table 4–4 ■ CULTURAL ASSESSMENT GUIDELINES

1. Know your own cultural attitudes, values, beliefs, and practices. This is essential to presenting a nonjudgmental attitude.
2. Be aware that regardless of good intentions, everyone has cultural baggage that ultimately results in ethnocentrism (i.e., the tendency to view one's own culture as superior to others). We all have prejudices but we are not necessarily racist.
3. Recognize that it's easier to understand those whose cultural heritage is similar to our own and to view those who are unlike us with suspicion and mistrust.
4. Maintain a broad, open attitude. Expect the unexpected. Enjoy surprises.
5. Avoid seeing all people as alike. Avoid cultural stereotypes, such as all blacks eat soul food or are uneducated and on welfare, or all Chinese like rice.
6. Always question the reason for any behavior. The best way to understand people from diverse cultural backgrounds is to discuss commonalities and differences.
7. Recognize that folk healing may be practiced side by side with Western biomedicine: for example, a traditional healer and a medical doctor may be treating an individual simultaneously. Don't settle for a single explanation but look for multiple dimensions.
8. If an explanation is given that you don't understand, ask for clarification. Be inquisitive. Most people respond positively to questions that arise from genuine concern and interest. Remember that "yes" in response to questions such as "Do you understand?" does not necessarily mean the individual understands. Self-reliance or pride might be at the foundation of the response.
9. Take care not to label what you don't understand, and don't make assumptions.
10. Be yourself. There are no right or wrong ways to learn about cultural diversity.

Adapted from Andrews M. Changing faces: Nursing in a multicultural society. Paper presented at the Genesee Valley Nurses Association Symposium, Rochester, NY, 1991.

tural differences may be improperly diagnosed (Sue and Sue 1990).

In the United States, clinicians use criteria set forth in the *Diagnostic and Statistical Manual of Mental Disorders, third edition, revised* (DSM-III-R) to arrive at a medical psychiatric diagnosis. The authors of the DSM-III-R suggest that caution be used when these criteria are applied to a person from an ethnic or a cultural group different from that of the clinician's to ensure that these criteria are culturally valid: "It is important that the clinician not employ DSM-III-R in a mechanical fashion, insensitive to differences in language, values, behavioral norms, and idiomatic expressions of distress. . . . The clinician working in such settings should apply DSM-III-R with open-mindedness to the presence of distinctive cultural patterns and sensitivity to the possibility of unintended bias because of such differences."

When an experience or behavior is entirely normative for a particular culture (e.g., the experience of hallucinating the voice of the deceased in the first few weeks of bereavement in various Native American groups, or trance and possession in states occurring in culturally approved ritual contexts in much of the non-Western world), it should not be regarded as pathological. Culture-specific symptoms of distress, such as particular somatic symptoms associated with distress in members of different ethnic and cultural groups, may create difficulties in the use of DSM-III-R or DSM-IV criteria because the psychopathology is unique to that culture or because the DSM-III-R or DSM-IV categories are not based on extensive research with non-Western populations (APA 1987, 1991).

For example, a religious client observed mumbling, with arms waving in the air, may be witnessing or communicating with God, but the culturally insensitive nurse might mislabel this behavior as hallucinatory or indicative of mental illness, as illustrated in the following case.

Vignette

Mr. Kay, a 78-year-old African American from South Carolina, is admitted to the hospital for the third time in six weeks with a complaint of severe respiratory distress. Although he has a history of emphysema, his color is good and his arterial blood gas findings are all within normal limits. Mr. Kay insists that he is in acute respiratory distress and demands oxygen therapy. His physician, recognizing his severe anxiety, orders oxygen therapy in an attempt to decrease Mr. Kay's anxiety level.

A review of Mr. Kay's history reveals that Mr. Kay has become increasingly anxious and depressed about his physical condition. He became dependent on oxygen therapy during his last hospital stay, and his physician, unable to wean him from the oxygen, prescribed home oxygen therapy. At home, Mr. Kay was restless, irritable, and difficult to get along with. He believed his physician did not know what he was doing and was using him as a guinea pig. He constantly complained about odors in his home, which he believed negatively affected his breathing. He accused his wife, a nonsmoker, of smoking in the house. Mr. Kay also refused to bathe himself, and rather than walk the few paces to the bathroom, he used a urinal.

Once admitted, Mr. Kay demands that the nurses bathe and feed him. One day, after his pastor has visited him, the nurses observe him mumbling to himself and waving his hands in the air. The only words they can make out are "Thank you, oh thank you. Even if you don't, I know you can. I'm ready." Because they cannot understand what he is saying, they assume he is hallucinating and request a psychiatric consultation.

What the nurses did not realize was that Mr. Kay was praying and carrying on a conversation with God. He was asking God to heal him. Furthermore, he told God that even if He didn't heal him, he believed He had the power to do so. He also told God he was ready to die because he had given himself to the Lord years ago.

Because the nurses did not understand the role that "witnessing" plays in African American culture, they mistakenly diagnosed Mr. Kay as psychotic. Although Mr. Kay was not hallucinating, he could have benefited from a consultation with a psychiatric liaison nurse. Such a nurse could have helped Mr. Kay recognize the effect that anxiety had on his illness and could have aided him in developing ways to cope more effectively with his anxiety and his illness.

The following sections give a brief overview of some cultural groups and some of the mental health problems they experience.

AFRICAN AMERICANS

Throughout this chapter, we make a concerted effort to use the term *African American* whenever possible. Although *black* is a less awkward term when used in a narrative context, it does not convey the positive sense of a person's heritage or identify the cultural homeland as well as the term *African American*.

African Americans, who now number 30 million, have a unique history. They are the only group of people in the United States who were brought forcibly to this country, separated from their families (nuclear and extended), and stripped of their identity and dignity. More than 300 years of exploitation and oppression followed. The oppression of African Americans continued into the postslavery era, when racist actions against individuals and families only exacerbated the harm done during the slavery period.

Historical evidence suggests that strong family ties bound African Americans together during the confusion that followed the Civil War. To adapt to pressures of slavery and discrimination, African American families developed the ability to persevere, organize, and succeed despite the odds. According to Staples (1985, p. 1011), "traditional family life remains the one viable option for Black Americans of all socioeconomic strata because it is less subject to the vagaries of race than any other institution in American life."

Today, in addition to the continuous challenges and pressures of racism and oppression, African American families face other threats to their family stability. Such threats include poverty (31% of African American families struggle for their daily survival), widespread substance abuse, teenage pregnancy, communicable diseases, and violent crimes. Wilson and Stith (1991) express concern that the traditional values and coping mechanisms of African American families may not be adequate to deal with these threats to family stability, however temporary.

Despite all these challenges, the African American family is surviving. Approximately 90% of college-educated African American men are married and living with their spouses (Staples 1985). Sixty-nine percent of African American families are not poor.

The presence of strong social support systems may be the only characteristic that distinguishes African Americans who are able to cope with the problems of life from those who are unable to cope (Lyles and Carter 1982). Although the African American family has many support systems, the two primary ones throughout history have been the church and the kin network (Malson 1982). The importance of church and kinship is consistent with the African values of sharing, affiliation, and spirituality.

The African American church is the root of social support for the African American family (Lyles and Carter 1982). Its members are respected and are able to excel in the struggle for survival, expression, participation, meaning, and fulfillment. The church helps to maintain family solidarity while also allowing for the expression of anger, distress, and pain (Lyles and Carter 1982).

Additionally, the African American church has provided a deep sense of spirituality to African Americans. The church and spirituality provide support plus an adaptive mechanism for coping with stress that must be recognized and incorporated into the therapeutic process (Boyd-Franklin 1989). A common method of treating illnesses for some African Americans is prayer, or the laying-on of hands. Prayer bands made up of missionaries from the Christian church or of clergy often visit the sick rooms of parishioners and offer a prayer of deliverance. These individuals deserve the same privacy and courtesy given to the priest who brings the sacraments to clients who are Roman Catholic.

Extended family relationships provide a second important source of support for African American families. From a very early age, African American children are taught to respect and revere older adults. Although unrelated by blood, family friends are often called auntie, uncle, cousin, brother, or sister. Calling an adult by his or her first name is usually not allowed. African American coworkers often become part of the extended family. These relationships may be especially important when coworkers experience prejudice on the job. Their mutual support provides a buffer to the psychological stressors they encounter in their work world. This extended support system needs to be considered in helping African American families cope effectively with illness.

Influence of the Majority Culture

Jones (1985) asserts that the traditions of the majority in the United States have had a major influence on African Americans and that many have adopted the values, mores, and orientation of the majority culture (p. 366):

> Black psychotherapy patients demonstrate a wide range of variability with regard to their adoption of majority culture interests and values, with varying degrees of associated internal conflict. The therapist aims for the goal of helping the patient make choices which are compatible temperamentally and which can be integrated with a positive black identity

Influence of the Traditional African American Culture

As previously mentioned, the church and the kin network have been two of the most important support systems throughout African American history, and they serve as sources of survival. Jones (1985) offers data to support his belief that several other aspects of African American culture serve as sources of adaptation as well. These include a flexible concept of time, a well-developed ability to use affect, and a general sensitivity to others. Obviously, African Americans will vary in the extent to which they are influenced by African American traditions. However, a nurse who has a knowledge of this culture "can help clients to use aspects of these traditions to deal with internal conflicts and to facilitate personal growth" (Jones 1985, p. 366).

African Americans and Mental Health Concerns

Very few research studies have been conducted on emotional disorders in African Americans. Neal and Turner (1991) suggest several reasons for this:

1. Failure of African Americans to volunteer for research studies

2. Disinterest on the part of researchers
3. Different patterns of help-seeking behavior among African Americans
4. Existence of relatively few African American researchers

To overcome these difficulties, Neal and Turner suggest that researchers abandon traditional methods of recruiting subjects (e.g., newspaper ads, television spots, and waiting for subjects to walk into clinics) and instead recruit within African American churches, schools, and other social organizations, because personal contact seems to be an important factor in a successful recruitment effort. Furthermore, because African Americans tend to seek help from agencies located within the African American community, collaborative efforts need to take place.

ANXIETY DISORDERS. The current literature on anxiety disorders in African Americans is scarce (Neal and Turner 1991). For example, in the last five years, only two studies have addressed the issue of panic disorder in African Americans. These studies indicate that in African Americans there is a higher incidence of anxiety disorders such as isolated sleep paralysis, symptoms of post-traumatic stress disorder, and simple phobias.

RAPE. Wyatt (1991) found no significant differences in the prevalence of reported rape incidents between African American women and their white counterparts. African American women, however, were significantly less likely to disclose incidents involving sexual assault. Wyatt suggests that long-established patterns of nondisclosure of rape have often been reinforced by historical, societal, and legal attitudes about racial and ethnic groups. Furthermore, the anticipated lack of community and societal support may be another important factor in African American women's hesitancy to disclose rape. Wyatt also states that "there is a possibility that African American women may not perceive themselves as rape victims. Their experience meeting the criteria of 'real rape' has implications for the disclosure of incidents, as well as the initial and lasting effects of sexual victimization." It is possible that African American women, because of the historical context of rape (i.e, the sexual exploitation of slaves for more than 250 years and a long-held belief that African Americans were not worthy of being protected from rape and its consequences), may find it difficult to believe that society has had a change of heart and now believes African Americans have a right not only to be protected from rape but also to be treated with respect and compassion after an assault occurs. Wyatt suggests that incidents of rape and its effect on survivors need to be investigated within the sociocultural and environmental context of the occurrence. Within that context, the strategies for recovery and the prevention of revictimization should evolve.

SCHIZOPHRENIA. African Americans have been consistently misdiagnosed and overdiagnosed as having schizophrenia (Snowden and Cheung 1990; Jones and Gray 1986; Adebimpe 1981). Jones and Gray suggest that the general causes of misdiagnosis include "overreliance on the classic thought disorder symptoms as pathognomonic of schizophrenia, . . . cultural differences in language and mannerisms, difficulties in relating between black patients and white therapist, and the myth that blacks rarely suffer from affective disorders" (p. 61). Therapists who do not understand the African Americans' use of language, behavioral mannerisms, and style of relating may consider these behaviors indicative of pathology. "Language not understood is often considered evidence of thought disorder; styles of relating are sometimes misinterpreted as disturbances of affect; and unfamiliar mannerisms are considered bizarre. These mistakes are unavoidable" (Jones and Gray 1986). Grier and Cobbs (1968), in their revolutionary book *Black Rage*, suggest that certain behaviors such as "paranoia," when seen in African Americans, may actually be "adaptive" rather than pathological. Because of the long history of abuse by the dominant society, African Americans must constantly be on guard to avoid being hurt and to protect themselves from a variety of abuses.

A well-informed, culturally sensitive nurse will be able to act as a client advocate and to question the misinterpretation of behaviors. In this way, nurses can help to reverse the trend of overdiagnosing African Americans as having schizophrenia. Furthermore, nurses who use this approach will be able to intervene more effectively with African American clients.

DEPRESSION. Historically, mood disorders have been underdiagnosed in African Americans (Jones and Gray 1986; Snowden and Cheung 1990). Jones and Gray suggest several reasons for this:

1. Problems in diagnosing mood disorders in general
2. The stereotypical belief that African Americans rarely suffer from depression
3. The fact that depressed African Americans may experience delusions and hallucinations more frequently than whites and therefore be diagnosed as having a thought disorder rather than depression

Hu et al. (1991) examined the use of mental health emergency services, inpatient care, individual outpatient visits, and case management by members of ethnic groups. Using a sample of 27,000 persons, they found that "utilization by Blacks appears especially problematic, because this group appears to rely more on emergency service and less on case management and outpatient care."

ALCOHOLISM. Alcoholism and other drug abuse has taken a considerable toll on the African American community. Neeley and Grant (1990), citing the US Department of Health and Human Services statistics, state that chemical dependency is a major reason for the overall shorter life expectancy (5.6 years) of African Americans compared with whites. The authors also report that according to the National Black Alcoholism Council, alcoholism is the number one health problem leading to disease and death among African Americans. Bell et al. (1990, p. 5) discuss the relationship between chemical abuse and dependency and the problems experienced by African American communities:

All major problems experienced by black communities —crime, unemployment, poverty, school drop outs, unplanned teenage pregnancies, etc.—are made worse by alcohol and drug abuse and drug dependency. In some cases chemical abuse is the cause of the other problems; in other cases chemical abuse exacerbates existing problems.

Crime and violence go hand in hand with the illicit drug trade. Bell et al. (1990, p. 6) state that "tragically, addiction and criminal activity have become rites of passage in many black communities. They are a quick and visible method to secure stature in a peer reference group." The challenge today is to provide a full range of culturally relevant chemical dependency treatment options to African American clients. Treatment options need to address African Americans' unique needs, in addition to providing conventional intervention for chemical dependency.

In traditional African societies, chemical dependency was not a problem. "Tradition and widely understood social norms and rules dictated the very circumscribed role of alcohol in community life. Those norms dictated when, where, how, and how much alcohol was to be consumed. Drinking to the point of intoxication, for instance, was almost universally despised" (Gossett 1988, p. 2). African Americans were able to adhere to these traditional values throughout their period of enslavement and during the period of the Reconstruction. Gradually, starting around the early 1900s, political, social, and economic factors combined to influence the use of alcohol and other drugs by African Americans. Gossett believes that the African American community needs to examine the traditional African culture, in which chemical dependency was not a problem, and identify strategies employed by that culture to prevent chemical abuse.

The next step is for African American communities to set up "multiple-help agencies to interact with clients in non-threatening, familiar surroundings. Prevention and treatment, drug-free recreational outlets, and culturally specific therapeutic alternatives are possible, must be made available, and are necessary for the attainment of 'quality sobriety'" (Gossett 1988, p. 22).

Box 4–1 is based on 11 strategies that family therapists can employ to better provide culturally sensitive care to African Americans. These same strategies have been modified for use by nurses in increasing the effectiveness of their nursing care.

Vignette

Ms. Lane, an attractive 17-year-old white nursing student, is assigned to care for Jamie, a 15-year-old African American boy who was admitted to the emergency department the previous evening with a gunshot wound in the right shoulder.

In the morning report, Ms. Lane learns that Jamie was injured during a store robbery. During the night shift, he did not receive relief from the analgesic. Jamie became upset, sobbed loudly, and angrily questioned why he had to wait so long for pain medication. He insisted numerous times that the night nurse call the doctor. Ms. Lane is to prepare Jamie for follow-up x-rays and surgery for an open reduction.

When Ms. Lane enters his room to prepare him for surgery, she finds him with four of his adolescent friends, who abruptly stop talking. One young man leans over and whispers something to another, and they all chuckle aloud. Ms. Lane quickly leaves the room without uttering a sound. Her nursing instructor finds her pacing outside the client's room, obviously upset. When asked if her client is ready for the x-rays and surgery, she tells the instructor she is afraid to re-enter the room because she thinks the young men visiting Jamie are gang members. They make her feel uncomfortable and intimidated—she is sure they are dangerous.

During the course of the conversation with the instructor, Ms. Lane admits that she has made the following assumptions:

1. Jamie was shot while robbing a grocery store and was therefore dangerous, as were his friends.
2. She, like the night nurse, would have a difficult time with Jamie.
3. His friends were gang members because they were all dressed alike.
4. Their loud voices meant they were angry and therefore a threat to her.
5. When they were whispering, they were talking about her.

Box 4–1. GUIDELINES FOR RELATING TO AFRICAN AMERICANS

1. Become aware of the historical and current experience of being black in America.
2. Consider value and cultural differences between black Americans and other American ethnic groups and how your personal values influence the way you (practice nursing).*
3. Consider the way your personal values influence the way you view both the presenting problem and the goals (of nursing intervention).
4. Include the value system of the client in the goal-setting process. Be sensitive to spiritual values and the value of the family and the church.
5. Be sensitive to variations in black family norms due to normal adaptations to stress, and be flexible enough to accept these variations.
6. Be aware of how ineffective verbal and nonverbal communication due to cultural variation in communication can lead to premature termination of (the nurse-client relationship). Become familiar with nonstandard or Black English, and accept its use by clients.
7. Consider the client's problems in the larger context. Include the extended family or other significant individuals and larger systems in your thinking, if not in your (actual intervention).
8. Be aware of your client's racial identification, and do not feel threatened by your client's cultural identification with his or her own race.
9. Learn to acknowledge and be comfortable with your client's cultural differences.
10. Consider the appropriateness of specific therapeutic models of intervention to specific black families. Do not apply interventions without considering unique aspects of each family.
11. Consider each black family and each black family member you treat as unique.

Adapted from Wilson LL, Stith SM. Culturally sensitive therapy with black clients. Journal of Multicultural Counseling and Development, 19:32, 1991.

*Phrases in parentheses indicate modifications of the guidelines for use by nurses.

The instructor is able to help Ms. Lane separate the facts from the assumptions and to apply cross-cultural considerations:

1. Jamie, a customer in the store, was shot while attempting to stop the robbery.
2. The young men, although friends, are not gang members. They are all solid students with good grades.
3. Being typical adolescents, they could not help but notice that their friend's nurse was just slightly older than they were and pretty besides. They were snickering about how embarrassed Jamie would feel having her give him a pain shot.

ASIAN AMERICANS

The Asian American population, totaling about 5 million people, is composed of at least 29 distinct subgroups, including Filipinos, Chinese, Koreans, Vietnamese, Asian Indians, and Japanese. It is difficult to provide the student with generalizations about Asian Americans because between subgroups there may be a multiplicity of values, religious beliefs, and languages. Furthermore, within any subgroup, "individuals diverge on variables such as migration or relocation experiences, degree of assimilation or acculturation, identification with the home country, facility with their native and English languages, family composition and intactness, amount of education, and degree of adherence to religious beliefs" (Wong 1985, as cited by Sue and Sue 1990, p. 189). Tsui and Schultz (1985) believe that although there is considerable variability among the groups that make up the Asian American population, similarities, such as specified roles within the family, deference to authority, hierarchical family structure, and emotional restraint, do exist.

Pacific Islanders and Asian Americans have had to meet numerous challenges in their struggle to become full-fledged American citizens. These include

1. Conflict between their traditional Buddhist and Confucian philosophies and the dominant Christian religion
2. Oriental Exclusion Acts, which were passed in the early part of the twentieth century to stop the migration of Asians into America
3. Laws that were enacted to prevent Asian Americans from purchasing land and other assets
4. Difficulty in learning the English language
5. In the case of Japanese Americans, deprivation of their property and civil rights during World War II (Goldman 1984)

Although some Pacific Islanders and Asian Americans have fared well despite these difficulties, others have not. The contemporary image that Asian Americans are "model minorities" and do not experience any difficulties in society is challenged by Sue and Sue (1990, p. 191):

A closer analysis of the status of Asian Americans does not support their success story. First, reference to the higher median income of Asian Americans does not take into account (a) the higher percentage of more than one wage earner in Asian than in white families, (b) an equal prevalence of poverty despite the higher median income, (c) lower poverty assistance and welfare than the general population, and (d) a discrepancy between education and income.

Three variables that support the thesis that Asian Americans may not enjoy the degree of success that society claims they have achieved are (1) level of education, (2) living conditions, and (3) use of mental health facilities.

Education

Although some Asian Americans have achieved a high level of education, many are undereducated. Many have had difficulty mastering the English language. This has been true even for college students. Sue and Sue (1990) state that more than 50% of Asian American students entering the University of California failed to pass an English examination and needed to take remedial English courses. A bilingual background is a major contributor to their difficulty with the English language; however, the Asians' strong cultural injunctions against assertiveness, the shame and disgrace felt by students at having to take such courses, and the isolation imposed on this group by a racist society are equally strong forces in their performance (Sue and Sue 1990, p. 191).

Living Conditions

Another serious problem for Asian Americans is the deplorable living conditions that exist in Chinatowns, Manilatowns, and Japantowns in San Francisco and New York City. Often these are ghetto areas with prevalent unemployment, poverty, health problems, and juvenile delinquency (Sue and Sue 1990). This is the side of these popular tourist attractions that the visitor rarely sees but that is a reality for the citizens of these communities.

Viewing Asian Americans as "model minorities" has several negative consequences that must be addressed (Sue and Sue 1990, p. 192):

1. These stereotypes reassert the erroneous belief that any minority can succeed in a democratic society if the minority group members work hard enough.
2. The Asian American success story is seen as a divisive concept used by the Establishment to pit one minority group against another by holding one group up as an example to others.
3. The success myth has prevented many Asian American communities from receiving the necessary moral and financial commitment due them as a struggling minority with unique concerns.

Asian Americans and Mental Health Concerns

The incidence of mental illness in the Asian American population has not been well documented. Because of this, it is difficult to discuss specific illnesses such as schizophrenia. Instead, we address certain culture-specific manifestations of mental illness in Asian Americans. According to Westermeyer (1985), Asian Americans suffer from certain "culture-bound" syndromes (i.e., trance-like or behavioral disturbances that are found in unusually high frequencies in certain societies). Westermeyer offers the following examples of these culture-bound syndromes:

- *Latah* in Southeast Asian women: Minimal stimuli elicit an exaggerated startle response, often with swearing.
- *Anthropophobia* among the Japanese, especially men: Involves easy blushing, anxiety with face-to-face contact, and fear of rejection.
- *Koro*, especially in Asian men: Consists of the fear that the penis will withdraw into the abdomen, causing death.
- *Amok* among Southeast Asian men: Involves sudden mass assault, usually including homicide and sometimes the death of the perpetrator.

The emotions and behaviors (e.g., anxiety, fear, social isolation, deviant behavior, and undirected violence) that seem to underlie these culture-bound syndromes are seen cross-culturally as well.

Asian Americans tend to view their illnesses as physical instead of psychological; therefore, they tend to exhibit numerous somatic complaints (Collins et al. 1992). Asians tend to believe that physical problems cause emotional distress, and they look to health professionals to take care of the physical problems. Nurses working with Asian American clients, as with any client who complains of somatic distress, should try hard to relieve the physical discomfort (e.g., the constipation that often accompanies depression).

Use of Mental Health Services

Asian Americans are underrepresented in the mental health system (Snowden and Cheung 1990; Hu et al. 1991). An example of the use of public mental health agencies found that "Asians had a lower probability than whites of using emergency, inpatient, and case management services, and a higher probability of using individual outpatient services" (Hu et al. 1991, p. 1434). Even though Asian Americans are infrequently admitted to inpatient units, once they are admitted, they have a longer stay, on average, than their white counterparts. "Relatively low rates of severe pathology would help to explain the infrequent use of inpatient care by Asian/Pacific Americans: this possibility cannot be evaluated at present. The lack of reliable knowledge about the true prevalence of disorder among . . . Asian/Pacific Americans represents a gap in our knowledge base that must be closed" (Snowden and Cheung 1990, p. 352).

Nursing Interventions

To provide culturally sensitive nursing care to Asian Americans and Pacific Islanders, nurses need to apply principles of intervention that integrate cultural knowledge and cultural sensitivity. Two processes that are basic to therapeutic intervention are credibility and giving. *Credibility* refers to the client's perception of the therapist as an effective and trustworthy helper. *Giving* is the client's perception that something was received from the therapeutic encounter (Sue and Zane 1987). Knowing a person's culture can help the nurse to be perceived as an effective and trustworthy helper, as long as the nurse can avoid confusing the cultural values of the client's ethnic group with those of the client.

Vignette

A 57-year-old Asian man is found by the nurse to be praying excessively. Periodically, while praying, he calls out the name Michael, gets up, takes flowers from the bedside vase, and lays them on the window sill. The staff is convinced that he is obsessive, compulsive, and hallucinating. They have devoted considerable effort to attempts to alter his behavior.

What the staff did not realize is that sacrificial offerings are normal for some Asians. In this case, the client was engaged in a normal ritual, offering flowers in sacrifice to St. Michael for the return of his health.

LATINO AMERICANS

Some controversy exists over the correct way to address individuals who live in the United States but come from Puerto Rico, Mexico, Cuba, El Salvador, the Dominican Republic, or other Latino American countries. In this chapter, we refer to such individuals as Latinos or Latino Americans. The student should know that certain groups prefer other terms, such as "Mexican American," "Spanish American," "La raza" (the race), and "Hispanic American."

The Latino population numbers about 14.6 million. The largest single subgroup is Mexican Americans (9 million). Three million Latinos are from Puerto Rico, and 1 million come from Cuba.

Latinos are overrepresented among the poor, have high unemployment, and often live in substandard housing (Sue and Sue 1990). Sue and Sue describe Latinos as having the following characteristics:

1. Respect for family and family values, and strong family loyalties. There is cooperation between family members as opposed to competition.
2. The large extended family, which includes persons who are not blood relatives, such as the maid-of-honor, best man, and godparents, is a major source of support for Latinos—Latinos will seek help from the extended family before seeking professional help.
3. Latino families are hierarchical in form and give special authority to the elderly, parents, and men. Fathers assume primary authority, and children are expected to be obedient.
4. Gender roles are clearly delineated, and the sexual activity of adolescent girls is severely restricted.
5. Catholic religious beliefs are viewed as a source of strength. Influenced by their Catholic religion, Latinos believe that sacrifice is helpful to salvation, being charitable is a virtue, and wrongs done to one are to be endured.

It is important to keep in mind that depending on the degree to which they have been acculturated, Latino clients will vary in how many of these characteristics they display. Nurses who work with Latino Americans will notice many differences within a specific subgroup (e.g., Mexican Americans) and between subgroups (e.g., between Mexican Americans and Puerto Ricans).

Latino Americans and Mental Health Concerns

Much of the distress experienced by Latino Americans is in response to external stressors, such as poverty, poor housing, and the need to learn the English language in order to communicate needs. A review of the writings of several authors identified a number of guidelines on how to relate to Latino Americans. Nurses will find these guidelines, which are found in Box 4–2, helpful in their practice.

Box 4–2. GUIDELINES FOR RELATING TO LATINO AMERICANS

1. Be respectful and warm when you introduce yourself. Pronounce the client's name correctly. If you are unsure of the correct way to pronounce the client's name, ask the client and then make a concerted effort to pronounce it correctly.
2. Explain what your role is as a nurse or psychiatric nurse, and explain the concept of confidentiality.
3. Ask clients to explain their problems as they see them, in their own words.
4. Summarize what the client has said to make certain that you understand the problems and to let the client know that you have understood.
5. Ask the client to tell you which problems she or he sees as most important.
6. With the client's help, establish goals.
7. Recognize the importance of family members, and discuss the possibility of involving family members in treatment.
8. Provide necessary assistance in developing and maintaining environmental supports.
9. Explain the nursing interventions you will use and how they will help the client to achieve his or her goals.

Adapted from copyright © Sue DW, Sue D. Counseling the Culturally Different. Theory and Practice, 2nd ed. New York: John Wiley & Sons, 1990. Reprinted by permission of John Wiley & Sons, Inc.

Use of Mental Health Services

Several scholars have examined the use of mental health services by Latinos. Collins et al. (1992) examined the effect of culture on consultation with a psychiatric liaison in a general hospital setting. The rate of referral was lower for Latinos than for African Americans, whites, or Asian Americans. The authors state that they cannot account for the decreased rate of consultation referral in Latinos, but they suggest several possible explanations:

1. Physicians may not refer Latinos because they perceive mental problems as being highly stigmatizing for this population.
2. Because Latinos underutilize mental health services, physicians may perceive them as needing fewer referrals.
3. Latinos' reliance on family, religious beliefs, and folk remedies for support instead of on mental health services may influence physicians' decisions to refer.
4. Primary physicians may underestimate the need for psychiatric intervention because of the language barrier.

When Latinos were referred, it was for evaluation of depression and suicide. This increased number of referrals did not reflect a higher frequency of mood disorders in this population, however. Instead, the psychiatric consultants found a significantly higher frequency of adjustment disorders in Latinos than in whites or African Americans. When Hu et al. (1991) studied the use of mental health services, they found that Latinos, compared with whites, had a higher probability of using case management intervention, a lower probability of using emergency services, and an equal probability of using inpatient facilities.

Some reasons Latinos as well as other ethnic minorities do not fare well in the mental health system include (1) the lack of bilingual therapists, (2) stereotypes that therapists have about clients from different cultural backgrounds, (3) discrimination, and most importantly, (4) failure of therapists to provide culturally sensitive forms of treatment (Sue and Zane 1987).

To overcome these difficulties, scholars have suggested matching clients with therapists who are better able to respond to the unique needs of ethnic populations. According to Sue and Zane (1987):

> Applying the concept of match, or fit, at the client-therapist level has generally meant that (a) more ethnic therapists who presumably are bilingual or are familiar with ethnic cultural values should be recruited into the mental health field, (b) students and therapists should acquire knowledge of ethnic cultures and communities, and (c) traditional forms of treatment should be modified because they are geared primarily for mainstream America. These tasks have been difficult and problematic to achieve. For example, it can be difficult to recruit Hispanics who are fluent in Spanish because graduate schools are often reluctant to admit students if their English verbal skills are low.

Vignette

A Latino adolescent girl is admitted to an empty bed in a semiprivate room. Her roommate is a 17-year-old white girl. The Latino girl's parents are obviously upset: they are crying and speaking angrily to their daughter in Spanish. Both clients have overdosed on unknown drugs and are being held for observation and psychiatric consultation. The mother of the white client abruptly gets up, draws the curtain, and rings for the nurse. She asks to have her daughter transferred to another room immediately. The Latino family overhears her mumble something about Puerto Ricans and her daughter's need to be with someone with whom she can relate. "For heaven's sake," the mother tells the nurse, "they can't even speak English."

The Latino client took the overdose because she had just broken up with her boyfriend, whom she said she loved and did not want to live without. The white client, who had been molested by her stepfather, said she was "sick and tired of fighting off her stepfather's advances and would rather be dead." The white client's mother refused to believe that her husband had molested her daughter.

Although these two clients have ethnic differences, there are commonalities. For example, they are both troubled teenagers who are at the same developmental stage.

The nurse should also be aware of cross-cultural communication differences. For example, speaking one's native language is not unusual when individuals are upset, although it may be considered threatening to some.

NATIVE AMERICANS

Native Americans, our country's "first peoples," now number more than 1 million. Approximately 50% of Native Americans live on reservations. The US government officially recognizes 511 distinct tribes, and the states recognize another 365 Native American tribal communities (LaFromboise and Nixon 1988). As do other cultural groups, Native Americans show immense variation in their costumes, religious practices, languages, and family structures. Furthermore, the extent of their acculturation into the larger society varies from group to group and from individual to individual.

Hobus (1990) studied the Lakotas, the fifth largest Native American population per capita in the United States. He found that when elders from the reservation were placed in culturally unacceptable environments, such as predominantly white nursing homes, stress and feelings of abandonment were experienced by clients, and devastation and guilt were experienced by the families.

Epperley (1991) asserts that despite the great variation that exists among Native American cultures, certain traits distinguish Native Americans from their white counterparts. Epperley revised Bryde's list of distinguishing Native American characteristics:

1. Native Americans tend to be present oriented; they are not concerned with time.
2. They value generosity and sharing.
3. They have respect for age.
4. They prefer cooperation to competition.
5. They try to live in harmony with nature.

Native American culture has special attributes that affect the ability of Native Americans to cope with problems. For example, great importance is placed on the family and the extended family network. The cohesiveness of Native American communities continues despite the severe social and economic pressures they have experienced. Finally, Native Americans have a holistic view of the universe: they see the importance of harmony between the mental, emotional, physical, and spiritual dimensions.

Native Americans and Mental Health Concerns

"Conquest, religious persecution, forced assimilation, land allotment, broken trust, open ridicule, and the boarding school experience . . . have created a legacy: a legacy whose primary contribution to the new generations has been personal emotional problems created by the transmission of cultural shame and self-hate" (Gale 1990, p. 13). Epperley (1991) identifies some of the most common manifestations of these phenomena seen in Native American youth. Common emotional disorders and related problems include (1) developmental disorders, (2) post-traumatic stress disorder, (3) identity disorder, (4) depression, (5) suicide, (6) anxiety, (7) substance abuse, and (8) behavioral disorders. A brief discussion of these disorders follows.

DEVELOPMENTAL DISORDERS. Almost 10% of Native American school-age children have some sort of developmental disability, and they have a higher rate of learning disabilities than that seen in other minority groups. Epperley (1991) suggests that the high prevalence of otitis media and fetal alcohol syndrome may contribute to this problem.

POST-TRAUMATIC STRESS DISORDER. Native American children suffer from "secondary post-traumatic stress disorder" (Epperley 1991): that is, they have reactive behaviors that they have learned from parents, grandparents, and great-grandparents who suffer from post-traumatic stress disorder. Some of the traumas that these elders have suffered include forced acculturation; incarceration on reservations; involuntary confinement at boarding schools; and individual traumas such as beatings, premature deaths of loved ones, and sexual abuse.

IDENTITY DISORDER. Native Americans frequently have difficulty forming a positive self-image because they must blend together the white and Native American world views.

DEPRESSION. Depression is a serious health problem for Native Americans: more than 50% of Native American adolescents report serious depressive symptoms; 40% of the patients seen daily at Indian Health Service clinics have conditions related to depression; and many of Native Americans' behavioral, developmental, and substance abuse problems have depression as the underlying problem (Epperley 1991).

SUICIDE. The statistics underscore the magnitude of the problem of suicide among Native American adolescents. Suicide is the second leading cause of death for Native American adolescents. The number of deaths from suicide is four times higher for Native American children aged 10 to 14 than for children of the same age of any other culture in the United Sates. Of these adolescents who have attempted suicide, 75% receive no mental health treatment (Epperley 1991).

ALCOHOLISM. The majority of Native Americans are not alcoholics and they do not abuse alcohol (Gale 1990). However, alcoholism is still a serious problem for Native Americans. The alcoholism mortality rate is still about four times greater for Native Americans than for the general US population. "Between 1978 and 1985, the Native American mortality rate from alcoholism . . . decreased from 54.5 to 26.1 per 100,000" (Gale 1990). Gale cites a study suggesting that acute and chronic alcoholism among Native Americans frequently masks the symptoms of primary depression. Furthermore, alcoholism exacerbates other mental health–related problems such as suicide, sexual assault, family violence, homicide, and child abuse. Alcoholism affects individuals, families, and communities and has biological, psychological, sociocultural, developmental, and spiritual ramifications. A holistic approach, then, makes the most sense. Native Americans, because of their belief in wholeness and in the interrelatedness of parts, should respond well to a treatment model that employs a holistic approach. Such an approach is outlined in a resource booklet published by the Native American Development Corporation: this type of holistic treatment model is presented in Box 4–3.

Nursing Interventions

The suggestions offered earlier in this chapter for the nurse to use when working with clients from culturally diverse populations are applicable to Native Ameri-

---

Box 4–3. GUIDELINES FORMULATED BY NATIVE AMERICANS FOR INTERVENING WITH ALCOHOL OR OTHER DRUG PROBLEMS

1. First, we need to recognize and utilize the changing attitudes in our communities. We need to continue to spread the belief that tribal people have a choice about alcohol and drugs. We need to promote and demonstrate the idea that abstinence is an acceptable option.

2. We need to ensure that individuals who choose not to use alcohol and drugs are not left isolated and lonely. . . . We need to continue offering and promoting dry drum pow-wows, sobriety campouts, and chemical-free celebrations of life.

3. We must continue to accept responsibility for our own sobriety. We must network our strategies and accomplishments.

4. We need to review our cultural strengths. We need to recognize and utilize our family and community systems. We must review our parenting skills and technique and develop, where we feel it is necessary, parent training programs. We need to call on our holistic orientations.

5. We need, too, to look at our cultural heritage and our behaviors and identify those aspects that may be helping to perpetuate alcoholism and drug abuse.

6. Finally, we must maintain an optimism. We must recognize our successes.

Adapted from Gale N. Pass the Word. Washington, DC: The Native American Development Corporation, 1990.

---

cans as well. By following these suggestions, the nurse will be able to respond to each client as an individual and to provide culturally sensitive nursing care.

Vignette

Mr. Simon, a Navajo Indian, is admitted to a local hospital emergency room with a two-month history of lingering headaches, visual disturbances, and ataxia. He believes that his symptoms have significantly wor-

sened during the past two days. Shortly after his arrival but before he is evaluated by the nursing or medical staff, Mr. Simon drifts off into a deep sleep. His wife denies that he has been drinking. Although no alcohol is detected on his breath, the emergency room physician, after briefly reviewing his chart, asks Mr. Simon's wife if he has been depressed lately. His wife replies that he has not. The physician, assuming Mr. Simon to be intoxicated, tells the nursing staff he will evaluate Mr. Simon after he sleeps it off.

An hour later, on the insistence of Mr. Simon's wife, the nurse practitioner who has been following Mr. Simon's case on the nearby reservation is called. She convinces the physician that Mr. Simon is probably not intoxicated because he despises alcohol. In her opinion, he is presenting with progressively worsened symptoms and needs a neurological consultation. Within one hour, Mr. Simon is in the operating room having a brain tumor removed. He does well postoperatively.

Much is to be learned by the emergency room staff with regard to their handling of the situation:

1. The staff's stereotypical views about Native Americans prevented them from providing quality care. In fact, these views nearly cost Mr. Simon his life.

2. The staff later admitted they had assumed that Mr. Simon was a heavy drinker who had probably been depressed.

3. It is common knowledge that the incidence of alcoholism and culturally induced depression is much higher for Native Americans than for white Americans. However, what the staff did not realize is that drinking alcohol is considered antithetical to the Navajo way of life.

Summary

This chapter has discussed various aspects of nursing a culturally diverse population. One of the hallmarks of nursing is that clients are seen as holistic beings with biological, psychological, sociocultural, developmental, and spiritual dimensions. When nurses respond to clients in stereotypical ways and ignore important data, such as a person's cultural background, they do an immense disservice to the individual and to the profession of nursing. Furthermore, if nurses formulate their responses to a member of a certain cultural group based on generalizations about that group and if they do not address individual differences, they will not be successful in meeting the client's needs.

There is a richness in the multiplicity of customs and beliefs that exist in this country. Whenever possible, nurses should expose themselves to cultures that are different from their own. They should be open to new ideas and to different ways of doing things. They should become aware of their biases and prejudices and try to limit the negative effect they may have on relationships with clients. Nurses should view cultural diversity as an opportunity for them to grow and to enrich their nursing practice.

References

Adebimpe VR. Overview: White norms and psychiatric diagnosis of black patients. American Journal of Psychiatry, 138:279, 1981.

American Psychiatric Association. Diagnostic and Statistical Manual of Mental Disorders, 3rd ed, revised (DSM-III-R). Washington, DC: American Psychiatric Association, 1987.

American Psychiatric Association. DSM-IV Options Book: Work in Progress. Washington, DC: American Psychiatric Association, 1991.

American Nurses' Association. 1988. As quoted in 1988 National Sample Survey. Bethesda, MD: US Department of Health and Human Services, 1988.

American Nurses' Association Statistics Report. 1979. As quoted in 1979 National Sample Survey. Bethesda, MD: US Department of Health and Human Services, 1979.

Andrews M. Changing faces: Nursing in a multicultural society. Paper presented at the Genesee Valley Nurses Association Symposium, Rochester, NY, 1991.

Bell P, Moore B, Peterson D. Developing Chemical Dependency Services for Black People: A Manual. Minneapolis: Institute on Black Chemical Abuse, 1990.

Boyd-Franklin N. Black Families in Therapy: A Multisystems Approach. New York: Guilford Press, 1989.

Bullough VL, Bullough B. Health Care for Other Americans. New York: Appleton-Century-Crofts, 1982, pp 102–107.

Collins D, Dimsdale J, Wilkins D. Consultation/liaison psychiatry utilization patterns in different cultural groups. Psychosomatic Medicine, 54:240, 1992.

DeSantiss L. A profile of cultural diversity in nursing practice. Cultural Connections, Council of American Nurses Association, 8(2), 1988.

Epperley LA. Protecting our youth—Preserving our future. Sovereignty's impact on children in need of treatment. Paper presented at Sovereignty Symposium IV, The Circles of Sovereignty, Oklahoma City, OK, 1991.

Gale N. Pass the Word. Washington, DC: Native American Development Corporation, 1990.

Giger JN, Davidhizar R. Transcultural nursing assessment and method for advancing nursing practice. International Nursing Review, 37(1):199, 1990.

Goldman HH. Review of General Psychiatry. California: Lange Medical Publications, 1984.

Gossett VR. Alcohol and Drug Abuse in Black America: A Guide for Community Action. Minneapolis: Institute on Black Chemical Abuse, 1988.

Grier WH, Cobbs PM. Black Rage. New York: Basic Books, 1968.

Hobus R. Living in two worlds: A Lakota transcultural nursing experience. Journal of Transcultural Nursing, 2:33, 1990.

Hu T, Snowden LR, Jerrell JM, et al. Ethnic populations in public mental health: Services, choice, and level of use. American Journal of Public Health, 81(11):1429, 1991.

Johnson SD. Toward clarifying culture, race, and ethnicity in the context of multicultural counseling. Journal of Multicultural Counseling and Development, 18(1):41, 1990.

Jones AC. Psychological functioning in Black Americans: A conceptual guide for use in psychotherapy. Psychotherapy, 22(25):363, 1985.

Jones E, Gray B. Problems in diagnosing schizophrenia and affective disorders among blacks. Hospital and Community Psychiatry, 1(37):61, 1986.

LaFromboise TD, Nixon DN. American Indian mental health policy. American Psychologist, 43:388, 1988.

Leininger M. A new generation of nurses discovers transcultural nursing. Nursing and Health Care, 8(5):5, 1989.

Leininger M. Cultural concepts in nursing. Journal of Transcultural Nursing, 2(1):52, 1990.

Leininger M. Leininger's Acculturation Health Care Assessment Tool for Cultural Patterns in Traditional or Non-Traditional Lifeways. Journal of Transcultural Nursing, 2(2):40, 1991.

Lyles M, Carter J. Myths and strengths of the black family: A historical and sociological contribution to family therapy. Journal of the National Medical Association, 74(11):1119, 1982.

Malson M. The social support system of black families. Marriage and Family Review, 5(4):37, 1982.

Neal A, Turner S. Anxiety disorders research with African Americans: Current status. Psychological Bulletin, 109(3):400, 1991.

Neeley A, Grant D. Social Policy Prevention Handbook. A Community-Based Alcohol and Drug Prevention Strategy. Minneapolis: Institute on Black Chemical Abuse, 1990.

Osborne O, Carter C, Pinkleton N, et al. Development of African American curriculum content in psychiatric and mental health nursing. In Chunn J, Dunston P, Ross-Sheriff F (eds). Mental Health and People of Color: Curriculum Development and Change. Howard University Press, Washington, DC: 1983, pp 335–375.

Sands RF, Hale SL. Enhancing cultural sensitivity in clinical practice. Journal of National Black Nursing Association, 2(1):54, 1987.

Smith PZ. International student depression during cultural adjustment: Two counseling approaches and strategies. Paper presented at Mid-South Educational Research Association 18th Annual Meeting, Little Rock, AR, 1989.

Snow L. Sorcerers, saints and charlatans: Black folk healers in urban America. Culture, Medicine and Psychiatry, 2:69. In Tripp-Reimer T, Lively S. Cultural Considerations in Therapy, 191, 1978.

Snowden LR, Cheung FK. Use of inpatient mental health services by members of ethnic minority groups. American Psychologist, 3:347, 1990.

Spector RE. Health and illness in the black community. In Cultural Diversity in Health and Illness. Spector RE (ed): New York: Appleton-Century-Crofts, 1985, pp 141–159.

Staples R. Changes in black family structure: The conflict between family ideology and structural conditions. Journal of Marriage and Family, 47:1005, 1985.

Sue DW, Sue D. Counseling the Culturally Different. Theory and Practice, 2nd ed. New York: John Wiley & Sons, 1990.

Sue S, Zane N. The role of culture and cultural techniques in psychotherapy. A critique and reformulation. American Psychologist, 1:37, 1987.

Tsui P, Schultz GL. Failure of rapport: When psychotherapeutic engagement fails in the treatment of Asian clients. American Journal of Orthopsychiatry, 55:561, 1985.

Valuing Diversity: Communicating Across Cultures. Teachers' Training Guide No. 3. San Francisco: Copeland Griggs Productions Inc., 1987, pp 1–13.

Wenger AF. Transcultural nursing and health care issues in urban and rural contexts. Journal of Transcultural Nursing, 4(2):4, 1992.

Westermeyer J. Psychiatric diagnosis across cultural boundaries. American Journal of Psychiatry, 142(7):798, 1985.

Where the minorities are the majority. Democrat and Chronicle, Rochester, NY. September 17, 1991.

Wilson LL, Stith SM. Culturally sensitive therapy with black clients. Journal of Multicultural Counseling and Development, 19:32, 1991.

Wyatt GE. The sociological context of African American and white American womens' rape. Journal of Social Issues, 48(1):77, 1991.

Self-study Exercises

1. Define the following terms:

    A. Race

    _____

    B. Ethnicity

    _____

    C. Culture_____

    D. Folk healer_____

2. What, if anything, can you do to assist others in better understanding the health needs of a diverse clientele?

3. List two ways in which you can improve communication across cultures.

4. Describe your multicultural experiences with someone not of European descent. Can you identify cultural values that may be health care barriers?

5. Briefly describe what you would include in a nursing care plan that takes into consideration clients' values, health needs, cultural practices, and language.

6. Identify three nursing approaches that could improve access to services for culturally diverse clients.

7. How would you develop a resource pool of culturally sensitive individuals with whom health care professionals could consult in addressing client needs?

8. In your workplace, has management articulated a need for diversifying the work force? For example, are there people of color in positions at all levels? If so, do they participate in policy-making decisions? Once hired, do they leave your institution at a faster rate than other employees?

9. Do you feel comfortable openly discussing issues of race, ethnicity, and diversity in your health care institution? If not, can you identify strategies that would enable you to accomplish this?

CHAPTER 5

Evolution of Nursing in Psychiatric Settings

Hildegard E. Peplau with second
edition revisions by Suzanne Lego

OUTLINE •

KEY TERMS, CONCEPTS, AND PEOPLE • • • • • • • • • •

The key terms, concepts, and people listed here also appear in bold where
they are defined or discussed in this chapter.

HARRIET BAILEY

DOROTHEA DIX

FLORENCE NIGHTINGALE

*NURSING: A SOCIAL POLICY
    STATEMENT*

HILDEGARD E. PEPLAU

PHENOMENA RELEVANT TO
    PSYCHIATRIC NURSING

LINDA RICHARDS

OBJECTIVES ■

After studying this chapter, the student will be able to

1. Recognize major components in the work of other health care providers working
   in various psychiatric settings.
2. Know available contemporary guidelines for use in providing psychiatric nursing
   care.
3. Briefly discuss two trends in psychiatric nursing.

4. Place contemporary nursing within a perspective of the historical development of psychiatric nursing.
5. Recognize the role psychiatric nursing has played in the development of nursing as a whole.
6. Appreciate the gradual evolution of the work role of nurses in psychiatric settings in the light of changing societal circumstances.

Overview of Nursing in Today's Psychiatric Settings

NATURE OF THE WORK ROLE OF NURSES WITH PSYCHIATRIC PATIENTS

Nurses consider themselves enhancers of healing and health, primarily through the use of noninvasive, humanistically oriented nursing practices. In caring for the mentally ill, nurses need to understand, theoretically, those internal processes that have become dysfunctional. Nursing practices address these manifestations, when observed in their many patterns and variations, to try to set these processes in a functional direction. These efforts by nurses help patients develop their capacity for intellectual and interpersonal competencies, such as focusing attention, describing experiences, and naming feelings. These nursing interventions are provided in all nurse-patient interactions: in informal contacts in the hospital and in structured relationships in which various therapeutic and psychotherapeutic modalities are used.

Psychiatric patients additionally receive services from other health care providers—physicians, psychologists, social workers, occupational and recreational therapists, and others. It is generally nurses who plan a patient's daily schedule in accordance with the total treatment plan and the patient's interests. Thus, nurses schedule and often coordinate the services of other health care providers so that patients make the best use of them. Nurses accept responsibility for carrying out the prescriptions of physicians for medications and treatments; they are also accountable for verifying the need for and accuracy of such prescriptions. Nurses are active members of interdisciplinary groups that plan, record, review, and evaluate patient care and provide peer-review evaluations of each other's work.

Psychiatric inpatients are residents in a facility. Their around-the-clock activities of daily living are the responsibility of nurses. All of the amenities and necessities of social living within an institution that has

highly specialized educative and therapeutic aims are also the concern of nurses. Nurses consult family members about supplies patients need and about plans for their release from the hospital. Nurses are responsible for ensuring that the patients' living environment is clean and safe; on these matters they consult with patients and the housekeeping, maintenance, security, and fire departments when necessary. Patients' overall health is related to nutrition; thus, nurses observe patients' dietary habits—at meals and in between—and take steps to educate patients about good nutrition. Many psychiatric patients tend to be isolated; nurses help and support them in establishing friendships with other patients.

Specially prepared psychiatric nurses (usually MSNs) take a nursing history and make periodic assessments of patient patterns of difficulty and progress toward their resolution. In addition, psychiatric nurses

- Provide situational counseling (e.g., arbitrating disputes among patients)
- Conduct short-term scheduled counseling sessions
- Provide individual, group, or family psychotherapy in a series of scheduled sessions
- Engage in biofeedback training and behavior modification
- Participate in "token economics"
- Use hypnosis, psychodrama, and other modalities

Health teaching is another role of nurses. Health teaching encompasses both experiential teaching (using an experience described or acted out by a patient) and didactic teaching (e.g., classes on sex education, anxiety, and stress management).

The interactions of patients with each other and with the staff members are of special interest to nurses. It is in this milieu that patients frequently seek partners with whom they can establish relationships that are illness maintaining and, therefore, comfortable and anxiety relieving (Benfer and Schroeder 1985). Studying such pattern interactions and intervening in them are complex features of the work of psychiatric nurses. Managing structured aspects of the milieu, such as location of patients, rules of living, and ward governmental meetings, is part of the work of nurses.

All staff are involved in careful recording of observations, for these records are of particular importance in studying a patient's progress. They also have legal implications.

All of the foregoing components of the work of nurses in psychiatric settings can be sorted into roles or modalities for viewing nurses' work in an organized way (Table 5–1). The division of work among nursing personnel, according to education, can similarly be shown.

RELATION BETWEEN WORK ROLE AND EDUCATION

Education determines the kind and scope of work that a particular nurse is capable of performing competently. This is not to say that work experience lacks value; however, educational credentials assure the

Table 5-1 ■ WORK OF NURSES IN PSYCHIATRIC SETTINGS	
ROLES OR MODALITIES*	**EXAMPLES**
"Mother surrogate"	Bathing, dressing, feeding, toileting, warning, disciplining, sleep routines
Technical	Assisting with medications and medical treatment; giving enemas, catheterizing, performing other nursing procedures (e.g., temperature, pulse, and respiration; blood pressure)
Socialization agent	Activities of daily living, ward games, grooming advice, promoting friendships
Health teaching Experiential Didactic (classes)	Eating habits, individual problems Stress management, anxiety, sex education, sessions for families of patients
Taking a nursing history	On admission
Preparing, revising nursing care plan, evaluation	
Assignment of nursing personnel to patients; evaluation	
Discharge planning and follow-up	
Coordination	Rounds, preparing patient schedules, scheduling patient appointments, health team meetings
Milieu	Study and record milieu interactions among patients, at ward government meetings, and during visitor-patient interactions
Relaxation therapy	
Recording	
Behavior modification	Token economics, individual schedules
Counseling	Situational Patient-patient disputes Incidents of violence Short term therapy Scheduled interview sessions (up to 6)
Individual psychotherapy	Scheduled sessions (more than 6)
Group psychotherapy	Scheduled sessions
Family psychotherapy	Scheduled sessions of a patient with family members
Biofeedback	
Hypnosis	
Psychodrama	
Liaison/consultation	
Other	

* Psychiatric nursing faculty should advise students of those nursing performances for which their nursing education has fully prepared them.

public that a nurse has successfully completed systematic, supervised study at a particular level that distinguishes a range of nursing competence. Nurses whose work experience exceeds their level of education should seek higher-level academic credentials.

THEORY. *The central feature of nursing education programs is theory—concepts and processes that explain the phenomena nurses observe in varied manifestations during clinical practice.* The theory that a nurse is able to recall and use during a particular nurse-patient interaction defines whether the nurse's response to the patient will set up a corrective pull in a direction favorable for the patient. *Concepts that explain anxiety, conflict, hallucinations, delusions, dissociation, self-system disturbances, language-thought disorders, and problems relating to attention or perception are of particular relevance for psychiatric nurses.* It is not enough for a nurse to know about these phenomena; the nurse must also grasp the mechanism or process of the phenomena—what they are, how they work, purposes and functions they have served and still provide for the patient, and their many variations in the patterning of presentation in behavior. Such in-depth knowledge is acquired through course work, reading and study, and most particularly, clinical experience. For students in psychiatric nursing, that clinical experience consists primarily of nurse-patient relationship studies, regularly scheduled interviews with psychiatric patients over a substantial period of time, followed by supervisory review of the details of interaction data with a qualified psychiatric nurse faculty member. In such lengthy review sessions, theory application by the student, for the purposes of explaining phenomena and determining constructive responses to the patient, is examined, developed, and verified. Obviously, the length and depth of the studies and the numbers of different patients studied in this manner will differ substantially among associate, baccalaureate, master's, and doctoral students who are studying nursing practice in psychiatric settings. At each successive level of education in nursing, the scope and complexity of psychiatric phenomena increase (or should increase), as does the number of explanatory concepts that the nurse masters. The nurse's competence in using these concepts is tested, as is the nurse's ability to constructively use increasingly complicated modalities and techniques of psychiatric nursing practice. These significant differences in education determine the level of competence in psychiatric nursing of a particular nurse.

PRACTICAL TECHNIQUES. Nursing education also includes practical techniques, which have already been more or less fully accepted for their usefulness. Practical techniques, such as bathing, feeding, planning games and other diversional or recreational activities, and helping patients establish friendships with other patients, require limited theory, if any. They rest on age-old social practices, common sense, and long traditions in nursing. Technical procedures, such as giving medications, assisting in medical treatments, or carrying out nursing procedures, are theory based but have been tested empirically over many years. Principles that guide their use include efficiency, accuracy, economy of resources, and safety for patients. The practical techniques and procedures used in psychiatric nursing are few and are the same as those used in general nursing. These practices may have to be adapted according to the psychiatric condition of a patient, such as when a patient experiences feelings of suspicion and ideas of persecution.

Violence is an increasing problem in psychiatric settings. Patients are admitted to public mental hospitals when they are dangerous to themselves and others. Methods of anticipating violent outbursts—recognizing cues and early intervention—require that nurses working psychiatric settings also know ways to protect themselves from injury and how to restrain patients when necessary.

PROMOTING SELF-CARE. The emphasis in psychiatric nursing is on promoting self-care rather than doing things for patients that they are able to do or can learn to do. Except in rare situations, all patients are ambulatory and physically able to meet basic self-care needs. Failure to do so suggests psychological problems, such as low self-esteem, rebellion against authority, felt and learned helplessness, and long-standing dependency claims. These aspects of self-care difficulties require a theoretical understanding of a particular patient's dilemmas so that nursing approaches to the problems can be designed. There are no research-tested nursing interventions that, for example, can be used with a patient who refuses to bathe or does not bathe regularly that will simultaneously help to resolve both the physical and psychological problems. One theory holds that if the behavior is changed first, progress is made on underlying problems. Psychiatric patients who do not attend to their basic needs require psychiatric nursing that helps meet those needs while minimizing dependency claims. The patient's objections to bathing can be talked about during the bathing scene and in other formal and informal nurse-patient contacts.

TALKING WITH PATIENTS. The following general principle is useful when applied in clinical work: *Anything that goes on may be talked about; events that are discussed are more likely to be understood; understanding is a basis for changing one's behavior.* Conversely, any behavior that is not talked about but merely acted out is most likely subject to highly private, autistic interpretation by the patient and may well contribute to the psychopathology and its maintenance.

Another general principle follows: *Language influences thought; thought influences actions; feelings are emotional re-*

Table 5–2 ■ INTELLECTUAL AND INTERPERSONAL SKILLS REQUIRED FOR PSYCHIATRIC NURSING

SKILL	DESCRIPTION
Observation	Acting as detached spectator or participant; being empathetic; sensing hunches
Interviewing	Performing situational counseling and short term therapeutic counseling: • Listening, hearing details and communicated messages • Giving disciplined attention to sustain a focus or to pursue a trend • Assessing patient data for patient's ability to focus, describe, and pursue relevant details • Selecting relevant verbal inputs to promote description and continuity of thought in patient • Controlling nurse verbalizations—quantity, quality, confidentiality, purpose of therapy, and timing of inputs
Self-reflection	Auditing and editing one's own behavior during nurse-patient relationships
Recording	Reporting is narrative and systematic; audio- and videotaping of nurse-patient data; recording for purposes of review, analysis, and study
Data analysis	Decoding; abstracting themes, trends, and patterns; seeing relationships and connections; processing patient data as nurse hears them
Formulation	Summarizing succinctly and accurately; generalizing—inferences, working hypotheses, and nursing diagnoses; revising
Theory application	Formulating frameworks; explaining observed phenomena; choosing interventions
Planning	Establishing short and long term goals; ensuring discharge continuity and follow-up
Validation	Verifying inferences with another nurse; consensually validating inferences of patients
Foreseeing	Predicting upcoming problems of patients and possibilities and opportunities for change; foreseeing short and long term possible effects of current nursing actions
Evaluation	Assessing short and long term effects of nursing actions on problems of patients
Arbitrating	Resolving disputes of patients so neither patient loses
Anticipatory intervention	Preparing for prepanic, previolent, or presuicidal behavior

From Peplau HE. List of intellectual and interpersonal basic skills. Nursing Times 83:1, 1987. Reproduced by kind permission of Nursing Times, where this table first appeared in an article on January 7, 1987.

sponses that arise in relation to thoughts and actions taken within events in which a person is a participant.

On the basis of the two foregoing principles, it can be argued that talking with patients is the most important component of the work of psychiatric nurses. Such talk, however, is not of the same quality as that in social conversations that a nurse might have outside of the clinical setting. Different purposes are served. In the clinical setting, the focus is one-way—on the life of the patient. The aims include helping patients to recall, describe, and clarify past experience and to put it in a new and more constructive perspective. The nurse listens, asks questions, seeks details, and so forth. Nurses who use the patient's time to talk about themselves or their own experiences put the patient in the position of audience, watcher, and listener. Discussions with patients are guided not by social aims such as the nurse's being liked, gaining a friend, or being complimented but by a theoretical understanding of how patients' talking develops their intellectual and interpersonal competencies and increases their self-understanding. Table 5–2 summarizes basic intellectual and interpersonal skills required for the practice of psychiatric nursing.

THEORIES RELEVANT TO PSYCHIATRIC NURSING

Psychiatric nurses generate theories for psychiatric nursing through scholarship and research. Smoyak and Rouslin (1982) described these efforts:

> From 1952 onward, psychiatric nursing textbooks took a decided turn toward educated scrutiny of clinical work. With the publication of Peplau's book, *Interpersonal Relations in Nursing*, no subsequent psychiatric nursing text could ignore the influence of some notion of 'nurse-patient relationship,' the 'therapeutic interview' or the 'participant observer' role of the psychiatric nurse. The nurse was now to be seen as an active, knowledgeable, knowledge-seeking therapeutic agent in work with patients. In one way or another, the impact of Peplau's introduction of an interpersonal concept of psychiatric nursing was reflected in books in the 1950's and 1960's such as the following: Kalkman's *Introduction to Psychiatric Nursing*, Mereness and Karnosh's *Psychiatry for Nurses*, Burton's *Personal, Impersonal and Interpersonal Relations*, Schwartz and Schokley's *The Nurse and the Mental Patient*, Muller's *The Nature and Direction of Psychiatric Nursing*, Hofling and Leininger's *Basic Psychiatric Concepts in Nursing*, Orlando's *The Dynamic Nurse-Patient Relationship*, Armstrong and Rouslin's *Group Psychotherapy in Nursing Practice*. Burd and Marshall's *Some Clinical Approaches in Psychiatric Nursing*, Hays and Larsen's *Interacting with Patients*, Bermosk and Mordan's *Interviewing in Nursing*, Manaser and Werner's *Instruments for the Study of the Nurse-Patient Relationship*, and Ujhely's *Determinants of the Nurse-Patient Relationship*.*

At a conference titled The State of the Art of Psychiatric Nursing, which was sponsored by the National Institute of Mental Health (NIMH) and Rutgers University, a critical assessment of psychiatric nursing developments from 1946 to 1974 was made and published (Huey 1975). Since then, there has been a proliferation of journal articles and textbooks on psychiatric nursing. However, much research still needs to be conducted, particularly in defining the phenomena that fall within the scope of psychiatric nursing. These phenomena are currently being identified by an American Nurses' Association (ANA) task force. Meanwhile, there are psychiatric nursing and psychosocial nursing diagnoses in current publications of taxonomies of nursing (Gebbie and Lavin 1972). The **phenomena** for which psychiatric nurses can provide therapeutic benefit also include processes such as attention, perception, memory, language-thought, the self-system and hallucinations, delusions, ideas of reference, sus-

piciousness, incorporated identities, loneliness, depression, and others. *For these phenomena, nurses need theories—concepts and processes—*that define the mechanisms of these disorders: what they are, how they arise and function, their distortions and how they occur, the purposes served in maintaining the dysfunctional patterns, and so forth.

Nurses generate psychiatric nursing theories in two ways. The first is scholarly study, reformulation, and empirical testing in clinical work of any theory published by any established science—physical, social, or applied sciences. Nurses have access to all published scientific literature. Concepts drawn from these sources become nursing theory when they are applied to nursing phenomena. The second way nursing theory is developed is from the results of nursing research. Nurses have a profound practical responsibility, as their interactions with patients may be around the clock. These interactions should be directed by theoretical understanding of psychopathology so that the nursing actions will help correct the patient's difficulties rather than participate in illness maintenance.

Nurses work with other health care providers within psychiatric services. Although psychiatric nurses use nursing theories in their work, they need to know and appreciate the theoretical orientations of their psychiatric colleagues. It is fair for any nurse working in a psychiatric facility to say, "I am interested and would appreciate it if you would share with me a brief overview of the theoretical orientation you use in your work with patients." By the same token, nurses ought to be able to state their own theoretical orientation simply and clearly.

Many theoretical frameworks are currently in use in psychiatric settings. Some professionals may use one exclusively, having an orientation to the work of Freud, Jung, Adler, Horney, Sullivan, Kohut, or one of many other psychiatric theorists. Some, if not most, psychiatrists or other professionals are eclectic in orientation. The following paragraphs provide brief descriptions of prevailing theoretical frameworks.

DESCRIPTIVE THEORIES. Descriptive theories of psychiatry primarily provide names for diagnostic categories of mental diseases and identify or describe the accompanying symptoms. Historically, most psychiatric nursing textbooks have followed this framework.

INTRAPERSONAL THEORIES. Intrapersonal theories present concepts to explain phenomena that purportedly occur within an individual. "Spectator observation" is used to notice the behavior of the individual being studied, without reference to others or to context. Many of Freud's intrapsychic concepts —id, ego, libido, repression—are intrapersonal constructs.

---

*Reprinted by permission of Slack Incorporated, Thorofare, NJ.

INTERPERSONAL THEORIES. Interpersonal theories include concepts that define "what goes on between two or more people, all but one of whom may be completely illusory" (Sullivan 1947). Thus, hallucinations would be described as an interaction between a patient and an autistically invented illusory figure, the interaction being a pattern-integration serving a purpose for the patient. The nurse-patient interaction would also be studied, by "participant observation," to notice relations, for instance, between nurse inputs and patient responses, and vice versa. Object relations theory and self-psychology are theoretical frameworks emphasizing the impact of early caregiver-infant and -child interactions on later behavior. The nurse observes the impact of the patients' relationships with the family, other patients, and the nurses themselves.

SYSTEMS THEORIES. Systems theories explain interactions among parts of a whole—a family, members of an inpatient milieu, or an organization. Pattern interactions, strategies used to maintain them, formal and informal rules of organization, and the privileges of the system and how they are gained would be among the phenomena studied.

SOCIAL SCIENCE THEORIES. Social science theories—psychology, social psychology, sociology, anthropology, and others—are derived from studies of some aspect of individual or collective human behavior, each discipline generally having areas and methods that are of special interest.

OTHER MEMBERS OF THE MENTAL HEALTH TEAM

There are about 250 different health care occupations. Not all of them are represented in psychiatric institutions, but they are available in general hospitals having inpatient psychiatric units. The following are very brief descriptions of the *major* unique functions of coworkers and colleagues who work alongside nurses in psychiatric settings.

PSYCHIATRISTS. Psychiatrists provide psychiatric diagnoses of patients for the official records and prescribe medications and medical treatments such as electroshock—which they administer. Some also provide psychotherapy.

PSYCHOLOGISTS. Psychologists administer psychological and other tests and therefore contribute to psychiatric diagnoses; some direct behavior modification and biofeedback programs; most engage in psychotherapy.

SOCIAL WORKERS. Social workers usually take an intake history and confer with families about admission, economic status, welfare problems, and discharge. Some also provide psychotherapy.

OCCUPATIONAL THERAPISTS. Occupational therapists generally provide various activities, based on the needs of the patients, for diversion, to increase attention span, to release emotions, to develop hand-eye coordination, and so forth. Some may also provide vocational or work training or activities to help patients develop a hobby.

RECREATIONAL THERAPISTS. Recreational therapists provide socializing group activities, physical exercise programs, diversion, and so forth.

DANCE THERAPISTS. Dance therapists use bodily movement as a medium of expression of self and feelings and to release inhibitions in patients.

ART THERAPISTS. Art therapists employ art materials both to encourage externalization of difficulties symbolically, through art forms, and to release and use creative capacities of the patients.

CLERGY. The clergy provide religious solace, instruction, continuation of patients' religious interests, counseling about religious conflicts, last rites, and so forth. Some also provide psychotherapy.

SETTINGS IN WHICH NURSES PRACTICE WITH PSYCHIATRIC PATIENTS

The number and kinds of settings in which health care of psychiatric patients is provided have been increasing since the 1970s. Only the major settings are briefly described here.

PUBLIC MENTAL HOSPITALS. The patient population of public mental hospitals established by state governments has changed. Deinstitutionalization, which began in the 1970s, has reduced the patient population considerably by returning patients to their families, by transferring them to nursing homes, and by shifting some to the status of homeless street people. Although there are still some older "chronic" patients, now there seem to be an increasing number of young persons admitted to mental hospitals, many of whom act out violence. In the past several decades, these institutions have been employing an increasing number of master's-prepared clinical specialists in psychiatric nursing. Associate degree nurses, therefore, have opportunities in these hospitals to work under the supervision of well-prepared clinical nurses.

PSYCHIATRIC UNITS IN GENERAL HOSPITALS. Psychiatric units may be specialized for children, adolescents, adults, alcohol or drug abusers, and other problems or problem populations. The advantage for the patient is access to all of the assessment technology usually associated with a modern hospital. Some units are psychotherapeutically oriented; some are more biomedical in their treatment approaches. Units associated with university teaching hospitals tend to be well staffed and generally engaged in research.

COMMUNITY MENTAL HEALTH CENTERS. Community mental health centers began to develop rapidly in 1963 as a "bold, new approach in attacking the societal problem of mental illness." Some centers have inpatient units as well as many outpatient services. Psychiatric nurses, especially clinical specialists, are employed for inpatient care and to provide psychotherapy. This is the setting in which most psychiatric nurses work.

OTHER FACILITIES. Psychiatric nurses are employed in many other psychiatric facilities: specialized centers for the treatment of alcohol and drug abuse, shelters for abused women or children, psychiatric clinics (most often attached to general hospitals), crisis intervention hotlines and walk-in clinics, day and night care centers, sheltered workshops for discharged patients or persons who are mentally retarded, Veterans Administration hospitals, the military, prisons, and many others.

PRIVATE PRACTICE. Since the mid-1960s, psychiatric nurses have engaged in private practice, particularly clinical specialists who hold a graduate degree and are eligible for or hold ANA certification in their specialty. Some psychiatric nurses practice independently, alone or in group practice with other nurses; others are in joint practice with other mental health professionals. Their practices include individual, group, or family psychotherapy, and other specialized services.

UNDERSTANDING THE HISTORY OF PSYCHIATRIC NURSING

History serves many important purposes. New opportunities and challenges arise with each era. Events occurring in those times create new contexts in which choices are made, either actively or by default. The narrative of history is rooted in such events. History consists not only of facts, dates, and circumstances but also of trends, themes, and patterns that characterize those situations. One purpose of history is to pinpoint trends in the forward movement of people —of nurses—in society.

The history of psychiatric nursing is about the struggles, choices, and progress that nurses have made over the many years of its development. It is the story of the continuities—the beginnings, and the forward steps that were taken by psychiatric nurses in the United States to get to their present position in nursing and society. The whole history of psychiatric nursing has not yet been told. It is a long story —much longer than what is presented in this chapter,

which primarily contains highlights in the development of psychiatric nursing in the United States.

There are always lessons to be learned from history. One such lesson comes from very courageous nurses, working in psychiatric hospitals, who were willing to take a stand on unpopular issues of their day. At the turn of the twentieth century and earlier, psychiatric nursing was an unpopular field of work. It shared the general stigma attached to mental illness and to the institutions that cared for psychiatric patients.

Another lesson is that after World War II, when a change in attitude toward the mentally ill occurred, the nursing profession was able to rise to this challenge. It was able to pursue opportunities promised in the provisions of the National Mental Health Act of 1946. Nursing's readiness occurred not so much by design but rather as a consequence of the persistence of a few psychiatric nursing leaders. In earlier years, at the beginning of organized nursing, they had spoken out, persuaded, and therefore helped to shape the general direction taken by the nursing profession. Their perspective, eventually adopted by the profession, was to include psychiatric nursing as an important component of the whole of nursing.

It is not the lessons per se that have contemporary relevance but rather the fact that struggle, persistence, and choice shaped nursing's future. All nurses, wittingly and unwittingly, are in the same way agents of change and are therefore participants in shaping nursing for today and for the future. Fresh opportunities arise, political winds inside and outside the profession shift and blow in new directions, social forces impinge in new ways, all allowing or forcing choices that nurses make, individually and collectively. Such choices shape and reshape nursing.

Nursing leaders and all other nurses are in one way or another participants in the drama of making nursing's history. It is out of this ongoing history-making process that the present role of psychiatric nursing has emerged. Nurses who know the history of psychiatric nursing gain a sense of the cohesion and continuity that exists between the work of their nursing forebears and their own present-day work. The future of psychiatric nursing can be more clearly determined when its past is appreciated; that future lies in the hands of the present generation of nurses—especially those who care deeply about the needs of the mentally ill.

FUTURE TRENDS IN PSYCHIATRIC NURSING

THE DECADE OF THE BRAIN. The years falling between 1990 and 2000 have been called the decade of the brain. Researchers are increasingly interested in brain anatomy and physiology and its relationship to behavior and to mental illness. The simplest theory is that these factors are the cause of behavior or of mental illness. A more sophisticated view is that a relationship between these factors may or may not exist and that it is difficult to determine what triggers changes in the brain. By the same token, although neuroactive drugs may help a patient, we do not know the role the *mind* plays in bringing about behavioral change in patients. We know that the likelihood of a drug's effectiveness may depend on the feelings or emotions of the patient (Lego 1992).

The trend in psychiatry toward biological, physiological, biochemical, and genetic explanations of psychiatric phenomena is sometimes referred to as the biomedicalization of psychiatry. In the history of medicine, this thrust is not entirely new; such efforts have been made by physicians since the seventeenth and eighteenth centuries, if not earlier (Scull 1981). Quite probably, in the next several decades there will be new medical treatments for psychiatric patients well beyond the present pharmaceutical management, including new forms of brain surgery (Valenstein 1986). No doubt some nurses will go along with this trend, providing the nursing required with more technological medical practices. It is hoped that other psychiatric nurses will continue the development of their already well-established psychotherapeutic nursing practices. In fact, the movement of psychiatrists in a biochemical direction creates a vacuum that can be filled by psychiatric nurses interested in the psychosocial needs of patients.

FUTURE SETTINGS. In the future, more and more psychiatric nurses will practice outside hospitals. Because inpatient hospitalization is so expensive, hospital stays are short or are avoided, if possible. As the population of elderly, chronically ill patients increases, the need for community-based resources will expand. The number of people with mental illness is not shrinking, however; consequently, patients will increasingly be treated in outpatient clinics, in day hospitals, and at home, through home visits or telephone therapy (Melton and Smoyak 1992).

THE AGING POPULATION. In 50 years, one in five Americans will be over 65. The problems of loss, increased dependency, and loneliness will continue to produce depression, paranoia, and other neurotic conditions in the aging population. Psychiatric nurses will spend a large percentage of their time with geropsychiatric patients.

ACQUIRED IMMUNODEFICIENCY SYNDROME. The human immunodeficiency virus (HIV) has produced an epidemic in the United States unparalleled in modern times. The psychological consequences are enormous for persons who fear they are HIV positive

(sometimes called the "worried well"), those who are indeed HIV positive, those who have acquired immunodeficiency syndrome (AIDS) or AIDS-related complex, the families and friends of those infected, and caregivers. Psychiatric nurses will spend a great deal of time helping persons in all of these categories.

DRUG AND ALCOHOL ABUSE. Drug abuse in the United States has also reached epidemic proportions. Health care costs attributed to illicit drug abuse total more than $60 billion annually. Ten to 12% of the total work force uses alcohol or drugs daily. Five million Americans are addicted to cocaine. Nurses in urban outreach centers report that nearly every patient they see uses drugs or alcohol. Psychiatric nurses in the future will need to spend much time with these patients. In fact, nursing of clients with substance abuse has become a subspecialty in the field.

THE HOMELESS AND THE CHRONICALLY MENTALLY ILL. Not since the Great Depression have there been so many homeless people living on the streets and eating in soup kitchens. There are an estimated 2 million homeless persons in the United States. Of these, two fifths are mentally ill. Psychiatric nurses are steadily becoming more involved in outreach centers, shelters, and soup kitchens, where clients are assessed and encouraged to accept treatment.

REIMBURSEMENT. Legislation has been introduced in the US Senate to reimburse nurses as Medicaid and Medicare providers. If these bills are passed into law, the health care of the poor and aged in the United States could be revolutionized. Psychiatric nurses would undoubtedly spend time in nursing clinics organized to treat these largely underserved populations. Even if this bill is not passed, it is highly likely that some form of national health insurance will be adopted in the next decade. If so, nurses are likely to be considered reimbursable providers.

Brief History of Psychiatric Nursing

EARLY DEVELOPMENT: PRE–WORLD WAR II

Exploring the Integration of Psychiatric Nursing Training into Basic Nursing Programs

In 1909, the ASSTS appointed the Sectional Committee of the Committee on Education. Members included Sara Parsons, Amy Hilliard, Linda Richards, and Elizabeth May—all nurse leaders who championed the cause of the mentally ill and promoted the development of psychiatric nursing. The committee recommended "affiliations" of general hospital students in psychiatric hospitals for three to nine months in their third year of training. There was not universal agreement on this recommendation; in fact, it took several decades before theory and clinical practice in psychiatric nursing were included in generic nursing education for all basic nursing students. The committee also proposed use of a list of books on "nursing the insane," all of which were written by non-nurses, for there were as yet no psychiatric nursing textbooks written by nurse authors.

The crucial question of whether to include affiliations in psychiatric nursing in all basic curricula was discussed at length many times during the first half of the twentieth century. The question was crucial because inclusion of this component of nursing meant that nursing would then become one whole comprehensive field of nursing practice. General hospitals that conducted training schools did not, as a rule, accept psychiatric patients. Sending students away for several months of training in a psychiatric hospital suggested at least some erosion of the basic school's authority over them and possibly of the student's loyalty to the basic school. Parents were apprehensive, too, for they tended to share the prevailing social fear of mental patients. Training schools were generally viewed as safe, protective places that kept close watch on the "young girls" who entered them. Nevertheless, during the period between 1909 and 1943, when many schools opened, there were an increasing number of efforts toward favorable resolution of the question (Oderkirk 1985). Neuropsychiatric casualties (69,394) among those who served in World War I (1914–1918) helped to force the issue toward resolution.

Each of the three curriculum guides (1917, 1927, 1937) published by the National League for Nursing Education (NLNE), now the National League for Nursing (NLN), suggested, in succession, a greater emphasis on psychiatric nursing. In 1920, the first textbook on psychiatric nursing, *Nursing Mental Diseases*, written by **Harriet Bailey,** a nurse, was published. Postgraduate courses offered by mental hospitals began to be provided—14 in 13 states by 1929—suggesting that registered nurses had a need left unfilled by their basic nursing programs. The grading committee reported that 88% of nursing students had less than two months' experience in psychiatric nursing services—73% had not yet spent one day with a psychiatric patient (Committee on the Grading of Nursing Schools 1934). Meanwhile, by 1930, more than half of the beds of all hospitals were for mentally ill patients. Moreover, these were the years of the Great Depression (1929–1935), when unemployment

of nurses was excessive. Nurses were needed in public mental hospitals; however, in that era, training schools prepared for "private duty nursing." In big-city general hospitals, staff nursing was provided by student nurses, not by registered nurses. Mrs. Robb called it "free labor" (Robb 1897).

Evolution of the Nurse's Role

The history of nursing is full of attempts to define the work role of nurses. In the earlier eras, the emphasis was mostly on the character of the student nurse. Patience, tact, and honesty were prime virtues. The morality of nurses was a major concern. Obedience and loyalty to the hospital were expected. Richards has described how students worked from 5:30 A.M. to 9 P.M., when they left to sleep in rooms adjacent to the wards in which they worked. The students had no evenings out, no study time, and no recreation; they were overworked, were poorly fed, and had no supervision. Twice each year they went to church (Richards 1949). The "born nurse" was a person of impeccable moral character. The injunction toward moral character was buttressed by long lists of "duties of the nurse," do's and don'ts, things nurses should, or must, do or not do. Some "shoulds" were even called "principles." Staff nurses were called "general duty nurses."

In the 1930s, the profession conducted a major study of the activities of nurses (Johns and Pfefferkorn 1934) that led to the publication of long lists of activities of nurses in various positions, such as general duty nurse, head nurse, supervisor, and instructor. These activities then began to appear in job descriptions and in activity-oriented definitions of nursing (Henderson 1961).

A decade or so later, the ANA embarked on a massive study of functions that similarly provided long lists of functions connected with various nursing positions in employment situations. A publication resulted from this effort (Hughes 1958).

In the 1950s and 1960s, the sociological concept of *role* entered the picture. Discussion and publications began to describe the work role and subroles of nurses. As can be seen from the foregoing accounts, the movement in describing the work of nurses has been from concrete duties toward more abstract ideas, such as role.

In 1972, exactly one century after the training schools for nurses began in 1872, New York State adopted a revised Nursing Practice Act that is having far-reaching impact on nursing. In 1980, the ANA publication **Nursing: A Social Policy Statement** proposed a definition of nursing in terms of a trend—already evident in licensing laws in many states—that originated with the New York act. In the ANA publication, nursing is defined as "the diagnosis and treatment of human responses to actual and potential health problems" (ANA 1980). This definition represents a paradigm shift—a reformulation of the question "what do nurses do?" to "what *phenomena* do nurses fix, correct, ameliorate, relieve, or prevent by addressing nursing practices to them?" (Fig. 5–1).

The work role of nurses in mental hospitals has evolved somewhat along the lines similar to those just described. Attendants in psychiatric institutions before and during the nineteenth century were called "cell keepers" and later "custodial attendants." Tucker, a nurse, decried the use of chains, iron chairs, handcuffs, straps, crib beds, and other primitive devices to restrain patients. Nurses were taught to use isolation, rest, diet, persuasion, and suggestion, with appeals to the intellect and willpower of the patient. One nurse said: "We have to study, if we study blindly." That was the problem—limited knowledge, if any, about the

phenomena observed by nurses, which, through nursing practices, they were expected to help correct in a way favorable for patients. In the absence of definitive nursing knowledge, nurses carried out medical prescriptions, assisted in medical treatments, provided recreational and diversional activities, often served as companions to patients, and promoted "habit training"—all within a framework of optimism, leniency, and patience.

LATER DEVELOPMENT: POST–WORLD WAR II

Wars produce profound social changes. World War II had a far-reaching impact on nursing, particularly on psychiatric nursing. During the war there were enormous shortages of physicians, stateside and in both theaters of war. Consequently, registered nurses had out of necessity to take on far greater authority and

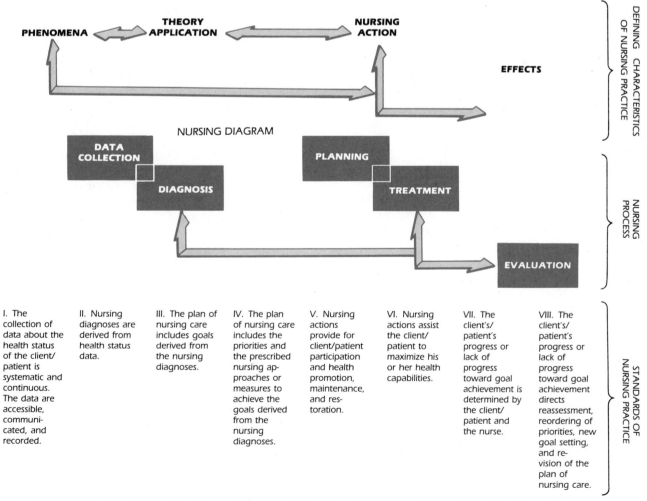

Figure 5–1. *Defining characteristics of nursing practice: relationship to the nursing process and the standards of nursing practice. (Reprinted with permission. Nursing: A Social Policy Statement.* ©1980, American Nurses' Association, Washington, DC.)

responsibility than ever before. Never again would nurses be satisfied with their previous "handmaiden" status. The thrust toward professionalization of the occupation of nursing moved steadily and more swiftly after World War II. Psychiatric nursing developed rapidly and provided considerable leadership in the profession as a whole during the four decades between the end of World War II and the publication of this book.

There were many psychiatric casualties during World War I. Public opinion, not universally sympathetic, attributed these "breakdowns" to problems ranging from weak willpower to cowardice. During and after World War II, public opinion turned on a new idea, namely "that everyone has his breaking point." During the war there were many efforts to treat "combat fatigue" and other psychiatric casualties, often just behind the lines of battle. Nurses participated in such medical treatments as narcosynthesis, subcoma insulin therapy, and thiopental sodium (Pentothal) interviews.

After the war, the high rate of psychiatric casualties aroused public generosity and gave rise to unprecedented federal legislation intended to improve the nation's mental health (Organizing Committee for the 40th Anniversary Commemoration 1986):

3 July 1946	National Mental Health Act signed by President Harry S. Truman
1 April 1949	National Institute of Mental Health established
28 July 1955	Mental Health Study Act signed by President Dwight D. Eisenhower
2 August 1956	Health Amendments Act signed by President Dwight D. Eisenhower
31 October 1963	Mental Retardation Facilities and Community Mental Health Centers Construction Act signed by President John F. Kennedy
8 November 1966	Narcotic Addiction Rehabilitation Act signed by President Lyndon B. Johnson
31 December 1970	Comprehensive Alcohol Abuse and Alcoholism Prevention, Treatment, and Rehabilitation Act signed by President Richard M. Nixon
21 March 1972	Drug Abuse Office and Treatment Act
And others	

In the half-century before World War II, the development of psychiatric nursing was greatly influenced by prevailing norms: descriptive psychiatry, hospital financing and control of training schools, largely physician control of content of teaching, a somewhat tenuous relationship between psychiatric nursing and nursing as a whole field, and a paucity of well-educated psychiatric nurse leaders. In 1943, with funds allocated under the Bolton Act, three university-sponsored courses in psychiatric nursing were started. By 1956, there were 28 university programs—20 on the master's level, two in schools of public health, and six at the undergraduate level (which soon were phased out). There are currently over 100 graduate programs in psychiatric nursing at the master's and doctoral levels.

Advanced Psychiatric Nursing Education

Between 1946 and the 1970s, funds available under the National Mental Health Act provided support for academic-based programs in advanced psychiatric nursing and for the preparation of teachers and supervisors, with stipends for students. The GI Bill, which provided support for education of World War II veterans, also enabled many registered nurses who had served their country to enter academic study. Furthermore, many states provided scholarships, particularly for nurses employed in public mental hospitals. In other words, in the late 1940s, there was generous support for the development of psychiatric nursing and for the education of nurses. However, there were many constraints. There were exceedingly few psychiatric nurses who had the proper credentials to qualify as academic faculty.

There were enormous challenges to defining "advanced psychiatric nursing" and to determining new directions to be taken in teaching graduate students. There were very few psychiatric nursing textbooks, and none that addressed advanced practice until the Burd-Marshall book was published in 1963 (Osborne 1984; Burd and Marshall 1963).

Integration of Psychiatric Nursing Training into Basic Nursing Programs

Affiliations in psychiatric nursing continued to progress. By 1944, basic experience was offered by 54% of the schools, but the prevailing idea was that the purpose of the exposure was to enrich general nursing practice. On June 21, 1952, the NLN—acting on a petition from a group of psychiatric nurses—established the Interdivisional Council on Psychiatric and Mental Health Nursing. On January 21, 1953, the NLN adopted a recommendation that basic programs in nursing should prepare students for beginning positions in the care of all patients—including psychiatric patients. Thus, seven decades after the McLean school started a training school, psychiatric nursing was finally and fully accepted as a part of the whole of nursing. In the 1950s, schools of nursing in mental hospitals began closing at a fairly rapid rate. They had served a worthy purpose.

In this same period, the attendants in psychiatric hospitals began to be threatened by the encroachment of developments in psychiatric nursing. Training programs to develop the attendant's occupation in competition for nurse positions were being set up. There were two major workshops, which included physicians, psychiatric nurses, social scientists, and attendants, to discuss this matter—the first in 1951 in Peoria, and the second in 1952 in Manteno, Illinois. In 1953, the NLN declared that psychiatric attendants and aides were nursing personnel who were to be supervised by registered nurses.

To promote interprogram consultation, develop some cohesion, and reduce isolation, meetings of directors of graduate programs in psychiatric nursing were held. Although many issues and concerns were debated in these meetings, the major question was whether psychiatric nurses should be prepared to provide psychotherapy for patients. In 1955, Rutgers University obtained an NIMH grant in support of preparation of only "clinical specialists in advanced psychiatric nursing"; all other programs at that time included teaching or supervision in addition to advanced nursing practice in their one-academic-year programs. The Rutgers program required two academic years of study plus one month and prepared nurses for individual, group, and family psychotherapy. Many academic programs eventually followed this pattern.

In 1952, the NIMH made grants of funds available to virtually all schools of nursing to enable them to employ a psychiatric nurse faculty member as "integrator." The purpose was to help all clinical faculty to include basic sociopsychiatric concepts in their teaching. The aim was to sensitize all nurses to the psychosocial stresses inherent in all illness experiences of patients, not to reduce, replace, or obviate the basic clinical educative experience students had with psychiatric patients. This latter effect occurred, however, in some schools in which faculty seemingly did not recognize the continuing need for more nurses as staff nurses and clinical specialists in psychiatric facilities.

Further Developments in Psychiatric Nursing

In the mid-1950s, various psychotropic drugs became available for medicating psychiatric patients, particularly for the relief of anxiety. Simultaneously, Smith, Kline, and French laboratories supported production of a film in 1958 titled *Psychiatric Nursing: The Nurse-Patient Relationship*. This film, which received several awards, encouraged nurses to talk with patients, inasmuch as the new medications made patients more accessible for therapeutic communication. Smith, Kline, and French distributed this film to virtually all schools of nursing and psychiatric hospitals at no cost to them. Before the 1950s, nurses generally were not encouraged to talk with patients—they were to keep busy "doing something."

In less than two decades after the Mental Health Act funds became available, developments in psychiatric nursing began to proceed more rapidly. In 1963, two journals addressed to the specific interests of psychiatric nurses began publication: *Perspectives in Psychiatric Care* and the *Journal of Psychiatric Nursing* (since renamed *Journal of Psychosocial Nursing and Mental Health Services*). In 1967, the ANA Division on Psychiatric and Mental Health Nursing published the *Statement on Psychiatric and Mental Health Nursing Practice*, which was revised in 1976. This statement provides a definition of psychiatric nursing, its roles, and its scope. The ANA division also issued *Standards of Psychiatric and Mental Health Nursing Practice* in 1982. This statement was further revised in 1994. (See inside front cover.) In the 1980s, the ANA sponsored a "phenomena project" defining the nursing diagnoses of interest to psychiatric nursing. Table 5–3 summarizes many of the historic contributions to psychiatric nursing.

Summary

The history of psychiatric nursing in the United States is just over one century old. In that short time, a basic work role has evolved, specialization has developed, and considerable influence has been exercised on nursing as a whole. The field has expanded in scope of practice, in numbers and kinds of practitioners, and in the variety of services and facilities in which psychiatric nursing is practiced. The continuing development of psychiatric nursing, however, depends on present-generation nurses becoming interested and competent in this component of nursing practice and in the preparation of many more psychiatric nurse clinical specialists and researchers.

Table 5-3 ■ SUMMARY OF CONTRIBUTIONS TO PSYCHIATRIC AND MENTAL HEALTH NURSING

PSYCHIATRIC NURSING LEADER	CONTRIBUTION
Pre-1860	
—	Nursing care for the young, ill, and helpless historically has existed as long as the human race. Care was given by family members, relatives, servants, neighbors, members of religious orders or humanitarian societies, or by convalescing patients or prisoners.
1860	
Florence Nightingale	Established Nightingale School at St. Thomas Hospital in London after Crimean War and worked with untrained women caring for soldiers. *Founder of modern-day nursing.*
1860–1880	
—	Emphasized maintaining healthful environment, personal hygiene, cleanliness, and healthful living habits, such as adequate nutrition, exercise, and sleep so that nature could heal. Emphasized kindness toward patients along with custodial care.
Linda Richards	*First graduate nurse and first psychiatric nurse in the United States.* After study under Miss Nightingale, organized nursing services and educational programs in Boston City Hospital and in several state mental hospitals in Illinois.
Dorothea Dix	*Worked to reform psychiatric care in mental hospitals* and to correct overcrowding and the insufficient number of physicians and attendants.
1882	
—	First school to prepare nurses to care for acutely and chronically mentally ill opened at McLean Hospital, Waverly, Massachusetts, through collaboration of Linda Richards and Dr. Edward Cowles.
1890–1930	
—	Nurses recognized by some administrative psychiatrists in state and private hospitals for their preparation. Nurses relieved of menial housekeeping chores to engage in physical custodial care of patients. Role primarily to assist physician or carry out procedures for physical care. Few psychological nursing skills. Psychologically concerned with maintaining kind, tolerant attitude and humane treatment.
1920	
Harriet Bailey	*First nurse educator to write a psychiatric nursing text, Nursing Mental Disease,* 1920. She wrote of the importance of a nurse's knowing mental illness and of teaching mental health nursing, and she worked for student experiences in psychiatry. She argued for more holistic care of patients.
1937	
—	The incorporation of psychiatric nursing was recommended by the National League for Nursing for inclusion in basic nursing curriculum.

PSYCHIATRIC NURSING LEADER	CONTRIBUTION
1946	
—	National Mental Health Act passed, authorizing establishment of National Institute of Mental Health, with funds and programs to train professional psychiatric personnel, conduct psychiatric research, and aid in development of mental health programs at the state level. Provided impetus for psychiatric nursing as a specialty.
1950–1960	
—	Nurse's role included physical care and medications and maintenance of therapeutic milieu. Less emphasis on physical restraints.
Ruth Matheney Mary Topalis	Emphasized importance of milieu therapy and the nurse's using this intervention.
1952	
Hildegard E. Peplau	*Formulated first systematic theoretical framework in psychiatric nursing; presented in Interpersonal Relations in Nursing, 1952.* Emphasized that nursing is an interpersonal process and that psychological techniques and theoretical concepts are essential to nursing practice. Emphasized steps in nurse-patient relationship: 1. Nurse helps patient examine situational factors through observation of behavior. 2. Nurse helps patient describe and analyze behavior. 3. Nurse formulates with patient connections between feelings and behavior. 4. Nurse encourages patient to improve interpersonal competence through testing new behavior. 5. Nurse validates with patient when new behavior is integrated into personality structure. Psychoanalytical, interpersonal, and communication theories used by nurses.
1953	
—	*The Therapeutic Community,* by Maxwell Jones in Great Britain, laid basis for movement in United States toward therapeutic milieu and nurse's role in this therapy.
1956	
—	National Conference on Graduate Education in Psychiatric Nursing introduced concept of psychiatric clinical nurse specialist. Theoreticians begin to differentiate functions based on master's level of preparation in nursing.
1957	
June Mellow	*Introduced second theoretical approach to psychiatric nursing, called Nursing Therapy, using psychoanalytical theory in one-to-one approach with schizophrenic patient. Emphasized providing corrective emotional experience rather than investigating pathological processes or interpersonal developmental processes in order to facilitate integration of overwhelmed ego.*
1958	
—	American Nurses' Association established Conference Group on Psychiatric Nursing.

Table continued on following page

PSYCHIATRIC NURSING LEADER	CONTRIBUTION
1959	
—	Accredited schools of nursing had to have own psychiatric nursing curriculum and instructor, per National League for Nursing. Could no longer buy services of hospitals to supply education.
1960–1970	
Hildegard E. Peplau Gertrude Ujhely Joyce Travelbee Shirley Burd Loretta Bermosk Joyce Hays Catherine Norris Gertrude Stokes Anne Hargreaves Dorothy Gregg Sheila Rouslin	Nursing leaders emphasized importance of self-awareness and use of self, nurse-patient relationships therapy, therapeutic communication, and psychosocial aspects of general nursing. Peplau formulated the manifestations of anxiety and steps in anxiety intervention, now used by all health care professions. All of these nursing leaders developed various psychological concepts into operational definitions for use in nursing.
1960	
Ida Orlando	*Initiated term* nursing process *and began to delineate its components.* Presented general theoretical framework for all nurse-patient relationships, with focus on client ascertaining meaning of behavior and explaining help needed. Wrote the classic book *The Dynamic Nurse-Patient Relationship,* 1961.
—	Comprehensive Community Mental Health Act passed, 1960; provided impetus for nurses moving from hospital to community setting.
1961	
Anne Burgess Donna Aguilera	Engaged in crisis work and short term therapy as well as in long term therapy. *Applied crisis theory to psychiatric nursing.*
Hildegard E. Peplau	Promoted *primary role of nurse as psychotherapist or counselor* rather than as mother surrogate, socializer, or manager.
1960–65	
Sheila Rouslin Suzanne Lego	Opened private practices in psychotherapy.
1967	
—	American Nurses' Association presented Position Paper on Psychiatric Nursing, endorsing role of clinical specialist as therapist in individual, group, family, and milieu therapies.
—	American Nurses' Association, Division in Psychiatric and Mental Health Nursing Practice published first *Statement on Psychiatric Nursing Practice.*
1970–1980	
Sheila Rouslin	*Certification of clinical specialists in psychiatric nursing begun* by Division of Psychiatric Mental Health Nursing, New Jersey State Nurses' Association, *because of her leadership.* Later, certification developed by American Nurses' Association.
Shirley Smoyak	*Client defined as individual, group, family, or community;* nurse defined as family therapist. Expanding role of psychiatric nurse.

Table 5–3 ■ SUMMARY OF CONTRIBUTIONS TO PSYCHIATRIC AND MENTAL HEALTH NURSING *Continued*

PSYCHIATRIC NURSING LEADER	CONTRIBUTION
Gwen Marram Irene Burnside	*Group and family psychotherapy by graduate-prepared nurses emphasized by nursing leaders.*
Carolyn Clark —	*Systems framework was used increasingly* by psychiatric nurses. Change agent, health maintenance, and research roles emphasized in latter half of decade.
Bonnie Bullough	*Legal and ethical aspects of psychiatric care emphasized.*
Madeleine Leininger —	*Care of whole person reemphasized. Introduced implications of cultural diversity for mental health services and psychiatric treatment.*
Hector Gonzales Doris Mosley Paulette D'Angi	Practice as autonomous member of team and in independent or private practice increased in latter half of decade. Work with citizens, consumer groups, and consumer organizations increased toward end of decade.
1976	
—	American Nurses' Association Division of Psychiatric and Mental Health Nursing Practice published revised *Statement on Psychiatric and Mental Health Nursing Practice.*
1978	
—	President's Commission Report of 1978 concluded that effects of deinstitutionalization and discharge of patients to community facilities have not worked as expected because of lack of financial, social, medical, and nursing resources and lack of coordination of services.
1980s	
Anne Burgess	*Formulated theory of victimology,* based on extensive studies of adult and child victims of rape and abuse, child victims of neglect, and family violence of incest and battering. *Described rape trauma syndrome, silent rape trauma, and compounded reactions to rape.*
Lee Ann Hoff	*Expanded crisis theory to be used in nursing practice. Contributed to theory of suicidology.* Described battering syndrome after research on battered women and battered elderly.
1982	
—	American Nurses' Association Executive Committee and Standards Committee, Division of Psychiatric and Mental Health Nursing Practice, published *Standards of Psychiatric and Mental Health Nursing Practice.*
1987	
Maxine E. Loomis Anita W. O'Toole Marie Scott Brown Patricia Pothier Patricia West Holly S. Wilson	Began the development of a classification system for Psychiatric and Mental Health Nursing, first published in *Archives of Psychiatric Nursing*, 1(1):16–24, 1987.
Judith Krauss	Became the first editor of a new journal, *Archives of Psychiatric Nursing.*
1990	
Suzanne Lego	Opened the first psychoanalytical training program admitting nurses only, at Columbia University School of Nursing.

Adapted from Murray RB. The nursing process and emotional care. *In* Murray RB, Huelskoetter MMW (eds). Psychiatric Mental Health Nursing—Giving Emotional Care, 3rd ed. Norwalk, CT: Appleton & Lange, 1991, pp 94–97.

References

American Nurses' Association. Nursing: A Social Policy Statement. Kansas City, MO: American Nurses' Association, 1980.

Benfer BA, Schroeder PJ. Nursing in the therapeutic milieu. Bulletin of the Menninger Clinic, 49(5):451, 1985.

Burd SF, Marshall MA. Some Clinical Approaches to Psychiatric Nursing. New York: Macmillan Publishing Company, 1963.

Committee on the Grading of Nursing Schools. Nursing Schools Today and Tomorrow: Final Report of the Committee on the Grading of Nursing Schools. New York, 1934.

Gebbie K, Lavin MA (eds). Classification of Nursing Diagnosis: Summary of the Second National Conference. St. Louis: Clearinghouse, 1972.

Henderson V. Basic Principles of Nursing Care. Geneva: International Council of Nurses, 1961.

Huey FL (ed). Psychiatric Nursing 1946 to 1974: A Report on the State of the Art. New York: American Journal of Nursing Company, 1975.

Hughes EC. Twenty Thousand Nurses Tell Their Story. Philadelphia: JB Lippincott, 1958.

Johns E, Pfefferkorn B. An Activity Analysis of Nursing. New York: Committee on the Grading of Nursing Schools, 1934.

Lego S (ed). The American Handbook of Psychiatric Nursing. Philadelphia: JB Lippincott, 1984.

Lego, S. Biological psychiatry and psychiatric nursing in America. Archives of Psychiatric Nursing 6(3):147, 1992.

Melton, MC, Smoyak, S. Telephone therapy: Call for help. Journal of Psychosocial Nursing 30(4):29, 1992.

Oderkirk WW. Setting the records straight: A recount of late nineteenth-century training schools. Journal of Nursing History, 1(1):30, 1985.

Organizing Committee for the 40th Anniversary Commemoration. 40th Anniversary of the National Mental Health Act. Organizing Committee, 1986.

Osborne OH. Intellectual traditions in psychiatric-mental health nursing: A review of selected textbooks. Journal of Psychosocial Nursing, 22(11):27, 1984.

Richards AJ. Reminiscences of Linda Richards: America's First Trained Nurse. Philadelphia: JB Lippincott, 1949.

Robb IH. Nursing in the smaller hospitals and in those devoted to the care of specialized forms of disease. Proceedings, p 59, 1897.

Scull A (ed). Madhouses, Mad-doctors, and Madmen: The Social History of Psychiatry in the Victorian Era. Philadelphia: The University of Pennsylvania Press, 1981.

Smoyak S, Rouslin S. Introduction. In Smoyak S, Rouslin S (eds). A Collection of Classics in Psychiatric Nursing Literature. Thorofare, NJ: Charles B. Slack, 1982.

Sullivan HS. Conceptions of Modern Psychiatry. Washington, DC: William Alanson White Institute, 1947.

Valenstein ES. Great and Desperate Cures: The Rise and Decline of Psychosurgery and Other Radical Treatments for Mental Illness. New York: Basic Books, 1986.

Further Reading

Albee GA, et al. The mental health disciplines. Hospital and Community Psychiatry, 27(7):492, 1976.

Bailey H. Nursing Mental Disease. New York: Macmillan Publishing Company, 1920.

Boorstin DJ. The Discoverers. New York: Random House, 1983.

Bridges DC. A History of the International Council of Nurses, 1899–1964: The First 65 Years. Geneva: International Council of Nurses. Philadelphia: JB Lippincott, 1967.

Carpenter M. Asylum nursing before 1914: A chapter in the history of labor. In Davis C (ed). Rewriting Nursing History. London: Croom Helm, 1980.

Chappell EA, McDonald TC. Containing madness. Colonial Williamsburg, Spring, 1985.

Dato C, Rafferty M. The homeless mentally ill. International Nursing Review, 32(6):170, 1985.

Fiesta J. Look beyond your state for your standards of care. Nursing '86, 16(8):41, 1986.

Mericle B. The male as psychiatric nurse. Journal of Psychosocial Nursing, 21(11):30, 1983.

Packard FR. Some Account of the Pennsylvania Hospital of Philadelphia from 1751–1956. Philadelphia: Pennsylvania Hospital, 1957.

Painter D, Painter TK. Building innovative nursing departments in turbulent times. Nursing Economics, 3:73, 1985.

Pappas NA. The public hospital: Its place in Williamsburg. Colonial Williamsburg, Summer, 1985.

Peplau HE. Historical development of psychiatric nursing: A preliminary statement of some facts and trends. In Smoyak SA, Rouslin S (eds). A Collection of Classics in Psychiatric Nursing Literature. Thorofare, NJ: Charles B. Slack, 1982.

Proceedings of the Fifth Annual Convention of the National League of Nursing Education. New York: NLN, 1899.

Roberts MM. American nursing: History and interpretation. New York: Macmillan Publishing Company, 1954.

Rosenfeld P. Nursing education: Statistics you can use. Nursing and Health Care, 7(6):329, 1986.

Rouslin S. Coping with chronic helpfulness. In Smoyak S, Rouslin S (eds). A Collection of Classics in Nursing Literature. Thorofare, NJ: Charles B. Slack, 1982.

Snively MA. A uniform curriculum for training schools. Proceedings, p. 24, 1895.

Tomes N. Little world of our own: The Pennsylvania Hospital training school for nurses 1895–1907. In Leavitt JW (ed). Women and Health in America. Wisconsin: University of Wisconsin Press, 1984.

Zwilling SS. Inside the public hospital. Colonial Williamsburg, Spring, 1985.

Self-study Exercises

Write a short answer to the questions that follow:

1. Name as many components of the total work role of nurses in psychiatric settings as you can. Indicate those for which your education has prepared you for competent functioning.

2. Name two ways in which nursing theory can be generated.

3. Cite two principles useful in practice with psychiatric patients. State why you accept them as important.

4. Name four to five theoretical frameworks that are used by providers of psychiatric services.

5. Identify six to eight other mental health care providers, and name one major unique function each performs in psychiatric settings.

6. What do you think will be your position as a practicing nurse with regard to the relation between psychiatric nursing practice and the biomedicalization of psychiatry?

7. If you had a family member or a friend who was seeking psychotherapy, would you refer that family member or friend to a qualified psychiatric nurse clinical specialist for psychotherapy? Justify your position.

8. What was the major method for getting psychiatric nursing included into all basic nursing curricula? When was it first proposed? When was it finally accomplished?

9. Who was the nurse author of the first textbook for psychiatric nurses? In contemporary terms, what is problematic about the book's title?

10. Discuss four future trends that will influence the practice of nursing and psychiatric nursing in particular.

11. In what year did the NLN recommend that all schools of nursing prepare all nursing students for beginning positions in psychiatric nursing?

Basic Concepts in Psychiatric Nursing

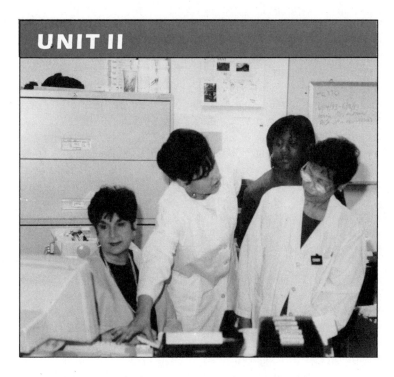

UNIT II

It is good to rub and polish our brains against those of others.

MICHEL DE MONTAIGNE

A Nurse Speaks

by John A. Payne

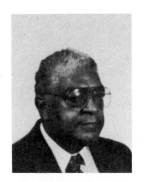

Forty years ago psychiatry was practiced in an environment vastly different from the one in which it is practiced today. Most patients were treated in large state hospitals, which were like small towns with their own store, restaurant, churches, farms, power plant, carpentry shop, and buildings housing thousands of patients and staff. There were buildings for admission and for treatment, infirmaries, chronic quiet units, and chronic disturbed units.

As nursing students, we were taught to care for patients who were receiving sedation, insulin shock, electric shock, malaria therapy, continuous hydrotherapy, wet packs, supraorbital lobotomies, physical restraints, and seclusion. All of these treatments were designed to make the patients more amenable to psychotherapy, to calm them, or for the safety of themselves or others. The disturbed wards were usually noisy and very active places in which patients acted out their psychoses both physically and vocally. Care for these patients was mostly custodial and involved keeping them clean, fed, safe, and calm.

I distinctly remember one patient who was almost continuously kept in seclusion because of bizarre and aggressive behavior. He would not keep his clothes on, could not safely use eating utensils, and roared like a lion. Because of his behavior, he was frequently referred to as the Lion Man.

Keeping him clean and fed was a major project for the staff and always required several people. It was a frustrating experience because we all wanted to help him and see him behave in a more acceptable manner.

During the Korean War, I was away in the Air Force for four years. For three years I was a part of a system that treated young men for psychiatric problems by using many of the same modalities that were used in the state hospitals. The treatment there was somewhat more successful than that provided in the state hospitals because most of the men's visible signs of psychoses were of recent origin, having been caused by the stress of basic training or the stress of being in battle.

In my fourth year, psychotropic drugs were introduced. We began to use them very cautiously on our patients, with very limited success. As the doctors became more familiar with the drugs and increased the dosages, the results showed much improved behavior with most patients. Gradually no patients were being put into packs, and the hydrotherapy room was seldom used.

After being discharged from the Air Force, I returned to the hospital in which I had trained. As I went to the different buildings, I was surprised to see that here too there had been a decrease in the use of the old treatment modalities. Patients for the most part appeared much calmer; no patients were in seclusion all of the time, not even the Lion Man.

One day, while I was walking on the grounds with one of the charge attendants, he asked me if I knew who a patient sitting on a bench talking with another patient was. I said, "No. Who is he?" "That is the guy we used to call the Lion Man." What a change! The attendant told me that they had given him Thorazine and that within one week he was out of seclusion and keeping his clothes on. Gradually he began to socialize with staff and other patients. Within one month he was playing checkers, and within one year he was granted ground privileges. Truly, the psychotropic drugs revolutionized the treatment of psychiatric patients.

Some psychotherapeutic modalities that had been used in smaller settings began to be used in the state hospitals. Group therapy, milieu therapy, and remotivation therapy became the vogue, and with this the role of nursing became a more therapeutic one.

During President Kennedy's tenure in office, the Community Mental Health Bill was passed. This provided funds for moving the treatment of patients from the large state hospitals to the local hospital. Two things were significant about this legislation. First, all levels and modalities of treatment had to be provided to all residents within a specific "catchment area." Second, all disciplines (including nursing) had to be represented on the treatment team.

States passed patients' bills of rights that released into the community thousands of patients who had spent many years in state hospitals. A part of the movement that was never adequate was the provision of group homes and follow-up supervision. This has led to our present situation of many actively psychotic ex-patients wandering our streets as homeless citizens. A change is going to come, and nursing is going to be an important part of that change. For now we have nurses in ever-increasing numbers who are becoming psychotherapists and psychiatric nurse practitioners. They will be leaders in providing care themselves and through mental health or psychiatric technicians—for nursing is still the only discipline that is proficient in providing 24-hour care to people in need.

Communication: The Clinical Interview and the Nurse-Client Relationship

Elizabeth M. Varcarolis with
contributions by Mattie Collins and
Judith Sutherland

OUTLINE •

KEY TERMS AND CONCEPTS ◆ ◆ ◆ ◆ ◆ ◆ ◆ ◆ ◆ ◆ ◆ ◆ ◆ ◆ ◆

The key terms and concepts listed here also appear in bold where they are defined or discussed in this chapter.

ACTIVE LISTENING

COMMUNICATION MODEL (BERLO'S)

CONFIDENTIALITY

CONTRACT

COUNTERTRANSFERENCE

EMPATHY

EXPLORING

FEEDBACK

INTIMATE RELATIONSHIP

MEDIUM

MESSAGE

NONTHERAPEUTIC (NONHELPFUL)
  TECHNIQUES

NONVERBAL COMMUNICATION AND
  BEHAVIORS (PROCESS)

ORIENTATION PHASE

PARAPHRASING

PROCESS RECORDINGS

RECEIVER

REFLECTING

RESTATING

SENDER

SOCIAL RELATIONSHIP

STIMULUS

TERMINATION PHASE

THERAPEUTIC ENCOUNTER

THERAPEUTIC (HELPFUL) TECHNIQUES

THERAPEUTIC RELATIONSHIP

TRANSFERENCE

USE OF SILENCE

VERBAL COMMUNICATION (CONTENT)

WORKING PHASE

OBJECTIVES ■

After studying this chapter, the student will be able to

1. Define the five components in Berlo's communication model.
2. Identify three personal factors that can impede accurate communication.
3. Identify two environmental factors that can impede accurate communication.
4. Discuss the differences between verbal and nonverbal communication and identify five areas of nonverbal communication.
5. Identify four techniques that enhance communication and discuss what makes them effective.
6. Identify four techniques that hinder communication and discuss what makes them ineffective.
7. Contrast and compare the purpose, focus, communication styles, and goals for (a) a social relationship, (b) an intimate relationship, and (c) a therapeutic relationship.
8. Define and discuss the role of empathy and positive regard on the part of the nurse in a nurse-client relationship.
9. Discuss four steps in the process of empathy according to Shackelford.
10. Identify two attitudes and four actions that may reflect the nurse's positive regard toward a client.
11. Summarize the three stages of the nurse-client relationship.
12. Discuss the purpose of clinical supervision.
13. Name four areas of concern the nurse should address during the first interview.
14. Identify four client behaviors a nurse can anticipate and discuss possible nursing interventions for each behavior.

Effective communication is the foundation for a therapeutic nurse-client relationship. Communication is the medium through which the nursing process is realized. In this chapter, a review of the basics of communication is presented, followed by a discussion of the nurse-client relationship and an introduction to a special form of communication—the clinical interview.

Communication

Simply put, communication is the process of sending a message to one or more persons. One way of thinking about the process of communication is a **communication model,** which identifies the parts of an inter-

action. Berlo's model has five parts: stimulus (referent), sender, message, medium (channel), and receiver (Berlo 1960).

The **stimulus** begins communication. For example, the stimulus can be a need for information, comfort, or advice. A stimulus in a nurse might be the perception that the client is feeling discomfort or confusion. A stimulus in a client could be the experience of anxiety, despair, or pain.

The **sender** initiates interpersonal contact. The **message** is the information sent or expressed to another. The clearest messages are those that are well

Portions of this chapter first appeared in Communication in Health Care: The Human Connection in the Life Cycle, 2nd ed. St. Louis: CV Mosby, 1983. We thank Dr. Mattie Collins for generously sharing her insights and ideas.

organized and expressed in a manner familiar to the receiver. The message can be sent through a variety of **mediums.** A message can be sent through an auditory (hearing), a visual (seeing), or a tactile (touch) medium. For example, a person may send a very clear message through silence, body language, or a hug, as well as through the stated word.

The **receiver** receives and interprets the message. Often the message from the sender may act as a stimulus to the receiver. The receiver may then respond to the sender by giving **feedback** to the sender. The nature of the feedback often indicates whether the meaning of the message sent by the sender has been correctly interpreted by the receiver. When the receiver gives feedback to the sender, communication becomes reciprocal. Communication is most effective when the message sent is the same as the message received.

Figure 6–1 shows this simple model of communication. However, communication is a *complex* process involving a variety of personal and environmental factors that can distort both the sending and the receiving of messages.

Personal factors that can impede accurate transmission or interpretation of messages include emotional factors (e.g., knowledge levels and language use) and social factors (e.g., differences in culture, ethnic background, and language).

Environmental factors include physical factors (e.g., background noise, lack of privacy, and uncomfortable accommodations) and social factors (e.g., the presence of others and the expectations of others).

Effective communication in helping relationships depends on the nurse's knowing what he or she is trying to convey (the purpose of the message), communicating what is really meant to the client, and comprehending the meaning of what the client is intentionally or unintentionally conveying (Collins 1983). The success of such an interdependent activity can be evaluated by the degree to which each person understands what was communicated and can show the other person that the message was understood.

Communication consists of verbal and nonverbal elements. It is said that communication is roughly 10% verbal and 90% nonverbal (Shea 1988). Therefore, learning to be an effective communicator means using both verbal and nonverbal cues.

VERBAL COMMUNICATION

Verbal communication consists of all words a person speaks. We live in a society of symbols, and our supreme social symbol is words. Talking is our most common activity, our public link with one another, the primary instrument of instruction, a need, an art, and

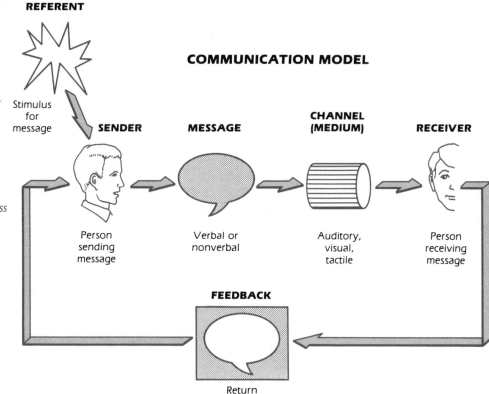

Figure 6–1. *The reciprocal process of communication.*

one of the most personal aspects of our private life. When we speak we

1. Communicate our beliefs and values
2. Communicate perceptions and meanings
3. Convey interest and understanding *or* insult and judgment
4. Convey messages clearly *or* convey conflicting or implied messages
5. Convey clear, honest feelings *or* disguised, distorted feelings

Even if the nurse and client have the same cultural background, the mental image they have of a word may not be exactly the same. Although they believe they are talking about the same thing, the nurse and client may in reality be talking about two quite different things. Words are the symbols for emotions as well as for mental images. For example, the word *trip* shows the manner in which differences in mental images can produce misunderstanding. If a nurse says to a client, "I heard you had some trip," the client will define *trip* according to the images that he or she has formed of the word from speaking, reading, writing, and listening. Depending on the client's past experience, the nurse's statement could convey interest or insult. Did the nurse think that the client stumbled and fell? Traveled to another city? Experimented with a drug? Reflecting the rapid, widespread changes in our society, words often change meanings and are therefore best interpreted in accordance with the company they keep (Collins 1983).

Conversation between persons of different cultures can be confusing if one statement simultaneously conveys different messages. One message is the *explicit* message (i.e., the precise or literal meaning of the sentence); the other message is the *implicit* message (i.e., the meaning that the speaker wishes to convey at the moment). In some cultures, the question, "Why don't you drop in sometime?" is not a request for a visit. If it were a true invitation, a specific date and hour would be set. However, someone from a different background may take the speaker at his or her word and create an embarrassing situation for all concerned. That a person can say one thing and at the same time mean another may be baffling to someone unfamiliar with the way a particular culture uses words. Many remarks are no more than social phrases: "Nice day, isn't it?" or "Hi, how are you?" These remarks are made in passing, and the speaker neither expects to discuss the weather seriously nor really wants to know how someone is. More information must be communicated either verbally or nonverbally to make the statement personally relevant (Collins 1983).

NONVERBAL COMMUNICATION

Nonverbal behaviors are the behaviors displayed by an individual, in contrast to the actual content of speech (Shea 1988). Tone of voice and the manner in which a person paces speech are examples of **nonverbal communication.** Other common examples of nonverbal cues are facial expressions, body posture, amount of eye contact, eye cast (emotion expressed in the eyes), hand gestures, sighs, fidgeting, yawning, and so forth.

INTERACTION OF VERBAL AND NONVERBAL COMMUNICATION

Communication thus involves two radically different but interdependent kinds of symbols: the deliberate impressions that one *gives* and the less deliberately controlled impressions that one *creates*. The first type involves the *spoken word*, which is the best friend of our public selves. Verbal assertions can be skillfully used to distort, conceal, deny, and generally disguise true feelings. The second type, *nonverbal behaviors*, covers a wide range of human activities, from body movements to responses to the messages of others. How one listens and uses silence and sense of touch may also convey very important information about the private self that is not available from conversation alone (Collins 1983).

Table 6–1 lists some types of nonverbal behaviors. Some nonverbal communication seems to be inborn and is similar across cultures (e.g., facial expressions). Other types of nonverbal behaviors, such as how close people stand to each other to speak, depend on cultural conventions. Some nonverbal communication is formalized and has very specific meanings (e.g., the military salute or the Japanese bow).

Therefore, an interaction consists of both verbal and nonverbal messages. Often people have more conscious awareness of their verbal messages and less awareness of their nonverbal behaviors. The verbal message is sometimes referred to as the **content** of the message, and the nonverbal behavior is called the **process** of the message. *When the content (verbal message) is congruent with (agrees with) the process (nonverbal behavior), the communication is more clearly understood and is considered healthy.* For example, if a student says that it is important to earn high grades and proceeds to buy the text, read the notes, and study systematically, the content message is consistent with the process, or the nonverbal behaviors.

If, however, the verbal message is not reinforced or is in fact contradicted by the nonverbal behavior, the message is confus-

Table 6–1 ■ NONVERBAL BEHAVIORS

POSSIBLE BEHAVIORS	EXAMPLE
Body Behaviors	
Posture, body movements, gestures, and gait	The client is slumped in a chair, puts her face in her hands, and occasionally taps her right foot.
Facial Expressions	
Frowns, smiles, grimaces, raised eyebrows, pursed lips, licking lips, and tongue movements	The client grimaces when speaking to the nurse; when alone, the client smiles and giggles to himself.
Eye Cast	
Angry, suspicious, and accusatory looks	The client's eyes are hardened with suspicion.
Voice-Related Behaviors	
Tone, pitch, level, intensity, inflection, stuttering, pauses, silences, and fluency	The client talks in a loud, sing-song voice.
Observable Autonomic Physiological Responses	
Increase in respirations, diaphoresis, pupil dilation, blushing, and paleness	When the client mentions discharge, she becomes pale, her respirations increase, and her face becomes diaphoretic.
General Appearance	
Grooming, dress, and hygiene	The client is dressed in a wrinkled shirt and his pants are stained; the client's socks are dirty, and he wears no shoes.
Physical Characteristics	
Height, weight, physique, and complexion	The client appears grossly overweight, and the client's muscle tone appears flabby.

ing. If the student who stated that it was important to earn high grades did not purchase the text, did not clarify questions from the notes, and did not study, the student would be sending out two different messages. Conflicting messages are known as double or mixed messages.

Nurses can be trained to become aware of a client's verbal and nonverbal communication. Nurses can compare the client's dialogue with the client's nonverbal communication to gain important clues about the client's real message.. What persons do may either express and reinforce or contradict what they say. Thus, as in the saying "actions speak louder than words," actions often tell the true meaning of a person's intent, whether it is conscious or unconscious. The meaning of the nonverbal cues depends on the context of the situation, the client, and the total pattern of both nonverbal and verbal behavior. The cues need to be considered together to form an accurate interpretation. The greater the cultural distance between the nurse and the client, the greater the probability of miscommunication (Collins 1983).

TECHNIQUES THAT ENHANCE OR HINDER COMMUNICATION

The goals of the nurse in the mental health setting are to help the client

1. Identify and explore problems relating to others
2. Discover healthy ways of meeting emotional needs
3. Experience satisfying interpersonal relationships
4. Feel understood and comfortable

Once specific needs and problems have been identified, the nurse can work with the client on increasing problem-solving skills, learning new coping behaviors, and experiencing more appropriate and satisfying ways of relating to others.

To do this, the nurse needs to have a sound knowledge of communication skills. Therefore, the nurse needs to become more aware of his or her own interpersonal techniques. The nurse is then better able to eliminate nonhelpful (nontherapeutic) techniques and to apply additional responses that maximize nurse-client interactions. Appropriate techniques are neither therapeutic nor nontherapeutic in and of themselves. They can, when used in the context of respect and genuine interest, greatly facilitate open communication.

Peplau's book *Interpersonal Relations in Nursing* (1952) and her groundbreaking article "Interpersonal techniques: The crux of psychiatric nursing" (1962) are the classic writings that defined nurses' understanding of the relationship between nurse and client.

Hays and Larson (1963) discussed and compiled from various sources and the works of various theorists examples of **therapeutic (helpful)** and **nontherapeutic (nonhelpful) techniques,** which are basic to communication skills used by mental health personnel today. These communication techniques are used throughout the nurse-client relationship.

Techniques that are deemed nontherapeutic are often used in social relationships, but they may impede communications during a therapeutic relationship.

Table 6–2 identifies techniques that may enhance communication. In the description of the technique and the examples given, students may recognize some techniques that they already use. Throughout this book, in case studies and in the text, examples of verbal communication are given. Students can identify various therapeutic techniques as they read and learn to recognize and apply them in their practice.

Table 6–3 identifies techniques that may hinder communication and make understanding between two people difficult.

Students new to a mental health setting can become aware of their own communication patterns, identify their responses, and increase their ability to alter responses in order to maximize open communication. Some important therapeutic techniques are discussed further in the next sections: (1) clarifying techniques, (2) the use of silence, and (3) active listening.

Clarifying Techniques

Understanding depends on clear communication, which is aided by the nurse's verifying with a client the nurse's interpretation of the client's messages. The nurse must request feedback on the accuracy of the message he or she receives from both verbal and nonverbal cues. The use of clarifying techniques assists both participants in identifying major differences in their frame of reference, giving them the opportunity to correct misperceptions before they cause any serious misunderstandings. The client who is asked to elaborate on or to clarify vague or ambiguous messages needs to know that the purpose is to promote mutual understanding.

PARAPHRASING. For clarity, one might use **paraphrasing:** that is, one might restate in newer and fewer words the basic content of a client's message. Using simple, precise, and culturally relevant terms, one may confirm without delay the interpretation of the client's previous message before the interview proceeds. By prefacing statements with a phrase such as "I am not sure I understand" or "In other words, you seem to be saying," the nurse helps the client form a clearer perception of what may be a bewildering mass of details. After paraphrasing, the nurse must validate the accuracy of the restatement and its helpfulness to the discussion. The client may confirm or deny the perceptions through nonverbal cues or by directly responding to a question such as, "Was I correct in saying that . . . ?" As a result, the client is made aware of the fact that the interviewer is actively involved in the search for understanding.

RESTATING. With **restating,** the nurse mirrors the client's overt and covert messages. Thus, this technique may be used to echo feeling as well as content. Restating differs from paraphrasing in that it involves repetition of the same key words the client has just spoken. If a client remarks, "My life has been full of pain," additional information may be gained by restating, "Your life has been full of pain." The purpose of this technique is to more thoroughly explore subjects that may be significant. However, too frequent and indiscriminate use of restating might be interpreted by clients as disinterest or inattention. It is very easy to overuse this tool and become mechanical. To inappropriately parrot or mimic what another has said may be perceived as poking fun at the person, making this nondirective approach a definite drawback to comunication. To avoid overuse of restating, the nurse can combine restating with direct questions that encourage descriptions: "Tell me about how your life has been full of pain."

REFLECTING. Another key to understanding is **reflecting** the feelings that messages convey. The interviewer describes briefly to the client the apparent meaning of the emotional tones of his or her verbal and nonverbal behavior. For example, to reflect a client's feelings about his or her life, a good beginning might be, "You sound like you have had many disappointments." Sharing *observations* with a client shows acceptance. The nurse helps make the client

Table 6–2 ■ TECHNIQUES THAT ENHANCE COMMUNICATION

DISCUSSION	EXAMPLE
Using Silence	
Gives the person time to collect his or her thoughts or to think through a point.	Encouraging a person to talk by waiting for the answers.
Accepting	
Indicates that the person has been understood. The statement does *not* necessarily indicate agreement but is nonjudgmental. However, nurses do *not* imply they understand when they do *not* understand.	"Yes." "Uh-huh." "I follow what you say."
Giving Recognition	
Indicates awareness of change and personal efforts. Does not imply good or bad, or right or wrong.	"Good morning, Mr. James." "You've combed your hair today." "I notice that you shaved this morning."
Offering Self	
Offers presence, interest, and a desire to understand. Is *not* done to get the person to talk or behave in a specific way.	"I would like to spend time with you." "I'll stay here and sit with you awhile."
Offering General Leads	
Allows the other person to take direction in the discussion. Indicates that the nurse is interested in what comes next.	"Go on." "And then?" "Tell me about it."
Giving Broad Openings	
Clarifies that the lead is to be taken by the client. However, the nurse discourages pleasantries and small talk.	"Where would you like to begin?" "What are you thinking about?" "What would you like to discuss?"
Placing the Events in Time or Sequence	
Puts events and actions in better perspective. Notes cause-and-effect relationships and identifies patterns of interpersonal difficulties.	"What happened before?" "When did this happen?"
Making Observations	
Calls attention to person's behavior, e.g., trembling, biting nails, restless mannerisms. Encourages the person to notice the behavior in order to describe thoughts and feelings for mutual understanding. Helps with mute and withdrawn persons.	"You appear tense." "I notice you're biting your lips." "You appear nervous whenever Mr. X enters the room."
Encouraging Description of Perception	
Increases nurse's understanding of client's perceptions. Talking about feelings and difficulties can lessen the need to act them out inappropriately.	"What do these voices seem to be saying?" "What is happening now?" "Tell me when you feel anxious."
Encouraging Comparison	
Brings out recurring themes in experiences or interpersonal relationships. Helps the person clarify similarities and differences.	"Has this ever happened before?" "Is this the way you felt when . . . ?" "Was this something like . . . ?"
Restating	
Repeats the main idea expressed. Gives the client an idea of what has been communicated. If the message has been misunderstood, the client can clarify it.	C: I can't sleep. I stay awake all night. N: You have difficulty sleeping?

Table continued on following page

Table 6-2 ■ TECHNIQUES THAT ENHANCE COMMUNICATION *Continued*

DISCUSSION	EXAMPLE
Reflecting	
Directs questions, feelings, and ideas back to the client. Encourages clients to accept their own ideas and feelings. Acknowledges the client's right to have opinions and make decisions and encourages clients to think of themselves as capable people.	C: What should I do about my husband's affair? N: What do you think you should do? C: My brother spends all of my money and then has the nerve to ask for more. N: This causes you to feel angry?
Focusing	
Concentrates attention on a single point. Is especially useful when the client jumps from topic to topic. If a person is experiencing a severe or panic level of anxiety, the nurse should *not* persist until the anxiety lessens.	"This point seems worth looking at more closely."
Exploring	
Examines certain ideas, experiences, or relationships more fully. If the client chooses not to elaborate, the nurse does *not* probe or pry. In such a case, the nurse respects the client's wishes.	"Tell me more about that." "Would you describe it more fully?" "Give me an example of one time you thought everyone hated you."
Giving Information	
Makes available facts the person needs. Supplies knowledge from which decisions can be made or conclusions can be drawn. For example, the client needs to know the role of the nurse, the purpose of the nurse-client relationship, and the time, place, and duration of the meetings.	"My purpose for being here is . . . " "This medication is for . . . "
Seeking Clarification	
Helps clients clarify their own thoughts and maximizes mutual understanding between the nurse and the client.	"I'm not sure I follow you." "What would you say is the main point of what you just said?"
Presenting Reality	
Indicates what is real. The nurse does not argue or try to convince the client, just describes personal perceptions or facts in the situation.	"I don't see anyone else in the room." "That was the sound of a car backfiring." "Your mother is not here; I am a nurse."
Voicing Doubt	
Undermines the client's beliefs by not reinforcing the perceptions.	"Isn't that unusual?" "Really?" "That's hard to believe."
Seeking Consensual Validation	
Clarifies that both the nurse and the client share mutual understanding of communications. Helps clients become clearer about what they are thinking.	"Tell me whether my understanding agrees with yours." "Are you using this word to convey . . . ?"
Verbalizing the Implied	
Puts into concrete terms what the client implies, making the client's communication more explicit.	C: I can't talk to you or anyone else. It's a waste of time. N: Do you feel no one understands?
Encouraging Evaluation	
Aids the client in considering people and events within his or her own set of values.	"How do you feel about . . . ?" "Does this contribute to your comfort?"

Table 6–2 ■ TECHNIQUES THAT ENHANCE COMMUNICATION *Continued*	
DISCUSSION	**EXAMPLE**
Attempting to Translate into Feelings	
Responds to the feelings expressed, not just the content. Often termed "decoding."	C: I am dead. N: Are you saying that you feel lifeless? Does life seem meaningless to you?
Suggesting Collaboration	
Emphasizes working with the client, not doing things for the client. Encourages the view that change is possible through collaboration.	"Perhaps you and I can discover what produces your anxiety."
Summarizing	
Brings together important points of discussion to enhance understanding. Also allows the opportunity to clarify communications so both nurse and client leave the interview with the same ideas in mind.	"Have I got this straight?" "You said that . . . " "During the past hour you and I have discussed . . . "
Encouraging Formulation of a Plan of Action	
Allows clients to identify alternative actions for interpersonal situations they find disturbing, e.g., when anger or anxiety are provoked.	"What could you do to let anger out harmlessly?" "Next time this comes up, what might you do to handle it?"

Reprinted with the permission of Macmillan Publishing Company from *Interacting with Patients* by Joyce Samhammer Hays and Kenneth Larson. Copyright © 1963 Macmillan Publishing Company.

aware of his or her feelings and encourages the client's ownership of them: for example, the nurse may tell a client, "You look sad." Perceiving that the nurse's concern may parallel his or her own, a client may more spontaneously share feelings.

EXPLORING. An important technique that enables the nurse to examine important ideas, experiences, or relationships more fully is **exploring.** For example, if a client tells the nurse that he does not get along well with his wife, the nurse would want to further explore this area.

- "*Tell me* more about your relationship with your wife."
- "*Describe* your relationship with your wife."
- "*Give me an example* of you and your wife not getting along."

Asking for an example can greatly clarify a vague or generic statement made by another person.

MARY: No one likes me.
NURSE: Give me an example of *one* person who doesn't like you.

JIM: Everything I do is wrong.
NURSE: Give me an example of *one* thing you do that you think is wrong.

Use of Silence

In many cultures in our society and in nursing, there is an emphasis on action. In communication, we tend to expect a high level of verbal activity. Many students and practicing nurses find that when the flow of words stops, they become uncomfortable. The effective **use of silence,** however, is a good communication technique.

Silence is not the absence of communication; *silence is a specific channel for transmitting and receiving messages.* The practitioner needs to understand that silence is a significant means of influencing and being influenced by others.

In the initial interview, the client may be reluctant to speak because of the newness of the situation, the strangeness of the nurse, self-consciousness, embarrassment, or shyness. Talking is highly individualized: some find the telephone a nuisance, whereas others believe they cannot live without it. The nurse must recognize and respect individual differences in styles and tempos of responding. How else can nurses learn of another's nature and their own but by courtesy, care, and time? Quiet persons, persons with a language barrier or speech impediment, the elderly, and persons who lack confidence in their ability to express themselves may be communicating through

Table 6–3 ■ TECHNIQUES THAT HINDER COMMUNICATION

DISCUSSION	EXAMPLE
Reassuring	
Underrates a person's feelings and belittles a person's concerns. May cause clients to stop sharing feelings if they think they will be ridiculed or not taken seriously.	"I wouldn't worry about . . . " "Everything will be alright." "You're doing fine."
Giving Approval	
Indicates what the client is doing now is "good" and implies that not doing it is "bad." When praise is given, potential learning may be hindered because the client then seeks to gain the nurse's approval rather than to focus on the steps of learning.	"That's good." "I'm glad you . . . "
Rejecting	
May make client feel rejected by the nurse because he or she is unable to express personal thoughts and feelings. Thus, the client avoids sharing thoughts or feelings to avoid the risk of further rejection.	"Let's not discuss . . . " "I don't want to hear about . . . "
Disapproving	
Implies that the nurse has the right to judge the client's thoughts or actions. Further implies that the client is expected to please the nurse. If the client's behavior is extreme or hurtful, the nurse should not label the behavior.	"That's bad . . . " "I'd rather you wouldn't . . . " "You are upset now. We can't allow you to do this."
Agreeing	
Denies clients an opportunity to change their point of view.	"That's right." "I agree."
Disagreeing	
May make a person defensive. Defending one's ideas often tends to strengthen them. If a client has delusional thinking, defending such thinking prevents the exploration of feelings or refocusing energies into more productive activities or interactions.	"I don't believe that." "I disagree with that."
Advising	
Conveys that the nurse knows best and that clients cannot think for themselves. Fosters dependency and denies clients the right to think through their own problems.	"I think you should . . . " "Why don't you . . . "
Probing	
May make clients feel used and valued only for the information they can give. Most people resent persistent personal questions.	"Tell me about your dislike for your wife."
Challenging	
Tends to expand and strengthen client's beliefs, especially if their beliefs serve an unmet need. Clients become more defensive and block attempts to discuss unmet needs.	"If you're dead, how come your heart is beating?"
Testing	
Indicates that the nurse feels the client needs help. Instead of asking questions such as "Can you remember?," the nurse could say, "Tell me what took place."	"What day is this?" "Do you know what kind of hospital this is?"

Table 6–3 ■ TECHNIQUES THAT HINDER COMMUNICATION *Continued*

DISCUSSION	EXAMPLE
Defending	
Implies that the client has no right to express his or her impressions, opinions, or feelings. Defending could also imply to the client that the nurse is taking the others' side against the client.	"I am sure he only meant to help you." "No one around here would lie to you."
Requesting an Explanation	
May be intimidating. Actually, if people knew why they were losing weight or were anxious, they could probably deal with the situation. It is better to ask people to describe *what* is occurring rather than *why* it is occurring.	"Why do you feel this way?" "Why did you do that?"
Indicating an External Source	
May have two detrimental outcomes: it encourages the use of projection (the devil made me do it) and it negates the client's responsibility for his or her own thoughts or actions. It is better to ask, "What events led up to that conclusion?"	"What would make you say that?" "Who told you that you were God?" "What made you do that?"
Expressing Belittling Feelings	
Is evident when the nurse is unable to empathize or understand another point of view. When a nurse tells a client to "buck up" or "cheer up," the client's feelings or experiences are being belittled. This can cause a person to feel "small" or "insignificant." It is more useful to say, "You must feel upset" or "Would you like to talk about it?"	C: "I wish I was dead." N: "Everyone gets down once in awhile." *or* "I know just what you mean." *or* "I get that way sometimes."
Making Stereotypical Comments	
Lacks value in the nurse-client relationship. Encourages empty responses by the client.	"It's for your own good." "Keep your chin up." "I'm fine, how are you?"
Giving Literal Responses	
Indicates the nurse's inability to understand the client's experience. Prevents the nurse's working with the client to describe feelings.	C: I'm an Easter egg. N: What a shame. You don't look like an Easter egg. C: They are looking into my head with a TV. N: What channel?
Using Denial	
Blocks avenues of discussion. Clients are blocked from identifying and exploring their difficulties.	C: I am nothing. N: Of course you're something. Everybody is something.
Interpreting	
Although a psychiatrist may interpret directly, the nurse is not prepared to deal with a client's unconscious perceptions.	"What you really mean is . . . " "Unconsciously you're saying . . . "
Introducing an Unrelated Topic	
Happens when the nurse changes the topic when a threatening or anxiety-provoking topic is brought up. It is important for the nurse to become aware of what precipitates these occurrences.	C: I'd like to die. N: Did you have any visitors this weekend?

Reprinted with the permission of Macmillan Publishing Company from Interacting with Patients by Joyce Samhammer Hays and Kenneth Larson. Copyright © 1963 Macmillan Publishing Company.

their silences a need for support and encouragement in acts of self-expression (Collins, 1983).

Although there is no universal rule concerning how much silence is too much, silence has been said to be worthwhile only as long as it is *"serving some function and not frightening to the patient"* (Schulman 1974). Knowing when to speak during the interview is largely dependent on the nurse's perception about what is being conveyed through the silence. Sometimes the topic under discussion has been exhausted; if the comments or an open-ended question may stimulate conversation in another direction. Icy silence may be an expression of anger and hostility. Being ignored or "given the silent treatment" is recognized as an insult and is a particularly hurtful form of communication.

Silence may also indicate emotional blocking. A client who feels pressured to talk about a subject that is too painful or delicate may react by changing the subject or by looking away with stony silence as a form of defiance or resistance. The nurse can intervene in a sure-footed manner against resistance only when the relationship has a reservoir of trust and intimacy that can help it withstand the strain. Timing is essential: the more positive experiences the participants have had together over time, the greater the likelihood that the client will make painful disclosures. If the relationship has not reached the stage of mutual trust, more may be gained if the client's unreadiness is respected and the conversation is not pursued along the lines that evoked the initial reaction. Silence can communicate strength and support by allowing the client to regain composure and to continue the conversation at a more comfortable level. *Thus, silence can show respect for the client's right to choose the nature, circumstances, and the degree of openness in communication* (Collins 1983).

Successful interviewing may be largely dependent on the nurse's "will to abstain"—refrain from talking more than necessary. Silence may provide meaningful moments of reflection for both participants. It gives each an opportunity to contemplate thoughtfully what has been said and felt, to weigh alternatives, to formulate new ideas, and to gain a new perspective of the matter under discussion. If the nurse waits to speak and allows the client to break the silence, the client may share thoughts and feelings that might otherwise have been withheld. Nurses who feel compelled to fill every void with words often do so because of their own anxiety, self-consciousness, and embarrassment. When this occurs, the nurse's need for comfort tends to take priority over the needs of the client.

On the other hand, prolonged and frequent silences by the nurse may hinder an interview that requires verbal articulation. Although the untalkative nurse may be comfortable with silence, this mode of communication may make the client feel used and like a fountain of information to be drained dry. Moreover, without feedback, the client has no way of knowing whether what he or she said was understood. The verbal patterns of nursing students have been demonstrated to correlate with communication competence (Johnson 1964). The *appropriate* use of verbal techniques of interviewing helped the students focus more directly on clients' needs and to elicit more emotional responses. Nurses who value silence highly may need to reassess the impact of nonverbal communication on the interviewing process. Without such a reassessment, there may be minimal use of the creative potential of mutuality, or working with the client toward goals (Collins 1983).

Active Listening

Active listening is listening attentively and responding relevantly. This kind of listening can be of considerable help to persons working through a problem. Listening creates an interpersonal situation of maximal involvement that may allow clients to experience themselves more fully and freely. In the search for understanding, the nurse observes the client's total network of communication, both verbal and nonverbal messages. In turn, caring and concern for the client may be communicated by acknowledging understanding of messages (Collins 1983).

Listening helps strengthen the client's ability to solve personal problems. To realize an objective, whether it is relief from tension or gaining information, one usually has to place one's thoughts in some semblance of order to be able to explain the problem more readily to others. By giving the client undivided attention, the nurse communicates that the client is not alone but with someone who is working along with the client to understand and help. This kind of intervention enhances self-esteem and encourages the client to direct energy toward reaching the discussion objectives. Serving as a "sounding board," the nurse listens as the client tests thoughts by voicing them aloud. This form of interpersonal interaction often enables the client to clarify thinking, link ideas, and tentatively decide what should be done and how best to do it (Collins 1983).

The Helpful Nurse-Client Relationship

TYPES OF RELATIONSHIPS

The nurse-client relationship is often loosely defined within a hospital setting, but a therapeutic relationship incorporating principles of mental health nursing is more clearly defined and differs from other relationships. In a helpful or therapeutic nurse-client relationship, there is an awareness that such a relationship develops over time and goes through specific stages. It is also acknowledged that *specific phenomena occur during the process of the relationship.*

A relationship is an interpersonal process that involves two or more people. Throughout life, we meet people in a variety of settings and share a variety of experiences. With some individuals, we develop relationships on either a short or a long term basis. The kinds of relationships we enter into vary with different people. Generally, they may be defined as (1) social, (2) intimate, or (3) therapeutic in nature.

Social Relationships

For the purpose of this text, a **social relationship** can be defined as a relationship that is primarily initiated for the purpose of friendship, socialization, enjoyment, or accomplishing a task. Mutual needs are met during social interaction: for example, participants share ideas, feelings, and experiences. Communication skills used in this type of relationship include giving advice and, sometimes, meeting basic dependency needs, such as loaning money and helping with jobs. Often the content of the communication remains superficial. During social interactions, roles may shift. Within a social relationship, there is little emphasis on the evaluation of the interaction.

Students often struggle with requests by clients to "be my friend." When this occurs, the nurse should make it clear that the relationship is a therapeutic (helping) one. This does *not* mean that the nurse is not "friendly" toward the patient at times. It does mean, however, that the nurse follows the guidelines stated later regarding a therapeutic relationship: essentially, the focus is on the client. The client's problems and concerns are explored and potential solutions are discussed by both client and nurse, and solutions are implemented by the client.

Intimate Relationships

An **intimate relationship** occurs between two individuals who have an emotional commitment to each other. Those in an intimate relationship usually react naturally to each other. Often the relationship is a partnership whereby each member cares about the other's needs for growth and satisfaction. Within the relationship, mutual needs are met and intimate desires and fantasies are shared. Short and long range goals are usually mutual. Information shared between these individuals may be personal and intimate. People may want an intimate relationship for many reasons, such as procreation, sexual or emotional satisfaction, economic security, social belonging, and reduced loneliness. Although transference and countertransference phenomena occur, they are usually not recognized or dealt with within the relationship. Depending on the style, level of maturity, and awareness of both parties, evaluation of the interactions may or may not be ongoing.

Therapeutic Relationships

The **therapeutic relationship** between nurse and client differs from both a social and an intimate relationship in that the nurse maximizes his or her communication skills, understanding of human behaviors, and personal strengths in order to enhance personal growth in the client. The focus of the relationship is on the client's ideas, experiences, and feelings (Smitherman 1982). Inherent in a therapeutic (helping) relationship is the nurse's focus on significant personal issues introduced by the client during the clinical interview. The nurse and the client identify areas that need exploration and periodically evaluate the degree of change in the client. *The roles do not change, and the relationship is consistently focused on the client's problems.* Communication skills and knowledge of the stages and phenomena occurring in a therapeutic relationship are crucial tools in the formation and maintenance of that relationship. Within the context of a helping relationship:

1. The needs of the client are identified.
2. Alternate problem-solving approaches are taken.
3. New coping skills may develop.
4. Behavioral change is encouraged.

King (1971) describes a therapeutic relationship as a learning experience for both client and nurse. She identifies four actions that must take place between nurse and client:

1. An initial action by the nurse
2. A reaction response from the client
3. An interaction in which the nurse and the client assess client needs and define goals
4. A transaction in which a reciprocal relationship is finally established to achieve relationship goals

FACTORS THAT ENHANCE GROWTH IN OTHERS

Rogers (1967) identified three personal characteristics that aid in the promotion of change and growth in clients: (1) congruence (genuineness), (2) empathy, and (3) positive regard (Rogers and Truax 1967).

Congruence

Rogers uses the word *congruence* to signify genuineness or an awareness of one's own feelings as they arise within the relationship, and the ability to communicate them when appropriate. Essentially, it is the ability to meet "person to person" in a therapeutic relationship, and it is conveyed by such actions as not hiding behind the role of nurse, listening to and communicating with others without distorting their messages, and being clear and concrete in communications with clients. Congruence connotes the ability to use therapeutic communication tools in an appropriately spontaneous manner, rather than rigidly or in a parrot-like fashion.

Empathy

Empathy is the ability to see things from the other person's perspective and to communicate this understanding to the other person. LaMonica (1980), a nurse researcher who developed a valid empathy instrument, defines empathy.

> Empathy signifies a central focus and feeling with and in the client's world. It involves (1) accurate perception of the client's world by the helper, (2) communication of this understanding to the client and (3) the client's perception of the helper's understanding.

Some researchers propose that empathy develops through experience in age-related stages in the same manner as other human development (Alligood 1992). Alligood identified two types of empathy in the nursing literature and in literature from other disciplines: basic and trained empathy.

The first type, basic empathy, is a basic human attribute sometimes referred to as natural or raw empathy. The second type, trained empathy, is empathy that can be learned in relation to clinical practice.

People often confuse the term *empathy* with *sympathy*. Sympathy is the actual sharing of another's feelings, and consequently experiencing the need to reduce one's personal distress. When a helping person is "feeling sympathy" with another, objectivity is lost, and the ability to assist the client in solving a personal problem ceases. For example, a friend tells you her mother was just diagnosed with inoperable cancer. Your friend then begins to cry and pounds the table with her fist.

- *Sympathetic response*: "I know exactly how you feel. My mother was hospitalized last year and it was awful. I still get upset just thinking about it." You go on to tell your friend about the incident.
- *Empathetic response*: "How upsetting this must be for you. How frustrating you must feel when you

are powerless to do anything about her diagnosis." You sit with your friend in silence a few moments.

Positive Regard

Positive regard implies respect. It is the ability to view another person as being worthy of caring about and as someone who has strengths and achievement potential. Respect is usually communicated not directly in words but indirectly by actions.

ATTITUDES. One attitude that a nurse might have that conveys respect is willingness to work with the client. That is, the nurse takes the client and the relationship seriously. The experience is not viewed as "a job," "part of a course," or "time spent talking" but rather as an opportunity to work with people to develop their own resources and actualize more of their potential in living.

ACTIONS. Some actions that manifest an attitude of respect are attending, suspending value judgments, and helping clients develop their own resources.

Attending. *Attending* refers to an intensity of presence, or being with the client (Egan 1982). Some nonverbal behaviors that reflect the degree of attending are the nurse's body posture (leaning forward toward the client, arms comfortably at sides), degree of eye contact, and degree of relaxation during the interaction.

Suspending Value Judgments. Nurses should not judge a client's thoughts, feelings, or behaviors using their own value systems. For example, if a client is taking drugs or is sexually promiscuous, the nurse might recognize that these behaviors are hindering the client from living a more satisfying life or from developing satisfying relationships. However, labeling these activities as "bad" or "good" is not useful. Rather, the nurse focuses on exploring the behavior of the client and works toward identifying the thoughts and feelings that influence this behavior. Judgmental behavior on the part of the nurse will most likely interfere with further exploration. Egan (1982) cites the following example:

CLIENT: I am really sexually promiscuous. I give in to sexual tendencies whenever they arise and whenever I can find a partner. This has been going on for at least three years.

NURSE: So, letting yourself go sexually is part of the picture also.

In this example, the nurse focuses on the client's behaviors and the possible meaning these behaviors might have to the client. The nurse does not introduce personal value statements or prejudices regarding promiscuous behaviors.

Helping Clients Develop Resources. The nurse becomes aware of clients' strengths and encourages them to work at their optimum level of functioning. The nurse does not act for clients unless absolutely necessary, and then only as a step toward helping them act on their own.

CLIENT: This medication makes me so dry. Could you get me something to drink?

NURSE: There is juice in the refrigerator. I'll wait here for you until you get back.

or

I'll walk with you while you get some juice from the refrigerator.

CLIENT: Could you ask the doctor to let me have a pass for the weekend?

NURSE: Your doctor will be on the unit this afternoon. I'll let her know that you want to speak with her.

Consistently encouraging the client to use his or her own resources helps minimize the client's feelings of helplessness and dependency and also validates the client's potential for change.

APPLICATION OF EMPATHY TO THE NURSE-CLIENT RELATIONSHIP

Sutherland (1985) developed a conceptual model of empathic nursing. This model is a four-phase process composed of identification, introjection, intervention, and evaluation.

PHASE I: IDENTIFICATION. In identification, the nurse uses cognitive skills to assess what is happening with the client. This critical scrutiny involves analysis of the following four major client-oriented categories:

1. *Appearance–physical state.* The nurse assesses and interprets the client's general appearance and physical status.
2. *Behavioral–emotional state.* The nurse assesses and interprets the client's behavior and emotional status as expressed in verbal and nonverbal messages.
3. *Physical–emotional state.* The nurse assesses and interprets a combination of information communicated by the client's general physical status and expressed emotional status.
4. *Behavioral–physical–emotional state.* The nurse assesses complex information related to the client's behavior and physical and emotional status.

PHASE II: INTROJECTION. Introjection occurs after the nurse has completed the assessment of the client through cognitive processing. Based on the information obtained from phase I, the nurse internalizes the information and resonates emotionally with the client's experience. Introjection is indicated by the nurse's expression of her feelings relative to the client's experience or the nurse's expression of the client's feelings. Introjection acts as a catalyst for nursing action.

PHASE III: INTERVENTION. Intervention occurs when the nurse takes action and intervenes as a result of the information obtained from the cognitive phase (identification) and based on an emotional understanding of the meaning that the experience has for the client (introjection). The most common interventions arising from this cognitive and affective process are

- *Restorative.* The nurse satisfies a client's need and restores or attempts to restore the client to a new physical state, a new emotional state, or both. This intervention evokes change in the client's status through various nursing care strategies.
- *Consolatory.* The nurse seeks to provide comfort. Physical or verbal actions are instituted to bring comfort, peace, and consolation to the client.
- *Sustentative.* The nurse sustains or supports the client. The intervention involves a variety of strategies aimed at maintaining the client's present physical or emotional status. Emotional support is provided through encouragement and instillation of hope.
- *Validative.* The nurse acknowledges verbally or nonverbally the client's emotional state or experience. Validative interventions are advocative of the client's experience.
- *Explorative.* The nurse seeks to obtain more information from the client by direct verbal inquiry.

PHASE IV: EVALUATION. Evaluation involves a continuous assessment of the client's response to nursing interventions. If client responses are congruent with the interventions, they lend support to the process of empathic care provided by the nurse. Accurate identification of the client's status combined with an understanding of the meaning the experience has for the client results in accurate nursing interventions. The most frequent responses from clients based on the previously cited interventions are

- *Metamorphic.* A verbal or nonverbal message indicates a change in the client's physical, emotional, or mental status as a result of a nursing intervention.
- *Gratuitous.* A verbal or nonverbal expression of gratitude or pleasure results from a nursing intervention.
- *Compliant.* The client agrees verbally or behaviorally to a nursing intervention.
- *Protective.* The client expresses a caretaking feeling for the nurse.

Clinical Example

Identification

Behavioral—Emotional

NURSE: She looked so sad and forsaken as she sat with bent head, hands folded on her knee, and no outward sign of suffering, until I saw great tears roll down her cheeks and drop on to the floor.

Introjection

Nurse's Feelings

NURSE: I felt so sad when I saw her utter dejection and very touched by her open expression of pain.

Intervention

Validative

NURSE: You seem to be feeling very sad right now. Cry if you need to.

Consolatory

NURSE: I will stay here with you.

Restorative

NURSE: I would like to hear about what is troubling you when you are ready to talk.

Evaluation

Gratuitous

PATIENT: Thank you. I need to talk to someone about this.

Metamorphic

PATIENT: I feel so much better. Just as though a terrible weight has been taken off my shoulders.

Therefore, the conceptual model of nurse empathy embraces the concepts of congruence, empathy, and positive regard proposed by Rogers. Congruence is the process of relating to the client with a demeanor and response appropriate to that client's experience. The nurse is congruent with the client when the nurse accurately assesses the client's status, experiences on an emotional (empathic) level what the situation means to the client, and responds appropriately (intervenes).

Empathy is the ability to experience what the other person is feeling. It is dependent on the cognitive process of accurate assessment of the client while internalizing and resonating with the client's emotional experience.

Positive regard is expressed in the entire process of empathic nursing care by the nurse's actively attending to the client's situation and by the nurse's action-oriented behaviors in service to the client.

The Clinical Interview

The clinical interview is not a random meeting between nurse and client. It is a systematic attempt to understand the relation of psychopathology to emotional conflicts (MacKinnon and Michels 1971).

The clinical interview differs from the intake interview, or the assessment interview, which is described in Chapter 8 as part of the nursing process. In most cases, by the time a student meets with a client for the first time, the intake interview has already been recorded. In the hospital setting, the intake interview is often recorded in the chart by the physician. However, during the clinical rotation, it is not uncommon for the student to obtain important data from the client that can be added to the data base.

The content and the direction of the clinical interview are decided by the client. The client leads. The nurse employs communication skills and active listening (identifying what the client says as well as what the client does not say) to better understand the client's situation. The nurse also observes how congruent the content (what the client says) is with the process (what the client does). During the clinical interview, the nurse provides the opportunity for the client to reach goals mentioned earlier: (1) identify and explore problems relating to others, (2) discuss healthy ways of meeting emotional needs, (3) experience a satisfying interpersonal relationship, and (4) feel understood and comfortable.

Communication and interviewing techniques are acquired skills. Nurses learn to increase their ability to use communication and interviewing skills through practice and supervision by a more experienced clinician. One method of increasing communication and interviewing skills is by reviewing clinical interactions exactly as they occur. This process offers students the opportunity to identify themes and patterns in their own communication, as well as in their client's communication. The student also learns to deal with a variety of situations that arise in the clinical interview.

Perhaps the best way of reviewing nurse-client interactions is by viewing a videotape, which reveals the nonverbal as well as the verbal communications between both parties. The second-best method of capturing the interaction between nurse and client is through an audiotape recording. Unfortunately, these methods are often not possible.

The use of **process recordings** is a popular way to examine the student's and the client's communication and to identify patterns. Process recordings have some disadvantages because they rely on memory and are subject to distortions. However, they can be a useful tool for identifying communication patterns. It is usually best if the student can write down notes verbatim (word for word) in a private area immediately after the interaction has taken place. Sometimes, a clinician takes notes during the interview. This practice also has disadvantages. One disadvantage is that it may be distracting for both the interviewer and the client, and some clients (especially those with a paranoid disorder) may resent or misunderstand the nurse's intent. Table 6–4 shows a segment of a process note. The nurse records his or her words and the client's words, identifies whether the responses are therapeutic or not, and recalls his or her emotions at the time.

Students new to the psychiatric setting often say they feel overwhelmed by the severity of some of the clients' problems and that they feel responsible for "doing something" to positively affect the emotional health of the client. It may help to know that numerous studies show the strength of the therapist-client relationship to be more important for a successful therapeutic outcome than a variety of other factors. Nicholi (1988) states that studies have borne out that the "therapist's ability to convey an intrinsic interest in the patient has been found to be more important than his position, appearance, reputation, clinical experience, training, and technical or theoretical knowledge." This finding does not negate the importance of clinical training, skill, or experience. It does, however, emphasize the need for the nurse to convey genuine interest in another human, without being patronizing or condescending.

Anxiety during the first interview is to be expected, as in any meeting between strangers. Clients may be anxious about their problems, about the nurse's reaction to them, about their treatment, and so forth.

Students may be anxious about the client's reaction to them, their ability to provide help, what the instructor will think of them, and how they will do compared with their peers (MacKinnon and Michels 1971).

Students have many concerns when entering the psychiatric unit for the first time. Two common concerns are (1) how to begin the interview and (2) what to do in response to specific client behaviors. The following section offers some basic guidelines for the first interview, identifies some common problems in clinical situations, and offers possible solutions.

HOW TO BEGIN THE INTERVIEW

SETTING. Effective communication could take place almost anywhere. However, because the quality of the interaction, whether in a clinic, ward, or office, depends on the degree to which the nurse and client feel safe and secure, establishing a setting that enhances the feelings of security can enhance the helping relationship. A specific location such as a conference room or a quiet part of the unit that has relative privacy but is within view of others is ideal.

SEATING. In all settings, chairs need to be placed so that conversation can take place in normal tones of voice and so that eye contact can be comfortably maintained or avoided.

INTRODUCTIONS. In the orientation phase, students tell the client who they are, the name of their school, the purpose of the meetings, and how long and when they will be meeting with the client. The issue of confidentiality is also covered at some point during the initial interview. The nurse can then ask the client how he or she would like to be addressed. This question accomplishes several tasks (Shea 1988):

1. It conveys respect.
2. It gives the client direct control over an important ego issue. (Some clients do not like to be called by their last names, and others do not like to be called by their first names.)
3. The nurse may learn something about the client when his or her preference is revealed.

HOW TO START. Once introductions have been made, the nurse can turn the interview over to the client by using one of a number of open-ended statements (Shea 1988; MacKinnon and Michels 1971):

- *Where should we start?*
- *Tell me a little about what has been going on with you.*
- *What are some of the stresses you have been coping with recently?*
- *Tell me a little about what has been happening in the past couple of weeks.*

Table 6-4 ■ SEGMENT OF A PROCESS NOTE

NURSE	CLIENT	COMMENTS	FEELINGS
"Good morning, Mr. L."		*Therapeutic.* Giving recognition. Acknowledging a client by name can enhance self-esteem and communicates that the client is viewed as an individual by the nurse.	
	"Who are you and where the devil am I?" *Looks around with a confused look on face—quickly sits on edge of bed.*		
"I am Mrs. V. I am a student nurse from X college, and you are at Mt. Sinai Hospital. I would like to spend some time with you today."		*Therapeutic.* Giving information. Informing the client of facts needed to make decisions or come to realistic conclusions. *Therapeutic.* Offering self. Making oneself available to the client.	
	"What am I doing here? How did I get here?" *Spoken in a loud, demanding voice.*		
"You were brought in by your wife last night after swallowing a bottle of aspirin. You had to have your stomach pumped."		*Therapeutic.* Giving information. Giving needed facts so client can orient himself and better evaluate his situation.	
	"Oh . . . yeah." *Silence for two minutes. Shoulders slumped, Mr. L. stares at the floor and drops his head and eyes.*		
"You seem upset, Mr. L." "What are you thinking about?"		*Therapeutic.* Making observations. He looks sad. *Therapeutic.* Giving broad openings in an attempt to get at his feelings.	
	"Yeah, I just remembered . . . I wanted to kill myself." *Said in a low tone almost to himself.*		
"Oh Mr. L., you have so much to live for. You have such a loving family."		*Nontherapeutic.* Defending. *Nontherapeutic.* Introducing an unrelated topic.	I felt overwhelmed. I didn't know what to say—his talking about killing himself made me nervous. I could have said, "You must be very upset" (verbalizing the implied) or "Tell me more about this" (exploring).
	"What do you know about my life? You want to know about my family? . . . My wife is leaving me, that's what." *Faces nurse with an angry expression on his face and speaks in loud tones.*		
"I didn't know. You must be terribly upset by her leaving."		*Therapeutic.* Reflective. Observing angry tone and content of client's message and reflecting back client's feelings.	

- *Perhaps you can begin by letting me know what some of your concerns have been recently.*
- *Tell me about your difficulties.*

Communication can be facilitated with the appropriate use of offering leads (e.g., "Go on"), statements of acceptance (e.g., "Uh-huh"), or other conveyances of the nurse's interest.

TACTICS TO AVOID. The nurse should avoid some behaviors (Moscato 1988):

- Do not argue with, minimize, or challenge the client.
- Do not praise the client or give false reassurance.
- Do not interpret to the client or speculate on the dynamics of the client's problem.

- Do not question the client about sensitive areas.
- Do not try to "sell" the client on accepting treatment.
- Do not join in attacks the client launches on his or her mate, parents, friends, or associates.
- Do not participate in criticism of another nurse or any other staff member.

WHAT TO DO IN RESPONSE TO CLIENT BEHAVIORS

Often, students new to the mental health setting are concerned about being in situations that they may not know how to handle. These concerns are universal and often arise in the clinical setting. Table 6–5 identifies common client behaviors, such as crying, asking the nurse to keep a secret, or threatening to commit suicide. The table gives an example of an appropriate response, the rationale for the response, and a possible verbal statement. Read the table, paying particular attention to the *rationales* for responses. The exact words will depend on the situation, but understanding the rationale will help the student apply the information in future situations.

PHASES OF THE NURSE-CLIENT RELATIONSHIP

The ability of the nurse to engage in interpersonal interactions in a goal-directed manner for the purpose of assisting clients with their emotional or physical health needs is the foundation of nursing practice (Hagerty 1984).

The nurse-client relationship is synonymous with a professional helping relationship. The behaviors described by Mauksch and David (1972), which have relevance to many health care workers, including nurses, are as follows:

1. *Accountability.* The nurse assumes responsibility for the conduct and consequences of the task. As the originator of the tasks, the nurse is fully answerable for them.
2. *Primacy of client interest.* The interest of the client, not that of other health care workers or of the institution, is given first consideration. The nurse's role is that of client advocate.
3. *Scientific competence.* The criteria on which the nurse bases his or her conduct are principles of knowledge and appropriateness to the specific situation, as well as the latest knowledge made available from research. This, however, involves self-awareness and a "modicum" of mental health on the part of the nurse.

4. *Supervision.* Validation of performance quality is through regularly scheduled supervisory sessions. Supervision is conducted either by a more experienced clinician or through discussion with the nurse's peers in professionally conducted supervisory sessions.

Nurses interact with clients in a variety of settings, such as emergency rooms, medical-surgical units, maternity and pediatric units, clinics, community settings, schools, and client homes. Nurses who are sensitive to the client's needs and have effective assessment and communication skills can significantly help the client confront present problems and make future choices.

Sometimes, the type of relationship that occurs may be informal and not extensive, such as when the nurse and client meet for only a few sessions. However, even though it is brief, the relationship may be substantial, useful, and important for the client. This limited relationship is often referred to as a **therapeutic encounter** (Hagerty 1984).

At other times, the encounters may be of longer duration and more formal, such as in inpatient settings, mental health units, crisis centers, and mental health centers. This longer time span allows the development of a therapeutic nurse-client relationship. The therapeutic nurse-client relationship is the medium through which the nursing process is implemented (Hagerty 1984).

Three distinctive phases of the nurse-client relationship are generally recognized: (1) the orientation phase, (2) the working phase, and (3) the termination phase. Although various phenomena and goals are identified for each phase, they often overlap from phase to phase.

Orientation Phase

The **orientation phase** can last for a few meetings or can extend over a longer period, depending on the client's psychopathology, the complexity of the client's problems, the comfort and experience of the nurse, and other variables.

The first time the nurse and the client meet, they are strangers to each other. When strangers meet, whether or not they know anything about each other, they interact according to their own backgrounds, standards, values, and experiences. This fact—that each person has a unique frame of reference—underlies the need for self-awareness on the part of the nurse.

As the relationship evolves through a series of ongoing reactions, each participant may elicit in the other a wide range of positive and negative emotional

Table 6–5 ■ COMMON CLIENT BEHAVIORS AND NURSE RESPONSES

POSSIBLE REACTIONS BY NURSE	USEFUL RESPONSES BY NURSE
What to Do If the Client Cries	
The nurse may feel uncomfortable and experience increased anxiety or feel somehow responsible for making the person cry.	The nurse should stay with the client and reinforce that it is all right to cry. Often, it is at this time that feelings are closest to the surface and can be best identified. "You seem ready to cry." "You still are upset about your brother's death." "What are you thinking right now?" The nurse offers tissues when appropriate.
What to Do If the Client Asks the Nurse to Keep a Secret	
The nurse may feel conflict because the nurse wants the client to share important information but is unsure about making such a promise.	The nurse *cannot* make such a promise. The information may be important to the health or safety of the client or others. "I cannot make that promise. It might be important for me to share it with other staff." The client then decides whether to share the information or not.
What to Do If the Client Leaves Before the Session Is Over	
The nurse may feel rejected, thinking it was something that he or she did. The nurse may experience increased anxiety or feel abandoned by the client.	Some clients are not able to relate for long periods of time without experiencing an increase in anxiety. On the other hand, the client may be testing the nurse. "I will wait for you here for 15 minutes, until our time is up." During this time, the nurse does *not* engage in conversation with any other client or with the staff. When the time is up, the nurse approaches the client, tells him or her the time is up, and restates the day and time the nurse will see the client again.
What to Do If Another Client Interrupts During Time with Your Selected Client	
The nurse may feel a conflict. The nurse does not want to appear rude. Sometimes the nurse tries to engage both clients in conversation.	The time the nurse had contracted with a selected client is that client's time. By keeping their part of the contract, nurses demonstrate that they mean what they say and that they view the sessions as important. "I am with Mr. Rob for the next 20 minutes. At 10 A.M., after our time is up, I can talk to you for five minutes."
What to Do If the Client Says He Wants to Kill Himself	
The nurse may feel overwhelmed or responsible to "talk the client out of it." The nurse may pick up some of the client's feelings of hopelessness.	The nurse tells the client that this is serious, that the nurse does not want harm to come to the client, and that this information needs to be reported to other staff. "This is very serious, Mrs. Lamb. I do not want any harm to come to you. I will have to report this to the other staff." The nurse can then discuss with the client the feelings and circumstances that led up to this decision (refer to Chapter 21 for suicide intervention).
What to Do If the Client Says She Does Not Want to Talk	
The nurse new to this situation may feel rejected or ineffectual.	At first, the nurse might say something to this effect: "It's all right. I would like to spend time with you. We don't have to talk."

Table 6–5 ■ COMMON CLIENT BEHAVIORS AND NURSE RESPONSES *Continued*

POSSIBLE REACTIONS BY NURSE	USEFUL RESPONSES BY NURSE
	The nurse might spend short, frequent periods of time (e.g., five minutes) with the client throughout the day.
	"Our five minutes is up. I'll be back at 10 A.M. and stay with you five more minutes."
	This gives the client the opportunity to understand that the nurse means what he or she says and is back on time consistently. This also gives the client time between visits to assess the nurse and perhaps feel less threatened.
What to Do If the Client Seeks to Prolong the Interview	
Sometimes, clients will open up dynamic or "juicy" topics right before the interview time is up. This is often done to test or manipulate the nurse.	The nurse sets limits and restates and reinforces the original contract.
The nurse might feel tempted to extend the scheduled time or might not want to hurt the client's feelings.	The nurse states that they will use the issues for the next session.
	"Our time is up now, Mr. Jones. This would be a good place to start at our next session, which is Wednesday at 10 A.M."
What to Do If the Client Gives the Nurse a Present	
The nurse may feel uncomfortable when offered a gift.	Possible guidelines

The meaning needs to be examined. Is the gift
  1. A way of getting better care?
  2. A way to maintain self-esteem?
  3. A way of making the nurse feel guilty?
  4. A sincere expression of thanks?
	If the gift is expensive, the best policy is perhaps to graciously refuse.

	If the gift is inexpensive and
	  Is given *at the end* of hospitalization in which a relationship has developed, graciously accept.
	  Is given *at the beginning* of hospitalization, graciously refuse.

	"Thank you, but it is our job to care for our clients. Are you concerned that some aspect of your care will be overlooked?"
	If the gift is money, it may be best to graciously refuse.

reactions (Bonnivien 1992). The stirring up of feelings in the client by the nurse is referred to as **transference,** and the stirring up of feelings in the nurse or therapist by the client is referred to as **countertransference.** The nurse is responsible for identifying these two phenomena.

TRANSFERENCE. **Transference** is the process whereby a client unconsciously and inappropriately displaces (transfers) onto individuals in his or her current life those patterns of behavior and emotional reactions that originated with significant figures from childhood. Although the transference phenomenon occurs in all relationships, transference seems to be intensified in relationships with authority. Because the process of transference is accelerated toward a person in authority, physicians, nurses, and social workers are all potential objects of transference. It is important to realize that the client may experience thoughts, feel-

ings, and reactions toward a health care worker that are realistic and appropriate; these are *not* transference phenomena.

Common forms of transference include the desire for affection or respect and the gratification of dependency needs. Other transferential feelings the client might experience are intense feelings of hostility, jealousy, competitiveness, and love. Requests for special favors (e.g., cigarettes, water, extra time within the session) are concrete examples of transference phenomena (MacKinnon and Michels 1971).

COUNTERTRANSFERENCE. **Countertransference** refers to the tendency of the nurse to displace onto the client feelings caused by people in the nurse's past. Frequently, the client's transference to the nurse will evoke countertransference feelings in the nurse. For example, it is normal to feel angry when attacked persistently, annoyed when frustrated unreasonably, or

·flattered when idealized. A nurse might also feel omnipotent or very important when depended on exclusively by a client (Bonnivien 1992).

If the nurse feels either a very strong positive or negative reaction to a client, the feeling may signal a countertransferential process in the nurse. A common sign of countertransference in the nurse is overidentification with the client. In this situation, the nurse may have difficulty recognizing or understanding problems the client has that are similar to the nurse's own. For example, a nurse who is struggling with an alcoholic family member may feel disinterested, cold, or disgusted toward an alcoholic client. Other indications of countertransference are when the nurse gets involved in power struggles, competition, or arguing with the client (MacKinnon and Michels 1971). Box 6–1 identifies some common emotional reactions that might indicate countertransference by the nurse.

This identification of and working through various transference and countertransference issues is crucial for growth and positive change in the client. These issues are best dealt with by the use of supervision, either supervision by a more experienced professional or peer supervision. Regularly scheduled supervision or peer supervision sessions provide the opportunity for increased self-awareness, increased clinical skills, and increased growth on the part of the nurse, as well as of the client.

ESTABLISHING TRUST. A major emphasis during the first few encounters with the client is providing an atmosphere in which trust can grow. As in any relationship, trust is nurtured by demonstrating congruence and empathy, developing positive regard, showing consistency, and offering assistance in alleviating the client's emotional pain or problems.

Box 6–1. POSSIBLE COUNTERTRANSFERENCE REACTIONS

- Wandering thoughts and feelings of detachment
- Feelings of impatience or insensitivity toward the client
- Feelings of envy
- Sexual or aggressive fantasies about the client
- Overconcern for the client between sessions
- Power struggles with the client
- Dreams about the client
- Intrusiveness or use of controlling actions with the client
- Overidentification with the plight or happiness of the client

---

During the orientation phase, four important issues need to be addressed: (1) the parameters of the relationship, (2) the formal or informal contract, (3) confidentiality, and (4) termination.

The Parameters of the Relationship. The client needs to know about the nurse (who the nurse is and what the nurse's background is) and the purpose of the meetings. For example, a student might furnish the following information.

STUDENT: Hello, Mrs. James. I am Nancy Rivera from Orange Community College. I am in my psychiatric rotation, and I will be coming to York Hospital for the next 10 Thursdays. I would like to spend time with you each Thursday if you are still here. We can use that time to discuss areas of your life that are a concern or that you might like to change.

The Formal or Informal Contract. Contracts emphasize the client's participation and responsibility because the contract shows that the nurse does something *with* the client rather than *for* the client (Collins 1983). The **contract,** either stated or written, contains the place, time, date, and duration of the meetings. During the orientation phase, the client may begin to express thoughts and feelings, identify problems, and discuss realistic goals. Therefore, the mutual agreement on goals is also part of the contract. If the goals are met, the client's level of functioning will return to a previous level or at least improve from the present level. If fees are to be paid, the client is told how much they will be and when the payment is due.

STUDENT: Mrs. James, we will meet at 10:00 A.M. each Thursday in the music room, for 45 minutes, from September 15th through November 16th. We can use that time for further discussion of your feelings of loneliness and anger with your husband and to explore some things you could do to make things better for yourself.

Confidentiality. The client has a right to know who else will know about the information he or she shares with the nurse. The client needs to know that the information may be shared with specific people, such as a clinical supervisor, the physician, the staff, or other students in conference. The client also needs to know that the information will *not* be shared with the client's relatives, friends, or others outside the treatment team, except in extreme situations. If information must be given to others, this is usually done by the physician, according to legal guidelines (refer to Chapter 3). The nurse must be aware of the client's right to **confidentiality** and must not violate that right.

STUDENT: Mrs. James, I will be sharing some of what we discuss with my nursing instructor, and at times I may discuss certain concerns with my peers in conference or with the staff. However, I will *not* be sharing this information with your husband or any other members of your family without your permission.

Termination. Termination begins in the orientation phase. It may be mentioned when appropriate during the working phase as well, if the nature of the relationship is time limited (e.g., 10 sessions). The date of the termination phase should be clear from the beginning. In some situations, the nurse-client contract may be renegotiated when the termination date has been reached. In other situations, when the therapeutic nurse-client relationship is an open-ended one, the termination date is not known.

STUDENT: Mrs. James, as I mentioned earlier, our last meeting will be on November 16th. We will have nine more meetings after today.

During the orientation phase and later, clients often unconsciously employ "testing behaviors." These behaviors may be used to test the nurse. The client wants to know if the nurse will

- Be able to set limits when the client needs them
- Still show concern if the client acts angry, babyish, unlikable, and so on
- Still be there if the client is late, leaves early, won't speak, and more

Table 6–6 identifies some testing behaviors and possible responses by nurses.

Working Phase

Moore and Hartman (1988) identify specific tasks of the working phase of the nurse-client relationship:

1. Maintain the relationship
2. Gather further data
3. Promote the client's problem-solving skills, self-esteem, and use of language
4. Facilitate behavioral change
5. Overcome resistance behaviors
6. Evaluate problems and goals and redefine them as necessary

During the **working phase,** the nurse and client together identify and explore areas in the client's life that are causing the client problems in living. Often, the client's ways of handling situations stem from earlier ways of coping devised in order to survive in a chaotic and dysfunctional family environment. Although certain coping methods may have worked for the client at an earlier age, they now interfere with the client's interpersonal relationships and prevent the client from attaining current goals. Because the client's dysfunctional behaviors and basic assumptions about the world are often defensive in nature and because the client is unable to change his or her dysfunctional behavior at will, most of the problem behaviors or thinking continues because of unconscious motivations and needs that are out of the client's awareness.

The nurse can work with the client to identify these unconscious motivations and assumptions that keep the client from finding satisfaction and reaching his or her potential. The describing and often the re-experiencing of old conflicts awakens high levels of anxiety in the client. The client may use various defenses against anxiety and displace his or her feelings onto the nurse. Therefore, during the working phase, intense emotions such as anxiety, anger, self-hate, hopelessness, and helplessness may surface. Behaviors such as acting out anger inappropriately, withdrawing, intellectualizing, manipulating, denying, and others are to be expected.

During the working phase, strong transferential feelings may appear. The emotional responses and behaviors in the client may also awaken strong countertransferential feelings in the nurse. *The nurse's awareness of personal feelings and reactions to the client is vital for effective interaction with the client.* Common transferential feelings and reactions that nurses experience in response to different behaviors and situations are discussed in the planning component of each of the clinical chapters (Chapter 11–25).

The development of a strong working relationship can allow the client to experience increased levels of anxiety and demonstrate dysfunctional behaviors in a safe setting, as well as to try out new and more adaptive coping behaviors.

Termination Phase

Termination is discussed during the first interview. During the working stage, the fact of eventual termination may also be raised at appropriate times. Six reasons for terminating the nurse-client relationship have been identified (Campaniello 1980):

1. Symptom relief
2. Improved social functioning
3. Greater sense of identity

Table 6–6 ■ TESTING BEHAVIORS USED BY CLIENTS

CLIENT BEHAVIOR	CLIENT EXAMPLE	NURSE RESPONSE	RATIONALE
Shifts focus of interview *to* the nurse, *off* the client.	"Do you have any children?" or "Are you married?"	"This time is for you." If appropriate, the nurse could add: 1. "Do *you* have any children?" or "What about your children?" 2. "Are you married?" or "What about your relationships?"	The nurse refocuses back to the client and the client's concerns. The nurse sticks to the contract.
Tries to get the nurse to take care of him or her.	"Could you tell my doctor . . . "	"I'll leave a message with the ward clerk that you want to see him." or "You know best what you want him to know. I'll be interested in what he has to say."	1. The nurse validates that the client is able to do many things for him- or herself. This aids in increasing self-esteem.
	"Should I take this job . . . "	"What do you see as the pros and cons of this job?"	2. The nurse *always* encourages the person to function at the highest level, even if he or she doesn't want to.
Makes sexual advances toward the nurse, e.g., touching the nurse's arm, wanting to hold hands or kiss nurse.	"Would you go out with me? . . . Why not?" or "Can I kiss you? . . . Why not?"	"I am *not* comfortable having you touch (kiss) me." The nurse briefly reiterates the nurse's role: "This time is for you to focus on your problems and concerns." If the client stops: "I wonder what this is about?" 1. Is the client afraid the nurse won't like him or her? 2. Is the client trying to take the focus off of problems? If the client continues: "If you can't cease this behavior, I'll have to leave. I'll be back at (time) to spend time with you then."	1. The nurse needs to set clear limits on expected behavior. 2. Frequently restating the nurse's role throughout the relationship can help maintain boundaries. 3. Whenever possible, the meaning of the client's behavior should be explored. 4. Leaving gives the client time to gain control. The nurse returns at the stated time.
Continues to arrive late for meetings.	"I'm a little late because (excuse)"	The nurse arrives on time and leaves at the scheduled time. (The nurse does not let the client manipulate him or her or bargain for more time.) After a couple of times, the nurse can explore behavior, e.g.: "I wonder if there is something going on you don't want to deal with?" or "I wonder what these latenesses mean to you?"	1. The nurse keeps the contract. Clients feel more secure when "promises" are kept, even though clients may try to manipulate the nurse through anger, helplessness, and so forth. 2. The nurse doesn't tell the client what to do, but nurse and client need to explore what the behavior is about.

4. More adaptive defenses
5. Accomplishment of goals
6. Impasse in therapy that the nurse is unable to resolve

In addition, forced termination may occur, such as when the student completes the course objectives. The **termination phase** is the final phase of the nurse-client relationship. Important reasons for the student to address the termination phase of the relationship have been identified (Phillips 1968):

1. Termination is a phase of the therapeutic nurse-client relationship, and without it the relationship remains incomplete.
2. Feelings are aroused in both the client and the student with regard to the experience they have had; when these feelings are recognized and shared, the client learns that it is acceptable to feel sadness and loss when someone he or she cares about leaves.
3. The client is a partner in the relationship and has a right to see the nurse's needs and feelings regarding their time together and the ensuing separation.
4. Termination can be a learning experience; the client can learn that he or she is important to at least one person.
5. By sharing the termination experience with the client, the nurse demonstrates caring for the client.

Termination often awakens strong feelings in both nurse and client. Termination of the relationship between the nurse and the client signifies a loss for both, although the intensity and meaning of termination may be different for each. If a client has unresolved feelings of abandonment or loneliness, or feelings of not being wanted or of being rejected by others, they may be reawakened during the termination process. The termination process can be an opportunity for the client to express these feelings, perhaps for the first time.

It is not unusual to see a variety of client behaviors that indicate defensive maneuvers against the anxiety of separation and loss. For example, a client may withdraw from the nurse and not want to meet for the final session or may become outwardly hostile and sarcastic, accusing the student nurse of using the client for his or her "own gains," like a "guinea pig," as a way of deflecting the awakening of anger and pain rooted in past separations. Often, a client will deny that the relationship had any impact or deny that ending the relationship evokes any emotions whatsoever. Regression is another behavioral manifestation; it may be seen in increased dependency on the nurse or in an increase in prior symptoms.

It is important for the student to work with the client to bring into awareness the feelings and reactions the client may be experiencing in relation to separations. If a client denies that the termination is having an effect (assuming the nurse-client relationship was strong), the student may say something like, "Good-byes are difficult for people. Often they remind us of other good-byes. Tell me about another separation in the past." If the client appears to be displacing anger, either by withdrawing or by displacing overt anger onto the nurse, the nurse may use generalized statements, such as, "People may experience anger when saying good-bye. Sometimes they are angry with the person who is leaving. Tell me about how you feel about me leaving." Students need to give thought to their last clinical experience with their client and to work with their instructor to facilitate communication during this time.

Summarizing the goals and objectives achieved in the relationship is part of the termination process. Reviewing situations that occurred during the time spent together and exchanging memories can help validate the experience for both nurse and client and facilitate closure of that relationship.

A common response students have is feeling guilty about terminating the relationship. These feelings may be manifested in students' giving the client their telephone number, making plans to get together for coffee after the client is discharged, continuing to see the client afterward, or exchanging letters. Students need to understand that such actions may be motivated by their own sense of guilt or misplaced feelings of responsibility, not by concern for the client. Indeed, part of the termination process may be to explore client plans for the future: where to go for help in the future, which agencies to contact, and which specific resource persons are available (e.g., social workers and job counselors).

During the student affiliation, the nurse-client relationship exists for the duration of the clinical course only. The termination phase is just that. Thoughts and feelings the student may have about continuing the relationship are best discussed with the instructor or shared in conference with peers, because these are common reactions to the student's experience.

Summary

Communication is a complex, reciprocal process. This chapter dealt with some of these complexities by discussing techniques that can enhance or hinder the communication process.

Berlo's communication model was reviewed, and the various components in this model were identified (stimulus, sender, message, medium, receiver, and feedback). Various personal and environmental factors that can impede accurate transmissions or interpretations of messages were listed, such as emotional factors, physical factors, intellectual factors, and social factors.

During nurse-client interactions, both verbal and nonverbal levels of communication exist. Communications also contain a *content* or subject dimension and a *process* dimension. Emphasis was placed on the nurse's ability to be aware of both levels to maximize communication and minimize the continuation of nonproductive behaviors on the part of the client.

Techniques that may enhance or hinder communications were presented. The student is urged to become familiar with these techniques, to be able to identify personal communication patterns, and to know when changes in responses may be appropriate.

The nurse-client relationship was discussed. Factors that differentiate a therapeutic relationship from a social relationship and an intimate relationship were outlined. Personal strengths in the nurse that can enhance growth in others—namely genuineness, empathy, and positive regard—were discussed, and examples were given.

Phases of the nurse-client relationship were presented: the orientation phase, the working phase, and the termination phase. The processes of transference and countertransference were defined. Basic guidelines for the first interview were discussed, and potential clinical situations were identified, with suggestions for nursing actions.

References

Alligood MR. Empathy: The importance of recognizing two types. Journal of Psychosocial Nursing, 30(3):15, 1992.

Berlo DK. The Process of Communication. San Francisco: Reinhart Press, 1960.

Bonnivien JF. A peer supervision group: Put countertransference to work. Journal of Psychosocial Nursing, 30(5):5, 1992.

Campaniello JA. The process of termination. Journal of Psychiatric Nursing and Mental Health Services, 18:29, 1980.

Collins M. Communication in Health Care: The Human Connection in the Life Cycle, 2nd ed. St. Louis: CV Mosby, 1983.

Egan, G. The Skilled Helper. Monterey, CA: Brooks/Cole, 1982.

Gass W. Learning to talk. University Magazine, 21, 1979.

Hagerty BK. Psychiatric-Mental Health Assessment. St. Louis: CV Mosby, 1984.

Hays JS, Larson KH. Interacting with Patients. New York: Macmillan Publishing Company, 1963.

Johnson B. The relationship between verbal patterns of nursing students and therapeutic effectiveness. Nursing Research, 13:339, 1964.

King IM. Toward a Theory for Nursing. New York: John Wiley & Sons, 1971.

LaMonica E. Validity of empathy instruments. Health, Education and Welfare Research Project Grant No. 5R01 NU00640 (December 1, 1977 through February 29, 1980).

MacKinnon RA, Michels R. The Psychiatric Interview in Clinical Practice. Philadelphia: WB Saunders, 1971.

Mauksch G, David M. Prescription for survival. American Journal of Nursing, 72:2189, 1972.

Moore JC, Hartman CR. Developing a therapeutic relationship. In Beck CK, Rawlins RP, Williams SR (eds). Mental Health-Psychiatric Nursing. St. Louis: CV Mosby, 1988.

Moscato B. The one-to-one relationship. In Wilson HS, Kneisel CS (eds). Psychiatric Nursing, 3rd ed. Menlo Park, CA: Addison-Wesley Publishing Company, 1988.

Nicholi AM. The therapist-patient relationship. In Nicholi AM (ed). The New Harvard Guide to Psychiatry. Cambridge, MA: The Belknap Press of Harvard University, 1988.

Peplau HE. Interpersonal Relations in Nursing. New York: New York: GP Putnam & Sons, 1952.

Peplau HE. Interpersonal techniques: The crux of psychiatric nursing. American Journal of Nursing, 62:50, 1962.

Phillips B. Terminating a nurse-patient relationship. American Journal of Nursing, 68(9):1941, 1968.

Richardson S, Dowhrenwend B, Klein D. Interviewing: Its Forms and Functions. New York: Basic Books, 1965.

Rogers CR (ed). The Therapeutic Relationship and Its Impact. Madison: University of Wisconsin Press, 1967.

Rogers CR, Truax CB. The therapeutic conditions antecedent to change: A theoretical view. In Rogers CR (ed). The Therapeutic Relationship and Its Impact. Madison: University of Wisconsin Press, 1967.

Sutherland J. The nature and evolution of phenomenological empathy in nursing: A historical treatment. Unpublished doctoral dissertation, University of Texas at Austin, 1985.

Shea SC. Psychiatric Interviewing: The Art of Understanding, Philadelphia: WB Saunders, 1988.

Schulman ED. Intervention in Human Services. St. Louis: CV Mosby, 1974.

Smitherman C. Nursing Action for Health Promotion. Philadelphia: FA Davis, 1982.

Further Reading

Hall ET. Excerpts from an interview conducted by Carol Travis. Geo, 25(3):12, 1983.

Haney W. Communication and Organizational Behavior. Chicago: Richard D. Irwin, 1967.

Lego S. Individual therapy. In Lego S (ed). The American Handbook of Psychiatric Nursing. Philadelphia: JB Lippincott, 1984, pp 197–205.

Parkinson MH. Therapeutic interaction. In Sorensen KC, Luckmann J. Basic Nursing: A Psychophysiologic Approach, 2nd ed. Philadelphia: WB Saunders, 1986.

Ushvendra K. Verbal responses for nurses to patients in emotional-laden situations in public health nursing. Nursing Research, 16:365, 1967.

Wahlous S. Family Communication. New York: Macmillan Publishing Company, 1974.

Wolberg L. The Technique of Psychotherapy. New York: Grune & Stratton, 1977.

Self-study Exercises

True or false

1. _____ A stimulant is the medium by which a message is sent.
2. _____ Feedback can indicate if a message has been correctly interpreted.
3. _____ Communication is a reciprocal process.
4. _____ Emotional factors, intellectual factors, and social factors play no part in accurate transmission or interpretation of communications.

5. _____ Content expressed in the nurse-client interaction refers to what the client has already spoken.

6. _____ Process messages that are expressed in the nurse-client interaction refer to nonverbal communications.

Place a V (verbal) or an N (nonverbal) next to the appropriate communication.

7. _____ Hair is uncombed and stringy; clothes have food stains.

8. _____ Person states that his body feels heavy.

9. _____ Person licks her lips and grimaces while talking to the nurse.

10. _____ Person writes the nurse a note before she leaves for the day.

Place a T (therapeutic) or an N (nontherapeutic) next to the appropriate communication and name the response.

11. _____ I know exactly how you feel. R _____

12. _____ I am not sure I understand what you mean. R _____

13. _____ I noticed you changed into a different dress this evening. R _____

14. _____ You should call the doctor and tell him these pills make R _____
you dizzy.

15. _____ Tell me more about your bad dream. R _____

16. _____ STUDENT: I had to repeat Nursing I, and for a long time
I felt like a failure.
TEACHER: That must have been very painful for you. R _____

17. _____ I observed several strengths that you bring to this difficult R _____
situation.

Place an S (social), an I (intimate), or a T (therapeutic) next to the corresponding behaviors.

18. _____ The relationship is initiated primarily for socialization, enjoyment, and friendship.

19. _____ The relationship is initiated between two people who have an emotional commitment to each other.

20. _____ Sharing ideas, feelings, and experiences is part of the relationship.

21. _____ The focus of the relationship is on the ideas, experiences, and feelings of just one party in the relationship.

22. _____ Content may be superficial; giving advice or meeting certain dependency needs may be appropriate.

23. _____ Evaluation of specific stated goals is ongoing within the life of the relationship.

24. _____ Mutual fantasies and goals that meet mutual needs are an integral part of the relationship.

25. _____ The relationship is equal (on the same level).

True or false

26. _____ Transference is the attribution (projection) of feelings, wishes, and attitudes originally thought and felt regarding significant others in the client's life to the nurse.

27. _____ It is important for the nurse to be tuned in to personal feelings when the nurse works with a client and to use these feelings to understand the client's experience better.

28. _____ Strong and intense (positive or negative) feelings in the nurse toward the client are referred to as countertransference feelings.

Write a short answer to the questions that follow:

29. You are spending time with a young woman who is depressed. She tells you she wants to kill herself. What two actions can you take?

30. You approach a middle-aged man, introduce yourself, and tell him your purpose and where you are from. When you mention to him that you would like to spend time with him, he looks down and does not respond. You become anxious. Name three actions you can take.

Place an O (orientation), a W (working), or a T (termination) next to the appropriate phase of the nurse-client relationship.

31. _____ Some regression and mourning may occur, although the client has reached a point of satisfaction, security, and competence in his or her life.
32. _____ The nurse assesses the client's level of psychological functioning, and both begin to identify problems and set realistic goals.
33. _____ The client begins to seek connections between actions, thoughts, and feelings; takes a more active role in problem solving; and tries out alternative coping behaviors.
34. _____ The nurse summarizes the objectives achieved in the relationship.

CHAPTER 7

Communication Within Groups

Catherine M. Lala

OUTLINE

KEY TERMS AND CONCEPTS

The key terms and concepts listed here also appear in bold where they are defined or discussed in this chapter.

ACTING OUT
BEHAVIORAL GROUP THERAPY
DIFFERENTIATION OF SELF
EGO STATES
FLOODING
GAMES
HETEROGENEOUS GROUP
HETEROGENEOUS TEAM GROUP
HOMOGENEOUS GROUP
INSIGHT

RESISTANCE
SCAPEGOAT
SCRIPTS
SELF-HELP GROUP
STROKES
SYSTEMATIC DESENSITIZATION
TRANSACTIONS
TRIANGLE
UNIVERSALITY

OBJECTIVES ■

After studying this chapter, the student will be able to

1. Define basic concepts used in group therapy.
2. Identify basic concepts of family therapy.
3. Describe the different roles group members may adopt within a group.
4. Discuss the approaches to group therapy for
   A. Psychoanalytically oriented groups
   B. Transactional analysis groups
   C. Therapeutic milieu groups
   D. Behavioral group therapy
   E. Self-help groups
   F. The family as a group
5. Compare and contrast the guidelines for establishing an inpatient versus an outpatient therapy group.
6. Name one behavior group members display in (a) the uncertainty phase, (b) the overaggressive phase, (c) the regression phase, and (d) the adaptation phase of group therapy.
7. Act out one intervention for a group member who
   A. Monopolizes a group
   B. Complains but rejects help
   C. Chronically helps others
8. Discuss three useful interventions a group leader would use when leading (a) a group for people with schizophrenia and (b) a group for people with a mental disorder and a substance abuse problem (dual diagnosis).

All humans, in order to live, strive for some personal connections in life. Infants are particularly sensitive to nonverbal behaviors, such as perceived tenderness in touch. As growing children master language, they interpret verbal and nonverbal behaviors according to the frame of reference used within the family. Language defines thought. As individuals mature through experiences with significant role models and peers, they become members of school, social, or work groups, which gives them a sense of belonging to the larger society. Failure, then, to experience positive group interactions leads to feelings of isolation and loneliness. Patients frequently use their experience in a group to help them find the way to resolve problems and to develop interpersonal skills, thereby increasing personal growth and fulfillment, and perhaps to redefine a satisfying emotional connection with others (Clarke 1993).

However, many people are reluctant to join therapy groups and are initially fearful of being judged or of revealing personal information. Yalom (1983) states that "patients often enter therapy with the disquieting feeling that their misery is unique or that they alone have certain frightening or unacceptable impulses or fantasies." In the group, patients hear others share similar concerns, fantasies, and life experiences. The disconfirmation of the feeling of uniqueness offers considerable relief and a "welcome-to-the-human-race" experience. This concept is the curative factor of **universality.** Universality is one of 10 curative factors of group therapy described by Yalom (1985) that can guide therapeutic interventions. Yalom's other curative factors of group therapy are

1. **Imparting of information.** Some groups, such as Alcoholics Anonymous or psychotherapy groups, help members learn about their symptoms, their interpersonal dynamics, and how working through problems in a trusting atmosphere leads to growth as an adult or individual.
2. **Instillation of hope.** Groups can instill hope in patients who are demoralized or pessimistic. Group members can gain hope from others with similar problems who have made positive changes in their lives through therapy.
3. **Altruism.** Learning that they can be useful to others leads members to value themselves more, prevents morbid self-absorption, and promotes self-growth.
4. **Corrective recapitulation of the primary family group.** The member is influenced in the group by his or her history. For example, the patient initially

perceives the behavior of other members as being like that of the patient's siblings and the behavior of the group leader as being like that of the patient's parents. When neither the members nor the leader responds as siblings or parents have in the past, the patient begins to gain insight into his or her own behavior (Naegle 1993). Through feedback and exploration, early conflicts can be resolved and growth can then take place.

5. **Development of socializing skills.** Group members can develop new socializing skills and can learn to correct maladaptive behavior through ongoing group interactions.

6. **Imitative behavior.** Imitative behavior is a powerful therapeutic tool through which a patient identifies with the healthier aspects of the other group members or the leader and learns to imitate behaviors the patient wishes to develop (Wolfe 1993).

7. **Interpersonal learning.** Interpersonal learning in the group experience is gradually transferred to other situations in the person's life outside the group.

8. **Group cohesiveness.** This relates to bonding or solidarity of the group members, the feelings of "we" instead of "I," and that members are of value to each other. Cohesiveness is shown by regular group attendance and the ability to communicate a full range of feelings (e.g., anger to joy) without the group's disintegrating.

9. **Catharsis.** Catharsis is the expression of feelings in a nonthreatening atmosphere, particularly intense negative as well as positive emotions.

Psychiatric nurses have many opportunities for observation and intervention. In primary psychiatric nursing, the nurse-patient relationship is the cornerstone of all therapeutic nursing interactions. Within a group setting, the nurse observes, interprets, and facilitates the patient's relationships with others. The nurse-patient relationship often affects a client's motivation and ability to feel safe in any kind of group. The experience in group therapy can motivate patients to continue in outpatient treatment.

The Nurse as a Group Educator

Nurses can teach groups of patients about managing chronic illness or specific rehabilitation or about preventive health care. Some examples of group teaching in a community setting are conducting seminars on nutrition for senior citizens or stress management seminars, or organizing an exercise program. Many wellness programs directed and coordinated by nurses are an opportunity for increased nursing visibility in the community. Many facilities welcome new speakers and opportunities for new knowledge for their participants. With the increasing cost of health care, groups can be seen as an economical solution to health care, as well as an opportunity to decrease social isolation.

The Nurse as a Group Therapist

Nurses began to develop a role as leaders of group therapy in the 1960s (Armstrong and Rouslin 1963). Peplau believes that as group therapists, nurses should function along with other health professionals, such as psychiatric social workers, psychologists, and psychiatrists, in the role of group psychotherapist.

Individuals conducting group psychotherapy need specific education and experience. For nursing, the American Nurses' Association (ANA) sets the standard of graduate study, which includes the necessary theory, supervision, and clinical practice. On the bachelor's and associate's levels, nurses need to have an understanding of group therapy and process and may be actively involved in leading therapeutic groups.

Training through college courses, workshops, and ongoing clinical supervision is essential. Psychiatric clinical specialists can serve as role models and mentors for nurses desiring to learn about many types of groups. Group therapy always uses a theoretical base; this base is one that the leader believes in and is educated in.

Nurse group therapists need to have individual or peer-group supervision. In supervision, the nurse reviews the process of therapy with a more experienced therapist or with peers. Group work provides a rich learning environment. All psychotherapeutic work with patients, whether it is individual, couple, family, child, group, or any other type of psychotherapy, requires interpersonal learning with a senior clinician trained in that particular therapy (Critchley and Maurin 1985). Supervision is a relationship between supervisor and supervisee that helps the supervisee become more therapeutic. The ANA's Standards of Psychiatric and Mental Health Nursing Practice states that "the nurse participates in peer review and other means of evaluation to assure quality of nursing care provided by nurses for clients." Clinical supervision should be ongoing throughout the nurse's experience as a group leader.

THE NURSE AS COTHERAPIST

The use of a cotherapist can benefit the beginning group therapist: for example, a cotherapist may be helpful for handling escalating anger, when a patient decides to leave the group, or when a patient threatens to commit suicide. It is advantageous for the therapist and cotherapist to discuss their theoretical frameworks beforehand to establish if the frameworks are the same or compatible.

The cotherapists need to communicate about the group process and content as often as the group meets, both before and after each group session. Both therapists need to be aware of their reactions to each other. Feelings of competition or disagreement concerning interventions often emerge.

Feeling of Therapist	Possible Therapist Behavior	Improved Therapeutic Behavior
1. Feels left out, not understanding where the cotherapist is "leading" a patient.	1. Begins to tell group members personal information.	1. Clarifies with the other therapist his or her confusion. Provides a model for other patients.
2. Has the same problem as a group member.	2. Asks the cotherapist in the group for a solution.	2. Works through the problem in own supervision, joins therapy group on the outside.

Basic Concepts of Groups

Groups are based on different models and theoretical orientations. However, they have in common the following (Morgan 1973):

1. *Group acceptance.* Individuals feel they are respected, accepted by, and belong to the group.
2. *Reality testing.* Group members can monitor each person's reactions and behaviors, providing feedback in an open and nonthreatening manner.
3. *Universality.* Group members feel secure when they realize that they do not have unique problems and are not so different from other persons.
4. *Ventilation.* Group therapy provides an opportunity for ventilation of various emotions that would otherwise remain bottled up.

5. *Intellectualization.* Members gain insight into their problems by learning to examine or explore symptoms in themselves, as well as in other group members.
6. *Altruism.* Members give advice, support, and encouragement to one another.
7. *Transference.* The individual develops an emotional attachment to another person, such as the therapist or members of the group.
8. *Interactions.* Group therapy provides group members with the opportunity to assert themselves to improve communication skills with others outside the group.

Basic Roles of Group Members

The following are some roles that individuals adopt when participating in a group. Each member may adopt more than one role.

- Opinion giver—states beliefs or values
- Opinion seeker—asks for clarification of beliefs or values
- Information giver—offers facts or personal experience
- Information seeker—asks for facts pertinent to what is being discussed
- Initiator—proposes new ideas on how the goal can be reached or how to view the problem
- Elaborator—expands on the idea of another; takes the idea and works out what would happen if it was adopted
- Coordinator—brings together ideas and suggestions
- Orientor—keeps the group focused on goals or questions the direction taken by the group
- Evaluator or critic—examines possible group solutions against group standards and goals
- Clarifier—checks out what someone said by restating or questioning
- Recorder—acts as the group's memory (e.g., takes notes)
- Summarizer—pulls together related ideas, restates suggestions, and offers decisions or conclusions

Box 7–1 identifies terminology central to group work.

Box 7-1. TERMS CENTRAL TO GROUP WORK

Group content—all that is said in the group

Group process—constant movement as members seek to reduce tensions that arise when people attempt to have their individual needs met while working to meet group goals; also includes all nonverbal behavior, such as yawning, facial expressions, and body posture.

Confrontation—the process whereby problems or conflicts that have been covert are brought into the open

Covert content—the deeper, underlying meaning of messages or what is happening in the group

Closed group—membership is restricted; no new members are added when others leave

Dynamics—the ebb and flow of power and energy within a group

Feedback—letting group members know how they affect each other

Hidden agenda—individual, subgroup, or leader goals that are at cross-purposes to the group's goals

Cohesiveness—the bond between members of a group, measured by the group's willingness to work toward common goals; members' sense of identification with the group

Conflict—open disagreement among members; may be positive, indicating involvement with the task, or negative, indicating frustration with an impossible task or intergroup conflict

Open group—a group in which new members are added as others leave

Subgroup—an individual or a small group that is isolated within a larger group and functions separately; members of a subgroup may have more loyalty, similar goals, or perceived similarities to one another than they do to the larger group

Types of Groups and Group Therapies

At present, there are many approaches to the group therapy method of treatment. Major types of groups and group therapies include

1. Psychoanalytically oriented group psychotherapy
2. Transactional analysis group therapy
3. Therapeutic milieu groups
4. Behavioral group therapy
5. Self-help groups
6. The family as a group

Other groups include problem-solving groups and children's groups. These last two are not covered in this chapter.

PSYCHOANALYTICALLY ORIENTED GROUP PSYCHOTHERAPY

The premise underlying psychoanalytical group psychotherapy is that early interactions are believed to play a part in problems people have as adults. According to psychoanalytical theory, there must be a healthy balance between the id, ego, and superego if an individual is to achieve satisfaction and competence in the areas of activity, work, play, and personal relationships.

Therapists use a variety of concepts in psychoanalytical work. Important concepts include (1) transference, (2) countertransference, (3) resistance, (4) acting out, and (5) insight. Transference and countertransference were introduced in Chapter 6, pages 133 to 136. Resistance, acting out, and insight are discussed in the following paragraphs.

Resistance is the unconscious use of thoughts, feelings, or behaviors that help clients avoid changing their view of reality. "A member of the group who does not accept the group in the first place . . . may simply walk out when things get unpleasant, not show up for sessions, or consistently come late to group" (Edelwich and Brodsky 1992).

Acting out occurs when unconscious wishes, needs, conflicts, and feelings are expressed in actions rather than words. For example, a woman who is married to a controlling husband may act out her unconscious anger toward her husband by entering into an extramarital affair.

Insight occurs when the patient connects unconscious feelings, wishes, and conflicts to conscious behavior. An experience of emotional understanding can change both behaviors and underlying feelings.

Table 7–1 ■ PSYCHOANALYTICAL GROUP THERAPY			
TARGET POPULATION	**GOALS**	**THERAPIST'S ACTIVITY**	**FREQUENCY AND DURATION**
People with • Anxiety disorders • Conversion disorders • Dysthymia • Behavioral problems (e.g., overeating, drinking, and smoking) • Relationship problems • Features of borderline personality disorder	*Overall goal:* Reconstruction of personality dynamics 1. Remove, modify, or retard existing symptoms 2. Mediate disturbed patterns of behavior 3. Promote positive personality growth and behavior	1. Challenges defenses 2. Interprets unconscious conflicts and dreams 3. Makes use of transference and countertransference phenomena	*Meets:* 1–3 times per week *For:* 1–3 or more years

The role of the therapist is to stimulate group interaction and group analysis of the interaction. The therapist does not do anything for the group members that they can do for themselves. The group leader helps make group members aware of defensive ways in which individual group members function and helps move patients toward emotional insight by "poking and prodding" at their defense mechanisms. In a psychoanalytical therapy group, members may be in individual therapy with the leader. Basic overall goals for psychoanalytical group therapy, as shown in Table 7–1, are (Wolberg 1977)

- To remove, modify, or retard existing symptoms
- To mediate disturbed patterns of behavior
- To promote positive personality growth and behavior

TRANSACTIONAL ANALYSIS GROUP THERAPY

Eric Berne, MD, developed the group modality of transactional analysis (TA), which is a unified, systematic, and observable theory of personality and social dynamics that incorporates concepts from psychoanalysis and ego psychology. TA is a method of examining the interactions between people that organizes information derived from analyzing interpersonal transactions. TA uses specific words that have the same meaning for everyone who is using them. This use of specific words or language is clearly one of the most important components of the system. According to TA enthusiasts, agreement on the meanings of words and agreement on what to examine are the two keys that have unlocked the door to the mysteries of why people do what they do (Harris 1969).

Concepts used in TA include (1) ego states, (2) transactions, (3) strokes, (4) games, and (5) scripts.

Ego states refer to parts of the personality identified by consistent feelings and behavior patterns.

These ego states consist of the parent, the child, and the adult. Essentially, the child represents the (archaic) elements of the personality that are fixed in early childhood. The adult is the part of the personality that objectively appraises reality. Finally, the parent is the part of the personality that reflects the client's parents' values (Kaplan and Sadock 1991). Table 7–2 gives examples of ego states.

Transactions are the stimuli from one person that produce responses in another. For example, a husband tells his wife that he wishes she would keep the house in better order.

Strokes show recognition of a person, either through touch or verbalizations. Recognition is a basic human need and a way to validate an individual's existence. Strokes are based on a need for affirmation from another to prevent sensory or emotional deprivation. A person may elicit strokes through various behaviors such as withdrawal, rituals, activities, games, or intimacy. The order of these behaviors indicates increasing interpersonal involvement and therefore an increase in the stroke value (Berne 1966). Strokes can be either positive, negative, conditional, or unconditional. They are conditional when something is done in order to receive them and unconditional when the person receives them for just being.

Games are series of repetitive and stereotyped transactions with hidden messages directed toward another person's weakness. They result in a negative stroke (payoff) for the player.

Scripts are ways of living that were prescribed by early parental influence. These messages of "how to be" or "how not to be" result in feelings of being "OK" or "not OK" (Goulding et al. 1979).

In TA groups, data are collected by the group leader during the group treatment session (Table 7–3). The leader helps members analyze the data so that they can recognize "game playing" and how they employ their various ego states (parent, adult, and child) and thereby learn to take responsibility for themselves.

Table 7–2 ■ THE EGO STATES OF TRANSACTIONAL ANALYSIS

PARENT	ADULT	CHILD
Definition		
Attitudes, beliefs, and behaviors learned as a child from parents, or parental messages continuing in the client's mind	Objective, rational, and realistic behaviors that deal with facts	Impulses, basic needs, desires, and feelings learned as a child and acted out in the here-and-now
Functions		
Sets limits, preaches, teaches, protects, supports, reassures self and others; may be *nurturing* or *critical*	Solves problems, weighs possibilities and probabilities, based on past and present experiences; is always *rational*	Acts intuitively; experiences intimacy, pleasure, pain, and other feelings
Decisions		
Imitative	Informed	Impulsive
Statements		
"You should"; "I'll never"	"I think"; "I figure"	"I want"; "I can't"

From Craig J, Kirkpatrick T. Transactional analysis. In Lego S (ed). The American Handbook of Psychiatric Nursing. Philadelphia: JB Lippincott, 1984.

The therapist bases his or her interventions on the premise that the patient has a built-in drive toward health, mental as well as physical. The therapist's task is to locate the healthy areas in each person's personality, to nurture them, and to strengthen their potential. The therapist does not cure anyone but rather works with group members to facilitate the desired change (Berne 1966).

The therapist strives toward (McNeel 1977)

- Fostering a nurturing environment where learning and changing are fun

- Modeling in actions and words the philosophy and values of the theoretical model

- Helping individuals claim power and take control of and responsibility for their choices

THERAPEUTIC MILIEU GROUPS

Therapeutic milieu groups aim to help increase patients' self-esteem, decrease social isolation, encourage appropriate social behaviors, and re-educate patients in basic living skills. These groups are often led by occupational or recreational therapists, although nurses frequently colead such groups. Examples include recreational, creative arts, and self-care groups (Table 7–4).

Recreational Groups. Recreational groups focus on teamwork, learning how to spend leisure time, and increasing self-esteem by completing a project. Nostalgia groups encourage patients to talk about earlier years and about the good things in life. Exercise groups let patients experience physical and psychological release through physical exercise and games.

Table 7–3 ■ TRANSACTIONAL ANALYSIS GROUP THERAPY

TARGET POPULATION	GOALS	THERAPIST'S ACTIVITY	FREQUENCY AND DURATION
People with • Anxiety disorders • Conversion disorders • Dysthymia • Behavioral problems (e.g., overeating, drinking, and smoking) • Relationship problems	*Overall goal:* Alteration of behavior through conscious control 1. Alter a behavior or way of thinking that is causing difficulty in living *and/or* 2. Alter old internal conflicts and distortions 3. Help individuals take responsibility for their choices	1. Challenges defenses 2. Gives personal responses rather than advice 3. Teaches clients to recognize ego states (child, parent, adult) during transactions, games, and scripts	*Meets:* 1–3 times per week *For:* 1–3 years

	Table 7-4 ■ **THERAPEUTIC MILIEU GROUPS**		
MILIEU GROUPS	**TARGET POPULATION**	**GOALS**	**FREQUENCY AND DURATION**
Activity groups (hospital) • Recreational: current events, nostalgia, exercise, horticulture, pets, crafts • Self-care: reality, cooking, grooming, discharge group, community meeting • Creative arts: art, dance/movement, poetry, psychodrama, music, bibliotherapy • Self-awareness: feeling, men's group, women's group • Education: stress reduction, skills training, medication groups, assertiveness training, ways to increase self-esteem	The psychiatric patient in the hospital or in a day treatment program	*Overall goal:* Increase in self-esteem 1. Help patients manage time 2. Increase cooperation 3. Teach specific knowledge, skills, or both related to patient's illness, treatment, or interpersonal communication (psychoeducational)	*Meets:* Once per week or more, often depending on the program

Creative Arts Groups. The goal of creative arts therapy is for patients to get in touch with feelings and emotions through books, poems, music, and dance. Dance therapy, art therapy, and music therapy are helpful to patients who are demonstrating withdrawn behaviors and are not amenable to "talk" therapy. These groups are led by specially trained therapists.

Self-Care Groups. Examples of self-care groups include cooking groups, activities of daily living or grooming groups, medication groups, and client government groups. These types of groups educate patients and provide an opportunity for staff members to assess a patient's ability to function in areas such as planning, budgeting, and basic skills needed for living. Psychiatric nurses are the ideal professionals to teach in a medication education group for long term self-management care. Sharing a concrete and objective "here-and-now" subject such as medication information in a group setting can also facilitate discussion of feelings of stigmatization, alienation, helplessness, and loss of self-control (Kuipers et al. 1988).

BEHAVIORAL GROUP THERAPY

Behavioral group therapy can help members of a group to eliminate certain undesirable behaviors. This type of group is led by a professional trained in behavioral therapy. The group is generally homogeneous (e.g., clients have the same phobias or the same compulsions). Behavioral therapy seeks to bring about change by altering the client's environment or the client's response to the environment.

The principles of behavioral therapy are guided by the tenets of behavioral theory. According to behavioral theorists, (1) the frequency of a specific behavior is influenced by a negative stimulus, a positive stimulus, or both, (2) events are associated when they occur together, and (3) through teaching and role-modeling, new behaviors can be learned.

During behavioral group therapy, basic behavioral techniques such as systematic desensitization or other anxiety-reducing behaviors such as flooding are used. (Refer back to Chapter 2 for other behavioral therapy techniques.)

Systematic desensitization involves having a patient gradually approach the feared object or situation while the patient is in a state of relaxation. **Flooding** is the process of saturating the patient with the anxiety-producing experience, without allowing the patient to escape. This causes the patient to experience the anxiety, and usually within five to 20 minutes, the anxiety decreases.

During behavioral group therapy, clients discuss each person's problems, such as phobia, and how they interfere with the quality of life. Each week, at the end of the session, the therapist gives clients individual homework assignments designed to help them overcome their undesirable behaviors. Clients are expected to complete their assignments and to report the results the following week. The homework begins with small, easy steps and progressively becomes more difficult.

An example of desensitization in a group in which all members have a fear of elevators would start with the leader talking group members through an imagined elevator ride. Next, the leader would walk them

Table 7–5 ■ BEHAVIORAL GROUP THERAPY			
TARGET POPULATION	**GOALS**	**THERAPIST'S ACTIVITY**	**FREQUENCY AND DURATION**
People with specific symptoms they want to modify, e.g.: • Phobias • Sexual problems • Passivity • Smoking • Overeating	*Overall goal:* Relief of a specific symptom or change in a specific behavior	1. Works to create new defenses 2. Uses an active and directive approach 3. Uses techniques of behavioral modification	*Meets:* 1–3 times per week *For:* 6–12 sessions or more

to the elevator, and the next step would be getting into the elevator. A subsequent step would be having the door close and immediately reopen, and then allowing clients to get out. Eventually, they would ride the elevator up one floor, then up several floors.

During these short, progressive steps, the group members would be encouraged to use stress reduction techniques throughout the experience. Group support and encouragement are important aspects of behavioral group therapy (Table 7–5).

SELF-HELP GROUPS

Self-help groups are based on the premise that people who have experienced a particular problem are able to help others who have the same problem. Nurses may serve as resource persons for these groups and need to be aware of the many self-help groups available in order to refer clients. Self-help groups consist of persons who have a common problem, and individuals learn that they are not alone in having a particular problem. These groups provide members with support, and members may help others by telling their stories and providing alternative ways to both view and tackle problems.

A prototype for many self-help groups is the 12-step program developed by Alcoholics Anonymous (AA). The first step is admitting that one has a problem (e.g., alcohol or drug abuse, overeating, or gambling). The first meeting is an open or general meeting at which several members tell their stories. Later, clients go to small group discussion meetings, which are at a more intimate level, and members work through more of the 12 steps. Refer to Chapter 23 for the 12 steps of AA. A key element of self-help groups is mutual support. In AA, members may choose a sponsor on whom they can call if they feel compelled to drink.

AA is supportive in nature, and the goal is to maintain sobriety through group support, shared experiences, and faith in a power greater than themselves. AA and groups patterned after AA (e.g., Narcotics

Anonymous and Overeaters Anonymous) are led by group members. Often, one member makes a presentation and other members share their experiences. To acknowledge one's experience verbally is to "take ownership" of a problem. In a study done by Sheeren (1988), recovering alcoholic members of AA were asked to complete a questionnaire to assess the occurrence of relapse and its correlation to their level of involvement in the AA program. The findings showed that the greater the member involvement in AA, the lower the chance for relapse to occur. The most significant area of involvement was in reaching out to other members of AA for help and making use of a sponsor (Sheeren 1988). Self-help groups such as these are spreading rapidly, and new ones are constantly being formed.

Not all self-help groups use the 12-step method, but all support groups are organized around one particular problem or crisis that has been experienced by all members of that group. A nurse may be included as a group member and be asked to speak as a resource person, but unless the nurse has personally overcome the problem group members have, the nurse would not be asked to lead the group.

Strategies employed by group leaders include promoting dialogue, self-disclosure, and encouragement among members (Kane et al. 1990). Concepts used in support groups include psychoeducation, self-disclosure, and mutual support. These groups can also (1) prevent physical, emotional, or social health problems, (2) improve an individual's or a family's quality of life, and (3) provide education necessary to further develop the member's potential.

Clinical Example
Bob and Jill, a married couple, are having difficulty conceiving a child. Their infertility is affecting their marriage, and they are depressed and angry. They begin to attend a RESOLVE group in which everyone is having the same difficulty. Through the group process, they explore their options for having children or living child-free. Bob and Jill realize they are not alone,

	Table 7-6 ■ SELF-HELP GROUP THERAPY		
TARGET POPULATION	**GOALS**	**THERAPIST'S ACTIVITY**	**FREQUENCY AND DURATION**
People who have experienced a common tragedy, crisis, illness, or self-destructive behavior, e.g.: *Support groups* • Bereavement: for those who have experienced the loss of a loved one • Rape: for those who have been raped • Cancer: for those families and patients coping with the ramifications of cancer and its treatment • RESOLVE: for couples experiencing infertility *Self-help groups* • Alcoholics Anonymous (AA) —the prototype • Gamblers Anonymous (GA) • Overeaters Anonymous (OA) • Narcotics Anonymous (NA) • Co-Dependents Anonymous	*Overall goal:* Provision of support and encouragement of positive coping behaviors 1. Decrease feelings of isolation 2. Provide mutual support 3. Provide psychoeducation and health education 4. Reduce stress 5. Help people cease self-destructive behaviors or come to terms with an overwhelming event or situation	1. May or may not have a specific leader 2. Strengthens existing defenses 3. Is actively involved in the group process 4. Provides information to educate and give direction	*Meets:* Once or more per week *For:* Indefinite period of time, ongoing and open membership

and through the group, they gain insights that help them deal with their anger and depression.

Two examples of groups initiated by nurses include a support group for parents who have a child with a terminal illness or who had a child who died and one for anorexics (Staples et al. 1990). Other self-help groups or support groups include Weight Watchers, Parents Without Partners, and the National Alliance for the Mentally Ill. Characteristics of these groups are peer support, group teaching, counseling, and using shared experiences (Table 7–6).

THE FAMILY AS A GROUP

The family differs from other therapeutic groups in that a family is a naturally formed group. The traditional family is the nuclear family, whose members are related by blood or marriage. Today's society is broadening the concept of family to include those a person lives with, such as same-gender parents. The family is looked on as a unit, an emotional system. Individual problems are often viewed as by-products of the family system. The main goal of family therapy is to change the dysfunctional patterns in the family system into more functional patterns, thereby improv-

ing the functioning and quality of life for all members of the system. The "sick" member or the "identified patient" is thought to be the one who "signals" that a family is in crisis or dysfunctional. Groups and families have many similar dynamics. The approach and aims of family therapy are often similar to those of group therapy. Family therapy is ideally done in the home.

Family therapists employ a variety of therapeutic styles. In general, all family therapists define and clarify the relationship between the spouses and relationships between generations. The family therapist is someone with specific family therapy training. Family therapists come from a variety of disciplines and base their clinical work on any given number of theorists. For example, system theorists, such as Murray Bowen, view the family as consisting of emotional and relationship systems (Jones 1980); structural theorists describe the family as an open system governed by a set of invisible rules or laws that evolve over a period of time (Minuchin 1974); and interactionalists study the behavior and communication patterns among and between family members (Haley 1976; Satir 1984). Certain phenomena seem to occur within families.

A **triangle** is the dynamic equilibrium of a three-person system influenced by anxiety. If anxiety is low, a relationship between two people can be calm and comfortable. When anxiety or conflict is high, a third person becomes involved in the tension of the twosome, creating a triangle (Kerr and Bowen 1988). An example of a triangle is when a married couple contemplating divorce ask their 13-year-old daughter for her opinions on how to solve their problems.

Differentiation of self is the amount of independent emotional and intellectual functioning in a person. Defining one's own values and beliefs, without fluctuating in times of stress, is taking an "I" position. For example, a married woman with two children in college desires to return to school, even though she is afraid her husband, who is extremely controlling, will become angry with her.

A **scapegoat** is often the child who acts out the family's dysfunction. The scapegoat's difficult behavior may help keep the family together (Barker 1992). The scapegoat may be seen first, but family therapy may be called for. An example of a scapegoat is a kindergarten-age boy who will not join in play activities. Further investigation reveals that his parents have been fighting almost daily and are talking about divorce.

Family Therapy in Recovery from Alcoholism. Clinical reports and research studies have begun to direct increased attention toward the importance of the family's involvement in successful rehabilitation from alcoholism. With alcoholism identified as a family illness, clinicians indicate that recovery is partially contingent on a family's ability to renegotiate patterns of interacting and functioning without alcohol. The degree to which a family is able to make these necessary adjustments may determine the extent to which rehabilitation will be maintained by the alcoholic. Moreover, it may have a bearing on the health and survival of the entire family system (Captain 1989).

Family therapy for all recovering families is not a realistic goal. Captain (1989) states that if a family is not motivated or has limited financial resources, family therapy is not an option. In this case, family-centered nursing services are more appropriate and necessary. "The nurse can . . . assume multiple roles using the nursing process as the framework for intervention." The family is seen as a system. Change in one member of the family system means another member needs to change in order to keep the family together. The family can evolve toward healthier behaviors.

Multiple-Family Group Therapy. Multiple-family group therapy is often used in an inpatient setting in which several families meet as a group with one or more therapists (Table 7–7). This allows communication to take place among several families, and often a member of one family who is uninvolved in another family's emotional system can observe patterns in that other family. This person also feels more free to state these observations. Families can identify with other families and their problems and can recognize maladaptive behavior. Often, family members may see their own problems reflected in the problems of other families. The common fears, anger, resentment, and guilt experienced in each family are perceived and shared with others (Lacquer 1972).

Establishing a Psychotherapy Group

This section discusses general guidelines for starting a psychotherapy group, as well as specifics for establishing inpatient and outpatient groups.

	Table 7–7 ■ MULTIPLE-FAMILY GROUP THERAPY		
TARGET POPULATION	**GOALS**	**THERAPIST'S ACTIVITY**	**FREQUENCY AND DURATION**
Families with a hospitalized family member	*Overall goal:* Improvement in family functioning 1. Understand that the "patient's" problem not only affects the family but is often precipitated and perpetuated by the family 2. Improve patient and family communication 3. Increase awareness of the interaction and communication occurring in the family 4. Clarify family roles	1. Creates a supportive milieu for therapy: a nonjudgmental atmosphere, stimulation and expression of pathology, encouragement of verbalization, and reality testing 2. Provides a role model for constructive interaction 3. Attempts to develop introspection in the family by • Examining how members of the group relate • Encouraging alternatives • Resolving how to continue working within the group	*Meets:* Once per week as long as the family member is hospitalized and one month or more after discharge

GENERAL GUIDELINES

The ideal number of patients in a psychotherapy group is seven to 10. More than 10 members is not recommended because the group will subdivide, which will be counterproductive. Too large a group can also create more opportunities for acting out as opposed to working through.

Members should vary in age, gender, race, and psychodynamics. The presence of both male and female members helps members work through personal issues with persons of both genders. People have different personalities and coping styles, which helps members "try on" another member's way of dealing with an issue. Groups that have a mixture of personalities, coping styles, and pychodynamics are often referred to as **heterogeneous groups.** There is a trend in some areas to have all-women's or all-men's groups. These groups focus on unique gender-specific issues.

Types of patients who should not be included in psychotherapy groups include acutely psychotic persons, persons with antisocial personality disorder, those experiencing drug or alcohol withdrawal, those who are actively using drugs or alcohol, and those who are violent. However, schizophrenic patients can greatly benefit from particular modes of group therapy. Persons diagnosed with antisocial personality disorder should not be included in groups because they are often disruptive to a psychotherapy group and are unable to relate in a way helpful to themselves or others (Lego 1984). There are, however, special groups that may benefit people with antisocial traits. Other groups are effective for schizophrenics and people with addictions. These groups are discussed later.

Group therapy may take place in an inpatient or an outpatient setting. Table 7–8 outlines the basic differences between inpatient and outpatient group therapy.

ESTABLISHING AN INPATIENT GROUP

One popular method of structuring an inpatient therapy group is by focusing on the here-and-now (Yalom 1985). The group therapist should

1. Provide instruction about the relevance of the here-and-now. Begin with a brief orientation for

---

Table 7–8 ■ DIFFERENCES BETWEEN OUTPATIENT AND INPATIENT GROUP THERAPY

OUTPATIENT GROUPS	INPATIENT GROUPS
1. The group has a stable composition.	1. The group is rarely the same for more than one or two meetings.
2. Patients are carefully selected and prepared.	2. Patients are admitted to the group with little prior selection or preparation.
3. The group is homogeneous regarding ego function, although conflicts and issues differ.	3. The group has a heterogeneous level of ego functioning.
4. Motivated, self-referred patients make up the group; therapy is growth orientated.	4. Patients are ambivalent, often there because they are in crisis and therapy is compulsory; therapy is relief oriented.
5. Treatment proceeds as long as required: 1–2 years, 50–100 meetings.	5. Treatment is limited to the hospital period: 1–3 weeks, with rapid patient turnover.
6. The boundary of the group is well maintained, with few external influences.	6. Continuous boundary interface with the milieu occurs.
7. Group cohesion develops normally, given sufficient time in treatment.	7. There is no time for cohesion to develop spontaneously; group development is aborted at an early stage.
8. Therapy is private.	8. Patients are open to observation and scrutiny by the milieu.
9. The leader allows the process to unfold; there is ample time to set group norms.	9. The group leader's structuring of the group is critical; passive analytical approaches lead to group disintegration.
10. No extragroup contact is encouraged.	10. Patients sleep, eat, and live together outside of the group; extragroup contact is endorsed.

From Leszcz M. Inpatient groups. In Frances AJ, Aoles RE (eds). Psychiatric Update, Volume 5. Washington, DC: American Psychiatric Press, 1986.

new patients: state that patients enter the hospital for different reasons and that everyone can benefit from examining how he or she relates to other people. Group members and the therapist or therapists provide feedback. Members have important and painful problems other than interpersonal ones, but given the often short duration of inpatient hospitalizations, these problems may need to be addressed more in individual therapy.

2. Provide spatial boundaries. No table is used. The group meets in the same place each time.

3. Start and end the session on time. Encourage patients and other therapists not to interfere with group time. Obtain administrative support.

4. Encourage patients to stay, but do not lock the door. If a patient attempts to leave, ask him or her what is going on. Try to connect the behavior to a feeling. For example, a patient who stated the day before that she isolates herself when she is feeling depressed will need encouragement to stay. If the patient still leaves, follow up with the patient after the group therapy session.

5. Be directive and decisive. For example, if a manic person monopolizes the group, tell the patient to stop talking and to listen to others.

6. If a patient threatens to act out physically (e.g., by striking somebody), tell the patient, "You may talk about your anger, but you cannot act on it in this group." Get help if the patient becomes increasingly threatening, and escort the patient from the room. Follow up after the group session, and do not allow the patient back until the reason for the threatening behavior has been explored with the patient's primary therapist.

An example of a basic protocol for an inpatient group could be:

1. Orientation or preparation (3–5 minutes)
2. Agenda go round—each member offers a personal agenda for the meeting (20–30 minutes)
3. Agenda "fitting"—the therapist tries to fit agendas together
4. Review

In many inpatient settings, the group leader is often not the client's primary therapist. Information is obtained from the patient, the primary therapist, and the chart. The nurse should keep in mind that the patient's ease in communicating in the group setting is often based heavily on his or her feelings of comfort with the group leader.

Many patients have difficulty understanding that group therapy is indeed therapy, and they tend to feel that they need more individual therapy. If the nurse therapist encounters this attitude, it is helpful to acknowledge that it is not unusual for the patient to feel this way and that the patient may be concerned about revealing information, experiencing rejection, or reliving a humiliating group experience. It is helpful to remind patients of the confidentiality of anything discussed in group therapy in order to build trust.

The nurse should encourage patients to discuss individual group issues with their therapists. If the patient brings up any issues in group therapy that impact on his or her safety, such as suicide, the nurse must discuss this with the patient's therapist, the treatment team, or both.

It is often of little value for the patient or the group for the nurse to mandate patient attendance or for the patient to use group therapy as a means of gaining a privilege, such as to obtain a day pass. Patients must take responsibility for their own needs. Better-functioning patients will attend a group session with regularity if it is run effectively and if the entire staff values group sessions and encourages patients. Yalom (1983) states that "patients who are . . . sincerely interested in doing something about their mental health gradually assimilate the ward values and soon have a difficult time justifying to themselves their failure to attend." Yalom advocates mandatory attendance on inpatient units for heterogeneous team groups and homogeneous groups. "The clinical facts of life are that if these groups were not mandatory, a significant proportion of patients would not attend. Patients who are withdrawn, frightened, depressed, hopeless, or drowsy because of medication would, if given a choice, opt to remain in their rooms, and an effective ward program would not be feasible" (Yalom 1983).

A modification of group psychotherapy is therapy with the **heterogeneous team group.** A heterogeneous team group is one to which patients are assigned according to their order of admission instead of their suitability for a specific group. An advantage of this practice is that all patients are assigned to a group and are expected to attend group therapy. A disadvantage is that it is often difficult to lead sessions with such a group because of the wide range of psychopathological conditions of the group members. Often, members may be too ill during the first few days of hospitalization to receive any benefit from therapy.

A **homogeneous group** is one in which all members have the same diagnosis and similar levels of functioning. An example is a group composed of people with schizophrenia. The advantages of the homogeneous group are that it provides more specific and appropriate therapy for persons who are disoriented and delusional and may be hallucinating and that it provides preparation for ongoing group work. One disadvantage of running both heterogeneous team groups and homogeneous groups on the same unit is that this practice can lead to further divisiveness on the inpatient unit.

Table 7-9 ■ OUTPATIENT PSYCHOTHERAPY GROUPS

NURSING ACTION	THEORETICAL RATIONALE
All prospective members are seen at least once individually before admission to the group. (The more times they are seen, the better.)	A tie will develop between the patient and the nurse. This tie will help the patient stay in the group, even as anxiety increases.
Clients are seen in group sessions and individual sessions as well.	Group psychotherapy produces anxiety, which spills over at times outside the group. This anxiety can motivate clients to explore their own reactions in individual sessions.
Before entering the group, the client is not prepared for what happens in the group session or who will be there. Only a general statement is made, such as, "The group is a place to discuss feelings, problems, or reactions."	If the client knows a great deal about the group in advance, spontaneous reactions are lost to exploration. These spontaneous reactions are "grist for the therapeutic mill."
Group members are not told about new members before the new members appear.	The spontaneous or irrational response of group members to the new member is useful for exploring (e.g., this may be reminiscent of the birth of a sibling).
Group members sit in chairs in a circle. No table is used, and no one sits on the floor.	All members should be visible to one another. This increases anxiety slightly, which leads to more irrational behavior and its subsequent observation. It also aids in the observation of nonverbal communication, which can then be explored.
The leader changes seats each session, causing other members to shift seats.	Members should not be able to find a comfortable "niche" in which to hide.
Weekly sessions last 1½ hours, and daily sessions last at least 1 hour.	When groups meet only once a week, resistance builds between sessions, and it may take 45 minutes for work to begin. When groups meet daily, resistance is lower.
Sessions begin and end on time.	Clients pace their reactions according to this time frame. This pacing in itself is interesting to note (e.g., when a client reports in the last 5 minutes that he has quit his job).
The same leader leads the group.	Group process is based on a balance of forces that takes the leader into account. Changing leaders seriously changes this balance and makes interaction more superficial.
Observers do not sit in the group.	This disturbs the ongoing balance and process, causing more superficiality.
Open-ended groups are more effective than time-limited groups. The group continues indefinitely, with replacements made as members leave.	When members know there are only a certain number of sessions left, they remain more controlled and superficial.

From Lego S. Group therapy. In Lego S (ed). The American Handbook of Psychiatric Nursing. Philadelphia: JB Lippincott, p 208, 1984.

Open inpatient psychotherapy groups do not usually pass through all stages of group development. An inpatient may be in group therapy for only two or three sessions. Although open therapy is of limited value for the patient and the group, the patient can still gain from even a single session (Yalom 1985). Most patients have never been part of a group: with group therapy, patients have the opportunity to feel they belong to something, often for the first time in their lives. With open psychotherapy groups, the inpatient group therapist must consider the life of the group to be only a single session (Yalom 1985). The therapist must be efficient, be active, and offer something useful for as many patients as possible during that session.

ESTABLISHING AN OUTPATIENT GROUP

Table 7-9 identifies specific nursing actions and rationales for organizing an outpatient psychotherapy group. Nurses often run outpatient psychotherapy groups in clinics, in community health units, and in private practice.

All prospective members are seen at least once individually before they are admitted to the group. The more times they are seen, the better. The rationale for this is that a close tie will develop between the patient and the nurse; this tie will help the patient remain in the group longer when the patient becomes anxious. In contrast to pregroup preparation in an inpatient group, in an outpatient group the patient is often not prepared for what happens in group therapy or who will be there. Only a general statement is made (e.g., "The group is a place to discuss feelings, problems, or reactions") (Lego 1984). Setting general goals, such as wanting closer relationships, improvement in one's work life, and relief of painful symptoms, is useful. It may be unrealistic to set goals that are too specific. Goal setting that is too specific is antithetical to the natural process of developing ongoing intimate relationships. Patients often have very specific conscious goals that for a time are unobtainable because of unconscious factors.

Phases of Group Development

In long term outpatient groups, four phases of development are identified. These phases are (1) uncertainty, (2) overaggression, (3) regression, and (4) adaptation.

UNCERTAINTY PHASE

During this initial orientation phase, group members are anxious and want to carve out a place for themselves. They are often angry at the leader for not providing enough structure but are afraid to say so. Instead, they may make comments in group therapy in hopes that the leader will get the hint. The leader will often see attrition during this phase. Lego (1984) identifies specific client behaviors that emerge during this initial phase. Behaviors and leader interventions for these behaviors are described in Table 7–10.

OVERAGGRESSIVE PHASE

During the overaggressive phase, hostility inevitably develops toward the leader. This hostility is usually based on clients' projection of unrealistic, magical attributes on the leader. Unconsciously, many members crave dependency and may first attempt to create and then destroy the authoritarian figure, in this case the group leader. In psychoanalytical terms, this transference reaction is necessary in order for clients to work out their feelings of dependency. Some individuals only feel powerful by assailing others who are perceived as being more powerful. Other patients feel resentful that they are not the "favored one" in the group; sometimes, the group leader is viewed as deceitful. In addition, members begin to feel attracted to each other and try at the same time to avoid these feelings of closeness by being aggressive. Table 7–11 identifies some common behaviors seen during this phase.

Both new and experienced therapists need support to endure this phase and become, in Peplau's terms, the "participant observer" (O'Toole and Welt 1989). Group therapists need supervision in order to work through their feelings. In participant observation, the nurse observes not only patients' behaviors, reactions, and feelings but also her or his own.

REGRESSION PHASE

During the regression phase, people are more able to experience genuine feelings of dependency, anger, fear, jealousy, longing, and anxiety. Group members take more risks with one another by exposing their feelings, and they no longer need to feel in control. Personal feelings such as dependency, longing, and anger become more acceptable.

ADAPTATION PHASE

When group members reach the adaptation phase, they are able to accept one another despite their weaknesses and faults. As a result, defenses are lowered, and in this atmosphere of acceptance, members are able to explore their conflicts more openly. This mutual acceptance can, however, be a problem if members become too tolerant of each other's problems and problem behaviors and cease to offer important observations and feedback that a member can use as a basis for change. Therefore, the leader is responsible for keeping a sense of objectivity and for staying alert when members begin to use self-defeating defensive behaviors. An example of this type of behavior is when an unemployed member who has been making progress in finding a new job begins to avoid coming to group therapy.

A universal experience for patients is difficulty with relationships, and the group experience enables members to realize they are not alone with this problem and that change is possible. Even patients who do not say a word may pick up valuable information about

BEHAVIOR	EXAMPLE	LEADER INTERVENTION
Table 7–10 ■ OUTPATIENT GROUP—UNCERTAINTY PHASE		
Initial anxiety	Pacing the floor. Leaving and returning. Excessive intellectualization. Organization of a "group plan."	Comment about the anxiety. Question what members fear happening in the group.
Demands on leader to explain the purpose of therapy or provide a structure	"Do we begin now?" "What is supposed to happen here?" "How does this work?"	Communicate to members that it is their group ("Let's see how things go").
Competition	Members compare past group experience, past number of years in psychotherapy, knowledge of the leader, and so forth.	Point out that competition is taking place. Be careful to communicate that it is not wrong and should not necessarily stop just because it has been noted.
Excessive politeness	Members feel anxious and angry about the lack of structure from the leader, but they are afraid to show this. Instead, they react with inappropriate kindness. One member may say to a monopolizer, "You certainly are talkative today."	Note the covert feeling and ask if it is present ("Are you a little irritated by all that talking?"). Encourage openness rather than politeness.
Silence	All members sit for 5 minutes staring at the floor or occasionally glancing at each other.	Comment on the silence ("I guess everyone is afraid to start"). Comment on some nonverbal behavior ("Mary, I notice you're staring at John. Do you wish he'd speak?").
Questions about the leader's personal life, qualifications, and competence	A member asks, "Are you a mother?" A member asks, "Are you an MD?"	"No. Are you afraid I won't know how to care for you because I'm not?" "No, I'm a psychiatric nurse. Are you afraid I won't know enough to do things right?"
Avoidance of involvement in the group	A schizophrenic member talks to voices instead of to other group members. Members intellectualize about their problems. Members adopt roles that were used in their families to reduce anxiety but that are not appropriate in the current group (e.g., the buffoon, the boss, the incompetent person, and the ingenue).	Comment that these are methods to avoid reacting emotionally to the current group. Explore why this is feared and avoided.
	The leader is seen as a "savior" with all the answers.	Explore why a "savior" is necessary.
	The leader is seen as using power to manipulate or humiliate members and as having a secret reason for every comment or move.	Explore the meaning of these ideas in the context of members' lives.

From Lego S. Group psychotherapy. In Haber J, et al (eds). Comprehensive Psychiatric Nursing, 2nd ed. New York: McGraw-Hill, p. 212, 1982.

clear communication and validation of feelings. People may be silent in groups for various reasons. For some, marked conflicts about their own aggression may mean they cannot undertake the self-assertion inherent in speaking. Perfectionists may be afraid of not being able to get the words out properly. Some fear attack from a particular member and only speak in the absence of that member.

Descriptions of Challenging Patients in Groups

A number of defensive behaviors used by some clients interfere with their attaining satisfaction in their lives.

At the same time, these behaviors can be disruptive to a group process and the development of group cohesion.

SPECIFIC BEHAVIORS

Specific defensive and nonproductive behaviors or roles that some people play out may become evident during the process of group psychotherapy. However, the therapist must carefully assess the group's readiness to have the therapist interpret such behavior for them. Patients are not always ready to hear insights, no matter how accurate these insights are. Premature interpretations can be ineffective and can impede therapy by misdirecting attention from the therapeutic

BEHAVIOR	EXAMPLE	LEADER INTERVENTION
Criticism of one another	One member who is very lonely but who leads the life of the happy, sophisticated swinger is critical of another member whose isolation and loneliness are all too stark and evident.	Ask whether the "swinger" is reminded of herself by the isolated member. Explore their similarities and the resultant anxiety.
	One member becomes enraged when another acts stubborn and impenetrable.	Ask whether there was someone else in the member's life that he could not "get through" to.
Anger at one another for using one's own defenses in a clumsy way	One obsessional member begins sentences with, "Please don't think I'm trying to be controlling . . . ." Another obsessional member says, "Don't warn us so obviously. It only calls our attention to the fact that you are!"	Point out the dynamic that people feel their own defenses should be used only in their own unique way and are spoiled or "exposed" if used "incorrectly."
Ganging up	One member who is secretly anxious about almost everything arrives late at the group session each week, giving various weak excuses. He refuses to acknowledge that he might have wanted to miss part of a session or that he wanted to stir everyone up.	Examine and explore both sides of the process, why the member is so provocative as well as why members cannot resist being provoked.
Hostility toward the leader	A client distorts the leader's behavior ("You do nothing to help us").	Accept members' hostility in a nondefensive way. Avoid a win-lose approach.
	A client points out real eccentricities of the leader ("You are too compulsive!").	Acknowledge weaknesses and eccentricities freely. It is often a great relief to members to see that the leader is human and does not mind if this shows.

Table 7–11 ■ OUTPATIENT GROUP—OVERAGGRESSIVE PHASE

From Lego S. Group psychotherapy. In Haber J, et al (eds). Comprehensive Psychiatric Nursing, 2nd ed. New York: McGraw-Hill, p. 213, 1982.

work (Yalom 1983). The patient who monopolizes the group, the patient who complains but continues to reject help, and the patient who chronically helps others and avoids his or her own issues are all using behaviors that defend against the underlying issues.

The Patient Who Monopolizes the Group

This person's compulsive speech is an attempt to deal with anxiety. As the patient sees group tension grow, the patient's level of anxiety rises and the patient's tendency to speak increases even more. Therefore, no one else gets a chance to be heard, and eventually other group members lose interest and begin to withdraw.

Example
Holly is the most talkative member of the group until the nurse intervenes. Initially, Holly talks at length about her early experiences relating to the deaths of both her mother and father and to having to live with her grandparents. The other members of the group become bored with the same old story and drift off. They have heard these stories multiple times, not only in group therapy but also during other activities.

Intervention. The leader asks group members why they have permitted the monopolizer to go on and on. This serves to validate the other members' feelings of anger. After the group members become angry, they may see how they, too, are responsible for allowing themselves to be victimized. Some members may be angry at the therapist for pointing out their passivity, but they may subsequently realize that they are responsible adults with the right to say what they feel. They may then discuss their fears of being assertive or of hurting the feelings of the monopolizer. Placing responsibility on the group members also takes the therapist out of the authoritative position.

Group members may need help disclosing their own feelings and responses. The therapist encourages statements such as, "When you speak this way, I feel . . . ." The therapist helps by saying feelings are not right or wrong but simply exist. People feel less defensive with "I feel" statements than they do with "you are" statements. They help members feel part of the group, not alienated from it.

The Patient Who Complains but Continues to Reject Help

The patient who complains but continues to reject help continually brings environmental or somatic problems to the group and often describes them in a manner that makes them seem insurmountable; in fact, the client appears to take pride in the insolubility of his or her problems. The client seems entirely self-centered. The group's attempts to help the person are continually rejected. The person who uses these tactics usually has highly conflicting feelings about his or her own dependency. Any notice from the therapist temporarily increases the client's self-esteem; on the other hand, the client has a pervasive mistrust toward all authority figures. Most patients who complain but continue to reject help were subjected to severe deprivation early in their lives. For example, they may be orphans or those who were emotionally and physically abused.

Example

Michelle is always complaining about how horrible her relationship with her boyfriend is, and she manages to get the entire group worked up over this. Members tell her to leave him, not to spend all her time with him, and not to spend all her money on him, but each week she reports a new escapade or crisis. In every session, the group members become concerned and offer encouragement, advice, and solutions. Each time, the group becomes angry at her lack of change, and she is frustrated by her own inability to change. She asserts that the group is not helpful.

Intervention. The therapist agrees with the content of the patient's pessimism and maintains a detached affect. If the patient stays in the group long enough and the group develops a sense of cohesion, the therapist helps this individual recognize the pattern of his or her relationships. The therapist encourages the patient to look at her or his "yes, but" behavior.

The Patient Who Chronically Helps Others

The patient who chronically helps others is one who is overly helpful to others in an effort to defend against his or her own intense dependency needs. Because these dependency needs were never met during early childhood, clients are left with intense longings and unmet dependency needs as adults. These clients secretly wish that others would fulfill their wishes. They further have a need to have others treat them in a hostile way. Therefore, chronic helpers become masochistic in their dealings with others. Essentially, there is no way anyone can fulfill their intense dependency needs. Their dependency is so great because they have subordinated all of their own needs to the needs of others. These people deny their

own anger and needs and often tend to marry persons who cannot meet their dependency needs and who reject them through physical or emotional abuse or neglect (Light 1974).

Example

Sally always has a solution or a suggestion for everyone else's problem. She is adept at keeping the focus off herself and is always trying to "help" others in various ways. Psychodynamically, this allows her to avoid her own problems and to avoid making changes.

Intervention. The therapist helps clients experience their dysfunctional patterns of helpfulness and helps them experience their true feelings. The therapist could state how helpful this client has been to others in the group and then remark on the client's reluctance to ask for something personal from the group. The therapist could explore whether the patient fears being rejected or feels he or she does not have any right to seek help from the group. A patient's behavior in the group is usually symbolic of the patient's behavior outside the group.

SPECIFIC DSM-III-R CATEGORIES

Group psychotherapy is appropriate for patients with many DSM-III-R diagnoses. However, for people with the diagnosis of antisocial personality disorder or those with paranoid personality disorder, for example, insight-oriented group psychotherapy is usually not appropriate. In addition, people with borderline personality disorders are not appropriate therapeutic candidates for the beginning group therapist.

Antisocial Personality Disorder

Some of the DSM-III-R criteria that support not including patients with antisocial personality disorder in insight-oriented group psychotherapy include

- Failure to conform to social norms with respect to lawful behavior (e.g., stealing)
- Impulsiveness
- Disregard for the truth, as indicated by repeated lying, use of aliases, or conning
- Lack of remorse for actions
- Tendency to use others for their own satisfaction

People with antisocial personality disorders may benefit from a "tough love" group in which there is constant, open confrontation of wrongdoing. Such a group is here-and-now oriented and generally does not promote long-lasting change. The patient usually does not gain insight but may conform to peer pressure. The patient can benefit from a tough love group because it is action oriented and is a homogeneous group. Self-help groups such as AA, if appropriate, can be of help. This beneficial effect may be due to the absence of a leader, because the presence of a leader elicits feelings of resistance to authority. The antisocial patient is self-serving and may consistently prevent the group from achieving any cohesion by the constant overt or covert "stirring up" of others. Refer to Chapter 16 for further discussion of people with antisocial personality disorder.

Paranoid Personality Disorder

People with strong paranoid traits consistently expect to be exploited or harmed by others and are reluctant to confide in others because they feel any information they share will be used against them. They therefore usually avoid or soon drop out of group psychotherapy. Other personality traits that make it difficult for a paranoid person to benefit from group psychotherapy include the following:

- They are easily slighted and quick to react with anger or to counterattack.
- They read hidden, demeaning, or threatening meanings into benign remarks or events.
- They maintain grudges or are unforgiving of insults or slights.

Refer to Chapter 16 for a more in-depth discussion of people with paranoid personality disorder.

Borderline Personality Disorder

As mentioned previously, many people with the diagnosis of borderline personality disorder can gain insight in a psychotherapy group; however, because of their marked manipulativeness and self-destructive traits, they are not appropriate group therapy candidates for new group leaders. Their rage may not be tolerated in a group setting. However, the use of a cotherapist could be helpful as long as the therapists acknowledge they could be played against each other through this patient's defense mechanism of splitting. One problem encountered in group psychotherapy with a client who has borderline personality disorder is that the person with this disorder may become anxious as the group atmosphere becomes more cohesive, thereby increasing the potential for splitting the group. The benefit of group psychotherapy for this

type of patient is that the patient may become less regressed in the group situation than in individual sessions because the group pressures the patient to work things through instead of using avoidance and denial. For patients who are impulsive and action oriented (particularly those who are self-destructive), the action orientation of a group, as opposed to one-to-one psychotherapy sessions, is often appealing (Leszcz 1989).

Group members serve as a "mirror" and reflect back to the impulsive or self-destructive person how his or her actions affect the group.

The use of projective identification and exaggerated anger in a group setting by the patient with borderline personality disorder is often a paradox and a defense. For example, a male patient who stated that he wanted to learn to be close to others persisted in "tearing down" a female patient who had asked the group for acknowledgment after she achieved a significant professional goal. After several group sessions, the man stated that he could not tolerate seeing this woman ask the group for recognition, which acknowledged her need for the group. He attacked her in the same fashion that he feared being attacked for his own neediness and his need of the group. He projected onto her his own contemptibility for his dependent, needful self, and he adopted the position of ruthless persecutor, much as his parents had done with regard to his neediness. He elicited from the group intense hostility for his treatment, instead of the increased closeness he had said he wanted. Thus, he created the very atmosphere he dreaded (Leszcz 1989).

The group therapist gently pointed out to the man that his criticizing actually served to distance him from others. The therapist then proceeded to ask him if someone significant in his past had criticized him excessively.

At the same time, the group therapist acknowledged the risk that the woman took in asking for acknowledgment from the group. The group therapist neutralized the attack by indicating that the behaviors are reminiscent of not feeling acknowledged (by parents) or of actually being rejected. The man desired the recognition he never received from his parents.

THERAPY FOR SPECIAL POPULATIONS

Two populations that some therapists have found amenable to alternative types of group therapy are persons with schizophrenia and persons with mental illness along with substance abuse.

Persons with Schizophrenia

A helpful form of therapy for persons with schizophrenia is therapy in a supportive group. In supportive group work, the goals are to help patients better adapt to the environment by focusing on reality and to help them learn new behaviors to decrease isolation. The therapist needs to note early indications of the emergence of psychotic symptoms, which may indicate a need to change the patient's treatment program. For example, nursing interventions aimed at decreasing anxiety may be implemented, or antipsychotic medication may need to be changed.

When psychotic patients enter a group, the dynamics that develop can mobilize psychotic resistances, which then become the dominant group feature (Cohn 1988). Frosch (1983) states that the major anxiety against which psychotic patients defend is "annihilation anxiety"—fear of dissolution of an already fragile self. At first, unacceptable aspects of the self are often projected onto the therapist in malignant forms. It is the therapist's task to help the patient perceive projected parts of his or her self as benign and useful rather than dangerous (Cohn 1988). To place a psychotic patient in group therapy is to challenge the core around which defenses are constructed —that is, the need to avoid new experiences. There are several theoretical modalities to guide group interventions. Table 7–12 identifies some of the goals of supportive group work for schizophrenic clients. The following sections discuss other orientations to group work with a schizophrenic population.

PSYCHOANALYTICAL APPROACH
Concepts

1. A stable and realistic point of emotional reference is established and maintained in the group.
2. The group leader is a resource person who "uses tenderness . . . maintains an attitude of dignity and respect, helps to pinpoint anxieties, decode delusions and symbolic communication, and brings into awareness dissociated material. The leader encourages open expression of emotions and acknowledges that the experience of anger is OK. The group leader is always thinking 'one step ahead' of the group" (Lego 1987).
3. Because of the symbolic nature of schizophrenic communication, the emphasis of interpretation is placed more on process than on content. The therapist and the group members need to remind themselves frequently that the distortions of communication are needed by the schizophrenic to make it possible for this patient to function at all (Geller 1963).

INTERPERSONAL APPROACH
Concept

1. Loneliness is one of the central problems schizophrenics face (Fromm-Reichman 1954). "Fearing that their aggressive impulses would lead to destruction of the object . . . they withdraw" (Kahn 1984).

Techniques

1. Questions directed to the therapist are directed to other members. Extremely withdrawn members may be given homework. Members are asked to rank the group and decide how they can improve it, if needed.
2. The therapist interprets transference reactions.
3. The therapist should use humor. Psychotic patients will mirror fear that is manifested by the therapist. Similarly, patients will be calmed by a therapist who feels relaxed and in good spirits. Laughter provides catharsis.

Table 7–12 ■ SUPPORTIVE GROUP THERAPY FOR PERSONS WITH SCHIZOPHRENIA

TARGET POPULATION	GOALS	THERAPIST'S ACTIVITY	FREQUENCY AND DURATION
• Schizophrenic patients • Psychotic clients • Chronically mentally ill clients • Patients with organic mental disorders	*Overall goal:* Better adaptation to environment 1. Decrease isolation 2. Increase involvement in group activities 3. Promote discussion relative to immediate life events and feelings in the group 4. Detect problems early 5. Focus on reality testing	1. Strengthens existing defenses 2. Is actively involved in the group process 3. May give advice and direction 4. Models appropriate behavior 5. Creates a safe environment	*Meets:* Once weekly *For:* 6 months or longer

HETEROGENEOUS GROUP APPROACH
Concepts

1. The person with schizophrenia should be incorporated and integrated into a heterogeneous group that represents a cross section of the unit.
2. The person with schizophrenia is often more tuned in to the emotions of others and emotionally laden group themes than other patients. Higher-functioning patients often use intellectualization and denial, avoiding here-and-now interactions.
3. Schizophrenic members may also provide meaningful feedback to other group members as to how others relate in the here-and-now.

   For example, in a group in which two women persisted in whispering to each other despite the nurse therapist's attempt to share their material with the group, a schizophrenic member who perceived the leader's frustration stated, "Hey, we can't get any work done around here!"

When a schizophrenic client's contribution to a group is acknowledged, the client experiences, often for the first time, the sense of being helpful and accepted by others.

Techniques

1. The therapist encourages schizophrenic member(s) to give feedback to the group as to how group members relate in the here-and-now.
2. The therapist acknowledges the feedback from the schizophrenic member(s) as being valuable.
3. The therapist is active and supportive, provides structure, and clarifies the purpose of the group.

HOMOGENEOUS GROUP APPROACH
Concepts

1. Maintaining a homogeneous population allows for a clearer focus on topics relevant to all group members, and cohesiveness is easier to achieve.
2. Cognitive approaches are useful for dealing with hallucinations and have relevance for most group members.
3. Participation in a structured homogeneous group for schizophrenics may result in a successful group experience for many of these patients by providing group tasks the group is capable of completing and that assist in identifying the interpersonal patterns that tend to get the person in an "unfortunate position" (Kanas 1988).

   Some examples of group tasks are

- Nonintrusive, "safe" self-disclosure exercises
- Sentence completion exercises about personal strengths
- Exercises aimed at improving reality testing
- Sharing techniques of coping with hallucinations

Persons with a Mental Disorder and Substance Abuse (Dual Diagnosis)

Some inpatient psychiatric units recognize the importance of treating a person for both substance abuse and his or her mental illness. The addition of dual-diagnosis groups for patients diagnosed with both types of disorder is increasing with the recognition that substance abuse often exacerbates psychiatric symptoms and that the actual substance abuse is not detected unless there is an accurate assessment.

Persons with a mental disorder and substance abuse have increased in number, particularly in urban and suburban areas (Office of Mental Health News 1991). A special program was started at Buffalo General Hospital in New York in 1988 after it was noted that 40% of patients using the emergency services were dual-diagnosis patients. Many of these clients were in crisis; had a history of resistance to treatment, denial of problems, and noncompliance with medication; were impulsive; and were concerned only with their immediate needs. This special program uses counselors who are available 24 hours a day and who have training in crisis intervention. The program continues to grow.

Edelwich and Brodsky (1992) advocate the use of group counseling, instead of group therapy, for drug and alcohol abusers. The rationale is that group counseling

- Is more action and task oriented.
- Emphasizes problem solving and decision making rather than gaining insight. Group counseling has as its primary objectives behavioral change and skill acquisition.
- Is interactive, with an adherence to group process that is . . . as rigorous as that of group psychotherapy (Edelwich and Brodsky 1992).

It is recommended that the group leader have a background in group process, reality therapy, and rational-emotive therapy (Ellis and Harper 1975). Glasser (1985) describes four basic needs people have and gives questions the leader can use to assess each member in relationship to these needs. These basic needs include those for (1) relationships and belonging, (2) self-esteem, power, and control, (3) fun and recreation, and (4) freedom and choices.

The need for relationships and belonging

- *Who are the important people in your life?*
- *How intimate are these relationships?*
- *Who can you talk to when you have a problem?*

Table 7–13 ■ EXAMPLE OF A SCHEDULE FOR A DRUG AND ALCOHOL EDUCATION GROUP		
TIME	**TOPIC**	**OBJECTIVE**
Week 1 Monday	Addiction • What it is • What it is not	To identify parallels of addiction and mental illness
Friday	Introduction to recovery	To define recovery To identify parallels of addiction and mental illness in recovery
Week 2 Monday	Introduction to relapse	To define relapse
Friday	Distortions in thinking and feeling	To identify thoughts and feelings that lead to reuse
Week 3 Monday	The 12 steps	To identify a common framework to confront and aid in the recovery process
Friday	Physical aspects	To identify harmful effects of substances To identify dangers of medication and alcohol combinations To define cross-addiction
Week 4 Monday	Preventing relapse	To define relapse prevention strategies To develop one fail-safe plan

The need for self-esteem, power, and control

- *What do you want that you're not getting?*
- *What have you done in the past several days that improves your image of yourself?*

The need for fun and recreation

- *When was the last time you had fun?*
- *How has your having fun in the past hurt other people?*

The need for freedom and choices

- *What choices do you have in your life?*
- *What would you do if things did get better for you?*

Some goals of groups composed of persons who have a mental disorder and substance abuse are to (Lala et al. 1992)

1. Provide education about the processes of alcoholism, substance abuse, and addiction.
2. Offer clients the opportunity to explore their issues with addiction.
3. Identify issues related to relapse and discuss relapse prevention strategies.
4. Encourage and motivate clients to use outpatient resources.

Many people are in the precarious position of using alcohol or other substances of abuse while balancing a job, managing their family life, or both. Often, the use of substances, including alcohol, is a symptom of underlying low self-esteem, depression, or unresolved grief and loss. The use of the substance may not be discovered until a crisis erupts, such as a divorce or a car accident in which someone is hurt as a result of drunk driving. Because of the guilt and shame often associated with substance abuse by a person who was previously viewed as competent and judicious, a comprehensive treatment program is advocated, such as a 30-day alcohol or substance rehabilitation treatment program. People need to be motivated to stay in these programs. These programs offer a multitreatment approach using individual, group, family, and spiritual therapies.

Terence Gorski (1988) developed the CENAPS model of relapse prevention, a cognitive system that covers chemical addictions and dependencies, as well as relapse prevention, by using cognitive, affective, behavioral, and situational techniques. Gorski advocates the involvement of spouses, older children, friends, and sponsors.

Table 7–13 gives an example of how a drug or alcohol education group may be structured and the kinds of issues such a group addresses.

Summary

Nurses have multiple opportunities for professional, creative, and thoughtful work in groups. The beginning group therapist is encouraged initially to use modalities such as medication education group work on the inpatient psychiatric unit in order to become familiar with group dynamics, task roles, and psychiatric diagnoses. The use of advanced practitioners, such as clinical nurse specialists, is recommended for ongoing clinical supervision and role-modeling. Leading other groups, such as behavioral, TA, and family therapy groups, requires specialized training and education. Beginning group therapists may benefit from observing such groups.

When working with groups, the nurse identifies the theoretical base he or she feels most comfortable working with. To prepare patients adequately for therapy in an inpatient, insight-oriented psychotherapy group, the nurse needs to assess patients and to give them a cognitive structure of what to expect. The focus is on the here-and-now and on relationships. The group psychotherapist is always active, analyzing both the group process and content, and continually strives to link the universal aspects of clients' common issues. The group becomes a microcosm of the inpatient unit, and the therapy group may be the first group a patient has belonged to.

Outpatient groups provide therapy for a longer period of time, may be less structured, and tend to have the same members over a longer period of time. These outpatient, insight-oriented psychotherapy groups usually have open membership. The nurse therapist in an outpatient group may see the patient for individual therapy as well. The group therapist usually provides less structure and less preparation than the inpatient therapist and has more time to see the group develop through the phases of uncertainty, overaggression, regression, and adaptation.

The learning challenges of working with complex persons with mental disorders in groups, such as persons with borderline personality disorder, persons with schizophrenia, and persons with both a mental disorder and substance abuse, are presented using various frameworks. For persons with substance abuse, one of the goals of group work is to increase the client's responsibility for him- or herself.

This chapter presented some of the groups in which nurses can become experts, either as educators or therapists. Different characteristics of inpatient and outpatient therapy groups were presented. Self-care groups such as medication education, women's, and men's groups were also identified.

References

American Nurses' Association. Standards of Practice for Psychiatric/ Mental Health Nursing Practice. Kansas City, MO: American Nurses' Association, 1982.

American Psychiatric Association. Diagnostic and Statistical Manual of Mental Disorders, 3rd ed, revised (DSM-III-R). Washington, DC: American Psychiatric Association, 1987.

Armstrong S, Rouslin S. Group Psychotherapy in Nursing Practice. New York: Macmillan Publishing Company, 1963.

Barker P. Basic Family Therapy. New York: Oxford University Press, 1992.

Beeber A. Psychotherapy with schizophrenics in team groups: A system model. American Journal of Psychotherapy, 45:78, 1991.

Berne E. Principles of Group Treatment. New York: Oxford University Press, 1966.

Captain C. Family recovery from alcoholism: Mediating family factors. Nursing Clinics of North America, 24:55, 1989.

Clarke L. Personal communication, The University of Vermont School of Nursing, Burlington, VT, 1993.

Cohn B. Keeping the group alive: Dealing with resistance in a long term group of psychotic patients. International Journal of Group Psychotherapy, 38(3):319, 1988.

Craig J, Kirkpatrick T. Transactional analysis. In Lego S (ed). The American Handbook of Psychiatric Nursing. Philadelphia: JB Lippincott, 1984.

Critchley D, Maurin J. The Clinical Specialist in Psychiatric Mental Health Nursing. New York: John Wiley & Sons, pp 178–198, 1985.

Edelwich J, Brodsky A. Group Counseling for the Resistant Client. New York: Lexington Press, 1992.

Ellis A, Harper R. A New Guide to Rational Living. North Hollywood: Wilshire, 1975.

Fromm-Reichman F. Psychotherapy of schizophrenia. American Journal of Psychiatry, 11:410, 1954.

Frosch J. The Psychotic Process. New York: International Universities Press, 1983.

Geller J. Group psychotherapy in the treatment of schizophrenia syndromes. Psychiatric Quarterly, 63:1, 1963.

Glasser W. Control Theory. Scranton, PA: Harper Collins, 1985.

Glasser W. Reality Therapy. New York: Harper & Row, 1965.

Gorski T. A Guide for Relapse Prevention and the Staying Sober Workbook—A Serious Solution for the Problem of Relapse. Independence, MO: Independence Press, 1988.

Goulding M, et al. Changing Lives Through Redecision Therapy. New York: Brunner-Mazel, 1979.

Haley J. Problem Solving Therapy. San Francisco: Jossey Bass, 1976.

Harris T. I'm O.K.—You're O.K. New York: Harper & Row, 1969.

Jones S. Family Therapy: A Comparison of Approaches. Bowie, MD: Robert J. Brady Company/Prentice Hall, 1980.

Kahn EM. Group treatment interventions for schizophrenics. International Journal of Group Psychotherapy, 34(1):149, 1984.

Kanas N. Therapy groups for schizophrenics—patients on acute care units. Hospital and Community Psychiatry, 39(5):546, 1988.

Kane CF, DiMarino E, Jiminez M. A comparison of short-term psychoeducational supports for relatives coping with chronic schizophrenia. Archives of Psychiatric Nursing, 4(6):343, 1990.

Kaplan HI, Sadock BJ. Synopsis of Psychiatry, 6th ed. Baltimore: Williams & Wilkins, 1991.

Kerr M, Bowen M. Family Evaluation. New York: WW Norton, 1988.

Kuipers J, et al. Designing a psychiatric medication education program. Journal of Rehabilitation, July-Sept:55, 1988.

Lacquer HP. Mechanisms of change in multiple family therapy. In Sager CJ, Kaplan HS (eds). Progress in Group and Family Therapy. New York: Brunner-Mazel, 1972.

Lala C, Shannison S, Williams G. Drug/Alcohol Education Group Outline. Albany Medical Center, unpublished, 1992.

Lego S. Group psychotherapy. In Haber J, et al (eds). Comprehensive Psychiatric Nursing, 2nd ed. New York: McGraw-Hill, 1982.

Lego S. The American Handbook of Psychiatric Nursing. Philadelphia: JB Lippincott, 1984.

Leszcz M. Inpatient groups. In Frances AJ, Aoles RE (eds). Psychiatry Update. Washington, DC: American Psychiatric Press, p. 729, 1986.

Leszcz M. Group psychotherapy of the characterologically difficult patient. International Journal of Group Psychotherapy, 39(3):311, 1989.

Light N. The chronic helper in group therapy. Perspectives in Psychiatric Care 12:129–139, 1974.

McNeel J. Seven components of redecision therapy. In Barnes G (ed). Transactional Analysis After Eric Berne. New York: Harper's College Press, 1977.

Minuchin S. Families and Family Therapy. Cambridge, MA: Harvard University Press, 1974.

Morgan AJ, Moreno JW. The Practice of Mental Health Nursing: A Community Approach. Philadelphia: JB Lippincott, 1973.

Naegle M (ed). Substance Abuse Education in Nursing, vol III. New York: National League for Nursing. Press Publication No. 15-2464, 1993.

Office of Mental Health News, New York State, Summer, 1991.

O'Toole A, Welt S. Interpersonal Theory in Nursing Practice: Selected Works of Hildegard Peplau. New York: Springer Publishing Company, 1989.

Satir V. Conjoint Family Therapy. Palo Alto: Science Behavior Books, 1984.

Sheeren M. The relationship between relapse and involvement in Alcoholics Anonymous. Journal of Studies on Alcohol, 29:104, 1988.

Staples N, et al. Anorexia nervosa support group: Providing transitional support. Journal of Psychosocial Nursing, 28(2):6, 1990.

Wolberg LR. The Technique of Psychotherapy, 3rd ed. New York: Grune & Stratton, 1977.

Wolfe M. Group modalities in the care of clients with drug and alcohol problems. In Naegle MA (ed). Substance Abuse Education in Nursing, Vol III. New York: National League for Nursing Press, pp 6–7, 1993.

Yalom I. Inpatient Group Psychotherapy. New York: Basic Books, 1983.

Yalom I. The Theory and Practice of Group Psychotherapy. New York: Basic Books, 1985.

Flaskerud J. Psychiatric nurses' needs for AIDS information. Perspectives in Psychiatric Care, 25(3,4):3, 1989.

Harman R. Recent developments in gestalt group therapy. International Journal of Group Psychotherapy, 34(3):473, 1984.

Johnson D, et al. Group psychotherapy with schizophrenic patients: The pairing group. International Journal of Group Psychotherapy, 36(1): 1986.

Josephs L, Dorman L. The application of self-psychology principles to long term group therapy with schizophrenic patients. Group, 9:3, 1985.

Kapur R, et al. Group psychotherapy in an acute inpatient setting. Psychiatry, 49: 1986.

Klein R, Carroll R. Patient characteristics and attendance patterns in outpatient group psychotherapy. International Journal of Group Psychotherapy 36(1):115, 1986.

Kohut H. Analysis of the Self. New York: International Universities Press, 1971.

Kuipers J, et al. Designing a psychiatric medication education program. Journal of Rehabilitation, 54(3):55, 1988.

Lacquer HP. Multiple family therapy and general systems theory. International Psychiatric Clinics, 7:99, 1970.

Lego S. Masochism: Implications for psychiatric nursing. Archives of Psychiatric Nursing, 6(4):224, 1992.

Minkoff KMD. Parallels Between Alcoholism Addiction and Major Mental Illness: Active Use and Stages of Recovery. Woburn, MA: Choate Symnes Health Services, 1990.

Munzer J. Acting out—communication or resistance? International Journal of Group Psychotherapy, 16:434, 1977.

Peplau H. Interpersonal Relations in Nursing. New York: Springer Publishing Company, 1989.

Piccinino S. The nursing care challenge: Borderline patients. Journal of Psychosocial Nursing, 28(4):22, 1990.

Slavson SR. Introduction to Group Psychotherapy. New York: The Commonwealths Press, 1943.

Tansey B. Understanding Countertransference: From Projective Identification to Empathy. Hillside, NJ: Analytic Press, 1987.

Van Sevellen G, et al. Nursing-led group modalities in a psychiatric inpatient setting. A program evaluation. Archives of Psychiatric Nursing, 5(3):128, 1991.

Van Sevellen G, Poster EC, Ryan J, et al. Methodological concerns in evaluating psychiatric nursing care modalities and proposed standard group protocol format for nurse led groups. Archives of Psychiatric Nursing, 6(2):117, 1992.

Witt T. Transference and countertransference in group therapy settings. Journal of Psychosocial Nursing and Mental Health Services, 20(2):31, 1982.

Further Reading

Bateson G, et al. Toward a theory of schizophrenia. In Jones S. (ed). Family Therapy: A Comparison of Approaches. Maryland: Prentice Hall, 1985.

Bowen M. Family psychotherapy. From the workshop The Family as a Unit of Study and Treatment. American Journal of Orthopsychiatry, 31:40, 1961.

Collins-Colon T. Do it yourself—Medication management for community based clients. Journal of Psychosocial Nursing, 28:6, 1990.

Collison C, Miller J. The role of family re-enactment in group psychotherapy. Perspectives in Psychiatric Care, 23(2):74, 1985.

Delgado M. Hispanics and psychotherapy groups. International Journal of Group Psychotherapy, 33(4):503, 1983.

Erikson E. Childhood and Society. New York: WW Norton, 1963.

Self-study Exercises

Match each group term with the correct definition.

1. _____ Ebb and flow of power or energy
2. _____ Group in which new members are added as others leave
3. _____ Process by which a problem that has been hidden is brought into the open
4. _____ Deeper, underlying meaning of messages of what is happening in the group
5. _____ All that is said in a group
6. _____ The nonverbal actions that vary depending on the level of anxiety in meeting individual goals while working to meet group goals

A. Group content

B. Group process

C. Subgrouping

D. Covert content (communication)

E. Confrontation

F. Open group

7. _____ Two or more individuals in a group that join together. They may have more loyalty to each other than they do to the larger group.

G. Closed group

H. Dynamics

8. _____ Membership is restricted and often time limited.

Select the correct answer.

9. The primary goal of the inpatient group therapist is

   A. To focus on the here-and-now
   B. To examine interpersonal relationships within the group
   C. To be proactive and create a structure for the group
   D. All of the above

10. Countertransference is

   A. The patient's feelings or reactions toward the therapist
   B. The therapist's feelings or reactions toward the patient
   C. Underlying meaning in group interaction
   D. The content of an interaction

True or false

11. _____ For treatment of an alcoholic to be successful, it is helpful for the alcoholic's family to receive some kind of family therapy.

12. _____ For the family of an alcoholic, family-centered nursing services can be just as effective as family therapy.

13. _____ Corrective recapitulation of the primary family group means that group members will relate to each other as they did to members of their own nuclear family.

14. _____ Some theorists believe that there are rules in family systems that are not always discussed.

Match each group role with the correct definition.

15. _____ Asks for clarification of beliefs and values

A. Scapegoat

16. _____ Checks out what someone said by questioning and restating

B. Identified patient

17. _____ Keeps the group focused on goals and questions directions

C. Orientor

18. _____ Acts out family dysfunction

19. _____ Is seen as the person in the family who most needs treatment

D. Clarifier

20. _____ States beliefs and values

E. Opinion seeker

F. Opinion giver

Select the correct answer.

21. In TA groups, ego states are defined as

   A. Parent, child, and adult
   B. Id, ego, and superego
   C. Games, scripts, and strokes
   D. None of the above

22. Self-help groups

    A. Can use a nurse as a leader or group member only if she or he has had a similar problem and has resolved it
    B. Often meet without a designated leader
    C. Provide mutual support
    D. All of the above

23. Self-help groups, such as AA, Co-Dependents Anonymous, and the National Alliance for the Mentally Ill, can

    A. Prevent physical, emotional, or social health problems
    B. Improve an individual's or a family's quality of life
    C. Provide education to develop an individual's potential
    D. All of the above

True or false (If false, correct the statement.)

24. _____ A patient should not be included in an inpatient group if he or she can only attend two sessions. _____

_____

25. _____ Confidentiality is essential in all aspects of inpatient group therapy, even if a patient reveals suicidal thoughts. _____

_____

26. _____ Group members are encouraged to stay, even when they want to leave, once the group session has started. _____

27. _____ The group therapist encourages a patient to talk about his or her feelings if the patient threatens to do something violent. _____

_____

Select the correct answer.

28. In the uncertainty phase

    A. Members want to carve out a place for themselves
    B. Attrition is common
    C. Silence may pervade
    D. All of the above

29. In the overaggressive phase

    A. Hostility toward the group therapist is common
    B. It is particularly important for the group therapist to be aware of her or his own feelings of anger
    C. The therapist needs to ask a member who criticizes another if the member is reminded of him- or herself
    D. All of the above

30. In a group of persons with schizophrenia, it is most important for

    A. The process to be analyzed more than the content
    B. The expression of anger to be validated as OK
    C. The therapist to understand that anxiety can increase auditory hallucinations
    D. All of the above

CHAPTER 8

The Nursing Process in Psychiatric Settings

Elizabeth M. Varcarolis

OUTLINE •

KEY TERMS AND CONCEPTS ◆ ◆ ◆ ◆ ◆ ◆ ◆ ◆ ◆ ◆ ◆ ◆ ◆ ◆ ◆

The key terms and concepts listed here also appear in bold where they are defined or discussed in this chapter.

ASSESSING BEHAVIOR
Echopraxia
Waxy Flexibility
Akathisia
Dyskinesia

ASSESSING THOUGHT PROCESSES
Tangential
Flights of Ideas
Neologisms
Confabulation
Looseness of Association

ASSESSING PREOCCUPATIONS IN
    THOUGHT CONTENT
Hallucinations
Delusions

Obsessions
Rituals
Phobias

GENERAL SYSTEMS THEORY

HOLISTIC MODEL

MASLOW'S HUMAN NEEDS THEORY

NURSING DIAGNOSIS

INTERVENTION
Psychotherapeutic Interventions
Health Teaching
Activities of Daily Living
Somatic Therapies
Therapeutic Environment
Psychotherapy

OBJECTIVES ■

After studying this chapter, the student will be able to

1. Identify the components of each of the five steps in the nursing process.
2. Discuss what is meant by the "process" of psychiatric assessment.
3. Summarize the contents of the *Client History* and the *Mental and Emotional Status* of the psychiatric nursing assessment.
4. Explain five functions of the nursing diagnostic system.
5. Predict when a problem becomes a nursing diagnosis.
6. Illustrate the three components of the nursing diagnosis.
7. Write an effective goal including the three criteria discussed in this chapter.
8. Explain three principles the nurse follows in planning nursing actions to meet goals.
9. Give two examples for each of the six areas of psychiatric nursing intervention.
10. Outline three areas of concern when validating a plan of care.
11. Discuss two components of the evaluation process.
12. Recognize four possible outcomes after reassessment of the care plan.

The nursing process is an adaptation of the scientific method. This problem-solving process is used today by many professions and encourages clinical care based on scientific and systematic decision making rather than on rote tasks and randomly applied nursing interventions. The use of a scientific and systematic process for planning effective patient care helps to distinguish nursing as a profession, as opposed to a trade solely composed of technical skills (Hagerty 1984).

The terms *nursing process* and *nursing diagnosis* first appeared in the nursing literature in the early 1950s. The process of defining and operationalizing these concepts continued to evolve during the 1960s and 1970s through contributions by many nursing scholars. The first formalized presentation of the nursing process was presented by Yura and Walsh in 1967 and consisted of four steps: assessment, planning, intervention, and evaluation (Yura and Walsh 1983). Later, nursing diagnosis was included as a separate step, apart from assessment, resulting in the five accepted steps used today: assessment, diagnosis, planning, intervention, and evaluation. The components of each step are presented in Figure 8–1.

Assessment is done for the purpose of identifying client problems and formulating nursing diagnoses. Planning includes identifying desired outcome criteria in the form of long and short term goals. Goals give direction for effective nursing actions. The nurse, often with input from the patient, determines the interventions that will result in the desired outcomes. The process of evaluating whether the outcome criteria have been obtained is the fifth phase of the process. If the goals have not been met, then reassessment and replanning may be necessary.

The nurse must determine if necessary data are available, the diagnosis is correct, the goals realistic and obtainable, and the interventions appropriate for meeting the goals.

These five steps help to operationalize the ongoing nursing process. In reality, these steps often overlap. The nurse continually assesses and analyzes data, identifies needs, resets goals, and brings various appropriate nursing skills into play. Evaluation of these activities is ongoing.

Today, the nursing process is the basic framework for nursing practice. The nursing process has been used as a basis for the following:

1. Criteria for certification
2. Legal definition of nursing, as reflected in many states' nurse practice acts
3. The National Council of State Boards of Nursing licensure examination (NCLEX-RN) format since July 1982

The nurse uses the nursing process when evaluating the client at any point on the health-illness continuum. A client may be an individual, a family, a group, or a community. Assessment is made on many levels: physical, social, emotional, intellectual, spiritual, and cultural. Nursing diagnosis and planning of interventions may include primary, secondary, or tertiary interventions, depending on the specific needs and environment of the client.

The actions of the nurse are based on a number of accepted theoretical frameworks: (1) a holistic model, (2) Maslow's human needs theory, and (3) the general systems theory.

The **holistic model** supports the assessment, diagnosis, planning, intervention, and evaluation of care

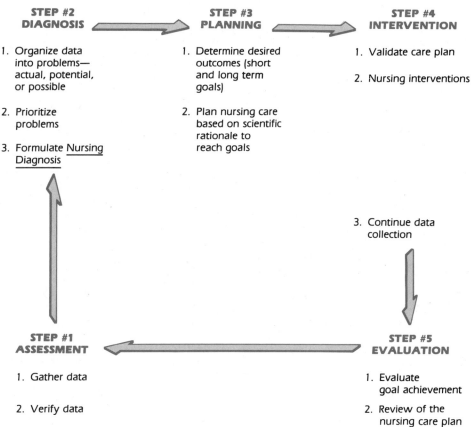

Figure 8–1. *Components of the nursing process.*

for the total person. The holistic approach considers the client's physical, emotional, social, spiritual, intellectual, and cultural stresses and their impact on the whole individual (Bower 1982).

Human needs theory is most basic to the nursing process. When an individual's ability to meet a need is interrupted, a problem exists. Maslow (1962) has outlined our basic needs in a hierarchy familiar to all nurses:

1. Hunger, thirst, sex, and survival
2. Safety, self-preservation, security
3. Belongingness and love
4. Social esteem and self-respect
5. Self-actualization

Recognition of unmet needs is made evident from information the nurse has gathered in the assessment. An unmet need constitutes a problem. The problems nurses are most involved with are in the areas of physical and emotional health. Problems are formulated into nursing diagnoses and are listed in order of priority. Assessment, planning, interventions, and evaluation are ongoing until an acceptable alternative for dealing with the unmet need or problem is found.

General systems theory recognizes the impact a person's internal and external environments have on personal health. All things belong to a matrix of complex systems, and individuals are constantly being in-

fluenced and affected by the systems of which they are a part. External systems include family, community, and regional and national influences. Internal systems include body systems, organs, cells, chemical elements, and atoms.

Each level of systems is composed of subsystems. For example, internal systems, such as the respiratory, digestive, reproductive, and immune systems, are all part of the larger system, the human body. Nursing is a subsystem of an external system, the health care system, which is made up of other subsystems, such as medicine, dentistry, pharmacology, and social work. Any change in one system or subsystem can have a profound impact on related systems. Therefore, a thorough assessment takes into account both the internal and the external systems of the client. Nursing diagnoses and interventions address both the internal and the external environments for optimum total patient care.

There are many nursing frameworks that may be used as guides when making a nursing assessment, such as those of Rogers (1970), Riehl and Roy (1980), and Orem (1980). However, the holistic approach, Maslow's human needs theory, and general systems theory are inherent to the nursing process.

Psychiatric and mental health nursing practice bases nursing judgments and behaviors in an accepted theoretical framework. The importance of a theoretical framework has been supported by the Standards of Psychiatric and Mental Health Nursing, developed by the ANA.

Theory

All psychopathology will be presented within the framework of the nursing process. The most recent and prevalent theories of etiology will be presented for the clinical syndromes discussed in the clinical chapters (11–25).

Assessment

Although high levels of anxiety and maladaptive behaviors are commonly seen by the practitioners of psychiatric nursing, these phenomena are encountered in all areas in the health care setting. Depression, suicidal thoughts, anger, disorientation, delusions, and hallucinations are frequently encountered on medical-surgical wards and obstetrical and intensive care units, as well as in emergency rooms, clinics, and pediatric settings. The **assessment** of the client's psychosocial status is a part of any nursing assessment, along with the assessment of the client's physical health.

The nursing process is a cyclical one. Assessment is ongoing and continues throughout the planning, intervention, and evaluation phases. The initial assessment often clarifies the client's immediate needs. As the nurse works further with the client, the data base is enlarged, and other problems may become evident.

Psychiatric nursing assessment is done within the framework of the psychiatric interview. The assessment interview in psychiatric nursing is often done in the psychiatric inpatient units; however, it can be done in many settings: emergency rooms, medical-surgical units, intensive care units, crisis units, community mental health centers, private practice, homes, and schools. The time given for the interview varies, depending on the clinical setting and the circumstances of the client. During emergencies, immediate intervention is often based on a minimal amount of data. A scheduled psychiatric interview and psychosocial assessment in a more structured setting allows more time for a more elaborate assessment. At other times, completing the assessment process may involve many interviews.

The purpose of the psychiatric assessment (Hagerty 1984) is to

1. Assess a person's current level of psychological functioning
2. Establish a trusting rapport
3. Understand how previous modes of coping contributed to the person's psychosocial development
4. Formulate a plan of care

Although the nurse might obtain a lot of needed data from the physician's assessment, the nurse's primary source for data collection is the client. There may be times when the client is unable to assist with the assessment. For example, if the client is severely delusional, mute, comatose, or extremely confused, then secondary sources would be used. Secondary sources include members of the family, friends, neighbors, police, other members of the health team, medical records, and laboratory results. Both primary and secondary sources need to be used during assessment.

PROCESS OF THE PSYCHIATRIC NURSING ASSESSMENT

If the nursing process is the framework for nursing practice, *the therapeutic relationship is the medium through which the nursing process is implemented.* Although the client is the focus, the nurse and the client work together to reduce anxiety, relieve pain, satisfy unmet needs, and promote optimum functioning. Assisting a person toward optimum functioning is accomplished through three levels of nursing intervention:

- Preventive (primary intervention)
- Restorative (secondary intervention)
- Rehabilitative (tertiary intervention)

Underlying these three levels of nursing intervention are certain premises (Bower 1982):

1. Individuals have the right to decide their destiny and to be involved in decisions that affect them.
2. Nursing intervention is designed to assist individuals to meet their own needs or to solve their own problems.
3. The ultimate goal of all nursing action is to assist individuals to maximize their independent level of functioning.

The development of the therapeutic relationship is a crucial factor in the implementation of the nursing process. As discussed in Chapter 6, the optimum use of communication skills and therapeutic use of self affect all phases of the nursing process. This is especially true during the assessment phase.

When assessment occurs during the initial interview, the nurse and the client are essentially strangers. Both experience anxiety, as in any other meeting between strangers. The interviewer's anxiety may stem from the client's self-perception of the interviewer's ability (or inability) to help the client. If the interviewer is a nursing student, anxiety regarding the instructor's evaluation becomes an added dimension. Clients' anxiety centers on their problems, the nurse's view of the clients, and what is ahead for them in treatment (MacKinnon 1971).

Both client and nurse bring to their relationship their total background experiences. These experiences include cultural beliefs and biases, religious attitudes, educational background, and occupational and life experiences, as well as attitudes regarding sexual roles. These attitudes, beliefs, and values influence the nurse's interactions with clients. It is important for nurses to be aware of their biases and values and not feel compelled to impose their personal beliefs on others. Although the nurse shares perceptions and alternatives with the client, the goal is to work with the client so that decisions and actions taken are the right ones for the client. Theoretically, this sounds easy, but often it is not. When beginning practitioners share their perceptions and thoughts with a more experienced nurse, unrecognized biases and value judgments often become evident. **Experience and supervision help a nurse separate what is important to the client from any bias that might impede mutually agreed-on goals.**

Although the purpose of the psychiatric assessment is to gather data that will help clarify the client's situation and problem, this is best done in an atmosphere of minimal anxiety. Therefore, if an individual becomes upset, defensive, or embarrassed regarding any topic, the topic should be abandoned. The nurse can acknowledge that this is a subject that makes the client uncomfortable and can suggest that it would best be discussed when the client feels more comfortable. It is important that the nurse not probe, pry, or push for information that is difficult for the client to discuss. The purpose of an assessment is to gather data pertaining to the client's problem, *not* to collect a lot of data.

CONTENT OF THE PSYCHIATRIC NURSING ASSESSMENT

The actual assessment consists of (1) gathering data and (2) verifying the data.

Gathering Data

The use of a standardized nursing assessment tool facilitates the assessment process. Many assessment forms are available for use. Most health care systems and schools of nursing have their own assessment tool; however, even though an assessment tool is used, it is best to gather information from the client in an informal fashion, with the nurse clarifying, focusing, and exploring pertinent data with the client. This method allows clients to state their perceptions in their own words and enables the nurse to observe a wide range of nonverbal behaviors. When the order and the questions on the assessment tool are too rigidly applied, spontaneity is reduced. Assessment is a skill that is learned over a period of time. The development of this skill is enhanced by practice, supervision, and patience. A personal style of interviewing congruent with the nurse's personality develops as comfort and experience increase.

The basic components of the psychiatric nursing assessment include (1) client history and (2) mental and emotional status.

The client's history is the *subjective* part of the assessment. The focus of the history is the client's perceptions and recollections in three broad areas: presenting problem, current lifestyle, and briefly, the client's life (family, friends, education, and work experience) (Eisenman and Dubbert 1978).

The mental and emotional status is the *objective* part of the assessment. The nurse observes the person's physical behavior and nonverbal communication, appearance, speech patterns, thought content, and cognitive ability.

The assessment covers social, physical, emotional, cultural, cognitive, and spiritual aspects of an individual. It elicits information about the systems in which a person operates. To conduct such an assessment, the nurse should have fundamental knowledge of growth and development and of basic cultural and religious practices, as well as pathophysiology, psychopathology, and pharmacology.

Figure 8–2 at the end of the chapter shows a sample assessment tool that covers the following areas:

I. CLIENT HISTORY
    I. General History of Client
        Data include the client's age, sex, and culture.

        With whom does the client live? Who is the client's family? Whom does the client trust? Who cares for the client? Information regarding the constellation of the client's family helps the nurse determine the client's role in the family. How does the client's illness affect the family members? What level of education does the client have?

Religious beliefs can provide an important source of strength for many clients. What are the specific values and norms with which the individual identifies?

II. Presenting Problem

A. In the client's own words, what is happening that needs changing? What was the reason for seeking treatment? Has the client experienced any recent traumatic events? Has anything like this experience happened before?

B. Are there recent difficulties or alterations in relationships? Is the person functioning at his or her usual level? Is the client having difficulty thinking or problem solving?

C. Can the client identify increased feelings of depression, anxiety, suspiciousness, or hopelessness? Is the person feeling overwhelmed or confused? How does the person describe his or her feelings at this moment?

D. What kind of somatic changes has the individual noticed? Are there changes in bowel patterns, sleep, and eating habits? Has the person gained or lost weight recently?

III. Relevant History—Personal

A. Were there any previous hospitalizations and illnesses? Did the client perceive past medical attention as helpful? What prescribed or over-the-counter medications does the client take?

B. What was the client's educational background, including positive or negative perceptions?

C. What is the client's occupational background, including the person's present place of employment? If the client is not employed, what kind of job would the client prefer?

D. Who are the client's friends? With whom does the client identify? Describe a usual day.

E. What are the client's sexual patterns? Does the person have problems or concerns related to sexual habits or orientation?

F. What are the person's interests and abilities? What kinds of activities give the client pleasure? What is the client good at?

G. Does the person overeat or undereat? What drugs does the person take? How often? How many alcoholic drinks does the person take per day or per week? At what age did use of drugs begin? Does the client identify any of these habits as problematic?

H. How does the client cope with stress? What does the client usually do when upset? With whom can the client talk? What coping mechanism does the client find the most helpful?

IV. Relevant History—Family

A. Who was important to the client during childhood? Was there any physical or sexual abuse? Did the parents drink? Who was in the home during the client's childhood?

B. How does the client describe adolescence?

C. Was there use or abuse of drugs or alcohol by family members? What was the effect on the family?

D. Who had physical or mental problems in the family? Describe the problems.

E. Are there any unusual or outstanding events the client wishes to mention?

2. **MENTAL AND EMOTIONAL STATUS**

A. Appearance

What does the client look like? How is the client dressed? Is the client well groomed or are hair and nailbeds dirty? Does the client appear neat or disheveled? How does the client relate to the interviewer? Is eye contact maintained? Describe the client's posture? Draw a picture in words.

B. Behavior

Describe the motor activity: restless, agitated, lethargic? What kind of mannerisms and facial expressions does the client use when talking? Does the client show signs of **echopraxia, waxy flexibility, akathisia,** or **dyskinesia?** Table 8–1 defines these and other abnormal motor behaviors.

C. Speech

Is the client's speech intelligible and clear, or does he or she mumble or speak fast and forcefully? Are there barriers to communications, such as confusion or delusions?

D. Mood

What mood does the client convey to the nurse? Hostile? Grandiose? Helpless?

E. Affect

What is the client's presenting affect? Is the affect appropriate, bizarre, bland, apathetic, or overly dramatic?

F. Thought Process

1. Describe the characteristics of the person's responses. Does the client change the topic often **(tangential)**? Are the client's responses appropriate to the questions asked? Does the client jump from topic to topic so that it is difficult to follow the thought process **(flights of ideas)**? Does the client make up words **(neologisms)** or make up events to fill periods of time **(confabulation)**? Is there an illogical stream of thought **(loose-**

Table 8–1 ■ ABNORMAL MOTOR BEHAVIORS

DEFINITION	EXAMPLE
Echopraxia	
Repeating the movements of another person.	Every time the nurse would move or gesture with her hands, the client would copy her gestures.
Echolalia	
Repeating the speech of another person.	The nurse said to the client, "Tell me your name." The client responded, "Tell me your name, tell me your name."
Waxy Flexibility	
Having one's arms or legs placed in a certain position and holding that same position for hours.	The nurse lifted the client's arm to check the pulse, and the client left his arm extended in the same position.
Parkinson-like Symptoms	
Making mask-like faces, drooling, and having shuffling gait, tremors, and muscular rigidity. Seen in people who are on antipsychotic medication, such as phenothiazines.	The nurse noticed that the client's face held no emotion. He walked very stiffly, leaning forward, almost robot-like.
Akathisia	
Displaying motor restlessness, feeling of muscular quivering; at its worst, patient is unable to sit still or lie quietly.	The client's leg kept jiggling up and down when he talked to the nurse. When his feet were still, his arm would jiggle constantly during the interview.
Dyskinesia	
Having distortion of voluntary movements, such as involuntary muscular activity (e.g., tic, spasm, or myoclonus).	The client had a marked facial tic around his mouth, which was distracting to the nurse during the interview.

ness of associations) or blocking of ideas? Table 8–2 defines these and other disordered characteristics.

2. Cognitive Ability

Assessment of language skills and reading and writing abilities can prove helpful in distinguishing between functional psychosis and organic psychosis (Hagerty 1984). Not all clients require cognitive testing in depth. If, however, a client exhibits disorganized thinking and bizarre behavior, formal testing of cognitive functions may be ordered.

G. Thought Content
1. What central themes are important to the client?
2. Does the client have a good self-concept? What does the client like most about him- or herself? What does the client want to change?
3. Does the client have insight into the presenting problem? Is the client aware of the existing or potential problems?
4. Is there suicidal or homicidal ideation? If the client has suicidal thoughts, what is his suicide potential (see SAD PERSONS Scale, Chapter 21)? If the client is homicidal, or

suicidal, have any past attempts at either been made? Has anyone in the client's family attempted to, or succeeded in, killing someone?
5. Does the client's thought content contain any particular **preoccupations,** such as **hallucinations, delusions, obsessions, rituals, phobias,** religiosity, grandiosity, or feelings of worthlessness? (See Table 8–3 for a more detailed discussion of these preoccupations.)

H. Reality Orientation
1. Time

Can the person tell the nurse the day, the month, and the year?
2. Place

Can the client tell you where he or she is? If the client is in a hospital, have the client name and give the location of the hospital.
3. Memory

Questions such as, "Who is the President?" or "What were you doing last week?" are good tests of recent memory.

I. Level of Anxiety

From the data and observations of the client, the nurse assesses the client's level of anxiety

Table 8–2 ■ SUMMARY OF ABNORMAL THOUGHT PROCESSES

DEFINITION	EXAMPLE
Tangentiality	
Association disturbance in which the speaker goes off the topic. When it happens frequently and the speaker does not return to the topic, interpersonal communication is destroyed.	The nurse asked the client to talk more about his family. The client continuously left the topic and talked about boats, animals, his apartment, and so forth. Each time the nurse tried to help the client to focus, he would go off on another topic.
Neologisms	
Words a person makes up that only have meaning for the person himself, often part of a delusional system.	"I am afraid to go to the hospital because the *norks* are looking for me there."
Looseness of Association	
Thinking is haphazard, illogical, and confused. Connections in thought are interrupted. Seen mostly in schizophrenic disorders.	"Can't go to the zoo, no money, Oh . . . I have a hat, these members make no sense, man . . . What's the problem?"
Flights of Ideas	
Constant flow of speech in which the person jumps from one topic to another in rapid succession. There is a connection between topics, although it is sometimes hard to identify. Characteristically seen in manic states.	"Say babe, how's it going . . . Going to my sister's to get some money . . . money, honey, you got any bread . . . bread and butter, staff of life, ain't life grand? . . ."
Blocking	
Sudden cessation of a thought in the middle of a sentence. Person is unable to continue his train of thought. Often sudden new thoughts crop up unrelated to the topic. Can be disturbing to the individual.	"I was going to get a new dress for the . . . I forgot what I was going to say."
Circumstantiality	
Before getting to the point or answering a question, the person gets caught up in countless details and explanations.	"Where are you going for the weekend, Harry?" "Well I first thought of going to my mother's, but that was before I remembered that she was going to my sister's. My sister is having a picnic. She always has picnics at the beach. The beach that she goes to is large and gets crowded. That's why I don't like that beach. So I decided to go someplace else. I thought of going to my brother's house. He has a large house on a quiet street . . . I finally decided to stay home."
Perseveration	
Involuntary repetition of the same thought, phrase, or motor response to different questions or situations. Associated with brain damage.	N: How are you doing, Harry? H: Fine, nurse, just fine. N: Did you go for a walk? H: Fine, nurse, just fine. N: Are you going out today? H: Fine, nurse, just fine.
Confabulation	
Filling in a memory gap with detailed fantasy believed by the teller. The purpose is to maintain self-esteem and is seen in organic conditions, such as Korsakoff's psychosis.	The nurse asked Harry, who spent the weekend at home, what he did that weekend. "Well, I just came back from California after signing a contract with MGM for a film on the life of Roosevelt. We had the most marvelous tour of the studio . . . went to lunch with the director . . ."
Word Salad	
Mixture of words and phrases that have no meaning.	"I am fine . . . apple pie . . . no sale . . . furniture store . . . take it slow . . . cellar door . . ."

Table 8–3 ■ PREOCCUPATIONS IN THOUGHT CONTENT

DEFINITION	EXAMPLE
Hallucinations — *Sensory Perceptions*	
A sense perception for which no external stimuli exist. Hallucinations can have an organic or a functional etiology.	
Visual: Seeing things that are not there.	During alcohol withdrawal he kept shouting, "I see snakes on the walls."
Auditory: Hearing voices when none are present.	"I keep hearing my mother's voice telling me I am bad. She died a year ago."
Olfactory: Smelling smells that do not exist.	"I smell my stomach rotting."
Tactile: Feeling touch sensations in the absence of stimuli. (Also referred to as haptic.)	A paranoid man feels electrical impulses "from outer space" entering his body and controlling his mind.
Gustatory: Experiencing taste in the absence of stimuli.	A paranoid woman tastes poison in her food while eating at her son's wedding.
Delusions	
A false belief held to be true even with evidence to the contrary. Three common delusions follow:	
Persecution: The thought that one is being singled out for harm by others.	An intern believes that the chief of staff is plotting to kill him to prevent the intern from becoming too powerful.
Grandeur: The false belief that one is a very powerful and important person.	A newly admitted patient told the nurse that he was God, and he was here to save the world.
Jealousy: The false belief that one's mate is going out with other people. The person may take everyday occurrences for "proof."	Sally "knew" that her husband, Jim, was being unfaithful. Even when Sally's brother swore he and Jim really did play pool Friday nights, Sally declared Jim's not being home then was her "proof."
Obsessions	
An idea, impulse, or emotion that a person cannot put out of his or her consciousness. Can be mild or severe.	A young mother, Jane, told the nurse that she was hounded by constant thoughts that something terrible was going to happen to her baby. She knew that this was crazy, but she could not get the thought to stop.
Rituals	
Repetitive actions that people must do over and over until either they are exhausted or anxiety is decreased. Often done to lessen the anxiety triggered by an obsession.	Jane stated to the nurse the only way she could temporarily get these obsessions to cease was to say three "Hail Mary's" and knock on wood twice to reassure herself that "nothing terrible was happening."
Phobias	
An intense irrational fear of an object, situation, or place. The fear persists even though the object of the fear is perfectly harmless and the person is aware of the irrationality.	Although she was aware that cats would not harm her, Mary was deathly afraid of cats and refused to visit her sister and friends who had cats.

as mild, moderate, severe, or panic level. Knowing the level of anxiety helps the nurse identify appropriate approaches to intervention (see Chapter 9 for criteria in assessing level of anxiety).

After the nurse has concluded the assessment, it is useful for the nurse to briefly summarize pertinent data with the client. The summary provides the client with the reassurance that he or she has been heard, and it allows the client the opportunity to clarify any misinformation (Eisenman and Dubbert 1978). The client should be told what will happen next. For example, if the initial assessment takes place in the hospital, the nurse should tell the client who else he or she will be seeing. If the initial assessment was conducted by a psychiatric nurse in a mental health clinic, the nurse should let the client know when and how often they will meet to work on the client's problems. If the nurse feels a referral is necessary (e.g., to a psychiatrist, social worker, or physician), the nurse should discuss this with the client.

Verifying Data

It is necessary that the nurse validate data obtained from the client with secondary sources. Whenever possible, *family members* should be a part of the assessment. Is there anything going on in the family that is affecting the family? It is important for the nurse to understand how the family views the client. How does the family define the problem? How do the client's problems affect the family? What does the family think might help the client? Who else in the family is having difficulty? Does the client perceive his or her problems and behavior in the same way the family does?

Friends and *neighbors* can be important sources of information. They may verify or contradict the client's self-perception and actions. They may add information that the client did not think relevant.

Often, *police officers* are the ones who bring clients into the psychiatric emergency rooms. It is important for the nurse to know as much as possible about exactly what the client was doing that warranted police intervention. Was the client suicidal or homicidal? Was anyone hurt?

Other members of the *health team* are important sources of information and data verification. Many members of the health team will have contact with the client on admission to the hospital. The psychiatrist or psychologist, social worker, psychiatric nurse, recreation therapist, therapy aides, and student nurses can add to the nurse's data base. Observations from all health team members are important for making a thorough assessment. Often the client has been admitted previously. Are the circumstances and symptoms the same as previously, more intense, less intense? Are circumstances totally different on this admission?

Old charts and *medical records* can help validate information the nurse already has or can add new information. Medical history can aid in assessing physical losses and stress and can alert the staff to potential medical problems. If the client has been admitted to a psychiatric unit in the past, information about the client's previous level of functioning and behavior gives the nurse a baseline for making clinical judgments. Is the client functioning at a higher or lower level than previously? Does the client cope with anxiety in similar ways or use different coping skills at present? Is the reason for the client's present admission similar to that for past admissions or not? What were the previous precipitating events that led to admission?

Laboratory reports can provide useful information. When the body's chemistry is abnormal, personality changes and violent behaviors can result. For example, abnormal liver enzymes can explain irritability, depression, and lethargy. People who have chronic renal disease often suffer from the same symptoms when their blood urea nitrogen and electrolyte levels are abnormal. People with endocrine diseases, like diabetes, can have changes in mood and level of consciousness related to sugar and insulin levels.

Nursing Diagnosis

Nursing diagnosis is a crucial component in the nursing process because the diagnosis directs nursing actions and provides the focus for evaluating outcomes (Kim 1985).

The development of the concept of nursing diagnosis has been controversial and stormy. Nursing authors have written to support and differentiate nursing diagnosis from medical diagnosis since the 1950s. The National Group for the Classification of Nursing Diagnosis met for the first time in 1973 and has since been renamed the North American Nursing Diagnosis Association (NANDA). Under the leadership of this group, the development of nursing diagnosis continues. Table 8–4 identifies accepted nursing diagnoses under assessment categories.

Because nurses are increasingly faced with caring for culturally diverse populations, there is increasing need for nursing diagnoses and subsequent care to be planned around unique cultural health care beliefs, values, and practices. Awareness of individual cultural beliefs and health care practices can help nurses minimize "labeling" of clients. This unintentional stereotyping sets up barriers for optimum health care intervention and benefit to the patient (Geissler 1991) (see Chapter 4).

WHY A NURSING DIAGNOSTIC SYSTEM?

The use of a unified classification system among nurses helps to identify nurses' independent functions. A formalized diagnostic system can perform many functions for the practice of nursing. Some of the purposes served by nursing diagnoses follow:

1. Help define the practice of nursing
2. Provide nurses with a common frame of reference
3. Improve communication among staff members and between facilities
4. Help define a body of unique nursing knowledge
5. Differentiate nursing from medicine
6. Facilitate intraprofessional and interprofessional communications
7. Make nurses more accountable for care
8. Assist educators and students in focusing on nursing phenomena rather than on medical phenomena

Table 8-4 ▪ NURSING DIAGNOSIS FUNCTIONAL HEALTH PATTERNS

Health perception–health management pattern
Altered health maintenance
Ineffective management of therapeutic regimen
Noncompliance (specify)
Health-seeking behaviors (specify)
High risk for infection
High risk for injury (trauma)
High risk for poisoning
High risk for suffocation
Altered protection

Nutritional-metabolic pattern
Altered nutrition: high risk for more than body
   requirements *or* high risk for obesity
Altered nutrition: more than body requirements
Altered nutrition: less than body requirements
Ineffective breast-feeding
Effective breast-feeding
Interrupted breast-feeding
Ineffective infant feeding pattern
High risk for aspiration
Impaired swallowing
Altered oral mucous membrane
High risk for fluid volume deficit
Fluid volume deficit
Fluid volume excess
High risk for impaired skin integrity
Impaired skin integrity
Impaired tissue integrity (specify type)
High risk for altered body temperature
Ineffective thermoregulation
Hyperthermia
Hypothermia

Elimination pattern
Constipation
Colonic constipation
Perceived constipation
Diarrhea
Bowel incontinence
Altered urinary elimination pattern
Functional incontinence
Reflex incontinence
Stress incontinence
Urge incontinence
Total incontinence
Urinary retention

Activity-exercise pattern
High risk for activity intolerance
Activity intolerance (specify level)
Fatigue
Impaired physical mobility (specify level)
High risk for disuse syndrome
Total self-care deficit (specify level)
Self-bathing–hygiene deficit (specify level)
Self-dressing–grooming deficit (specify level)
Self-feeding deficit (specify level)
Self-toileting deficit (specify level)
Diversional activity deficit
Impaired home maintenance management
Dysfunctional ventilatory weaning response (DVWR)
Inability to sustain spontaneous ventilation
Ineffective airway clearance
Ineffective breathing pattern

Impaired gas exchange
Decreased cardiac output
Altered tissue perfusion (specify)
Dysreflexia
High risk for peripheral neurovascular dysfunction
Altered growth and development

Sleep-rest pattern
Sleep-pattern disturbance

Cognitive-perceptual pattern
Pain
Chronic pain
Sensory-perceptual alterations
Unilateral neglect
Knowledge deficit (specify)
Impaired thought processes
Decisional conflict (specify)

Self-perception–self-concept pattern
Fear (specify focus)
Anxiety
Hopelessness
Powerlessness (severe, low, moderate)
Self-esteem disturbance
Chronic low self-esteem
Situational low self-esteem
Body image disturbance
High risk for self-mutilation
Personal identity disturbance

Role-relationship pattern
Anticipatory grieving
Dysfunctional grieving
Disturbance in role performance
Social isolation
Impaired social interaction
Relocation stress syndrome
Altered family processes
High risk for altered parenting
Altered parenting
Parental role conflict
Caregiver role strain
High risk for caregiver role strain
Impaired verbal communication
High risk for violence

Sexuality-reproductive pattern
Sexual dysfunction
Altered sexuality patterns
Rape-trauma syndrome
Rape-trauma syndrome: compound reaction
Rape-trauma syndrome: silent reaction

Coping–stress-tolerance pattern
Ineffective coping (individual)
Defensive coping
Ineffective denial
Impaired adjustment
Post-trauma response
Family coping: potential for growth
Ineffective family coping: compromised
Ineffective family coping: disabling

Value-belief pattern
Spiritual distress (distress of human spirit)

From Gordon M. Manual of Nursing Diagnosis 1993–1994. St. Louis, MO: Mosby–Year Book, 1993.

WHAT IS A NURSING DIAGNOSIS?

There are a number of definitions for **nursing diagnosis** in the literature. The following three definitions are among the most widely accepted:

1. Gordon defines nursing diagnosis as an "actual or potential health problem which nurses, by virtue of their education and experience are capable and licensed to treat" (Gordon 1982).
2. Shoemaker's definition of a nursing diagnosis is "a clinical judgment about an individual, family, or community which is derived through a deliberate, systematic process of data collection and analysis. It provides the basis for prescriptions for definitive therapy for which the nurse is accountable. It is expressed concisely and it includes the etiology of the condition when known" (Shoemaker 1984).
3. Carpenito defines nursing diagnosis as "a statement that describes a health state or an actual or potential alteration in one's life processes (physiological, psychological, sociocultural, developmental and spiritual). The nurse uses the nursing process to identify and synthesize clinical data and to order nursing interventions to reduce, eliminate, or prevent (health promotion) health alterations which are in the legal and educational domain of nursing" (Carpenito 1991).

Common threads among these definitions are evident. The following seven assumptions can be drawn from these three definitions:

1. Health problems or alterations in a client's life process can be actual or potential.
2. A client can be an individual, a family group, or a community.
3. Health problems can be physiological, psychological, sociocultural, developmental, or spiritual.
4. The health problems are identified through a systematic process of data collection and data analysis.
5. The clinical judgment made from the assessment provides the basis for nursing interventions (primary, secondary, or tertiary).
6. The intervention and treatment are prescribed within the educational and legal domain of nurses, by way of licensure.
7. The statement of the problem is expressed concisely and includes the etiology when known.

A nursing diagnosis has three structural components (Gordon 1982):

1. Problem (unmet need)
2. Etiology (probable cause)
3. Supporting data (signs and symptoms)

The *problem*, or unmet need, describes the state of the client at present. Problems that are within the nurse's domain to prescribe and treat are termed *nursing diagnoses*. The nursing diagnostic title states what should change. For example:

Altered thought processes

Etiology, or probable cause, is linked to the diagnostic title with the words *related to*. Stating the etiology or probable cause tells what needs to be done to effect the change and identifies causes that the nurse can treat through nursing interventions.

Altered thought processes:
related to psychological conflicts

Supporting data, or signs and symptoms, state what the condition is like at present.

Altered thought processes: related to psychological conflicts
Supporting data that validate diagnosis:

- Client's thinking has slowed down.
- Client complains of trouble with memory.
- Client complains of difficulty concentrating.

A nursing diagnosis can reflect an actual, high-risk, or possible problem.

An *actual* problem means that the problem has been clinically identified by the supporting data. For example:

Self-esteem disturbance: related to recent divorce
Supporting data that validate diagnosis:

- Client shows signs of weeping and despair.
- Client withdraws from social contacts.
- Client states, "I feel like half a person."

A nursing diagnosis of a *high-risk* problem suggests a problem that is likely to occur if nursing intervention is not ordered. For example:

High risk for violence: related to aggressive behaviors
Supporting data that validate diagnosis:

- Client becomes physically aggressive when drinking.
- Client states, "I know I drink too much . . . but I can't stop."
- Client has been arrested twice for disorderly conduct while drinking.

A nursing diagnosis of a *possible* problem alerts the nurse that a problem may be present but that more data are needed. For example:

Possible altered family processes: related to mother having to go to work to support children's education
Supporting data that validate diagnosis:

- Husband had been against mother working in the past.
- There are insufficient finances to support education for two children.

WHEN IS A PROBLEM A NURSING DIAGNOSIS?

Nursing consists of three levels of nursing functioning, each determined by the type of problem. These levels of nursing functions are (1) *dependent*, (2) *interdependent*, and (3) *independent*. Carpenito (1991) clarifies the dependent dimension as follows: dependent nursing functions occur when there is a clinical medical problem, and the diagnosis and prescription of treatment come under the direct responsibility of the physician. Nursing practices in clinical medical problems are dependent actions prescribed by the physician. Medical problems are not within the legal or educational realm of the nurse to diagnose or to treat.

Information from the following vignette will be used to illustrate the three levels of nursing functions.

Assessment

Mr. Saltzberg is a 47-year-old man, the father of two boys, aged seven and nine. He is admitted to the hospital because of depression. Two months ago his business failed. Mr. Saltzberg states, "I built that business up from nothing; now I am left with nothing." He states he has been feeling depressed and "I just want to be alone."

He has been anorexic and has lost 19 pounds in the past two months. He weighs 140 pounds and is 10 pounds under his range for normal body weight, 150–165 pounds. He has no interest in sex or any other activity. Family history reveals that his father suffered from depression and attempted suicide at age 60.

He appears unkempt—his clothes are wrinkled, and he has not shaved for three days. He sits slumped in the chair, facing the interviewer but seldom making eye contact, and keeps his head down. His speech is slow, and his mood is depressed. His thinking has slowed down. He states, "I can't think."

He admits that the idea of suicide has occurred to him. His wife states that he just sits and stares into space all day, keeping to himself. She states that this is the first time she has ever known him to react like this, and that his behavior is greatly upsetting the whole family. Mrs. Saltzberg is very upset and states that she feels overwhelmed without his help and support. The children are confused and upset and miss doing things with their father. The family has not gone to temple, the movies, or sports activities—all of which are important events for this family—for two months.

Mr. Saltzberg was seen by the psychiatrist on the unit and was given the DSM-IV diagnosis of dysthymic disorder (depressive neurosis).

In this case, a *dependent* nursing function would be administering medication prescribed by the psychiatrist.

DSM-IV Diagnosis
Dysthymic disorder (depressive neurosis)
Medical Order
Elavil, 75 mg at bedtime
Nursing Interventions
Administer Elavil, 75 mg at bedtime (dependent function)

Interdependent nursing functions refer to problems on which health care professionals collaborate to prescribe and treat. Carpenito describes these problems as *clinical nursing problems*. For example:

DSM-IV Diagnosis
Dysthymic disorder (neurotic depression)
Medical Order
Elavil, 75 mg at bedtime
Clinical Nursing Problem
At risk for orthostatic hypotension (common side effect of prescribed medication)
Nursing Order

1. Take blood pressure and pulse on both arms in standing, sitting, and supine positions.
2. Have client dangle legs by side of bed before getting up.

Independent nursing functions involve actual, potential, or possible clinical problems or situations that are the direct responsibility and under the influence of the nurse. Problems or situations that call for independent nursing interventions are termed *nursing diagnoses* (Carpenito 1991). Independent nursing interventions are aimed at preventing or alleviating identified problems.

The nurse meets with Mr. Saltzberg and makes an initial assessment. The nurse speaks with Mrs. Saltzberg, verifies her assessment, and adds it to the data base. Information is shared with other staff, and the admitting notes by the psychiatrist are read.

The analysis of the data consists of (1) organizing the data into problems (actual, high risk, or possible), (2) prioritizing problems, and (3) formulating nursing diagnoses.

After the nurse assesses Mr. Saltzberg, the data are organized into problems and placed in order of priority. Three major problem areas are identified:

1. Risk of suicide
2. Inadequate nutrition
3. Disrupted family functioning

From these problem areas, three nursing diagnoses are formulated:

1. High risk for self-directed violence: suicide related to multiple losses
   Supporting data that validate diagnosis:

   - Client states, "I have nothing left to live for."
   - Client has suffered a great loss.
   - Father attempted suicide at age 60.
   - Client states he has had vague thoughts of killing himself.

2. Altered nutrition: less than body requirements, related to apathy and poor self-concept
   Supporting data that validate diagnosis:

   - Client has suffered a 19-pound weight loss in two months.
   - He is 10 pounds under his recommended weight range.
   - He refuses to eat prepared meals.
   - He states he has no appetite.

3. Altered family process: related to an ill family member
   Supporting data that validate diagnosis:

   - Since the client's illness, the family has not participated in usual family activities.
   - Wife and husband have not shared usual activities involving companionship since illness.
   - Wife states that she feels overwhelmed without the husband's help and support.

Planning

A clearly stated nursing care plan is the most effective means of assuring clients that their needs are heard and their problems are being addressed (Yura and Walsh 1983). When possible, the nurse works with the client to identify problems and to plan care. Planning care is also done collaboratively with other health care workers, as well as individually.

In order to design a care plan that is appropriate and workable, it is necessary to have a direction of care. Planning a direction of care consists of deciding in advance what to do, who is to do it, and what is needed to get the job accomplished.

Planning involves (1) determining desired outcomes (short and long term goals) and (2) identifying appropriate nursing care based on scientific principles or rationales designed to reach stated goals.

DETERMINING THE DESIRED OUTCOMES

For each nursing diagnosis, outcome criteria are established. *Outcome criteria* are the behaviors or situations hoped for after the implementation of nursing interventions designed to remedy or lessen the problem identified in the nursing diagnosis. Therefore, the nurse sets client-centered goals for nursing care aimed at alleviating the client's problems. Clearly stated goals give direction to nursing actions. There are two categories of goals: long term goals and short term goals. *Long term goals* are the hoped-for outcomes that reflect the maximum level of client health that can be reached realistically by nursing interventions. *Short term goals* are the intermediate goals that assist the client in achieving the long term goals.

Each goal is derived from only one nursing diagnosis. Goals should be realistic and acceptable to the client. An appropriate goal meets the following criteria (Atkinson and Murray 1990):

1. It is stated in observable or measurable terms.
2. It indicates client outcomes.
3. It has a specific time set for achievement.
4. It is short and specific.
5. It is written in positive terms.

The following is a generally held formula for writing goals (Atkinson and Murray 1990):

Goal = Patient Behavior + Criteria of Performance + Time + Conditions (if needed)

Patient behavior refers to observable activities that the patient will demonstrate in response to effective treatment. For example:

- Client *will state.*
- Client *will name.*
- Client's *anxiety* level *will decrease.*

The *criteria of performance* refer to how well, how long, how far, how much, and by when the behavior or situation will be altered. Therefore, the criteria include a measure of performance and a realistic deadline by which the behavior or situation will be altered. For example:

- Client will name *three things he likes about himself.*
- Client will name *three alternative actions he can take when feeling hopeless.*
- Client's anxiety level will decrease from *severe to moderate.*

The *time* frame includes a time or date to clarify how long it would realistically take to reach the level of functioning stated in the goal.

- *Within two weeks*, client will name three things he likes about himself.
- *By June 1*, client will name three alternative actions he can take when feeling hopeless.
- *By 8:00 P.M. tonight*, client's anxiety level will decrease from severe to moderate.

The conditions refer to circumstances under which the behavior or situation will be altered. Not all goals need conditions. For example:

- Client will remain safe while in the hospital *with the help of the staff.*
- By 8:00 P.M., the client's anxiety level will decrease from severe to moderate *with the aid of medications.*

Referring to the nursing diagnoses formulated for Mr. Saltzberg, the nurse sets long and short term goals. The goals for the second nursing diagnosis are provided here as an example.

Nursing Diagnosis: Altered nutrition: less than body requirements, related to apathy and poor self-concept

Long Term Goal	Short Term Goal
1. By discharge, client will be within normal body weight range (150–165 pounds).	1. Client will gain two pounds per week while in the hospital. Present weight (date) is 140 pounds.

IDENTIFYING INTERVENTIONS NECESSARY TO HELP CLIENTS ACHIEVE GOALS

The nurse writes a set of interventions appropriate for reaching each goal. Each stated goal should include numerous nursing interventions, which should be seen as instructions for all people working with the client. These instructions, written in the Kardex, aid in the continuity of care for the client and are points of information for all members of the health team. When the short term goals are reached and charted, as reflected on the Kardex, a picture of the client's progress is evident. The nurse considers specific principles when planning care. Nursing interventions planned for meeting a specific goal should include the following principles (Atkinson and Murray 1990):

1. *Safe*: They must be safe for the client.
2. *Appropriate*: They must be compatible with other therapies as well as with the client's personal goals and cultural values.
3. *Effective*: They should be based on scientific principles.
4. *Individualized nursing care*: They should be realistic: that is, (1) be within the capabilities of the client's age, physical strength, condition, and willingness to change; (2) be based on the number of staff available; (3) reflect the level of experience and ability of the staff; and (4) use available equipment and resources.

The nurse plans the interventions to meet the goals set for Mr. Saltzberg. Development of one goal for Mr. Saltzberg follows:

Nursing Diagnosis: High risk for self-directed violence: suicide related to multiple losses

Long Term Goal: By discharge, client will state he wants to live.

Short Term Goal	Nursing Intervention
1. Client will remain safe while in the hospital, with the aid of staff.	1a. Remove all items that could potentially be used as weapons, e.g., belts, ties, shoelaces, razors, plastic bags.
	1b. Assess immediate degree of suicidal risk, and ask client if he is thinking of killing himself.
	1c. Check client every 15 minutes, and keep him in view at all times.
	1d. Observe for any signs of suicidal indicators: sudden sense of well-being, giving away prized possessions, making out a will.
	1e. Spend time with client for 15 minutes, three times a day.
	1f. Recognize suicide as realistic option.
	1g. Document all assessments, interactions, and interventions.

Refer to the working care plan for Mr. Saltzberg (Nursing Care Plan 8–1), which includes the rationale for each nursing intervention.

Intervention

Implementation of nursing care includes three basic areas: (1) validating the care plan, (2) giving nursing care, and (3) continued data collection.

VALIDATING THE NURSING CARE PLAN

It is sound practice for less experienced staff members or students to review their care plans briefly with more experienced staff members (team leader, colleague, instructor, or head nurse). Often, experienced nurses have parts or all of their care plans reviewed by other professionals. By having the care plan reviewed, quality of care can be maximized. This reviewing process is called validating the care plan. Areas of concern include the following (Atkinson and Murray 1990):

- Does the plan ensure the client's safety?
- Is the plan based on sound scientific principles?
- Are the nursing diagnoses supported by the data?
- Does the goal contain time criteria and client behavior for evaluation?
- Can the planned nursing action realistically assist the client in achieving the intended goal?
- Are the client's priorities being considered?

Nursing care plans are often transferred to a Kardex, although the working nursing care plan (see Nursing Care Plan 8–1) may be condensed. Ideally, new plans of care are discussed in team meetings that take place once or twice a week among the staff. Sharing plans of care with other staff members allows for further input and suggestions. This helps to ensure commitment of all staff toward the stated goals.

GIVING NURSING CARE IN THE PSYCHIATRIC SETTING

Six areas of **intervention** are generally identified in psychiatric nursing: psychotherapeutic interventions, health teaching, activities of daily living, somatic therapies, therapeutic environment, and psychotherapy.

Psychotherapeutic Interventions

Psychotherapeutic intervention is usually carried out by a nurse minimally prepared as a generalist in psychiatric and mental health nursing. Some of the interventions include reinforcing functional coping pat-

terns, employing problem-solving and communication skills, and using other members of the health team to help evaluate the outcome of interventions. The dialogue in Box 8–1 illustrates the use of psychotherapeutic interventions.

Health Teaching

Health teaching includes identifying health education needs of the client and teaching basic principles of physical and mental health. The following vignette illustrates health teaching:

While working with the client on creating alternatives to his present solution, the nurse notes that family communications seem to break down when the client is faced with an issue that threatens his self-image. Mr. Saltzberg states that the family is usually able to talk about personal concerns. However, when the business started to falter, Mr. Saltzberg began to think of himself as a failure. He felt ashamed and impotent, and he isolated himself from his family emotionally, hiding his feelings. Thus, he increased his feelings of isolation and helplessness. As anxiety increases, the ability to solve problems decreases. Eventually, Mr. Saltzberg felt overwhelmed and defeated.

The nurse intervenes to suggest alternative interpersonal communication skills Mr. Saltzberg can use within the family to minimize feelings of hopelessness and helplessness when problems arise. The nurse suggests to Mr. Saltzberg that the family and nurse meet together so that he can "practice" sharing personal feelings. Illness or problems of one family member usually affect all family members. By having the family meet together and work on important issues with some degree of safety and guidance, problems can be minimized. For example, the family may decide to encourage Mr. Saltzberg to talk things out when he seems preoccupied or upset. Discussing problem situations as a family can help put situations into a realistic perspective, provide a variety of alternative actions, and decrease feelings of isolation and helplessness. The family may also identify outside resources that could prove helpful, for example, religious counseling and sympathetic relatives and friends.

Activities of Daily Living

Activities of daily living include an individual's developmental and intellectual levels, as well as emotional state and physical limitations.

The nursing interventions aimed at increasing Mr. Saltzberg's physical care center on nutrition. Mr. Saltz-

Nursing Care Plan 8-1 ■ A DEPRESSED INDIVIDUAL: MR. SALTZBERG

NURSING DIAGNOSIS

High risk for self-directed violence: suicide related to multiple losses

Supporting Data

- States, "I have nothing left to live for"
- Has suffered a great loss
- Father attempted suicide at age 60
- Admits to vague thoughts of killing himself

Long Term Goal: By discharge, the client will state he wants to live.

Short-Term Goal	Intervention	Rationale	Evaluation
1. Client will remain safe while in the hospital, with the aid of the staff.	1a. Remove all possible weapons, e.g., belts, ties, shoelaces, razors, plastic bags.	1a. Minimizes potential for self-harm.	Goal Met Client states he no longer thinks of killing himself; has been working on plans for the future in business and with his family.
	1b. Assess immediate degree of suicide risk, and ask client if he is thinking of killing himself.	1b. Evaluates level of suicidal potential to determine the degree of suicide precautions.	
	1c. Check client every 15 minutes, and keep him in view at all times.	1c. Maximizes client's safety and lets him know he is cared for.	
	1d. Observe for any signs of suicidal indicators: displaying a sudden sense of well-being, giving away prized possessions, making out a will.	1d. Notes nonverbal clues necessary for assessing suicidal ideation.	
	1e. Spend time with client for 15 minutes, three times a day.	1e. Provides the opportunity to build rapport and trust with client. Client senses others are concerned and feel he is worthwhile. Forms the foundation for problem solving and sharing.	
	1f. Recognize suicide as realistic option; do not discredit.	1f. Acknowledges that situation is serious; can give client a feeling he is understood.	

	1g. Observe for signs of orthostatic hypotension and dizziness from medication.
	  a. Check blood pressure lying down and standing
	  b. Instruct to dangle feet before getting out of bed
		1g. Prevents injury from falls.	

	1h. Document all assessments, interactions, and interventions.	1h. Ensures communication among all health team members and for legal purposes.	

berg will gain two pounds per week while in the hospital.

Getting an anorexic person to eat takes creative thinking and patience. In implementing the plan of care for Mr. Saltzberg, the nurse first finds out whether there are any religious or medical dietary restrictions. Mr. Saltzberg states that he eats only kosher foods and that he does have food preferences. These preferences are special dishes his wife makes for him at home.

By working with Mr. Saltzberg and contacting other members of the health team and family, the nurse sets up optimum conditions for increasing Mr. Saltzberg's weight. The doctor is first contacted to approve Mrs. Saltzberg's bringing in foods from home. The dietitian is contacted to visit Mr. Saltzberg. Kosher foods are requested, and food preferences are listed. Mrs. Saltzberg is contacted and agrees to make foods her husband especially likes and that she feels will tempt him

Box 8–1. PSYCHOTHERAPEUTIC INTERVENTIONS

Short Term Goal: Client will name three personal strengths that have worked for him in the past.

Interaction	Rationale
NURSE: You mentioned everything coming down on you when your business began to fail.	Placing the event in time and sequence, validating the precipitating event.
CLIENT: Yes . . . everything I had worked for was lost. That business was my whole life. Everything I did was for my business. It was my baby.	
NURSE: You lost a great deal. You said it was like your baby?	Reflecting and showing empathy. Restating.
CLIENT: Yeah, well, I had dreamed of it for years. My brother lent me some money, but it was my idea, and I did most of the work to get it going.	
NURSE: It seems to me that building up a business from scratch takes a lot of work and know-how.	Pointing out realities and assisting to clarify strengths.
CLIENT: Oh yes, I was never afraid of hard work. I used to be good at figuring my way out of a tight spot. Now . . . I don't know . . . Ever since that automated shop came in, I couldn't keep up with those prices. Everything caved in . . . It doesn't seem to matter anymore.	
NURSE: What doesn't seem to matter?	Clarifying.
CLIENT: Me . . . being a success . . . being somebody. I guess now I'll never be anybody.	
NURSE: Are you saying that you equate what happens in business with your personal worth?	Validating client's perception.
CLIENT: Yes . . . I mean . . . no, I just felt so awful when everything caved in . . . I felt so responsible.	
NURSE: Responsible?	Restating.
CLIENT: Yeah . . . responsible to my family.	
NURSE: How did your family react?	Giving broad openings.
CLIENT: Well . . . I really didn't say too much to them. I didn't want to worry them . . . I guess I was afraid.	
NURSE: Afraid?	Restating.
CLIENT: Yeah. That they would think I was no longer a success now that the business was failing.	
NURSE: You were afraid they would see you as a failure if the business ran into trouble?	Reflecting.

CLIENT:	I don't know . . . the business was such a great success in the beginning.	
NURSE:	What do you think made the shop so successful in the beginning?	Encouraging the client to realistically appraise his strengths.
CLIENT:	Well, I worked very hard . . . and I am good at knowing what people want. Everyone always says I have a unique way of marketing and advertising.	
NURSE:	You are conscientious, observant of others, and creative.	Restating what the client has said. At this point the client can agree or clarify what he meant.
CLIENT:	Well . . . yes, but what does it matter now?	
NURSE:	In what other ways could you use these qualities?	Encouraging client to problem-solve.
CLIENT:	Huh . . . I hadn't thought about other ways . . . *Silence* Sam Cohn . . . well . . . Sam . . . he always wanted me to come in with him. I always wanted my own place though.	
NURSE:	Well, that is one possibility. We talked this morning about some of your strengths and maybe this afternoon we can talk some more about other ways you can use these strengths in the future.	Summarizing and encouraging collaboration in setting future goals.
CLIENT:	Yeah . . . some other possibilities.	

to eat. The nurse works with Mr. Saltzberg, and it is agreed that during the three times he meets with her each day, he will eat a high-caloric snack.

The importance of follow-up care, community resources, and suicide prevention centers is also a vital part of the nurse's health teaching for Mr. Saltzberg and his family when planning discharge.

Somatic Therapies

One of the nurse's responsibilities relating to **somatic therapies** includes the observations and judgments made concerning the effects of drugs and other somatic treatments.

One of the nurse's dependent functions is the administration of medications to clients. There are many nursing responsibilities associated with administering medications to clients. An important responsibility is to observe the client's reaction to the medication for known side effects and toxic effects.

Mr. Saltzberg is taking amitriptyline (Elavil), and the nurse notes in her care plan to watch for signs of orthostatic hypotension, a common side effect. Her interventions include checking his blood pressure when he is lying down and when he is standing, and instructing him to dangle his feet before getting out of bed.

Therapeutic Environment

A **therapeutic environment** is an extremely important consideration for the nurse working with a client. The client should feel comfortable and safe and that help is available. A positive environment can greatly affect a client's outlook and ability to solve problems. Not all clients at all times can make use of the therapies available to them. However, a therapeutic environment can influence the choices a client makes.

A safe therapeutic environment for Mr. Saltzberg is the highest priority when he is first admitted to the unit. A person who is feeling overwhelmed and in a great deal of emotional pain often has difficulty figuring out ways to solve his problems. Sometimes suicide appears to be the only solution at the time. Mr. Saltzberg has suffered a great loss, is a male, and is over 45 years old; his father had attempted suicide at age 60; Mr. Saltzberg is clinically depressed. All of these factors place him at high risk for suicide. (See Chapter 21 for assessing a person's suicide risk.)

A safe environment is arranged for by providing Mr. Saltzberg with close observation and setting limits. All potential weapons are removed, and he is put on suicide precautions. Suicide precautions entail checking the client every 15 minutes and keeping him in view at all times. He is also observed for any behaviors that might indicate thoughts of suicide, such as a sudden sense of well-being, giving away possessions, or making out a will.

These nursing interventions occur within the framework of building a relationship with Mr. Saltzberg. The nurse sets aside at least 15 minutes three times per day for Mr. Saltzberg. The *content* includes sitting, talking, walking, planning, and engaging him in recreational activities—whatever seems the most useful to Mr. Saltzberg at the time. The *process* is providing the presence of a person who is interested in the client's situation, is willing to work on issues in a nonjudgmental and nonthreatening manner, and is able to provide important resources when needed.

Psychotherapy

A nurse qualified to work with a client as a psychotherapist is prepared at the master's level or higher. Most nurses who engage in **psychotherapy** have obtained certification through the ANA. Certification entails performing many hours of supervised clinical work and passing the certification exam, as well as achieving of specific educational credentials. A nurse may specialize in working with adults, children, or adolescents, although many nurses prefer working as family therapists.

If at the time of discharge Mr. Saltzberg wants to explore further his motivations, coping patterns, life goals, and emotional responses that kept him from meeting his goals, referral to a therapist would be appropriate.

CONTINUED DATA COLLECTION

Data collection is an ongoing process throughout all the phases of the nursing process. While observing Mr. Saltzberg, one nurse noted that he had difficulty sharing problems with his family when his self-esteem was threatened. During these times, family communications broke down, and family members became confused and isolated. The added data directed future nursing intervention.

Evaluation

Evaluation is often the most neglected part of the nursing process. Ideally, evaluation should be part of each phase in the nursing process. Evaluation of a care plan involves two basic steps: (1) evaluation of goal achievement and (2) review of the nursing care plan (Atkinson and Murray 1990).

EVALUATING GOALS ACHIEVED

There are three possible outcomes when goals are evaluated: goal met, goal not met, goal partially met. The nurse develops the statement of evaluation and documents the client's behavior to determine whether the goal has been met. Diagrammatically, evaluation of goal achievement appears as follows (Atkinson and Murray 1990):

$$\text{EVALUATION} = \begin{array}{l} \text{Goal Met} \\ \text{Goal Not Met} \\ \text{Goal Partially Met} \end{array}$$

Whether the goal is met or only partially met, actual patient behaviors should be added as evidence. For example, evaluation of the goals set by the nurse for Mr. Saltzberg's third nursing diagnosis might be:

Nursing Diagnosis: Altered family process related to an ill family member

Long Term Goal: By discharge, client and family will discuss and identify three outside supports available to them all.

Short Term Goal	Evaluation
1. By 6/11, client will meet with family and discuss feelings each member is experiencing related to client's illness.	1. 6/11—Goal met. Family was able to share with client and each other their own experiences. Client stated he felt very supported and cared for. Wife and children stated they felt relieved to talk about things together again like a family.
2. By 6/21, client and family will plan two family activities they wish to resume.	2. 6/21—Goal met. Client suggested that he and his wife go to the movies once a week, as they had in the past. Client agreed to go with his sons to Little League practice at least three times per month.

3. By 6/28, family will discuss resources and supports they feel are important to the family unit.

3. 6/30—Goal met. Family states that going to temple and talking to their family rabbi was special to them. They mentioned certain family friends in whom they could confide and two relatives who were especially close to the family. The wife asked if there was a women's support group in her area. "Now that the boys are growing, maybe I'll go back to work. It would be helpful to see how other women manage."

client's status. Reassessment of a client's care plan with other members of the nursing staff can aid in the creation of a more effective plan.

REVIEW OF THE NURSING CARE PLAN

The nurse continuously collects data during the planning and implementation of nursing interventions. After evaluating the client-centered goals, it is often necessary to re-evaluate why some goals were not met, and, if some goals were met, whether the nursing diagnoses or goals are still an appropriate focus of nursing care for a particular patient. For example, do the nursing diagnoses still have the same order of priority, or are there new diagnoses and goals that must be set to assure effective, safe, and appropriate nursing interventions?

The following are five possible outcomes that could occur after the care plan is reviewed (Atkinson and Murray 1990):

- Priorities may change, and the order of nursing diagnoses will change.
- New data may point to the need for new diagnoses, goals, and nursing actions.
- When a goal is met and the problem no longer exists, a nursing diagnosis is dropped after appropriate documentation on either the client's records or the Kardex or both.
- At other times, although a goal might be met, the problem still exists. If a number of short term goals need to be set to achieve a long term goal, the nurse would choose another goal reflecting the client's progress and ability.
- When a goal is not met or is only partially met, reassessment is done to identify and write a more successful plan. The problem with an unsuccessful plan can be an incorrect nursing diagnosis, unrealistic goals, ineffective nursing measures planned to meet goals, or a change in the

Summary

The nursing process is an adaptation of the problem-solving process used by many professions. Inherent in the nursing process are three theoretical frameworks: (1) the holistic model, (2) Maslow's human needs theory, and (3) general systems theory.

The *primary* source of assessment is the client. The psychiatric nursing assessment is done within the psychiatric interview. *Secondary sources* of information include the family, neighbors, friends, police, and other members of the health team. The *process* component of the interview, use of communication skills and the therapeutic use of self, have a great impact on the resulting relationship. Both the nurse's and the client's anxiety levels need to be acknowledged, as do personal biases and value judgments. The *content* of the interview includes gathering subjective data (client history) and objective data (mental or emotional status). An assessment tool is provided, and charts defining motor behaviors and thought content are included in this chapter. Assessment tools are useful and can help the nurse focus the interview. When the nurse develops skill and becomes more comfortable in this role, the interview becomes less formal without sacrificing important data. The two major components of the assessment process are (1) gathering data and (2) verifying the data. Verifying the data is done by checking with secondary sources of information.

The nursing diagnosis is a crucial phase in the nursing process. The nursing diagnosis performs a number of functions: it defines the practice of nursing, improves communication between staff, assists in accountability for care, differentiates nursing from medicine, and so forth. A nursing diagnosis consists of (1) an unmet need or problem, (2) an etiology or probable cause, and (3) supporting data. A problem becomes a nursing diagnosis when it falls under the independent functions of nursing practice—areas the nurse is trained and licensed to treat. A nursing diagnosis can be stated as an actual, potential, or possible problem.

Planning nursing care involves (1) determining desired outcomes and goals and (2) planning nursing actions to reach those goals. A goal should be measurable, indicate desired outcome, have a set time for achievement, and be short and specific. Goals identify the direction for nursing care. Planning nursing action to achieve the goals includes using specific principles:

the plan should be safe, based on scientific rationale, realistic, and compatible with other therapies.

The implementation of psychiatric care involves (1) verifying the care plan, (2) giving nursing care, and (3) conducting continuous data collection. The nurse validating the care plan asks these questions: Is the plan safe? Is it based on scientific principles? Do the data support the nursing diagnosis? Are priorities correct? Practice in psychiatric nursing encompasses six areas: psychotherapeutic interventions, health teaching, activities of daily living, somatic therapies, therapeutic environment, and psychotherapy. For the purposes of

evaluation, data collection continues throughout the nursing process.

The evaluation of care involves (1) evaluation of goal achievement and (2) review of the nursing care plan. The nurse judges the goal to be met, not met, or partially met. Supporting data are included to clarify the evaluation. Review of the care plan is done periodically. The nurse decides whether priorities in diagnosis need changing, new diagnoses need to be added, new interventions are needed to meet goals, and whether diagnosis, goals, interventions, and plans are currently appropriate.

ASSESSMENT TOOL

1. **Client History**

   I. GENERAL HISTORY OF CLIENT
   Name _____ Age _____ Sex _____
   Racial and ethnic data _____
   Marital status _____
   Number and ages of children/siblings _____
   Living arrangements _____
   Occupation _____
   Education _____
   Religious affiliations _____

   II. PRESENTING PROBLEM

   A. Statement in the client's own words of why he or she is hospitalized or seeking help

   _____
   _____
   _____
   _____

   B. Recent difficulties/alterations in
      1. Relationships
      2. Usual level of functioning
      3. Behavior
      4. Perceptions or cognitive abilities

   C. Increased feelings of
      1. Depression   4. Being overwhelmed
      2. Anxiety   5. Suspiciousness
      3. Hopelessness   6. Confusion

   D. Somatic changes, such as
      1. Constipation   4. Weight loss or gain
      2. Insomnia   5. Palpitations
      3. Lethargy

   III. RELEVANT HISTORY—PERSONAL

   A. Previous hospitalizations and illnesses _____

   B. Educational background _____

   C. Occupational background
      1. If employed, where? _____
      2. How long at that job? _____
      3. Previous positions and reasons for leaving _____
      4. Special skills _____

   D. Social patterns
      1. Describe friends _____
      2. Describe a usual day _____

Figure 8–2. *Comprehensive nursing assessment tool.*

E. Sexual patterns
    1. Sexually active? _____
    2. Sexual orientation _____
    3. Sexual difficulties _____

F. Interests and abilities
    1. What does the client do in his or her spare time? _____
    2. What is the client good at? _____
    3. What gives the client pleasure? _____

G. Substance use and abuse
    1. What psychotropic drugs does the client take? _____
       How often? _____ How much? _____
    2. How many drinks of alcohol does the client take per day? _____
       Per week? _____
    3. Does the client identify use of drugs as a problem? _____

H. How does the client cope with stress?
    1. What does the client do when he or she gets upset? _____
    2. Whom can the client talk to? _____
    3. What usually helps to relieve stress? _____
    4. What did the client try this time? _____

IV. RELEVANT HISTORY—FAMILY

A. Childhood
    1. Who was important to the client growing up? _____
    2. Was there physical or sexual abuse? _____
    3. Did the parents drink or use drugs? _____
    4. Who was in the home when the client was growing up? _____

B. Adolescence
    1. How would the client describe his or her feelings in adolescence? _____
    2. Describe the client's peer group at that time _____

C. Use of drugs
    1. Was there use or abuse of drugs by any family member? _____
       Prescription _____ Street _____ By whom? _____
    2. What was the effect on the family? _____

D. Family physical or mental problems
    1. Who in the family had physical or mental problems? _____
    2. Describe the problems. _____
    3. How did it affect the family? _____

E. Was there an unusual or outstanding event the client would like to mention? _____

2. Mental and Emotional Status

A. Appearance
    Physical handicaps _____
    Dress appropriate _____ Sloppy _____
    Grooming neat _____ Poor _____
    Eye contact held _____ Describe posture _____

B. Behavior **(see Table 8–1)**
    Restless _____ Agitated _____ Lethargic _____
    Mannerisms _____ Facial expressions _____ Other _____

C. Speech
    Clear _____ Mumbled _____ Rapid _____ Slurred _____ Constant _____ Mute or
    silent _____ Barriers to communications _____ Specify (e.g., client has delusions or is confused, with-
    drawn, or verbose) _____

D. Mood
    What mood does the client convey? _____

E. Affect
    Is the client's affect bland, apathetic, dramatic, bizarre, or appropriate? Describe _____

Illustration continued on following page

F. Thought process **(see Table 8–2)**
  1. Characteristics
     Describe the characteristics of the person's responses: Flights of ideas _____ Looseness of association _____ Blocking _____ Concrete _____ Confabulation _____
     Describe _____
  2. Cognitive ability
     Proverbs: Concrete _____ Abstract _____
     Serial sevens: How far does the client go? _____ Can the client do simple math? _____
     What seems to be the reason for poor concentration? _____
     _____

G. Thought content
  1. Central theme: What is important to the client? _____
     Describe _____
  2. Self-concept: How does the client view him- or herself? _____
     What does the client want to change about himself? _____
  3. Insight? Does the client realistically assess her symptoms? _____
     Realistically appraise her situation? _____
     Describe _____
  4. Suicidal or homicidal ideation? _____ What is suicide potential? _____ Family history of suicide or homicide attempt or successful completion? _____
     Explain _____
     Preoccupations **(see Table 8–3).** Does the client have hallucinations? _____ Delusions _____
     Obsessions _____ Rituals _____ Phobias _____ Grandiosity _____ Religiosity _____
     Worthlessness _____ Describe _____

H. Reality orientation
   Time: _____
   Place: _____
   Person: _____
   Memory: _____

I. Level of Anxiety
   Mild   Data _____
   Moderate Data _____
   Severe   Data _____
   Panic   Data _____

References

Atkinson LD, Murray ME. Understanding the Nursing Process, 4th ed. New York: Member of Maxwell Macmillan Pergamon Publishing Corporation, 1990.

Bower FL. The Process of Planning Nursing Care. St. Louis: CV Mosby, 1982.

Carpenito LJ. Nursing Diagnosis: Application to Clinical Practice, 4th ed. Philadelphia: JB Lippincott, 1991.

Eisenman EJP, Dubbert PM. Mental health assessment interview. In Backer, et al (eds). Psychiatric/Mental Health Nursing: Contemporary Readings. New York: D Van Nostrand Company, 1978.

Geissler EM. Nursing diagnosis of culturally diverse patients. International Nursing Review, 38(5):150, 1991.

Gordon M. The concept of nursing diagnosis. Nursing Clinics of North America, 14:487, 1979.

Gordon M. Historical perspective: The national group for classification of nursing diagnosis. In Kim MJ, Moritz DA (eds). Classification of Nursing Diagnoses. New York: McGraw-Hill Book Company, 1982.

Gordon M. Manual of Nursing Diagnosis 1993–1994. St. Louis, MO: Mosby–Year Book, 1993.

Hagerty BK. Psychiatric Mental Health Assessment. St. Louis: CV Mosby, 1984.

Kim MJ. Without collaboration, what's left? American Journal of Nursing, 85:281, 1985.

MacKinnon RA, Michels R. The Psychiatric Interview in Clinical Practice. Philadelphia: WB Saunders, 1971.

Maslow AH. Toward a Psychology of Being, 2nd ed. New York: D Van Nostrand Company, 1962.

Orem D. Nursing Concepts of Practice. New York: McGraw-Hill Book Company, 1980.

Riehl J, Roy C (eds). Conceptual Models for Nursing Practice. New York: Appleton-Century-Crofts, 1980.

Rogers M. An Introduction to the Theoretical Basis of Nursing. Philadelphia: FA Davis, 1970.

Shoemaker J. Essential features of nursing diagnosis. In Kim MJ, et al (eds). Classification of Nursing Diagnoses. Proceedings of the Fifth National Conference. St. Louis: CV Mosby, 1984.

Yura H, Walsh MB. The Nursing Process—Assessing, Planning, Implementing, Evaluating, 4th ed. Norwalk, CT: Appleton-Century-Crofts, 1983.

Further Reading

American Nurses' Association. Standards of Psychiatric and Mental Health Nursing Practice. Kansas City, MO: American Nurses' Association, 1982.

Atkinson LD, Murray ME. Understanding the Nursing Process, 4th ed. New York: Pergamon Press, 1990.

This is an excellent reference for students for applying the theories of the nursing process to the clinical setting. The authors break down the nursing steps in the nursing process very concretely. There is frequent use of diagrams and examples to take the student through each step. The instructions make the process very comprehensible and easy to use, minimizing the errors often made when the process is applied to the clinical setting.

Barry PD. Psychosocial Nursing Assessment and Intervention. Philadelphia: JB Lippincott, 1990.

Coombs RA, et al. Perceptual Psychology: A Humanistic Approach to the Study of Persons. New York: Harper & Row, 1976.

Dettmore D. Spiritual care: Remembering your patients' forgotten needs. Nursing 84, 14:46, 1984.

This short article encourages nurses to assess and intervene in an area of great importance to many clients. It validates how real the need is for spiritual care and emphasizes that nurses are often the only ones who can intervene while the client is hospitalized.

Douglas DJ, Murphy EK. Nursing process, nursing diagnosis and emerging taxonomies. In McCloskey JC, Grace HK (eds). Current Issues in Nursing. Boston: Blackwell Scientific Publications, 1981.

Fickeissen J. Getting certified. American Journal of Nursing, 86:265, 1985.

Field LL. The implication of nursing diagnosis in clinical nursing practice. Clinics of North America, 14:497, 1979.

Geltrust KV, et al. Applied Nursing Diagnosis Guides for Comprehensive Care Planning. New York: John Wiley & Sons, 1985.

Lesse S. Anxiety—Its Components, Development and Treatment. New York: Grune & Stratton, 1970.

Lesse S. The relationship of anxiety to depression. American Journal of Psychotherapy, 36:332, 1982.

McFarland GK, Wasli EL, Gerety EK. Nursing Diagnosis and Process in Psychiatric Mental Health Nursing, 2nd ed. Philadelphia: JB Lippincott, 1992.

An updated and well-researched practical guide for nurses planning care for people with behavioral problems. Nursing diagnoses used most often in mental health nursing are well developed and include nursing interventions for ritualistic behaviors, seclusion, restraints, and social skills management.

Maloney EM. The nursing process. In Haber, et al (eds). Comprehensive Psychiatric Nursing, 2nd ed. New York: McGraw-Hill Book Company, 1982.

Newman MA. Nursing diagnosis: Looking at the whole. American Journal of Nursing, 84:1496, 1984.

Tartaglia MJ. Nursing diagnosis: Keystone of your care plan. Nursing 85, 15:34, 1985.

Townsend MC. Nursing Diagnoses in Psychiatric Settings: A Pocket Guide for Care Plan Construction, 2nd ed. Philadelphia: FA Davis, 1991.

Excellent guide for planning nursing interventions, employing many of the nursing diagnoses used in psychiatric settings. Gives a brief, concrete overview of theory.

Weber S. Nursing diagnosis in private practice. Nursing Clinics of North America, 14:533, 1979.

Webster M. Psychiatric nursing assessment. In Lego S (ed). The American Handbook of Psychiatric Nursing. Philadelphia: JB Lippincott, 1984.

Self-study Exercises

Name the components for each of the steps in the nursing process.

1. Assessment

   A. Gather data
   B. Verify Data

2. Diagnosis

   A. Organize data
   B. Prioritize Problems
   C. Formulate Nsg Dx

3. Planning

   A. Determine short & long term goals
   B. Plan Nsg care

4. Intervention

   A. Validate care Plan
   B. Nsg interventions
   C. Continue data Collection

5. Evaluation

   A. Evaluate goal achievement
   B. Review Nsg care Plan

Label each of the behaviors described with one of the following parts of the psychiatric interview: P (process), C-H (content: history), and C-M/E (content: mental/emotional).

6. _____ Nurse approaches client, lets him know when the interview will be, how long it will be, and what it will entail.

7. _____ Nurse asks the client to explain what he sees as his problem and what he thinks might help him at this time.

8. _____ Is the client able to assess his symptoms realistically?

9. _____ When the nurse is assessing the client's sexual orientation, the client becomes defensive, evasive, and anxious. The nurse goes on to another topic.

10. _____ The nurse concludes the client is confabulating, since he says he went to England over the weekend, and he has been hospitalized for a month.

11. _____ The nurse asks the client how he usually copes with stress.
12. _____ The nurse asks the client what he values. Are there religious beliefs that are particularly important to him?
13. _____ When explaining the saying, "Don't put all your eggs in one basket," the client states that if you do that, and the basket drops, you won't have any eggs left.

Situation

Ms. Jamison is a 25-year-old woman who came to the hospital because voices told her to kill herself, and she became very frightened. She appears tense. Her posture is rigid, her respiration rapid, and she states she has not eaten for three days. When asked what she usually does when she gets upset, she states that she used to talk to her mother, but her mother died a year ago. Since then, she has been extremely lonely. She tells the nurse she does not have any friends and works part-time as a temporary secretary. She says her voices started a week after her mother died. "They used to be friendly voices, but now they want me to die." She has an aunt and a brother but is hesitant to contact them. She states, "They don't really need my problems . . . they have busy lives." She says she is frightened about the voices and is afraid she might obey them. She asks the nurse to help her.

Questions 14 through 19 refer to the preceding situation. The questions are organized according to the steps of the nursing process.

14. There are a number of diagnoses the nurse could choose. Formulate one nursing diagnosis for Ms. Jamison. Include the problem statement, probable etiology, and supporting data.

    A. The diagnostic title: What should change? _____
    B. The etiology or possible cause related to: _____
    C. Supporting data to validate diagnosis:
        -
        -
        -

15. State at least one long term goal and two short term goals, using all four criteria for setting an effective goal.

    A. *Long term:* _____
    B. *Short term:* _____
    C. *Short term:* _____

16. When planning nursing care for Ms. Jamison, list four principles you would consider.

    A. _____   B. _____
    C. _____   D. _____

Ms. Jamison is to be discharged tomorrow. She tells the nurse that the voices no longer tell her to kill herself and do not seem as threatening. She stated that she would like to continue seeing the nurse therapist in the clinic and plans to continue visiting her brother on weekends but does not feel up to trying any other activity at this time, although she completes her self-care. She is able to explain to the nurse the dose and time of the medications and the side effects.

17. For the following goals, state whether the goal was met, not met, or partially met, and give the supporting data.

Long term goal: By discharge, client will state she no longer hears threatening or frightening voices.

A. Goal: _____ Supporting data: _____
_____

Short term goal: Within two weeks, the client will be able to name three sources of support (church, community health center, women's group, relatives, neighbors) that she is comfortable using.

B. Goal: _____ Supporting data: _____
_____

Short term goal: Client will complete self-care while in the hospital, with the aid of medication and a daily therapy session with the nurse.

C. Goal: _____ Supporting data: _____
_____

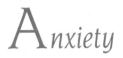

CHAPTER 9

Anxiety

Elizabeth M. Varcarolis

OUTLINE

THEORY
Psychodynamic Theory
Behavioral Theory
Biological Theory

ASSESSMENT
Assessing Levels of Anxiety
Assessing Relief Behaviors
    Interpersonal Relief Behaviors
    Intrapsychic Relief Behaviors—
      Defense Mechanisms
Assessing Circumstances Surrounding
  Increases in Anxiety

NURSING DIAGNOSIS
PLANNING
Content Level—Planning Goals
Process Level—Nurses' Reactions and
  Feelings

INTERVENTION
Psychotherapeutic Intervention
Health Teaching
Somatic Therapies
Psychotherapy

EVALUATION

CASE STUDY: WORKING WITH A
PERSON IN MODERATE LEVELS OF
ANXIETY

CASE STUDY: WORKING WITH A
PERSON IN SEVERE LEVELS OF
ANXIETY

SUMMARY

KEY TERMS AND CONCEPTS

The key terms and concepts listed here also appear in bold where they are defined or discussed in this chapter.

ACTING OUT BEHAVIORS

ACUTE ANXIETY (STATE)

ANXIETY

CHRONIC ANXIETY (TRAIT)

DEFENSE MECHANISMS
Compensation
Conversion
Denial
Displacement
Identification
Introjection
Projection
Rationalization
Reaction-Formation
Regression
Repression

Sublimation
Suppression
Undoing

EMPATHY

FEAR

MILD, MODERATE, SEVERE, AND
  PANIC LEVELS OF ANXIETY

NORMAL ANXIETY

PRIMARY ANXIETY

SECONDARY ANXIETY

SELECTIVE INATTENTION

SOMATIZING

OBJECTIVES ■

After studying this chapter, the student will be able to

1. Identify one contribution made by each of the following etiological theories of anxiety that can be used in nursing practice:
   A. Psychodynamic theory
   B. Learning theory
   C. Biological theory
2. Compare and contrast the meanings of the following concepts:
   A. Anxiety and fear
   B. Primary and secondary anxiety
   C. Acute and chronic anxiety
3. Discuss what is meant by normal anxiety.
4. Define the term *empathy*.
5. Name and give an example of each step in the operational definition of anxiety.
6. Select six defense mechanisms and give examples of both adaptive and maladaptive ways they are used.
7. Write three characteristics (perceptual field, ability to learn, or other defining characteristics) for a person in each of the following levels of anxiety:
   A. Mild
   B. Moderate
   C. Severe
   D. Panic
8. Give two examples of basic goals for a person in each of the following levels of anxiety:
   A. Mild to moderate
   B. Severe to panic
9. Discuss various nursing interventions, including rationales for a person in each of the following levels of anxiety:
   A. Mild to moderate
   B. Severe to panic

Anxiety is a universal human experience. It is an everyday component of our lives and a stranger to no one. Anxiety is the most basic of emotions and is part of all emotions. It is the basic ingredient in the most unpleasant emotions, such as grief, jealousy, and anger, as well as in those emotions that lead to our peak experiences, such as love and joy.

Behavior stems from anxiety. A basic principle in psychiatric nursing is, *"all behavior is purposeful, meaningful, and can be understood"* (Burd 1968). Dysfunctional behavior is often a defense against anxiety. When behavior is recognized as dysfunctional, interventions to reduce anxiety can be initiated by the nurse. As anxiety decreases, dysfunctional behavior will frequently decrease and vice versa.

Anxiety is experienced on four levels: mild, moderate, severe, and panic. It can be broken down into three categories—normal, acute, and chronic—and it can be operationally defined.

Hildegard Peplau, one of the first nurse theorists, identifies anxiety as one of the most important con-

cepts in psychiatric nursing. Nurses can use the concept of anxiety to explain many clinical observations. Peplau has conceptualized an anxiety model useful to the practice of nursing. Conceptualizing anxiety using Peplau's model has led to principles that serve as guides in nursing intervention (Burd 1968). This conceptual basis of anxiety can be used by nurses as a framework to guide therapeutic approaches to clients inside and outside the hospital setting.

Anxiety can be defined as a feeling of apprehension, uneasiness, uncertainty, or dread resulting from a real or a perceived threat whose actual source is unknown or unrecognized. Physiological responses to anxiety and fear are similar. However there are important distinctions between anxiety and fear.

First, there is general agreement that **fear** is a reaction to a specific danger, whereas anxiety is a vague sense of dread from an unspecified danger (May 1983). The body reacts in similar ways physiologically, however, to both anxiety and fear.

Second, an important distinction between anxiety

and fear is that anxiety attacks us at a deeper level than fear. Anxiety invades the central core of the personality. It erodes the individual feelings of self-esteem and personal worth that contribute to a sense of being fully human (Chapman and Chapman 1980).

Normal anxiety is a healthy life force that is necessary for survival. It provides the energy needed to carry out the tasks involved in living and striving toward goals. Anxiety motivates people to make and survive change. It prompts constructive behaviors, such as studying for an examination, being on time for job interviews, preparing for a presentation, and working toward a promotion.

Acute anxiety is precipitated by an imminent loss or change that threatens an individual's sense of security. Acute anxiety may be seen in performers before a concert. For example, Barbra Streisand admits to experiencing acute anxiety before live concerts. Patients preparing for surgery often experience acute anxiety. The death of a loved one can stimulate acute anxiety when there is great disruption in one's life. In general, crisis involves the experience of acute anxiety. Acute anxiety is also referred to as **state anxiety.**

In acute anxiety, emotional arousal triggers the sympathetic branch of the autonomic nervous system (which causes the fight-or-flight response), as well as the endocrine system. Behavioral responses to stress and anxiety are affected by age, sex, culture, and lifestyle. In contrast, the physiological response is more predictable and essentially the same whether the stress is physical, psychological, or social (Lesse 1982). The *fight-or-flight response* may be useful in emergencies, but when it becomes chronic, pathophysiological changes (e.g., high blood pressure, ulcers, cancer, and cardiac problems) and various psychological symptoms or syndromes may occur.

The *relaxation response*, identified by Herbert Benson (1975), is the opposite of the fight-or-flight response. It is caused by the parasympathetic branch of the nervous system and can stabilize the disruptive effects of the fight or flight response (Aron and Aron 1980). The objective, behavioral, and subjective experiences of the fight-or-flight response and the relaxation response are compared in Table 9–1.

Chronic anxiety is anxiety that the person has lived with for a period of time. Ego psychologists suggest

Table 9–1 ■ FIGHT-OR-FLIGHT RESPONSE VERSUS THE RELAXATION RESPONSE	
FIGHT-OR-FLIGHT RESPONSE (Sympathetic Branch—Epinephrine/ Norepinephrine)	**RELAXATION RESPONSE** (Parasympathetic Branch—Acetylcholine)
Objective Findings	
1. Increased heart rate 2. Increased blood pressure 3. Increased oxygen consumption 4. Peripheral vasoconstriction 5. Sweat gland stimulation (hands, feet, axillae) 6. Pupil dilation 7. No endorphin release 8. Minimal or absent slow alpha waves on EEG; no theta waves 9. Increased blood lactate levels (associated with high anxiety) 10. Increased blood glucose, free fatty acid, and cholesterol levels	1. Decreased heart rate 2. Decreased blood pressure 3. Decreased oxygen consumption 4. Peripheral vasodilation 5. No sweat gland stimulation 6. Pupils normal or constricted 7. Increase in endorphin levels (body's natural opiate) 8. Increase in slow alpha and theta waves on EEG (associated with feelings of well-being) 9. Decrease in blood lactate levels (associated with lowered anxiety) 10. Sufficient blood glucose, free fatty acid, and cholesterol levels for normal body functioning
Behavioral Manifestations	
Frequent urination, restlessness, sleeplessness, hostility, motor incoordination, repetitive questioning, disorganized speech, and scattered thoughts	Comfortable posture, speech clear, intact thinking process, and effective and purposeful behavior
Subjective States	
Tension, fear, frustration, difficulty concentrating, "pressured," shaky, or jittery feeling, confusion, desire to flee, butterflies in stomach, nausea, irritability, depression, and pounding heart	Increased sense of well-being, greater ability to cope with stress, refreshed feeling, more energy, and increased concentration

Data from Benson 1975; Gellhorn and Kiely 1972; Snyder 1977; Varcarolis 1984.
EEG = electroencephalogram.

that in a nurturing environment, the developing personality incorporates the parents' positive attributes, thus allowing the child to tolerate anxiety. When conditions for personality growth are less than adequate, positive values may not be incorporated, and the child may become anxiety-ridden, a state that often covers up overwhelming, angry, and hostile impulses (Sullivan 1953). A child may demonstrate chronic anxiety by a permanent attitude of apprehension or by overreaction to all unexpected environmental stimuli. In the adult, chronic anxiety may take the form of chronic fatigue, insomnia, discomfort in daily activities, and discomfort in personal relationships. Poor concentration may interfere with effective work functioning. When the subjective feelings of anxiety become too overwhelming, anxiety is unconsciously placed out of awareness (repressed) and is expressed in behavioral characteristics or symptoms. **Trait anxiety** is another name for chronic anxiety.

Understanding the types, levels, and defensive patterns used in response to anxiety is basic to psychiatric nursing care. This understanding is essential for assessing and planning interventions to lower a client's level of anxiety, as well as one's own, effectively. With practice, one becomes more skilled at identifying levels of anxiety and defenses used to alleviate it, as well as at evaluating the possible stressors contributing to increases in a person's level of anxiety.

This chapter elaborates basic concepts regarding anxiety used by all nurses in all clinical settings. Common psychotherapeutic interventions are introduced for mild to moderate and severe to panic levels of anxiety. Brief case studies of a person in moderate levels of anxiety and a person in severe levels of anxiety are presented to illustrate the theoretical component through use of the nursing process. Figure 9–1 presents a conceptual framework for anxiety.

Theory

Anxiety is a response to a stressful situation. Stress can be defined as a perceived threat to an expectation, thereby triggering anxiety. The result is some form of relief behavior (Knowles 1981). Therefore:

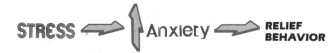

Stress can be psychological, social, or physical. Anxiety can be an appropriate or inappropriate response and can result in healthy relief behaviors or psychiatric symptoms (Lesse 1982). Thus, anxiety may be experienced as a (1) *symptom* involving a subjective feeling of apprehension or nervousness, (2) *syndrome* involving both psychic and somatic symptoms, or (3) *primary disease*, such as generalized anxiety disorder or phobic disorder. As a symptom or syndrome, anxiety may be "normal" in certain circumstances. Anxiety may be "abnormal" when its severity is inappropriate or when it occurs in inappropriate circumstances (Cameron 1985).

There is no one etiological theory of anxiety that explains all the clinical and biological data. Various theories have made contributions to possible etiological factors in the development of anxiety. Three major theories are (1) psychodynamic, (2) behavioral, and (3) biological.

PSYCHODYNAMIC THEORY

Chapters 1 and 2 discuss in detail the major personality theories and therapies. Here we briefly review them in relation to the concept of anxiety.

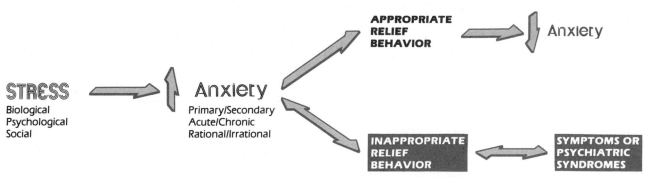

Figure 9–1. *Conceptualization of psychiatric symptoms or syndromes along the anxiety continuum.*

Freud proposed that anxiety is the result of *unconscious* psychic conflicts. When these *intrapsychic conflicts*, or forbidden impulses (sexual or aggressive), threaten to become conscious, anxiety is experienced. Anxiety then becomes a *signal* to the ego to take defensive action to repress anxiety. When these defense mechanisms are successful, anxiety is lowered and a sense of security returns. However, if the conflict is intense and the anxiety level high, the defense mechanisms might be experienced as symptoms, such as phobias, regression, or ritualistic behaviors.

Harry Stack Sullivan believed that anxiety resulted from *interpersonal conflicts* rather than from an intrapsychic process. Sullivan stated that anxiety is linked to the anxiety experienced in infancy and early childhood. The infant's first experiences with emotional discomfort and acute anxiety become the prototype for future emotional distress. For example, a child reared by hostile and rejecting parents may later react with painful anxiety when treated in a cold or critical manner by another individual. Past experiences leave people vulnerable to anxiety in the present, and specific events or interpersonal exchanges can trigger underlying anxiety (Chapman and Chapman 1980). Two principles basic to nursing practice are based on Sullivan's theory of anxiety.

First, anxiety can be communicated interpersonally. Anxiety is communicated from one person to another via empathy (Sullivan 1953). **Empathy** is the ability to feel for and with another and to understand the other's experience. An example of anxiety transferred from person to person via empathy is what may occur in mass crisis situations. In mass crisis situations, people in high levels of anxiety need to be attended to first to avoid the spread of anxiety, which could lead to group panic and confusion. (See Chapter 6 for a discussion of the process of empathy.)

Second, anxiety is an energy (Peplau 1968). We cannot see anxiety in others; instead, behavior expresses the anxiety that a person feels. No one wants to experience uncomfortable levels of anxiety. Relief behaviors are those that discharge the energy of anxiety. Familiar behaviors, such as movement, talking, and meditation, are examples of relief behaviors used to lessen the experience of anxiety.

Rollo May (1983) states, "Anxiety is the apprehension cued off by a threat to some value that the individual holds essential to his existence as a personality." These threats comprise those to biological integrity, such as food or shelter, and those to psychological well-being, such as loss of respect or freedom. A person experiencing an unconscious conflict may become anxious, although the reason for the anxiety may not be known. People modify their relationships with others constantly to keep anxiety as low as possible, thereby maintaining a feeling of emotional security.

Anxiety caused by psychological factors (intrapsychic or interpersonal conflicts) is referred to as **primary anxiety** (Rockwell 1982).

BEHAVIORAL THEORY

The success of behavioral therapy techniques in the treatment of phobias and obsessive-compulsive behaviors gives support to the theory that anxiety is a result of a learned, or conditioned, response (Curtis 1985). According to behavioral theory, anxiety results from a system of responses to a particular stimulus. Over a period of time, an individual develops a learned, or conditioned, response to certain stimuli. This assumption has given rise to the concept that anxiety can be learned and unlearned as a result of experience. Some behavioral therapists have regarded Freud's *signal* theory as identical to that of the learned conditioned response (Curtis 1985). Chapter 14 discusses behavioral interventions used effectively in the treatment of certain anxiety disorders, such as phobias.

BIOLOGICAL THEORY

There is an increasing body of knowledge supporting the hypothesis that manifestations of anxiety may be due to physiological abnormalities. Diagnostic decisions need to be made when one is confronted with anxiety symptoms to determine whether the anxiety is (1) secondary to a medical disorder, (2) secondary to a pervasive psychiatric disorder, such as depression, or (3) a primary anxiety disorder, such as a phobia (Curtis 1985).

In up to 40% of cases, anxiety may be a warning of an underlying physiological process (Hall 1980). That is, the anxiety is caused by a physical disease or abnormality, *not* by an emotional conflict. Anxiety secondary to a physical condition is termed **secondary anxiety.** For example, people with certain neurological disorders (multiple sclerosis, brain tumor), endocrine disorders (thyroid, pituitary), circulatory disorders (anemia, coronary insufficiency), and other disorders may experience anxiety due to physiological processes (Rockwell 1982; Kaplan and Sadock 1991).

Several promising studies have focused on the neuroanatomy and biochemistry of normal and pathological anxiety states. (Chapter 14 identifies specific studies relevant to anxiety disorders.) Although these preliminary investigations do not show conclusive cause-and-effect relationships at present, it is a rich field for future research (Kaplan and Sadock 1991).

Assessment

Assessing the presence of problematic levels of anxiety may or may not be easy. For example, a person in *acute* anxiety may demonstrate obvious signs and symptoms of distress and may be experiencing the anxiety subjectively: "I feel so upset." Or, a person might not be aware of experiencing anxiety; instead, the anxiety might be repressed from conscious awareness but expressed in some other form of relief behavior. For example, a woman who is unaware of experiencing anxiety related to feelings of inadequacy might be *displacing* her anxiety as anger toward her family. A man who is unaware of experiencing anxiety related to low self-esteem might *compensate* by drinking or taking drugs to feel better temporarily. Established patterns of dealing with anxiety may be observed by noting specific relief behaviors a person uses.

The nursing assessment of the anxious client should include information about the (1) level of anxiety, (2) relief behaviors used to minimize the subjective experience of anxiety, and (3) circumstances surrounding increases in anxiety.

ASSESSING LEVELS OF ANXIETY

Levels of anxiety range from mild to moderate to severe to panic. Peplau's (1968) classic delineation of these four levels of anxiety is based on Harry Stack Sullivan's work. Assessment of a client's level of anxiety is basic to therapeutic intervention in any setting —psychiatric, hospital, or community. Determination of specific levels of anxiety can be used as guidelines for intervention (Table 9–2). Anxiety is experienced on a continuum from mild to moderate to severe to panic, and overlapping can and does occur. Use Table 9–2 as a guide for your observations.

MILD. Mild anxiety occurs in the normal experience of everyday living. The person's ability to perceive reality is brought into sharp focus. A person sees, hears, and grasps more information, and problem solving becomes more effective. A person might display such physical symptoms as slight discomfort, restlessness, irritability, or mild tension-relieving behaviors, such as nail-biting, foot or finger tapping, or fidgeting.

MODERATE. As anxiety escalates, the perceptual field narrows, and some details are excluded from observation. The person in moderate anxiety sees, hears, and grasps less information than someone not in that state. Individuals may experience **selective inattention,** in which only certain things in the environment are seen or heard unless they are brought to the person's attention. Although the ability to think clearly is hampered, learning and problem solving can still take place, though not at an optimum level. At the moderate level of anxiety, the person's ability to problem solve is greatly enhanced by the supportive presence of another. Physical symptoms include tension, pounding heart, increased pulse and respiration rate, perspiration, and mild somatic symptoms (gastric discomfort, headache, urinary urgency). Voice tremors and shaking might be noticed.

Mild or moderate anxiety levels can be constructive because anxiety can be viewed as a signal that something in the person's life needs attention (Chapman and Chapman 1980).

SEVERE. The perceptual field of a person experiencing severe anxiety is greatly reduced. A person in severe anxiety may focus on one particular detail or many scattered details. The person may have difficulty noticing what is going on in the environment, even when it is pointed out by another. Learning and problem solving are not possible at this level, and the person may be dazed and confused. Behavior is "automatic" and aimed at reducing or relieving anxiety. The person may complain of increased severity in somatic symptoms (headache, nausea, dizziness, insomnia), trembling, and pounding heart. The person may also experience hyperventilation and a sense of impending doom or dread.

PANIC. Feelings of panic are very painful. Panic is the most extreme form of anxiety and results in markedly disturbed behavior. The person is not able to process what is going on in the environment and may lose touch with reality. The behavior that results may be confusion, shouting, screaming, or withdrawal. Hallucinations, or false sensory perceptions, such as seeing people or objects that are not there, may be experienced by people in panic levels of anxiety (refer to Chapter 19). Physical behavior may be erratic, uncoordinated, and impulsive. Automatic behaviors are used to reduce and relieve anxiety, although such efforts may be ineffective. Acute panic may lead to exhaustion. Table 9–2 identifies levels of anxiety in relation to (1) perceptual field, (2) ability to learn, and (3) physical and other defining characteristics.

Table 9-2 ■ ANXIETY LEVELS			
MILD	**MODERATE**	**SEVERE**	**PANIC**
Perceptual Field			
Perceptual field can be heightened	Perceptual field narrows. Person grasps less of what is going on.	Perceptual field greatly reduced.	Unable to focus on the environment.
Is alert and can see, hear, and grasp what is happening in the environment.	Can attend to more *if pointed out by another* (selective inattention).	Focus is on details or one specific detail. Attention is scattered.	Experiences the utmost state of terror and emotional paralysis. Feels he "ceases to exist."
Can identify things that are disturbing and are producing anxiety.		Completely absorbed with self.	In panic, hallucinations or delusions may take the place of reality.
		May not be able to attend to events in the environment *even when* pointed out by others.	
		In severe and panic levels of anxiety, the environment is blocked out. It is as if these events are not occurring.	
Ability to Learn			
Able to effectively work toward a goal and examine alternatives.	Able to solve problems but not at optimum ability.	Unable to see connections between events or details.	May be mute or have extreme psychomotor agitation leading to exhaustion.
	Benefits from guidance of others.		
Mild and moderate levels of anxiety can alert the person that something is wrong and stimulate appropriate action.		**Severe and panic levels prevent problem solving and finding effective solutions. Unproductive relief behaviors are called into play, thus perpetuating a vicious cycle.**	
Physical and Other Characteristics			
Slight discomfort	Voice tremors	Ineffective functioning	Experience of terror and dread
Attention-seeking behaviors	Change in voice pitch	Inability to concentrate	Immobility or severe hyperactivity
Restlessness	Difficulty concentrating	Confusion	Dilated pupils
Irritability or impatience	Shakiness	Purposeless activity	Pallor
Mild tension-relieving behavior, such as foot or finger rapping, lip chewing, or fidgeting	Repetitive questioning	Sense of impending doom	Unintelligible communication or inability to speak
	Somatic complaints, such as urinary frequency and urgency, headache, backache, or insomnia	More intense somatic complaints, such as dizziness, nausea, headache, and sleeplessness	Severe shakiness
	Increased respiration rate	Hyperventilation	Sleeplessness
	Increased pulse rate	Tachycardia	Severe withdrawal
	Increased muscle tension	Withdrawal	Hallucinations or delusions likely
	More extreme tension relieving behavior, such as pacing and banging hands on table		

Data from Chapman and Chapman 1980; McFarland and Wasli 1984; Peplau 1968.

ASSESSING RELIEF BEHAVIORS

Interpersonal Relief Behaviors

Anxiety and defenses against anxiety are a necessary part of human life. Peplau (1968) has identified four major patterns of reducing and relieving anxiety:

1. Acting-out behaviors
2. Somatizing
3. "Freezing to the spot"
4. Learning and problem solving

ACTING-OUT BEHAVIORS. Acting-out behaviors are those that originate on an unconscious level to reduce anxiety and tension. Anxiety is displaced from one situation to another in the form of observable behavioral responses. Some examples follow:

Anger can be used to conceal thoughts or feelings that threaten to trigger anxiety. Anger distracts an individual from threatening thoughts and feelings. Anger can effectively remove the focus from the self and redirect attention to something or someone in the environment. The verbal expression of appropriate or inappropriate anger makes an individual feel more powerful and in control, and not as helpless or vulnerable.

Crying can at times be an effective relief from tension and painful feelings. When a person is crying, feelings are close to the surface, thereby enabling a person to identify what he or she is feeling.

Laughter can afford a partial relief of tension. Laughter can express conscious and unconscious psychological meanings and may mask feelings like hostility, fear, despair, triumph, or relief.

Both crying and laughter give the individual a sense of control. They also assist in the repression of anxiety-producing threats.

Physical and verbal abuse distracts the person from threatening realizations. By lashing out at others, the individual transfers the focus from personal doubts and insecurities to some other person or object.

SOMATIZING. To somatize is to experience an emotional conflict as a physical symptom. When attention is focused on bodily complaints, underlying anxiety and interpersonal difficulties can be kept out of awareness. Physical discomfort can be used to distract one from threatening emotional anguish. Therefore, the energy of anxiety is internalized physiologically (Chapman and Chapman 1980). For example, a person might experience a headache or backache as a distraction from interpersonal conflicts.

"FREEZING TO THE SPOT." "Freezing to the spot" involves withdrawal and depression. Withdrawal is a reaction in which psychic energy is withdrawn from the environment into the self in response to anxiety. An example of severe withdrawal is seen in the catatonic schizophrenic (Chapter 19). A person with catatonia may sit for days or months if psychotrophic drugs are not provided. Investment in the environment is lost while the person is in a withdrawn state.

LEARNING AND PROBLEM SOLVING. Learning takes place when anxiety is recognized and the unconscious unmet need identified. This process is often referred to as "talking it out" and "figuring it out" and involves talking about the anxiety-producing event and determining the feelings that result from a threat or an unmet expectation (Peplau 1968). When painful feelings or unsatisfying behaviors can be discussed with a caring person in a counseling situation, alternative and more satisfying solutions can be evaluated.

Intrapsychic Relief Behaviors— Defense Mechanisms

Defense mechanisms are intrapsychic relief behaviors used by everyone. They serve to lower anxiety, maintain ego function, and protect self-esteem. Defense mechanisms can be classified as relief behaviors because they lessen or relieve anxiety. High levels of anxiety can disturb problem solving and learning as well as perception and functioning. Unconscious defensive maneuvers are mobilized so that an individual can continue to meet personal and social goals in acceptable ways. All defense mechanisms are mobilized by the ego, with the exception of regression. In regression, the ego itself (personality) is relegated to a less mature, although more comfortable, mode of operation. Most defense mechanisms are mobilized by the ego on an unconscious level. A notable exception is suppression, which uses the conscious mind.

Adaptive use of defense mechanisms helps people lower anxiety to achieve goals in acceptable ways. Maladaptive use of defense mechanisms may lead to distortions in reality and self-deception that can interfere with individual growth and interpersonal satisfaction. Determination of effective use of defense mechanisms is based on frequency, intensity, and duration of use.

A review of some of the most commonly used defense mechanisms is presented subsequently. Refer to Table 9–3 for illustrations of mild and maladaptive examples of each.

REPRESSION. Repression is the exclusion of unpleasant or unwanted experiences, emotions, or ideas from conscious awareness. "Forgetting" the name of a former husband and "forgetting" an appointment to discuss poor grades are examples. Repression is considered the cornerstone of the defense mechanisms, and it is the first line of psychological defense against anxiety.

SUBLIMATION. Sublimation is an unconscious process of substituting constructive and socially acceptable activity for strong impulses that are not acceptable in their original form. Usually these impulses are sexual or aggressive in nature. A man with strong hostile feelings becomes a butcher, or he may be involved with rough contact sports. A person who is unable to experience sexual activity may channel this energy into a creative activity, like painting or gardening.

REGRESSION. In regression, the ego returns to an earlier, more comforting, although less mature way of behaving. For example, some adults who cannot have their own way pout and whine and behave in a manner that got them their own way as children. When regression is severe, a person may regress to an infantile level and be unable to care for his or her own needs.

DISPLACEMENT. Transfer of emotions associated with a particular person, object, or situation to another person, object, or situation that is nonthreatening is called displacement. The frequently used example, boss yells at man—man yells at wife—wife yells

Table 9-3 ■ DEFENSE MECHANISMS

MILD USE	MALADAPTIVE USE
Repression	
Man forgets wife's birthday after a marital fight.	Woman is unable to enjoy sex after having pushed out of awareness a traumatic sexual incident from childhood.
Sublimation	
Woman who is angry with her boss writes a short story about a heroic woman. By definition, use of sublimation is always constructive.	None
Regression	
Four-year-old with new baby brother starts sucking his thumb and wanting a bottle.	Man who loses a promotion starts complaining to others, hands in sloppy work, misses appointments, and comes in late for meetings.
Displacement	
Patient criticizes the nurse after his family failed to visit.	Child who is unable to acknowledge fear of his father becomes fearful of animals.
Projection	
Man who is unconsciously attracted to other women teases his wife about flirting.	Woman who has repressed an attraction toward other women refuses to socialize. She fears another woman will make homosexual advances toward her.
Compensation	
Short man becomes assertively verbal and excels in business.	Individual drinks when self-esteem is low to diffuse discomfort temporarily.
Reaction-Formation	
Recovering alcoholic constantly preaches about the evils of drink.	Mother who has an unconscious hostility toward her daughter is overprotective and hovers over her to protect her from harm.
Denial	
Man reacts to news of the death of a loved one: "No, I don't believe you. The doctor said he was fine."	Woman whose husband died three years ago still keeps his clothes in the closet and talks about him in the present tense.
Conversion	
Student is unable to take a final exam because of a terrible headache.	Man becomes blind after seeing his wife flirting with other men.
Undoing	
After flirting with her male secretary, a woman brings her husband tickets to a show.	Man with rigid and moralistic beliefs and repressed sexuality is driven to wash his hands when around attractive women to gain composure.
Rationalization	
"I didn't get the raise because the boss doesn't like me."	Father who thinks his son was fathered by another man excuses his malicious treatment of the boy by saying, "He is lazy and disobedient," when that is not the case.
Identification	
Five-year-old girl dresses in her mother's shoes and dress and meets daddy at the door.	Young boy who thinks a pimp in the neighborhood with money and drugs is someone to look up to.
Introjection	
After his wife's death, husband has transient complaints of chest pain and difficulty breathing—the symptoms his wife had before she died.	Young child whose parents were overcritical and belittling grows up thinking that she is not any good. She has taken on her parent's evaluation of her as part of her own self-image.

Table 9–3 ■ DEFENSE MECHANISMS *Continued*	
MILD USE	**MALADAPTIVE USE**
Suppression	
Businessman who is preparing to make an important speech that day is told by his wife that morning that she wants a divorce. Although visibly upset, he puts this incident aside until after his speech, when he can give the matter his total concentration.	A woman who feels a lump in her breast shortly before leaving for a three-week vacation puts the information in the back of her mind until after returning from her vacation.

at child—child kicks the cat, demonstrates a successive use of displaced hostility. The use of displacement is common but not always adaptive. Spouse, child, and elder abuse are often cases of displaced hostility.

PROJECTION. A person unconsciously rejects emotionally unacceptable features and attributes them to other people, objects, or situations through projection. This is the hallmark of "blaming" or "scapegoating," which is the root of prejudice. People who always feel that others are out to deceive or cheat them may be projecting onto others those characteristics in themselves that they find distasteful and cannot consciously accept.

Projection of anxiety can often be seen in systems (family, hospital, school, and business). In a family in which there are problems, often the child is "scapegoated," and the pain and anxiety within the family are projected onto the child: "the problem is Tommy." In a larger system in which anxiety and conflict are present, the weakest members are scapegoated; "The problem is the nurses' aides, the students, the new salesman" (Miller and Winstead-Fry 1982). When pain and anxiety exist within a system, projection can be an automatic relief behavior. Once the cause of the anxiety is identified, changes in relief behavior can ensue and the system can become more functional and productive.

COMPENSATION. Making up for deficits in one area by excelling in another to raise or maintain self-esteem is called compensation. An unsuccessful actor becomes a successful playwright, or a student with poor grades becomes outstanding in sports. These are two examples of adaptive compensation.

REACTION-FORMATION. In reaction-formation (also termed *overcompensation*), unacceptable feelings or behaviors are kept out of awareness by developing the opposite behavior or emotion. For example, a man who harbors hostility toward children becomes a boy scout leader.

DENIAL. Denial involves escaping unpleasant realities by ignoring their existence. A man might believe physical limitations would be a negative reflection on his "manhood." Therefore, a man may deny chest pains even though heart attacks run in his family because of the threat to his self-image as a man. A woman whose health has deteriorated because of alcohol abuse denies she has a problem with alcohol by saying she can stop drinking whenever she wants.

CONVERSION. Transforming anxiety on an unconscious level to a physical symptom that has no organic cause is called conversion. Often the symptom functions to obtain attention or as an excuse. For example, a professor develops laryngitis on the day he is scheduled to defend a research proposal to a group of peers.

UNDOING. Undoing makes up for an act or communication, e.g., giving a gift to "undo" an argument. A common behavioral example of undoing is compulsive handwashing. This can be viewed as cleansing oneself of a perceived unacceptable act or thought.

RATIONALIZATION. Rationalization is justifying illogical or unreasonable ideas, actions, or feelings by developing acceptable explanations that satisfy the teller as well as the listener. Common examples are, "If I had his brains then I'd get good grades also" or "Everybody cheats, so why shouldn't I?" Rationalization is a form of self-deception.

IDENTIFICATION. Identification is an unconscious mechanism used to protect the person against anxiety and loss by imitation of mannerisms or behaviors of a person or group. By identifying with the parent of the same sex, the child resolves his Oedipal conflict. Hero worship is a form of identification.

INTROJECTION. Introjection involves intense identification in which a person incorporates or takes into his or her own personality qualities or values of another person or group with whom or with which intense emotional ties exist. The use of introjection is frequently seen in the grieving process and serves to lessen the anxiety of separation temporarily by the mourner. The mourner may take on some of the physical symptoms or behavioral mannerisms of the deceased for a period of time as a way of "holding on" to the deceased.

SUPPRESSION. Suppression is the conscious denial of a disturbing situation or feeling. A student who has been studying for the state board examinations says, "I can't worry about paying my rent until after my exam tomorrow." A more destructive use of suppression would be, "I know my child is having trouble in school, but I just don't want to think about it."

ASSESSING CIRCUMSTANCES SURROUNDING INCREASES IN ANXIETY

The nurse can work with the client to determine what triggered an increase in anxiety if the precipitating stress has not already been identified. Understanding the steps that operationally define anxiety can help both nurse and client identify unmet needs and expectations. People are often not aware of the process of their thinking, especially in emotional areas. Sometimes, just determining the source of the behavior or feelings is sufficient to lower anxiety effectively. The steps that operationally define anxiety are as follows (Manaser and Warner 1964):

Steps	Examples
1. Expectation or need present (status, recognition, success).	1. Client expects nurse to talk to him after rounds.
2. Expectation or need not met (threat, or precipitating stress).	2. Nurse is unable to return to client's room.
3. Feelings of discomfort and uneasiness. Anxiety may be out of the individual's awareness.	3. This step often goes unnoticed. Step 4 follows immediately.
4. Relief behavior mobilized (e.g., withdrawal, anger, somatizing, crying).	4. Client accuses nurse of being "no good," lazy, and incompetent.
5. Relief behavior is rationalized but not understood.	5. "Nurses are just doctors' maids. They don't count anyway."

In the preceding example, the client's problem is not competent or incompetent nurses, but rather the threat to the client's need for recognition. The client's expectation was that the nurse would visit to talk to him. When the nurse did not return, the client felt slighted, thinking, "I'm not good enough for her to spend time with me." The "uneasy feeling" stemming from the unmet need for recognition was quickly transferred into relief behavior. In this example, *projection* occurred when the client's feelings of low self-esteem were transferred onto the nurse, for example, "She is no good." Projection temporarily lowers the subjective feelings of anxiety, thereby protecting self-esteem, but it does not help the situation. The client's need for recognition is still not met.

At times, nurses react to the relief behavior of clients rather than to the clients' needs. For example, after being told she is lazy, the nurse might get angry with the client. She could choose to spend less time with the client and rationalize her behavior by labeling him as difficult. Or, the nurse might recognize the client's reaction as relief behavior. The nurse could then explore further the unmet needs: "You seem so upset. You didn't seem upset at rounds. What happened to upset you?" This response opens the avenue for identifying unmet needs, clarifying misconceptions, and offering alternatives for clients to meet their own needs. This kind of response also prevents the nurse from personalizing the client's comments and becoming angry.

Thus far in this chapter, several concepts about anxiety have been introduced:

1. Anxiety can be *primary* (caused by interpersonal or intrapsychic conflicts) or *secondary* (caused by physical disorders or processes).
2. Anxiety is experienced on a continuum from *mild* to *moderate* to *severe* to *panic*. Each level has specific characteristics.
3. Anxiety can be *acute* (state) or *chronic* (trait) in nature.
4. Anxiety can be *operationally defined*. Briefly, a need or an expectation is not met, anxiety results, and relief behaviors occur and are then rationalized.
5. *Relief behaviors* can be viewed as interpersonal (*acting out, somatizing, withdrawal,* or *problem solving*) or intrapsychic (*defense mechanisms*).
6. *Anxiety* and *fear* are experienced in similar ways physically, but anxiety is said to be a response to an unknown or unconscious threat, and fear a response to a known or identified threat. Anxiety is more erosive to a person's sense of self than is fear.
7. One way to conceptualize anxiety is shown in Figure 9–1.

Nursing Diagnosis

Anxiety exists on a continuum from mild to panic. The nursing diagnosis of anxiety is made when there are supporting physical, emotional, and cognitive signs and symptoms of anxiety (Carpenito 1991). The diagnosis of anxiety is always qualified by the level of anxiety, such as mild, moderate, severe, or panic.

Evaluating perceptual field, ability to learn, and other defining characteristics helps nurses assess a person's anxiety level. Equally important to assess are the client's physiological reactions to anxiety. This is especially true on a medical-surgical unit in which high anxiety levels may be physiologically detrimental to a. person's health (increased blood pressure, increase in blood glucose, and more).

Without a clear idea of the client's anxiety level, the effectiveness of goals and interventions is minimized. The level of anxiety helps clarify the goal and suggests specific interventions. The "related to" component of the nursing diagnosis guides the formulation of goals and interventions. If the "related to" component involves primary anxiety, the goals and interventions might be different than if it involves secondary anxiety. Carpenito identifies three etiological or contributing risk factors that help identify the nursing diagnosis of anxiety:

1. *Situational* (personal or environmental) factors include failure, lack of recognition, hospitalization, death, and divorce.
2. *Maturational* (threat to developmental tasks) factors include sexual development, pregnancy, and adolescence. Anxiety arising from these areas would be considered primary anxiety, that is, anxiety caused by psychological stress.
3. *Pathophysiological* causes of anxiety include any that interfere with basic human needs (e.g., food, air, or comfort). Pathophysiological causes include factors in which anxiety is caused by a physical disease or abnormality, such as brain tumors, multiple sclerosis, ovarian dysfunctions, chronic infections, and rheumatoid arthritis. Anxiety arising from a physical disease or disorder is called secondary anxiety.

Planning

Planning involves more than just the identification of measurable and attainable goals. It should include the identification of personal reactions and feelings the nurse might experience in response to a client's feelings or behaviors. Sometimes, personal responses interfere with effective nursing care. Therefore, planning

should be done on the (1) content level (goals) and the (2) process level (nurses' reactions and feelings).

CONTENT LEVEL—PLANNING GOALS

Long and short term goals are often guided by the "related to" component of the nursing diagnosis. When planning these goals, the nurse considers both the contributing factors and the data that helped to formulate the actual nursing diagnosis. Because the goals and nursing diagnosis depend on the patient's level of anxiety, it is best to divide goals and interventions into those for persons in *mild to moderate* levels of anxiety and those for persons in *severe to panic* levels of anxiety.

Essentially, goals for people in *mild to moderate* levels of anxiety often include preventing further escalation of anxiety, decreasing anxiety levels, and facilitating effective problem solving, as shown in the following example.

Nursing Diagnosis: Anxiety (moderate): related to hospitalization, as evidenced by difficulty in concentrating, irritability, and stating "I don't know what the devil is going on here."

Long Term Goal	Short Term Goal
1. Client will state he understands the need for hospitalization and can describe purpose of diagnostic procedures.	1. By 4:00 P.M., the client will relate to the nurse what the doctor has told him regarding his need for hospitalization.
	2. By 6:00 P.M., the client will describe the tests he is having after health teaching by the nurse.
	3. Client will name two staff members with whom he can discuss his concerns when questions arise.

Goals for people in *severe to panic* levels of anxiety may center on physical safety, such as protection from aggressive drives and physical neglect. Lowering levels of anxiety is crucial, although interventions for lowering anxiety may be different for a person in severe to panic levels of anxiety than for someone in mild to moderate levels.

Nursing Diagnosis: Anxiety (severe): related to loss of spouse, evidenced by 16-pound weight loss, insomnia, and withdrawal

Long Term Goal	Short Term Goal
1. Client will remain physically healthy while going through grieving process.	1. Within two days, the client will discuss feelings of grief with one other person.
	2. Within one week, the client will spend one hour per day with a friend, neighbor, or group in activities (shopping, church, visiting).
	3. Client will gain one to two pounds per week until baseline weight is achieved by 6/14.
	4. Client will sleep six hours per night by 6/1.
	5. Client will state she has three important support people or groups available while going through the grieving process.

PROCESS LEVEL—NURSES' REACTIONS AND FEELINGS

Nurses are constantly working with people in high-stress situations, an environment that results in high levels of anxiety. Anxiety can be experienced by clients, clients' families, and health care workers. Mild to moderate anxiety reactions are commonly seen in clients on the medical and surgical units, as well as in the obstetrical and gynecological and pediatric settings. Severe to panic levels of anxiety can also be seen in the general hospital setting, but they are most often observed in the psychiatric setting.

Working with people in high levels of anxiety can be uncomfortable and intimidating at times for all staff members, but especially for students new to the psychiatric setting. Because anxiety is communicated from person to person through the process of empathy (Sullivan 1970), some anxiety will be experienced by nurses working with clients in any hospital setting.

At times, the nurse may find that before he or she is ready to interact with a client, personal feelings need to be sorted out so that therapeutic communication between nurse and client can be at its most effective. Identifying levels of anxiety in the client and

in oneself, and dealing with strong and sometimes confusing countertransferential feelings triggered by certain client behaviors can all be greatly facilitated by working closely with the instructor.

The discussion of feelings and reactions and problem solving is a process that is ongoing in the practice of psychiatric nursing (see Chapter 6). In most hospitals, staff on psychiatric units have regularly scheduled supervisory sessions in which client-staff interactions are discussed, and intervention strategies are planned and evaluated. These meetings may take the form of peer group supervision, supervision with a psychiatric clinical nurse specialist, or joint sessions with medical and nursing staff.

Each clinical chapter in this book (Chapters 11–25) will discuss common reactions and countertransferential feelings experienced by health care workers when dealing with specific behaviors.

Intervention

Perhaps one of the most helpful and meaningful experiences for a person in uncomfortable levels of anxiety is a calm and caring human presence. The calmness of another helps deflect some of the anxious person's own anxiety. The feeling that someone cares helps lessen the feelings of isolation and aloneness and offers a connection to stability.

Specific nursing interventions will always be based on assessment of the client's specific needs, and many of the interventions suggested for people in mild to moderate levels of anxiety are also appropriate for people in other levels of anxiety and vice versa. Guidelines that can be helpful in planning care for anxious clients are provided subsequently.

PSYCHOTHERAPEUTIC INTERVENTIONS

MILD TO MODERATE ANXIETY LEVELS. A person in mild to moderate levels of anxiety is still able to problem-solve; however, the ability to concentrate decreases as anxiety increases. The nurse can help the client focus and solve problems with the use of specific communication techniques, such as employing open-ended questions, giving broad openings, and exploring and seeking clarification. These techniques can be useful to a client experiencing mild to moderate anxiety. The nurse is aware of both the content and the process levels in the client's communication. Closing off topics of communication and bringing up irrelevant topics are both avoided.

Table 9–4 ■ NURSING INTERVENTIONS AND RATIONALES: MILD TO MODERATE LEVELS OF ANXIETY

INTERVENTION	RATIONALE
Nursing Diagnosis: Moderate anxiety related to situational event or intrapsychic conflict, as evidenced by increase in vital signs, moderate discomfort, narrowing of perceptual field, and selective inattention	
1. Help client identify anxiety. "Are you uncomfortable right now?"	1. Validate observations with client, name anxiety, and start to work with the client to lower anxiety.
2. Anticipate anxiety-provoking situations.	2. Escalation of anxiety to more disorganizing level is prevented.
3. Use nonverbal language to demonstrate interest, e.g., lean forward, maintain eye contact, nod your head.	3. Verbal and nonverbal messages should be consistent. The presence of an interested person provides a stabilizing focus.
4. Encourage the client to talk about his or her feelings and concerns.	4. When concerns are stated out loud, problems can be discussed.
5. Avoid closing off avenues of communication that are important for the client. Focus on the client's concerns.	5. When staff anxiety increases, "changing the topic" or "offering advice" is common but not useful to the client.
6. Ask questions to clarify what is being said. "I'm not sure what you mean. Give me an example."	6. Increased anxiety results in scattering of thoughts. Clarifying helps the client identify thoughts and feelings.
7. Help the client identify thoughts or feelings prior to the onset of anxiety. "What were you thinking right before you started to feel anxious?"	7. Help client identify the unmet expectations or needs.
8. Discuss the client's expectations or needs and the difference between the expectation and the outcome.	8. When differences between expectation and outcome can be clarified, alternatives for meeting needs can be explored.
9. Encourage problem solving with the client.	9. Encouraging clients to explore alternatives increases sense of control and decreases anxiety.
10. Assist in developing alternative solutions to a problem.	10. Role-play when possible. Encourage the client to try out alternative solutions.
11. Explore behaviors that have worked to relieve anxiety in the past.	11. Encourage mobilization of successful coping mechanisms and strengths.
12. Provide outlets for working off excess energy (e.g., walking, ping pong, dancing).	12. Physical activity can provide relief of built-up tension.
13. Choose reassurance carefully. Not "Everything will be all right," but "You seem upset, let me stay with you for a while."	13. False reassurance may increase feelings of alienation or not being understood. Everything may not turn out all right; this blocks communication. Acknowledging concern and offering presence can increase feelings of security and decrease anxiety.

Reducing the anxiety level and preventing escalation of anxiety to more distressing levels can be aided by a calm presence, recognition of the anxious person's distress, and willingness to listen. Evaluation of effective past coping mechanisms is useful.

Often the nurse can assist the client in considering alternatives to problem situations and offer activities that may temporarily relieve feelings of inner tension.

Table 9–4 offers concrete examples of appropriate nursing interventions and rationales for patients in mild to moderate levels of anxiety.

SEVERE TO PANIC ANXIETY LEVELS. A person in severe to panic levels of anxiety is unable to solve problems and may have a poor grasp of what is happening in the environment. Unproductive relief behaviors may take over, and the person may not be in control of his or her actions. Extreme regression or running about aimlessly may be behavioral manifestations of the person's intense pain. The nurse is concerned with the client's safety and, at times, the safety of others. Physical needs (e.g., fluids and rest) have to be met to prevent exhaustion. Anxiety reduction measures may take the form of removing the person to a quiet environment, where there is minimal stimulation, and providing gross motor activities to drain off some of the tension. The use of medications may have to be considered, but both medications and restraints should be used only after other more personal and less restrictive interventions have failed to decrease anxiety to safer levels. Although communication may be scattered and disjointed, themes can often be heard, and the nurse can address these themes. The feeling that one is understood can decrease the sense of isolation and also reduce anxiety.

Because the person in severe to panic levels of anxiety is unable to solve problems, communication techniques suggested for the person in mild to moderate levels of anxiety are not always effective. Because clients in severe to panic anxiety levels are out of control, they need to know that they are safe from

Table 9–5 ■ NURSING INTERVENTIONS AND RATIONALES: SEVERE TO PANIC LEVELS OF ANXIETY

INTERVENTION	RATIONALE
Nursing Diagnosis: Severe to panic levels of anxiety related to severe threat, as evidenced by verbal or physical acting out, extreme immobility, sense of impending doom, inability to differentiate reality (possible hallucinations or delusions), and inability to problem-solve	
1. Maintain a calm manner.	1. Anxiety is communicated interpersonally. The quiet calm of the nurse can serve to calm the client. The presence of anxiety can escalate anxiety in the client.
2. Always remain with the person in severe to panic levels of anxiety.	2. Alone with immense anxiety, a person feels abandoned. A caring face may be the only contact with reality when confusion becomes overwhelming.
3. Minimize environmental stimuli. Move to a quieter setting and stay with the client.	3. Further escalation of anxiety to self and to others in the setting is prevented.
4. Use clear and simple statements and repetition.	4. A person has difficulty concentrating and processing information with severe to panic levels of anxiety.
5. Use a low-pitched voice.	5. A high-pitched voice can convey anxiety.
6. Reinforce reality if distortions occur, e.g., seeing objects that are not there or hearing voices when no one is present.	6. Anxiety can be reduced by focusing in on, and validating, what is going on in the environment.
7. Listen for themes in communication.	7. In severe to panic levels of anxiety, verbal communication themes may be the only indication of the client's thoughts or feelings.
8. Attend to physical needs when necessary, e.g., warmth, fluids, elimination, pain relief, and need for family contact.	8. High levels of anxiety may obscure client's awareness of physical needs.
9. Because safety is an overall goal, physical limits may need to be set. Speak in a firm, authoritative voice, "You may not hit anyone here. If you can't control yourself, we will help you."	9. A person who is out of control is often terrorized. Staff must offer the client and others protection from destructive and self-destructive impulses.
10. Provide opportunities for exercise, e.g., pacing with nurse, punching bag, or ping pong.	10. Physical activity helps channel and dissipate tension and may temporarily lower anxiety.
11. When a person is constantly moving or pacing, offer high-caloric fluids.	11. Prevent dehydration and exhaustion.
12. Assess person's need for medication or seclusion after other interventions have been tried.	12. Prevent exhaustion and physical harm to self and others.

their own impulses. *Firm, short, and simple statements are useful.* Reinforcing commonalities in the environment and pointing out reality when there are distortions can also be useful interventions for the severely anxious person. Table 9–5 suggests basic nursing interventions for the client in severe to panic levels of anxiety.

HEALTH TEACHING

Examples of health teaching for clients who experience anxiety include relaxation techniques, progressive muscle relaxation (PMR), and biofeedback. Nurses at any level of preparation can be trained in these techniques, which can then be taught to the client in any setting. The techniques are taught to clients with the consent of the client's doctor because there are some contraindications.

Nurses today are playing a larger and larger role in teaching patients alternative methods of handling stress. By using these techniques, patients can positively affect the course or severity of some physical disorders. Nurses use the relaxation techniques mentioned subsequently in all areas of nursing practice. For example, a study of preoperative cardiac catherization patients showed that relaxation techniques could reduce the amount of preoperative medication (diazepam [Valium]) needed (Warner et al. 1992). Relaxation techniques are used successfully by nurses in critical care areas to help patients cope with their symptoms and treatment (Health 1992). Relaxation techniques and PMR are taught to elderly clients to help treat areas of anxiety, altered comfort, or sleep pattern disturbances (Weinberger 1991).

Herbert Benson (1975) outlined specific techniques that enable most people to elicit what he referred to as the "relaxation response." Essentially, these tech-

---

Box 9–1. BENSON'S RELAXATION TECHNIQUES

Practicing this exercise for 15–20 minutes once or twice daily can produce desired results. It may take a number of weeks or a few months before positive benefits are noticed. The essential ingredients for triggering the parasympathetic response (relaxation response) are

1. A *quiet environment*—External distractions can inhibit relaxation.
2. An *object to dwell on*—Mediators use a mental device to help them elicit deep stages of relaxation. Such a mental device can be a word (e.g., ohm, peace, love) repeated silently over and over. A mental device helps distract the mind from logical thought and prepare for deeper levels of relaxation and "letting go." When distracting thoughts occur, and they will initially, the person is told to push them aside gently. The following advice is given, "Tell each thought you will take care of it later, and go back to the mental device or sound."
3. A *passive attitude*—This can be extremely difficult for people in our culture. Many feel they should be accomplishing some task and may initially view sitting quietly as a waste of time. Once benefits are forthcoming, however, many people regard achieving the relaxation response as one of their most important accomplishments.
4. A *comfortable position*—A sitting position with hands resting on thighs is suggested. Lying down may lead to sleep. Sitting cross-legged can interfere with circulation, and if position is uncomfortable, the discomfort will distract from the process of relaxation.

Sometimes this exercise is referred to as centering. Many nurses, as well as other health care professionals, find this tool useful in dealing with job stress.

---

niques teach the client how to switch from the sympathetic mode (fight-or-flight response) of the autonomic nervous system to a state of relaxation (the parasympathetic mode) (Box 9–1).

Many students find that by using these techniques on a regular basis, they are able to reduce exam anxiety and increase concentration and retention. Although many of these stressors cannot be removed, the level of stress can be reduced. Altering personal perception of an experience and learning new coping skills can be achieved through stress reduction techniques. Feelings of anxiety and stress can be decreased by a student's choice to become actively involved in stress reduction techniques (Davidhizer 1991). Students are encouraged to teach friends and family members these techniques. Practicing with others can enhance results.

For those who are unable to use Benson's techniques, biofeedback can bring about the same results.

Reducing the chronic fight-or-flight response of the sympathetic nervous system can

1. Alter the course of certain medical conditions (e.g., high blood pressure, arrythmias, migraine headaches) (Kolb and Brodie 1982)
2. Decrease the need for certain medications (e.g., analgesics, antihypertensives) (Morris 1979)
3. Diminish or eliminate unhealthy behaviors (e.g., drug addictions, insomnia, overeating) (Aron and Aron 1980)

4. Increase cognitive functions (e.g., concentration and learning ability) (Morse 1977)

Benson's relaxation techniques have been used successfully in conjunction with meditation and visual imagery treating numerous disorders, such as diabetes, high blood pressure, migraines, cancer, and peptic ulcers.

Any client who is to be taught relaxation techniques should do so only with the knowledge and consent of his or her physician. Snyder (1984) cautions against the use of relaxation techniques with certain clients. For example:

1. Depressed persons may experience further withdrawal.
2. Hallucinating and delusional patients may lose contact with reality altogether.
3. The toxic effects of some medications may be enhanced.
4. Some patients in pain may have a heightened experience of pain corresponding to the increase in body awareness.

Other techniques to induce relaxation have been developed. Some have an inward focus. These techniques include meditation, visual imaging, hypnosis, and therapeutic touch. Others have an external focus. These include (1) PMR and (2) biofeedback.

PROGRESSIVE MUSCULAR RELAXATION. PMR is a technique that can help patients achieve deep relaxation. The premise behind PMR is that deep relaxation can occur when muscle contraction is almost completely eliminated. Jacobson, who first developed PMR, devised a program of instruction wherein systematic tensing and releasing of various muscles and learning to discriminate between sensations of tension and relaxation occur. The technique can be learned and practiced in hospitals for patients with a variety of conditions.

Many training sessions are usually needed for mastery of PMR. As mentioned, for best results the student should receive live instruction and proceed only with the approval of a physician.

SOMATIC THERAPIES

People in acute levels of anxiety may benefit from temporary use of medication to reduce anxiety. One group of drugs used for this purpose is called the anxiolytic (antianxiety) agents. One of the most popular groups of anxiolytics in current use is the benzodiazepines. Diazepam (Valium) and chlordiazepoxide hydrochloride (Librium) are two commonly used drugs in this group that are effective in relieving symptoms of anxiousness, agitation, and tension. These drugs should always be used with caution and on a short term basis because of their ability to lead to physical dependence. Refer to Chapter 14 for actions, side effects, and toxic effects and Chapter 24 for signs of withdrawal from and intoxication by anxiolytic agents.

People in chronic anxiety who have severe to panic levels may benefit from a neuroleptic (antipsychotic) agent. These drugs are effective in altering thought disorders and reducing psychotic behaviors. For example, haloperidol (Haldol) is an effective drug used to reduce assaultive behavior and to treat thought disorders. Refer to Chapter 19 for a discussion of the neuroleptic drugs.

BIOFEEDBACK. Biofeedback (discussed earlier) is another somatic therapy that is used for people who suffer from disorders of chronic intermittent anxiety. Relaxation through biofeedback is achieved when an individual learns to control physiological mechanisms that are ordinarily outside of one's awareness and control. Awareness and control are accomplished by monitoring body processes, such as muscle tone, heart rate, and brain waves, with mechanical devices. During this time, the client is presented with signal lights that intensify with tension and dim with relaxation. The client learns to use the signals to produce a relaxed state. With practice, an individual can invoke the relaxation state at will.

PSYCHOTHERAPY

Nurses trained at the master's level may use many different therapies when working with clients who experience uncomfortable levels of anxiety. Two common modalities of therapy are psychotherapy and behavioral therapy. Psychotherapy helps people understand their experience by identifying unconscious conflicts and developing more productive and satisfying coping behaviors.

Behavioral therapists focus on the client's problematic behavior and work with the client to modify or change the behavior. One very effective behavioral approach for people with high levels of anxiety is called desensitization. An overview of behavioral therapy is given in Chapter 2 (see also Chapter 14 on anxiety disorders.)

Evaluation

Because interventions for a person in mild to moderate levels of anxiety often center on decreasing anxiety, preventing future escalation of anxiety, and facilitating effective problem solving, specific goals for reaching these desired outcomes are evaluated.

Interventions for a person in severe to panic levels of anxiety often center on ensuring physical safety, such as protecting the client from aggressive drives and personal neglect. Therefore, evaluation of the specific goals that identify the status of the client's physical safety is needed. Once these goals are met, further goals and interventions focus on reducing anxiety to a more moderate level. Whenever possible, the client works with the nurse to plan future goals and identify potential solutions to problems.

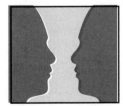

Case Study: Working with a Person in Moderate Levels of Anxiety

Donna James, a 24-year-old recently married woman, had been brought to the hospital for vaginal bleeding during her fourteenth week of pregnancy. The medical team was unable to save the baby. Ms. James had learned about the loss of her baby early that morning.

That evening, after dinner trays had been served, Jane Johnson, the evening nurse, went in to check Ms. James's vital signs. She found the dinner tray untouched and Ms. James crying. Ms. Johnson introduced herself and said, "You're crying. Can I help?" Ms. James started talking rapidly in a high-pitched voice, asking the nurse several times when she could go home. She said, "I didn't know I'd be so upset." Ms. James's pulse rate was 112, and her respiration rate, 26. She stated that she was not hungry and had a terrible headache. The nurse checked her for signs of shock and bleeding, but the physical assessment findings were normal.

Assessment

From her data, the nurse assessed Ms. James's anxiety level as moderate: she had repeatedly asked the same question in a high-pitched voice; she had an increase in pulse and respiration rates; she was crying; and she complained of lack of appetite and a headache. Further assessment and intervention could increase Ms. James's comfort and prevent her anxiety from escalating. The nurse told Ms. James that she understood that she was very upset. She told Ms. James that when she was finished taking her other patient's vital signs in 15 minutes, she would be back to spend 15 minutes with her.

OBJECTIVE DATA

1. Increase in pulse and respiration rates (pulse, 112; respiration, 26)
2. Change in voice pitch
3. Crying—relief behavior
4. Repetitive questioning

SUBJECTIVE DATA

1. "I didn't know I'd be so upset."
2. "I have a terrible headache."
3. "I'm not hungry."

Nursing Diagnosis

From her data, Ms. Johnson devised the following nursing diagnosis:

1. Anxiety (*moderate*), possibly related to termination of pregnancy (situational crisis), as evidenced by crying and somatic complaints.

However, more data would be needed.

Planning

Because general goals focus on decreasing anxiety, preventing further escalation of anxiety, and facilitating effective problem solving for a person in a moderate level of anxiety, Ms. Johnson proposed the following short term goal:

1. Client's anxiety level will be mild by 11:00 P.M., with the aid of nursing interventions.

The nurse planned to spend time with Ms. James to assess her concerns further. Ms. James needed to discuss her feelings and concerns further and mobilize some of her usual coping patterns.

Intervention

When Ms. Johnson returned, she pulled the curtain around the bed. She leaned forward and sat where eye contact was possible. The nurse told Ms. James she had 15 minutes to spend with her. At first, Ms. James's talk shifted from topic to topic, and it was difficult for the nurse to identify Ms. James's feelings.

Dialogue	Therapeutic Tool/Comment
N: I came back because you looked so upset. MS. J: Yes . . . the baby . . . we wanted the baby, but my husband says we can have more . . . he's quite right, I guess. My mother-in-law blames the whole thing on me . . . says I'm too irresponsible and that we can't afford a family right now. I did want the	baby . . . my husband is so worried about all the bills. He just got a job last month, you know. He couldn't come to see me because he is working overtime. My mother-in-law phoned, but I could tell she wanted to get off the phone. Initially, the nurse provides privacy and decreases the environmental stimuli.

Continued on following page

Case Study: Working with a Person in Moderate Levels of Anxiety *(Continued)*

The nurse demonstrates concern for Ms. James by:
A. Making the observation that she understands that Ms. James is upset.
B. Coming back at the time she had indicated.
C. Letting Ms. James talk about how she is

feeling. She did not assume what Ms. James was feeling or why. She neither cut Ms. James off nor offered advice.
D. Letting Ms. James talk, listening for themes.

At first the nurse sat with Ms James, nodding and listening carefully to what was being said and listening for themes. The nurse waited until she had more data, then began to redirect and comment on what was being said.

Dialogue	Therapeutic Tool/Comment
N: It sounds as if there is a lot going on, but no one seems available for you now.	The nurse listens to the content of what Ms. James is saying and tries to focus on the themes.
MS. J: My husband is a good man, he's very concerned with the bills. We were just starting to save some money (*begins to cry*).	Crying can be a healthy release of tension. It is an excellent time to identify feelings because at that time feelings are close to the surface.
N: Tell me what you're feeling right now.	
MS. J: Lonely . . . I feel so alone.	
N: What usually helps you when you're feeling lonely?	The nurse assesses past coping mechanisms that have been helpful.
MS. J: My husband . . . talking to my husband. He's my best friend.	
N: Since he's not here now, perhaps it will help if we talk.	Nurse offers her assistance.

The nurse and Ms. James continued to talk. Ms. James talked about the lack of support she felt from her mother-in-law and her feelings of being left alone by her husband because of his new job. They talked together about the possibility of Ms. James finding a part-time job that would help the financial situation. Ms. James would have an opportunity to be a part of a social network other than her immediate family if she worked. The nurse wondered if the actual loss of the baby was only a part of what was bothering Ms. James, who explained that once the bleeding had started, they had prepared themselves for the loss.

After 15 minutes, the nurse said that

their time was up, but that she would come back before the end of the shift at 11:00 P.M., and she would spend 10 more minutes with her. The nurse asked Ms. James about her headache. Ms. James said that she felt much better and that her headache was gone. She appeared more relaxed and her vital signs had returned to baseline. Her voice was softer and more natural, and she was no longer easily distracted. Ms. James stated she felt she was now able to get some rest.

When the nurse went back at 11:00 P.M., Ms. James was asleep. When the nurse reported off, she asked the day shift to evaluate the need for further referrals before discharge.

Evaluation

The goal was set that Ms. James's anxiety level would be reduced to mild by 11:00 P.M. with the aid of nursing intervention. This was an appropriate and realistic goal set within a realistic time frame, and most important, it was measurable.

The nurse noted that one of Ms. James's

somatic complaints (headache) was gone, her vital signs were back to baseline, her speech was no longer rapid and forced, her thoughts were more coherent, and she was now asleep. The nurse determined that the stated short term goal was met.

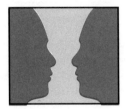

Case Study: Working with a Person in Severe Levels of Anxiety

Tom Michaels, a 63-year-old man, came into the emergency room (ER) with his wife, Anne, who had taken an overdose of sleeping pills and antidepressant medications. Ten years before, Anne's mother had died, and since that time she had suffered several episodes of severe depression with suicidal attempts. She had needed hospitalization during these episodes. Anne Michaels had just been released from a psychiatric unit two weeks previously for another bout of depression and threatened suicide.

Tom Michaels had long established a routine of giving his wife her antidepressant medications in the morning and her sleeping medication at night and keeping the bottles hidden when he was not at home. Today, he had forgotten to hide the medications before he went to work. His wife had taken the remaining pills from both bottles with large quantities of alcohol. When Tom returned home for lunch, Anne was comatose.

In the ER, Anne suffered a cardiac arrest and was taken to the intensive care unit (ICU).

Mr. Michaels appeared very jittery. He moved about the room aimlessly. He dropped things, such as his hat, medication card, and keys. His hands were trembling, and he looked around the room bewildered. He appeared unable to focus on any one thing. He said over and over in a loud, high-pitched voice, "Why didn't I hide the bottles?" He was wringing his hands, and he began stamping his feet, saying, "It's all my fault. Everything is falling apart."

Other people in the waiting room appeared distracted and alarmed by his behavior. He appeared oblivious to his surroundings.

Assessment

Mr. Brown, the psychiatric nurse clinician working in the ER, came into the waiting room and assessed Mr. Michaels's behavior as indicative of a severe anxiety level. After talking with Mr. Michaels briefly, Mr. Brown felt nursing intervention was indicated.

The nurse based his conclusion on the following assessment of the client:

OBJECTIVE DATA

1. Unable to focus on anything
2. Purposeless activity (walking around aimlessly)
3. Oblivious to his surroundings
4. Confused and bewildered
5. Unproductive relief behavior (stomping, wringing hands, dropping things)

SUBJECTIVE DATA

1. "Everything is falling apart."
2. "Why didn't I hide the bottles?"

Nursing Diagnosis

Mr. Brown formulated the following nursing diagnosis:

1. *Anxiety* (*severe*) related to the client's perception of responsibility for his wife's coma and possible death, as evidenced by inability to focus, confusion, and the feeling that "everything is falling apart."

Planning

Mr. Brown thought that if he could lower Mr. Michaels's anxiety to a moderate level, Mr. Michaels could work with him to get a clear picture of his situation and place the events in a more realistic perspective. He also thought that Mr. Michaels needed to talk to someone and share some of his pain and confusion and sort out what he was feeling. Mr. Brown identified two short term goals:

1. Client's anxiety will decrease to moderate levels by 4:00 P.M.
2. Client will talk about his feelings and plans by 4:00 P.M.

Continued on following page

Intervention

The nurse took Mr. Michaels to a quiet room in the back of the ER. The nurse introduced himself to Mr. Michaels and said he noticed that Mr. Michaels was upset. He said, "I will stay with you." At first, Mr. Michaels found it difficult to sit down, and he continued his pacing around the room. Mr. Brown sat quietly and calmly, listening to Mr. Michaels's self-recriminations. The nurse listened carefully to what Mr. Michaels was saying and what he was not saying, to identify themes.

After a while, Mr. Michaels became calmer and was able to sit next to the nurse. The nurse offered him orange juice, which he accepted and held tightly.

Mr. Brown spoke calmly, using simple, clear statements. He used communication tools that were helpful to Mr. Michaels in sorting out his feelings and naming them.

Dialogue	Therapeutic Tool/Comment
MR. M: Yes . . . yes . . . I forgot to hide the bottles. She usually tells me when she feels bad. Why didn't she tell me?	
N: You think that if she had told you she wanted to kill herself you would have hidden the pills?	The nurse asks for clarification on Mr. Michaels's thinking.
MR. M: Yes, if I had only known, this wouldn't have happened.	
N: It sounds as if you believe you should have known what your wife was thinking without her telling you.	Here the nurse clarifies Mr. Michaels's expectations that he should be able to read his wife's mind.
MR. M: Well . . . yes . . . when you put it that way . . . I just don't know what I'll do if she dies.	

When the nurse thought that Mr. Michaels had discussed his feelings of guilt, he asked Mr. Michaels to clarify his thinking about his wife's behavior. Mr. Michaels was able to place his feelings of guilt in a more realistic perspective. Next Mr. Brown brought up another issue—the question of whether Mr. Michaels's wife would live or die.

Dialogue	Therapeutic Tool/Comment
N: You stated that if your wife dies, you don't know what you will do.	Reflecting.
MR. M: Oh God, (Mr. Michaels begins to cry) I can't live without her . . . she's all I have in the world. *Silence.*	
N: She means a great deal to you.	The nurse reflects Mr. Michaels's feelings back to him.
MR. M: Everything. Since her mother died, we are each other's only family.	
N: What would it mean to you if your wife died?	The nurse asks Mr. Michaels to evaluate his feelings about his wife.
MR. M: I couldn't live by myself, alone. I couldn't stand it. (*Starts to cry again.*)	
N: It sounds as if being alone is very frightening to you.	The nurse restates in clear tones Mr. Michaels's experience.
MR. M: Yes . . . I don't know how I'd manage by myself.	
N: A change like that could take time adjusting to.	The nurse validates that if Mr. Michaels's wife died it would be very painful. At the same time, he implies hope that Mr. Michaels could work through the death, in time.
MR. M: Yes . . . it would be very hard.	

214

Again, the nurse gave Mr. Michaels a chance to sort out his feelings and fears. The nurse helped him focus on the reality that his wife might die and encouraged him to express fears related to her possible death. After a while, the nurse offered to go up to the ICU with Mr. Michaels to see how his wife was doing. On arrival at the ICU, Mrs. Michaels, although still comatose, was stabilized and breathing on her own.

After arrival at the ICU, Mr. Michaels started to worry about whether he had locked the door at home. The nurse encour-aged him to call neighbors and ask them to check the door. At this time, Mr. Michaels was able to focus on everyday things. The nurse made arrangements to see Mr. Michaels the next day when he came in to visit his wife.

The next day, Mrs. Michaels regained consciousness, and she was discharged one week later. At the time of discharge, Mr. and Mrs. Michaels were considering family ther-apy with the psychiatric nurse clinician once a week in the outpatient department.

Evaluation

The first goal was to lower anxiety from se-vere to moderate within a given period of time. The nurse could see that Mr. Michaels had become more visibly calm: his trem-bling, wringing of hands, and stomping of feet had ceased, and he was able to focus on his thoughts and feelings with the aid of the nurse.

The second short term goal set for Mr. Michaels was that he would talk about his feelings and plans within a given period of time. Mr. Michaels was able to identify and discuss with the nurse feelings of guilt and fear of being left alone in the world if his wife should die. Both these feelings were overwhelming him. He was also able to make tentative plans with the nurse for the future.

Summary

Anxiety is the most basic of all emotions, and it is an integral part of all emotions. Dysfunctional behavior stems from anxiety. As an everyday component of life, anxiety can facilitate learning and the attainment of goals. It can also lead to ineffective and unsatisfying behaviors. The outcome depends upon the level of anxiety, the choice of relief behaviors, and the inter-vention and guidance received. Anxiety is triggered by a threat to biological safety or psychological security (May 1983).

Anxiety is an energy, and it can be communicated interpersonally via empathy from one person to an-other. Anxiety can be triggered by a psychological conflict (primary anxiety) or a biological cause (sec-ondary anxiety). Anxiety can be experienced on four levels: mild, moderate, severe, and panic. Steps in the operational definition of anxiety follow:

1. Expectation (need) held
2. Expectation not met and felt as a threat
3. Uneasiness or anxiety felt
4. Relief behavior mobilized
5. Relief behaviors rationalized

Relief behaviors can alter anxiety levels through various patterns of behavior and defense mechanisms.

Stress can be psychological, social, or biological. Anxiety can be rational or irrational, and the relief behavior can be adaptive or can take the form of symptoms or syndromes (see Fig. 9–1).

Physiologically, the body reacts to anxiety and fear by the arousal of the sympathetic nervous system. Specific symptoms include rapid heartbeat, increased blood pressure, increased pulse rate, diaphoresis, peripheral vasoconstriction, restlessness, repetitive questioning, feelings of frustration, and difficulty con-centrating.

The nurse learns to assess (1) the level of anxiety, (2) the relief behaviors used, and (3) the circum-stances surrounding the escalation of anxiety. For ex-ample, anxiety is assessed as mild to moderate or severe to panic. Different levels may indicate the need for different goals and nursing interventions. Relief behaviors can be interpersonal (acting out, somatiz-ing, freezing to the spot, or problem solving) or intra-psychic (defense mechanisms).

Anxiety is not a constant state. It can be concep-tualized on a continuum. Anxiety follows specific prin-ciples, and these principles can be used as guides to planning effective nursing care. Specific nursing inter-ventions are useful to people in moderate levels of anxiety, and other nursing interventions are useful to those experiencing severe to panic levels of anxiety. The ability to evaluate personal levels of and reactions to anxiety is a process that can be learned. The ability to assess personal anxiety, as well as the anxiety of others, enables the nurse to increase his or her effectiveness in interpersonal exchanges with clients, peers, and others. Applying the conceptual model of anxiety while implementing the nursing process was illustrated in two case studies.

References

Aron A, Aron B. The transcendental meditation program's effect on addictive behavior. Addictive Behaviors, 5:5, 1980.

Benson H. The Relaxation Response. New York: William Morrow & Company, 1975.

Burd SF. Effects of nursing intervention in anxiety of patients. In Burd SF, Marshall MA (eds). Some Clinical Approaches to Psychiatric Nursing. New York: MacMillan Publishing Company, 1968.

Cameron OG. The differential diagnosis of anxiety: Psychiatric and medical disorders. Psychiatric Clinics of North America: Symposium on Anxiety Disorders, 8(1), March 1985.

Carpenito LJ. Handbook of Nursing Diagnosis, 3rd ed. Philadelphia: JB Lippincott, 1991.

Chapman A, Chapman M. Harry Stack Sullivan's Concepts of Personality Development and Psychiatric Illness. New York: Brunner/Mazel, 1980.

Curtis CC. Anxiety and anxiety disorders: Toward a conceptual reorientation. Psychiatric Clinics of North America: Symposium on Anxiety Disorders, 8(1), March 1985.

Davidhizer R. How to stay sane as a student of nursing. Imprint, 38(4):96,1991.

Hall R. Anxiety. In Hall R (ed). Psychiatric Presentations of Medical Illness. Jamaica, NY: Spectrum Publications, 1980.

Heath AH. Imagery: Helping ICU patients control pain and anxiety. Dimensions of Critical Care Nursing, 11(1):57, 1992.

Kaplan HI, Sadock BJ. Synopsis of Psychiatry (6th ed.). Baltimore: Williams & Wilkins, 1989.

Knowles RD. Managing anxiety. American Journal of Nursing, 81(1), 1981.

Kolb LC, Brodie HKH. Modern Clinical Psychiatry, 10th ed. Philadelphia: WB Saunders, 1982.

Lesse S. Relationship of anxiety to depression. American Journal of Psychotherapy, 36:332, 1982.

Manaser JC, Warner AM. Instruments for the Study of Nurse-Patient Intervention. New York: MacMillan Publishing Company, 1964.

May R. Anxiety and stress. In Seyle H (ed). Seyle's Guide to Stress Research, vol 2. New York: Scientific and Academic Editions, 1983.

McFarland GK, Wasli EL. Nursing care of patients with psychiatric mental health problems, mild, moderate, severe, panic anxiety. In Kim MJ, et al (eds). Pocket Guide to Nursing Diagnosis. St. Louis: CV Mosby, 1984.

Miller S, Winstead-Fry P. Family Systems Theory in Nursing Practice. Reston, Virginia: Reston Publishing Company, 1982.

Morris C. Relaxation therapy in a clinic. American Journal of Nursing, 79:1958, 1979.

Morse D, et al. A physiological and subjective evaluation of meditation, hypnosis, and relaxation. Psychosomatic Medicine, 39:305, 1977.

Peplau HE. A working definition of anxiety. In Burd S, Marshall M (eds). Some Clinical Approaches to Psychiatric Nursing. New York: Macmillan Publishing Company, 1968.

Rockwell D. Anxiety and related disorders. In Donlon P, Rockwell D (eds). Psychiatric Disorders, Diagnosis and Treatment. Bowie, MD: Robert J. Brady Company, 1982.

Snyder SH. Progressive relaxation as a nursing intervention: An analysis. Advances in Nursing Science, 6:47, 1984.

Sullivan HS. The Interpersonal Theory of Psychiatry. New York: WW Norton & Company, 1953.

Sullivan HS. The Psychiatric Interview. New York: WW Norton & Company, 1970.

Warner CD, et al. The effectiveness of teaching relaxation techniques to patients undergoing elective cardiac catheterization. Journal of Cardiovascular Nursing, 6(2):66, 1992.

Weinberger R. Teaching the elderly stress reduction. Journal of Gerontologic Nursing, 17(10):23, 1991.

Yura H, Walsh MB. The Nursing Process. Connecticut: Appleton-Century-Crofts, 1983.

Further Reading

American Psychiatric Association. Diagnostic and Statistical Manual of Mental Disorders, 3rd ed, revised (DSM-III-R). Washington, DC: American Psychiatric Association, 1987.

Benson H. The Relaxation Response. New York: The Hearst Corporation, 1975.

Benson demonstrates how the use of the relaxation response can alter the body's physiological reactions to stress. He outlines the simple steps a person can follow to elicit the relaxation response. Benson's scientific work had a marked influence in further stress research and in the therapeutic use of the relaxation response in a variety of physical and behavioral problems, i.e., cancer, high blood pressure, phobias, and alcoholism. The relaxation response is taught by health care professionals to clients routinely in a variety of health care settings and is in common use by laymen as an effective tool to combat stress and increase a person's sense of well-being.

Bruch H. Eating Disorders: Obesity, Anorexia Nervosa and the Person Within. New York: Basic Books, 1973.

Chapman AH. Textbook of Clinical Psychiatry, 2nd ed. Philadelphia: JB Lippincott, 1976.

Crowe RR. Mitral valve prolapse and panic disorder. Psychiatric Clinics of North America: Symposium on Anxiety Disorders, 8(1), March 1985.

Curtis CC. New findings in anxiety. A synthesis for clinical practice. Psychiatric Clinics of North America: Symposium on Anxiety Disorders, 8(1), March 1985.

Engel GL. A unified concept of health and disease. Perspectives in Biology and Medicine, 3:459, 1960.

Freedman A, Kaplan H, Saddock B. Modern Synopsis of Comprehensive Textbook of Psychiatry, vol 11. Baltimore: Williams & Wilkins Company, 1976.

Hagerty BK. Psychiatric-Mental Health Assessment. St. Louis: CV Mosby, 1984.

Jimerson S. Anxiety. In Haber J, et al (eds). Comprehensive Psychiatric Nursing, 2nd ed. New York: McGraw-Hill Book Company, 1982.

Lentz JR. Therapy with clients with organic brain syndromes. In Beck, et al (eds). Mental Health–Psychiatric Nursing: A Holistic Life-Cycle Approach. St. Louis: CV Mosby, 1984.

May R. The Meaning of Anxiety. New York: Ronald Press, 1950.

A book that had a tremendous impact on the psychiatric community and is still regarded as a reference as well as a classic. May contributed to the theoretical understanding of anxiety and its experience from cultural, philosophical, biological, and psychological standpoints.

National League for Nursing. Programmed instruction, anxiety recognition and intervention. American Journal of Nursing, 65(9), 1965.

Peck MS. The Road Less Traveled. New York: Simon and Schuster, 1978.

Peplau HE. Working definition of anxiety. In Burd S, Marshall M (eds). Some Clinical Approaches to Psychiatric Nursing. New York: Macmillan Publishing Company, 1968.

This classic work by Hildegard Peplau provides nurses with a clear and meaningful understanding of the components of anxiety (definition, etiology, effects, and levels) and offers a theoretical base for the practice of psychiatric nursing. Peplau is very much influenced by the works of Harry Stack Sullivan and has adapted Sullivan's interpersonal approach to the practice of psychiatric nursing.

Schwartz M, Schockley E. The Nurse and the Mental Patient. New York: John Wiley & Sons, 1956.

Self-study Exercises

True or false. If false, change the statement to make it true.

1. _____ The concepts that anxiety (1) is an energy and (2) can be communicated interpersonally come from *psychodynamic theory*.
2. _____ Secondary anxiety originating from physiological abnormalities or processes is consistent with *behavioral/learning theory*.
3. _____ Anxiety is a learned response, and learned responses to anxiety can be unlearned. This is a basic premise of *biological theory*.

Matching

4. _____ A feeling of dread resulting from a threat whose source is unknown.
5. _____ Anxiety precipitated by an imminent loss or change.
6. _____ Anxiety that a person has lived with for a long time and that possibly results from inadequate nurturing.
7. _____ Anxiety that is triggered by a physiological process or dysfunction.
8. _____ The ability to feel for and with another and understand the other's experience.

A. Fear

B. Primary anxiety

C. Chronic anxiety

D. Empathy

E. Normal anxiety

F. Anxiety

G. Secondary anxiety

H. Acute anxiety

Match the steps in the operational definition of anxiety.

9. _____ Need or expectation exists.
10. _____ Need or expectation not met.
11. _____ Anxiety ensues.
12. _____ Relief behavior.
13. _____ Behavior-rationalized.

A. Momentary uneasiness

B. For approval and praise

C. Nurse calls in sick

D. "They don't need me anyway"

E. Head nurse doesn't commend nurse for job well done

Matching

14. _____ Physical disability having no organic base.
15. _____ Self-righteous man always finding fault in everyone else, never in himself.

A. Somatizing

B. Displacement

16. _____ Student who is angry at the teacher picking
a fight with a friend.
    C. Undoing

17. _____ Physical disability in which emotions play a
significant role.
    D. Conversion

18. _____ Knocking on wood to prevent an untold
event after speaking of a bad omen.
    E. Projection

Complete the statements by filling in the appropriate information.

19. Jean unconsciously harbors intense feelings of hostility toward her roommate, who is always flirting with her dates. However, Jean is always extremely sweet and giving to her roommate in interpersonal exchanges. She is using the defense mechanism of _____ .

In questions 20–25, identify levels of anxiety.

20. Rosa is extremely agitated. She is pacing up and down, complaining of nausea and headache, and is unable to concentrate on anything but her lost cat. She is in _____ level of anxiety.

21. Neil is having difficulty taking in what is going on around him since he heard his promotion was denied. His heart is pounding, and his hands are diaphoretic. He finds a friend, who helps him look at his situation and figure out his alternatives. He is in _____ level of anxiety.

22. Gary tells his neighbors that he has been chosen by God to bring peace to the world and that God speaks to him all the time. He is too disorganized to work at a steady job but sometimes helps neighboring farmers harvest their crops. He is in chronic _____ level of anxiety.

23. Denise is told she has been chosen to compete in the final rounds of the championship spelling bee in her state. She starts planning her strategy by making up study time schedules and lists of words to go over, and she becomes very intent on her goal of doing her best. She is in _____ level of anxiety.

24. A man who is to have open heart surgery in the morning starts to complain of palpitations and nausea, has difficulty articulating, and his speech jumps from one topic to the next. He can hardly take in what is going on around him unless it is pointed out to him. He is in _____ level of anxiety. State three interventions that would be useful to this client and give the rationale for each intervention.

A. _____   R _____

_____   _____

B. _____   R _____

_____   _____

C. _____   R _____

_____   _____

25. A woman comes into the emergency room after having been beaten by a mugger. She is incoherent, says she feels like she is going to die, vacillates between periods of withdrawal and crying and screaming. She is in acute _____ level of anxiety. State at least three interventions a nurse could use with a person in this level of anxiety and give the rationale for each intervention.

A. _____   R _____

_____   _____

B. _____   R _____

_____   _____

C. _____   R _____

_____   _____

CHAPTER 10

Anxiety and the Mental Health Continuum as a Conceptual Framework

Thomas Wenzka

OBJECTIVES ■

After studying this chapter, the student will be able to

1. Visualize a relationship among different levels of anxiety along the mental health continuum and selected psychiatric syndromes.
2. Identify two symptoms associated with each disorder described in this overview.
3. For each disorder identified in the illustrations, identify two priorities of nursing care.

Students new to a psychiatric setting have many valid questions and concerns. Several general and specific concerns are addressed in Chapter 6 in The Clinical Interview. Other concerns voiced by students often include the following:

- *What unexpected behaviors or statements might the client present?*
- *Will my own behavior betray inexperience?*

- *Will the staff expect skills and knowledge that I haven't yet mastered?*

Before students enter the psychiatric clinical setting for the first time, an overview of possible behavior manifestations of anxiety (whether biologically, situationally, or psychologically induced) can be useful. Several illustrations are presented to help the student better consolidate the information presented.

Management of Anxiety by the Nurse

The concept of anxiety and the mental health continuum offer a framework to help beginning practitioners understand the behavioral challenges that the psychiatric nurse routinely encounters. The client in crisis, or the client diagnosed according to the DSM-III-R, can be expected to exhibit behaviors and experience needs that can be understood in terms of the levels and types of anxiety the individual is experiencing. The psychiatric disorder may reflect the client's maladaptive responses to stress and anxiety, or the client's anxiety may result from the biological or psychological sequelae of a psychiatric disorder. The client with a specific syndrome or disorder tends to display certain patterns of behavior that typify the particular syndrome or disorder.

Anxiety acted out by one or more clients on a unit is likely to affect the anxiety level of other clients in the treatment community. The nurse observes anxiety's effect on the therapeutic milieu. Interventions aimed at the needs of the community contribute to the treatment plans of each individual. An example is a community meeting composed of clients and staff specifically called to discuss how one client's recent loss of control may be contributing to an increase of anxiety and feelings of insecurity in other clients on the unit.

For assisting the beginning practitioner, this chapter briefly describes the most outstanding characteristics of specific mental disorders commonly treated on acute inpatient psychiatric units and discussed in Units III through VI of this text. The use of the mental health continuum presented along the four levels of anxiety provides a framework for understanding behaviors and disorders. Using this framework, selected common nursing approaches specific to management of anxiety and behavior associated with particular psychiatric syndromes are identified (Fig. 10–1). The beginning practitioner's own anxiety can be reduced by this overview of psychiatric disorders and the general goals of psychiatric nursing staff. The ensuing chapters more fully describe the care of clients experiencing these crises and disorders.

Unit III: Acute Anxiety

CRISIS AND CRISIS INTERVENTION

When acute anxiety escalates in response to stress and a person's usual relief behaviors (defense mechanisms) are no longer able to control disorganizing levels of anxiety, a crisis can ensue. (See Chapter 11.) A crisis is usually precipitated by an overwhelming event or events in a person's life, and these events can be identified. Crisis intervention increases the likelihood that the person will return to a precrisis level of functioning. Without support, a person in severe levels of acute anxiety may experience confusion and personality disorganization. The anxiety can become chronic if it is not reduced in a short time (4–6 weeks). A true crisis situation is a psychiatric emergency. People with high levels of chronic mental disorders are also susceptible to crisis, and the crisis model can be adapted effectively with clients who have long term emotional problems.

Assisting the client to resolve a crisis may result in benefits beyond the relief of anxiety for the individual with chronic anxiety. The client's resultant experience of success and control can bolster self-esteem and enhance insight.

FAMILIES IN CRISIS: FAMILY VIOLENCE

Child abuse, spouse abuse, and elder abuse signal a family in crisis. Victims of physical, sexual, and emotional abuse face stressors that understandably can overwhelm their usual coping abilities. (See Chapter 12.) The acute crisis may or may not be resolved in a manner that fosters healthy lifetime patterns of coping. People who develop maladaptive coping responses often have had to use the best means available at the time to survive overwhelming stress. Even the perpetrators of abuse are highly likely to have been victimized themselves. Maladaptive behaviors clearly require intervention and correction for the cycle of violence to be broken. The mental health nurse often has the opportunity to assist an individual dealing with acute anxiety stemming from crisis; it is hoped that the need for the client to later struggle with the long term effects of chronic anxiety can be bypassed. All too commonly, the nurse encounters an abused person only after chronic anxiety and maladaptive coping have solidified as permanent behavioral patterns. Interventions are then aimed at assisting clients to observe their maladaptive patterns and to make changes that lead to more satisfying and growth-enhancing behaviors. Client safety is always an overall goal. Rape, or sexual assault, is discussed in Chapter 13 as another example of crisis.

Unit IV: Moderate to Severe Levels of Chronic Anxiety

ANXIETY DISORDERS

Central to anxiety disorders is the unconscious attempt to ward off chronic anxiety by refocusing on thoughts or behaviors that distract the individual from

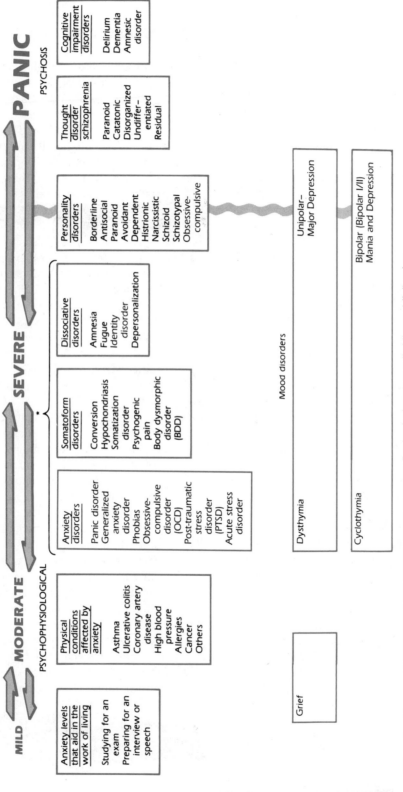

MILD ⇄ MODERATE ⇄ SEVERE ⇄ PANIC

PSYCHOPHYSIOLOGICAL

PSYCHOSIS

Anxiety levels that aid in the work of living

Studying for an exam
Preparing for an interview or speech

Physical conditions affected by anxiety

Asthma
Ulcerative colitis
Coronary artery disease
High blood pressure
Allergies
Cancer
Others

Anxiety disorders

Panic disorder
Generalized anxiety disorder
Phobias
Obsessive-compulsive disorder (OCD)
Post-traumatic stress disorder (PTSD)
Acute stress disorder

Somatoform disorders

Conversion
Hypochondriasis
Somatization disorder
Psychogenic pain
Body dysmorphic disorder (BDD)

Dissociative disorders

Amnesia
Fugue
Identity disorder
Depersonalization

Personality disorders

Borderline
Antisocial
Paranoid
Avoidant
Dependent
Histrionic
Narcissistic
Schizoid
Schizotypal
Obsessive-compulsive

Thought disorder schizophrenia

Paranoid
Catatonic
Disorganized
Undiffer-entiated
Residual

Cognitive impairment disorders

Delirium
Dementia
Amnesic disorder

Mood disorders

Grief

Dysthymia

Cyclothymia

Unipolar–Major Depression

Bipolar (Bipolar I/II) Mania and Depression

*These disorders are currently classified by presenting clinical symptoms. Previously they were called "neurotic" disorders.

Figure 10–1. *Mental health continuum.*

221

underlying conflicts. Recent research provides evidence that many of the anxiety disorders have biological correlates. Experiences such as panic or phobias are perceived by the client as troublesome, frightening, and intrusive.

Clients suffering from such disorders are most frequently able to continue functioning in their usual roles but often experience moderate to severe anxiety, impaired relationships, and lack of fulfillment. These disorders do not commonly cause debilitating symptoms or require hospitalization unless they are associated with self-destructive behaviors. Such may be the case for the victim of physical or sexual abuse who for years has repressed related memories and feelings. The nurse assists the client in learning skills and in safely attempting healthier interpersonal behaviors. Refer to Figure 10–2 for a summary of these points.

SOMATOFORM AND DISSOCIATIVE DISORDERS

As is the case with anxiety disorders, somatoform and dissociative symptoms are often viewed as unconscious attempts to cope with chronic anxiety. The symptoms of somatization and dissociation are thought to divert attention away from traumatic memories or unconscious conflicts. These unconscious defenses at first serve as survival behavior in the face of unbearable trauma but become maladaptive over time. (See Chapter 15.)

The diagnostic process for a *somatoform disorder* involves ruling out a physical disorder. In a somatoform disorder, the client experiences physical symptoms, but no organic pathological process can be identified. In addition, a connection with a severe stressor can often be identified. The client with such a disorder is not "faking" the symptom: the symptoms are very real to the client. However, the client does obtain certain allowances, excuses, or advantages, called secondary gains, because of the physical symptoms.

The client with a *dissociative disorder* loses track of certain life memories, of personal identity, or of customary sense of self. Other thought processes are intact, but the client uses defenses to keep out of conscious awareness traumatic memories that may be threatening to emerge into consciousness.

Assisting the client to address the underlying conflict or sources of anxiety *may* be within the realm of nursing, depending on decisions made by the mental health team and the education and training of staff members. The nurse, in collaboration with the mental health team, supports the client's development of more effective coping skills. The nurse supports healthy aspects of the client's identity and enhances the client's perception of the therapeutic environment as safe and secure (see Fig. 10–2).

PERSONALITY DISORDERS

"Personality traits are enduring patterns of perceiving, relating to, and thinking about the environment and oneself, and are exhibited in a wide range of important social and personal contexts" (APA 1987). If these traits are maladaptive and rigid and cause significant impairment in occupational and interpersonal functioning or personal distress, a personality disorder is suspected. (See Chapter 16.) These characteristics are often present from childhood.

The personality traits of people with personality disorders are *ego-syntonic*: that is, they are part of the person's personality and self-concept and are not experienced as undesirable. For example, a person with an antisocial personality disorder may *not* experience his or her lying, cheating, stealing, or aggressive sexual behavior as a problem, or have any desire to change or to relate differently to others. These characteristics are part of the person's integral personality makeup and are accepted by the person as part of his or her self-concept. When those with personality disorders are in conflict with others, they assume others are at fault.

Although all of the personality disorders are introduced in this text, the borderline, antisocial, and paranoid personality disorders are discussed in depth. Not all of the personality disorders are severe; however, people with borderline, antisocial, and paranoid disorders are more likely to be hospitalized than are people with other personality disorders. Nurses are often in situations that call for interventions in antisocial, borderline, and paranoid acting-out behaviors in any hospital setting. People with one of these disorders can cause constant upheaval and disruption in hospital units by pitting staff against staff and clients against staff. Staff members are often left confused and angry until the dynamics of the interactions are clarified and team interventions are initiated.

Nursing measures may need to be largely directed toward the needs of the therapeutic community when clients with borderline, antisocial, or paranoid personality disorders or traits are admitted to an inpatient mental health unit. *Consistent limits on the behaviors of the client with such a disorder and frequent, patient involvement by staff* are necessary to prevent the destructive social consequences of manipulation and undermining, which are common behaviors in these disorders. Beginning practitioners are cautioned to seek close guidance and feedback from staff and instructors while working with clients who have such personality disorders (see Fig. 10–2).

	ANXIETY DISORDERS	SOMATOFORM AND DISSOCIATIVE DISORDERS	PERSONALITY DISORDERS
STRESS ↓ **ANXIETY** ↓ **RELIEF BEHAVIORS** ↓	Biological/Psychological	Psychological/Environmental	Biological/Environmental/ Psychological
RELIEF BEHAVIORS	Increased anxiety and rigidity in thinking and behaving	**Somatoform**—Attention on bodily functions, which distracts the individual from painful or repressed issues **Dissociative**—Inability to recall events or parts of one's past or to be aware of parts of one's personality	Lifelong pattern of socially unacceptable behaviors based solely on one's own needs and dominating one's coping style; behaviors are not seen by client as a problem of his or her own (ego–syntonic)
ASSOCIATED SYMPTOMS THAT CHARACTERIZE THIS DISORDER	Moderate to severe: • Phobias • Obsessive–compulsive behaviors (OCD) • Panic attacks • Generalized anxiety • Flashbacks of traumatic events (PTSD)	**Somatoform**—Multiple physical complaints, pain, paralysis, and other persistent bodily complaints that have no physical cause **Dissociative** • Blanks out period of time (amnesia) • Travels to distant places and forgets one's past (fugue) • Has multiple personalities (DID)	• Lack of insight regarding consequences of behaviors • Little motivation for change
UNHEALTHY OUTCOMES FREQUENTLY ASSOCIATED WITH THIS DISORDER	• Moderate to severe emotional discomfort • Usually able to function in everyday life but not to optimum level	• Disrupted interpersonal relationships • Inability to function at job • Anxiety and depression may be part of the clinical picture	Social rejection, legal problems, and chaos caused in social settings, including treatment setting
MAJOR AREAS OF NEED TO BE ADDRESSED BY NURSING	• Reduction of anxiety • Teaching of stress reduction skills • Assistance in the development of more appropriate coping skills • Medication teaching	• Reduction of anxiety • Development of more adaptive coping skills • Enhancement of personal identity • Enhancement of emotionally safe physical environment	• Limits on destructive actions • Limits on manipulation of others • Limits on actions taken without regard for consequences • Consistency among staff in enforcing limits • Assistance in learning about consequences of behaviors

Figure 10–2. *Moderate to severe levels of chronic anxiety.* OCD = *obsessive-compulsive disorder;* PTSD = *post-traumatic stress disorder;* DID = *dissociative identity disorder.*

Unit V: Severe to Panic Levels of Chronic Anxiety

ALTERATIONS IN MOOD: DEPRESSION

Depression is characterized by a long-lasting episode of lowered mood, including overwhelming feelings of anhedonia, despair, negativity, and low self-esteem. A loss or a series of losses for which the client has not grieved in a healthy manner frequently compound this state. Included in depression are sleep disturbances, poor appetite, lack of energy or interest, and an inability to experience pleasure (anhedonia). Suicidal thoughts and attempts may accompany depression. The client is often withdrawn from others and demonstrates nonassertiveness and passivity in relationships while maintaining a hidden hostility. (See Chapter 17.)

The mental health nurse first attends to helping the

	DEPRESSION	ELATION/MANIA
STRESS ↓ **ANXIETY** ↓ **RELIEF BEHAVIORS** ↓	Biochemical/Psychological	Biochemical/Psychological
	• Withdrawal from others, from own angry feelings, from self, and from environment • Regression	Reaction–formation in which elation, hyperactivity, and exaggerated sense of self–importance mask underlying depression
ASSOCIATED SYMPTOMS THAT CHARACTERIZE THIS DISORDER ↓	• Low self–esteem • Poor physical care of self • Sleep and eating disturbances • Passive expressions of hostility • Low energy levels • Anhedonia (inability to experience pleasure)	• Overactivity • Delusions of grandeur • Poor attention span • Bizarre use of makeup, jewelry, and clothing • Intrusion into space of others • Too busy to eat, sleep, or rest • Impulsivity and poor judgment
UNHEALTHY OUTCOMES FREQUENTLY ASSOCIATED WITH THIS DISORDER	• Suicide attempts • Alienation from others • Weight loss • Failure to assertively call attention to own needs • When severe, failure to meet own basic needs or perform in usual roles	• Exhaustion • Inadvertent harm to self or others • Sexual acting out • Negative reactions by others • Long term physical, social, and financial consequences
MAJOR AREAS OF NEED TO BE ADDRESSED BY NURSING	• Protection from self–harm • Basic hygiene and nutrition needs • Assertiveness training • Ventilation of anger related to losses • Teaching of positive self–statements • Medication teaching	• Provision of food, fluid, rest, sleep, and basic safety • Guarding client from impulsive decisions and from anger of others in the environment • Medication teaching and follow–up care when possible

Figure 10–3. *Severe to panic levels of chronic anxiety.*

client meet basic physiological and safety needs and later reinvolves the client in social interactions. In individual and group therapies, the client is assisted in observing and correcting maladaptive responses, especially in practicing more assertive communications and attempting more healthy self-appraisals. Figure 10–3 summarizes these points. Nursing is responsible for monitoring desired and adverse effects of medications.

ALTERATIONS IN MOOD: ELATION

Clients with *bipolar disorders* experience episodes of mood change, swinging into elation or mania and then swinging into either a depressive or a normal state. (See Chapter 18.) During a manic episode, the client experiences elation, feelings of great importance and power, and an energy for exciting projects and adventures. The nurse observes overactivity, unrealistic expressions of self-importance, and an exaggerated sense of ability in the client. Often seen are sexual indiscretions; bizarre and colorful dress; lack of time for sleep, rest, food, or fluids; intrusiveness into the space and privacy of others; and reckless behaviors. The nurse plans for ways to protect the client from exhaustion, excessive demands on physiological systems, and behaviors reflecting poor social and personal judgment.

As the client's mania diminishes, the nurse helps the client cope with the consequences of reckless behaviors, such as huge debts or legal problems resulting from uncontrolled spending or checks written on overdrawn accounts. Mania is often seen as the apparent opposite of depression. Medications used to treat bipolar disorders require close monitoring and detailed teaching of the client and family by the nurse. Figure 10–3 summarizes these points.

SCHIZOPHRENIC DISORDERS

Schizophrenia is the major type of psychosis (or thought disorder) that nurses encounter. (See Chapter 19.) The main feature of schizophrenia is bizarre and suspicious thought processes not based in reality. The process of schizophrenia, thought to be biologically or structurally induced, results in altered perceptions of reality (hallucinations) that further compound the person's ability to analyze problems, plan, or maintain motivation to accomplish life goals, or even to solve everyday problems. Maladaptive behaviors include marked use of regression, withdrawal from others and from the environment, and projection. Nurses may need to assist regressed clients to become motivated and organized sufficiently to bathe, toilet, and feed themselves. Clients who have remained regressed for long periods may, when they are thinking more clearly as a result of medication therapy, require planned rehabilitation to learn simple personal, social, and financial survival skills of everyday life. Extreme withdrawal, as seen in catatonic clients, may call for nursing efforts that gradually and painstakingly build trust between nurse and client through creative and patient use of nonverbal and verbal communication skills. Massive projection, as seen in paranoid clients, calls for the nurse to communicate simply and clearly to paranoid clients. Staff members need to monitor the effects of their own communication with highly suspicious clients, who often misinterpret reality (delusions), which can seem quite bizarre and even frightening for both the nurse and the client. Beginning practitioners often feel a sense of gratification, how-

ever, when a client finally experiences more comfort in interpersonal contact.

Care for schizophrenic clients includes strategies to relieve social isolation, inhibit bizarre social behaviors, and cope with the effects of joblessness, homelessness, and despair that too often lead to suicide, disease, or victimization. The client also needs information about medication regimens, which can be complicated in terms of side effects and measures for managing the side effects (Fig. 10–4).

COGNITIVE IMPAIRMENT DISORDERS

Cognitive impairment disorders are characterized by changes in thought, mood, personality, and behavior secondary to temporary or permanent alterations in the structure or biochemical function of the brain. (See Chapter 20.) These disorders are often referred to as organic mental syndromes or disorders. Cognitive impairment disorders (1) are traceable to cell damage from toxic substances, trauma, or disease processes, (2) have neurological symptoms that often accompany the mental symptoms, and (3) when the cause is irreversible, have symptoms that are likely to persist or worsen. For many clients, anxiety can be generated by the perception of change, loss, and inability to successfully employ formerly helpful coping behaviors. The combination of this anxiety with organically based changes in mood, loss of control over behavior, and loss of memory can greatly distress the client and the client's family.

Nursing care aims to assist the client to cope and retain or regain maximum independence within the limits of the loss of mental functioning. Safety must be balanced against independent functioning, and the family's coping should be supported. The nurse's skills in assessment, especially that involving the neurological system, play a vital role in accurate medical diagnosis and interdisciplinary team planning (see Fig. 10–4).

Unit VI: Self-destructive Defenses Against Anxiety

SUICIDE

Suicide receives special attention because of its finality and complexity. It involves an interplay of feelings, behaviors, social interaction, and cultural expression active in all the mental disorders. (See Chapter 21.)

	SCHIZOPHRENIA	COAGULATION IMPAIRMENT DISORDERS
STRESS ⬇ **ANXIETY** ⬇	Biochemical/Genetic/Environmental	Neuron interference or death of neurons
RELIEF BEHAVIORS ⬇	• Withdrawal from reality into inner world • Suspiciousness, extreme regression, and projection	• Withdrawal • Regression • Emotional outbursts • Occasional violence
ASSOCIATED SYMPTOMS THAT CHARACTERIZE THIS DISORDER ⬇	• Distorted perceptions, hallucinations, delusions, and bizarre behaviors • Stifled emotional expression • Interpersonal withdrawal • Lack of motivation • Inability to solve problems and perform other thinking skills	• Neurological deficits • Lack of ability for self–care • Memory deficits • Loss of own identity
UNHEALTHY OUTCOMES FREQUENTLY ASSOCIATED WITH THIS DISORDER	• Inability to care for self • Suicide • Homelessness and chronicity with a deteriorating course	• Accidental harm to self • Wandering without sense of direction or place • Deterioration to the point of requiring total care • Exhaustion of family
MAJOR AREAS OF NEED TO BE ADDRESSED BY NURSING	• Assistance with basic human needs • Establishment of trust with others • Clarification of reality • Communication that is mutually understood • Medication teaching and measures to encourage compliance	• Monitoring for safety • Assistance in most aspects of self–care • Promotion of independence within limitations of safety and ability • Promotion of ventilation of anger related to major losses • Provision of information and support for family caregivers

Figure 10–4. *Common mental disorders.*

Although frequently uncomfortable with the task at first, students must quickly learn to ask the client directly whether self-destructive thoughts or intent is present when risk factors or clues indicate that possibility. The nursing staff forms the most immediate line of defense against the client's acting on suicidal urges. The strength of the nurse-client relationship is often the principal factor that encourages the client to attempt more adaptive problem solving.

PEOPLE WHO DEPEND ON ALCOHOL AND OTHER DRUGS

Treatment for people with chemical dependency may occur on specialized inpatient units, on mental health units, in outpatient settings, or on medical or surgical units in the general hospital. (See Chapters 23 and 24.) All nurses work directly with addicted persons, whatever the setting. Even the nursery nurse assists in

	ADDICTIONS	EATING DISORDERS
STRESS ▼ **ANXIETY** ▼	Environmental/Psychological	Psychological/Environmental
RELIEF BEHAVIORS ▼	• Avoidance of anxiety through chemical alteration of mood and thought • Denial and rationalization	• Compulsive attention to weight control, compulsive eating, or both • Sense of control obtained through this behavior
ASSOCIATED SYMPTOMS THAT CHARACTERIZE THIS DISORDER ▼	• Poor judgment • Personality changes or deficits (poorly developed coping skills) • Family dysfunction • Low self–esteem • Guilt and anxiety	• Extreme weight loss or gain • Bingeing and purging pattern (bulimia) • Distorted body image (anorexia) • Family dysfunction • Client with anorexia is often a high achiever • Compulsive exercise (anorexia)
UNHEALTHY OUTCOMES FREQUENTLY ASSOCIATED WITH THIS DISORDER	• Loss of health, job, and family • Suicide or accidental injury to self and others • Legal complications	• Death from starvation (anorexia) • Damage to mouth and esophagus from vomiting (bulimia) • Failure to address family or personal conflicts
MAJOR AREAS OF NEED TO BE ADDRESSED BY NURSING	• Safety during detoxification • Teaching of coping skills • Provision of self–help and spiritual resources to aid recovery	• Maintenance of adequate weight to support life (anorexia) • Encouragement of healthy patterns of food intake without creation of power struggles • Encouragement of insight and coping skills

Figure 10–5. *Self-destructive defenses against anxiety.*

detoxification of addicted newborns and struggles with the needs and defenses of the addicted mother. Much of the challenge for many beginning practitioners involves developing an attitude that is professionally nonjudgmental in dealing with addicted persons.

The addicted person has limited resources for anxiety management because of chronic avoidance of anxiety through the use of mood-altering chemicals. As a result of the avoidance of anxiety and healthy problem solving, normal developmental stages and tasks are circumvented. An underdeveloped personality results, frequently bolstered by massive use of denial and rationalization. Personal and social functioning are disrupted. Family relationships are severely impaired; other family members are found to be engaged in unhealthy patterns of self-defense. Physical safety and health are endangered. Thinking, perception, and judgment are distorted.

The nurse guides the client safely through detoxification. During the ensuing rehabilitation, the nurse enhances the client's development of insight and more healthy responses to anxiety (Fig. 10–5).

EATING DISORDERS

Clients with eating disorders maladaptively exercise control over anxiety through compulsive patterns of eating or weight control. (See Chapter 25.) The client with anorexia nervosa diets and exercises to an extreme, despite dangerous weight loss. This client, typically an intelligent and overachieving young woman, perceives her body as obese, despite obvious evidence to the contrary. While avoiding a power struggle, the nurse must plan interventions to help the client survive what can be a life-threatening illness. The client with bulimia nervosa binges and then purges. Nursing care promotes physical health as well as measures to help the client understand family dynamics that contribute to increased anxiety. Healthier means of reducing anxiety are taught (see Fig. 10–5).

Summary

This chapter presents an overview of the clinical chapters to be covered in this text within the framework of the anxiety and mental health continuum. The illustrations conceptualize the role of stress (biological, psychological, or social) leading to increased levels of anxiety (either primary or secondary, acute or chronic) associated with crises, selected disorders, or psychiatric syndromes. Brief glimpses of unhealthy responses to anxiety and related threats to well-being associated with these disorders are presented. Major responsibilities of the psychiatric nurse, especially those that have relevance for the beginning practitioner, are introduced. The illustrations can be used as a guide for those new to the clinical setting, to identify specific behaviors for selected disorders, and to focus on critical areas for planning nursing care.

The concept of anxiety, the mental health continuum and the steps in the nursing process are the conceptual models for the presentation of the clinical chapters in this text. It is hoped that these models will be an effective format for students to organize the vast amount of psychiatric mental health material they are given to assimilate in a short time.

References

American Psychiatric Association. Diagnostic and Statistical Manual of Mental Disorders, 3rd ed, revised (DSM-III-R). Washington, DC: American Psychiatric Association, 1987.

Self-study Exercises

Match the disorder (right column) with the major features of the mental disorder (left column).

1. ___C___ Lifelong characteristics that clash with societal norms or cause client to be "different"
2. ___F___ Phobias, compulsions
3. ___A___ Interpersonal withdrawal, low self-esteem, poor self-care
4. ___D___ Hyperactivity, grandiose thoughts, poor judgment, sexual acting out
5. ___B___ Physical symptoms with no organic basis
6. ___H___ Compulsive attention to weight control, purging
7. ___e___ Suspiciousness, distortion of reality, hallucinations
8. ___I___ Memory deficits, lack of ability to care for self, emotional changes
9. ___G___ Denial, rationalization, use of chemicals to alter moods or thoughts

A. Mood disorder: depression

B. Somatoform disorders

C. Personality disorders

D. Mood disorder: elation

E. Schizophrenia

F. Anxiety disorders

G. Addictions

H. Eating disorder

I. Organic mental disorders

Circle all correct answers.

10. The nurse should consider suicide a high risk for the client with

    A. Organic mental disorder
    B. Eating disorder
    C. Anxiety disorder
    D. Depression

11. The client most likely to require assistance with activities of daily living is the client diagnosed with

    A. Anxiety disorder
    B. Personality disorder
    C. Schizophrenia
    D. Eating disorder

12. The nurse assigned to work with an individual with a personality disorder should be especially aware of the client's

    A. Effect on others in the therapeutic environment
    B. Need for help with meeting basic human needs
    C. Distorted perception of reality
    D. Need for protection during detoxification

13. The client who is addicted is likely to deal with anxiety by using which defense mechanisms?

    A. Regression and withdrawal
    B. Rationalization and denial
    C. Reaction-formation and isolation
    D. Projection and regression

14. The client with elation (mania) needs protection from inadvertent self-harm caused by

    A. Poor judgment
    B. Compulsive behaviors
    C. Passive expressions of hostility
    D. Wandering without sense of direction or place

15. The client with anorexia may require which of the following interventions at mealtime?

    A. Monitoring and encouragement without a power struggle
    B. Assistance with organizing mealtime behavior while promoting independence
    C. Providing foods in small amounts that can be eaten "on the run"
    D. Assistance with trusting that the food is safe to eat

PART TWO

FOUNDATIONS IN PRACTICE: THE ANXIETY CONTINUUM

PEOPLE IN ACUTE ANXIETY

UNIT III

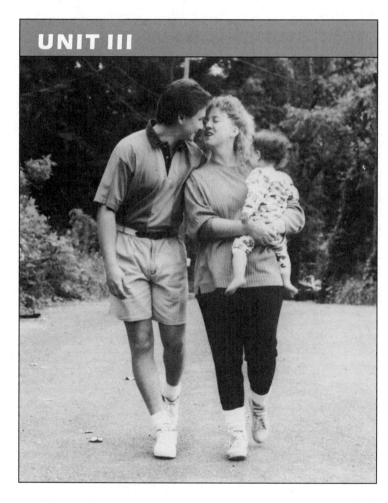

Grief can take care of itself, but to get the full value of a joy you must have somebody to divide it with.

MARK TWAIN
PUDD'NHEAD WILSON'S NEW
CALENDAR (1894)

A Nurse Speaks

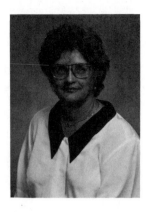

by L. Sharon Shisler

As the coordinator of a psychiatric liaison service in a general hospital, I had the opportunity to assist a variety of hospitalized patients in crisis.

Ms. Dolorum

The oncology nursing staff asked me to see Ms. Dolorum, a 27-year-old African-American woman who had been told that she had a recurrence of her breast cancer. She was observed to be crying at frequent intervals, saying she didn't know what she was going to do, and having difficulty sleeping. The nursing staff had attempted to decrease her anxiety, but she continued to cry, making the nurses feel anxious and helpless.

Ms. Dolorum was open to discussing her feelings. She described her sense of disappointment and anger at being cheated of her chance to finally live: she had acquired a small business through an inheritance, completed her college education, and enjoyed buying old, inexpensive furniture for her new apartment. I validated her feelings by saying how understandable her anger and feelings were. I stated that now, just as she is ready to really start living, she perceives the rug being pulled out from under her.

I was surprised when she enthusiastically agreed with my observation but still remained very anxious. Many other attempts at identifying the sources of her anxiety were unsuccessful, until I finally asked when she had felt a similar sense of extreme anxiety. She said she felt just as she had the time she confronted her grandfather with sexually molesting her. She continued nonstop to describe her feelings of fear and anger at him and hurt and anger at the lack of protection by other family members. She then sighed deeply, appeared much more relaxed, thanked me, and asked if she could take a nap, since she had not been sleeping very well.

Mrs. Fish

Mrs. Fish, a 35-year-old white woman, was assessed as being extremely anxious before minor surgery. While I sat at her bedside, Mrs. Fish described her dread of losing control during the anesthesia, a fear stemming from the fact that her aunt had died during open heart surgery. Knowing that Mrs. Fish was a painter and very graphic in her descriptions, I used a minirelaxation response with visualization. I said, "See the brush painting soft, cooling strokes on the paper, breathing with each stroke." Surprisingly, Mrs. Fish rapidly became drowsy and fell asleep. I asked the nurse what preoperative medication gave such a prompt sedative effect. She replied that she was waiting for me to come out of the patient's room before she gave preoperative medicine because she did not want to disturb our talk.

Mr. Carmichael

Mr. Carmichael, a 45-year-old homeless man with a diagnosis of chronic schizophrenia, was pacing back and forth in the psychiatric observation room. He would not permit me to talk with him until his voice, Jehovah, would give him permission to listen to me.

My own anxiety began to increase. One reason was that Mr. Carmichael was tapping his head on the walls as he paced back and forth. Another reason was that he was not letting me conduct the interview the way I wanted. However, he did grant me permission to sit down as he paced.

The turning point came when the aide asked him to pick up some of his belongings from the floor and put them in a plastic bag for safekeeping. Considering him to be in an acute state, I asked him if I could assist him and he allowed me to place his belongings in the plastic bag.

In my mind, I could hear the aide saying that I was catering to the patient: "He should pick up his own clothes and you are allowing him to remain out of control." I also had the urge to stop him from tapping his head on the wall, but at the same time I knew he required a sense of self-control and observed that he was not actually harming himself. I decided that I would have to let him pace the interaction.

Because I was limited in direct intervention with Mr. Carmichael, I focused on my own anxiety. I practiced a quick breathing technique matching my breathing with his, and waited. His looseness of associations decreased, his pacing slowed, and he said he would need to be here about 20 days. Eventually, "Jehovah" seldom interrupted our discussion and Mr. Carmichael cooperated and asked for his medication.

After three days, Mr. Carmichael was ready for discharge: he was oriented, coherent in thought, and taking his neuroleptic medications, and he had washed his clothes and bathed. Before he left, he shook my hand and thanked me for caring.

Webster's Dictionary defines a privilege as a "right, a benefit or advantage granted to an individual or a group of people not enjoyed by others," but cautions that "sometimes privilege can be detrimental." The privilege to enter the therapeutic space requires vigilance, compassion, external support, and inner resources on the part of the nurse. Safeguards need to be used to prevent the nurse from getting too close and losing objectivity or getting too distant and becoming cold and aloof.

Nurses enter that intimate space with the potential for therapeutic outcomes, but they need to proceed with discretion and not mishandle the trust and power when the patient is in a vulnerable position.

I feel grateful that my mother guided me toward nursing. I am pleased with the many opportunities that nursing has granted me in working with patients and their families.

CHAPTER 11

Crisis and Crisis Intervention

Elizabeth M. Varcarolis

OUTLINE

THEORY
Types of Crisis
Phases of Crisis
Aspects of Crisis That Have Relevance for
Nurses

ASSESSMENT
Assessing the Client's Perception of the
Precipitating Event
Assessing Situational Supports
Assessing Personal Coping Skills

NURSING DIAGNOSIS

PLANNING
Content Level—Planning Goals
Process Level—Nurses' Feelings and
Reactions

Personal Qualities That Enhance
Nursing Effectiveness
INTERVENTION
Psychotherapeutic Interventions
EVALUATION
CASE STUDY: WORKING WITH A
PERSON IN CRISIS
CRISIS INTERVENTION WITH THE
CHRONICALLY MENTALLY ILL CLIENT
Potential Crisis Situation for a Person
with Chronic Mental Health Problems
Adapting the Crisis Model to Meet the
Needs of a Person with Chronic
Mental Health Problems
SUMMARY

KEY TERMS AND CONCEPTS

**The key terms and concepts listed here also appear in bold where they are
defined or discussed in this chapter.**

ADVENTITIOUS CRISIS

CRISIS

MATURATIONAL CRISIS

PHASES OF CRISIS

SITUATIONAL CRISIS

PRIMARY CARE

SECONDARY CARE

TERTIARY CARE

OBJECTIVES

After studying this chapter, the student will be able to

1. Define the three types of crises and give an example of each.
2. Diagram Caplan's four phases of crisis.
3. State at least six aspects of crisis that have relevance for nurses involved in crisis
   intervention.
4. Identify three areas to assess during crisis, with two sample questions for each
   area.
5. List three qualities the nurse can develop that can greatly enhance effective crisis
   intervention.

6. Identify two of the four common problems health care professionals may have when starting crisis intervention, and discuss at least two interventions for each problem.
7. Compare and contrast the differences among primary, secondary, and tertiary intervention, including appropriate intervention strategies.
8. Identify four situations that can precipitate a crisis in an individual with chronic mental health problems.
9. Name four potential crisis situations common in the hospital setting that a client may face.

A crisis is an overwhelming emotional reaction to an event, and not necessarily to the threatening situation or event itself. One person may perceive a stressful event as disastrous, whereas another person may view the same event as a challenge. For example, one woman upon finding that she is pregnant may experience anxiety and depression, whereas another woman will feel joy and excitement. Stress by itself does not constitute a crisis, but often a stressful event precipitates a crisis.

Life events, such as marriage, job promotion, death of a spouse, or loss of job, can be viewed as potential crises and may lead to psychological or physical illness (Holmes and Masuda 1972). Refer to Figure 11–1 for an assessment tool that measures the stress level of life events. Anxiety usually characterizes the reaction to crisis, but other emotions, such as depression, anger, and fear, may also be involved (Taylor 1986).

The crisis itself is not a pathological state, and being in crisis is not pathological. It is a struggle for equilibrium and adjustment when problems are perceived as insolvable. Crisis presents both a danger to personality organization and a potential opportunity for personality growth. The outcome depends on how the individual deals with the crisis and what outside supports are available at the time the crisis occurs.

As anxiety escalates in response to a stressful event, relief behaviors are elicited. When a person's usual defense mechanisms are not able to lower or maintain anxiety, personality disorganization and interferences with daily living may follow. When the ability to cope with specific stresses is hampered, anxiety may rise to severe or panic levels and may therefore interfere with problem solving. The person experiencing a psychiatric emergency needs immediate help, which is termed *crisis intervention*. Basic steps in the development of a crisis can be conceptualized as follows:

Essentially, a **crisis** is a temporary state of disequilibrium (high anxiety) in which a person's usual coping mechanisms or problem-solving methods fail. Crisis can result in personality growth or personality disorganization, depending on personal and social supports available at the time of crisis.

Crisis and crisis intervention have the following features: (1) crisis intervention is short term; (2) it focuses on solving the immediate problem; (3) it aims to re-establish former coping patterns and problem-solving ability; and (4) the crisis is usually limited to a four- to six-week period of time—then an initial resolution will be made (Croushore et al. 1981; Robinson 1973).

Nurses, perhaps more than any other group, deal with people who are experiencing disruption in their lives. People often undergo increased amounts of stress and anxiety in the medicosurgical, pediatric, obstetrical, and emergency room settings, as well as in the formal psychiatric setting. Understanding what constitutes a crisis and possessing a basic knowledge of crisis intervention enable the nurse to cope effectively with potential and actual crisis situations. The ability to recognize a crisis and intervene in a timely manner can influence the quality and course of another person's life.

Theory

Crisis theory was developed in the early 1940s by Erich Lindemann, who conducted a classic study of the grief reactions of close relatives of victims in the Coconut Grove nightclub fire in Boston. This study

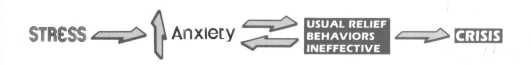

formed the foundation of crisis theory and clinical intervention. Lindemann observed that "acute grief was the normal reaction to a distressing situation" (Ewing 1978). He showed that preventive intervention in crisis situations could eliminate or decrease serious personality disorganization and devastating psychological consequences from the sustained effects of severe anxiety.

In the early 1960s, Gerald Caplan defined crisis theory and outlined crisis intervention. Since that time, our understanding of crisis and effective intervention has been refined and enhanced by competent clinicians and theorists.

In 1961, a report from the Joint Commission on Mental Illness and Mental Health spoke about the need for community mental health centers throughout the country (Levenson 1974). This report stimulated the establishment of crisis services, which are now an important part of mental health services in hospitals and communities.

The following areas are derived from established crisis theory and constitute a sound knowledge base for the application of the nursing process to a crisis. An understanding of these three areas of crisis theory enables application of the nursing process. These areas are (1) types of crisis, (2) phases of crisis, and (3) aspects of crisis that have relevance for nurses.

TYPES OF CRISIS

Three basic types of crisis situations have been identified:

1. Maturational
2. Situational
3. Adventitious

MATURATIONAL CRISIS. A process of maturation occurs throughout the life cycle. Erikson identified

eight stages of growth and development in which specific maturational tasks must be mastered. Each of these stages constitutes a crisis in personal growth and development. The eight stages and their tasks as defined by Erikson are reviewed in Table 11–1 (Erikson 1963). (Refer to Chapter 1 for other developmental theories.)

Each developmental stage can be referred to as a **maturational crisis.** When a person arrives at a new stage, formerly used coping styles are no longer appropriate, and new coping mechanisms have yet to be developed. For a period of time, the person is without effective defenses. This often leads to increased anxiety, which may be seen in variations in the person's normal behavior. Temporary disequilibrium may affect interpersonal relationships, body image, and social and work roles (Hoff 1989). Successful resolution of these tasks leads to development of basic human qualities. Erikson believes that how these crises are solved at one stage affects the ability to pass subsequent stages because each crisis provides the starting point for moving to the next stage. If a person lacks support systems and adequate role models, successful resolution may be difficult or may not occur. Unresolved problems in the past and inadequate coping mechanisms can adversely affect what is learned in each developmental stage. When a person is experiencing severe difficulty during a maturational crisis, professional intervention may be indicated.

Alcohol and drug addiction are examples of how progression through the maturational stages can be interrupted. This phenomenon is too often seen among teenagers today. After the addictive behavior is controlled (hopefully, by the late teens), the young person's growth and development will resume at the point at which it was interrupted. Therefore, at the time his or her addiction has been arrested, the older teenager, say, 19 years of age, could have the social and problem solving skills of a 14-year-old. Often

Table 11–1 ■ ERIKSON'S EIGHT STAGES OF GROWTH AND DEVELOPMENT AND THEIR MATURATIONAL TASKS		
STAGE	**AGE**	**PSYCHOLOGICAL TASK**
1. Infancy	0–1	Trust versus mistrust
2. Early childhood	1–3	Autonomy versus shame and doubt
3. Late childhood	3–6	Initiative versus guilt
4. School age	6–12	Industry versus inferiority
5. Puberty and adolescence	12–20	Ego identity versus role confusion
6. Young adulthood	20–30	Intimacy versus isolation
7. Adulthood	30–65	Generativity versus stagnation
8. Late adulthood	65–death	Ego integrity versus despair

these teens do not get treatment, and other problems worsen.

SITUATIONAL CRISIS. A **situational crisis** arises from an external rather than an internal source. Examples of external situations that could precipitate a crisis include loss of a job, death of a loved one, abortion, change of job, change in financial status, divorce, additional family members, pregnancy, and severe physical illness.

These situations were first referred to as "life events" by Holmes and Masuda (1972). Each event is assigned stress points, which, when totaled, may predict the risk for illness. A high point count can act as a predictor of physical or psychological illness. This *Life Events and Social Readjustment Scale* (see Fig. 11–1) can be a useful tool for evaluating potential crisis situations and for planning primary intervention.

Some authors refer to these events as critical life problems because these problems are encountered by most people during the course of their lives. Whether these events precipitate a crisis depends on such factors as the degree of support available from caring friends and family members, a person's general emotional status, and a person's ability to understand and cope with the meaning of the stressful event.

As in all crises or potential crisis situations, the stressful event involves a loss or change that threatens a person's self-concept and self-esteem. To varying degrees, successful resolution of a crisis depends on resolution of the grief associated with the loss.

ADVENTITIOUS CRISIS (CRISIS OF DISASTER). An **adventitious crisis** is not a part of everyday life but is unplanned and accidental. Adventitious crises may result from (1) natural disasters (e.g., floods,

---

LIFE EVENTS AND SOCIAL READJUSTMENT SCALE

DIRECTIONS:
Using yourself or a client as the subject, place a check mark on the line to the left of each event that has occurred in the subject's life during the past year. If the event has occurred more than once, place a check mark for each occurrence, then add up the accumulated points.

	Points			Points
1. Death of a spouse	100		24. Trouble with in-laws	29
2. Divorce	73		25. Outstanding personal achievement	28
3. Marital separation	65		26. Spouse beginning or stopping work	26
4. Jail term	63		27. Beginning or ending school	26
5. Death of a close family member	63		28. Change in living conditions	25
6. Personal injury or loss	53		29. Revision of personal habits	24
7. Marriage	50		30. Trouble with boss	23
8. Firing from work	47		31. Change in work hours or conditions	20
9. Marital reconciliation	45		32. Change in residence	20
10. Retirement	45		33. Change in schools	20
11. Change in health of family member	44		34. Change in recreation	19
12. Pregnancy	40		35. Change in church activities	19
13. Sexual difficulties	39		36. Change in social activities	18
14. New family member	39		37. Mortgage or loan less than $10,000	17
15. Business readjustment	39		38. Change in sleeping habits	16
16. Change in financial state	38		39. Change in number of family get-togethers	15
17. Death of a close friend	37		40. Change in eating habits	15
18. Change to different line of work	36		41. Vacation	13
19. Change in number of arguments with spouse	35		42. Christmas	12
20. Mortgage over $10,000	31		43. Minor violations of the law	11
21. Foreclosure of mortgage or loan	30			
22. Change in responsibilities at work	29		SUBJECT'S TOTAL _____	
23. Son or daughter leaving home	29			

FIND THE SUBJECT'S LIFE CRISIS LEVEL AMONG THE FOLLOWING:

150–199	Mild risk
200–299	Moderate risk
300 or more	Major risk

Figure 11–1. *Life events and social readjustment scale. (Adapted from Holmes TH, Masuda M. Psychosomatic syndrome. Psychology Today, April 1972, p 71.)*

fires, and earthquakes), (2) national disasters (e.g., wars, riots, and internment in concentration camps), and (3) crimes of violence (e.g., rape, murder, and spouse and child abuse).

Sometimes a person may experience two types of crisis situations simultaneously. For example, a 51-year-old woman may be going through a midlife crisis when her husband dies suddenly of cancer. Another example would be a 14-year-old girl who is forced to move away from her friends because of her father's job transfer to another state.

PHASES OF CRISIS

Caplan has identified four distinct **phases of crisis** (Caplan 1964):

1. A person confronted by a conflict or problem that threatens the self-concept responds with increased feelings of anxiety. The increase in anxiety stimulates the use of problem-solving techniques and defense mechanisms in an effort to solve the problem and lower anxiety.
2. If the usual defensive response fails, and if the threat persists, anxiety continues to rise and produce feelings of extreme discomfort. Individual functioning becomes disorganized. Trial-and-error attempts at solving the problem and restoring a normal balance begin.
3. If the trial-and-error attempts fail, anxiety can escalate to severe and panic levels, and the person mobilizes automatic relief behaviors, such as withdrawal and flight. Some form of resolution, e.g., compromising needs or redefining the situation to

make an acceptable solution, may be made in this stage.
4. If the problem is not solved, anxiety can overwhelm the person and lead to serious personality disorganization. This maladaptive response can take the form of confusion, immobilization with fear, violence against others, or suicidal behavior, as well as yelling or running about aimlessly (Robinson 1973; Hoff 1989).

Figure 11–2 is a diagram of the phases of crisis.

ASPECTS OF CRISIS THAT HAVE RELEVANCE FOR NURSES

The specific aspects of crisis theory that are basic to crisis intervention follow:

1. A crisis is self-limiting and is usually resolved within four to six weeks (Aguilera and Messick 1990; Croushore et al. 1981).
2. The resolution of a crisis results in one of three different functional levels. The person will emerge at a higher level of functioning, the same level of functioning, or a lower level of functioning.
3. The goal of crisis intervention is to maintain the precrisis level of functioning (Aguilera and Messick 1990).
4. The form of the resolution of the crisis depends on the actions of the subject and the intervention of others (Ewing 1978).
5. During a crisis, people are more open to outside intervention than they are at times of stable functioning (Ewing 1978). With intervention, the per-

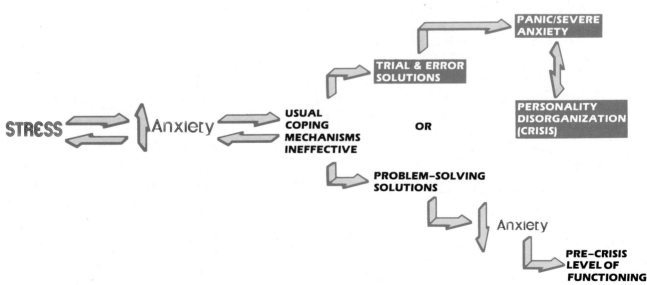

Figure 11–2. *Phases in the process of crisis.*

son can learn different adaptive means of problem solving to correct inadequate solutions.

6. The person in a crisis situation is assumed to be mentally healthy and to have functioned well in the past *but* is presently in a state of disequilibrium.
7. Crisis intervention deals with the person's present problem and resolution of the immediate crisis only (Aguilera and Messick 1990). Dealing with material not directly related to the crisis can take place at a later time. Crisis intervention deals with the "here and now."
8. The nurse must be willing to take an active, even directive, role in intervention, in direct contrast to what occurs in conventional therapeutic intervention techniques, which stress a more passive and nondirective role (Aguilera and Messick 1990).
9. Early intervention probably increases the chances for a better prognosis.
10. The client is encouraged to set realistic goals and plan an intervention that is focused on the current situation.

Assessment

A person's equilibrium may be adversely affected by one or more of the following: (1) an unrealistic perception of the precipitating event, (2) inadequate situational supports, or (3) inadequate coping mechanisms (Aguilera and Messick 1990; Ewing 1978). Assessing these factors when a crisis situation is evaluated is crucial because data gained from the assessment are used as guides for both the nurse and the client to set realistic and meaningful goals, as well as to plan possible solutions to the client's problem situation.

After determining whether there is a need for external controls because of suicidal or homicidal ideation or gestures, the nurse assesses three main areas: the client's perception of the precipitating event, the client's situational supports, and the client's personal coping skills.

ASSESSING THE CLIENT'S PERCEPTION OF THE PRECIPITATING EVENT

The nurse's initial task is the assessment of the individual and the problem. The more clearly the problem can be defined, the better the chance that an effective solution will be found.

SAMPLE QUESTIONS TO ASK (Croushore et al. 1981; King 1971)

- *Has anything particularly upsetting happened to you within the past few days or weeks?*
- *What was happening in your life before you started to feel this way?*
- *What leads you to seek help now?*
- *Describe how you are feeling right now.*
- *How does this problem affect your life?*
- *How do you see this problem affecting your future?*

Laura, a 15-year-old girl, is brought to the emergency room after slashing her wrists. She was found by her mother, who had returned home early from a date. Her mother called the police, and they rushed Laura to the hospital. After Laura is seen by the medical personnel, she is interviewed by the psychiatric nurse working in the emergency room. The nurse speaks calmly. She introduces herself and tells Laura she would like to spend some time with her. The nurse states that she can see that Laura is upset. She makes the observation that things must be very bad if she wants to kill herself. Laura sits slumped in a chair with her hands in her lap and her head hanging down. There are tears in her eyes.

Example: Assessing Laura's Perception of the Precipitating Event

NURSE: Laura, tell me what has happened to make you feel like killing yourself.

LAURA: I can't . . . I can't go home . . . no one cares or believes me . . . I can't go through it again.

NURSE: Tell me what you can't go through again, Laura.

Laura starts to cry, shaking with sobs. The nurse sits quietly for a while, offers Laura some tissues, then speaks:

Laura tell me what is so terrible. Let's look at it together.

After a while, Laura starts telling the nurse that when she was nine, her mother had a boyfriend. When her mother was out of the house, the boyfriend would touch her and eventually forced her to have sex with him. He threatened Laura that if she told, he would kill her. When she was 11, the boyfriend moved south. Two weeks ago, Laura's mother told her the old boyfriend was coming back to live with them. Laura, terrified, told her mother what had happened years ago, but her mother refused to believe her and called her a liar. Her mother said that if it came to a choice between Laura and the boyfriend, the mother would take the boyfriend.

ASSESSING SITUATIONAL SUPPORTS

The client's support systems are assessed to determine the resources available to the person. Does the stressful event involve important people in the support system? Is the client isolated from others or are there family and friends who can provide the vital support? Family and friends may be called upon to aid the individual by offering material or emotional supports, for example, lending money, offering services, or being available to give affection and understanding. If these resources are not available, the therapist acts as a temporary support system while relationships with individuals or groups in the community are established.

SAMPLE QUESTIONS TO ASK (Aguilera and Messick 1990)

- With whom do you live?
- To whom do you talk when you feel upset?
- Whom can you trust?
- Who is available to help you?
- Where do you go to church, school, or other community-based activities?

Example: Assessing Laura's Situational Supports

NURSE: Laura, who can you go to, do you have any other family?

LAURA: No. My dad left when I was six. We stay pretty much alone. My mom doesn't allow my brother and me to play with other kids.

NURSE: Do you have anyone you can talk to?

LAURA: No, I really don't have any friends. All the other kids think I'm stuck-up. I don't fit in too well, I guess. My mom would never let me go out anyway; there's always things to do at home.

NURSE: What about church, or your teachers at school?

LAURA: The teachers are nice and all, but I can't tell them things like this. They wouldn't believe me either.

ASSESSING PERSONAL COPING SKILLS

In crisis situations, it is important to evaluate the person's level of anxiety. Common coping mechanisms may be overeating, drinking, smoking, withdrawing, seeking out someone to talk to, yelling, fighting, or engaging in other physical activity (Croushore et al. 1981). The potential for suicide or homicide must be assessed. If the patient is suicidal, homicidal, or unable to take care of personal needs, hospitalization should be considered (Aguilera and Messick 1990).

SAMPLE QUESTIONS TO ASK

- What do you usually do to feel better?
- Did you try it this time? If so, why do you think it didn't work?
- Have you thought of killing yourself or someone else?
- Has anything like this ever happened before?
- What do you think might happen now?

Example: Assessing Laura's Personal Coping Style

The nurse learns that Laura does very well in school, especially in math. Laura explains that when she studies, she can forget her problems and get lost in other worlds. Getting good grades also has another reward: it is the only time her mother says anything nice about her. Her mother boasts to her boyfriends about how bright her daughter is.

NURSE: What would you think would help your situation?

LAURA: I don't want to die . . . I just don't know where to turn.

The nurse tells Laura that she wants to work with her to find a solution, and that she is concerned for Laura's safety and well-being.

Nursing Diagnosis

A person in crisis may exhibit various behaviors that may indicate a number of human problems. For example, when a person is in crisis, the nursing diagnosis *ineffective individual coping* is often evident. Because anxiety levels may escalate to moderate or severe levels, the ability to solve problems is usually impaired, if it is present at all. Ineffective individual coping may be evidenced by inability to meet basic needs, inability to meet role expectations, alteration in social participation, use of inappropriate defense mechanisms, or impairment of usual patterns of communication. Possible "related to's" for ineffective individual coping could include situational crises, inadequate support systems, maturational crises, multiple life changes, inadequate coping methods, unrealistic perceptions, and unmet expectations (Doenges and Moorehouse 1988).

Altered thought processes may be evidenced by altered attention span, distractibility, or disorientation to time, place, person, circumstance, and events. Altered thought processes in a crisis situation could be "related to" psychological conflicts or impaired judgment.

Because change in one member of a family most always affects all members of a family, *altered family process* is probable. Altered family process can be "related to" a situational or developmental crisis of one or more members. Altered family process may be evidenced by subjective data regarding confusion or objective data identified by the nurse. For example, the family may no longer be able to help each other or the member in crisis in meeting physical or emotional needs. The family may have difficulty being able to adapt or respond to the changes or traumatic experience of the member in crisis. The family's ability to make decisions or accomplish developmental tasks may be impaired. Communications may become confused, and inability to express feelings may be evident.

Anxiety (moderate/severe/panic) is always present, and the nurse works with the client to lower the anxiety to a level at which the client is able to start problem solving and making effective plans for dealing with the crisis situation. Anxiety can be "related to" many etiologies, such as situational or maturational crises, threat to self-concept, threat to or change in health status (role functioning or socioeconomic status), and physiological factors (hyperthyroidism or use of some medications).

Example: Nursing Diagnosis—Laura

The assessment of Laura's (1) perception of the precipitating event, (2) situational supports, and (3) personal coping skills gives the nurse enough data to formulate two diagnoses and to work with Laura in setting goals and planning interventions.

The nurse formulates the following goals:

1. *Anxiety (moderate/severe):* related to rape-trauma syndrome, as evidenced by ineffectual problem solving and feelings of impending doom.
2. *Ineffective family coping:* compromised, related to inadequate understanding by Laura's mother.

Planning

Planning involves planning on the (1) content level and (2) process level. Planning on the content level includes setting realistic goals with the person in crisis and identifying actions that will meet these goals. Planning on the process level involves identifying personal feelings or behaviors that would diminish effective interventions.

CONTENT LEVEL—PLANNING GOALS

Planning realistic goals is done with the client. Goals are made to fit within the person's cultural and personal values. Without the client's involvement, the goals may be irrelevant to what would be acceptable solutions to that person's crisis. For example, the nurse who suggests to a woman to leave her husband because he beats her may find that the woman has different goals. The basic goal in all potential crisis situations is to resolve the presenting problem and to support the person in crisis in an attempt to regain a normal level of functioning. Defining realistic goals gives the client a sense of control, which can decrease the impact of the crisis. The nurse and the client plan together acceptable means of meeting these goals.

The client—not the nurse—solves the problem. The nurse helps the client refocus to gain new perspectives on the situation. The nurse supports the client during the process of finding constructive ways to solve or cope with the problem. The client is involved in setting both the long term and the short term goals, as well as in planning intervention.

PROCESS LEVEL—NURSES' FEELINGS AND REACTIONS

All types of people may be involved in helping individuals in crisis. For example, people from various professional backgrounds are trained in crisis intervention—police, teachers, welfare workers, clergy, social workers, psychologists, as well as nurses. Crisis intervention is often practiced unwittingly by people without formal training, such as bartenders, concerned bystanders, friends, and neighbors. People can play a crucial role in the successful resolution of a crisis by responding spontaneously with concern and caring.

Beginning practitioners in crisis intervention often face common problems that must be worked through before they become comfortable and competent in the role of a crisis counselor. Four of the more common problems are the counselor's (1) needing to be needed, (2) setting unrealistic goals for clients, (3) having difficulty dealing with the issue of suicide, and (4) having difficulty terminating. Refer to Table 11–2 for examples and results of these problems, appropri-

Table 11–2 ■ COMMON PROBLEMS FACED BY BEGINNING PRACTITIONERS

EXAMPLES	RESULT	INTERVENTIONS	OUTCOME
Problem 1. *Counselor needing to feel needed.* Feels total responsibility to "care for" or "cure" client's problems.			
The nurse • Allows excessive phone calls between sessions • Gives direct advice without sufficient knowledge of client's situation • Attempts to influence lifestyle of client on a judgmental basis	Client becomes more dependent on nurse and relies less on own abilities. Nurse reacts to client's not getting "cured" or taking advice by projecting feelings of frustration and anger onto the client.	The nurse • Evaluates with an experienced professional nurse's needs versus client's needs • Discourages dependency by the client • Encourages goal setting and problem solving by the client • Takes control only if suicide or homicide is a possibility	Client is free to grow and problem-solve own life crises. Nurse's skills and effectiveness grow as comfort with role and own goals are clarified.
Problem 2. *Counselor setting unrealistic goals for clients.* Goals become nurse's goals and not mutually determined goals for the client.			
The nurse • Expects physically abused woman to leave battering partner • Expects man who abuses alcohol to stop drinking when loss of family or job is imminent	Nurse feels anxious and responsible when expectations are not met. Anxiety resulting from feelings of inadequacy are projected onto the client in the form of frustration and anger.	The nurse • Examines with an experienced professional realistic expectations of self and client • Re-evaluates client's level of functioning and works with the client on his level • Encourages setting of goals by client	Nurse's ability to assess and problem solve increases as anger and frustration decrease. Client feels less alienated, and a working relationship can ensue.
Problem 3. *Counselor having difficulty dealing with suicidal client.*			
Nurse selectively inattends by • Denying possible clues • Neglecting to follow up on verbal suicide clues • Changing topic to less threatening subject when self-destructive themes come up	Client is robbed of opportunity to share feelings and find alternatives to intolerable situation. Client remains suicidal. Nurse's crisis intervention ceases to be effective.	The nurse • Assesses her own feelings and anxieties with the help of an experienced professional • Evaluates all clues or slight suspicions and acts on them, for example, "Are you thinking of killing yourself?" If yes, the nurse assesses a. Suicide potential b. Need for hospitalization	Client experiences relief in sharing feelings and evaluating alternatives. Suicide potential can be minimized. Nurse becomes more adept at picking up clues and minimizing suicide potential.
Problem 4. *Counselor having difficulty terminating* after crisis has resolved.			
Nurse tempted to work on other problems in the client's life in order to prolong contact with the client	Nurse steps into territory of traditional therapy without proper training or experience.	The nurse • Works with an experienced professional to a. Explore own feelings regarding separations and termination. b. Reinforce crisis model. Crisis intervention is a preventive tool, not psychotherapy.	Nurse becomes better able to help client with his feelings when own feelings are recognized. Client is free to go back to his life situation or request appropriate referral to work on other issues of importance to him.

Data from Finkelman AW. The nurse therapist: Outpatient crisis intervention with the chronic patient. Journal of Psychosocial Nursing and Mental Health Services, 8:27, 1977; Wallace MA, Morley WE. Teaching crisis intervention. American Journal of Nursing, 7:1484, 1970.

ate interventions, and desired outcomes. It is crucial in beginning crisis intervention that supervision be made available as an integral part of the training process. The supervisor should be an experienced professional who could be a peer, teacher, or supervisor.

Personal Qualities That Enhance Nursing Effectiveness

Nurses need to monitor personal feelings and thoughts constantly when dealing with a person in crisis. It is important to recognize one's own level of anxiety to prevent closing off the expression of painful feelings by the client. Because a client's situation or anxiety level may trigger uncomfortable levels of anxiety in the nurse at times, the nurse tends to repress such feelings to maintain personal comfort. When the nurse is not aware of personal feelings and reactions, the nurse may unconsciously prevent the expression of the painful feelings in the client that are precipitating the nurse's own discomfort. Thus, closing off feelings in the client can render the nurse ineffective. However, specific personal attributes in the nurse can contribute favorably to the outcome of an individual in crisis (Donlon and Rockwell 1982).

CARING. The caring nurse has profound respect for the human condition and believes that the person in crisis should have the opportunity to ease his or her pain and to alter his or her situation. A cold and technical approach will bring little success with a person in crisis.

LISTENING. This specifically refers to

1. Hearing what the client says and does not say in the conversation
2. Monitoring what goes on in the interaction between the client and the nurse
3. Identifying one's own feelings during the interaction with the client

Listening is facilitated by looking at the person who speaks. Feedback can be given by clarifying what the person is saying. This is done by repeating a short summary to the patient, who agrees with or corrects the nurse's impression. Refrain from judging or moralizing, but try to understand the other person's experience. The importance of having someone listen during a difficult time is described in the poem "Listening" (Box 11–1).

CREATIVITY AND FLEXIBILITY. A helping person must be able to look at another person's crisis situation from various angles and to work with the client to find possible solutions. Each individual is unique, and one's perception of the situation is filtered through cultural, family, and personal traditions and beliefs. The possible alternatives must be compatible with these traditions and beliefs. What is helpful for one person is often not appropriate for another. There are no simple solutions for people in crisis. The nurse must be able to view the situation from the client's perspective (have empathy) and work with the client to identify alternatives that will be effective in lowering anxiety and facilitating normal functioning.

Example: *Planning the Intervention with Laura*

A social worker is called. Laura, the nurse, and the social worker meet together. All agree that Laura

---

Box 11–1. LISTENING

When I ask you to listen to me
  and you start giving me advice,
  you have not done what I asked.

When I ask you to listen to me
  and you begin to tell me why I shouldn't feel
    that way,
  you are trampling on my feelings.

When I ask you to listen to me
  and you feel you have to solve my problems,
  you have failed me, strange as that may seem.

Listen! All I asked was that you listen . . .
  not talk or do—just hear me.
    Advice is cheap; 10 cents will get you both
      Dear Abby and
    Billy Graham in the same newspaper.
    And I can do for myself; I'm not helpless.
    Maybe discouraged and faltering, but not
      helpless.

When you do something for me that I can and
  need to do
  for myself, you contribute to my fear and
    weakness.
  But, when you accept as a simple fact that I
    do feel what I feel
      no matter how irrational, then I can quit
        trying to convince
    you and get about the business of under-
      standing what's
    behind this irrational feeling.
    And when that's clear, the answers are
      obvious and I don't
    need advice.

Irrational feelings make sense when we understand what's
  behind them.
  Perhaps that's why prayer works, sometimes,
    for some people
      because God is mute, and he doesn't give
        advice or
    try to fix things. He just listens and lets you
    work it out for yourself.

So please listen and just hear me. And, if you
  want to talk,
    wait a minute for your turn; and I'll listen to
    you.

                        ANONYMOUS

should not be in the home if the boyfriend returns. The nurse then meets with Laura and her mother; however, Laura's mother continues to berate Laura for lying. She states that she does not care what Laura says, she has her own life to live. She says if Laura doesn't like it, she can move out. The nurse and Laura set three goals together:

1. *A safe environment will be found for Laura before the boyfriend comes to live with the mother.*
2. *At least two support systems will be made available to Laura within 24 hours.*
3. *Continued evaluation and support will be available until the immediate crisis is over (six to eight weeks).*

After talking with the nurse and the social worker, Laura seems open to the possibility of going to a foster home. She also agrees to talk to a counselor at her school. The nurse sets up an appointment when she, Laura, and the counselor can meet. The nurse will continue to see Laura twice a week.

Intervention

Crisis intervention has two basic thrusts. First, external controls may be applied for protection of the person in crisis if the person is suicidal or homicidal. Second, anxiety reduction techniques are used, so that inner resources can be put into effect.

During the initial interview, the person in crisis first needs to gain a feeling of safety. Solutions to the crisis may be offered, so that the client is aware of other options. Feelings of support and hope will temporarily diminish anxiety. The nurse needs to play an active role by indicating that help is available. Help is conveyed by the competent use of crisis skills and genuine interest and support. It is *not* conveyed by the use of false reassurances and platitudes, such as "everything will be all right."

Crisis intervention requires a creative and flexible approach by the use of traditional and nontraditional therapeutic roles. The nurse may act as educator, adviser, and model.

PSYCHOTHERAPEUTIC INTERVENTIONS

There are three levels of nursing care in crisis intervention. Psychotherapeutic nursing interventions in crisis are directed toward these three levels of care: primary, secondary, and tertiary.

PRIMARY CARE. Primary care promotes mental health and reduces mental illness in order to decrease the incidence of crisis. On this level the nurse can:

1. Work with an individual to recognize potential problems by evaluating the stressful life events the person is experiencing.
2. Teach an individual specific coping skills such as decision-making, problem-solving, and assertiveness skills, and meditation and relaxation skills, to handle stressful events.
3. Assist an individual to evaluate the timing or reduction of life changes in order to decrease the negative effects of stress as much as possible. This may involve working with a client to plan environmental changes, make important interpersonal decisions, and rethink changes in occupational roles.

SECONDARY CARE. Secondary care establishes intervention during an acute crisis to prevent prolonged anxiety from diminishing personal effectiveness and personality organization. The nurse works with the client to assess the client's problem, support systems, and coping styles. Desired goals are explored, and interventions are planned. Secondary care lessens the time a person is mentally disabled during a crisis. Secondary level care occurs in hospital units, emergency rooms, clinics, or in mental health centers, usually during daytime hours.

TERTIARY CARE. Tertiary care provides support for those who have experienced and are now recovering from a disabling mental state. Social and community facilities that offer tertiary intervention include rehabilitation centers, sheltered workshops, day hospitals, and outpatient clinics. Primary goals are aimed at facilitating optimum levels of functioning and preventing further emotional disruptions. People with chronic mental problems are often extremely susceptible to crisis, and community facilities provide the structured environment that can help prevent problem situations.

Example: Performing Secondary Crisis Intervention with Laura

The nurse meets with Laura twice weekly during the next four weeks. Laura is motivated to work with the social worker and the nurse to find another place to live. The nurse suggests several times that Laura start to see a counselor in the outpatient clinic after the crisis is over, where she can talk about some of her pain. Laura is not interested, however, and said she will talk to the school counselor if she needs to talk.

Three weeks after the attempted suicide, foster placement is found for Laura. The couple seems very interested in Laura, and Laura appears happy about the attention she is receiving.

Evaluation

Goals are compared with the outcomes for the effectiveness of the crisis intervention. This is usually done four to eight weeks after the initial interview, although it can be done in a shorter time frame. If the intervention has been successful, the person's level of anxiety and ability to function should be at precrisis levels. Often, a person chooses to follow up additional areas of concern, and referral to other agencies for more long term work is made. Crisis intervention often serves to prepare a person for further treatment (Ewing 1978).

Example: Evaluating Laura's Crisis

After six weeks, Laura and the nurse decide that the crisis is over. Laura remains aloof and distant. The nurse evaluates Laura as being in a moderate amount of emotional pain. Laura feels she is doing well, however, and she feels more secure and accepted. She is satisfied with the way things are, and again states that if she has any problems she will see her school counselor.

Postscript

Two years later, Laura is continuing to do well in school and is planning to go to a local community college for computer programming. Laura gets along well with her foster parents, and plans are being made for adoption. Laura remains aloof. She has no close friends and continues to throw her energy into her studies. For the present, she is getting pleasure from her academic accomplishments, and she has security and warm attention in her new home environment. If at a later date she decides there are other things for her to work out, she knows the resources in the community that she could contact.

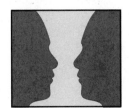

Case Study: Working with a Person in Crisis

Ms. Greg, the psychiatric nurse consultant, was called to the neurological unit. Ms. Greg was told that Mr. Raymond, a 43-year-old man with Guillain-Barré syndrome, was presenting a serious nursing problem, and the staff requested a consult.

The head nurse said that Mr. Raymond was hostile and sexually abusive to the nursing staff. His abusive language, demeaning attitude, and angry outbursts were having an adverse effect on the unit as a whole. The nurses stated that they felt ineffective and angry and that they had tried to be patient and understanding; however, nothing seemed to get through to him. The situation had affected the morale of the staff, and the nurses felt that the quality of their care was affected.

Mr. Raymond, a Native American, was employed as a taxicab driver. Six months before his admission to the hospital, he had given up drinking after years of episodic alcohol abuse. He was engaged to a woman who visited him every day.

He needed a great deal of assistance with every aspect of his activities of daily living. His muscle weakness had progressed such that he was essentially paralyzed. At the time the consult was made, he could breathe on his own, but he had to be turned and positioned every two hours. He was fed through a gastrostomy tube.

Assessment

Ms. Greg gathered data from Mr. Raymond and the nursing staff and spoke with Mr. Raymond's fiancee.

MR. RAYMOND'S PERCEPTION OF THE PRECIPITATING EVENTS

During the initial interview, Mr. Raymond spoke to Ms. Greg angrily, using profanity and making lewd, sexual suggestions. He also talked with anger about needing a nurse to "scratch my head and help me blow my nose." He still could not figure out how his illness suddenly developed. He said the doctors told him that it was too early to know for sure if he would recover completely but that the prognosis was good.

MR. RAYMOND'S SUPPORT SYSTEM

Ms. Greg spoke with Mr. Raymond's fiancee. Mr. Raymond's relationships with his fiancee and with his Native American culture group were strong. With minimal ties outside this group, both Mr. Raymond and his fiancee had little knowledge of outside supportive agencies.

Continued on following page

MR. RAYMOND'S DEFENSE SYSTEM

Mr. Raymond came from a male-dominated society in which the man was expected to be a strong leader. His ability to be independent with the power to affect the direction of his life was central to his perception of being accepted as a man.

Mr. Raymond felt powerless, out of control, and enraged. He was handling his anxiety by displacing these feelings onto the environment, namely, the staff and his fiancee. The redirection of anger temporarily lowered his anxiety, and it distracted him from painful feelings. When he intimidated others through sexual profanity and hostility, he felt temporarily in control and experienced an illusion of power. He used displacement to relieve his painful levels of anxiety when he felt threatened.

Mr. Raymond's use of displacement was not adaptive because the issues causing his distress were not being resolved. His anxiety continued to escalate. The effect his behavior was having on others caused them to move away from him. This withdrawal further increased his sense of isolation and helplessness.

Nursing Diagnosis

Based on her assessment, Ms. Greg formulated the following nursing diagnosis:

1. *Ineffective individual coping* related to inadequate coping methods, as evidenced by inappropriate use of defense mechanism (displacement)
   - Anger directed toward staff and fiancee
   - Profanity and crude sexual remarks aimed at staff
   - Frustration and withdrawal on the part of the staff
   - Continued escalation of anxiety

2. *Powerlessness* related to health care environment, as evidenced by frustration over inability to perform previously uncomplicated tasks
   - Angry over nurses having to "scratch my head and blow my nose"
   - Minimal awareness of available supports in larger community

3. *Ineffective staff coping* related to exhaustion of staff supportive capacity toward client, as evidenced by staff withdrawal and limited personal communication with client
   - Staff felt ineffective.
   - Morale of staff was poor.
   - Nurses believed that the quality of their care was adversely affected.

Planning

Ms. Greg spoke to Mr. Raymond and told him she would like to spend time with him for 15 minutes every morning and talk about his concerns. She suggested that there might be alternative ways he could handle his feelings, and community resources could be explored. Mr. Raymond gruffly agreed, "You can visit me, if it will make you feel better." They made arrangements to meet at 7:30 A.M. for 15 minutes each morning.

For each nursing diagnosis the following short term goals were set:

Nursing Diagnosis	Short Term Goal
1. *Ineffective individual coping* related to inadequate coping methods, as evidenced by inappropriate use of defense mechanisms (displacement)	1. Mr. Raymond will be able to name and discuss at least two feelings about his illness and lack of mobility (by the end of the week).
2. *Powerlessness* related to health care environment, as evidenced by frustration over inability to perform previous tasks	2. Mr. Raymond will be able to name two community organizations that could offer him information and support (by the end of two weeks).
3. *Ineffective staff coping* related to exhaustion of staff supportive capacity toward client, as evidenced by staff withdrawal and limited personal communication	3. Staff and nurse consultant will discuss reactions and alternative nursing responses to Mr. Raymond's behavior (two times within the next seven days).

Ms. Greg made out a nursing care plan (Nursing Care Plan 11–1) and shared it with the staff.

Intervention

The following morning, Ms. Greg went into Mr. Raymond's room at 7:30 A.M. and sat by his bedside. At first, Mr. Raymond's comments were hostile.

Dialogue	Therapeutic Tool/Comment
NURSE: Mr. Raymond, I'm here as we discussed. I'll be spending 15 minutes with you every morning. We could use this time to talk about some of your concerns.	Nurse offers herself as a resource, gives information, and clarifies her role and client expectations. Night was the most difficult time for Mr. Raymond. In early morning he would be the most vulnerable and open for therapeutic intervention and support.
MR. R: Listen sweetheart, my only concern is how to get a little sexual relief, get it?	
NURSE: Being hospitalized and partially paralyzed can be overwhelming for anyone. Perhaps you wish you could find some relief from your situation.	Nurse focuses on the process "need for relief" and not the sexual content. Encourages discussion of feelings.
MR. R: What do you know, Ms. Know-it-all? I can't even scratch my nose without getting one of those fools to do it for me . . . and half the time those bitches aren't even around.	
NURSE: It must be difficult to have to ask people to do everything for you.	Nurse restates what client says in terms of client's feelings. Continues to refocus away from the environment back to the client.
MR. R: Yeah . . . the other night a fly got into the room and landed on my face. I had to shout for five minutes before one of those bitches came in . . . just to take the fly out of the room.	
NURSE: Having to rely on others for everything can be a terrifying experience for anyone. It sounds extremely frustrating to you.	Nurse acknowledges that frustration and anger would be a normal and healthy response for anyone in this situation. Encourages client to talk about these feelings instead of acting them out.
MR. R: Yeah . . . it's a bitch . . . like a living hell.	

Ms. Greg continued to spend time with Mr. Raymond in the mornings. He was gradually able to talk more about his feelings of anger and frustration and was less apt to act with hostility toward the staff. As he began to feel more in control, he became less defensive about others caring for him.

After two weeks, Ms. Greg cut her visits down to two times a week. Mr. Raymond was beginning to get gross motor movements back but was not walking yet. He still displaced much of his frustration and lack of control on the environment, but he was better able to acknowledge the reality of his situation. He could identify what he was feeling and talk about those feelings briefly.

Dialogue	Therapeutic Tool/Comment
NURSE: You seem upset this morning, Mr. Raymond.	Nurse observes client's clenched fists, rigid posture, and tense facial expression.
MR. R: I had to wait 10 minutes for a bedpan last night.	
NURSE: And you're angry about that.	Nurse verbalizes the implied.
MR. R: Well, there were only two nurses on for 30 people, and the aide was on her break . . . You can't expect them to be everywhere . . . but still . . .	
NURSE: It's hard to accept that people can't be there all the time for you.	Nurse validates the difficulty of accepting situations one does not like when one is powerless to make changes.
MR. R: Well . . . that's the way it is in this place.	

Continued on following page

Case Study: Working with a Person in Crisis (Continued)

Ms. Greg met with the staff twice. The staff discussed their feelings of helplessness and lack of control stemming from their feelings of rejection from Mr. Raymond. They talked about their anger about Mr. Raymond's demeaning behavior, and their frustration about the situation. Ms. Greg pointed out to the staff that Mr. Raymond's feelings of helplessness, lack of control, and anger at his situation were the same feelings the staff was experiencing. Displacement of the helplessness and frustration by intimidating the staff gave Mr. Raymond the brief feeling of control. It also distracted him from his own feelings of helplessness.

The nurses had become more understanding of the motivation for the behavior Mr. Raymond employed to cope with moderate to severe levels of anxiety. The staff focused more on the client, and less on personal reactions. The staff decided together on two approaches they could try as a group. First, they would not take Mr. Raymond's behavior personally. Second, Mr. Raymond's feelings that were displaced would be refocused back to him.

Evaluation

After six weeks, Mr. Raymond was able to get around with assistance, and his ability to care for his activities of daily living was increasing. Although Mr. Raymond was still angry and although he still felt overwhelmed at times, he was able to identify more of his feelings. He did not need to act them out so often. He was able to talk to his fiancee about his feelings, and he lashed out at her less. He was looking forward to going home, and his boss was holding his old job.

Mr. Raymond contacted the Guillain-Barré Society, and they made arrangements for a meeting with him. He was still thinking about Alcoholics Anonymous but thought he could handle this problem himself.

The staff felt more comfortable and competent in their relationships with Mr. Raymond. The goals had been met. Mr. Raymond and Ms. Greg both felt that the crisis was over, and the visits were terminated. Mr. Raymond was given the number of the crisis unit. He was encouraged to call if he had questions or felt the need to talk.

Nursing Care Plan 11–1 ■ A PERSON IN CRISIS: MR. RAYMOND

NURSING DIAGNOSIS

Ineffective individual coping related to inadequate coping methods, as evidenced by inappropriate use of defense mechanisms (displacement)

Supporting Data

- Anger directed at staff and fiancee
- Profanity and crude sexual remarks aimed at staff
- Isolation related to staff withdrawal
- Continued escalation of anxiety

Long Term Goal: By discharge, Mr. Raymond will state he feels more comfortable discussing difficult feelings.

Short Term Goal	Intervention	Rationale	Evaluation
1. Mr. Raymond will be able to name and discuss at least two feelings about his illness and lack of mobility (by the end of the week).	1a. Nurse will meet with client for 15 minutes at 7:30 A.M. each day for a week.	1a. Night was usually the most frightening for the client; in early morning, feelings were closer to the surface.	Goal met Within seven days, Mr. Raymond was able to speak to nurse more openly about feelings of anger and frustration.
	1b. When client lashes out with verbal abuse, nurse will remain calm.	1b. Client perceives that nurse is in control of her feelings. This can be reassuring to client and can increase client's sense of security.	
	1c. Nurse will consistently redirect and refocus anger from environment back to the client, e.g., "It must be difficult to be in this situation."	1c. Refocusing feelings offers the client the opportunity to cope effectively with his anxiety and decreases the need to act out toward staff and fiancee.	
	1d. Nurse will come on time each day and stay for allotted time.	1d. Consistency sets the stage for trust and reinforces that client's anger will not drive nurse away.	

NURSING DIAGNOSIS

Powerlessness related to health care environment, as evidenced by frustration over inability to perform previous tasks

Supporting Data

- Angry over nurses having to "scratch my head and help me blow my nose"
- Minimal awareness of available supports in larger community

Long Term Goal: By discharge, Mr. Raymond will have contacted at least one outside community support.

Short Term Goal	Intervention	Rationale	Evaluation
1. By the end of two weeks, Mr. Raymond will be able to name at least two community organizations that can offer information and support.	1a. Nurse will spend time with the client and his fiancee. The role of specific agencies and how they may be of use will be discussed.	1a. Both client and fiancee will have the opportunity to ask questions with nurse present.	Goal met By end of 10 days, Mr. Raymond and his fiancee could name two community resources that they were interested in.
	1b. The nurse will introduce one agency at a time.	1b. Gradual introduction allows time for information to sink in and minimizes feeling of being pressured or overwhelmed.	At the end of six weeks, Mr. Raymond had contacted the Guillain-Barré Society.
	1c. The nurse will follow up but not push or persuade client to contact any of the agencies.	1c. Client is able to make own decisions once he has appropriate information.	

NURSING DIAGNOSIS

Ineffective staff coping related to feelings of helplessness, as evidenced by staff withdrawal and limited personal communication

Supporting Data

- Staff state they feel ineffective.
- Morale of staff is poor.
- Nurses state the quality of their care is adversely affected.

Long Term Goal: By the end of three weeks, staff will state interactions with Mr. Raymond are comfortable and effective.

Short Term Goal	Intervention	Rationale	Evaluation
1. Staff and nurse will meet for 15 minutes twice by the end of the week to discuss reactions and alternative nursing responses to Mr. Raymond's behavior.	1a. Specific time for staff meeting is set aside and participation is encouraged.	1a. Action gives message that meeting is serious and input from entire staff is needed to plan effective intervention.	Goal met By the end of seven days, staff had met twice to discuss feelings and reactions toward Mr. Raymond.
	1b. Staff is encouraged to identify commonalities in their feelings and how these feelings are affecting their level of care.	1b. Sharing can minimize feelings of isolation and guilt over angry feelings. Examining reactions to client behaviors and possible client motivation for behavior can facilitate staff problem solving.	Staff planned to redirect feelings back to client.
	1c. The nurse will support group planning of effective nursing actions.	1c. When anxiety is lowered, staff is able to discuss as a unit the aspects of the client's behavior they view as a problem. Interventions then can be carried out with consistency and mutual support.	Staff planned to make an effort to remember Mr. Raymond's remarks were a defensive reaction.
			By the end of six weeks, staff stated they felt more comfortable and competent in their care of Mr. Raymond.

Crisis Intervention with the Chronically Mentally Ill Client

The client with chronic mental health problems also experiences crises. The incidence of crisis may be increased in this population because of the nature of chronic mental illness. Crisis theory and intervention can be adapted successfully with clients who have long term mental illness. Five characteristics of people with chronic mental illness have been identified (Finkelman 1977):

1. Inadequate problem-solving ability
2. Inadequate communication skills
3. Low self-esteem
4. Poor success with endeavors such as work, school, family, and social relationships
5. Inpatient or outpatient treatment for at least two years

Although the client's illness is in the chronic state, there are healthy and unhealthy aspects of the client's personality. It is important to stress the healthy aspects of the client's personality, rather than the pathological aspects, during assessment of this client. Some of the major differences between the person who has chronic and severe difficulties in living and the mentally healthy person are outlined in Table 11–3.

POTENTIAL CRISIS SITUATION FOR A PERSON WITH CHRONIC MENTAL HEALTH PROBLEMS

People usually have a number of coping responses they use when there are stresses in their everyday world. Any kind of change in our routines or lives constitutes some degree of stress (see Fig. 11–1). For the person with limited abilities, even slight change might increase the potential for a full-blown crisis. Four common potential crisis situations for the chronically mentally ill patient have been identified (Finkelman 1977):

1. Change in treatment approaches, such as change in routine of treatment, therapist's absence due to vacation or illness, or change in appointment time.
2. Problems or changes at work, at school, or with the family, and anniversaries of significant or traumatic events in the person's life.
3. Lack of money, inadequate transportation, and problems meeting basic needs.
4. Sexual relationships for someone who is unsure about his or her own sexual identity are always a source of anxiety and can be compounded in the chronically ill client if there are other complications, for example pregnancy or impotence.

ADAPTING THE CRISIS MODEL TO MEET THE NEEDS OF A PERSON WITH CHRONIC MENTAL HEALTH PROBLEMS

Traditionally, crisis intervention refers to disequilibrium in the functioning of otherwise mentally healthy persons. The goal is to prevent temporary difficulty in functioning from progressing to severe personality disorganization. Intervention and support can aid the person in finding the way back to his or her previous level of functioning. People with chronic mental health problems, however, are readily susceptible to crisis. The nurse must be able to adapt the crisis model to this group. These adaptations include focusing on the client's strengths, modifying and setting realistic goals with the client, taking a more active

Table 11–3 ■ MENTALLY HEALTHY VERSUS CHRONICALLY MENTALLY ILL PERSON IN CRISIS

MENTALLY HEALTHY PERSON	LONG TERM MENTALLY ILL PERSON
1. Has realistic perception of potential crisis event.	1. Because of chronically high anxiety state, potential crisis event is usually distorted by minimizing or maximizing the event.
2. Has healthy ego boundaries, good problem-solving abilities.	2. Inadequate ego functioning assumes inadequate problem-solving abilities; nurse becomes more active in assisting the person with this task.
3. Usually has adequate situational supports.	3. Often the person has no family or friends and may be living an isolated existence.
4. Usually has adequate coping mechanisms. Defense mechanisms can be used as support to lower anxiety.	4. Because ego functioning in the chronic patient is poor, coping mechanisms are usually inadequate or poorly utilized.

Data from Finkelman AW. The nurse therapist: Outpatient crisis intervention with the chronic psychiatric patient. Journal of Psychosocial Nursing and Mental Health Services, 8:27, 1977.

role in the problem-solving process, and using direct interventions, such as making arrangements the person would ordinarily be able to make.

Summary

A crisis is not a pathological state but rather a struggle for emotional balance. A crisis can offer the opportunity for emotional growth, or it can lead to possible personality disorganization. Early intervention during a time of crisis greatly increases the possibility for a successful outcome. There are three types of crises: maturational, situational, and adventitious, as well as specific phases in the development of a crisis. Crisis and crisis intervention are based on certain assumptions:

1. A crisis is usually resolved within a period of four to six weeks.
2. Crisis intervention therapy is short term, from one to six weeks, and focuses on the present problem only.
3. Resolution of a crisis takes three forms. A person emerges at a higher level, at precrisis level, or at a lower level of functioning.
4. Social support and intervention maximize successful resolution.
5. Crisis therapists take an active and directive approach with the client in crisis.
6. The client takes an active role in setting goals and planning possible solutions.

Traditionally, crisis intervention is aimed at the mentally healthy person who is functioning well but is temporarily overwhelmed and unable to function. However, people who have chronic mental problems are also susceptible to crisis, and the crisis model can be adapted for their needs as well.

The steps in crisis intervention are consistent with the nursing process (assessment, nursing diagnosis, planning, intervention, and evaluation). Each has specific goals and tasks.

Specific qualities in the nurse that can facilitate effective intervention are a caring attitude, flexibility in planning care, and an ability to listen.

The nurse's ability to be aware of his or her feelings and thoughts is crucial in working with a person in crisis. The availability of peer supports and supervision to discuss the questions that normally arise is essential for the beginning crisis counselor. Learning crisis intervention is a process, and there are certain problems all health care professionals must deal with to improve their skills.

The basic goals of crisis intervention are to reduce the individual's anxiety level and to support the effort to return to a normal level of functioning.

References

Aguilera DC, Messick JM. Crisis Intervention Theory and Methodology, 6th ed. St. Louis: CV Mosby, 1990.

Caplan G. Symptoms of Preventive Psychiatry. New York: Basic Books, 1964.

Croushore T, et al. Using crisis intervention wisely. Philadelphia: Nursing 81 Books, Intermed Communications, 1981.

Doenges M, Moorehouse M. Nurses Pocket Guide: Nursing Diagnoses with Interventions, 2nd ed. Philadelphia: FA Davis, 1988.

Donlon PT, Rockwell DA. Psychiatric Disorders, Diagnosis and Treatment. Bowie, MD: Robert J. Brady Company, 1982.

Erikson E. Childhood and Society, 2nd ed. New York: Norton, 1963.

Ewing CP. Crisis Intervention as Psychotherapy. New York: Oxford University Press, 1978.

Finkelman AW. The nurse therapist: Outpatient crisis intervention with the chronic patient. Journal of Psychosocial Nursing and Mental Health Services, 8:27, 1977.

Hoff LA. People in Crisis: Understanding and Helping, 3rd ed. Menlo Park, CA: Addison-Wesley, 1989.

Holmes TH, Masuda M. Psychosomatic syndrome. Psychology Today, p 72, April 1972.

King JM. The initial interview: Basis for assessment in crisis intervention. Perspectives in Psychiatric Care, 6:247, 1971.

Levenson AI. A review of the Federal Community Mental Health Centers Program. In Arieti S, Caplan G (eds). American Handbook of Psychiatry, vol 2, 2nd ed. New York: Basic Books, 1974.

Robinson L. Psychiatric emergencies. Nursing 73, 7:43, 1973.

Taylor CM. Mereness' Essentials of Psychiatric Nursing, 12th ed. St. Louis: CV Mosby, 1986.

Wallace MA, Morley WE. Teaching crisis intervention. American Journal of Nursing, 7:1484, 1970.

Further Reading

Aguilera DC, Messick JM. Crisis Intervention Theory and Methodology, 6th ed. St. Louis: CV Mosby, 1990.

An important reference for all health professionals dealing with people in crisis. Now in its fifth edition, this text provides a comprehensive overview of crisis theory and intervention techniques by individuals and groups. The authors discuss the sociocultural factors that influence interventions, and outline in detail the problem-solving approach to intervention. A variety of situational crises are discussed and case examples are given, for example, rape, divorce, suicide, death, and grieving. Maturational crises from infancy to old age are well presented with helpful case studies. A chapter is also provided on the burn-out syndrome.

Barry PD. Psychosocial Nursing Assessment and Intervention. Philadelphia: JB Lippincott, 1984.

Caplan G. Principles of Preventive Psychiatry. New York: Basic Books, 1964.

Drawing from the work of Lindemann, his own experience, and that of others, Caplan lays down the theoretical basis for crisis that is in current practice today. Caplan identifies four distinctive phases of crisis. He maintains that crisis is not a pathological state but a predictable reaction of a person overwhelmed by problems that appear insolvable. He also identifies a number of aspects of crisis that have relevance for therapeutic intervention and are integral to the present-day practice of crisis intervention.

Coler MS, Hafner LP. An intercultural assessment of the type, intensity and number of crisis precipitating factors in three cultures: U.S., Brazil, and Taiwan. International Journal of Nursing Studies,28(3):223, 1991.

Doenges M, Moorehouse M. Nurse's Pocket Guide: Nursing Diagnoses with Interventions, 2nd ed. Philadelphia: FA Davis, 1988.

Flax JW. Crisis intervention with the young adult chronic patient. In Pepper B, Rygkewicz H (eds). New Dimensions for Mental Health Services: The Young Adult Chronic Patient. San Francisco, CA: Jossey-Bass, June 1982.

The young adult chronic client is increasingly coming to the attention of mental health care workers. This population appears to be growing and using more and more of the community health care facilities. Flax states that assessment of these clients can be difficult, since they present many problems. He outlines an assessment model including prerequisites for outpatient treatment. He presents a case study to illustrate his model of assessment and intervention. The article provides useful guidelines to a population that nurses will be dealing with in all areas of practice.

Lindemann E. Symptomatology and management of acute grief. American Journal of Psychiatry, 101:141, 1944.

Lindemann's classic study of the grief reactions of 101 persons, victims and relatives of those lost in the infamous Coconut Grove nightclub fire. The results of this study provide the foundation of crisis theory and crisis intervention. Lindemann identified grief as "the normal reaction to a distressing situation," and identified uniform and predictable stages in the grief reaction.

He proposed that appropriate intervention in an acute grief reaction (crisis) would minimize subsequent mental problems.

Murphy SA. After Mount St. Helens: Disaster stress research. Journal of Psychosocial Nursing and Mental Health Services, 22(7), 1984.

The author studied the adventitious crisis of the eruption of Mount St. Helens in terms of (1) the relationship between illness and presumed death of a loved one, (2) the effects of social supports and self-efficacy as influencing positive or negative outcomes of health, and (3) the perceived effects of the media on coping with the loss following a disaster. This nurse-author's research project is well written and points out important guidelines for psychiatric mental health workers in mass crisis situations.

Swanson AR. Crisis intervention. In Lego S (ed). The American Handbook of Psychiatric Nursing. Philadelphia: JB Lippincott, 1984.

A concise and thorough overview of crisis, including the basic concepts, facts and misperceptions, characteristics of crisis intervention, assumptions about people in crisis, developmental and situational crisis, and general and specific guidelines in crisis intervention. A helpful, quick reference with useful charts and tables.

Self-study Exercises

Match the situation with the type of actual or potential crisis.

1. _____ New baby is brought into household
2. _____ Person is raped
3. _____ Man celebrates 50th birthday
4. _____ House burns down
5. _____ Child or spouse is battered
6. _____ Girl becomes a teenager

A. Maturational

B. Situational

C. Adventitious

Place a T (true) or F (false) next to each statement. Correct the false statements.

7. _____ A crisis situation can last up to four months before it is resolved.
8. _____ The goal of crisis therapy is to have the person obtain a higher level of functioning.
9. _____ Crisis therapy deals with the person in the present situation and with the person's immediate presenting problems.
10. _____ A person in crisis has always had problems and does not cope well in his or her usual life situations.
11. _____ A crisis situation can offer the opportunity for personality growth, or the potential for personality deterioration.
12. _____ Intervention rarely has any effect in the resolution of a crisis.
13. _____ The nurse counselor must take a firm and direct approach with a person in crisis.
14. _____ It is necessary for the nurse counselor to do all the planning and make all the decisions for the person in crisis because the person is often too disorganized.

Write a short paragraph in response to the following:

15. After you determine whether a person is homicidal or suicidal, identify the three important areas in the assessment. Give examples of two questions in each area that need to be answered before planning can take place.

Complete the statements by filling in the appropriate information.

16. Three personal qualities that can enhance a nurse's effectiveness in a crisis are

A. _____

B. _____

C. _____

17. Three ways you can demonstrate concern and show that you are listening are

A. _____

B. _____

C. _____

18. Identify two self-interventions a nurse can use if problems arise when crisis counseling is started.

Problem	*Intervention*
A. Needing to feel needed	1. _____
	2. _____
B. Setting unrealistic goals	1. _____
	2. _____

Match the appropriate intervention to the appropriate level of intervention.

19. _____ Teach problem solving

20. _____ Attends rehabilitation center

21. _____ Assess precipitating events

22. _____ Teach assertiveness training

A. Primary

B. Secondary

C. Tertiary

Complete the statements by filling in the appropriate information.

23. Four experiences that could potentiate a crisis in a person with a chronic mental problem are

A. _____

B. _____

C. _____

D. _____

24. Four common crisis situations that a nurse may encounter in a general hospital are

A. _____

B. _____

C. _____

D. _____

CHAPTER 12

Families in Crisis: Family Violence

Kathleen Smith-DiJulio
Sally Kennedy Holzapfel

OUTLINE •

KEY TERMS AND CONCEPTS ◆ ◆ ◆ ◆ ◆ ◆ ◆ ◆ ◆ ◆ ◆ ◆ ◆ ◆ ◆

The key terms and concepts listed here also appear in bold where they are defined or discussed in this chapter.

ABUSE

ABUSE CYCLE

ABUSE-PRONE INDIVIDUAL

CRISIS SITUATION

CYCLE THEORY OF VIOLENCE
Acute Battering Stage
Honeymoon Stage
Tension-building Stage

ECONOMIC ABUSE

EMOTIONAL ABUSE

MEDICAL-NURSING RECORD

NEGLECT

PHYSICAL ABUSE
Battering
Endangerment

PRIMARY PREVENTION

SAFETY PLAN

SECONDARY PREVENTION

SEXUAL ABUSE

SHELTERS OR SAFE HOUSES

STAGES OF TREATMENT
Crisis Stage
Stage of Internal Change and Rebuilding

TERTIARY PREVENTION

TITLE XX OF THE 1974 SOCIAL
  SECURITY AMENDMENT ACT

VULNERABLE PERSON

OBJECTIVES ■

After studying this chapter, the student will be able to

1. Discuss the epidemiological theory of abuse in terms of stresses on the abuser, victim, and environment that could escalate anxiety to the point at which violence becomes the relief behavior.
2. List three characteristics of abusers.
3. Describe three characteristics of a vulnerable person.
4. List three physical and three behavioral indicators of physical abuse.
5. List three physical and three behavioral indicators of sexual abuse.
6. List two physical and two behavioral indicators of neglect.
7. List two physical and two behavioral indicators of emotional abuse.
8. Describe an example of economic abuse.
9. Briefly name and discuss three stages in the process of the cycle of violence that results in abuse.
10. List four areas of assessment in interviewing an abuse victim.
11. Identify pertinent nursing diagnoses for the victim and list supporting data from the assessment.
12. Identify pertinent nursing diagnoses for the abuser and list supporting data from the assessment.
13. Formulate two short term goals for both the victim and the abuser.
14. State three interventions that would be appropriate in dealing with both the victim and the abuser.
15. Compare and discuss primary, secondary, and tertiary levels of intervention, giving two examples of intervention for each level.
16. Discuss two common emotional responses by health personnel faced with situations of abuse.
17. Name and discuss three areas of intervention in the crisis stage of counseling an abuse victim.
18. Name and discuss three psychotherapeutic modalities that are useful for violent families.
19. Name three areas of evaluation in working with violent families.

It has been said that family violence is America's number one public health issue (Klingbeil 1991). The secondary effects of abuse, such as anxiety, depression, and suicide, can last a lifetime and are also health care issues. Abuse is common in childhood histories of juvenile delinquents, runaways, violent criminals, prostitutes, and those who in turn abuse their children, spouses, or parents (Bullock et al. 1989). Abuse in childhood can lead to later social and mental maladjustment throughout the life span. Abused adolescents report more psychopathological changes, poorer coping skills, higher incidence of multiple personality disorder, and poorer impulse control than do nonabused adolescents. Differences are also found in orientation to future vocational and educational goals as well as in peer realtionships (Kluft 1987). Box 12–1 identifies some of the sequelae of family violence.

Because interpersonal abuse occurs most often within families, it is not easy to document the actual incidence or prevalence of this problem. It has been estimated that half of all Americans have experienced violence in their families. Battering is the single largest cause of injury to women in the United States (Novello and Soto-Torres 1992). Between 1976 and 1987, the number of reports of child abuse and neglect increased 225% (Office of Maternal and Child Health 1989). Abuse of infants is one of the leading causes of postneonatal mortality (Ludwig and Kornberg 1992). It has been estimated that over 1 million older Americans annually, or more than one in 10 elderly persons living with a family member, are mistreated (Fulmer 1991).

Abusive families also include those with abuse in gay and lesbian relationships, sibling abuse, and parental abuse by children, as well as those in which spouse, child, and elder abuse occurs. Violence against children, women, and the elderly is declared to be wrong, but violence is acceptable on television, in movies, and even in schools. Such a double message makes it nearly impossible to make inroads against violence in America.

Yet violence within families is seldom recognized by outsiders, including nurses. The US Objectives for the Year 2000 call for the extension of "protocols for routinely identifying, testing and properly referring victims" seen in emergency departments and primary care settings (Public Health Service 1989). As of January 1993, the Joint Commission on Accreditation of Health Care Organizations requires emergency services and staff education in domestic violence and elder abuse as well as policies and procedures to give patients care and treatment.

The nurse is often the first point of contact for a victim of abuse. The time and energy spent may have future as well as immediate impact. *The American Nurse* highlighted the role of the nurse in trying to break the cycle of violence (Meierhoffer 1992). The Nursing Network on Violence Against Women was founded in 1985 during the first National Nursing Conference on Violence Against Women. The goal of the network is to provide a presence in the struggle to end violence in women's lives. Altering the pattern of violence against women can also affect child abuse because there are linkages between the two (National Coalition Against Domestic Violence 1988).

The general subject of violence in the United States must be addressed if long-lasting changes are to be made. It took until 1967 for all states to enact laws

---

Box 12–1. LONG TERM EFFECTS OF FAMILY VIOLENCE

People involved in family violence are found to have higher levels of

- Depression
- Suicidal feelings
- Self-contempt
- Inability to trust
- Inability to develop intimate relationships in later life

Victims of severe abuse are also at higher risk for experiencing recurring symptoms of post-traumatic stress disorder related to the unresolved trauma:

- Flashbacks
- Dissociation—out-of-body experiences
- Poor self-esteem
- Compulsive or impulsive behaviors (e.g., substance abuse, spending money, gambling, and promiscuity)
- Multiple somatic complaints

Children who witness abuse in their homes

- After the age of five or six show an indication of identifying with the aggressor and losing respect for the victim
- Are at greater risk for developing behavioral and emotional problems throughout their lives

Some mental and behavioral disorders are associated with abuse in childhood:

- Depressive disorders
- Post-traumatic stress disorder
- Dissociative disorders, the most severe of which is multiple personality disorder
- Self-mutilating behaviors in adolescence
- Phobias (agoraphobia, social and specific phobias)
- Antisocial behaviors
- Child or spouse abuse

Children or adolescents who mask their depression are more likely to have behavioral symptoms such as

- Failing grades
- Difficulty forming relationships
- Increased incidence of theft, police arrest, and violent behaviors
- Seductive or promiscuous behaviors
- Running away from home

against child abuse. The emphasis is on the protection of children through identification of abuse and provision of services to stabilize conditions for troubled families (Kreitzer 1981). It has only been since 1978 that battered women can expect to be somewhat protected in most communities. Laws against elder abuse lag even further behind.

The Senate Select Committee on Aging in 1978 began to hear testimony on abuse of older Americans. Although all states subsequently developed systems for investigating elder abuse, not all have mandatory reporting laws. As of 1989, 43 states had mandatory reporting laws, up from 16 states in 1980 (Elder abuse 1991). Awareness and public concern continue to grow. Laws and awareness are not enough to decrease the incidence of family violence in the United States, however. As long as families live in crisis and social changes are not forthcoming, the conditions for abuse are ripe.

One fourth of all children living in this country, the richest nation on earth, do not have adequate food. Parents raising children in poverty are not likely to have the skills or resources to teach their children to function effectively as adults. Family stress is constant. For example, some fathers of children living in poverty cannot financially support their families because of long term unemployment. Other fathers cannot be permanent family members without jeopardizing their families' public assistance payments, and therefore they cannot maintain their role as responsible adults.

Smaller family units, more working mothers and one-parent households, and a higher life expectancy have changed the character of the family structure and support for the older adult. It is frequently the "young-old" children who take care of their "old-old" parents. In addition, this sandwich generation is still coping with the demands of their own growing offspring and are just beginning to savor some long-awaited respite from them (Gelman 1985). Abuse as a

maladaptive response to acute anxiety can be conceptualized as in Figure 12–1.

Theory

Abuse is defined as the "willful infliction of physical injury or mental anguish and the deprivation by the caregiver of essential services" (Verwoerdt 1976). To be more effective in working with abuse victims, the nurse must have an understanding of conditions for abuse and types of abuse.

CONDITIONS FOR ABUSE

Abuse occurs across all segments of American society. A combination of three specific factors signals conditions for abuse in most instances. These factors are (1) an **abuse-prone individual,** (2) someone who by age or situation is a **vulnerable person,** that is, child, woman, elderly person, or mentally ill person, and (3) a **crisis situation.**

Abuse-prone Individuals

The most disconcerting aspect of abuse is that it is multigenerational. Abusers are frequently former abuse victims. Family histories of both the abused and the abuser often contain accounts of violence. The propensity for abuse is rooted in childhood and manifested by a general lack of self-esteem, satisfaction with life, and ability to assume adult roles (Wissow 1990).

Deficiencies in patterns of family functioning in households experiencing violence result from many factors. There has usually been lack of role modeling

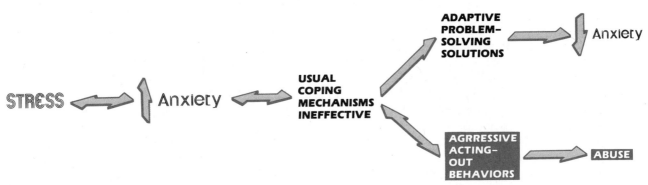

Figure 12–1. *Conceptualization of the process of intrafamily abuse.*

as well as lack of knowledge of characteristics of healthy relationships. There is uncertainty about what to expect realistically of self, spouse, or children. Abusers often consider their own needs to be more important than anyone else's and look to others to meet their needs. Because this is an ineffective way to meet needs, abusers come to believe that they are unable to have any effect or control over events inside and outside the family.

These same families, already highly stressed, often have even greater demands placed on them by geographical moves, job changes, and illnesses. Abusing families are also socially isolated from support systems. This isolation may be a result of mobility patterns, characteristics that alienate others, and social stresses that cut families off from potential and actual supports.

In addition to these general characteristics of abusers and abusing families, other specific characteristics are found either singly or in combination among all individuals involved in families affected by domestic violence (Box 12–2).

In *child abuse*, parents with a drug or an alcohol problem may be more likely to maltreat their children. The abuser is often a stepparent who projects hostility toward the new mate or mate's ex-spouse onto the child. At other times, the abuser may be a friend of the parent.

In *elder abuse*, growing evidence suggests that the caregiver may be a severely troubled individual with a history of antisocial behavior or instability. There is often a high level of dependence on the victim, and elements of exploitation may exist in these relationships (Pillemer and Prescott 1989).

For simplifying the discussion, the pattern of a husband abusing his wife is the model used here. Although there are cases of women assaulting their husbands, the incidence of this is much lower. Studies show that the majority of these women are attempting to protect themselves from abuse initiated by their spouses (Gelles and Straus 1988).

Men who batter believe in male supremacy, being in charge, and being dominant. "Acting out" physically makes them feel more in control, masculine, and powerful, which attests to their low self-esteem and insecurity. Extreme pathological jealousy is characteristic of batterers. Many refuse to let their wives work; others have their wives work in the same place they do so that they can monitor their wives' activities and friendships. Many accompany their wives to and from all activities and forbid them to have personal friends or to participate in recreational activities outside the home. Even with such restrictions, these men accuse their wives of infidelity. Many batterers maintain their possessiveness by controlling the family finances to

---

Box 12–2. CHARACTERISTICS OF ABUSING PARENTS

A history of abuse, neglect, or emotional deprivation as a child

Family authoritarianism—raise children as they were raised by their own parents

Low self-esteem, feelings of worthlessness, depression

Poor coping skills

Social isolation (may be suspicious of others)—few or no friends, little or no involvement in social or community activities

Involved in a crisis situation—unemployment, divorce, financial difficulties

Rigid, unrealistic expectations of child's behavior

Frequent use of harsh punishment

History of severe mental illness, such as schizophrenia

Violent temper outbursts

Looking to child for satisfaction of needs for love, support, and reassurance (often unmet because of parenting deficits in family of origin)

Projection of blame onto the child for their "troubles" (e.g., stepparent may project hostility toward new mate onto a child)

Lack of effective parenting skills

Inability to seek help from others

Perception of the child as bad or evil

History of drug or alcohol abuse

Feeling of little or no control over life

Low tolerance for frustration

Poor impulse control

Data from Warner CG (ed). Conflict Intervention in Social and Domestic Violence. Bowie, MD: Robert J Brady Company, 1981.

---

the extent that there is barely enough money for daily living. In their study, Else et al. (1993) found that men who commit domestic violence may be found among a larger pool of men with poor problem-solving skills; in addition, they seem to have borderline or antisocial personality traits and histories of abuse as children.

Individuals are more likely to engage in family violence (child, elder, or spouse abuse) when intoxicated. Alcohol may play a role in disinhibition for disregarding social rules that prohibit violence against children, women, and the elderly (Wissow 1990). Unfortunately, the consumption of alcohol and drugs is often used as a rationalization to excuse the behavior: for example, "He was drunk; he didn't know what he was doing." The fact is that when drug and alcohol use are reduced or eliminated, family violence still occurs (Delgaty 1985).

Both male and female batterers perceive themselves as having poor social skills. They describe their relationships with their spouses as being the closest they have ever known. They lack supportive relationships outside the marriage. When not being abusive, spouse abusers have been described as remorseful, child-like, and yearning to be nurtured (Swanson 1984). As mentioned, abusers of the elderly are more likely to have mental, emotional, or alcohol problems and to be financially dependent on the victims (Box 12–3).

The **abuse cycle** can be operationally defined as follows:

1. A person is brought up in an atmosphere devoid of love, affection, and security.
2. A sense of being valued and cared for never develops.
3. Tremendous needs for love and security are left unfulfilled.
4. Others (child, spouse) are sought to fill the void for love and acceptance.
5. When these unrealistic demands are unable to be met, feelings of rejection and anger are mobilized in the abuser.
6. Rage and helplessness, coupled with poor impulse control, lead to projection onto the vulnerable person (child, spouse, elder).

Table 12–1 summarizes the characteristics of batterers.

Vulnerable Person

The characteristics of the vulnerable battered mate and children are listed in Table 12–1. The dependency needs of elderly persons are usually what puts them at risk for abuse. Dealing with the problems of the elderly can be stressful for adult caregivers.

Violence often does not occur until after the legal marriage of couples who have lived together or dated for a long time (Gemmill 1982). Perhaps this reflects the notion of women as property legally bound to the husband by virtue of the marriage ceremony.

Pregnancy often serves to increase violence even further. One reason may be that the husband resents the added responsibliity that a baby requires; or he may resent the relationship that the baby will have with his mate. Violence also escalates when the wife makes moves toward independence, such as visiting friends "without permission," getting a job, or going back to school.

Box 12–3. CHARACTERISTICS OF ELDER ABUSERS

Physical and Psychological Abuse

The abuser may have

- A history of mental illness
- A recent decline in mental status
- Recent medical problems
- A financial dependence on the victim
- Shared living arrangements with the victim
- A history of alcohol or drug abuse
- Pathological family dynamics

Neglect

The abuser may

- Abuse alcohol or drugs
- Not live with victim
- Not have a decline in mental status
- Not have recent medical problems
- Not experience the victim as a source of stress

Financial Abuse

The abuser may

- Abuse alcohol or drugs
- Be a distant relative
- Be financially dependent on the victim
- Be greedy

Data from Wolf RS, Pillemer KA. Helping Elderly Victims: The Reality of Elder Abuse. New York: Columbia University Press, 1989; Wolf RS. Elder abuse: Scope, characteristics, and treatment. Nurse Practitioner Forum, 1(2):102, 1990.

Through no fault of his or her own, one child in the family may be singled out as the recipient of all parental hostility. The child may be rejected because she or he reminds the parents of someone they do not like (perhaps an ex-spouse), because the child is different from the parents' fantasy of what the child "should" be like, or because the child is a product of an unwanted pregnancy. The vulnerable child may be seen as "abnormal" because of a physical or mental infirmity or "difficult" because of being highly intelligent, uncooperative, or withdrawn (Ludwig and Kornberg 1992). Interference with emotional bonding between parents and child (e.g., with a premature birth or prolonged illness requiring hospitalization) has also been found to increase the risk of possible future abuse.

Table 12-1 ■ BEHAVIORAL CHARACTERISTICS OF DOMESTIC VIOLENCE

BATTERER	BATTERED MATE	ABUSED CHILDREN
Batterers are found in all socioeconomic, educational, ethnic, racial, and age groups Are psychologically, physically, and sexually abusive Use excessive minimization and denial	Battered mates are found in all socioeconomic, educational, ethnic, racial, and age groups Are psychologically, verbally, and physically abused, are frequently sexually abused Use excessive minimization and denial	Children are found in all socioeconomic, educational, ethnic, racial, and age groups Are psychologically abused and may be verbally, physically, and sexually abused Use excessive minimization and denial
Batterer Is Characterized By	**Battered Mate Is Characterized By**	**Abused Children Are Characterized By**
Poor impulse control, limited tolerance for frustration, unpredictable temper—rage; constantly demonstrates but often successfully masks anger	Long-suffering, martyr-like endurance of frustration, passive acceptance, internalized anger	Potential for limited tolerance for frustration, poor impulse control; may either externalize or internalize anger
Stress disorders and psychosomatic complaints; success at masking dysfunction varies with social sophistication and educational levels	Stress disorders and psychosomatic complaints, sadness, and depressions	Stress disorders and psychosomatic complaints; absences from school, predelinquent and delinquent behavior, sadness, and depression
Emotional dependency, subject to secret depressions known only to the family; high risk for codependency	Economic and emotional dependency; high risk for secret drugs and alcohol, home accidents; high risk for codependency	Economic and emotional dependency; high risk for alcohol or drug abuse, sexual acting out, running away, isolation, loneliness, and fear; high risk for excessive caretaking
Limited capacity for delayed reinforcement, very "now" oriented	Unlimited patience for discovery of "magic combination" in solving marital and abusive problems, "travels miles" on tiny bits of reinforcement	Combination of "now" orientation and continual hopefulness that situation will improve
Insatiable ego needs and qualities of childlike narcissism, not generally detectable to people outside family group	Uncertainty of own ego needs; defines self in terms of partner, children, family, job, and other external components	Shaky definition of self (grappling with child-like responses of parents for modeling); defines self in parenting role (role reversal)
Low self-esteem; perceived unachieved ideals and goals for self-disappointment in career, even if successful by others' standards	Low self-esteem, continued faith and hope that battering mate will get "lucky" break	Low self-esteem; seeing self and siblings with few options or expectations to succeed
Qualities that suggest great potential for change and improvement (i.e., makes frequent "promises" for the future)	Unrealistic hope that change is imminent, belief in "promises"	Combination of hope and depression that there is no way out; peer group or extended family may be most important contact, if available
Poor social skills; describes relationship with mate as closest he has ever known; remains in contact with his own family	Gradually increased social isolation including loss of contact with immediate family and friends	Increased social isolation, increased peer isolation, or complete identification with peers; poor social skills
Excessive jealousy and frequent accusations against mate; voicing great fear of abandonment or "being cheated on"; possessive, controlling, hovering, and harassing behavior	Inability to convince partner of loyalty, futility guarding against accusations of "seductive" behavior toward others; compliant, helpless, and powerless	Bargaining behavior with parents; attempts to prove self; compliant or rebellious; feelings of powerlessness, helplessness
Fearfulness that partner or children will abandon; fear of being alone	Constant fear and terror, which gradually become cumulative and oppressive with time	Constant fear and terror for their life as well as parents and siblings; confusion and insecurity (appetite and sleep disturbances)
Containment or confinement of mate and use of espionage tactics against her (i.e., checks mileage, times errands); cleverness depends on level of sophistication	Helplessly "allowing" containment, confinement, or restriction by mate; usually misinterpreted as caring behavior	Increasing deceptiveness, lying, excuses for outings, stealing, cheating, feeling trapped by parental dynamics
Use of invasive tactics; violates others' personal boundaries; rejects responsibility for failure (marital, familial, or occupational) or for violent acts	Gradually losing sight of personal boundaries for self and children; unable to assess danger accurately; accepts all blame	Poor definition of personal boundaries, violation of others' personal boundaries; accepts or projects blame
Belief that coercive behavior is aimed at securing the family nucleus ("for the good of the family")	Belief that transient acceptance of violent behavior will ultimately lead to long term resolution of family problems	Little or no understanding of the dynamics of violence; often assumes violence to be the norm
Absence of guilt or remorse on an emotional level, even after intellectual recognition	Emotional acceptance of guilt for mate's behavior; thinks mate "can't help it"; considers own behavior provocative	Self-blame (depending on age) for family feuding, separation, divorce, and internal conflicts
Generational history of abuse	Generational history of witnessing abuse in family or being abused	Continuation of abuse pattern in adult life

Table 12–1 ■ BEHAVIORAL CHARACTERISTICS OF DOMESTIC VIOLENCE *(Continued)*

Batterer Is Characterized By	Battered Mate Is Characterized By	Abused Children Are Characterized By
Frequent participation in pecking order battering	Participation in pecking order battering	Frequent participation in pecking order pattern (maims or kills animals, abuses siblings); often abuses parents in later years
Assaultive skills that improve with age and experience (increase in danger potential and lethality risks to family members over time)	"Creative" behavior that either diverts or precipitates mate's violence; but level of carelessness increases (judgment of lethality potential deteriorates) over time	Poor problem-solving skills; may use violence as problem-solving technique in school, with peers, with family (appears as early as preschool); demonstrates aggression or passivity
Demanding and often assaultive role in sexual activities; sometimes punishes with abstinence, at times experiences impotence	Poor sexual self-image, assumes that role is total acceptance of partner's sexual behavior; attempts at abstinence result in further abuse	Poor sexual image, uncertainty about appropriate behavior, confused model identification, immaturity in peer relationships
Increasingly assaultive behavior when mate is pregnant; pregnancy often marks the first assault	High risk for assaults or abuse during pregnancy	Higher risk for assaults during mother's pregnancy
Controlling mate by threatening homicide or suicide; often attempts one or both when partners separate (known to complete either or both)	Frequent contemplation of suicide; history of minor attempts, occasionally completes suicide or becomes a homicide victim; frequently wishes partner dead; occasionally completes homicide in self-defense	Heightened suicide risks and attempts; increased thoughts of suicide or murdering parents; prone to negligence and carelessness
Frequently using children as "pawns" and exerts power and control through custody issues; may kidnap or hold children hostage	Powerless in custody issues; lives in fear children will be "kidnapped," struggles to maintain rights of children and self; may use "underground" to escape	Feeling used and powerless in all decisions (age specific) regarding custody issues, including current or proposed living situation

Courtesy of Vicki D. Boyd, PhD, and Karil S. Klingbeil, MSW, ACSW, Seattle, Washington.

Crisis Situation

Anyone may be at risk for abuse in a situation that puts stress and strain on a family with an abuse-prone member. Stressful life events tax coping skills, leaving the abuse-prone person incapable of dealing with periods of increased stress. A person with good impulse control who can solve problems and has a healthy support system is less likely to resort to abusive behavior. A person who projects anger and frustration onto the environment in times of stress is at high risk for an abusive situation.

THE CYCLE OF VIOLENCE

Walker's (1979) **cycle theory of violence** was developed from a study of 400 women in violent families. It describes three stages of violence: the tension-building stage, the acute battering stage, and the honeymoon stage.

Tension-building Stage

The **tension-building stage** is characterized by such minor incidents as pushing, shoving, and verbal abuse.

Acute Battering Stage

During the **acute battering stage,** the abuser releases the built-up tension by brutal and uncontrollable beatings. The abuser is unable to control the degree of destructiveness inflicted on the victim. Severe injuries may result. The abuser usually has complete amnesia and does not remember what happened during the battering. The victim usually depersonalizes the incident and is able to remember the beatings in detail. After the beatings, both are in shock.

Honeymoon Stage

The **honeymoon stage** is characterized by kindness and loving behaviors. The abuser feels remorseful and apologetic and may bring presents, make promises, and generally tell the victim how much she or he is loved and needed. The victim usually believes the promises, feels needed and loved, and drops any legal proceedings or plans to leave that may have been initiated during the acute battering stage. Unfortunately, without intervention, the cycle will repeat itself. The honeymoon stage will fade away as tension starts to build.

Without treatment, violence never diminishes but almost always escalates in frequency and intensity.

With each repeat of the cycle, the beatings usually become more severe and the victim's self-esteem more and more eroded. The victim either believes the beatings were deserved or accepts the blame for them. This leads to feelings of depression, hopelessness, and immobilization.

TYPES OF ABUSE

Five specific types of abuse have been identified: (1) physical abuse, (2) sexual abuse, (3) emotional abuse, (4) neglect, and (5) economic abuse.

Physical Abuse

Physical battering and physical endangerment are two types of **physical abuse.** Physical **battering** refers to physical assaults, such as hitting, kicking, biting, throwing, and burning. Physical **endangerment** is reckless behavior toward a vulnerable person that could lead to serious physical injury (e.g., leaving an immobilized elderly person alone for long periods of time or allowing a child to play in an environment where toxic chemicals are within reach).

Sexual Abuse

Sexual abuse of children, usually by a father or step-father, is now reported in such numbers that it may well be the most common form of abuse of children. See Box 12–4 for forms of sexual abuse of children. Childhood sexual abuse destroys an individual's positive self-concept and interferes with the learning of self-care skills (Rew 1990). Child victims fail to develop either a positive sense of caring *about* themselves or a protective sense of caring *for* themselves. (Sexual abuse of adults is usually referred to as sexual assault or rape and is discussed in Chapter 13).

Emotional Abuse

Emotional abuse kills the spirit and the ability to succeed later in life, to feel deeply, and to make emotional contact with others. Emotional abuse can take the form of

- Terrorizing the victim through verbal threats
- Demeaning the victim's worth
- Blatant or subtle hostility and hate directed toward the victim
- Constantly ignoring the victim and his or her needs
- Consistent belittling and criticisms
- Withholding warmth or affection

Box 12–4. FORMS OF SEXUAL ABUSE OF CHILDREN

Touching, fondling, and physically exploring child's genitalia

Masturbation by male abuser against child's perineum, buttocks, abdomen, or thighs

Manual masturbation of abuser by child

All combinations of oral-genital contact between child of either sex and adult of either sex

Actual or attempted anal intercourse with child of either sex

Actual or attempted vaginal intercourse (without force)

Forceful attempt at vaginal intercourse, with local or general trauma

Exhibitionism

Voyeurism

Exploitation of children in preparation of sexually suggestive or pornographic materials

---

Data from Ghent WR, DaSylva NP, Farren ME. Family violence: Guidelines for recognition and management. Canadian Medical Association Journal, 132(5):545, 1985.

Neglect

Neglect can be physical, developmental, or educational. *Physical neglect* is failure to provide the medical, dental, or psychiatric care needed to prevent or treat physical or emotional illnesses. *Developmental neglect* is failure to provide emotional nurturing and the physical and cognitive stimulation needed to ensure freedom from developmental deficits. The physical consequences of child abuse are typically overshadowed by the associated disruption in the child's critical areas of development, such as trust, attachment, self-control, and moral and social judgments. Lack in these areas results in emotional and behavioral problems in abused children (Wolfe 1987). *Educational neglect* occurs when a child's caretakers deprive the child of the education provided in accordance with the state's education law. Adolescents are most often the victims of neglect as manifested by such things as abandonment, inattention to health care, inadequate supervision including permitting or condoning maladaptive behavior (e.g., substance abuse), deprivation of necessities, educational neglect, and emotional neglect (Wissow 1990). Neglect of the elderly is an especially disturbing phenomenon. Caregivers may withhold proper medical care, allow their elderly family member to live in unsafe conditions, and let them go without sufficient food or clothing.

Economic Abuse

Economic abuse refers to using another's resources, without permission, for one's personal gain. This can occur, for example, when family members deplete an elderly person's resources without the person's knowledge, as well as when an abusive husband squanders his wife's income or refuses to allow her access to money because he wants to maintain her dependence on him.

Assessment

Victims of abuse present in every health care setting including outpatient clinics, emergency departments, general hospitals, and nursing homes. Complaints may be vague and include sleep disorders, abdominal pain, headache, or menstrual problems. Sensitivity is required on the part of the nurse who might suspect abuse. Awareness of the nurse's feelings and attention to the process and setting of the interview are important to facilitating accurate assessment of physical and behavioral indicators of abuse.

ASSESSING THE NURSE'S FEELINGS

In all areas of psychiatric nursing and counseling, personal emotions and thoughts should be consciously available to the nurse. Strong negative feelings can cloud one's judgment and interfere with assessment and intervention no matter how well the nurse tries to cover or deny feelings. Perhaps more than in any other situation, intense and overwhelming feelings may be aroused in working with victims of abuse. Common reactions include (1) intense protective feelings and sympathy for the victim and (2) anger and outrage toward the abuser.

Intense feelings of sympathy and protectiveness triggered by the victim's pain and vulnerability may lead to "rescue fantasies" in the nurse. When this happens, the nurse projects personal emotional needs onto the victim, and the tendency is to be the "savior." When the rescue contract is not fulfilled, the victim is left more isolated than ever.

Outrage and anger toward abusers may lead to ignoring their needs. In the case of child abuse, parents' support and involvement in a treatment plan may be the best option for stopping abuse.

Interdisciplinary team conferences can be especially helpful in clarifying reactions and neutralizing intense emotions. Information from physicians, psychologists, nurses, and social workers can assist in refocusing efforts to work constructively with a family in crisis. Sharing perceptions and feelings with other professionals can help reduce feelings of isolation for nurses and lessen the feelings of responsibility for the victim.

THE PROCESS AND SETTING OF THE INTERVIEW

Important and relevant information about the family situation can be gathered from the conversations with the victim and, when appropriate, the abuser. Important interviewing guidelines are listed in Table 12–2.

A great deal of tact, understanding, and thought needs to go into planning an interview with the victim or suspected abuser. A person who feels judged or accused of wrongdoing is most likely to become defensive, and any attempts at changing coping strategies in the family are thwarted.

During interviewing, a calm and relaxed attitude is extremely important to lower their victim's anxiety. Sit near victims and spend some time establishing a rapport with them before focusing on the details of the abuse experience. Reassure them that they did not do anything wrong. The experience should be nonthreatening and supportive and not resemble a trial or inquisition. Questions that may be asked of children, for example, include

- *How did this happen to you?*
- *Who takes care of you?*
- *What do you do after school?*
- *Who are your friends?*
- *What happens when you do something wrong?*

Similar questions can be asked of female or elderly victims: for example, "How did this happen to you?" and "How do you and your spouse/caregiver resolve disagreements?"

An interview built on concern and carried out in an atmosphere that is nonjudgmental is most effective with an abuser. Such statements as "It must be difficult to care for three small children when there is little food in the house" or "Being responsible for two elderly parents without the help of family or friends must be hard on you" are useful for eliciting important data that help the nurse plan more effective alternatives and coping strategies. When the abuser is informed that a referral to Child/Adult Protective Services has been made, for example, it should be emphasized that the referral is not punishment but an attempt to safeguard the victim and obtain help for the family.

Table 12–2 ■ INTERVIEW OF AN ABUSER OR AN ABUSE VICTIM

DO'S	DON'TS
• Conduct the interview in private.	• Do *not* try to "prove" abuse by accusations or demands.
• Be direct, honest, and professional.	• Do *not* display horror, anger, shock, or disapproval of the abuser or the situation.
• Be understanding.	• Do *not* place blame or make judgments about the abuser or victim.
• Be attentive.	• Do *not* allow the victim to feel "at fault" or "in trouble."
• Inform the client if you must make a referral to Child/Adult Protective Services and explain the process.	• Do *not* probe or press for answers the victim is not willing to give.
• Assess safety and help reduce danger (at discharge).	• Do *not* conduct the interview with a group of interviewers.

Specific to Children	
• Tell the child that the interview is confidential.	• Do *not* force the child to remove clothing.
• Use language the child understands.	
• Ask the child to clarify words that you do not understand.	
• Tell the child whether any future action will be required.	

Questions that are open ended and require a descriptive response can be less threatening and elicit more relevant information than questions that are direct or can be answered yes or no. Some examples for parents of abused children follow.

- *What arrangements do you make when you have to leave your child alone?*
- *How do you punish your child?*
- *When your infant cries for a long time, how do you get him or her to stop?*
- *What does your child do that makes you cry?*

Openness and directness about the situation can strengthen the relationship with the victims. The following vignette illustrates the key points for a nurse assessing a woman in crisis at the initial interview as well as suggested follow-up.

Darnell Peters is a 42-year-old married woman in a relationship she describes as "being bad for a long time. We don't communicate." She is brought to the emergency department by ambulance with lacerations to her face and swollen eyes, lips, and nose. She tells the nurse that her husband had been in bed asleep for hours before she joined him. On getting into bed, she attempted to redistribute the blankets. Suddenly, he leaped from the bed, started punching her in the face, and began to throw her against the wall. She called for her 11-year-old son to call the police. The police arrived, called an ambulance, and took Mr. Peters to jail.

The nurse takes Ms. Peters to an individual examination room (to emphasize *confidentiality*) to *ask questions for ascertaining the whole problem*. Ms. Peters states that their relationship is always stormy. "He always is putting me down and yelling at me." He started hitting her five years ago when she became pregnant with her second and last child. The beatings have increased in intensity over the past year, and this emergency department visit is the fifth this year. Tonight is the first time she has ever called the police.

Ms. Peters is visibly upset. Periods of crying alternate with periods of silence. She appears apathetic and depressed. The nurse remains calm and objective. After Ms. Peters has finished talking, the nurse explores alternatives designed to help her reduce the danger when she is discharged. *"I'm concerned you will be hurt again if you go home. What options do you have?"* Acknowledging the escalating intensity of the violence, Ms. Peters is able to make arrangements with a shelter to take her and her two children in until after she has secured a restraining order.

The nurse carefully and completely charts the abuse referrals so that proper follow-up care can be given to assist Ms. Peters as she pursues legal action (see the section Maintaining Accurate Records).

For determining the need for further help, it is also useful to assess (1) level of anxiety and coping responses, (2) support systems, (3) family coping patterns, (4) abuse indicators, (5) suicide potential, and (6) drug and alcohol abuse.

ASSESSING THE LEVEL OF ANXIETY AND COPING RESPONSES

Nonverbal responses to history taking can be indicative of the victim's anxiety level. The identification of anxiety levels is described in Chapter 9. Hesitation, lack of eye contact, and vague statements, such as "It's been rough lately," indicate the victim is dealing with a problem that is difficult to talk about.

Agitation and anxiety bordering on panic are often present in abused women. They may be apprehensive of imminent doom, with good reason, as their husbands threaten violence, death, or mutilation. Because they live in terror, battered women remain vigilant, unable to relax or sleep. When they do sleep, they may have nightmares of danger and violence. Signs of the effect of living with chronic stress and severe levels of anxiety may be present, such as hypertension, irritability, or gastrointestinal disturbances.

The coping mechanisms many battered women employ to live in violent and terrifying situations often prevent the dissolution of the marriage. These coping mechanisms are in the form of beliefs or myths and are included in Table 12–3. Because of feelings of confusion, shame, despair, and powerlessness, victims may withdraw from interaction with others (Moss 1991).

Having elderly victims relate the events of an average day can supply essential information about how they are coping and clarify for the interviewer their experience of isolation. As a result of their isolation, their self-esteem plummets further, and any sense of control over their lives is lost. Self-blame is used as a temporary coping device. In an attempt to retain a sense of control, the victim thinks that if something had been done differently, the abuse would not have occurred. So the victim tries to be the perfect child, wife, mother, or parent. Eventually, all efforts fail, and a profound sense of powerlessness results. The victim begins to feel that the abuse is deserved and sees no options for escape, even if alternatives are present. A child and a dependent elderly person may in fact have no options without outside intervention. A pattern of learned helplessness may develop. Because solutions to the problem have failed in the past, further effort may cease.

Table 12–3 ■ MYTHS VERSUS FACTS: SPOUSE ABUSE

MYTH	FACT
1. The woman's behavior often causes the man to strike out at her.	1. The woman's behavior is *not* the cause of spouse abuse.
2. Men have the right to keep their wives in line.	2. No one has the right to beat or hurt another person.
3. Spouse abuse is a minor problem.	3. There is a *real* danger that a woman may be killed by a violent partner.
4. Battered women are masochistic and like to be beaten. (The abuse cannot be that bad or the woman would leave.)	4. Women do not like, ask, or deserve to be abused. Economic considerations are usually the only reason they stay.
5. Battered women come from poor working-class backgrounds and are usually poorly educated.	5. Studies show that battered women and batterers come from all socioeconomic, religious, and educational backgrounds.
6. The family is sacred and should be allowed to take care of its own problems.	6. Intervention in family violence is justified because it always escalates in frequency and intensity, can end in death, and is passed on to future generations.
7. Women who are abused tend to become helpless.	7. Women who are abused are not different from the rest of the population, except that most grew up with violence in their homes. After years of abuse, self-esteem is devastated.
8. Myths abused women believe: "I can't live without him." "If I hadn't done . . . , it wouldn't have happened." "He will change." "I stay for the sake of the children." "His jealousy and possessiveness prove he really loves me."	8. These myths are coping mechanisms women use to allay panic in a situation of random and brutal violence. They give the illusion of control and rationality.
9. Alcohol causes battering.	9. This myth offers an explanation and tolerance for battering. There are *no* excuses and it is *not* acceptable behavior. Alcohol use is correlated with battering but does not cause it!

ASSESSING SUPPORT SYSTEMS

The victim of abuse is usually in a dependent position, relying on the abuser (spouse, parent, other family member, or caregiver) for basic needs. In such situations, the victim may be or feel isolated from others. Contacts to the outside are often controlled by the abuser, which causes the victim to feel unconnected to other family members or friends. In addition, victims may feel unworthy and believe that no one else could possibly want anything to do with them, a reflection of their low self-esteem. Children's options are especially limited. Feelings of shame and disgrace also prevent victims from talking to others, including social agency supports or the criminal justice system. Assessing for support should focus on intrapersonal, interpersonal, and community resources.

ASSESSING FAMILY COPING PATTERNS

In assessing abuse in a family situation, the nurse must use great skill in questioning because the perpetrator may react with indifference or anger to such questions. The nurse must show a willingness to listen and avoid any judgmental tone during the interview. Questioning about memories of early family relationships can provide additional information about attitudes in the home. Find out about the family members' general income level and religious and cultural beliefs (Anderson and Thobaben 1984).

Attitudes about children, women, and the elderly and the roles and duties of each should be considered further. Notice whether the perpetrator views these roles in a negative light. In our society, responsibility for care of children and the elderly usually falls on the woman. If there are disputes, she is generally expected to mediate between the needs of her spouse and those of the child or older person. This burden may be difficult to bear physically and emotionally and may set her up for abuse. The problem is compounded if the husband refuses to share in the responsibility while feeling accountable. Living with children and older adults in the same household can cause frustration, stress, and anger. Abusive behavior (battered child, women, elderly syndrome) is linked to the way certain families cope with such situations.

ASSESSING ABUSE INDICATORS

PHYSICAL ABUSE. A series of minor complaints, such as headaches, dizziness, and "accidents," especially falls, may be covert indications of abuse. Overt signs of battering include bruises, scars, burns, and other wounds in various stages of healing, particularly around the head, face, chest, arms, abdomen, and genitalia (Haviland and O'Brien 1989). Signs of abuse may not be clearly manifested (Box 12–5). Injuries seen in emergency rooms and offices that should arouse the nurse's suspicion are included in Box 12–6. A physician's office or clinic may be one of the few places a battered woman or elder is allowed to go. Sickness is viewed as a legitimate excuse for seeking professional help. *If the explanation does not match the injury seen or if the patient minimizes the seriousness of the injury, abuse may be suspected.* The key to identification is a high index of suspicion.

Nonspecific bruising in older children is common. Any bruises on an infant less than six months old should be considered suspicious. A specific type of abuse to which young children are susceptible is shaking. They are more vulnerable because of their relatively large head size and weight; weak neck muscles; thin, friable central nervous system vasculature; and soft, less myelinated brain tissue. The baby who has been shaken may often present with respiratory problems. If the pulmonary examination is not normal, the possibility of rigorous shaking must be considered. Full bulging fontanels and a head circumfer-

---

Box 12–5. PHYSICAL SYMPTOMS INDICATING POSSIBLE SPOUSE OR ELDER ABUSE

Chief Complaints Without Physical Cause

- Headache
- Abdominal pain
- Insomnia
- Choking sensation
- Chest pain
- Back pain
- Dizziness
- "Accidents"

Presenting Problems (Signs of High Anxiety and Chronic Stress)

- Agitation
- Hyperventilation
- Panic attack
- Gastrointestinal disturbances
- Hypertension
- Physical injuries

Data from Swanson RW. Battered wife syndrome. Canadian Medical Association Journal, 130(6):709, 1984.

Box 12–6. PRESENTING INJURIES OF FAMILY ABUSE VICTIMS

In the Emergency Room

- Bleeding injuries, especially to the head and face
- Internal injuries, concussions, perforated eardrums, abdominal injuries, severe bruising, eye injuries, and strangulation marks on the neck
- Back injuries
- Broken or fractured jaws, arms, pelvis, ribs, clavicle, and legs
- Burns from cigarettes, appliances, scalding liquids, and acids
- Psychological trauma, anxiety, attacks of hyperventilation, heart palpitations, severe crying spells, and suicidal tendencies
- Miscarriages

In the Office or Clinic

- Perforated eardrums, twisted or stiff neck and shoulder muscles, headache
- Depression, stress-related conditions (e.g., insomnia, violent nightmares, anxiety, extreme fatigue, eczema, loss of hair)
- Talk of having "problems" with her husband or son, describing him as very jealous, impulsive, or an alcohol or drug abuser
- Repeated visits with new complaints

In Both Settings

- Observe child, spouse, or elder for signs of stress due to family violence: emotional, behavioral, school, or sleep problems and increased aggressive behavior

---

ence greater than the 90th percentile are also suggestive. Shaking can cause intracranial hemorrhage leading to cerebral edema and death (Ludwig and Kornberg 1992). Table 12–4 lists the physical and behavioral indicators of all types of physical abuse.

Ask directly, but in a nonthreatening manner, whether the injury has been caused by someone close to them. Observe the nonverbal response, such as hesitation or lack of eye contact, as well as the verbal response. Then ask specific questions, such as "When was the last time it happened?" "How often does it happen?" "In what ways are you hurt?"

Along with recognition of the indicators of physical abuse, nurses should note the alleged method of injury. Inconsistent explanations serve as a warning that

further investigation is necessary. Vague explanations, such as "she fell from a chair (a lap, down the stairs)," "the child was running away," or "the hot water was turned on by mistake," should alert the nurse to possible abuse (Ghent et al. 1985).

After the history of abuse has been ascertained, carefully document verbal statements as well as physical findings. Sketch a body map and draw areas of injury with accompanying explanation. If the patient consents, take Polaroid photos. If the beating has just occurred, ask the patient to return in a day or two for more photos; bruises may be more evident at that time.

SEXUAL ABUSE. Sexual abuse of children and dependent elders has been receiving more attention and concern. Unfortunately, there is a drastic lack of documentation by health care professionals of medical and social data in cases of sexual abuse. Nurses need to be familiar with the physical and behavioral indicators of sexual abuse as presented in Table 12–5. Once these indicators have been identified and the possibility of sexual abuse is suspected, appropriate action must be taken to protect the victim from further devastating emotional and physical effects of sexual abuse (Stanley 1989).

Ms. Randall, an 83-year-old, is admitted from an adult foster home for evaluation of deterioration in her mental status. She appears confused and disoriented and is not able to give a coherent history. Blood and urine are collected for diagnostic evaluation. The laboratory report noted semen in the urine. Adult Protective Services is called to begin an investigation into the adult family home.

EMOTIONAL ABUSE. Whenever physical or sexual abuse is occurring, emotional abuse occurs also. In addition, it may exist alone. With emotional abuse, low self-esteem, anguish, and isolation are instilled in place of love and acceptance. Emotional abuse is less obvious and more difficult to assess than is physical abuse. Intimidation or threats may be used to keep victims from revealing their plight, causing the victim to react to the nurse with passivity, withdrawal, or discounting. Table 12–6 lists the physical and behavioral indicators of emotional abuse.

NEGLECT. Neglect may stem from both benign and hostile causes. When a person does not meet another's needs because of a lack of resources, the neglect is benign. When the perpetrator is well intentioned, response to educational efforts is healthy and constructive. Education combined with support is sufficient to create positive change. Neglect may also stem from hostility, however, signaling a serious disturbance in the caregiving relationship. In such a case, education is not sufficient, and more rigorous inter-

Table 12–4 ■ PHYSICAL AND BEHAVIORAL INDICATORS OF PHYSICAL ABUSE

PHYSICAL INDICATORS	BEHAVIORAL INDICATORS
Unexplained bruises and welts of varying age: • On face, lips, mouth • On torso, back, buttocks, thighs • In various stages of healing • Clustered, forming regular patterns • Reflecting shape of article used to inflict (e.g., electrical cord, belt buckle) • On several different surface areas • Regular appearance after absence, weekend, or vacation • Human bites • Fingernail indentations Unexplained burns: • Small, circular burns—cigar or cigarette burns, especially on soles, palms, back, or buttocks • Immersion burns, sock-like, glove-like • Patterned like electrical burner, iron, etc. • Rope burns on arms, legs, neck, or torso Unexplained fractures or dislocations (especially in children under one year): • To skull, nose, facial structure • In various stages of healing • Multiple spiral fractures • Dislocation of shoulder or hip Unexplained lacerations or abrasions of varying age: • To mouth, lips, gums, eyes • To external genitalia Evidence of improper care: • Inappropriate restraining • Inappropriate administration of medications (e.g., drowsiness or confusion from sedatives) Other: • Bald patches on the scalp • Subdural hematoma in a child under two years • Retinal hemorrhage	Wary of adult contacts Apprehensive when other children cry Behavioral extremes: • Aggressiveness • Withdrawal Frightened of parents or constant effort to please parents Afraid to go home Reports injury by parents Monosyllabic speech Ability to withstand examination and painful procedures with little movement or crying Indiscriminate seeking of affection Goes to extremes (including misbehaving) to call attention to self Demonstration of fear by victim Excessive dependence of victim on caregiver "Blaming" of victim by caregiver (e.g., complaining that incontinence was a deliberate act)

Data from Heindl C, et al. The Nurse's Role in the Prevention and Treatment of Child Abuse and Neglect. Washington, DC: US Department of Health, Education, and Welfare, 1979. Publication No. 79-30202; Ebersole P, Hess P. Toward Healthy Aging. St. Louis: CV Mosby, 1990.

Table 12–5 ■ SUMMARY OF PHYSICAL AND BEHAVIORAL INDICATORS OF SEXUAL ABUSE

PHYSICAL INDICATORS	BEHAVIORAL INDICATORS
Difficulty in walking or sitting Vulvovaginitis Torn, stained, or bloody underclothing Pain or itching in genital area Bruises or bleeding in external genitalia, vaginal area, or anal area Venereal disease, especially in preteens Pregnancy Evidence of physical manipulation of the vagina Evidence of foreign body in the vagina In boys, pain on urination or penile swelling or discharge	Unwilling to change for gym or participate in physical education class Seductive behavior Withdrawal, fantasy, or infantile behavior (regression) Bizarre, sophisticated, or unusual sexual behavior or knowledge Phobias: • Fear of the dark, men, strangers, leaving the house Poor peer relationships Delinquent or runaway—severe acting out Profound personality change: • Depression, aggression, decline in school performance Reports sexual assault by caretaker Self-destructive behavior: • Alcohol or drug abuse • Attempted suicide

Data from Heindl C, et al. The Nurse's Role in the Prevention and Treatment of Child Abuse and Neglect. Washington, DC: US Department of Health, Education, and Welfare, 1979. Publication No. 79-30202.

Table 12-6 ■ PHYSICAL AND BEHAVIORAL INDICATORS OF EMOTIONAL ABUSE

PHYSICAL INDICATORS	BEHAVIORAL INDICATORS
Speech disorders Lag in physical development	Habit disorders (sucking, biting, rocking, head banging, feeding problems) Conduct disorder (antisocial, destructive, others) Difficulty in learning and living up to full potential Neurotic trait (sleep disorders, inhibition of play, unusual fearfulness) Psychoneurotic reaction (hysteria, obsessions, compulsion, phobias, hypochondriasis) Behavior extremes: • Compliant, passive • Aggressive, demanding • Agitated Expression of ambivalent feelings toward family Overly adaptive behavior • Inappropriately adult or inappropriately infantile • "On guard"—trying to please everyone Developmental lag (mental, emotional) Suicide attempt

Data from Heindl C, et al. The Nurse's Role in the Prevention and Treatment of Child Abuse and Neglect. US Department of Health, Education, and Welfare, 1979. Publication No. 79-30202.

ventions are needed to safeguard the child or older adult from permanent physical and emotional harm. Neglected children and elders often appear undernourished, dirty, and poorly clothed. Neglect is also manifested by inadequate medical care, such as lack of immunizations or untreated medical conditions. Specific physical and behavioral indicators of neglect are listed in Table 12-7.

ECONOMIC ABUSE. At times, money may serve as a motive for keeping the older adult at home, even if institutionalization is recommended. If the elderly are no longer able to care for their funds, the family may use some for their own personal purposes, thus restricting the older adult or not allowing the elder to

meet basic needs. When the elder is compelled to use all personal resources in return for care, abuse is occurring (Fulmer 1991).

ASSESSING SUICIDE POTENTIAL

An abuse victim may feel so trapped in a detrimental relationship yet so desperate to get out that suicide may be attempted. The threat of suicide may also be used by an emotionally abusive person in an attempt to manipulate the partner or spouse into caving in to demands (e.g., "Don't leave me or I'll kill myself." "I took all my pills. I said I would the next time you were late.").

Table 12-7 ■ PHYSICAL AND BEHAVIORAL INDICATORS OF NEGLECT

PHYSICAL INDICATORS	BEHAVIORAL INDICATORS
Consistent hunger, poor hygiene, inappropriate dress (for weather conditions) Consistent lack of supervision, especially in dangerous activities or for long periods Unattended physical problems or medical or dental needs • Missing false teeth, hearing aids, or eyeglasses • Gross pressure ulcers • Dehydration, weight loss, or malnourishment without an illness-related condition • Poor hygiene (e.g., uncut hair, decayed teeth, and overgrown toenails) • Scratching or picking at sores Abandonment Poor growth patterns: underweight, failure to thrive	Begging, stealing food Extended stays at school (early arrival and late departure) Constant fatigue, listlessness, or falling asleep in class; dull, inactive (in infants also) Alcohol or drug abuse Psychosomatic complaints Delinquency (e.g., thefts) Assumes adult responsibilities States there is no caretaker Lack of eye contact with caregiver

Data from Heindl C, et al. The Nurse's Role in the Prevention and Treatment of Child Abuse and Neglect. Washington, DC: US Department of Health, Education, and Welfare, 1979. Publication No. 79-30202; Ebersole P, Hess P. Toward Healthy Aging. St. Louis: CV Mosby, 1990.

A suicide attempt may be the presenting symptom in the emergency department. It has been estimated that 10% of abused women attempt suicide (Walker 1991). With sensitive questioning conducted in a caring manner, the nurse can elicit the abuse history (McLeer et al. 1989). Often the overdose will be with a combination of alcohol and other central nervous system depressants, tranquilizers, or sleeping medications that have been prescribed in previous visits to physicians' offices, clinics, or emergency departments.

When the crisis of the immediate suicide attempt has resolved, careful questioning to determine lethality is in order (see Chapter 21 for suicide assessment). For example, if the patient still feels that life is not worth living and has some pills at home that might be used, admission to an inpatient psychiatric unit must be considered. On the other hand, if the patient is talking about future plans and hanging in there "for the sake of the children," then outpatient referrals may be given, and the patient can be discharged. Each situation is dealt with individually.

ASSESSING DRUG AND ALCOHOL USE

A battered spouse or elder may self-medicate with alcohol or other drugs as a way of escaping a dreadful situation. The drugs are usually central nervous system depressants, such as benzodiazepines, prescribed by physicians in response to the battered victim's presentation with "vague" complaints. Alcohol and drug use also obviates a woman's responsibility in the battering situation: "I was intoxicated, I couldn't defend myself" or "I couldn't think clearly."

The level of intoxication can be determined by history, physical examination, and blood alcohol level. If the battered woman is intoxicated, allow her to sober up in the emergency department before instituting referral. Referral information will not be understood or assimilated if she is intoxicated. She should *not* be discharged with her husband.

The abused woman or elder may have a chronic alcohol or drug problem. This needs to be assessed (refer to Chapters 23 and 24) and appropriate treatment referrals need to be provided. Choices for treatment can include both inpatient and outpatient options.

MAINTAINING ACCURATE RECORDS

Because of the possibility of legal action, it is essential that the **medical-nursing record** contain an accu-

rate and detailed description of the victim's medical history, the psychosocial history of the family, and observations of the family interactions during the interviews. Especially important in documenting findings from initial assessment are (1) verbatim statements of both victim and perpetrators, if available, (2) a body map to indicate areas and types of injuries, and (3) physical evidence, when possible, of sexual abuse. Even if intervention does not occur at this time, the record is begun. The next provider will not have to stumble across the problem and will be in a better position to offer support.

Nursing Diagnosis

Nursing diagnoses can be many and varied for the abuse victim. There will most likely be a number of areas of concern and problems resulting from the abuse as well as the safety issue. Abuse is a situational crisis with attendant threats to the victim's physical, emotional, and psychological health and, ultimately, life. H*igh risk for injury, anxiety,* and *fear* are three diagnoses that apply. *Powerlessness* is a diagnosis that can be applied to any abused individual.

Abuse victims often think they have no control or influence over what happens to them. Feelings of helplessness, hopelessness, and powerlessness contribute to the diagnosis of *body image disturbances* and *self-esteem disturbances.* The crisis of family violence precipitates *altered family process* as the family system becomes less able to meet the emotional, physical, or security needs of its members.

Pain related to physical injury or trauma would most certainly take high priority and need immediate attention.

Planning

Planning interventions always includes planning on both (1) the content level and (2) the process level. The content level is the actual delineation of client-centered goals and designing of nursing interventions that facilitate meeting the goals. The process level of planning care involves the recognition of common reactions and emotions that may be evoked in health professionals by specific client behaviors. Awareness of how to deal effectively with strong feelings and reactions is important in maximizing care of the patient. Intense feelings, either positive or negative, can interfere with judgment, attitudes, and reactions to our patients, whether on a conscious or an unconscious level. Intense unexamined feelings toward patients can lead to power struggles, mutual lowering of self-esteem, and mutual withdrawal.

CONTENT LEVEL— PLANNING GOALS

With each nursing diagnosis, long term and short term goals are identified. They are directed toward the client and the abuser in specific circumstances. Diagnoses with possible goals for child, female, and elderly abuse victims are listed.

Altered family process related to the illness of one parent and difficulty with finances

Long Term Goals

- By (date), parents will state that group meetings with other parents who have battered are useful.
- Parents and child will share in two planned pleasurable activities twice a day when the child returns to the home.

Short Term Goals

- Within 24 hours, parents will be able to name and call three agencies that can help financially during the crisis.
- By the end of the first interview, parents will be able to name two places they can contact to discuss feelings of rage and helplessness.
- Within two weeks, parents will be able to name three alternative actions to take when feelings of helplessness and rage start to surface.

Altered family process related to inadequate marital relationship (applies when the battered woman chooses to stay with her mate)

Long Term Goals

- The batterer will state that he realizes he must change in order to stay with his family.
- The batterer will join and attend a group for spouses who batter.
- Within three months, the couple will state that they want to join a couples therapy group.
- The couple will be able to name three possible effects that family violence may have on their children.
- Within six months, the couple will state that the battering has ceased altogether.

Short Term Goals

- Client will state she is interested in knowing about family treatment modalities.
- Client will state that she no longer chooses to live in a situation with violence.
- Client will name three places she can call to receive counseling for herself, family, or batterer.

Altered family process related to demands of caring for a dependent elder

Long Term Goals

- Family members will seek counseling for behaviors by (date).
- Family members will state they will meet with the nurse on a weekly basis for counseling starting (date).
- Abuser will meet with other family members and discuss feelings on care of elderly by (date).
- Family members will meet together and discuss alternatives for care of the elderly by (date).
- Client and family will meet together and discuss resources and supports they feel are important to them by (date).
- Family members will demonstrate, instead of violence, two appropriate methods of dealing with frustration.

Short Term Goals

- Family members will meet together and discuss alternative ways of dealing with elderly client by (date).
- Family members will name two strategies for avoiding physical or emotional abuse of the client by (date).
- Family members will name two support services to whom they can turn for help by (date).
- One other family member will spend time with the elder and relieve abuser of caregiving duties by (date).

High risk for injury related to poor impulse control of mate

Long Term Goals

- Within three weeks, client will state that she believes she does not deserve to be beaten.
- Within three weeks, client will state that she has joined a women's support group or is having family counseling.
- Client will state that her living conditions are now safe from spouse abuse

or

- Within two months, client will state that she has found safe housing for herself and the children.

Short Term Goals

- After initial interview, client will name four community resources she can contact (hotlines, shelters, support groups).
- After initial interview, client will describe a safety plan to be used in future violent situations.
- Client will state her right to live in a safe environment.
- Client will state the dangers to her and her children in her home situation.
- Client will state she knows how to obtain a restraining order.

High risk for injury related to violent parent

Long Term Goals

- Child will know what plans are made for his or her protection and will state them to the nurse after decision is made by health care team.

Short Term Goals

- Child will be safe until adequate home and family assessment is made by (date).
- Child will be treated by physician and receive medical care for injuries within one hour.
- Child will participate with therapist (nurse, social worker, counselor) for the purpose of therapy and emotional support (art, play, group, or other) within 24 hours.

High risk for injury related to being a dependent elder

Long Term Goals

- Client will state that the caregiver has provided adequate food, clothing, housing, and medical care by (date).
- Client will be free of physical signs of abuse by (date).

Short Term Goals

- Client will state that he or she feels safer and more comfortable by (date)

or

- Client will ask to be removed from abusive situation by (date).
- Client will name one person who can be called for help by (date).

See Scherb (1988) for an example of a standardized care plan for suspected abuse and neglect of children.

PROCESS LEVEL—NURSES' REACTIONS AND FEELINGS

The more thought the nurse gives to the issue of domestic violence before encountering an abuse victim, the more effective is the subsequent interaction with the victim. Acknowledging accepted myths is the first step in at least putting them aside in working with an abused client, and it eventually allows counteracting them with facts. Myths have served to perpetuate acceptance of abuse (King 1989). Refer to Table 12–3 for some myths regarding spouse abuse and facts that counter them. Which of these are similar for abuse of children and elders?

Nurses are members of society and have been socialized to live within the social norms that contribute to the treatment of children, women, and the elderly as second-class citizens. Some nurses may still believe that it is acceptable for parents to hit children and for men to physically beat women. American society is violent, and some nurses may accept violence as a way of life. A nurse reacts to an abuse victim in large measure as a result of the way the nurse has been socialized. Some nurses have grown up in abusing households; some may currently live in abusive homes. Awareness of individual feelings and reactions facilitates caregiving in that the nurse can consciously and deliberately respond to the victim rather than get sidetracked into having to deal with personal reactions. Common responses of health care professionals to abuse are listed in Table 12–8 (Greany 1984; Delgaty 1985). These feelings need to be recognized when they arise and dealt with in supervision for therapeutic intervention to be maximized (Limandri 1987).

Awareness of personal feelings in response to the abuse victim stimulates examination of personal views toward violence and the status of children, women, and elders. Understanding the dynamics of abuse is crucial to effective nursing intervention. It is helpful as well as advisable for nurses working with people involved in family violence to review their cases with other professionals in peer supervision or with a clinical supervisor. Issues involving abuse usually evoke strong and frequently irrational feelings. Nurses need to sort out their own strong feelings through professional or peer supervision before they can work effectively with their clients.

Intervention

Nurses have a legal responsibility and are mandated to report suspected or actual cases of child abuse. At present, more than 40 states have mandatory report-

Table 12–8 ■ COMMON RESPONSES OF HEALTH CARE PROFESSIONALS TO ABUSE

FEELING	SOURCE
Anger	Anger may be felt toward the person responsible for the abuse, toward those who allowed it to happen, and toward society for condoning its occurrence through attitudes, traditions, and laws.
Embarrassment	The victim is a symbol of something close to home—the stress and strain of family life unleashed as uncontrolled anger.
Confusion	The victim challenges our cherished view of the family as a haven of safety and privacy.
Fear	A small percentage of batterers are dangerous to others.
Anguish	The nurse may have experienced family violence as a victim or a relative of a victim.
Helplessness	The nurse may want to do more, to eliminate the problem, to cure the victim.
Discouragement	Discouragement may result if no long term solution is achieved.

ing laws for elder abuse. When child or elder abuse is suspected, a report should be made to the protective agency designated by each state. The appropriate agency may be the state or county child welfare agency, law enforcement agency, juvenile court, or county health department. Each state has specific guidelines for reporting, including whether the report can be oral or written or both and specifying the time that can elapse after suspicion of abuse or neglect (stat, 24 hours, or 48 hours). Some states are examining similar mandatory requirements for spouse abuse.

An example follows of a case to report.

Two nurses who work in a family practice clinic are suspicious of child abuse. A 12-year-old girl has recurrent urinary tract infections. She is always accompanied to clinic visits by her father, who even goes into the bathroom with her when she is producing urine samples. He answers all questions for her even when they are directed toward her. He has recently refused the next diagnostic test for attempting to ascertain the reason for the recurrent infections. After pressure by the nurses, the physician agrees to ask the girl some questions in private. The nurses think he has discounted the problem, asked superficial questions, and dismissed their concern. They attempt to get the girl alone for a discussion, but to no avail. After consultation with clinical resources, they decide to report their concerns to Children's Protective Services. Subsequent investigation confirms the likelihood of sexual abuse, and the child is placed in temporary foster care with follow-up counseling. The father refuses treatment and four months later leaves the family.

This case illustrates that a reasonable basis for suspecting maltreatment, not proof, is all that is required to report. Nurses must attempt to maintain both an appropriate level of suspicion and a neutral, objective attitude. One can be too concerned and jump to conclusions (which is what the physician in this case thought the nurses were doing) or not concerned enough and rationalize an incomplete examination to avoid confrontation (which is what the nurses thought the physician was doing). Given these opposing stances, the case was reported, as required by law and ethical standards, and Children's Protective Services was given the opportunity to sort it out.

Immunity from criminal or civil liability is provided when reporting is mandated. There may be a risk to the ongoing health care relationship, but one must hold the victim's safety and health (mental, physical, and emotional) as most important (Stanley 1989).

Competency may be a consideration in an elder abuse situation. Unless incompetency has been established legally, elders have the right to self-determination. Some institutions and health care agencies have developed guidelines for dealing with actual or suspected abuse situations. These protocols list possible behaviors or conditions of the elderly and the most appropriate intervention. The establishment of such protocols is highly recommended because it gives support to the nurse's actions.

Primary prevention consists of those measures that are taken to prevent or reduce the occurrence of abusive situations. The aim of the interventions in primary prevention is to prevent maladaptive behaviors or disease by promoting optimum help. Identifying people at high risk, providing health teaching, and coordinating supportive services to prevent crises are examples of primary prevention.

Secondary prevention involves early intervention in abusive situations to minimize their disabling or long term effects. Nurses providing secondary prevention work with families and other members of the health care team to help those abusive families find alternative ways of dealing with stress. Community resources are mobilized (visiting nurse services, schools, clinics, homemaker agencies, Meals on Wheels, and more) to relieve overwhelming stress and to offer alternative outlets for emotions. Secondary prevention is often carried out in an outpatient setting. The following vignette illustrates a successful secondary prevention effort.

Billy J., four years old, is brought into the physician's office with second-degree burns on his right hand. Mary frequently babysits for Billy and his younger brother Jimmy, two, and older brother Tom, six. Mary appears apprehensive and states she is very concerned. Mary tells the nurse that the children have told her in the past that Billy's mother has threatened them with burning if they do not behave. Billy told her that once his mother had held his hands on a cold stove and told him if he was bad, she would burn him. Mary is shocked that Billy's mother would do such a thing, but at the same time, she mentions she feels guilty for "telling on Ms. J." Mary also states that the older brother told Mary what had happened but was afraid that if his mother found out, she would burn him also. Mary states she is aware that the mother hits the children, but she did not believe that anyone would burn her own child.

The nurse reports what happened to the physician, and the mother is called and asked to come to the office.

Billy appears frightened and in pain. The nurse asks Mary to come with Billy while she examines him.

NURSE: Tell me about your hand, Billy.
           Billy looks down and starts to cry.
NURSE: It's OK if you don't want to talk about it, Billy.
BILLY: *Not looking at the nurse, he says softly,* My mommy burned my hand on the stove.
NURSE: Tell me what happened before that happened.
BILLY: Mommy was mad because I didn't put my toys away.
NURSE: What does your mommy usually do when she gets mad?
BILLY: She yells mostly, sometimes she hits us. Mommy is going to be so mad at Tommy for telling.

NURSE: Tell me about the hitting.
BILLY: Mommy hits us a lot since daddy left us. *Billy starts to cry to himself.*

On examination, the nurse notices a ringed pattern of burns across Billy's right palm like the burner of an electric stove. There are blisters on the fingers. Billy appears well nourished and properly dressed. He is at his approximate developmental age except for some language delay.

Because of the physical evidence and history, there is strong suspicion of child abuse. Children's Protective Services is notified, and the family situation is evaluated for possible placement of Billy in protective custody. The initial evaluation concludes there is no indication of serious potential harm to the child and Billy should return home.

The mother, who was initially defensive, starts to cry and states, "I can't cope with being alone and I don't know where to turn." The intervention that the nurse facilitates centers around caring for Billy's immediate health needs; finding supports for the mother to help her cope with crises; providing a counseling referral for the mother to learn alternative ways of expressing anger and frustration; informing the mother of parents' groups; providing referrals to play groups or day care for the children to help increase their feelings of self-esteem and security; and providing a break from and perhaps some instruction in parenting for the mother.

Tertiary prevention involves interventions aimed at maintaining or reducing the severity of mental illness or handicaps resulting from chronic abusive trauma. Examples of offerings for tertiary care are general hospitals, psychiatric inpatient units, day care hospitals, adult family homes, foster homes, group homes, and shelters.

Two **stages of treatment** allow the most effective intervention, (1) the crisis stage and (2) the stage of internal change and rebuilding (Weingourt 1985).

The **crisis stage** includes (1) providing a safe atmosphere for reducing post-traumatic injury, (2) encouraging decision making, and (3) providing referral information.

Providing a Safe Atmosphere for Reducing Post-traumatic Injury

For example, if a woman abused by her spouse has no other alternatives within her own support system, **shelters or safe houses** are available in many communities. They are open 24 hours a day and can be accessed through hotline information, hospital emergency rooms, YWCAs, or the local office of the National Organization for Women (NOW). The address of the house is usually kept secret to protect the women from attack by their mates. Besides protection, many of these safe shelters provide important education and consciousness-raising functions. The woman should be given the number of the nearest available shelter, even if she decides for the present to stay with her husband. Referral phone numbers may be kept for years before the decision to call is made. Having the number all that time contributes to thinking about options.

If the woman chooses to stay, the next best approach is to help her develop a **safety plan,** a plan for a fast escape when violence recurs. Ask her to identify the signs of escalation of violence and to pick a particular sign that will tell her in the future "now is the time to leave." If children are present, they can all agree on a code word that, when spoken by their mother, means "it is time to go." If she plans ahead, she may be able to leave before the violence occurs. She should plan where she is going and how she will get there. Suggest that she have a bag already packed for herself and her children with a few articles of clothing, essential toiletry items, money for cab fare and phone calls, identification cards, insurance information, and a list of referral sources with their telephone numbers. (Many but by no means all communities have a 24-hour telephone number provided by the Domestic Abuse Warning Network, or help can be reached through a national hotline. People who answer the phone have information on the services available for battered women.)

Encouraging Decision Making

The abuse victim may have difficulty imagining options. It is useful to emphasize that people have a right to live without fear of violence or physical harm, without fear of assault. The role of the nurse is to support the victim and facilitate access to the legal system as appropriate. By listening, giving support, discussing options, and describing other ways of living, the nurse initiates an awareness of other possibilities.

Providing Referral Information

Battered women should also be given referrals to parenting resources that enable them to explore alternative approaches to discipline (i.e., no hitting, slapping, or other expressions of violence). It is distressing to see women in shelters use these methods with their children. Such behavior perpetuates the idea that violence solves problems and passes the problem of violence on to the next generation.

Individual counseling referrals and referrals for group therapy may also be given when available. Evaluating the need for referrals for the children may also be indicated if the children are in danger. Refer to Table 12–1 for the effects on children in homes where battering occurs.

Vocational counseling is another referral that may be appropriate. A list of programs for both men and women should be available to the client when indicated.

Specific referrals regarding emergency money and legal counseling should be made available to each woman. Emergency money is available through **Title XX of the 1974 Social Security Amendment Act.** These monies cover one month's rent and utilities, food for one month, emergency clothing, and emergency furniture. Legal assistance can take the form of an injunction, a civil suit, or criminal charges.

The **stage of internal change and rebuilding** includes focusing on rebuilding lives so destructive ways of relating are eliminated and self-esteem is elevated.

PSYCHOTHERAPEUTIC INTERVENTIONS

Effective interventions occur on multiple levels: individual, family, community, and social. Individual interventions are tailored to underlying psychological problems often resulting from childhood histories of victimization, coping deficiencies, stress-related symptoms, low self-esteem, or limited resources (intrapersonal as well as interpersonal). Family interventions may address marital discord and conflict, poor problem-solving abilities, responses to difficult child behavior, and methods for maximizing positive interactions among family members. Community interventions could be focused on socioeconomic conditions, support services for disadvantaged families, and job opportunities. Last, interventions directed to the social milieu would question, among other things, the acceptance of corporal punishment as a technique for guiding behavior in children, the unequal burden of caregiving responsibilities placed on women, and the low priority given to education and preparation for parenthood.

Psychotherapeutic interventions include crisis intervention and the promotion of growth. Children and vulnerable adults can have the state act in their interests because of limits in decision-making capabilities. Women must make the choice for themselves. Battered women are more successful at reversing their helplessness when they leave their husbands than when they remain and try to change their relationship.

Failures in interventions with abusive families are often due not to our lack or theirs but to deficits in the social, economic, and political systems in which we live. Being valued and protected as a child or elder and valued as a woman is not merely a privilege but a right. Our institutions often demonstrate the opposite (Pawl 1984).

HEALTH TEACHING

Health teaching is one of the most important aspects of primary prevention. The first line of intervention is prevention through teaching people additional ways of coping. In families at risk for violence (child, spouse, or elder), health teaching includes meeting with both the client and the family and discussing risk factors associated with violence. The client, caregiver, and family should learn to recognize behaviors and situations that might trigger abuse.

Normal developmental and physiological changes should be explained to enable family members to gain a more positive view of the child, woman, or older adult. This will help them avoid the often negative stereotyping of these groups. Gaining a more complete understanding can help family members broaden their insight and thus increase their compassion. They may then begin to anticipate new stress situations and be able to prepare for them before a crisis occurs.

Educating family members to analyze their respective roles and to develop suggestions for realignment or redistribution of responsibilities is important for effecting change in an abusive situation. The process would include assessing the need for role changes in all family members, identifying role conflicts, clarifying expectations, and strengthening the ability of family members to perform their individual roles.

Child abuse merits special attention here because being abused as a child is a predictor of being abusive as an adult. Recognition of an abuse-prone parent before abuse takes place is possible. Nurses who work on a maternity unit are often in a position to spot potential abusive situations in new mothers and to initiate appropriate interventions, including education about effective parenting techniques. Parents who stand out for special attention include

1. New parents whose behavior toward the infant is rejecting, hostile, or indifferent
2. Teenage parents, most of whom are children themselves and who require special help and guidance in handling the baby and discussing their expectations of the baby and their support systems
3. Retarded parents, for whom careful, explicit, and repeated instructions on caring for the child and recognizing the infant's needs are indicated

4. Parents who were abused as children or are abused by a spouse

Nurses can also recognize the vulnerable child. When it is known that specific children are at risk, referrals to community resources are in order. These may include emergency child care facilities, emergency telephone numbers, numbers of 24-hour crisis centers or hotlines, and respite programs in which volunteers take the child for an occasional weekend so that parents can get some relief. Public health nurses can

---

Box 12–7. FACTORS TO ASSESS DURING A HOME VISIT

For Child

Responsiveness to infant's crying
Responsiveness to infant's signals related to feeding
Caregiver's facial expressions in response to infant
Holding of the child
Playfulness of caregiver with infant
Type of physical contact during feeding
Temperament of the infant: average, quiet, or active
Parent's attitudes signaling possible warnings:

- Complaints of inadequacy as a parent
- Complaints of inadequacy of the child
- Fear of "doing something wrong"
- Attribution of badness to the newborn
- History of a destructive childhood
- Misdirected anger
- Continued evidence of isolation, apathy, anger, frustration, projection
- Adult conflict

Environmental conditions:

- Sleeping arrangements
- Child management
- Home management
- Use of supports (formal and informal)

Need for immediate services for situational (economics, child care), emotional, or educational information, that is:

- Sharing information about hotlines, babysitters, homemakers, parent groups
- Sharing information about child development
- Child care and home management

Continued

Box 12–7. FACTORS TO ASSESS DURING A HOME VISIT (*Continued*)

For Elder

Environmental conditions:

- House in poor repair
- Inadequate heat, lighting, furniture, or cooking utensils
- Presence of garbage or vermin
- Old food in kitchen
- Lack of assistive devices
- Locks on refrigerator
- Blocked stairways
- Victim lying in urine, feces, or food
- Unpleasant odors

Medication bottles:

- Medication not being taken as prescribed

Data from Pawl 1984; Ghent et al. 1985; Galbraith 1986; Elder abuse 1991.

---

make home visits. Home visits allow assessment of potential abuse situations in the crucial first few months of life. This early period is when the style of parent-child interactions is set for later life. Important factors the public health nurse can assess are noted in Box 12–7. Nurses in clinic and public health settings make such observations, which are fundamental in case-finding and evaluation.

THERAPEUTIC ENVIRONMENT

Whenever possible, the goal of intervention is to keep the family together. Interventions are geared toward stabilizing the home situation and maintaining a violence-free environment. Interventions offered would ideally leave options for growth, increase in self-esteem, and a higher quality of life for all family members.

Providing and maintaining a therapeutic environment in the home ideally involves three levels of help for abusing families (Taskinen 1984):

1. Provide the family with economic support and social services, such as family service agencies.
2. Arrange social support in the form of a public health nurse, lay home visitor, day care teacher, school teacher, social worker, respite worker, or any other potential contact person with a good relationship with the family.
3. Encourage and provide family therapy.

Day care centers for small children or elders can help relieve the caregiver. Homemakers, brought into the home to help with direct household assistance, can reduce feelings of being overwhelmed.

Amundson (1989) describes an intensive home-based crisis interaction and family education program developed by clinical nurse specialists in mental health nursing. The program accepts only families refered by Children's Protective Services in which at least one child is in imminent danger of being placed in foster, group, or institutional care. The goal is to prevent out-of-home placement of children through intensive, in-home intervention that teaches families new problem-solving skills for preventing future crises.

PSYCHOTHERAPY

Psychotherapy is carried out by a nurse who is educated at the master's level in psychiatric nursing and certified or eligible for certification. Therapy is most effective after crisis intervention, when the situation is less chaotic and tumultuous. A variety of therapeutic modalities are available for violent families.

Individual Therapy

The goals of individual therapy with a victim center on helping the person recognize feelings about being battered, about the self, and about options regarding the battering (McBride 1990). Expected outcomes include an increase in the victim's self-esteem and affirmation that no one deserves to be beaten.

Individual therapy is often indicated for the abuser as well, particularly when an individual psychopathological process is identified and sexual abuse has occurred. For example, a parent who is identified as psychotic, borderline, drug dependent, or depressed usually needs immediate and rigorous medical and psychiatric follow-up.

Family Therapy

Because family violence is a symptom of a family in crisis, each part of the family system needs attention. Also, because change in one member of the family system affects change in the whole system, support and understanding are needed by all members. One of the goals of therapy is to decrease the frequency and intensity of the abuse. Expected outcomes are that the abuser will recognize inner states of anger and learn alternative ways of dealing with anger. Intermediate goals are that members of the family will openly communicate and learn to listen to each other.

Group Therapy

Therapy groups provide assurances that one is not alone and that positive change is possible. Because many victims have been isolated over time, they have been deprived of validation and positive feedback from others. Working in a group can help diminish feelings of isolation, strengthen feelings of self-esteem and self-worth, and increase the potential for realistic problem solving in a supportive atmosphere.

Niksaitis (1985) accurately states that the real problem in a violent relationship is the abuser. The victim is the symptom of the problem. In the groups for men that batter, the men are taught to recognize signs of escalating anger and learn ways of channeling their anger nonviolently. Men who have never discussed problems with anyone before are encouraged to discuss their thoughts and feelings. Sharing with others who have similar problems can help minimize feelings of isolation and allow mutual problem solving for handling overwhelming feelings of pain, low self-esteem, and rage. These feelings often stem from some kind of loss. Untended mourning and grief (usually from childhood deprivations and victimization) get translated into anger, rage, abuse, and violence (Ewing 1987). Group therapy can help create a community of healing and restoration.

Self-help groups serve a vital function for many victims of abuse. Hotlines provide emergency resources and information on how to contact self-help groups within the community, such as Parents Anonymous.

Evaluation

Evaluation should be done by all members of the health care team on an ongoing basis. Because abuse is a symptom of a family in distress, diagnosis, interventions, and evaluation should be carried out by a multidisciplinary team. A team would ideally include a physician, a nurse, a social worker, an attorney, and perhaps a psychiatrist. Unfortunately, conditions are not always ideal.

Evaluating established goals can lead to new goals when old ones are reached or to changes in intervention if set goals have not been met. The goals set to change family interactions and to influence positively the incidence of abuse in the family are a primary focus of evaluation. Changes would be noted in decreased evidence of physical abuse or psychological abuse, in healthier coping patterns used by the victim or the family, or in support systems available. When these changes are positive, the nurse may continue to work with the family as a resource person or facilitator. When changes are not noted or are negative, the nurse works with the family to re-evaluate the goals and the interventions originally set for their attainment.

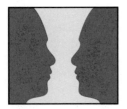

Case Study: Working with a Family Involved with Abuse

Mrs. Rob, an 84-year-old woman recently widowed, moved to her son's apartment three months ago. She had been living alone in her third-floor walk-up in the city. Because of her declining health, crime in the neighborhood, and three flights of stairs to climb, and with her son John's encouragement, she went to live with him. He and his wife, Judy, who have been married for almost 20 years, have five children aged six to 18, all living in a rather cramped three-bedroom apartment.

Mrs. Rob was being cared for by the visiting nurse to monitor her blood pressure and adjust her medication. Over a series of visits, the nurse, Ms. Green, noticed that Mrs. Rob was looking noticeably unkempt, pale, and withdrawn. While taking her blood pressure, the nurse observed bruises on Mrs. Rob's arms and neck. When questioned about the bruises, Mrs. Rob appeared anxious and nervous. She said that she had slipped in the bathroom. Mrs. Rob became increasingly apprehensive and stiffened up in her chair when her daughter-in-law, Judy, came into the room asking when the next visit was. The nurse noticed that Judy avoided eye contact with Mrs. Rob.

When the injuries were brought to Judy's attention, she responded by becoming angry and agitated, blaming Mrs. Rob for causing so many problems. She would not explain the reason for the change in Mrs. Rob's behavior or the origin of the bruises to the nurse. She merely commented, "I have had to give up my job since my mother-in-law came here. . . . It has been difficult and crowded ever since *she* moved in. The kids are complaining. We are having trouble making ends meet since I gave up my job. And my husband is not being any help at all."

Assessment

Ms. Green suspected that Mrs. Rob was in an abusive situation and spoke of the case with her team at the visiting nurse center. The nurse identified objective and subjective data that supported suspected elder abuse.

OBJECTIVE DATA

1. Physical symptoms of abuse (i.e., bruises, unkempt appearance, withdrawn attitude)
2. Stressful, crowded living conditions·
3. No eye contact between elder and daughter-in-law
4. Economic hardships leading to stress
5. No support for the daughter-in-law from rest of family for care of Mrs. Rob
6. Elder unable to make decisions

SUBJECTIVE DATA

1. Mrs. Rob states she "slipped in the bathroom," but physical findings do not support explanation
2. Daughter-in-law states, "It's been difficult and crowded ever since *she* moved in."
3. Mrs. Rob exhibits withdrawn and apprehensive behavior

Nursing Diagnosis

On the basis of the data, the nurse formulated the following nursing diagnoses:

1. *High risk for injury* related to increase in family stress, as evidenced by signs of abuse
   - Mrs. Rob states she slipped in the bathroom, but physical findings do not support that explanation
   - Physical symptoms of abuse present (bruises, unkempt appearance, withdrawn attitude)
   - Stressful, crowded living conditions

2. *Ineffective individual coping* related to helplessness, as evidenced by inability to meet role expectations
   - Mrs. Rob appears unkempt, anxious, depressed
   - Mrs. Rob exhibits withdrawn and apprehensive behavior
   - Mrs. Rob is unable to make decisions

3. *High risk for violence* related to increased stressors within a short period, as evidenced by probable elder abuse and feelings of helplessness
   - Judy states, "It's been difficult and crowded ever since *she* moved in."
   - No eye contact between Judy and Mrs. Rob
   - Signs and symptoms of physical abuse on elder
   - "My husband is no help at all."

4. *Ineffective family coping* related to unmet psychosocial needs of elder by son and daughter-in-law
   - Family not helping with care of mother-in-law, burden of care on Judy
   - Economic hardships leading to stress when Judy gave up job to care for Mrs. Rob

Planning

CONTENT LEVEL—PLANNING GOALS

The nurse discussed several possible goals with members of her team, giving attention to the priority of goals and to whether they are realistic in this situation.

Nursing Diagnosis	Long Term Goal	Short Term Goal
1. *High risk for injury* related to increase in family stress, as evidenced by signs of abuse 2. *Ineffective individual coping* related to helplessness, as evidenced by inability to meet role expectations	1. Mrs. Rob will be well nourished and free from signs of physical abuse by (date). 2. Mrs. Rob will have definite alternative plans for living situation by one month (date).	1. Mrs. Rob will name two persons she can call in case of further abuse in one week (date). 2a. Mrs. Rob will identify three personal strengths in one week (date). 2b. Mrs. Rob will make one decision about her future in two weeks (date). 2c. In three weeks (date), Mrs. Rob will state two

Continued on following page

Case Study: Working with a Family Involved with Abuse *(Continued)*

Nursing Diagnosis	Long Term Goal	Short Term Goal
		behavioral changes she will make.
3. *Risk for violence* by abuser related to increased stressors within a short period of time, as evidenced by probable elder abuse and feelings of helplessness	3. Judy will state she has control of feelings and is no longer abusing Mrs. Rob by one month (date).	3a. Judy will name three conditions that led to her loss of control with elder in one week (date). 3b. Judy will use three new coping behaviors within three weeks (date). 3c. Judy will seek counseling in three weeks (date). 3d. Judy will name three support services she can call in one week (date).
4. *Ineffective family coping* related to unmet psychosocial needs of elder by son and daughter-in-law	4. Mrs. Rob and family will meet together and discuss mutual expectations and actions they wish to share.	4a. Family members will meet with nurse on regular basis starting in one week (date). 4b. Family will identify supports and resources they feel are important to them in one week. 4c. One other family member will spend half a day per week with Mrs. Rob.

PROCESS LEVEL—NURSES' REACTIONS AND FEELINGS

Ms. Green has been in a number of situations with abusive families, but this was the first time she encountered elder abuse. She discussed her reactions with the other team members. She was especially angry at Judy, although she was able to understand the daughter-in-law's frustration. The team concurred with Ms. Green that there seemed to be potential for positive change with this family. If abuse does not abate, more drastic measures will need to be taken and legal services contacted.

Intervention

Elder abuse is a signal of a family in crisis. Ms. Green knew she had to address the needs of the whole family to effect change within the family system. She focused on Mrs. Rob's physical safety first, then on Mrs. Rob's strengths to work within the family system. It was evident that Judy was overwhelmed with multiple stressors, and interventions for her and the rest of the family were vital for effective change.

Ms. Green continued to meet with the family on a weekly basis. Interventions were mapped out, with input from the family. Although it was difficult at first to get the husband involved, he became more active when his feelings of helplessness and guilt began to fade. Ms. Green encouraged the children to participate, and many useful suggestions came from their observations and ideas.

This family seemed motivated to change their circumstances because all members were feeling overwhelmed and helpless. Although suggestions regarding outside services were initially met with some resistance, other services were contacted. Judy stated that she found weekly counseling a great help. The Friendly Visitors Service allowed Judy some time to herself each week. Refer to Nursing Care Plan 12–1 for specific interventions for this family.

Nursing Care Plan 12-1 ■ A FAMILY INVOLVED WITH ABUSE: Mrs. Rob

NURSING DIAGNOSIS

High risk for injury related to increase in family stress, as evidenced by signs of abuse

Supporting Data

- States that she slipped in the bathroom
- Physical symptoms of abuse (i.e., bruises, unkempt appearance, withdrawn attitude)
- Stressful, crowded living conditions

Long Term Goal: Mrs. Rob will be well nourished and free from signs of physical abuse by (date).

Short Term Goal	Intervention	Rationale	Evaluation
1. Client will state the abuse is decreased by (date).	1a. Assess severity of signs and symptoms of abuse and potential for further injury on weekly visits.	1a. Determines need for further intervention.	Goal met Client says she is no longer abused in family situation.
	1b. Discuss with client factors leading to abuse and concern for physical safety.	1b. Validates situation is serious and increases client's knowledge base.	
2. In one week client will name two persons she can call in case of further abuse.	2. Discuss with client support services such as hotlines and crisis units to call in case of emergency situation.	2. Maximizes client's safety through use of support systems.	

NURSING DIAGNOSIS

Ineffective individual coping related to helplessness, as evidenced by inability to meet role expectations

Supporting Data

- Appears unkempt, anxious, depressed
- Exhibits withdrawn and apprehensive behavior
- Unable to make decisions

Long Term Goal: Client will have definite plans for alternatives to present living situation within one month.

Short Term Goal	Intervention	Rationale	Evaluation
1. Client will identify three personal strengths by (date).	1a. Approach client in positive, nonjudgmental manner.	1a. Encourages disclosure and development of relationship.	Goal partially met Client has identified personal strengths and made two behavioral changes. She has not made any definite plans for a change in living situation. She says she is feeling a little better about living with son's family.
	1b. Assist client to develop effective coping skills.	1b. Redirects self-assessment to positive skills.	
	1c. Assist client to identify personal assets.	1c. Can help increase self-esteem.	
2. Client will make one decision about the future by (date).	2a. Encourage client to examine situation and alternatives.	2a. When in a dependent situation, individuals may have difficulties making decisions.	
	2b. Reinforce client's use of problem-solving skills.	2b. Encourages client to function at optimum level.	
3. Client will state two behavioral changes to be carried out by (date).	3a. Explore with client ways to make changes.	3a. Directs assessment to positive areas.	
	3b. Assist client in making decisions for action for future.	3b. Can help improve self-esteem.	

NURSING DIAGNOSIS

High risk for violence by abuser related to increased stressors within a short period of time, as evidenced by aggressive behaviors

Supporting Data

- States, "It's been difficult and crowded ever since *she* moved in."
- No eye contact with Mrs. Rob
- Signs and symptoms of physical abuse on mother-in-law

Continued on following page

Nursing Care Plan 12–1 ■ A FAMILY INVOLVED WITH ABUSE: Mrs. Rob *(Continued)*

Long Term Goal: By (date), abuser will state that she has control over her feelings and is not abusing Mrs. Rob.

Short Term Goal	Intervention	Rationale	Evaluation
1. Abuser will name three conditions that contribute to her loss of control with Mrs. Rob by (date).	1. Nurse will meet with abuser and encourage problem-solving approach.	1. Develops abuser's abilities.	Goal met Abuser has not abused Mrs. Rob. Daughter-in-law states, "I feel better about dealing with stressful situations."
2. Abuser will have used three new coping behaviors with Mrs. Rob by (date).	2a. Encourage abuser to verbalize feelings about Mrs. Rob and understand what conditions lead to stress so that they can be avoided.	2a. Positive approach to deal with stress.	
	2b. Encourage development of alternative behaviors.	2b. Acceptable manner of dealing with stress.	
	2c. Reinforce positive approaches suggested by abuser.	2c. Increases abilities to deal with stress.	
3. Abuser will seek counseling by (date).	3. Encourage abuser's use of counseling, reinforcing benefits and needs gained from such a regular intervention.	3. Increases coping abilities.	
4. Abuser will name three support services she can call on and will have used one by (date).	4a. Explore with abuser available support services. Encourage use.	4a. Increases knowledge of resources.	
	4b. Initiate referrals for support services.	4b. Provides needed support.	

NURSING DIAGNOSIS

Ineffective family coping related to unmet psychosocial needs of elder by son and daughter-in-law

Supporting Data

- Family not helping with care of mother-in-law; it is being left to daughter-in-law, who states, "My husband is not being any help at all."
- Economic hardships leading to stress when wife gave up job to care for elder

Long Term Goal: Client and family members will meet together and discuss mutual expectations and actions they wish to share by (date).

Short Term Goal	Intervention	Rationale	Evaluation
1. Family members will meet for counseling with nurse on a regular basis by (date).	1a. Nurse will meet with family members and encourage problem solving of present situation.	1a. Family members have opportunity to verbalize their feelings about present situation, offering different perspectives.	Goal met Family members are meeting regularly.
	1b. Nurse will suggest that family members meet together on regular basis for problem solving and support.	1b. Family will solve problems together.	

Long Term Goal: Family members will share the responsibilities of caring for Mrs. Rob by (date).

Short Term Goal	Intervention	Rationale	Evaluation
1. Family will identify supports and resources they feel are important to them by (date).	1a. Nurse will assist family in identifying support services available, then select appropriate services.	1a. Support services can provide assistance to the family.	Goal partially met No other outside family member is providing the half-day respite for Mrs. Rob's immediate family. The family has identified support services and contacted one agency.
	1b. Nurse will contact suggested services for family when requested.	1b. Nurse can provide needed support and expertise.	

2. One other family member
will spend half a day per
week with Mrs. Rob by
(date).

2. Family will meet together
and discuss responsibility
for care of Mrs. Rob and
make suggestions for more
support by family members.
Nurse will act as facilitator
in discussion, if necessary.

2. Family will problem-solve
and explore avenues for
needed assistance.

Case Study: Working with a Family Involved with Abuse

Evaluation

Eight weeks after the nurse's initial visit, Mrs. Rob appeared well groomed, friendly, and more spontaneous in her conversation. She commented, "things are better with my daughter-in-law." No bruises or other signs of physical abuse were noticeable. She was considerably more outgoing and even took the initiative to contact an old friend. She had talked openly with her son and daughter-in-law about stress in the family. When her daughter-in-law, Judy, appeared tense, Mrs. Rob went out for a walk and returned to find the tension had lessened. Neither Mrs. Rob nor her family had initiated plans for alternative housing.

As a further result of the nurse's intervention, Judy was more in control of her emotions. Although she did on occasion yell at her mother-in-law, she felt this was no longer the same uncontrolled explosive anger. Verbalizing her feelings to her husband helped alleviate her frustrations. Judy was seeing a counselor at the hospital and was planning to look for a part-time job to "get out of the house."

The family members gradually began to communicate with one another. Mrs. Rob's other son and his family were contacted for assistance. Although this son had not yet offered to share some of the responsibility for taking care of his mother, he did agree to give some financial support. The family continued to meet with the nurse.

Summary

Abuse occurs across all age groups and can be predicted to occur with some accuracy by examining characteristics of abusers, vulnerable people, and situations in which abuse is more likely to occur. Abuse can be physical, sexual, emotional, economic, or caused by neglect. Emotional abuse can occur in isolation; however, where other types of abuse occur, emotional abuse also occurs. Child abuse continues the cycle of violence. The cycle of violence follows predictable stages; unless interventions are applied, violence will grow in frequency and intensity. Assessment includes identifying levels of anxiety, coping mechanisms, support system, the actual abuse, and suicide potential as well as alcohol and drug abuse.

Suspicion or actual evidence of abuse *must* be carefully documented and then reported to the appropriate authorities. Strong and irrational responses by health care professionals are common in working with abuse victims. Knowing about these reactions and how to reduce intense feelings increases the nurse's therapeutic effectiveness. Intervention occurs at primary, secondary, and tertiary levels. Primary intervention aims at preventing abuse and the use of violence as a coping strategy. Early recognition and secondary intervention in cases in which abuse has already occurred but is not an ingrained habit can greatly reduce the subsequent incidence of abuse. Tertiary intervention occurs as a last resort, in the worst cases of abuse, and when previous intervention techniques have failed. Evaluation and follow-up interventions are vital to the promotion of family growth and individual safety.

References

Amundson MF. Family crisis care: A home-based intervention program for child abuse. Issues in Mental Health Nursing, 10(3/4):285, 1989.

Anderson L, Thobaben M. Clients in crisis. Journal of Gerontological Nursing, 10(12):7, 1984.

Bullock LFC, et al. Breaking the cycle of abuse: How nurses can intervene. Journal of Psychosocial Nursing, 27(8):11, 1989.

Delgaty K. Battered women: The issues for nursing. The Canadian Nurse, 81(2):21, 1985.

Ebersole P, Hess P. Toward Healthy Aging. St. Louis: CV Mosby, 1990.

Elder abuse: Risk factors help identify victims, burned out caregivers. Geriatrics, 46(10):23, 1991.

Else L, et al. Personality characteristics of men who physically abuse women. Hospital and Community Psychiatry, 44(10):54, 1993.

Ewing WA. Domestic violence and community health care ethics: Reflections on systemic intervention. Family and Community Health, 10(1):54, 1987.

Fulmer T. Elder mistreatment: Progress in community detection and intervention. Family and Community Health, 14(2):26, 1991.

Galbraith M (ed). Elder Abuse: Perspectives on an Emerging Crisis, vol 3. Kansas City, KS: Mid-America Congress on Aging, 1986.

Gelles R, Straus M. Intimate Violence. New York: Simon & Schuster, 1988.

Gelman D, et al. Who's taking care of our parents? Newsweek, May 6, 1985, pp 61–68.

Gemmill FB. A family approach to the battered woman. Journal of Psychosocial Nursing and Mental Health Services, 20(9):22, 1982.

Ghent WR, DaSylva NP, Farren ME. Family violence: Guidelines for recognition and management. Canadian Medical Association Journal, 132:541, 1985.

Greany GD. Is she a battered woman? A guide for emergency response. American Journal of Nursing, 85(6):724, 1984.

Haviland S, O'Brien J. Physical abuse and neglect of the elderly: Assessment and intervention. Orthopaedic Nursing, 8(4):11, 1989.

King MC, Ryan J. Abused women: Dispelling myths and encouraging intervention. Nurse Practitioner, 14(5):47, 1989.

Klingbeil K. Keynote address at a conference on "Battering of Women," Seattle, WA, 1991.

Kluft RP. Multiple personality disorder: An update. Hospital and Community Psychiatry, 38:363, 1987.

Kreitzer M. Legal aspects of child abuse: Guidelines for the nurse. Nursing Clinics of North America, 16(1):149, 1981.

Limandri BJ. The therapeutic relationship with abused women. Journal of Psychosocial Nursing, 25(2):9, 1987.

Ludwig S, Kornberg AE (eds). Child Abuse: A Medical Reference. New York: Churchill Livingstone, 1992.

McBride AB. Violence against women: Implications for research and practice. Reflections, 16(3):19, 1990.

McLeer SV, et al. Education is not enough: A systems failure in protecting battered women. Annals of Emergency Medicine, 18(6):651, 1989.

Meierhoffer LL. Nurses battle family violence. The American Nurse, 24(4):1, 1992.

Moss VA. Battered women and the myth of masochism. Journal of Psychosocial Nursing, 29(7):19, 1991.

National Coalition Against Domestic Violence (NCADV). NCADV Statistics, May 1988. Washington, DC: The Coalition, 1988.

Niksaitis G. Therapy for men who batter: Interview. Journal of Psychosocial Nursing, 23:33, 1985.

Novello AC, Soto-Torres LE. Women and hidden epidemics: HIV/AIDS and domestic violence. The Female Patient, 17:17, 1992.

Office of Maternal and Child Health. Child Health USA '89. Washington, DC: US Department of Health and Human Services, 1989. Publication No. HRS-M-CH 8915.

Pawl JH. Strategies for intervention. Child Abuse and Neglect, 8(2):261, 1984.

Pillemer K, Prescott D. Psychological effects of elder abuse: A research note. Journal of Elder Abuse and Neglect, 1(10):65, 1989.

Public Health Service: Goals for Year 2000. Promoting Health/Preventing Disease: Year 2000 Objectives for the Nation, Draft for Review and Comment, September 1989. Washington, DC: US Department of Health and Human Services, 1989.

Rew L. Child sexual abuse: Toward a self-care framework for nursing intervention and research. Archives of Psychiatric Nursing, 4(3):47, 1990.

Scherb BJ. Suspected abuse and neglect of children. Journal of Emergency Nursing, 14(1):44, 1988.

Stanley SR. Child sexual abuse: Recognition and nursing intervention. Orthopedic Nursing, 8(1):33, 1989.

Swanson RW. Battered wife syndrome. Canadian Medical Association Journal, 10(6):709, 1984.

Taskinen S. The Finnish approach to helping personnel deal with child abuse and neglect. Child Abuse and Neglect, 8(1):113, 1984.

Verwoerdt A. Clinical Geropsychiatry. Baltimore: Williams & Wilkins, 1976.

Walker B. Domestic Violence: Identifying and Treating Victims in the Emergency Room. Seattle: King County Department of Public Health, 1991.

Walker L. The Battered Woman. New York: Harper & Row, 1979.

Warner CG (ed). Conflict Intervention in Social and Domestic Violence. Bowie, MD: Robert J. Brady, 1981.

Weingourt R. Never to be alone: Existential therapy with battered women. Journal of Psychosocial Nursing, 23:24, 1985.

Wissow LS. Child Advocacy for the Clinician: An Approach to Child Abuse and Neglect. Baltimore: Williams & Wilkins, 1990.

Wolf RS. Elder abuse: Scope, characteristics, and treatment. Nurse Practitioner Forum, 1(2):102, 1990.

Wolf RS, Pillemer KA. Helping Elderly Victims: The Reality of Elder Abuse. New York: Columbia University Press, 1989.

Wolfe DA. Child Abuse: Implications for Child Development and Psychopathology. Newbury Park, CA: Sage Publications, 1987.

Further Reading

Bohn DK. Domestic violence and pregnancy: Implications for practice. Journal of Nurse-Midwifery, 32(2):86, 1990.

Burgess AW, Hartman CR, Kelley SJ. Assessing child abuse: The TRIADS checklist. Journal of Psychosocial Nursing and Mental Health Services, 28(4):6, 1990.

Delunas LR. Prevention of elder abuse: Betty Neuman health care systems approach. Clinical Nurse Specialist, 4(1):54, 1990.

Douglass R. Domestic Mistreatment of the Elderly—Towards Prevention. Washington, DC: AARP, 1987.

The handbook concentrates on definitions and examples of abuse. The focus is also on prevention by the older adult and the community as a key to the problem of abuse. Methods of early planning are considered.

Flaherty EG, Weiss H. Medical evaluation of abused and neglected children. American Journal of Diseases of Children, 144:330, 1990.

Flynn EM. Preventing and diagnosing sexual abuse in children. Nurse Practitioner: American Journal of Primary Health Care, 12(2):47, 1987.

Fulmer T. Mistreatment of elders. Nursing Clinics of North America, 24(3):707, 1989.

Gill FT. Caring for abused children in the emergency department. Holistic Nursing Practice, 4(1):37, 1989.

Kurz D. Emergency department responses to battered women: Resistance to medicalization. Social Problems, 34(1):69, 1987.

Lewin L. Establishing a therapeutic relationship with an abused child. Pediatric Nursing, 16(3):263, 1990.

Moehling KS. Battered women and abusive partners: Treatment issues and strategies. Journal of Psychosocial Nursing and Mental Health Services, 26(9):9, 1988.

Mooney AJ. Physical child abuse. Orthopaedic Nursing, 8(1):29, 1989.

Moss VA, Taylor WK. Domestic violence: Identification, assessment, intervention. AORN Journal, 53(5):1158, 1991.

Quinn MJ, Tomita SK. Elder Abuse and Neglect. New York: Springer, 1986.

Clinical guide to identifying and treating the abused elder adult. Guidelines for assessment and treatment are presented in a clear and complete manner. Case examples add to the text's usefulness.

Ryan JM. Child abuse and the community health nurse. Home Healthcare Nurse, 7(2):23, 1989.

Select Committee on Aging. Elder Abuse. A Decade of Shame and Inaction. Washington, DC: US Government Printing Office, 1990. House of Representatives Committee Publication No. 101-175.

The handbook provides an update on the hearings by the United States Committee on Aging House of Representatives; the status of elder abuse in this country.

Wolf RS, Pillemer KA. Helping Elderly Victims: The Reality of Elder Abuse. New York: Columbia University Press, 1989.

This concise research-based book profiles a basis for reasons that staff development, identification, and intervention projects should be developed and funded to address the victims of elder abuse.

Self-study Exercises

Place T (true) or F (false) next to each statement.

1. _____ Abusers are usually sociopaths or psychotic.
2. _____ Women usually stay in abusive relationships because they are masochistic.
3. _____ Headaches, palpitations, stomachaches, backaches, and other somatic complaints are *not* signals that may indicate abuse.
4. _____ Low self-esteem is characteristic of the victim only, not of the abuser.
5. _____ Children from violent homes often use violence later in life to cope with stress.
6. _____ Anxiety, depression, and suicidal thoughts or attempts are often seen in abused women.
7. _____ You can usually tell whether people are in abusive situations by the way they present themselves in the world.
8. _____ Men often do not clearly remember their acts of violence and use denial and rationalization as coping mechanisms.
9. _____ Promises, gifts, and loving behavior are characteristic of the honeymoon stage of the cycle theory of violence.
10. _____ Most nurses believe they can really make a difference in the lives of abuse victims.
11. _____ Elder abusers are likely to have mental, emotional, or alcohol problems.
12. _____ All states have mandatory reporting laws on elder abuse.

Choose the answer that most accurately completes the statement.

13. Which factor can signal conditions for family abuse?

    A. A family illness
    B. A parent who has been drinking
    C. A child who is highly gifted in an "average to below-average" household
    D. A parent who comes from another country
    E. All of the above.

14. Of the following, circle common characteristics of abusing parents.

    A. Unrealistic expectations of child's behavior
    B. Lack of effective parenting skills
    C. Male
    D. Poor coping skills
    E. Alcoholic
    F. All of the above.

Match the example on the left with the type of abuse listed in the right column.

15. _____ "You no good slut. I wish you were never born."

16. _____ Joe says children don't know how to behave unless you give them good healthy spankings.

17. _____ Tom says life is the best teacher. His children don't need schools.

A. Physical battering

B. Physical endangerment

C. Sexual abuse

18. _____ As Sally ate her lunch at the park, she noticed a man near her with his penis sticking out of his pants.

D. Physical neglect

19. _____ Henrietta refused to get her child counseling even though it had been recommended by her child's teacher, the principal, and concerned friends.

E. Developmental neglect

20. _____ The playground equipment in George's backyard was in a dangerous state of disrepair. Yet eight of his children and neighborhood children continued to play on it. "They'll survive" was his attitude.

F. Educational neglect

21. _____ When Joannie misbehaved, she would get locked in her closet for hours at a time.

G. Emotional abuse

22. _____ Martha never played with her baby and rarely touched him, feeling that he could do just fine for himself.

Match the symptom listed in the left column with the type of abuse it indicates in the right column.

23. _____ Apprehensive when other children cry

A. Physical abuse

24. _____ Profound personality change

25. _____ Unusual fearfulness

B. Sexual abuse

26. _____ Constant fatigue

27. _____ Pain in genital area

C. Neglect

28. _____ Always begging kids at school for food; never seems to bring own lunch

D. Emotional abuse

29. _____ Bald patches on scalp

30. _____ Always careful of behavior; wants to please

Choose the most appropriate answer.

31. For assessing whether a child's safety or security needs are being met, which question would be appropriate to ask parents?

   A. What do you do when you get angry with your child?
   B. Did you graduate from high school?
   C. How did this happen?
   D. Describe your marriage.

32. Circle all of the following myths a woman may believe that keep her locked into an abusive relationship.

   A. She stays "for the sake of the children."
   B. "He will change."
   C. She deserves the beatings once in a while.
   D. No one has the right to harm or beat another.

33. Which of the following are coping devices used by women who are abused?

   A. Self-blame
   B. Rationalization
   C. Somatization
   D. Assertiveness

34. Of the following, circle all important areas to assess in a woman presenting with spouse abuse.

   A. Suicide potential
   B. Use of drugs or alcohol
   C. Woman's support system
   D. Ethnic background

35. In interviewing the child about the abuse episode, which question should be included?

   A. Do you like school?
   B. What happens when you do something wrong at home?
   C. Do you have any brothers or sisters?
   D. What is your favorite TV program?

36. Questioning the acceptance of violence in America and modeling nonviolent problem-solving strategies are examples of what level of intervention?

   A. Primary intervention
   B. Secondary intervention
   C. Tertiary intervention

Write brief responses in answer to the following.

37. List two possible nursing diagnoses for a victim of elder abuse and one goal for each.

   1. Nursing Diagnosis: _____
      Goal: _____
   2. Nursing Diagnosis: _____
      Goal: _____

38. List three common responses of nurses working with an elderly person who is abused that would warrant peer supervision or clinical supervision.

   1. _____
   2. _____
   3. _____

39. Identify three areas to assess for evaluating the effectiveness of intervention in an elder-abusing family.

   1. _____
   2. _____
   3. _____

State whether the following interventions are part of the crisis (C) stage or are more apt to be carried out during the stage of internal change (I) for a victim of spouse abuse.

40. _____ Encourage catharsis, explaining she is not alone and reassuring her that she is safe in the emergency department.
41. _____ Devise a safety plan for her.
42. _____ Explore options and encourage decision making.
43. _____ Start couples therapy with both husband and wife.
44. _____ Have children evaluated for emotional and cognitive effects of violent environment.
45. _____ Make referrals.
46. _____ Refer husband to groups for men who batter.

CHAPTER 13

Evidence of Maladaptive Responses to Crisis: Rape

Kathleen Smith-DiJulio

OUTLINE

KEY TERMS AND CONCEPTS

The key terms and concepts listed here also appear in bold where they are defined or discussed in this chapter.

BEHAVIORAL SELF-BLAME

COMPOUND REACTION

CONTROLLED STYLE OF COPING

EXPRESSED STYLE OF COPING

RAPE-TRAUMA SYNDROME
Acute Phase
Long Term Reorganization Phase

SILENT REACTION

OBJECTIVES

After studying this chapter, the student will be able to

1. Discuss and define the meaning of a sexual assault.
2. Name two reasons why rapes often go unreported.
3. List three common reactions to the first phase—acute phase—of the rape-trauma syndrome.
4. List three common reactions to the second phase—long term reorganization—of the rape-trauma syndrome.
5. List five areas to assess when working with a person who has been sexually assaulted.

6. List two long term goals and two short term goals for the nursing diagnosis rape-trauma syndrome.
7. Discuss five myths popularly believed about rape and its victims.
8. Discuss five psychotherapeutic techniques that are useful when working with a person who has been sexually assaulted.
9. Briefly discuss the nurse's role during the physical examination.
10. Briefly discuss the responsibilities of the nurse when a rape victim is discharged from the emergency room, and give three specific referrals.
11. Briefly discuss the nurse's role when staffing a rape-crisis hotline.
12. Name three outcomes that would signify successful interventions with a victim of sexual assault.

Rape can be one of the most devastating experiences a person lives through—if he or she lives. It is one of the most traumatic adventitious crises. Rape causes severe panic reactions and engulfs its victims in the fear of death. After being traumatized, the rape victim often carries the additional burden of shame, guilt, and embarrassment. Rape is an act of violence, and sex is the weapon used by the aggressor on the victim (Burgess and Holstrom 1974).

Rape is generally defined as *forced* and *violent* vaginal, anal, or oral penetration against the victim's will and *without* the victim's consent. The term "sexual assault" more accurately describes rape and is increasingly used in place of the word "rape."

It is extremely uncommon for a woman to rape another person; it is usually men who rape, and the majority of rape victims are women. Men are raped less frequently and are usually raped by heterosexual males, although the attacker may also be bisexual or homosexual.

The male victim is more likely to have physical trauma than is the female victim, to have been victimized by several assailants, and to be more unwilling to report the crime (Merck 1992). Homosexual rape occurs primarily in closed institutions, such as prisons and maximum-security hospitals. The dynamics are the same as those of heterosexual rape, and the male victim of rape experiences the same devastation and sequelae as female victims (Kaplan and Sadock 1991).

Although men are susceptible to rape and suffer the same sequelae as women, women are the more common victims. For this reason, this chapter will use the female pronoun throughout. However, the principles discussed are the same for all rape victims.

In 1987, more than 91,000 rapes were reported in the United States (US Department of Commerce 1989), a 35% increase from 1978 (Sampselle 1991).

Rape often goes unreported. It is estimated that only one of four to one of 10 rapes is reported (Kap-

lan and Sadock 1991). One major reason for the underreporting of rape is that the victim, as well as the rapist, goes on trial. Rape is the only crime in which the victim is required to prove innocence. Women victims have historically been held responsible for the occurrence of rape. A common belief was that if the victim had not, for example, been so careless, been drinking, been dressed so provocatively, or been out too late, she would not have been raped. Additionally, women have usually been required to show evidence of having attempted to resist rape.

The fact that a woman is more likely to be raped by someone she knows than by a stranger also inhibits reporting (Sampselle 1991). Being the target of abuse at the hands of someone she knows seriously compromises a woman's sense of self-worth. Often, victims are threatened with another attack or with death if they report the rape (Dubin and Weiss 1991).

Another reason that rapes go unreported is social taboos against talking about sex—especially forced, violent sex crimes. Men who are raped are less likely to report than women because of the general lack of social acceptance of sex between two men. Victims of rape are victimized not only by the crime itself but also by society's reactions. Personal anguish and grief also keep the person from seeking emergency medical care and reporting the crime.

Recent changes in awareness of what rape is and in laws governing sexual assault are largely due to the women's movement. Feminists have done a great deal to raise the consciousness of individuals and of American society as a whole to allow acceptance of the concept that women are people, not property, and should be accorded the same rights and privileges as men. Women are now also seen as equals in the marriage relationship, so laws are changing to allow a wife to bring rape charges against her husband. Formerly it was believed that a man was entitled to sex in a relationship, no matter how he got it. The women's movement has heightened awareness such

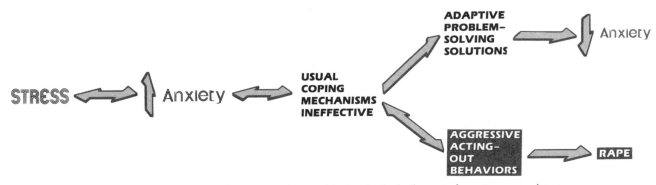

Figure 13–1. *Conceptualization of the process of aggressive acting-out behaviors in the development of rape-trauma syndrome.*

that gradual change in these perceptions is occurring. Through the planned application of feminist thought, nurses can effectively counteract social forces that sustain violence against women (Sampselle 1991).

Sexual assault as a maladaptive response to crisis is conceptualized in Figure 13–1.

Theory

Sexual assault may occur within the context of a social relationship that goes too far, and the rapist can be an acquaintance, a neighbor, a relative, or a total stranger. The assailant may use weapons, restraints, direct physical force, threats of physical harm, or other types of intimidation. Regardless of the methods employed to force the victim, the victim usually fears death during the assault. Most victims of rape suffer severe and long-lasting emotional trauma. Five features of the assault experience that contribute to psychological trauma have been identified by Abarbanel (1980):

1. The assault is sudden and arbitrary.
2. The assault is perceived as life threatening.
3. The main purpose of an assault is to violate the victim's physical integrity and render her helpless.
4. The assault forces the victim to participate in the crime.
5. The assault overwhelms normal coping strategies and renders the victim helpless to control her assailants. She becomes the victim of her assailant's rape and aggression.

Based on a landmark study of 92 rape victims, Burgess and Holstrom (1974) documented the existence of the **rape-trauma syndrome.** The rape-trauma syndrome comprises (1) an acute phase and (2) the long term reorganization process that occur following an actual or attempted sexual assault. Each phase has separate symptoms. Rape-trauma syndrome is a variant of post-traumatic stress disorder.

ACUTE PHASE OF RAPE-TRAUMA SYNDROME

The **acute phase** of rape-trauma syndrome occurs immediately following the assault and may last for a couple of weeks. This is the stage seen by hospital personnel in the emergency room. Nurses are the clinicians most involved in dealing with these initial reactions. During this phase, there is a great deal of disorganization in the person's lifestyle, and somatic symptoms are common. Burgess (1985) describes this disorganization in terms of impact reactions, somatic reactions, and emotional reactions. Refer to Table 13–1 for identifying symptoms of each reaction.

The most common initial reaction is shock, numbness, and disbelief. Outwardly, the person may appear self-contained and calm and make remarks such as "It doesn't seem real," or "I don't believe this really happened to me." Sometimes, cognitive functions may be impaired, and the traumatized person may appear extremely confused, have difficulty concentrating, and have difficulty with decision making. Or the person may become hysterical, restless, cry, or even smile. These reactions to crisis are typical, and they reflect cognitive, affective, and behavioral disruptions.

People who have experienced an emotionally overwhelming event may need to deny the event. Denial in this case is an adaptive and protective reaction and gives the person time to prepare for the reality of the event. Examples of denial may be found in such statements as "I don't want to talk about it," or "I just want to forget what happened."

LONG TERM REORGANIZATION PHASE OF RAPE-TRAUMA SYNDROME

The **long term reorganization phase** of rape-trauma syndrome occurs two or more weeks following the rape. Nurses who initially care for the victims can help

Table 13-1 ■ ACUTE PHASE OF RAPE-TRAUMA SYNDROME

IMPACT REACTION	SOMATIC REACTION	EMOTIONAL REACTION
Expressed style Overt behaviors ● Crying, sobbing ● Smiling ● Restlessness, agitation, hysteria ● Volatility, anger ● Hysteria ● Tenseness **Controlled style** Covert reactions ● Masked facies ● Calm, subdued appearance ● Shocked, numb, confused, disbelieving appearance ● Distractibility, difficulty making decisions	Evidenced within the first several weeks following a rape **Physical trauma** ● Bruises (breasts, throat, or back) ● Soreness **Skeletal muscle tension** ● Headaches ● Sleep disturbances ● Grimaces, twitches **Gastrointestinal** ● Stomach pains ● Nausea ● Poor appetite ● Diarrhea **Genitourinary** ● Vaginal itching ● Vaginal discharge ● Pain or discomfort	● Fear of physical violence and death ● Denial ● Anxiety ● Shock ● Humiliation ● Fatigue ● Embarrassment ● Desire for revenge ● Self-blame ● Lowered self-esteem ● Shame ● Guilt ● Anger

Data from Abarbanel 1980; Burgess 1985; Burgess and Holstrom 1974.

them anticipate and prepare for the reactions they are likely to experience. Reactions include the following (Abarbanel 1980; Burgess 1985; Burgess and Holstrom 1974):

1. Intrusive thoughts of the rape break into the victim's conscious mind during the day and during sleep. These thoughts include anger and violence toward the assailant. Flashbacks, (re-experiencing the traumatic event), dreams with violent content, and insomnia are common.
2. Increased motor activity follows, such as moving, taking trips, changing telephone numbers, and making frequent visits to old friends. This activity stems from the fear that the assailant will come back. Anxiety, mood swings, crying spells, and depression are likely to be observed.
3. Fears and phobias develop as a defensive reaction to the rape. Typical phobias include

● Fear of the indoors—if the rape occurred indoors
● Fear of the outdoors—if the rape occurred outdoors
● Fear of being alone—common for most women after an assault
● Fear of crowds—"Any person in the crowd might be a rapist"
● Fear of sexual encounters and activities—many women experience acute disruption of their sex life with husbands or boyfriends. Rape is especially upsetting for those with no prior sexual experience.

The consequences of assault may be severe and long term, including fear and anxiety, depression, suicide, difficulties with daily functioning and interpersonal relationships, sexual dysfunction, and somatic complaints (Schwartz 1991). One study (Bang 1991) of 168 women who had been raped an average of 13 years before found that

● 44% reported physical symptoms.
● 98% reported mental symptoms.
● 79% reported social symptoms.
● 11% had attempted suicide.
● 19% reported excessive use of alcohol, medications, or street drugs.
● Only 10% had sought help after the rape.

Assessment

Once the rape victim is at the emergency department, the attention she receives depends on the protocol of the particular hospital. Lederle et al. (1985) suggest the following interventions:

1. Provide immediate care and privacy.
2. Provide quality collection of evidence.
3. Conduct a physical examination.
4. Offer follow-up care.

The nurse talks with the victim, the family or friends who accompany the victim, and the police to gather as much data as possible for assessing the crisis.

The nurse assesses the (1) level of anxiety, (2) coping mechanisms used, (3) support systems available, (4) signs and symptoms of emotional trauma, and (5) signs and symptoms of physical trauma. Information obtained from the assessment is then analyzed, and nursing diagnoses are formulated.

ASSESSING THE LEVEL OF ANXIETY

Assessing, understanding, and evaluating the reactions and feelings of the victim following the rape are essential nursing skills. Because of the personal threat to the victim's sense of safety and security, the victim can be assumed to be experiencing acute anxiety. If nurses are sensitive to this fact, they will take their time with the patient. Support, reassurance, and appropriate therapeutic techniques can help diminish anxiety.

Depending on the individual's intrapersonal and interpersonal resources, the anxiety level may range from moderate to panic. (These levels are discussed in Chapter 9.) It is important to take cues from the patient. Do *not* initiate touching, as this may further increase the victim's anxiety level. If the victim reaches out and makes the first contact, then touch is acceptable.

The presence of a supportive, helpful person can assist in diminishing anxiety caused by the rape. If the victim is with a third party, obtain the victim's permission before taking a history in front of someone else. The third party should be there only for support, not to answer questions. If the third party interferes with the history-taking process or seems to make the victim uncomfortable, he or she should be asked to wait in another area.

ASSESSING COPING MECHANISMS USED

Everyone has ways of dealing with stressful situations. The same coping skills that have helped the victim through other difficult problems will be used in adjusting to the rape. In addition, new ways of getting through difficult times may be developed—for both the short term and the long term adjustment.

Behavioral mechanisms can be seen and therefore can be fairly easily assessed. Examples include crying, withdrawing, smoking, wanting to talk about the event, acting hysterical, confused, disoriented, or incoherent, and even laughing or joking. These behaviors are examples of an **expressed style of coping** (see Table 13–1).

Cognitive coping mechanisms are the thoughts people have that help them deal with high anxiety levels. If the victim is able to verbalize thoughts, the nurse will know what the victim is thinking. If not, the nurse can ask questions, such as "What do you think might help now?" or "What can I do to help you in this difficult situation?"

ASSESSING SUPPORT SYSTEMS AVAILABLE

The *availability, size,* and *utility* of a victim's social support system need to be assessed. The nurse asks the victim if there are family or friends with whom she feels safe and in whom she can confide. These people can be used to strengthen self-confidence and to assist the victim in resuming a normal style of living. However, nurses need to be aware that family, neighbors, and friends, generally the people considered as valuable supports, are the people most often involved in perpetrating the unwanted sexual experiences (Mims and Chang 1984). Pay careful attention to verbal and nonverbal cues the victim may be communicating regarding persons in her social network. For example, someone the victim knows may suggest that he or she has a spare room and the victim can spend the night there so she won't be alone, yet the victim seems hesitant. Be certain the source of the hesitancy is privately explored before railroading her into doing something that might be detrimental. The hesitancy could be due to increased anxiety and decreased ability to make decisions—or it could be due to fear of finding herself in another sexual assault situation. The following vignette illustrates this point:

Joyce, an 18-year-old, is brought to the emergency room by a concerned neighbor. She was found wandering aimlessly outside her house, sobbing, and muttering, "He had no right to do that to me." Because of Joyce's distraught appearance and her statement, the triage nurse suspects sexual assault and brings the victim to the office of the psychiatric nurse, Ms. Webster. Ms. Webster introduces herself, explains her role, and states that she is there to help. Ms. Webster then asks Joyce what happened. After careful, sensitive, nonthreatening questioning, Joyce divulges that she had been out with her boyfriend, who had raped her and then dropped her off at her house. Because no one else was at home and she was so upset and afraid, she did not go inside, and the neighbor, Mrs. Green, had seen her outside.

After the entire history and examination are completed, plans for discharge are discussed. Joyce states that no one will be home until Sunday night, two days away, and that she does not feel comfortable calling any friends because she does not want them to know what has happened. The neighbor, Mrs.

Green, had told the nurse earlier that Joyce could stay with her family.

NURSE:	Earlier, your neighbor, Mrs. Green, told me that you are welcome to spend the weekend with her family.
JOYCE:	(Loudly, sharply, with eyes wide) Oh, no, I couldn't do that.
NURSE:	You don't seem to like that idea.
JOYCE:	Oh, I just wouldn't want to bother them.
NURSE:	Mrs. Green seems quite concerned about your welfare.
JOYCE:	Oh, yes, she's very nice. (Pause)
NURSE:	But not someone you would want to spend the weekend with.
JOYCE:	Her children are too noisy. I've got homework to do.
NURSE:	You might not get the quiet you need to study. (Pause) Yet you also do not want to be alone.
JOYCE:	(Wringing a tissue in her hands, head hanging, soft voice) I can't go in that house anymore.
NURSE:	Something about being in that house disturbs you.
JOYCE:	Mr. Green (deep sigh, pause) used to . . . uh . . . take advantage of me when I used to babysit his children.
NURSE:	Take advantage?
JOYCE:	Yes . . . (sobbing) he used to force me to have sex with him. He said he'd blame it on me if I told anyone.
NURSE:	What a frightening experience that must have been for you.
JOYCE:	Yes.
NURSE:	I can see why you would not want to spend the night there. Let's continue to explore other options.

A suitable place to stay is finally arranged. Joyce is given counseling referrals that will help her deal with the process of reorganization from the current rape experience as well as begin to explore her feelings about past sexual abuse she has suffered at the hands of her neighbor.

ASSESSING SIGNS AND SYMPTOMS OF EMOTIONAL TRAUMA

Nurses work most frequently with rape victims in the emergency room soon after the rape has occurred. When the rape victim comes to the emergency room, the triage nurse makes the initial assessment. A special waiting area, separate from the general lobby,

should be provided. The victim should be admitted to the emergency room ahead of all patients except those with life-threatening emergencies. However, when extreme emotional or physical trauma is present, the victim should be immediately escorted to the treatment area. This kind of focused supportive attention helps the rape victim begin to feel safe and at ease. Some emergency departments provide sexual assault nurse examiners who are specially trained to meet the myriad needs of the sexual assault victim (Jezierski 1992).

The extent of the psychological and emotional trauma sustained by the victim may not be readily apparent from the victim's behavior (Antognoli-Toland 1985). If the person uses the **controlled style of coping** during the acute phase of the rape trauma (see Table 13–1), ill-informed staff may wonder whether the person was actually raped. That skepticism may be communicated to the victim, serving to increase anxiety and lower self-esteem. It is important to remember that despite the person's apparent response, *there is always psychological and emotional trauma experienced by a victim during and after an assault*. Nurses are *never* in the position of judging the validity of a rape.

A nursing history should be conducted and properly recorded. When obtaining a history, the nurse needs to determine only the details of the assault that will be helpful in addressing the immediate physical and psychological needs of the victim.

Allow the victim to talk at a comfortable pace. Pose questions in nonjudgmental, descriptive terms. Do not ask "why" questions. Relating the events of the rape will most likely be traumatic and embarrassing for the victim. The nurse should assess *the type of assault* in addition to the time, place, and circumstances of the assault. What occurred?

Fondling?
Oral penetration or attempted penetration?
Vaginal penetration or attempted penetration?
Rectal penetration or attempted penetration?
Ejaculation—Where? On or in the body?

If the victim expresses suicidal thoughts, the nurse should assess what precautions are needed by asking direct questions, such as "Are you thinking of harming yourself?" and "Have you ever tried to kill yourself before this attack occurred?"

ASSESSING SIGNS AND SYMPTOMS OF PHYSICAL TRAUMA

Most medicolegal evidence that must be collected is designed to document trauma. Practitioners must provide the best possible care and psychological support while collecting and preserving potentially crucial legal evidence (Braen 1989). Determination of the presence of sperm or semen may help to identify the assailant. The most characteristic physical signs of sexual assault are injuries to the face, head, neck, and extremities. Vaginal and perineal injury is absent in the majority of sexual assault victims. Most victims will have no evidence of sperm on physical examination, and they will have no evidence of trauma (Tintinalli 1985).

Other data that require careful documentation include location and dimensions of all bruises, fractures, lacerations, scratches, and inflammation of soft tissue and mucosae (Dubin and Weiss 1991). Medical evidence per se does not prove rape; it is only supportive evidence. Rape is a legal decision, not a medical diagnosis.

The nurse takes a brief gynecological history, including date of last menstrual period, likelihood of current pregnancy, and history of venereal disease. The victim should *not* be assumed to have had a pelvic examination prior to this event (Lederle et al. 1985). Many women have never had a pelvic examination; if the victim has not, the steps of the examination will need to be explained.

The victim has the right to refuse either a legal or a medical exam. *Consent forms must be signed for photographs, pelvic examination, and whatever other procedures might be needed to collect evidence and treat the victim.* During the pelvic examination, the nurse plays a crucial role in giving support to the victim and minimizing the trauma of the exam. A female nurse should stay in the room with the patient during the exam. The correct preservation of body fluids and swabs is essential, especially because new techniques, such as DNA fingerprinting (genetic fingerprinting), may identify the offender (Penning and Betz 1992). A water-moistened speculum is used to preserve all evidence.

Cultures of the urethra, vagina, and anus for gonococcus (GC) are obtained. A serological test is done for syphilis (serum VDRL). In many cases, prophylactic treatment, such as intramuscular procaine penicillin G or oral ampicillin (for those *not* allergic to penicillin) is given for venereal disease. However, routine administration of antibiotics is controversial because of evidence that the gonococcus organism may be becoming resistant to penicillin. Some experts suggest that venereal disease not be treated until it occurs. Others recommend using ceftriaxone (Rocephin) (Braen 1989).

More controversial is the routine use of diethylstilbestrol (DES) for postcoital contraception (except in cases of women already pregnant). The absolute effectiveness of postcoital contraception has not been determined. Statistics show that only 3–5% of women who are raped become pregnant as a result (Lederle et al. 1985). If the victim is likely to seek aftercare, she may want to wait to initiate intervention until results of a pregnancy test are obtained or until her next period is due to begin. If diethylstilbestrol is administered, close follow-up care should be provided to anticipate or eliminate complications, especially those associated with inadvertent pregnancy (Tintinalli 1985). When a rape counseling center is available, the counseling center staff should assume close and direct responsibility for directing patients for medical follow-up, regardless of emergency room treatment. In addition, to increase the victim's comfort, a shower and fresh clothing should be available to her immediately after the examination, if possible.

Although the medical examination helps determine whether any injury occurred, and although it is used to collect evidence for identification and prosecution of the rapist, the victim may feel that it is another violation of her body. Recognizing this, the nurse can explain the examination procedure in a way that will be reassuring and supportive to the victim. Allowing the victim to participate in all decisions affecting care helps her regain a sense of control over her life.

All data should be carefully documented. Documentation includes verbatim statements by the victim, detailed observations of emotional and physical status, and all results from the physical examination. All laboratory tests performed should be noted, and findings should be recorded as soon as they are available.

Nursing Diagnosis

Rape-trauma syndrome is the nursing diagnosis that applies to the physical and psychological effects resulting from an episode of rape. It includes an acute phase of disorganization of the victim's lifestyle and a long term phase of reorganization. The diagnosis has application regardless of the setting in which the victim is encountered. This syndrome comprises the following three subcomponents, with defining characteristics:

RAPE-TRAUMA SYNDROME. Rape-trauma syndrome can be divided into two phases.

- Acute phase (see Table 13–1)
- Long term phase: reorganization phase

Rape-Trauma Syndrome: Compound Reaction. **Compound reaction** can occur in victims who have had previous or current physical, emotional, or social difficulties and are suffering rape-trauma syndrome.

Symptoms include the following:

- All symptoms listed under *rape-trauma syndrome* (see Table 13–1)
- Reliance on alcohol or other drugs
- Reactivated symptoms of previous conditions, such as physical or psychiatric illness

Rape-Trauma Syndrome: Silent Reaction. Silent reaction is a complex stress reaction to rape, in which an individual is unable to describe or discuss the rape. Symptoms include the following:

- Abrupt changes in relationships with men
- Nightmares
- Increasing anxiety during the interview, such as blocking of associations, long periods of silence, minor stuttering, or physical distress
- Marked changes in sexual behavior
- Sudden onset of phobic reactions
- No verbalization of the occurrence of rape

Planning

Planning care for a person who has been the victim of a sexual assault includes planning on the (1) *content level* (planning goals) and the (2) *process level* (nurses' reactions and feelings).

CONTENT LEVEL—PLANNING GOALS

Client-centered goals for alleviating the victim's discomfort and distress originate from the nursing diagnosis. The goals are both short term and long term. Short term goals are those that the nurse and the victim can achieve while they are working together to relieve the symptoms exhibited during the acute phase of the rape-trauma syndrome. Long term goals are those that will allow the victim to begin to reorganize her life after the immediate crisis.

Examples of short term goals could be

1. Rape-trauma syndrome: acute phase. Victim will
   - Begin to express reactions and feelings about the assault before leaving the emergency room
   - Have short term plan for handling immediate situational needs
   - List common physical, social, and emotional reactions that often follow a sexual assault before she leaves the emergency room
   - Speak to community-based rape-victim advocate in emergency room

- State the results of the physical examination completed in the emergency department
- State she will keep follow-up appointment with nurse, rape-victim advocate, or social worker on (date)

2. Rape-trauma syndrome: long term reorganization phase. Victim will
   - Discuss need for follow-up crisis counseling and other supports by (date)
   - State that memory of the rape is less vivid and less frightening within three to five months
   - State that the physical symptoms (e.g., sleep disturbances, poor appetite, and physical trauma) have subsided within three to five months

PROCESS LEVEL—NURSES' REACTIONS AND FEELINGS

As members of society, nurses have been exposed to the various myths and judgments that exist about the event of rape and the victim of rape. Nurses' attitudes influence the physical and psychological care administered to rape victims, and knowing the myths and facts surrounding rape can increase nurses' awareness of their personal beliefs and feelings regarding rape. Nurses must examine these personal feelings and reactions prior to encountering a rape victim to minimize interference in caregiving. Nurses have their own perceptions and values to explore concerning rape before they can be objective in dealing with the perceptions of others. This process is the same as that described for caring for victims of other types of violence (see Chapter 12).

Belief in myths about rape is perpetuated by society's tendency to deny and minimize the perceived injury and to blame the victim for her own victimization. Acceptance of myths coincides with beliefs that women's social roles and rights should be more restricted than those of men (Costin 1985). Table 13–2 compares rape myths and facts.

Intervention

The experience of rape can be the most devastating experience in a woman's life and constitutes an *acute adventitious crisis*. It is a total violation of the person's body and will. Typical crisis reactions reflect cognitive, affective, and behavioral disruptions. In order for the victim to return to her previous level of functioning, it is necessary for her to mourn her losses, experience anger, and work through her terrifying fears.

Table 13–2 ■ RAPE: MYTH AND FACT

MYTH	FACT
1. Many women really want to be raped.	1. No women ask to be raped—no matter how they are dressed, what their behavior is, or where they are at any given time. No one asks to be hurt.
2. Most rapists are oversexed.	2. Sex is used as an instrument of violence in rape. Rape is an act of aggression, anger, or power.
3. Most women are raped by strangers.	3. 57% of rape victims are raped by someone they know and who is a part of their extended family.
4. No healthy adult female who resists vigorously can be raped by an unarmed man.	4. Most men can overpower most women because of differences in body build. Also the victim may panic, making her actions less effective than usual.
5. Most charges of rape are unfounded.	5. There is *no* evidence to show that there are more false reports for rape than for other crimes. Most rape victims do not even report the rape.
6. Rapes usually occur in dark alleys.	6. Over 50% of all rapes occur in the home.
7. Rape is usually an impulsive act.	7. Most rapes are planned; over 50% involve a weapon.
8. Nice girls don't get raped.	8. *Any* woman is a potential rape victim. Victims range in age from 6 months to 90 years.
9. There was not enough time for a rape to occur.	9. There is no minimum time limit that characterizes rape. It can happen very quickly.
10. Do not fight or try to get away because you will just get hurt.	10. There are no verifiable data to substantiate the theory that a victim will be injured if she tries to get away.
11. Only females are raped.	11. There is a growing number of male rape victims—not necessarily just men in prisons or in the homosexual community.
12. Rape is a sexual act.	12. Rape is a violent expression of aggression, anger, and need for power.

Data from Berkow 1982; Costin 1985; Helen 1984.

PSYCHOTHERAPEUTIC INTERVENTIONS

Nurses usually work with rape victims in the emergency room. However, the victim is often too traumatized, ashamed, or afraid to come to the hospital. For that reason, most communities provide telephone hotlines on a 24-hour basis. A discussion of psychotherapeutic interventions (1) in the emergency room and (2) on crisis hotlines follows.

Psychotherapeutic Interventions in the Emergency Room

Nurses' attitudes can have an important therapeutic impact on the victim's trauma. The most effective approach is to *maintain neutral behavior* with victims. This means that displays of shock, horror, disgust, surprise, disbelief, or any other emotion are not appropriate. *Provide nonjudgmental care* as well as *maximum emotional*

support to the victim. Crisis management of the rape victim is actually the practice of primary prevention of psychiatric disorders. Confidentiality is, of course, crucial in rape cases. Sexual assault cases are not to be discussed, except with medical personnel involved, without the victim's consent.

The most helpful things the nurse can do are to *listen* and to *let the victim talk.* When the nurse listens carefully and empathetically, the distress of the victim can be heard. A woman who feels understood is no longer alone; she then feels more in control of her situation. "A special dimension of listening and understanding is to help people bear the feelings they are trying to express. Sharing the pain is an emotionally strengthening experience for a person" (Burgess and Holstrom 1973).

Allowing the person to express negative affect and **behavioral self-blame** has been recognized as helpful. Behavioral self-blame is an adaptive, functional response to the psychological needs of rape victims (Damrosch 1985). The implication is not that the victim perceives herself to be the cause of the crime but that the person needs to restore control. Efforts to restore control are a positive response to victimization. Behavioral self-blame functions to help the person restore a sense of control.

Self-blame helps preserve one's belief in a just world in which people generally get what they deserve. Attributions to one's behavior (which is controllable) allows the victim to believe that similar experiences can be avoided in the future. Therefore, within this framework, self-blame serves to explain events that are otherwise incomprehensible.

When nurses fail to recognize the function of behavioral self-blame, they may try to dissuade the rape victim from beliefs that are helpful. Using reflective communication techniques (see Chapter 6) to respond to the psychological themes expressed by the victim is more helpful than discounting the victim's role. Examples of helpful and unhelpful responses follow:

A woman states, "I am so mad at myself. I should have never gone out tonight."

Helpful Response	Unhelpful Response
You believe if you had made a different decision earlier this evening, this wouldn't have happened.	Your actions had nothing to do with what happened.

Awareness that the expression of negative affect and behavioral self-blame may be quite helpful to the rape victim will enable nurses to avoid committing acts of *secondary victimization* (the process by which victims are victimized once again by others' reactions, including awkward or ineffective efforts to help) (Damrosch 1985).

If the victim consents, involve her support system, e.g., family or friends, and discuss with them the nature and trauma of sexual assault and possible delayed reactions the victim may experience. Unfortunately, significant relationships frequently deteriorate as a result of the crisis of rape. Reactions from significant others can range from indignation, to denial, to focusing blame on the victim. For this reason and because of the long term process of reorganization, follow-up care for the victim is strongly encouraged. Table 13–3 summarizes the main psychotherapeutic techniques used by the nurse working with a victim of rape.

When preparing the victim to go home, discuss follow-up procedures and give all referral information in writing. Referral to ongoing professional counseling resources and to community support groups, such as rape crisis services, should be routinely offered. Legal referrals (i.e., names of attorneys who specialize in rape cases and options for low-cost legal assistance) can also be given.

Table 13–3 ■ NURSING INTERVENTIONS AND RATIONALES: VICTIMS OF RAPE

INTERVENTION	RATIONALE
1. Do not leave person alone.	1. Prevents increase in isolation, escalation of anxiety.
2. Maintain neutral behavior.	2. Decreases emotional burden.
3. Provide nonjudgmental care.	3. Lessens feelings of shame and embarrassment
4. Maximize emotional support: • Stay with victim • Show concern for victim's needs	4. Prevents further disorganization: • Decreases potential for escalation of anxiety • Validates worth of person
5. Assure confidentiality.	5. Encourages sharing event and protects a person's self-concept and sense of control.
6. Encourage person to talk through empathetically listening.	6. Helps person sort out thoughts and feelings. Lowers anxiety by lowering feelings of isolation.
7. Allow negative expression of affect and behavioral self-blame.	7. Helps person gain a sense of control.
8. Encourage problem solving when anxiety lowers to moderate levels.	8. Increases person sense of control.
9. Engage support system (e.g., family and friends), when appropriate.	9. Provides warmth and feelings of safety when shock wears off and acute disorganization phase begins.
10. Emphasize that the person did the right thing in order to save his or her life.	10. Helps reduce guilt and maintain self-esteem.
11. Arrange for supportive follow-up.	11. Acknowledges that healing takes time.

Data from Burgess and Holstrom 1973; Damrosch 1985; Braen 1989.

The victim's emotional state and other psychological needs should be reassessed by phone or personal contact within 24–48 hours after discharge from the hospital. Repeat referrals should be made for needed resources or support services at this time. Effective crisis intervention and continuity of care require outreach activities and services beyond the emergency medical setting.

Follow-up visits should occur at least two, four, and six weeks after the initial evaluation. At each visit, the patient should be assessed for psychological progress, venereal disease, and pregnancy (Braen 1989).

Emergency departments try to provide comprehensive care and to inform victims of community resources. However, because traumatized people often cannot assimilate all of this information, many hospitals provide follow-up instructions detailing physical concerns, emotional reactions, legal matters, victim compensation, and ways that family and friends can help (Andrews 1992).

Psychotherapeutic Interventions on the Crisis Hotline

Nearly all communities provide 24-hour-a-day crisis telephone service. Some provide 24-hour-a-day hotlines for rape victims (e.g., Rape Relief in Seattle, Washington). The hotline may be used for information and referral, or as a prelude to a personal contact for future telephone counseling.

The phone counselor talks briefly with the person to determine where she is, what has happened, and what kind of help she needs. The counselor provides empathic listening, and the victim is further encouraged to go to the hospital and is advised *not to wash, change clothes, douche, brush teeth, or eat or drink anything,* all of which might destroy evidence. The victim is urged to call the police. The police and rape advocate can meet the victim at the emergency department. Over the phone, the counselor also can encourage the victim to make necessary decisions about communications with family and friends and can give information about what to expect from the hospital and the police. However, all of this communication is better done in person, if possible. The main focus of the telephone contact is on the immediate steps the victim may take. The counselor provides the necessary information for the victim to make decisions. Unfortunately, the victim frequently wishes to remain anonymous, and some do not want any immediate or follow-up counseling.

PSYCHOTHERAPY

Some people who are victimized by rape may be susceptible to a psychotic episode or an emotional disturbance so severe that hospitalization is required. Others whose emotional life may be so overburdened with multiple internal and external pressures may require individual psychotherapy. Most people, however, are eventually able to resume their previous lives after supportive services and crisis counseling. However, many of these victims carry with them a constant emotional trauma: flashbacks, nightmares, constant fear, phobias, and other symptoms associated with post-traumatic stress reaction (refer to Chapter 14).

Depression and suicide ideation are frequent sequelae of rape. Persistent depressive symptomatology is now recognized as an outcome of sexual trauma for some victims. In children who are sexually abused, depressive symptomatology can persist throughout their adult years. In their study of assault victims, Mackey et al. (1992) found that almost two thirds had some degree of depression a mean of 7.9 years after the assault. One factor that had a positive correlation with depression was nondisclosure of the assault to significant others because of concern about being stigmatized. Two other factors correlating with depression were the presence of children living with the victim and a pending civil lawsuit. Any exposure to stimuli related to the traumatic event may activate a re-experiencing of the traumatic state (Mackey et al. 1992).

Often, family and friends of victims of rape are unable or unwilling to be supportive. The long-standing cultural myth that women are the property of men still prevents family and friends from empathizing with the woman's severe psychic injury. She is, instead, often thought of as "devalued." Some clinicians are now offering other forms of therapy after the immediate crisis has lessened because the intrapsychic impact of the rape experience is so profound and can leave such devastating scars (Rose 1986; Ledray 1990).

Group therapy with other victims of rape has been very helpful for many people. Group therapy can make the difference between a person coming out of the crisis at a lower level of functioning or gradually adapting to his or her experience with an increase in coping skills (Gallese and Treuting 1981).

Evaluation

Completion of the process of reorganization after a rape crisis can be evaluated by assessing sleeping and eating patterns, presence or absence of phobias, motor behavior, relationships, self-esteem, and presence or absence of somatic reactions (DiVastro 1985). The victim is recovered if she is

1. Sleeping well, with only very few instances of episodic nightmares or broken sleep.

2. Eating as was her pattern before the rape.
3. Calm and relaxed or only mildly suspicious or restless.
4. Getting support from family and friends. Some strain might still be present in relationships, but it should be minimal.
5. Generally positive about herself. On occasion, doubts about self-worth may occur.

6. Free from somatic reactions. If mild symptoms persist and minor discomfort is reported, the victim should be able to talk about it and feel in control of the symptoms.

In general, the closer the victim's lifestyle is to the pattern that was present before the rape, the more complete the recovery has been.

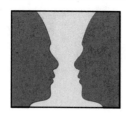

Case Study: Working with a Person Who Has Been Raped

Carol Smith, a 36-year-old single mother of two, went out one evening with some friends. Her children were at a slumber party and she "needed to get away and have a little rest and relaxation." She and her friends had gone bowling. Later in the evening, Carol was tired and ready to go home. One of the men who had joined the group offered to take Carol home. She had seen the man at the bowling alley before but did not know much about him. Not in the habit of going home alone with men she did not know, she hesitated. One of her friends, whom she trusted, told her it was OK to go with Jim because he was a nice man.

Jim drove Carol home. He then asked her if he could come into her house to use the bathroom before he drove the long distance to his house. Carol reluctantly agreed and sat on the living room couch. After using the bathroom, Jim sat next to Carol and began to kiss her and fondle her breasts. As Carol protested, Jim became more forceful in his advances. Carol was confused and frightened. She managed to get away from him briefly, but he began grabbing, squeezing, and biting her. He told her gruffly, "If you don't do what I say I'll break your neck." She screamed, but he proceeded to rape her. Jim became nervous that the noise would alert the neighbors and raced out of the house. A neighbor did in fact arrive just after Jim fled. The neighbor called the police and then brought Carol to the local hospital emergency room for a physical exam, crisis intervention, and support.

In the emergency room Carol was visibly shaken. She kept saying over and over, "I shouldn't have gone home with him, I should have fought harder, I shouldn't have let him do this."

The nurse took Carol to a quiet cubicle. She didn't want Carol to stay alone and asked the neighbor to stay with Carol. The nurse then notified the doctor and the rape-victim advocate. When the nurse came back, she told Carol that she would like to talk to her before the doctor came. Carol looked at her neighbor and then down. The nurse asked the neighbor to wait outside for awhile and told her that she would call her later.

CAROL: It was horrible. I feel so dirty.
NURSE: You have had a terrible experience. Do you want to talk about it?
CAROL: I feel so ashamed, I should have never let that man take me home.
NURSE: You think that if you hadn't gone home with a stranger this wouldn't have happened?
CAROL: Yes . . . I shouldn't have let him do it to me anyway, I shouldn't have let him rape me.
NURSE: You mentioned that he said he would break your neck if you didn't do as he said.
CAROL: Yes, he said that . . . he was going to kill me, it was awful.
NURSE: It seems you did the right thing in order to stay alive.

As the nurse continued to talk with Carol, Carol's anxiety level seemed to lessen. The nurse talked to Carol about the kinds of experiences rape victims often have and collected necessary information. She explained that the doctor would want to examine her and explained the procedure to her. She then asked Carol to sign a consent. While preparing Carol for examination, the nurse noticed bite marks and bruises on both breasts. She also noted Carol's lower lip, which was cut and bleeding. After the examination, Carol was given clean clothes and a place to shower.

Continued on following page

Case Study: Working with a Person Who Has Been Raped *(Continued)*

Assessment

The nurse organized her data into subjective and objective components.

OBJECTIVE DATA

1. Crying and sobbing
2. Bruises and bite marks on each breast
3. Lip cut and bleeding
4. Reported rape to the police

SUBJECTIVE DATA

1. "He was going to kill me."
2. "It was horrible . . . I feel so dirty."
3. "I shouldn't have let him rape me."

Nursing Diagnosis

The nurse formulated the following diagnosis:

1. Rape-trauma syndrome
   - "I shouldn't have let him rape me."
   - "He was going to kill me."
   - Crying and sobbing
   - Bruises and bites on both breasts
   - Reported rape to the police
   - "It was horrible . . . I feel so dirty."

Planning

CONTENT LEVEL—PLANNING GOALS

The nurse devised a plan of care for Carol, based on the nursing diagnosis and the nurse's training as a crisis counselor.

Nursing Diagnosis	Long Term Goals	Short Term Goals
1. *Rape-trauma syndrome*	1. Within five months Carol will state that she thinks less about the rape, is sleeping better, feels safer, and is functioning at her previous level.	1a. Carol will begin to express emotional reactions and feelings before she leaves the emergency room.
		1b. Carol will be able to list possible socioemotional reactions following sexual assault.
		1c. Carol will have written referrals for legal, medical, and crisis counseling before she leaves the emergency room.
		1d. Carol will have a follow-up appointment with the gynecology clinic and the rape advocate-counselor for weekly meetings before she leaves the emergency room.
		1e. Carol's anxiety level will go from severe to moderate before she leaves the emergency room.

PROCESS LEVEL—NURSES' REACTIONS AND FEELINGS

The nurse had worked with victims of rape before and had helped plan the hospital protocol. It had taken a while for her to be able to remain neutral as well as responsive, because her own anger at the assailant had initially gotten in the way. She also remembers a time when a woman came in stating that she was raped but was so calm, smiling, and polite that the nurse initially did not believe her story. She hadn't, at that point, examined her own feelings or dealt with the popular societal myths regarding rape. It was only later, when she had talked to more experienced health care personnel, that she learned that crisis reactions can seem bizarre, confusing, and contradictory.

The nurse learned that staying with the victim, encouraging the victim to express her reactions and feelings, and listening were effective methods of reducing the victim's feelings of anxiety. Once the nurse learned to let go of her personal anger at the attacker and her ambivalence toward the victim, her care and effectiveness improved greatly. All of this growth took time and support from more experienced nurses and other members of the health team.

Intervention	Carol stated that she felt more comfortable after taking a shower and talking to the nurse. She seemed less confused and better able to concentrate, and she began to discuss what she would tell her children. Specific interventions are found in Nursing Care Plan 13–1. It was decided that Carol's neighbor would stay with her overnight. Carol had an appointment the following week with the rape-victim advocate and with a gynecologist in the clinic. Carol was also given written information about legal counseling, crisis groups, and other community follow-up services for victims of rape. The nurse documented Carol's physical and emotional status, including verbatim responses, as well as the results of the physical examination and tests. The nurse called Carol the next morning and encouraged Carol to call her if she had any further questions.
Evaluation	Carol kept her appointment with the rape-victim advocate for counseling, as well as with the gynecologist at the clinic. She continued with the counseling for several months. For a period of time, she experienced acute anxiety attacks when she went out at night, and she had new locks put on all the windows and doors. After three months, she expressed interest in a group that was forming in the next town for women who had been raped; however, she stated that she didn't know if she could go because it started at 6:00 P.M. The counselor told her that arrangements could be made for a volunteer to take her there and back until she felt safer going out at night. After four months, Carol stated that she did feel safer and had been out at night twice in the past week. She was not comfortable yet, but stated that she was making progress. She told the counselor that she was not ready to date. The group had been a great help to her. She continued to call the nurse about once every two weeks and report on her progress. She told the counselor that the nurse had really "saved her life" and that she wasn't ready to let that support go. She was functioning well as a mother and in her job. After five months, the flashbacks ceased and she started sleeping throughout the night without nightmares.

Nursing Care Plan 13–1 ▪ A VICTIM OF SEXUAL ASSAULT: CAROL

NURSING DIAGNOSIS

Rape-trauma syndrome

Supporting Data

- "I shouldn't have let him rape me."
- "He was going to kill me."
- Sobbing and crying.
- Bruises and bites on both breasts.
- Reported rape to the police.
- "It was horrible, I feel so dirty."

Continued on following page

Nursing Care Plan 13–1 ▪ A VICTIM OF SEXUAL ASSAULT: CAROL *(Continued)*

Long Term Goal: Within five months, Carol will state that she thinks less about the rape, is sleeping better, feels safer, and is functioning at her previous level.

Short Term Goal	Intervention	Rationale	Evaluation
1. Carol will begin to express emotional reactions and feelings before she leaves the emergency room.	1a. Nurse remains neutral, non-judgmental, and assures Carol of confidentiality.	1a. Lessens feelings of shame and guilt and encourages sharing of painful feelings	1. <u>Goal met</u> Carol discussed feelings of shame, self-blame, and fear. Continues counseling with rape-victim advocate.
	1b. Nurse does not leave Carol alone.	1b. Deters feelings of isolation and escalation of anxiety	
	1c. Nurse allows negative expressions and behavioral self-blame—uses reflective techniques.	1c. Fosters feeling of control	
	1d. Nurse assures Carol she did the right thing to save her life.	1d. Decreases the burden of guilt and shame	
	1e. When anxiety level is down to moderate, nurse encourages problem solving.	1e. Increases Carol's feeling of control in her own life (when in severe and panic levels a person cannot problem solve)	
2. Carol will be able to list possible socioemotional reactions following sexual assault.	2. Nurse tells Carol of common reactions experienced by people in the long term reorganization phase, e.g., phobias, flashbacks, insomnia, and increased motor activity.	2. Helps Carol anticipate reactions and understand them as part of the recovery process	2. <u>Goal met</u> Carol was able to state five possible future reactions.
3. Carol will state that she will keep a follow-up appointment with the gynecology clinic and rape advocate or counselor before she leaves the emergency room.	3a. Nurse explains emergency room procedure to Carol.	3a. Lowers anticipatory anxiety	3. <u>Goal met</u> Carol kept appointments with gynecology clinic and rape advocate.
	3b. Nurse explains to Carol about the physical examination.	3b. Allows for questions and concerns; victim may be too traumatized and refuse	
	3c. Nurse has Carol sign consent form.	3c. Follow legal protocol	
	3d. Nurse (or female rape-victim advocate) stays with Carol during examination.	3d. Often decreases isolation and anxiety	
	3e. Nurse explains role of rape-victim advocate.	3e. Awareness of supports and why they are needed.	
	3f. Nurse gives results of gynecological and physical examination to Carol.	3f. Enables Carol to participate in decisions and to understand need for follow-up care	
	3g. Nurse documents all physical and emotional data (with verbatim remarks) and lists laboratory tests.	3g. Needed for both medical and legal follow-up	
4. Carol's anxiety level will lessen from severe to moderate before she leaves emergency room.	4a. Nurse gives written referrals for legal, medical, and crisis counseling.	4a. Minimizes increase in anxiety level	4. <u>Goal met</u> Carol was able to start making future plans and stated that she felt less anxious.
	4b. Nurse informs Carol he or she will call her tomorrow A.M.	4b. Validates concern for her feelings and safety	Carol called nurse to "check in." Nurse plans to have conferences with Carol.
	4c. Nurse makes plans such that Carol is not alone for a few days.	4c. Helps decrease anxiety and increase feelings of safety	

Summary

In recent years, rape victims have begun to receive the attention they deserve from the health care system—and the empathy and support they need. A rape victim experiences a wide range of feelings, which may or may not be exhibited. Feelings of fear, degradation, anger and rage, helplessness, and nervousness are common. Long term sequelae, such as sleep disturbances, disturbed relationships, flashbacks, depression, and somatic complaints are also common.

For the victim, the circumstances of the initial medical evaluation may be frightening and stressful. Police interrogation, repeated questioning by health professionals, and the physical examination itself all have the potential to add to the trauma of the sexual assault. Nurses, in their role of case managers, can serve to minimize repetition of questions and support the victim as she goes through the entire ordeal. Following resolution of the immediate crisis, victims require follow-up and, often, counseling to minimize the long term effects of the rape and to assist in an early return to a normal living pattern.

Although community resources may vary considerably, most metropolitan areas now have special programs to assist rape victims. Such assistance usually includes advice on the management of the acute crisis, as well as guidelines for the collection of evidence and preparation for trial should legal action follow.

References

Abarbanel G. Roles of the clinical social worker. *In* Warner CG (ed). Rape and Sexual Assault. Germantown, MD: Aspen Systems Corporation, 1980.

Andrews J. Sexual assault aftercare instructions. Journal of Emergency Nursing, 18(2):152, 1992.

Antognoli-Toland P. Comprehensive program for examination of sexual assault victims by nurses: A hospital-based project in Texas. Journal of Emergency Nursing, 11(3):132, 1985.

Bang L. Chronic health problems after rape. Tidsskrift for den Norske Laegeforening, 111(20):2525, 1991.

Berkow R (ed). The Merck Manual of Diagnosis and Therapy, 14th ed. Rahway, NJ: Merck Sharp & Dohme Research Laboratories, 1982.

Berkow R, Fletcher AJ (eds). The Merck Manual. Rahway, NJ: Merck Research Laboratories, 1992.

Braen GR. The adult female survivor of sexual assault. Hospital Medicine, 25(12):43, 1989.

Burgess AW. Rape trauma syndrome: A nursing diagnosis. Occupational Health Nursing, 33(8):405, 1985.

Burgess AW, Holstrom LL. The rape victim in the ER. American Journal of Nursing, 73(10):1740, 1973.

Burgess AW, Holstrom LL. Rape trauma syndrome. American Journal of Psychiatry, 131:981, 1974.

Costin F. Beliefs about rape and women's social roles. Archives of Sexual Behavior, 14(4):319, 1985.

Damrosch SP. Nursing students' assessments of behaviorally self-blaming rape victims. Nursing Research, 34(4):221, 1985.

DiVastro P. Measuring the aftermath of rape. Journal of Psychosocial Nursing, 23(2):33, 1985.

Dubin WK, Weiss KJ. Handbook of Psychiatric Emergencies. Springhouse, PA: Springhouse Corporation, 1991.

Gallese LE, Treuting EG. Help for rape victims through group therapy. Journal of Psychosocial Nursing and Mental Health Services, 19:20, 1981.

Helen M. Rape: Some facts, myths and responses. The Australian Nurses Journal, 13(8):42, 1984.

Jezierski M. Sexual assault nurse examiner: A role with lifetime impact. Journal of Emergency Nursing; 18(2):177, 1992.

Kaplan HI, Sadock BJ. Synopsis of Psychiatry, 6th ed. Baltimore: Williams & Wilkins, 1991.

Lederle DJ, DiGirolamo J, Poskins P. Rape crisis services. Illinois Medical Journal, 167(4):305, 1985.

Ledray LE. Counseling rape victims: the nursing challenge. Perspectives in Psychiatric Care, 26(2):21, 1990.

Mackey T, et al. Factors associated with long-term depressive symptoms of sexual assault victims. Archives of Psychiatric Nursing; 6(1):10, 1992.

Mims FH, Chang AS. Unwanted sexual experiences of young women. Journal of Psychosocial Nursing, 22(6):7, 1984.

Penning R, Betz P. Physical examination of the victim of alleged rape. Geburtshilfe und Frauenheilkunde, 52(1):59, 1992.

Rose DS. "Worse than death": Psychodynamics of rape victims and need for psychotherapy. American Journal of Psychiatry, 143:817, 1986.

Sampselle CM. The role of nursing in preventing violence against women. Journal of Obstetric, Gynecologic, and Neonatal Nursing, 20(6):481, 1991.

Schwartz IL. Sexual violence against women: Prevalence, consequences, societal factors, and prevention. American Journal of Preventive Medicine, 7(6):363, 1991.

Tintinalli JE. Clinical findings and legal resolution in sexual assault. Annals of Emergency Medicine, 14(5):447, 1985.

Further Reading

Bradford JM. Research on sex offenders. Psychiatric Clinics of North America, 6(4):715, 1983.

Brodyaga L. Rape and its victims: A report for citizens, health facilities, and criminal justice agencies. Washington DC: National Institute of Law Enforcement and Criminal Justice, Law Enforcement Assistance Administration, US Department of Justice, 1975.

Kim MJ, McFarland GK, McLane AM (eds). Pocket Guide to Nursing Diagnoses. St. Louis: CV Mosby, 1984.

Nelson C. Victims of rape: Who are they? *In* Warner CG (ed). Rape and Sexual Assault. Germantown, MD: Aspen Systems Corporation, 1980, pp. 9–20.

President's Task Force on Victims of Crimes. Washington DC: Government Printing Office, 1982. No. 82-24146.

Ruch LO, Chandler. Sexual assault trauma and trauma change. Women and Health, 8(4):5, 1983.

Warner CG (ed). Rape and Sexual Assault. Germantown, MD: Aspen Systems Corporation, 1980.

Self-study Exercises

Place a T (true) or an F (false) next to each statement.
The definition of rape:

1. _____ Is forced and violent vaginal or anal penetration.
2. _____ Can include forced genital contact, e.g., oral-genital contact.
3. _____ Cannot be used to describe relations between husband and wife.
4. _____ Is increasingly used to describe women assaulting men.

The truth regarding rape:

5. _____ Most rapists are oversexed.
6. _____ Do not fight or try to get away, for you will just get hurt.
7. _____ Most women who are raped "asked" for it.
8. _____ Rape is usually an impulsive act.

Place an A (acute phase) or an LT (long term reorganization phase) next to the symptoms most likely found in that phase.

9. _____ Skeletal muscle tension, e.g., headaches, twitches, and grimaces.
10. _____ Intrusive thoughts of the rape the woman is unable to control.
11. _____ A controlled style of handling trauma, e.g., calm and subdued, or numb and shocked.
12. _____ Phobias, e.g., fear of strangers, of being alone, of someone behind her, or of going out.
13. _____ Self-blame, shame, and guilt.
14. _____ Increased motor activity, e.g., taking trips, changing phone number, or moving to new location.
15. _____ Expressed style of handling trauma, e.g., crying, hysteria, tense, smiling, or sobbing.

Choose the letter that best answers the following questions.

16. When a person who has been sexually assaulted is assessed, all of the following are important considerations. Which of the following is *not* appropriate during the assessment in the emergency room:

    A. Do not touch the person, unless she reaches out for tactile support.
    B. Do not leave the person alone.
    C. If the person is extremely anxious, remove her to the treatment room or private place right away.
    D. The victim should not be seen until the emergency room is almost empty.

17. When helping with the physical part of the assessment, the nurse should be aware of all of the following except:

    A. The victim has the right to refuse a medical examination.
    B. The absence of sperm proves the absence of a rape.
    C. The physical examination should be carefully explained to the victim, and a nurse should stay with the person.
    D. Fresh clothes and a shower should be made available after the examination.

18. Choose the goal that is *not* a short term goal formulated for rape-trauma syndrome.

    A. Victim will experience reduction of anxiety before leaving the emergency room.

B. Victim will state short term plan for handling immediate situation.
C. Victim will begin to express reactions and feelings before leaving emergency room.
D. Victim will state that physical symptoms (e.g., sleep disturbances and poor appetite) have subsided.

19. Choose the intervention that is *not* a therapeutic technique for use with a victim of sexual assault.

   A. Never leave the woman alone.
   B. Allow negative expression and behavioral self-blame.
   C. Emphasize that the person did the right thing in order to save her life.
   D. Initiate touching the victim as a means of emotional support.

20. The main focus of the telephone contact in a rape crisis hotline is to

   A. Get the victim to prosecute her assailant.
   B. Find out where she is and get the police.
   C. Insist that she come to the hospital emergency room for further treatment.
   D. Provide information to facilitate the victim's decision making and help plan the next steps.

21. Which of the following is *not* a reason many rapes go unreported?

   A. The rape victim goes on trial as well as the rapist.
   B. Men are less likely to report rape because of strong reactions from society.
   C. Fear and anguish prevent people from seeking medical help and reporting the crime.
   D. Rape is not a crime.

Write brief responses in answer to the following.

22. Name four areas that the nurse carefully documents in the victim's chart.

   A. _____
   B. _____
   C. _____
   D. _____

23. Name four responsibilities of the nurse working with a victim of rape during a physical examination.

   A. _____
   B. _____
   C. _____
   D. _____

PEOPLE IN MODERATE TO SEVERE LEVELS OF CHRONIC ANXIETY

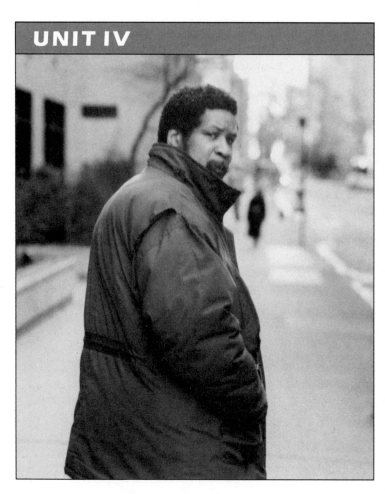

UNIT IV

The worst sin towards our fellow creatures is not to hate them, but to be indifferent to them; that's the essence of inhumanity.

GEORGE BERNARD SHAW
The Devil's Disciple (1901)

A Nurse Speaks

by Margaret R. Swisher

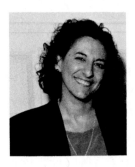

My first experience in mental health was on a substance abuse unit. Most of the patients abused alcohol; in 1976, only a few patients in a private psychiatric hospital were addicted to barbiturates or street drugs. The program was very structured and unified in its philosophy; I rarely questioned the path to recovery. These normal-looking individuals had a terrible disease, and we battled denial until the patients understood and began to work on their addiction. After two years, I moved to general psychiatry, unprepared for the diseases, the treatment, and the politics of chronic mental illness.

Many of the patients in the state hospital were schizophrenic. Everything I had read about the disease seemed inconsequential when I was actually confronted with the bizarre behavior of the patients. They shouted and argued with invisible people and occasionally punched each other. Some were like robots, unemotional and compliant, neither happy nor sad. Many patients had movement disorders due to neuroleptic medication. They twitched, they stumbled, they staggered down the corridors. They drooled and choked on their food. Treatment was a vague collection of busywork therapies and lots of television.

I felt confused and overwhelmed by schizophrenia. I watched patients like Wanda W., dressed in three layers of clothing, pace through the unit checking the ashtrays for cigarette butts. Her fingers had yellow and black stains from smoking. Always alone and roaming the grounds of the hospital, Wanda was preoccupied by a voice that whispered commands. What was I supposed to do for her? She seemed content. Did she really need motivation, plans for the future, or a relationship with me?

We started by talking about cigarettes. Wanda had a system for watching people who smoked and then finding their discarded butts. She kept them in a blue leather purse, which she stuffed into her coat pocket. "I need them," Wanda smiled and patted her pocket. I started making "rounds" with her as she searched the hospital grounds for smokers. Wanda, with her purse, three sweaters, and two pairs of pants, began looking for me in the morning. I smiled and waved to her and said, "I can see that you are waiting for me." Building trust was the simple act of listening to Wanda and acknowledging her without judgment or control. Should I have been telling her about the health effects of smoking and "redirecting" her to checkers? In time, I would.

Schizophrenia was beginning to make sense. You have to find a path inside the patient that reaches to the outside world. Perceptual distortions isolate the patient from social contact, and relationships deteriorate as the person withdraws in self-defense. Wanda would never be cured, but she could broaden her world. It was a slow process of offering her options and then walking her through the new behaviors.

Chronically mentally ill patients, many of whom are schizophrenic, are the most disenfranchised members of society. Most do not work, pay taxes, vote, or buy property. Many spend years in hospitals or outpatient programs, dependent on federal, state, and local funds for life. Organizations like National Alliance for the Mentally Ill (NAMI) provide a political voice, but friends move on, family members grow and change—the schizophrenic relapses and regresses. For the hospitalized patient, a mother or a brother may visit once a year, and ask cheerfully "How have you been?" Years pass, but the illness does not.

Today, I teach students about schizophrenia and answer the questions they ask when confronted with the disease. "What should I say?" "What should I do?" Listen. Find out what is important to the patient. Then, go walking.

CHAPTER 14

Anxiety Disorders

Helene S. Charron

KEY TERMS AND CONCEPTS

The key terms and concepts listed here also appear in bold where they are defined or discussed in this chapter.

AGORAPHOBIA

ANXIOLYTIC DRUGS/ANTIANXIETY
   DRUGS

COMPULSIONS

EGO-DYSTONIC/EGO-ALIEN

EGO-SYNTONIC

FLASHBACK

FLOODING

GENERALIZED ANXIETY DISORDER

GRADUATED EXPOSURE

MODELING

OBSESSIONS

PANIC DISORDER

PHOBIAS

POST-TRAUMATIC STRESS DISORDER

PRIMARY GAIN

SECONDARY GAIN

SIMPLE (SPECIFIC) PHOBIA

SOCIAL PHOBIA

SYSTEMATIC DESENSITIZATION

OBJECTIVES ▪

After studying this chapter, the student will be able to

1. Identify various theories of etiology associated with the anxiety disorders.
2. Formulate appropriate nursing diagnoses that can be used when working with a person with an anxiety disorder.
3. Propose realistic and measurable long term and short term goals for clients with anxiety disorders.
4. Discuss interventions that (a) reduce anxiety and ego-dystonic symptoms, (b) assist client to use more effective coping strategies, and (c) support client during ongoing therapy.
5. Evaluate the effectiveness of care based on established outcome criteria.
6. Identify examples of primary and secondary gain.
7. Analyze the value of ego-dystonic symptoms to the client.
8. Describe clinical manifestations of each anxiety disorder.
9. Identify ego defense mechanisms commonly associated with each anxiety disorder.
10. Identify psychiatric treatment modalities useful for each anxiety disorder.
11. Describe the nursing roles associated with each treatment modality.
12. Recognize feelings commonly experienced by nurses assigned to clients manifesting ego-dystonic symptoms.

As discussed in Chapter 9, ego defense mechanisms are unconsciously used by everyone as buffers against anxiety. This chapter focuses on a group of disorders that result when anxiety is not relieved by usual coping mechanisms. In these disorders, the individual resorts to multiple defense mechanisms, resulting in the development of rigid, repetitive, and ineffective behaviors. These disorders are classified in the *Diagnostic and Statistical Manual of Mental Disorders, third edition, revised* (DSM-III-R; APA 1987) as anxiety disorders and include:

1. Panic disorder
2. Phobic disorder
   a. Agoraphobia
   b. Social phobia
   c. Simple (or specific) phobias
3. Generalized anxiety disorder
4. Obsessive-compulsive disorder
5. Post-traumatic stress disorder

The common denominator among these disorders is that individuals experience a degree of anxiety that is so high it interferes with personal, occupational, or social functioning. Placement of these disorders on the mental health continuum can be seen in Figure 14–1.

Behaviors and symptoms observed among individuals experiencing anxiety disorders include

- *Overt anxiety*, with the unpleasant physical, psychological, and cognitive symptoms described in Chapter 9, e.g., palpitations, difficulty concentrating, and feelings of dread.
- *Phobias*, defined as excessive, irrational fears causing the individual to avoid the feared object or situation in order to control anxiety, e.g., fear of spiders (arachnophobia), fear of open spaces (agoraphobia), or fear of speaking in public (social phobia).

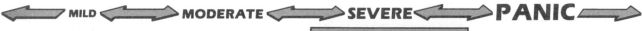

MILD	MODERATE	SEVERE	PANIC
Normal levels experienced by everyone	Psychophysiological disorders	**Anxiety disorders** Panic disorder Phobic disorder Agoraphobia Social phobia Simple (or specific) phobias Generalized anxiety disorder Obsessive-compulsive disorder Post-traumatic stress disorder	Psychoses Mood disorder Schizophrenia Organic mental disorder

Figure 14–1. *The mental health continuum for anxiety disorders.*

- *Obsessions*, defined as persistent and intrusive thoughts, impulses, or images that cannot be dismissed, e.g., believing that one's hands are full of germs or having obscene phrases that keep coming to mind.
- *Compulsions*, defined as ritualistic behaviors (e.g., handwashing or checking) or mental acts (e.g., praying or counting) that the person feels driven to perform.

Some symptoms experienced by individuals with anxiety disorders are termed **ego-alien** or **ego-dystonic,** that is, the individual recognizes them as strange or odd but is unable to do anything about them. For example, a person with a compulsion might state, "It's silly for me to do this checking and re-checking. It takes up so much of my time, but I can't help myself. If I don't check I get so anxious I can't stand it." Individuals experience feelings of dissatisfaction, unhappiness, and low self-esteem as a result of their ego-dystonic symptoms.

Individuals with **ego-syntonic** symptoms have behaviors or beliefs with which they are comfortable. However, others view these behaviors or beliefs as being strange. For example, a man who is highly suspicious might believe that the people in his neighborhood hate him. He does not feel that this belief is silly or strange because the idea that everyone hates him is compatible with his suspicious nature and his view of the world.

Why don't people who recognize a personal behavior as being "silly" stop performing that behavior? The clue to a person's powerlessness lies in such statements as, "I can't help myself. If I don't do it, I get so anxious I can't stand it!" Initially, these "silly" behaviors temporarily relieve anxiety; therefore, the behaviors are used again and again when anxiety occurs. Unfortunately, most ego-dystonic behaviors are effective in reducing anxiety for only a short time; therefore, the behavior must be repeated again and again (Fig. 14–2). A rigid pattern of repetition is established, and the individual does not have enough time or energy to try other ways of coping with the original stress.

When working with a client with an anxiety disorder, the nurse can often identify both primary and secondary gains achieved by the client. **Primary gain** refers to the anxiety relief resulting from the use of defense mechanisms and symptom formation. **Secondary gain** is defined as any benefit the individual obtains as a result of the behaviors, such as gaining attention, being able to avoid responsibility, having dependent needs met, or getting one's own way. Because the person's behavior actually reduces anxiety, it is often difficult for clients to give up their symptoms, maladaptive as they may be.

Theory

We are able to describe the symptoms of anxiety disorders, but little is actually known about the underlying causes. It's necessary to consider (1) biochemical, (2) genetic, (3) psychosocial, and (4) sociocultural factors.

BIOCHEMICAL FACTORS

Researchers are currently exploring possible biochemical causes for anxiety. Attention is being given to the brain stem, especially the locus ceruleus, because of its noradrenergic function; the limbic system, which may generate anticipatory anxiety; and the prefrontal cortex, which may be responsible for phobic avoidance.

Several interesting research findings hint at possible causes and treatments (Kaplan and Sadock 1991):

1. The brain's gamma-aminobutyric acid (GABA) system is believed to exert a "braking effect" on anxiety. GABA and GABA receptors seem to have a role in opening the chloride channels across cell membranes, producing a general inhibition of neuronal function. The effects of GABA seem to be potentiated by the benzodiazepine group of drugs.

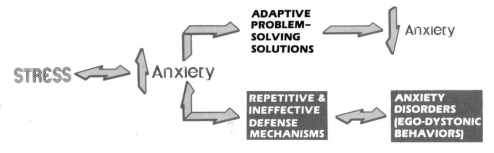

Figure 14–2. *Conceptualization of the process of developing anxiety disorders.*

2. The brain contains receptor or binding sites for antianxiety drugs. Anxiety-prone individuals may produce substances that interfere with the normal function of the binding sites (Hollander et al. 1988). Antianxiety drugs may lock into the receptor sites, thereby preventing these substances from disrupting normal brain physiology.

3. Individuals who have panic attacks tend to have higher levels of norepinephrine, suggesting an abnormality in the catecholamine system. Panic attacks occur spontaneously—they do not seem to be related to events or circumstances, unlike fear that is related to a specific object or event. Panic attacks may be related to a malfunction of the body's alarm system.

4. In about 70% of panic-prone individuals, panic attacks can be induced by infusing sodium lactate. Only 5% of control subjects are similarly affected (Kaplan and Sadock 1991). The chemical basis for this reaction seems to be that sodium lactate induces an abnormal increase of norepinephrine in panic-prone clients.

5. Panic-prone clients who are treated with imipramine (Tofranil), a tricyclic antidepressant, report fewer or no panic attacks. Tricyclic antidepressants exert a powerful noradrenergic effect on the locus ceruleus.

6. Monoamine oxidase inhibitors (MAOIs) are being used successfully to treat anxiety disorders, especially panic attacks and social phobias. MAOIs also exert noradrenergic effects on the locus ceruleus.

7. Obsessive-compulsive disorder (OCD) has been associated with excessive serotonin, a brain biogenic amine and synaptic neurotransmitter. Reduction in serotonin level, as occurs with the use of the tricyclic clomipramine (Anafranil), reduces obsessional thinking and compulsive behavior for many people (Simoni 1991).

8. Positron-emission tomographic scans have identified abnormal blood flow to the frontal lobes and basal ganglia in clients with OCD (Rapoport 1990).

As research reveals new findings, we must be alert to the possibility that these disorders may eventually be viewed more as physiological disorders than as psychological problems.

GENETIC FACTORS

Data from family and twin studies seem to support the idea that a predisposition to develop anxiety disorders may be partially hereditary. Kaplan and Sadock (1991) reported

- A 15–17% incidence of panic disorder among first-degree relatives of clients with panic disorders, compared with a 2.3% incidence in the control group.
- An 80–90% concordance of panic disorder in identical twins and a 10–15% concordance for fraternal twins.
- About 20% of first-degree relatives of agoraphobics have agoraphobia.
- Some 3–7% of individuals with OCD have first-degree relatives with the disorder.
- About 25% of the first-degree relatives of individuals with generalized anxiety disorder are affected.

PSYCHOSOCIAL FACTORS

Early theories about the development of anxiety disorders center around the idea that unconscious childhood conflicts are the basis for symptom development. *Freud* pictured anxiety as resulting from the threatened breakthrough of repressed ideas or emotions from the unconscious into consciousness. Examples would include

- Anxiety associated with guilt, if inner rules or standards are broken or high ideals are unmet
- Anxiety associated with losing the love of significant others (considered to have a relationship with agoraphobia in later life)
- Anxiety associated with the idea that the body or its parts may be injured
- Anxiety associated with dangerous impulses, such as hostility

Ego defense mechanisms are used by the individual to keep anxiety at manageable levels.

Table 14–1 defines and gives examples of defense mechanisms commonly used by individuals with anxiety disorders. These defense mechanisms produce behavior that is not wholly adaptive but nevertheless permits better adaptation than the more immature defenses, such as engaging in delusional projection, psychotic denial, or fantasy; turning against the self; or acting out. At the highly adaptive end of the continuum, more mature and desirable defenses, such as humor, altruism, suppression, and sublimation, are used by individuals who are happier and have a high level of mental health (Valliant 1986).

Harry Stack Sullivan placed anxiety in an interpersonal context. He believed that all anxiety is linked to the emotional distress caused when early needs go unmet and to the anxiety transmitted to the infant from the caregiver via the process of empathy. This initial anxiety becomes the prototype for what is experienced when unpleasant events occur in later life.

Learning theories provide another view. *Behavioral psychologists* see anxiety as a learned response that can

Table 14–1 ■ **DEFENSES USED IN ANXIETY DISORDERS**			
PHENOMENA	**DEFENSE**	**PURPOSE**	**EXAMPLE**
Phobias	Displacement	In phobias, anxiety is reduced when strong feelings about the original object are directed at a less threatening object and that object is avoided.	Client has abnormal fear of cats. In therapy, it is discovered that client is sexually attracted to sister-in-law.
Compulsions	Undoing	Performing a symbolic act cancels out an unacceptable act or idea.	Symbolic rituals, such as handwashing, cleaning, and checking. Handwashing removes guilt. Cleaning removes dirty thoughts. Checking protects against hostile thoughts.
Obsessions	Reaction-formation	Anxiety-producing unacceptable thoughts or feelings are kept out of awareness by the opposite feeling or idea.	Client with strong aggressive feelings toward husband repeatedly thinks the opposite ("I love him with all my heart") to keep feelings out of awareness.
	Intellectualization	The excessive use of reasoning, logic, or words is used to prevent the person from experiencing associated feelings.	Person talks in detail about his parents' funeral but is unable to feel the associated pain of loss.
Post-traumatic stress disorder	Isolation	Facts associated with an anxiety-laden event remain conscious, but associated painful feelings are separated from the experience.	Post-traumatic stress disorder client describes feeling "numb and empty inside."
	Repression	Unconsciously pushes an anxiety-producing idea or feeling out of awareness.	Man is unable to trust authority figures at work after taking orders from his commanding officer to kill civilians while in combat.

be unlearned. Some individuals may learn to be anxious from the modeling provided by parents or peers. For example, a mother who is fearful of thunder and lightning and who hides in closets during storms may transmit her anxiety to her children, who will continue to adopt her behavior even into adult life. Consequently, individuals can unlearn this behavior by observing others who react normally to a storm. Behaviorists contend that individuals may learn phobias as the result of a conditioning process.

Cognitive theorists take the position that anxiety disorders are caused by distortions in the way the individual thinks and perceives. *Albert Ellis* (1962) suggests that socially anxious people believe they must be approved of all the time by everyone. They must never make a mistake—when they do, they believe it is a catastrophe, and the ensuing response is acute anxiety.

SOCIOCULTURAL FACTORS

Reliable data on the incidence of anxiety disorders in both this and other cultures are sparse. Coleman and associates (1980) suggest that anxiety disorders and ritualistic behaviors are more commonly noted in societies with high technology. Dohrenwend and Dohrenwend (1974) found that anxiety disorders occur more frequently among urban populations than among rural ones. Some sociocultural variation in symptoms has been noted. For example, during panic attacks, Latino Americans and Northern Europeans are likely to experience sensations of choking, smothering, numbness, or tingling, as well as fear of dying. Agoraphobia is experienced more frequently by Northern Europeans and Americans (Global Heart of Panic 1990). Brown et al. (1990) mention that phobic disorders are more prevalent among blacks than whites. It is probably safe to infer that when a society undergoes rapid changes, the stress induced by the changes places the group at risk for the development of anxiety disorders.

THE CLINICAL PICTURE OF PANIC DISORDER

Symptoms essential for diagnosing a **panic disorder** include the presence of panic attacks (Fig. 14–3). The feelings of terror present during a panic attack are so severe that normal function is suspended, the perceptual field is severely limited, and misinterpretation of reality may occur. Severe personality disorganization is evident. Typically, panic attacks "come out of the blue" (i.e., suddenly and not necessarily provoked by stress), are extremely intense for three to 10 minutes, and then subside (Preston and Johnson 1991).

Persons experiencing a panic attack may believe they are losing their mind or having a heart attack. Individuals may feel dizzy or lightheaded, the heart may begin to pound, and they may not be able to catch their breath (Hollander et al. 1988). Attacks can be so intense that the individual is unable to tolerate the experience for a prolonged period. He or she typically pleads for help. Depression may complicate the symptoms in as many as 70% of cases.

Lisa is a 45-year-old teacher. She became overwhelmed in class when a student challenged her about a test score. She remembers this as her first panic attack. At the time, she felt that she was going to die, had palpitations, and started to perspire profusely. After that incident, she could not return to school. Even thoughts of teaching bring on great apprehension and fear.

THE CLINICAL PICTURE OF GENERALIZED ANXIETY DISORDER

The *DSM IV* criteria used for diagnosing generalized anxiety disorder can be reviewed in Figure 14–3. In addition to these manifest symptoms, other characteristics may be noted. Individuals with generalized anxiety disorder are chronic worriers, always "what if-ing" ("What if I fail the quiz?" "What if she doesn't like me?"). Decision making is difficult because of poor concentration and the dread of making a mistake. Worry over the physical symptoms being experienced is common, as is worry about inadequacies in interpersonal relationships. Initiating sleep is difficult because the individual worries about the day's events

and real or imagined mistakes, reviews past problems, and anticipates future difficulties. During sleep, nightmares about disastrous situations often occur. The individual may dream of being shot, of being chased and unable to run, of falling from high places, or of being choked. Generalized anxiety is a chronic condition. About 25% of these clients go on to develop panic disorders (Kaplan and Sadock 1991).

June is a 49-year-old legal secretary. She has been divorced for five years, and her only daughter is expecting her first child. Although the pregnancy is going well, June worries that something is wrong with the baby: "What if it's premature?" "What if it's deformed?" She is not sleeping well and is having difficulty concentrating at work, and her usual way of relaxing (gardening) doesn't interest her anymore. June has been a worrier for years. Over the past 17 months, she has experienced dizziness, sweaty palms, and irritability.

THE CLINICAL PICTURE OF PHOBIA

Characteristically, phobic individuals experience overwhelming and crippling anxiety when faced with the object of the phobia. Phobic people go to great lengths to avoid the feared object, situation, or activity. A phobic individual may not even be able to think about or visualize the object or situation without becoming severely anxious. The individual becomes more isolated, and life becomes more restricted as activities are given up to avoid contact with the feared object or situation.

The three classes of phobias are listed in Figure 14–3. **Agoraphobia** is the most common phobia for which people seek treatment. **Agoraphobia** is fear and avoidance of being in open spaces from which escape might be difficult. Although agoraphobic clients may think they are "going crazy," they do not exhibit psychotic symptoms. Agoraphobia can be debilitating and life constricting. Severely agoraphobic individuals may be unable to leave their homes. Panic attacks are commonly associated with this disorder.

Social phobias include fear of public speaking, fear of eating with others present, and fear of writing or performing in public. Social phobias may also involve general fears of saying foolish things or not being able to answer questions in public. Social phobias can cause considerable inconvenience and may result in substance abuse if the individual turns to alcohol or other drugs for reducing anxiety.

Simple (specific) phobias involve fear and avoidance of a single object, situation, or activity. Specific

PANIC DISORDER

1. Severe recurrent Panic Attacks

2. Sudden onset with intense apprehension and dread

3. At least four of the following symptoms:
   - Dyspnea
   - Chest discomfort
   - Dizziness
   - Hot or cold flashes
   - Tingling of hands or feet
   - Feelings of unreality
   - Palpitations
   - Syncope
   - Diaphoresis
   - Trembling
   - Fear of losing control, going crazy, or dying

POST-TRAUMATIC STRESS DISORDER

1. After experiencing a psychologically traumatic event, outside the range of usual experience (e.g., rape, combat, bombings, and kidnapping), the person re-experiences the event via recurrent and intrusive dreams or flashbacks

2. Emotional numbness, detachment, and estrangement may be used to defend against anxiety

3. May experience sleep disturbance, hypervigilence, guilt about surviving, poor concentration, and avoidance of activities that trigger memory of the event

PHOBIAS

1. Irrational fear of an object or situation that persists although the person may recognize it as unreasonable

2. Types include:
   - **Agoraphobia:** Fear of being alone in open or public places where escape might be difficult; may not leave home
   - **Social phobia:** Fear of situations in which one might be seen and embarrassed or criticized; speaking to authority figures, public speaking, or performing
   - **Specific phobia:** Fear of a single object, activity, or situation (e.g., snakes, closed spaces, and flying)

3. Anxiety is severe if the object, situation, or activity cannot be avoided

GENERALIZED ANXIETY DISORDER

1. Persists for at least six months

2. Symptoms present from three of the four following categories:
   - Motor tension (e.g., trembling, restlessness, inability to relax, and fatigue)
   - Autonomic hyperactivity (e.g., sweating, palpitations, cold clammy hands, urinary frequency, lump in throat, pallor or flushing, increased pulse, and rapid respirations)
   - Apprehensiveness (e.g., worry, dread, fear, rumination, insomnia, and inability to concentrate)
   - Hypervigilence (e.g., feeling edgy, scanning the environment, and distractability)

OBSESSIVE-COMPULSIVE DISORDER

1. Preoccupation with persistent intrusive thoughts (obsessions), repeated performance of rituals designed to prevent some event (compulsions), or both

2. Anxiety occurs if obsessions or compulsions are resisted and from being powerless to resist the thoughts or rituals

Figure 14–3. Diagnostic criteria for anxiety disorders. (Adapted from American Psychiatric Association. *Diagnostic and Statistical Manual of Mental Disorders, Fourth Edition, Revised.* (DSM-IV). Washington, DC: American Psychiatric Association, 1994.)

Table 14-2 ■ CLINICAL NAMES FOR COMMON PHOBIAS

CLINICAL NAME	FEAR
Acrophobia	Heights
Agoraphobia	Open spaces
Astraphobia	Electrical storms
Claustrophobia	Closed spaces
Glossophobia	Talking
Hematophobia	Blood
Hydrophobia	Water
Monophobia	Being alone
Mysophobia	Germs or dirt
Pyrophobia	Fire
Zoophobia	Animals

phobias usually do not cause the individual much difficulty because one can usually avoid a single object, such as snakes, closed spaces, darkness, cats, or spiders. Simple phobias are common in the general public.

It is acceptable to describe phobias in everyday language; however, Table 14–2 identifies specific terminology associated with them.

Jim is a 28-year-old agoraphobic. He used to live a very active life, often participating in thrill-seeking activities, like bungee jumping and skydiving. Jim's father died two years ago. Since that time, Jim has become more fearful of the outdoors. He has started a successful mail-order business from his home, which he shares with his mother. He gradually stops leaving the family home because of feelings of intense anxiety and the fear that he is going to die whenever he is away from home.

THE CLINICAL PICTURE OF OBSESSIVE-COMPULSIVE DISORDER

DSM-III-R and *DSM-IV* criteria for OCD are briefly described in Figure 14–3. Recent studies reveal that OCD occurs at rates 25–50 times greater than previous estimates (Whitley 1991). An **obsession** is a persistent intrusive thought or image that seems senseless to the individual but serves to lessen anxiety. An obsession is a thought or thoughts that are impossible to put out of one's mind. In true obsessions, the person considers the intrusive thought or

image to be ego-dystonic. **Compulsions** are senseless repetitive behaviors performed according to certain rules known to the client. The client performs the compulsive act to reduce or prevent some anxiety-laden event. Therefore, the act temporarily reduces high levels of anxiety. The individual usually realizes that the behavior is not connected in a realistic way with what it is designed to accomplish. Attempts to resist either the obsession or the compulsion cause the individual to feel increasingly anxious. Performing the action (compulsion) results in temporary relief of anxiety. Thus, the primary gain achieved by compulsive rituals can be seen as a temporary reduction of anxiety. Although obsessions can occur without accompanying compulsions, the two are often seen together.

"Normal" individuals may experience some manifestations of obsessions. Nearly everyone has had the experience of having a persistent tune run through his or her mind despite attempts to push it away. Also commonly experienced is a nagging doubt as to whether one has locked the door or turned off the stove. These obsessions often cannot be put to rest until the person goes back to check the door or stove, sometimes more than once. *The action of going back to check is the compulsion.* Obsessions that lead an individual into psychiatric care usually are more troublesome than these and usually center on issues of sexuality, violence, germs and dirt, or illness and death. People with mild obsessions think of themselves as worriers, whereas people with profound obsessions are deeply affected by them to the point of interpersonal, social, and economic dysfunction. Compulsions also exist on a continuum from mildly annoying to intricate, time-consuming rituals that interfere with the individual's

Table 14–3 ■ COMMON OBSESSIONS AND COMPULSIONS

TYPE OF OBSESSION	EXAMPLE	ACCOMPANYING COMPULSION
Doubt/need to check	"Did I turn off the stove?" repeatedly intrudes in the thinking of a woman who has recently gone from housewife to secretary.	Checks to see if appliance is turned off, returning home several times during each work day.
Sexuality	Young woman has recurrent thought when in presence of a man, "Pat his buttocks."	Avoids the presence of men if possible; if with men, excuses self to wash hands every 10–15 minutes.
Violence	Man repeatedly thinks the thought "I should kill her" when he sees blonde women.	Abruptly turns head away from women and squints eyes to try to avoid seeing blondes.
Germs or dirt	Woman ruminates, "Everything is contaminated."	Avoids touching all objects. Scrubs hands if she is forced to touch any object.
Illness or death	Adolescent boy repeatedly thinks, "My teeth are decaying."	Repeats ritual of brushing and flossing up to a dozen times an hour

TYPE OF COMPULSION	EXAMPLE	UNDERLYING OBSESSIVE THOUGHT
Counting	Man counts aloud each step he takes.	Counting will prevent mistakes and often serves to keep troublesome thoughts out of awareness.
Touching	Anorexic girl touches each doorknob she sees.	"Touch the knob or be a blob."
Washing or cleaning	Young woman repeatedly washes hands.	"Wash away my sins." Thought appeared following a sexual encounter with a married man.
Avoidance	Man uses a paper towel to touch objects touched by others.	"Maybe someone with AIDS touched it."
Doing or undoing	Woman walks forward, then backward, sits in a chair, then gets up and sits down again.	"Whatever I do has to be perfect or my husband won't love me"
Symmetry	Secretary lines up objects in rows on her desk, then realigns them repeatedly during the day.	"Secretaries who practice neatness never get fired."

AIDS = acquired immunodeficiency syndrome.

ability to function. Minor compulsions include behaviors such as "knocking on wood," crossing oneself when hearing bad news, or touching a lucky charm. Mild compulsions can be useful. For example, timeliness, orderliness, and reliability are valued traits in our society. Table 14–3 lists various types of obsessions and compulsions and gives clinical examples that show relationships between the two. Rapoport (1989) reports that most clients with OCD have more than one symptom and that many are able to conceal the problem for years by restricting their rituals to private hours.

At times, people engage in certain activities to excess, such as eating, sexual behaviors, gambling, or drinking, and may be labeled by others as "compulsive." These situations are different from true compulsions because the individual experiences the activity as pleasurable, although the consequences may not be (Hollander et al. 1988).

The obsessive-compulsive person is a perfectionist who finds it extremely difficult to admit to makng a

mistake or to having human failings. This need for perfection has its basis in the need to control self and others. At the extreme, such a person cannot make a decision for fear of being wrong. This doubting can be seen, for example, in the constant checking that the stove is turned off, the counting and recounting of a row of numbers, or the fastening of a button over and over to make sure it is done "correctly." Symptoms of depression are present in about 50% of these clients. This association between OCD and depression is one of the major areas of research suggesting a biological etiology.

Tom is 25 years old and is unaware of his anger and hostility. He has obsessive thoughts that he has killed someone, which worries him. Tom's compulsions are to keep checking that he has not hurt someone. He keeps opening and closing doors, looking for dead bodies. Tom thinks that someone he may have bumped into on the street is now dead, and he has to look for this person to see if this is true.

THE CLINICAL PICTURE OF POST-TRAUMATIC STRESS DISORDER

Symptoms experienced by individuals with **post-traumatic stress disorder** (PTSD) are identified in Figure 14–3. The three major features of PTSD are (1) re-experiencing the trauma through dreams and waking thoughts, (2) having emotional numbing to other life events and relationships, and (3) having symptoms of depression, poor concentration, and other cognitive difficulties.

PTSD has two subtypes: acute and chronic. The *acute disorder* is diagnosed when symptoms occur within six months of the trauma. The *delayed* or *chronic* type is diagnosed when the onset of symptoms is delayed at least six months. PTSD may occur following any psychologically traumatic event that is outside the range of usual experience, such as military combat, natural disasters (e.g., floods or earthquakes), man-made disasters (e.g., car or airplane crashes, bombings, or torture), and crime-related events (e.g., assaults, muggings, robberies, rapes, or hostage-taking). After a devastating disaster, 50–80% of the survivors may experience PTSD (Kaplan and Sadock 1991).

Exposure to a highly traumatic event predisposes an individual to the development of PTSD and signals a potential need for help in coming to terms with the experience. We learned all too well from the Korean and Vietnam wars that for combat veterans to resume a normal civilian life, they must come to terms with their war experiences. If resolution does not occur, PTSD can result. More recently, medical facilities are seeing more clients who have experienced sexual or physical abuse in childhood and are presenting with the same cluster of symptoms seen in PTSD (Schatzberg and Cole 1991). Particularly disturbing to clients are the intrusive symptoms, such as nightmares, **flashbacks,** and memories of traumatic events. Nightmares and flashbacks may be related to changes in catecholamine transmission, with the possibility existing that flashbacks are waking nightmares (Post-traumatic Stress: Part I 1991).

The hypervigilance experienced by most individuals with PTSD creates its own set of problems. PTSD victims seem to be attempting to prepare themselves for another traumatic event by being overly alert to danger. As a result, their bodies are in an almost permanent state of physiological arousal.

Because the symptoms of this disorder are not as well defined as those of other anxiety disorders, the disorder may go undiagnosed. The individual may seek relief by developing additional symptoms, such as physiological complaints (e.g., headaches, ulcers, or hypertension) or phobias, or by developing chemical dependence and abuse. Suicide attempts and intermittent psychotic episodes may occur, and problems existing before the traumatic event, such as impulsiveness or antisocial tendencies, may be intensified.

Difficulty in interpersonal relationships almost always occurs and may be manifested in many ways. The PTSD victim frequently states that he or she has turned off feelings and is empty inside. This psychic numbing protects the client from feelings associated with intense stress. Avoiding emotional attachment may become a learned response to protect the individual from experiencing the pain of multiple losses stemming from, for example, combat or natural disasters. Thrill-seeking behavior may also be noted. Thrill seeking allows feelings to surface and aggression to be mobilized. Spouse and child abuse may occur as part of PTSD. Struggles with bosses, family, and co-workers are frequent themes, as is having difficulty trusting others. The last is a recurrent theme among rape victims.

Barbara is a 22-year-old college student who was sexually assaulted by a family friend. She was wearing a bathing suit and has guilt feelings that somehow she is responsible for the rape. She excessively showers, sometimes for two hours at a time. She has nightmares about the rape, is fearful of going outside, and cannot return to school, fearing she will be raped again.

Assessment

Because clients with anxiety disorders are consumed by the need to keep anxiety at manageable levels, they have little time or energy to devote to personal growth or to developing mutually satisfying relationships with others. In fact, these people usually develop inflexible and maladaptive patterns of relating to people. Two of the more common patterns are (1) exhibiting excessive dependence on others and (2) using tactics to distance one's self from others. Behaviors associated with these two patterns of relating are described in Table 14–4.

Assessment should consist of the collection of physical, psychological, and social data. Anxiety is a mental and physical condition, with major symptoms resulting from stimulation of the autonomic nervous system. Therefore, before an anxiety disorder can be diagnosed, the clinician must rule out organic causes of anxiety (Dubin and Weiss 1991):

- Abuse of alcohol or drugs
- Symptoms that began in response to an illness
- Side effects from prescribed medications

Table 14-4 ■ INFLEXIBLE AND MALADAPTIVE PATTERNS OF RELATING

PATTERNS OF RELATIONSHIPS	CHARACTERISTIC BEHAVIORS
Dependence on others	1. Acts helpless. 2. Treats others as superior to self, is self-deprecatory. 3. Adopts others' opinions. 4. Is indecisive. 5. Seeks advice. 6. Submits or defers to others. 7. Seeks attention and approval. 8. Tolerates criticism poorly.
Distances self from others	1. Believes others are hostile. 2. Takes control of situations. 3. Displays anger when authority or opinions are questioned. 4. Employs manipulation. 5. Is demanding. 6. Rarely admits feelings. 7. Finds fault or blames others. 8. Rejects help. 9. Wants to be left alone. 10. Is aloof. 11. Withdraws or rebels when placed in dependent role. 12. Rejects advice. 13. Assumes moral superiority. 14. Treats others as inferior.

Specific symptoms should be noted, along with statements made by the client about his or her subjective distress. The nurse must use clinical judgment to determine the level of anxiety the client is experiencing (Refer to Chapter 9). External and internal stressors should be identified, if possible, and the degree to which the client's life is disrupted should be evaluated. Because clients with anxiety disorders usually remain in contact with reality, they are often able to collaborate, to some extent, with the nurse during the assessment. Suggestions for the kinds of questions the nurse can ask in order to gather and assess physical, psychological, and social data are presented in Table 14-5. The data collected about behaviors exhibited by individuals with anxiety disorders are usually markedly different from data collected about individuals with psychoses. Table 14-6 contrasts psychotic with nonpsychotic behaviors.

People who are experiencing anxiety disorders often resort to the use of ego defense mechanisms. The defense mechanisms being employed and the purpose they serve should be determined. Review Table 14-1 for commonly used defense mechanisms. Although it is difficult to pose specific questions to assess the use of defense mechanisms, their use may become apparent to the nurse during the course of interviews and observations.

Although violence is exhibited by only a small number of clients, the nurse must be aware that very high levels of anxiety may evoke the "fight-or-flight" response. The nurse must, therefore, assess the risk for aggression as well as for suicide. High levels of anxiety can be a debilitating illness, even resulting in a complete inability to function (Glod 1992). Suicide is often a possibility, and some believe that individuals with panic disorder may have as high a risk for suicide (or higher) as those with major depression (Weissman et al. 1989).

Nursing Diagnosis

Several nursing diagnoses should be considered for clients experiencing anxiety and ego-dystonic behaviors associated with anxiety reduction. Several etiological statements may be used for a nursing diagnosis of *anxiety*, including anxiety related to

- Exposure to phobic object
- Threat to self-concept
- Actual or perceived loss of significant other
- Actual or perceived change in socioeconomic status

Table 14–5 ■ NURSING ASSESSMENT: ANXIETY DISORDERS	
ASSESSMENT	**DATA-GATHERING STRATEGIES**
Physical Parameters	
Presence of anxiety	"Tell me what you are experiencing."
Potential to flee or fight	Observe appearance, behavior, posture, gait, and expression.
Impact of anxiety on physical functioning	Monitor pulse, respirations, sleep patterns, elimination, appetite, and energy level.
Psychological Parameters	
Understanding of illness	"What problems bring you here?" "Did this problem occur suddenly or over a period of time?" "Describe how you are feeling." Observe affect.
Mood	"How do you feel about yourself?"
Self-esteem	"What do you like and dislike about yourself?"
Normal coping ability	"When you experience stress, what do you do to decrease it?"
Defense mechanisms used	Observe and listen during interview. Note distractibility and vigilance.
Thought content or process	Note circumstantiality (many digressions before eventually concluding a thought) and blocking (sudden stopping of speech due to anxiety). "Are you preoccupied with any idea?" "Does one thought repeatedly force itself into awareness?" "Do you have any especially strong fears?"
Potential for suicide	If a client indicates feeling hopeless, helpless, or worthless, investigate whether he or she has considered suicide.
Social Parameters	
Characteristic patterns of relationships	"Describe your relationship with family/friends/peers."
Identification of stressors or threats to self-concept, role, values, social status, or support system	"What do you think might be causing this problem?" "What changes occurred in your life this past year?"
Ability to function	"How is this problem interfering with your life?"
	Investigate effects on work, school, church, hobbies, social activities, and sexual functioning.
Degree of strain in relationships	"Describe any strain on relationships with others this problem has caused." "How has this problem changed your relationship with . . . ?"
Secondary gains	Note benefits to client as result of symptoms.
Diversional activity	"What do you like to do for fun or recreation?"

- Change in status and prestige
- Lack of recognition from others
- Interference with ability to perform compulsions

Ineffective individual coping is a nursing diagnosis that may also have several different etiologies, such as

- Excessive negative beliefs about self
- Inadequate psychological resources
- Unsatisfactory support system

- Hypervigilance related to severe anxiety
- Severe or panic level of anxiety
- Ineffective use of defense mechanisms
- Compulsions related to need for excessive cleanliness
- Resistiveness associated with compulsivity

The diagnosis of *alteration in thought processes* as a result of severe or panic levels of anxiety must also be

Table 14-6 ■ NURSING ASSESSMENT: PSYCHOTIC VERSUS NONPSYCHOTIC BEHAVIORS

NONPSYCHOTIC BEHAVIOR	PSYCHOTIC BEHAVIOR
Appearance	
Usually unremarkable except for tension and autonomic symptoms	May look atypical, bizarre; grooming may be poor
Mood or Affect	
Usually appropriate to thought content; anxiety and depression are common	May be excessive, blunted, or inappropriate to thought
Perceptions	
Usually intact except in panic episodes	Altered; illusions and hallucinations are common
Thinking (cognition)	
Preoccupied with problems, may experience phobias, obsessions, indecisiveness, poor concentration, or sense of doom; able to abstract and perform math calculations except in severe anxiety	Decreased reality testing, delusions, concrete thinking, and loose associations
Secondary Gain	
Symptoms may provide benefits to client (e.g., attention)	Symptoms rarely provide secondary gains
Orientation	
Intact	Often impaired
Memory	
Usually intact except in panic	Often impaired
Insight	
Blames self for psychological problems	Denies illness; blames others for problems

considered. Multiple etiologies exist, and some are listed below:

- Inability to understand directions
- Pathological use of defense mechanisms
- Excessive use of reason and logic related to overcautiousness and fear of making a mistake
- Preoccupation with obsessive thoughts
- Disorganized thinking related to intense fear of a specific object, person, or situation

In *disturbance in self-esteem,* low self-esteem is nearly always present and may be related to inability to control ego-dystonic symptoms or to other reasons. *Powerlessness* related to inability to control symptoms may also be an appropriate diagnosis. A diagnosis of *altered role performance* is possible when assessment reveals inability to assume responsibilities associated with usual roles. *Risk for alterations in health maintenance* may also be related to phobias if ritualistic behavior or

excessive caution prevents the individual from seeking health care.

Planning

Planning occurs on two levels: (1) the content level—planning goals—and (2) the process level—dealing with nurses' reactions and feelings.

CONTENT LEVEL— PLANNING GOALS

Content planning involves establishing goals, outcome criteria, and interventions for a client. The client should actively participate in the process of goal set-

Table 14–7 ■ NURSING DIAGNOSES: ANXIETY DISORDERS

NURSING DIAGNOSIS	POSSIBLE GOAL AND OUTCOME CRITERIA
Anxiety related to unexpected panic attacks or related to re-experiencing traumatic events	Client will demonstrate psychological and physiological comfort by (date), as evidenced by • Pulse and respiration within normal parameters • Absence of symptoms associated with autonomic stimulation • Statement that anxiety has decreased
Ineffective individual coping related to excessive anxiety (related to distorted cognitive perception of problem)	Client will employ alternative coping resources by (date), as evidenced by • Appropriate balancing of dependence or distancing from others • Controlled expression of feelings • Successful use of problem-solving skills • Verbalization of ability to cope
Disturbance in self-esteem related to shame or guilt	Client will demonstrate improved self-esteem by (date), as evidenced by • Giving accurate, nonjudgmental self-assessment • Identifying personal strengths • Making positive statements about self • Reporting decreased shame or guilt
Disturbance in self-esteem related to change in role performance	Client will employ ability to perform in usual roles at pre-morbid level by (date), as evidenced by • Performing usual work and social activities and hobbies • Interacting with significant others in mutually supportive ways
Altered thought processes related to severe anxiety	Client will demonstrate ability to concentrate by (date). Client will report absence of obsessive thoughts by (date). Client will report experiencing, and will exhibit, mild to moderate anxiety in presence of phobic object by (date).
Diversional activity deficit related to preoccupation with symptoms	Client will use leisure time constructively by (date), as evidenced by • Listing diversional activities of interest • Participating in one diversional activity each day
Social isolation related to avoidance behavior, or related to shame associated with symptoms	Client will increase interaction with others by (date), as evidenced by • Interacting with a significant other or peer daily for 20 minutes • Participating in two group activities each week
Knowledge deficit related to dysfunctional appraisal of situation	Client will state relationship between anxiety and the developing of his or her symptoms by (date).
Sleep-pattern disturbance related to physiologic symptoms of anxiety	Client will express satisfaction with rest-sleep pattern by (date), as evidenced by • Verbalizing, "I slept well." Client will appear rested by (date), as evidenced by • Absence of yawning • Absence of dark circles under eyes
Self-care deficit related to ritualistic behavior	Client will independently perform bathing, hygiene, grooming, and dressing tasks by (date), as evidenced by clean, appropriate appearance.
Altered nutrition (less than body requirements) related to inability to stop performance of rituals	Client will maintain ideal body weight ±10 pounds, as evidenced by weekly weight graph.
Impaired skin integrity related to rituals of excessive washing or excessive picking at the skin	Client's skin will be intact, as evidenced by • Absence of chapping and excoriation • Absence of scratches or other self-inflicted lesions

ting whenever possible. By sharing decision making with the client, the nurse increases the potential for goal attainment. Shared planning is appropriate when working with the client with mild or moderate anxiety. When the client is in severe or panic levels of anxiety, the nurse takes a more active role. Sample goals and outcome criteria for several relevant nursing diagnoses can be seen in Table 14–7.

Nursing interventions for assisting a client who is experiencing mild to moderate and severe to panic levels of anxiety are discussed in depth in Chapter 9. Although interventions must be individualized to meet each client's unique situation, the planned strategies are geared toward the following objectives:

- Relieving the client's immediate distress
- Helping the client feel understood
- Assisting the client in identifying the source of the anxiety
- Identifying the client's strengths, coping skills, and resources, and supporting healthy aspects of the client's personality
- Supporting the client while new coping measures are learned
- Assisting the client in applying what is learned during therapy to his or her life situation
- Assisting the family in changing behavioral patterns that support the client's dysfunctional behaviors

PROCESS LEVEL—NURSES' REACTIONS AND FEELINGS

When the nurse has contact with an anxious client or with a client who uses ego-dystonic defenses to cope with anxiety, the nurse may experience strong feelings. Often, the anxiety originating in the client is experienced by the nurse empathically. Self-monitoring is vital to identify feelings originating in the nurse and those transferred to the nurse from the client. Without self-monitoring, peer supervision, or other interventions, the cycle shown in Figure 14–4 may develop. As the process continues, the result is an upward spiraling of anxiety in both the nurse and the client.

The nurse may experience feelings of frustration or anger while working with clients with anxiety disorders. For example, the rituals of the obsessive-compulsive client may frustrate the nurse's need to accomplish certain tasks within a given time. Communication with the obsessive-compulsive client can also be frustrating. These clients correct and clarify repeatedly. It is as though they cannot let go of any topic. If the nurse uses therapeutic communication techniques, such as reflection and paraphrasing, the client will take this opportunity to go over and

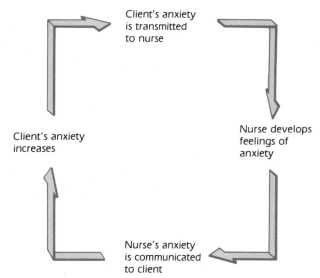

Figure 14–4. *The cycle of transmitting anxiety between the nurse and client.*

over material, often angrily implying that the nurse has not understood. The client may introduce detail after detail, although the conversation may become less and less clear. Communication requires much patience and the ability to provide clear structure. In caring for the phobic client, the nurse may become frustrated after realizing that both the client and the nurse regard the fear as exaggerated and unrealistic, but that the client is unable to overcome the avoidant behavior.

It is important to remember that *behavioral change is often accomplished very slowly.* The process of recovery is very different from that seen in a client with an infection who is given antibiotics and begins to demonstrate improvement within 24 hours. Nurses tend to become impatient with the anxious client and may feel frustrated or angry when the client does not make rapid progress. Negative feelings are easily transmitted to the client, who then feels increasingly anxious.

The nurse who feels anger or frustration may withdraw from the client both emotionally and physically. This does not go unnoticed by the client. The result is that the client feels greater anxiety. Therefore, a mutual withdrawal process may predominate. *Setting small, attainable goals can help prevent the nurse from feeling overwhelmed* by the client's slow progress and can help client gain a sense of control.

At the very least, the nurse often experiences increased tension and fatigue from mental strain when working with dependent and needy clients. Because the client's anxiety is controlled for only a short time by his or her ego-dystonic behaviors, client anxiety recurs, and the nurse is called on to intervene again and again. Unlike the client whose dressing needs to be changed twice a day, these clients require emotional bandaging many times a day.

It may be helpful for the nurse to consider the level of regression displayed by the client. If the client's behavior can be seen as regressive rather than perverse, staff can cope more easily. For example, dependence, excessive demands, and frequent reassurance seeking are behaviors associated with the unmet needs of infancy and early childhood. Excessive neatness, rituals, obsessions, and pickiness are behaviors related to the period of toilet training. It helps to remember that these behaviors provide us with clues to the identification of needs that must be met before the client can go on to develop more mature behaviors.

By having a clear understanding of the emotional pitfalls of working with clients with anxiety disorders, the nurse is able to minimize and avoid guilt associated with strong negative feelings. By examining personal feelings, the nurse is better able to identify what brought about the feelings and to act objectively and constructively to plan care.

Intervention

The nurse may encounter clients with anxiety disorders in numerous settings. Such clients may be seen on a medical-surgical unit, where the primary diagnosis will be associated with physical illness. A holistic approach necessitates consideration of psychological as well as physical needs. If the client's needs are difficult to meet or if a large amount of staff time is taken by the client, it may be wise to seek the assistance of the psychiatric liaison team (see Chapter 26).

Clients demonstrating anxiety disorders may be encountered in the psychiatric inpatient and outpatient settings, as well as in the home. Community health nurses and community mental health nurses often implement substantial portions of the long term treatment plan.

PSYCHOTHERAPEUTIC INTERVENTIONS

Nursing Care Plan 14–1 identifies generic nursing interventions for clients with anxiety disorders and gives a rationale for each intervention. The interventions in this plan may be considered the primary core of interventions for all clients with anxiety disorders. Specific interventions may be added to individualize care for clients with panic attacks, phobias, and PTSD (Nursing Care Plan 14–2). A nursing care for a person with OCD will be discussed subsequently.

HEALTH TEACHING

Clients often lack accurate knowledge about the effect of stress on the body and about the physiological components of anxiety. This information may be given separately or in conjunction with the teaching of relaxation techniques.

If a client is to receive anxiety-relieving medication, health teaching about desired effects and possible side effects must be carried out. Many antianxiety (anxiolytic) drugs are central nervous system depressants. The importance of strict adherence to prescribed dosage must be taught because the potential for dependence is high. Specific instructions to the client are discussed under Somatic Therapies.

ACTIVITIES OF DAILY LIVING

The client's ability to meet basic physical needs is often impaired by anxiety or the use of defenses against anxiety. Areas often affected are discussed subsequently.

NUTRITION AND FLUID INTAKE. Some anxious clients eat little. Ritualistic clients may be too involved with rituals to eat. Some phobic clients may be too afraid of germs to eat. On the other hand, some anxious clients seem hungry almost constantly. Nutritious diets with snacks need to be provided. Weighing the client frequently and keeping a record of food and fluid intake may be useful assessment tools.

PERSONAL HYGIENE AND GROOMING. Some clients are excessively neat and demonstrate time-consuming rituals associated with bathing and dressing. Sometimes, the rituals are repeated so often that the client may stay in the bathroom for hours. Maintenance of skin integrity may become a problem when rituals involve excessive washing, and the skin becomes excoriated and infected.

Some clients are indecisive about bathing or about what clothing to wear. For the latter, limiting choices to two outfits would be helpful. In the event of severe indecisiveness, simply presenting the client with the clothing to be worn may be necessary. The nurse may also need to remain with the client to give simple directions to "put on your shirt . . . now put on your slacks." Matter-of-fact support to assist the client in performing as much of the task as possible is effective. The client should be encouraged to express thoughts and feelings about self-care. This communication can provide a basis for later health teaching or for ongoing dialogue about the client's abilities.

ELIMINATION. Obsessive-compulsive clients may be so involved with the performance of rituals that they may suppress the urge to void and defecate.

Nursing Care Plan 14–1 ▪ A PERSON WITH ANXIETY DISORDER

NURSING DIAGNOSIS

Ineffective individual coping related to anxiety

Supporting Data

- Increased muscle tension and restlessness.
- Reports feeling apprehensive, jittery, and shaky.
- States, "No one seems to understand."
- Voice quivering, frequently diaphoretic, pulse elevated, skin pale, and pupils dilated.

Long Term Goal: Client will cope adaptively with anxiety.

Short Term Goal	Intervention	Rationale
1. Client will state that immediate distress is relieved by (date).	1a. Stay with client.	1a. Conveys acceptance and ability to give help.
	1b. Acknowledge the client's anxiety.	1b. Assists client in identifying feelings.
	1c. Speak slowly and calmly.	1c. Conveys calm and promotes security.
	1d. Use short, simple sentences.	1d. Promotes comprehension.
	1e. Assure client that you are in control and can assist him or her.	1e. Severe anxiety gives feeling of loss of control.
	1f. Give brief directions.	1f. Reduces indecision. Conveys belief that client can respond in healthy manner.
	1g. Decrease excessive stimuli and provide quiet environment.	1g. Reduces need to focus on diverse stimuli. Promotes ability to concentrate.
	1h. Walk with pacing client.	1h. Gives support while client uses anxiety-generated energy.
	1i. Increase level of supervision for acutely anxious client.	1i. Minimizes self-injury or loss of control.
	1j. Allow client to use defenses as long as physical well-being is not seriously jeopardized.	1j. Challenging defenses when client is acutely anxious causes further anxiety and may lead to panic.
	1k. After assessing level of anxiety, administer appropriate dose of anxiolytic agent, if warranted.	1k. Reduction of anxiety allows client to use coping skills.
	1l. Monitor and control own feelings.	1l. Anxiety is transmissible. Displays of negative emotion can cause client anxiety.
2. Client will state that he or she feels understood by nurse by (date).	2a. Listen.	2a. Conveys interest. Fosters trust. Provides tension relief. Permits data gathering. Identifies defenses.
	2b. Use empathy.	2b. Conveys concern. Helps client identify and accept feelings.
	2c. Focus on reality of present discomfort but not on ego-dystonic symptoms, e.g., rituals.	2c. Acknowledges client's distress but does not reinforce maladaptive behavior.
	2d. Encourage description of feelings.	2d. Facilitates identification of feelings.
	2e. Help client recognize anxiety.	2e. Overcomes denial and resistance.
	2f. Teach signs and symptoms of anxiety.	2f. Factual information promotes accurate perceptions and decreases excessive concern.
3. Client will be able to identify sources of anxiety by (date).	3a. Encourage to discuss preceding events.	3a. Identification of stressors promotes future change.
	3b. Link client's behavior to feelings.	3b. Promotes self-awareness.
	3c. Teach cognitive therapy principles: • Anxiety is the result of a dysfunctional appraisal of a situation. • Anxiety is the result of automatic thinking.	3c. Provides a basis for behavioral change.
	3d. Ask questions that clarify and promote logical thinking, e.g.,	3d. Helps promote accurate cognition.

Continued on following page

Nursing Care Plan 14–1 ■ A PERSON WITH ANXIETY DISORDER *(Continued)*

Short Term Goal	Intervention	Rationale
	"What evidence do you have?" "Explain the logic in that." "Are you basing that conclusion on fact or feeling?" "What's the worst thing that could happen?"	
	3e. Have client give alternative interpretations.	3e. Broadens perspective. Helps client think in a new way about problem or symptom.
	3f. Instruct client to refer to self by first name and comment on own anxiety or thoughts, e.g., "Steven's heart is beating fast." "Steven thinks everyone is looking at him now."	3f. Increases self-awareness while distancing self from own anxiety.
4. Client will identify strengths and coping skills by (date).	4a. Identify what has provided relief in the past.	4a. Provides awareness of self as individual with some ability to cope.
	4b. Give positive reinforcement for use of healthy behavior.	4b. Positively reinforced behavior tends to be repeated.
	4c. Have client write assessment of strengths.	4c. Increases self-acceptance.
	4d. Have client realistically assess weaknesses and state ways to convert them to strengths	4d. Weaknesses can become assets with careful work.
5. Client will use new effective coping strategies by (date).	5a. Provide support while new coping measures are learned.	5a–b. Promotes understanding of universality of feelings.
	5b. Accept client's feelings, especially anger, fear, guilt, or shame.	
	5c. Assist with practice of relaxation technique.	5c. Relaxation response is enhanced by frequent use. Competence in use increases self-esteem and feelings of being able to control symptoms.
	5d. Promote sleep with warm bath, warm milk, or sitting with client.	5d. Provides alternative to, and prevents overuse of, anxiolytics.
	5e. Provide full schedule of activities, especially familiar ones client has enjoyed in the past.	5e. Expands anxiety-generated energy constructively. Decreases self-preoccupation. Increases self-esteem by providing success experiences.
	5f. Give positive feedback for capabilities and competence.	5f. Enhances self-esteem.
	5g. Have client use positive "self-talk," e.g., "I can handle this" or "I can cope."	5g. Increases tolerance to anxiety.
6. Client will apply what is learned during therapy to life situation by (date).	6a. Provide opportunities to engage in normal (healthy) role behaviors.	6a. Strengthens role-taking and self-esteem.
	6b. Provide behavioral rehearsals for anticipated stressful situations.	6b. Predetermination of coping strategy and practice increases potential for success.
	6c. Discuss coping strategies client successfully employs.	6c. Reinforces use of healthy coping strategies.
7. Family will alter behavioral patterns that have been supportive of dysfunctional behavior by (date).	7a. Teach family to give reinforcement for use of healthy behaviors.	7a. Positively reinforced behaviors tend to be repeated.
	7b. Teach family not to take over roles normally reserved for client.	7b–c. Minimizes secondary gain.
	7c. Teach family to give attention to client, not to client's symptoms.	

Nursing Care Plan 14–2 ■ CLIENTS WITH PANIC DISORDER, PHOBIA, OR POST-TRAUMATIC STRESS DISORDER

PANIC DISORDER

NURSING DIAGNOSIS

Anxiety: panic attacks related to loss of significant other, unmet emotional needs, and negative thoughts about self

Client Goals	Intervention*	Rationale
1. Client's anxiety will decrease to moderate by (date).	1a. If hypercapnia occurs, instruct client to take slow, deep breaths. Breathe with client to obtain cooperation.	1a. Shifts focus from distressing symptoms.
	1b. Keep expectations minimal and simple.	1b. Anxiety limits ability to attend to complex tasks.
2. Client will gain mastery over panic episodes by (date).	2a. Help client connect feelings prior to panic attack with onset of attack: "What were you thinking about just before the attack?" "Can you identify what you were feeling just before the attack?"	2a. Physiologic symptoms of anxiety usually appear first as the result of a stressor. They are immediately followed by automatic thoughts, e.g., "I'm dying" or "I'm going crazy," which are distorted assessments.
	2b. Help client recognize symptoms as resulting from anxiety, not from a catastrophic physical problem, e.g., ● Explain physical symptoms of anxiety. ● Discuss the fact that anxiety causes sensations similar to physical events, such as a heart attack. *See the seven interventions in Nursing Care Plan 14–1.	2b. Factual information and alternative interpretations can help client recognize distortions in thought.

PHOBIAS

NURSING DIAGNOSIS

Fear related to a specific object or situation

Client Goals	Intervention	Rationale
1. Client will use adaptive coping strategies instead of avoidance by discharge.	1a. Determine type of phobia and when it first appeared.	1a. Determines whether phobia developed as a result of trauma, childhood experiences, or adult experiences.
	1b. Have client list consequences of contacting feared object.	1b. Isolates a specific fear associated with the object, e.g., a specific fear of flying may be a fear of being hurt in a plane crash. These data can aid the therapist using cognitive therapy.
	1c. Discuss concept that client may be afraid of own feelings and sensations, not of the object or situation.	1c. Casts doubt on the feared consequence of contact with the phobic object or situation.
	1d. Encourage client to practice techniques to promote relaxation and decrease physiologic sensations associated with fear or anxiety.	1d. Enhances client control over feelings and level of anxiety.
	1e. Do not force client to face phobic object or situation on own.	1e. The treatment decision to use flooding or implosion must be carefully considered.

Continued on following page

POST-TRAUMATIC STRESS DISORDER

Nursing Diagnosis

Post-traumatic response related to a specific event

Client Goals	Intervention	Rationale
1. Client will cope effectively with thoughts and feelings associated with traumatic events within six months.	1a. Assess the type of trauma, e.g., natural or human-induced.	1a. Victims of natural disasters experience less guilt. Victims of man-made disasters experience more humiliation and guilt.
	1b. Assess immediate post-trauma reaction and later coping.	1b. Numbing and denial are common. Knowing the range of behavior can help assess impact and meaning of trauma.
	1c. Assess functioning prior to event, including drugs and alcohol use.	1c. Knowing premorbid function may suggest additional diagnoses.
	1d. Assess use of drugs or alcohol since event.	1d. Attempts to self-medicate are common to reduce anxiety or induce sleep.
	1e. Explore shattered assumptions, e.g., "I'm a good person; why did this happen to me?" "This is a safe world."	1e. Victims need to find meaning in the event. Helplessness and anxiety result from lost feelings of safety.
	1f. Promote discussion of possible meanings of the event. Compare this situation with others that are worse.	1f. Helps client see self as less victimized, and his or her world as more understandable.
	1g. Suggest that client was not responsible for traumatic event but is responsible for learning to cope.	1g. Reduces powerlessness.
	1h. Encourage the use of social support system.	1h. Increases feelings of safety and of being understood.

Constipation and urinary tract infections may result. Interventions may include creating a regular schedule for taking the client to the bathroom.

SLEEP. Anxious clients frequently have difficulty sleeping, and ritualistic clients may perform their rituals to the exclusion of resting and sleeping. Physical exhaustion is a very real possibility for highly ritualistic clients. Clients suffering from generalized anxiety disorder and from PTSD often experience sleep disturbance from nightmares. Monitoring sleep and keeping a sleep record may be useful in establishing the diagnosis of sleep pattern disturbance and evaluating progress.

Ongoing assessment of the client's ability to perform self-care activities is important, as is the establishment of attainable goals. Several nursing diagnoses and goals related to activities of daily living can be reviewed in Table 14–7.

SOMATIC THERAPIES

Anxiolytics (antianxiety drugs) are used to treat the somatic and psychological symptoms of anxiety. Their use is a valuable adjunct to other therapies used to treat clients with anxiety disorders. When moderate to severe anxiety is reduced, clients are better able to participate in therapies directed at underlying problems. Several other classes of drugs, not normally thought of as anxiolytics, notably the tricyclic antidepressants (TCAs), monoamine-oxidase inhibitors (MAOIs), and beta-blockers, are now being considered as having the ability to effectively treat clients with selected anxiety disorders. See Table 14–8 for medications used in the treatment of anxiety disorders.

The anxiolytics classified as **benzodiazepines** should be used only on a short term basis because dependence and addiction develop rather easily. For example, dependency will occur if a client takes three to four times the normal daily dose over several weeks (Maxmen 1991). Because drugs from these classes have many side effects, clients receiving them should be assessed on an ongoing basis not only for anxiety level but also for side effects and untoward effects of the medication. The more common side effects of the benzodiazepines are listed by body system in Table 14–9. Because the **diphenylmethane antihistamines** such as hydroxyzine hydrochloride (Atarax) and hydroxyzine pamoate (Vistaril), produce no dependence, tolerance, or intoxication, they can be used for anxiety relief over long periods.

Table 14–8. ■ DRUG INFORMATION: TREATMENT OF ANXIETY DISORDERS

GENERIC NAME	TRADE NAME	USUAL DAILY DOSE (mg/day)	ACTION AND INDICATION
Benzodiazepines			
Alprazolam	Xanax	0.5–1.5	Increase GABA release and receptor binding at synapses. Show preferential effect on limbic system. (GABA is an inhibitory transmitter and slows turnover of other neurotransmitters.) Useful for short term treatment of anxiety *because dependence and tolerance develop quickly.*
Chlordiazepoxide	Librium	15–75	
Clonazepam	Klonopin	1.5–10	
Clorazepate	Tranxene	1.5–67.5	
Diazepam	Valium	4–30	
Lorazepam	Ativan	2–6	
Oxazepam	Serax	30–60	
Prazepam	Centrax	30–60	
Diphenylmethane antihistamines			
Hydroxyzine hydrochloride	Atarax	200–400	Depress subcortical centers. Produce *no dependence, tolerance, or intoxication.* Can be used for anxiety relief for indefinite periods.
Hydroxyzinepamoate	Vistaril	200–400	
Azaspirodecanediona			
Buspirone hydrochloride	Buspar	15–30	Alleviates anxiety. Less sedative than the benzodiazepines. Does not appear to produce physical or psychological dependence. *Requires up to three weeks or more to be effective.*
Beta-Adrenergic Blocker			
Propranolol	Inderal	30–80	Used to relieve physical symptoms of anxiety, as in stage fright. Acts by attaching to sensors that detect arousal messages.
Tricyclic Antidepressant			
Amitriptyline	Elavil	150–300	Used to prevent panic attacks, phobias, and PTSD. Act by regulating brain's reactions to serotonin. Clomipramine helpful for some in lowering obsessions in OCD.
Clomipramine	Anafranil	25–250	
Imipramine	Tofranil	150–300	
Monoamine oxidase inhibitors			
Phenelzine	Nardil	45–60	Used to treat panic disorders, phobias, and PTSD. Acts by blocking reuptake of norepinephrine and serotonin in central nervous system.

GABA = gamma-aminobutyric acid; OCD = obsessive-compulsive disorder; PTSD = post-traumatic stress disorder.

Buspirone (Buspar), a newer nonbenzodiazepine anxiolytic, does not cause dependence. Buspirone and the diphenylmethane antihistamines are well suited for addiction-prone individuals. Unlike the benzodiazepines, buspirone does not produce an immediate calming effect. Therefore, it cannot be used only as needed to relieve anxiety. Initial effects occur in one to two weeks, and full effects may take four to six weeks or longer. Buspirone is especially useful to treat generalized anxiety disorder, which tends to be a long term disorder. Clients taking this drug should be counseled to take the drug regularly for maximum effectiveness.

Panic disorders are currently being treated with TCAs,

Table 14-9 ■ DRUG INFORMATION: SIDE EFFECTS OF BENZODIAZEPINES

CENTRAL NERVOUS SYSTEM	CARDIOVASCULAR	BLOOD	GASTROINTESTINAL	OTHER
Drowsiness	Hypotension	Agranulocytosis, sore throat, fever	Dry mouth	Skin rash
Clumsiness	Palpitations		Nausea, vomiting	Pain at injection site
Blurred vision	Tachycardia	Thrombocytopenia, unusual bruising	Abdominal discomfort	Urinary retention
Slurred speech	Dizziness			Aggravation of narrow-angle glaucoma
Headache	Fainting			
Mental confusion				Menstrual irregularity
Disorientation				
Nystagmus				
Ataxia				
Agitation				
Sleep disturbance				
Psychological dependence				
Physical tolerance				

MAOIs, and selected benzodiazepines (Maxmen 1991). The TCAs and MAOIs are preferred because they are nonaddicting. The TCA of choice is imipramine. The nurse should warn the client that when imipramine is initiated, he or she may experience a sensation of being "speeded up" or jittery and may have insomnia. MAOIs are the second drug of choice, and phenelzine (Nardil) is preferred. An extremely important nursing consideration is that clients taking an MAOI must adhere to a special tyramine-free diet. See Chapter 17 for discussion of TCAs and MAOIs. The benzodiazepines of choice for panic disorder are alprazolam (Xanax) and clonazepam (Klonapin). Buspirone, on the other hand, seems to have no antipanic properties.

Agoraphobia has been reported to be successfully treated by the following drugs: benzodiazepines (e.g., alprazolam), TCAs (e.g., imipramine, amitriptyline, and clomipramine), and MAOIs (phenelzine [Nardil] and tranylcypromine [Parnate]). Social phobias are being successfully treated using beta-blockers, MAOIs, and TCAs. The beta-blockers, especially propranolol (Inderal), given two hours before an anxiety-arousing situation, such as a musical performance, have proven to be successful in controlling symptoms of anxiety. For clients who exhibit other more symptomatic social phobias, phenelzine, an MAOI, seems to be effective (Schatzberg and Cole 1991).

For the treatment of OCD, clomipramine (Anafranil), a serotonin reuptake inhibitor, is the current drug of choice (Schatzberg and Cole 1991). It is not, however, effective in all clients. In fact, it is effective in only about 50% of cases. Further, it seems to cause gradual improvement rather than immediate improvement, often taking six weeks to two months to reach maximum effectiveness. Clomipramine targets obsessions more than compulsions.

A relatively new serotonin reuptake inhibitor, sertraline (Zoloft), has been found to be effective in the treatment of both depression and OCD. It has a good side effect profile: low anticholinergic, sedative, and cardiac effects. The most prominent adverse reactions are gastrointestinal, including nausea, diarrhea, or dyspepsia (Berman et al. 1992). Another serotonin reuptake inhibitor drug currently used for OCD is fluoxetine (Prozac). All three drugs (clomipramine, sertraline, and fluoxetine) have antidepressant properties (Maxmen 1991).

The current literature offers no clear drug treatment for PTSD, but early research has suggested that both TCAs and MAOIs may be useful in some clients. TCAs are safer because many PTSD clients have substance abuse problems. Most positive findings stem from the antidepressants imipramine, fluoxetine, and doxepin (Sinequan). Propranolol (Inderal) may help with the persistent anger, vigilance, and significant distress on re-experiencing the trauma (Maxmen 1991).

Box 14-1 outlines specific nursing implications, including assessment considerations and client teaching needs associated with anxiolytic drug therapy.

THERAPEUTIC ENVIRONMENT

Most clients who demonstrate anxiety disorders can be treated successfully as outpatients. Severe anxiety

Box 14-1. NURSING IMPLICATIONS AND CLIENT TEACHING IN ANTIANXIETY DRUG THERAPY

Assessment

1. Identify other medications or drugs the client is taking.
2. Assess frequency of client requests for medication (many anxiolytics are schedule IV controlled substances).
3. Observe for indications that client is exceeding recommended dosage (e.g., ataxia, mental confusion, dizziness, slurred speech, and other symptoms of intoxication).
4. Observe for paradoxical excitation (e.g., restlessness, rage, and agitation). More common in elderly.
5. Observe for sleep disturbance: nightmares and vivid dreams may occur related to stage IV sleep suppression.
6. Assess change in urinary frequency, odor, or color, because urinary retention may occur.
7. Prior to initiating medication, record presence or absence of skin rash, flu-like symptoms, or bruising.
8. Obtain information about baseline sexual functioning because changes in libido or functioning may occur, causing client to discontinue medication without discussing with therapist.
9. Obtain information about menstrual regularity because irregularity may occur.

Client Teaching

1. Caution client not to increase dose or frequency of ingestion without prior approval of therapist.
2. Caution client that these medications reduce ability to handle mechanical equipment such as cars, saws, and machinery.
3. Caution client not to drink alcoholic beverages or take other antianxiety drugs because depressant effects of both will be potentiated.
4. Caution client to avoid drinking beverages containing caffeine because it decreases desired effects of drug.
5. Caution women to avoid becoming pregnant because taking benzodiazepines increases risk of congenital anomalies.
6. Caution new mothers taking benzodiazepines not to breast-feed because the drug is excreted in the milk and will have adverse effects on infant.
7. Teach clients taking monoamine oxidase inhibitors the details of tyramine-restricted diet (see Chapter 17).

Other Nursing Measures

1. Abrupt stoppage of benzodiazepines after three to four months of daily use may cause withdrawal symptoms, such as insomnia, irritability, nervousness, dry mouth, tremors, convulsions, or confusion.
2. Remain with client until medication is swallowed.
3. Take with, or shortly after, meals or snacks to reduce gastrointestinal discomfort.
4. Be alert for possible drug interactions:

   - Antacids may delay absorption.
   - Cimetidine interferes with metabolism of benzodiazepines, causing increased sedation.
   - Central nervous system depressants, such as alcohol and barbiturates, cause increased sedation.
   - Phenytoin serum concentration may build up because of decreased metabolism.

5. Lower doses should be considered for elderly clients.
6. Read drug literature carefully regarding reconstitution, storage, and administration of parenteral drugs.

   - Some drugs, such as hydroxyzine pamoate and diazepam, produce irritation at intramuscular injection sites.
   - Diazepam and chlordiazepoxide require slow intravenous injection.
   - Do not use if solution is cloudy or discolored.
   - Some drugs must be stored away from light.

7. When intramuscular injection is ordered, administer deeply and slowly into large muscle to minimize irritation and discomfort.
8. After intramuscular or intravenous administration, client should remain recumbent to minimize orthostatic hypotension.
9. Note contraindications of administration of individual drugs: for example, many benzodiazepines should not be given to clients in shock, clients with narrow-angle glaucoma, or clients with hepatic or renal disease.
10. Investigate complaints of sore throat or fever as possible symptoms of agranulocytosis.
11. Adopt positive attitude that medication will be effective.

or symptoms that interfere with the individual's health and well-being may cause the client to be hospitalized on a short term basis. When hospitalization is necessary, certain features of the therapeutic environment can be especially helpful to the client. These features include the following:

1. Structuring the daily routine to offer physical safety and predictability, thus reducing anxiety over the unknown
2. Providing daily activities to prevent constant focus on anxiety or symptoms
3. Providing therapeutic interactions
4. Evaluating and communicating the effects of the environment on the client to facilitate nursing care planning

PSYCHOTHERAPY

Professional accountability dictates that the nurse psychotherapist establish both a mechanism for peer review and a regular relationship with a professional colleague for the purpose of supervision and consultation. These actions help to ensure a high quality of care. Of particular importance is the need for the therapist to recognize and work through countertransferences that may develop.

The psychiatric nurse has several types of therapies from which to choose in treating a client with an anxiety disorder. In general, it seems that combinations of these treatment modalities may be more effective than single methods.

In all instances of treatment of anxiety disorders, it seems advisable to involve significant others in the treatment process. Often, the client has "trained" significant others to act in ways that support the use of symptoms, thus deriving secondary gains. For example, agoraphobics train others to shop for them. Families must unlearn these unhelpful behaviors in order to promote healthy behaviors on the part of the client. They may also need to learn how to assist the client to carry out treatment exercises.

Panic Disorder

In the treatment of panic disorder, researchers have concluded that cognitive restructuring is highly useful. When using *cognitive restructuring*, the therapist helps the client identify thoughts that arouse anxiety, look at the basis for these thoughts, and change them into more realistic thoughts (Hibbert 1984). Combining cognitive restructuring with applied relaxation training produces even better results (Barlow et al. 1984; Ost

1987). Applied *relaxation training* involves teaching relaxation techniques, and then helping the client apply the relaxation techniques at the first signs of anxiety to prevent escalation (see Chapter 9).

Working with a Client Who Has Panic Disorder

Dora, a 28-year-old pharmacist, lived at home and cared for her mother. Dora's father was cold and cruel to Dora during her childhood. After her mother's death, Dora admits feeling tense and irritable and is having trouble sleeping.

One night, Dora awakens gasping for breath. Her heart is pounding and she feels a tight sensation, like a band around her chest. Her pulse is 110 beats per minute, and she is dizzy. She fears she is going to die. She telephones her best friend, who finds her pacing, wringing her hands, and moaning. Dora seems totally disorganized. The friend takes Dora to the emergency room. After a thorough cardiac evaluation, Dora is kept overnight for observation. All diagnostic test results are normal, and she is discharged the next day. Over the course of the next three weeks, Dora has six attacks. The doctor suggests that because there is no apparent organic basis for these episodes, it is likely that they are caused by anxiety.

Imipramine is prescribed to block the panic attacks, and Dora is referred to a nurse psychotherapist. In outpatient therapy, she is encouraged to look at her present and past experiences to facilitate understanding of her symptoms. She becomes aware of intense anger toward her mother that has been repressed. She acknowledges longing for the warmth she has never received from her father. The immediate stressors in Dora's life are found to be losses: her mother's death and the impending retirement of a coworker of whom she is very fond. She is able to discuss and accept her feelings of loss, ambivalence, and anger associated with her life situation.

Dora's therapist encourages her to verbalize her thoughts and feelings about the panic attacks. She is instructed to keep a log to describe each attack: when the symptoms appear and end; the circumstances surrounding the attack, including her feelings, thoughts, the environment, and the interactions before, during, and after the attack; and the effectiveness of the strategies she uses to control the symptoms. Dora and the therapist use the log to help connect thoughts and feelings to the onset of panic attacks. The therapist uses supportive therapy techniques to bolster Dora's healthy coping strategies and her strengths.

The therapist offers her a choice of learning self-hypnosis, meditation, or progressive muscle relaxation techniques to help reduce anxiety and tension. Dora chooses progressive muscle relaxation and is taught to relax major muscle groups in a fixed order, beginning with the feet and working upward to her head. Progressive relaxation produces physiological effects that are opposite to those produced by anxiety, i.e., slow heart rate and neuromuscular stability (see Chapter 9).

After several weeks of practice using progressive relaxation, Dora reports that she is able to monitor her own tension level and invoke the relaxation response to reduce feelings of anxiety. Her panic attacks subside. Imipramine is gradually withdrawn without recurrence of the attacks.

Generalized Anxiety Disorder

Generalized anxiety disorder, a chronic disorder affecting 5% of the population, has been successfully treated by combining *cognitive therapy* (to identify and change anxiety-producing thoughts) with *relaxation training* (enabling gradual exposure to anxiety-producing situations) Butler et al. (1987).

Working with a Client Who Has Generalized Anxiety Disorder

Cameron, a 43-year-old pilot, seeks admission to the hospital, stating that for a month he has been unable to sleep without having a nightmare about a plane crash. The nightmares began shortly after he was passed over for promotion. After several nightmares, he begins to worry during his waking hours about the possibility of being involved in a plane crash. He experiences so much dread about flying that he grounds himself. He complains of constant fatigue. At the interview, he has shaky hands and sits tensely on the edge of the chair. His hands are cold, but facial perspiration is evident. Resting pulse is 100 beats per minute. As he describes his nightmares, he begins to hyperventilate. Admission for short term therapy is arranged.

Antianxiety medication is not prescribed because nursing measures are sufficient to reduce Cameron's anxiety to moderate levels during his first days on the unit. Cognitive therapy is begun. Cognitive therapy assumes that cognitive errors made by the client produce negative ideas, sometimes called schemas, that persist despite evidence to the contrary. As Cameron begins therapy, he reveals incidents in his childhood during which his father criticized him and told him that he would never amount to anything and that he never did anything right.

The therapist identifies the thought processes (that he would never be able to do anything right or be successful) and the faulty logic (that his father's saying this did not make it true) to Cameron and sets the stage for formulating hypotheses and testing them during therapy. The next step is to elicit Cameron's automatic thoughts: that is, distorted ideas that arise between an external event and the emotional reaction to the event. Cameron acknowledges that when he did not receive the promotion, he immediately thought, "My father was right. I can't do anything right so I'll never be successful." The next step involves the therapist and Cameron examining the validity of this automatic thought. Cameron comes to the conclusion that other explanations for not being promoted could exist. For example, he might not have met the length of service criterion for promotion. He is able to see that he is blaming himself for something that is actually outside of his control.

While engaging in cognitive therapy, Cameron is assigned homework. He is required to attend a full schedule of activities and to rate the amount of mastery and pleasure he achieves in each. He is also required to make a list of things in which he has achieved success. These behavioral techniques support the fact that he is, indeed, a capable person. He and the therapist also use role-playing to provide a behavioral rehearsal for an interview with his boss in which he will assertively seek information as to why he did not receive the promotion. Cameron had learned the technique of meditation in college, and he begins to use it again for relaxation. He also reinstitutes a regular exercise program of swimming daily. By discharge, he has re-evaluated his self-concept and is able to state positive self-attributes. He reports relief from excessive anxiety.

Phobias

Perhaps the most serious of the phobic disorders is agoraphobia. In the treatment of agoraphobia, Marchione et al. (1987) suggest that using cognitive therapy and exposure therapy together gives better results than using either modality alone. **Graduated exposure** or **desensitization** therapy are behavioral therapy techniques that desensitize the person by gradually introducing him or her to the feared object or situation in small doses with support. At the direction of the therapist, the client may be asked to imagine or visualize being in a public place. When the imagined encounters are tolerable for the client, he or she goes on to work through a hierarchy of real-life (in vivo) exposures, for example

1. Walking down a street away from home with a trusted person, then alone
2. Riding in a car with a trusted person
3. Entering a small shop to purchase one item
4. Going to a supermarket to purchase a small list of items
5. Attending a movie or play with a trusted person

Cognitive therapy for agoraphobics includes having the client monitor and record automatic thoughts, teaching the relationship of automatic thoughts and phobic behavior, and helping the client replace distorted cognitions with rational ideas. Training in assertiveness, social skills, and problem-solving techniques can also be effective.

SOCIAL AND SIMPLE PHOBIAS. Social and simple (specific) phobias also seem best treated with a combination of therapies. **Modeling** therapy, which involves a phobic person observing an individual model appropriate behaviors when exposed to the feared object or situation, has proven useful. Also effective is **systematic desensitization** therapy, which involves exposing the client to a predetermined sequence of real or imaginary anxiety-producing situations or objects arranged on a continuum from least to most frightening. *Relaxation techniques* are used at each level of the sequence to reduce the anxiety response. The basis for this treatment is the principle that anxiety is incompatible with relaxation; thus, relaxation can control anxiety. Graduated exposure has been used successfully in the treatment of fear of heights and flying (Walder et al. 1987). Adding *cognitive restructuring* to any of the above therapeutic strategies seems to enhance success (Mattrick and Peters 1988).

Working with a Client Who Has a Social Phobia

Tim, aged 22, a music theater major, seeks treatment for social phobia. He describes himself as a failure because for the past two months he has been fearful of performing on stage. He suffers severe anxiety attacks whenever he is scheduled to appear in a student production. Recently, he has become severely anxious whenever faced with classroom readings or singing solo in music class. His only recourse has been to avoid performing in public. He is now thinking about changing his major.

Outpatient treatment focuses initially on identifying events that preceded the development of the phobia. Tim relates that his father had strongly objected to his choice of a theater career, saying that he would be "contaminated" by contact with homosexuals. About a month before becoming phobic, Tim was propositioned by a homosexual classmate, whose advances he rejected. His phobia seems to be based on the fear that an audience would identify him as a homosexual and scorn his performance. Therapy focuses on exploration of values and Tim's own sexual role identity and on relieving guilt feelings about ignoring his father's wishes.

Graduated exposure therapy and use of propranolol are chosen to deal with the phobia itself. The therapist explains the difference between systematic or fantasy desensitization and in vivo graduated exposure. Tim decides that although in vivo graduated exposure might result in psychological discomfort, he prefers this approach. He is able to stand silently on stage, then sing and recite in an empty theater, followed by reading and singing solo in class, and after six weeks, performing again before an audience.

Obsessive-Compulsive Disorder

Relaxation and cognitive strategies have proved successful for some individuals with OCD. The combination of flooding and response prevention has also resulted in a good success rate (Moergen et al. 1987) and works in the following way.

A client obsessed with the thought that he will contract a fatal disease from contact with "dirty" items uses elaborate washing rituals whenever he touches or comes into contact with anything he considers dirty. The client is required to touch objects he considers dirty (**flooding** with the anxiety-producing stimulus) and then is not allowed to engage in the ritual washing (*response prevention*).

Flooding can extinguish anxiety as a conditioned response, and response prevention can eliminate the ritual. This technique is used after careful evaluation and in a controlled setting in the presence of trained personnel.

Thought-stopping techniques have proven helpful to some OCD clients. These techniques are similar to response prevention. The client is initially instructed to shout, "Stop!" when the obsessional thought occurs. Eventually, the client learns to give the command silently. Another useful thought-stopping technique is to place a rubber band on the client's wrist and instruct him or her to snap it whenever the obsessional thought occurs. Both techniques serve the purpose of helping the client dismiss the obsessive thought.

Working with a Client Who Has Obsessive-Compulsive Disorder

Tina, a 32-year-old single parent, seeks treatment for OCD. Tina was born 12 years after her older sister to parents who were aloof, perfectionistic, and morally strict. She often felt that she was an unwanted child. Tina, like her sister, majored in business administration in college. During her senior year, she became pregnant. She did not seek an abortion because she believed it morally wrong. The father of the baby became so anxious that he left the area. Tina, too embarrassed to return home, quit school to support herself and the child. She worked as a secretary, took courses at night, and presently holds a job in a prominent law firm. The only change in her life occurred several weeks ago, when a new secretary was hired for the office.

Recently, Tina has started to have intrusive thoughts that some harm would come to her daughter. Even though she knows these thoughts are irrational, the thought (obsession) persists. The only way Tina can reduce her anxiety is to check her daughter's safety (compulsion). She calls school hourly. She does not allow her daughter to play sports, she screens her daughter's friends, she monitors her activities, and generally tries to control her daughter's every move. Her daughter feels embarrassed about her mother's checking behavior.

Tina gets to the point where she hardly eats. She sleeps very little at night because of the need to go to her daughter's room to "check that she is safe." She states that she thinks that she is stupid for not being able to manage her life as well as her sister and for not being able to get rid of her senseless worries. She

is admitted for short term intensive therapy. Tina's nursing care plan is written shortly after admission to the unit (Nursing Care Plan 14–3).

During the hospital stay, her therapist avoids use of psychoanalytical techniques, which may promote an intellectual understanding of the illness but not help the person attain appropriate emotions or change behavior. Instead, the therapist stays active and energetic, intervening whenever Tina's conversation becomes rambling. Tina is able to identify a precipitating stressor, the hiring of the new secretary, who symbolizes the sister with whom she competed. She is able to acknowledge that hostile feelings might be transformed to excessive concern (reaction-formation) and might result in checking behaviors but denies having angry feelings toward her daughter or her parents.

Tina's therapist weighs the options of using response prevention or of gradually reducing Tina's ritualizing. Response prevention involves asking the

---

Nursing Care Plan 14–3 ■ A PERSON WITH OBSESSIVE-COMPULSIVE DISORDER: Tina

NURSING DIAGNOSIS

Ineffective individual coping related to unresolved conflict

Supporting Data

- Reported obsessive thoughts that daughter will be harmed
- Compulsive checking designed to ensure daughter's safety

Long Term Goal: Client will demonstrate ability to cope effectively without the use of obsessive-compulsive behavior by (date).

Short Term Goals	*Intervention*	*Rationale*	*Evaluation*
1. By (date), client will experience decrease in incidence of obsessive thinking and compulsive behavior, as evidenced by normal food and fluid intake, six hours of sleep per night, and no calls to school.	1a. Anticipate need for information; orient before client must ask and meet other needs promptly.	1a. Increases feelings of security.	Goals met Client states that she likes the idea that staff explains things to her; she states that she worries less.
	1b. Focus on client rather than on symptoms.	1b. Reinforces self-worth.	Client is able to adhere to a schedule.
	1c. Permit client to call school six times per day for two days, then four times per day for four days, twice daily for two days, and no calls thereafter.	1c. Allowing performance of ritual prevents panic.	Client states that it is hard to sit through meals when she feels she should check on her daughter. Eats snacks willingly. Two-pound weight gain in one week.
	1d. Firmly encourage client to attend and eat meals. Offer nutritious snacks between meals.	1d. Limits must be placed on behaviors that threaten health.	Client initiates sleep within 45 minutes but awakens more than 6 times nightly. She refuses sedation because it makes her feel groggy the next day.
	1e. Give warm milk and back rub at bedtime.	1e–f. Promotes relaxation and sleep.	
	1f. Offer sedation if client has not initiated sleep by midnight.		
	1g. Avoid hurrying client.	1g. Hurrying client increases anxiety and performance of rituals.	

Continued on following page

Nursing Care Plan 14–3 ■ A PERSON WITH OBSESSIVE-COMPULSIVE DISORDER: Tina *(Continued)*

Short Term Goals	Intervention	Rationale	Evaluation
2. By (date), client will state that she is able to dismiss obsessive thoughts and will acknowledge that compulsion is not acted on.	2a. Teach client to interrupt obsessive thoughts by snapping on rubber band on wrist. 2b. Give positive reinforcement for nonritualistic behavior.	2a–b. Gives control over obsessive thinking and compulsive rituals. Positive reinforcement promotes repetition of adaptive behavior.	<u>Goals met</u> By the sixth day, client states, "It's getting easier to ignore my obsessive thoughts."
3. Client will state relationship between anxiety and symptoms by (date).	3. Support efforts to explore what purpose the behavior serves.	3. Recognition of anxiety-provoking events is basic to teaching client to interrupt anxiety cycle.	Client states that her symptoms worsened when she learned that a new secretary had been hired for the office. Is able to see that the new secretary could be seen as a competitor, much as she views her sister.

NURSING DIAGNOSIS

Disturbance in self-esteem related to lack of perceived strengths

Supporting Data

● Verbalization of stupidity associated with not being able to manage life as well as sister can
● Statement that she is "stupid" for not being able to get rid of worrisome ideas

Long Term Goal: Client will verbalize positive self-perception by (date).

Short Term Goals	Intervention	Rationale	Evaluation
1. Client will list five good things about self by (date).	1. Encourage client to identify strengths.	1. Fosters realistic self-concept.	<u>Goals met</u> On seventh day, client talks with nurse about list of strengths.
2. Client will make realistic positive statements about self by (date).	2. Arrange for activities at which she can succeed. Give merited praise.	2. Raises self-esteem.	Client states that she sees that she copes well under difficult conditions as single parent.
3. Self-deprecatory statements will be absent by (date).	3. Avoid power struggles. Expect cooperation.	3. Power struggles increase anxiety. When client loses power struggle, esteem is lowered. When staff loses, anger is generated.	Skilled negotiation by nurse avoids power struggle.

NURSING DIAGNOSIS

Diversional activity deficit related to preoccupation with performance of rituals

Supporting Data

● Giving up all social activities

Long Term Goal: Client will balance work and pleasurable activity by (date).

Short Term Goals	Intervention	Rationale	Evaluation
1. Client will make list of things she used to enjoy by (date).	1. Encourage client to survey activities at which she was proficient and activities she enjoyed.	1. Reduces preoccupation with rituals. Provides anxiety relief. Fosters awareness that enjoyment is deserved.	<u>Goals met</u> Client lists activities she would enjoy. Attends activities as required but without enjoyment during the first week. Now shows enjoyment. Plans to take ceramics class after discharge and to attend single-parents social group.
2. Client will engage in assigned scheduled activity (date).	2. Expect participation.	2. Relieves guilt over attendance.	
3. Client will choose daily activities and participate by (date).	3. Encourage helping others during activities.	3. Lower anxiety.	

NURSING DIAGNOSIS

Altered family process **related to client dominating daughter**

Supporting Data

- Not allowing daughter to play sports
- Screening daughter's friends
- Monitoring daughter's activities to the point of calling school several times daily

Long Term Goal: Client will relate to daughter in parental fashion without excessive domination by (date).

Short Term Goals	Intervention	Rationale	Evaluation
1. Client will allow daughter appropriate social contacts and school activities by (date).	1. Using cognitive therapy techniques, evaluate "dangers" she imagines for her daughter.	1. Promotes reality.	Goal met Client states that she understands that the dangers are more in her own mind than actual. Signs permission for daughter to play intramural sports. Allows daughter to attend peer group party.

client to refrain from the compulsive behaviors altogether. The therapist opts for gradual reduction.

The therapist tries to help Tina accomplish the following:

1. Discriminate between thoughts and actions
2. Accept "forbidden" desires and "bad" thoughts as common to most people
3. Discriminate between real and imagined danger and act accordingly, especially as they relate to her daughter's activities
4. Achieve thought stopping by snapping a rubber band worn on her wrist whenever the obsessive thought begins

At the time of discharge, Tina is unable to get in touch with or discuss negative feelings toward her daughter or her parents. The progress she has made is noted in the evaluation section of the nursing care plan. On the day of discharge, Tina's physician decides to prescribe clomipramine (Anafranil) in the hope that her obsessive thoughts and compulsive behavior will remain under control.

Post-traumatic Stress Disorder

PTSD has been successfully treated by using *relaxation techniques* coupled with flooding, using recalled images of the traumatic event (Saigh 1987). In one case, a young boy who developed PTSD after a bombing that injured several people was treated by flooding in which he was directed to imagine scenes of injured people, to hear their shouts and moans, and to recall the smell of smoke.

Combined *cognitive* and *behavioral* strategies have also been used successfully to help individuals see the world as a more predictable and controllable place. Treatment strategies involve redefining the event by considering possible benefits from the experience, finding meaning and purpose in the experience, and changing behaviors to prevent the distressing symptoms of anxiety from recurring. Clients are also encouraged to seek self-help or support groups (Janoff-Bulman 1985).

Working with a Client Who Has Post-traumatic Stress Disorder

Jim is 21 when he returns home from combat in Vietnam. He is discharged without a reorientation period. He experiences feelings of alienation, indifference, and anger as he faces a society whose attitudes and moods he does not know. He becomes withdrawn and distrustful and describes himself as feeling dead inside. He is jumpy and irritable and often throws himself on the ground when he hears a loud noise. He begins drinking heavily, stating that it helps him relax and sleep, but nothing stops his nightmares. When his wife suggests that they have a baby, Jim becomes violent. He beats her and goes on a three-day drinking spree. When he quits his third job in three months, his wife leaves him. He attempts suicide and is sent to a Veterans Administration Hospital.

There, Jim joins a support group of veterans who have been in combat situations. He describes feeling as though someone finally understands him. Eventually, he reveals that his two best friends were killed when one of them held a booby-trapped baby. He reveals his intense feelings of guilt over surviving when his best friends were killed.

Because of Jim's history of alcohol abuse, benzodiazepines are not prescribed for anxiety relief. Hydroxyzine pamoate (Vistaril) is used, instead. In the support group, he begins to re-evaluate the logic of his guilt feelings. He slowly begins to display appropriate emotions and feelings of concern for group members. He learns the use of relaxation techniques, which are effective both in helping him resume sleep after experiencing a nightmare and in reducing his hypervigilance. Eventually, the nightmares diminish in frequency and stop. As his symptoms decrease, his abuse of alcohol also decreases. Four months after beginning therapy, Jim begins occupational counseling that leads to a job, and six months after beginning therapy, he begins marital counseling, leading to reconciliation with his wife.

Evaluation

Evaluation includes careful ongoing assessment of the client by the nurse for the purpose of monitoring progress toward goal attainment. Identified client care goals serve as the basis for evaluation. Whenever goals are not attained, the nurse should identify reasons for nonattainment. If new facts about the client come to light, the data base may be changed, and new nursing diagnoses may be established. Interventions, too, may change as a result of the evaluation. When problems are resolved, the plan must also reflect this progress. In general, evaluation of goal attainment for clients with anxiety disorders deals with questions such as the following:

- Is the client experiencing a reduced level of anxiety?
- Does the client recognize his or her anxiety?
- Can the client identify stressors?
- Have healthy coping strategies been mobilized for use?
- Are new coping strategies effectively used? Does the client exhibit behaviors associated with adequate self-esteem?
- Is the client able to engage in more satisfying interpersonal relationships?

Summary

Individuals suffering from anxiety disorders have several things in common:

- A clearly defined organic basis for the disorders cannot always be found, but an unresolved psychological conflict is often found.

- Many have sustained loss early in life or have been exposed to anxious adults.
- Although usually in touch with reality, the individual is usually not in touch with his or her real feelings.
- Great amounts of psychological energy and multiple defense mechanisms are used to deal with anxiety. The defense mechanisms are rarely able to accomplish the goal of permanent anxiety reduction.
- Rigid behavior patterns tend to be repeated whenever the individual is faced with stress and anxiety.
- Sufferers tend to recognize that their symptoms are odd or strange (ego-dystonic).
- Self-esteem and self-acceptance tend to be low.
- Altered patterns of relatedness are characteristic.
- These individuals may incite predictable negative feelings in staff who provide treatment. These feelings make it necessary for nurses to practice self-assessment and to be willing to accept supervision from another professional.

Several treatment modalities are useful: individual therapy, group therapy, behavior therapy, cognitive therapy, and pharmacotherapy. While complete "cure" is rare, clients can be helped to make more satisfactory changes in their lives.

The nurse caring for the client with anxiety disorders will have an opportunity to function in the roles of caregiver, teacher, communicator, and manager and will use the nursing process to provide comprehensive care for the client and his or her significant others.

References

American Psychiatric Association. Diagnostic and Statistical Manual of Mental Disorders, 3rd ed, revised (DSM-III-R). Washington, DC: American Psychiatric Association, 1987.

Barlow DH, et al. Panic and generalized anxiety disorders: Nature and treatment. Behavior Therapy, 15:431–449, 1984.

Berman I, Sapers BL, Salzmanc. Sertraline: A new serotonergic antidepressant. Hospital and Community Psychiatry, 43(7):671, 1992.

Brown DR, et al. Racial differences in prevalence of phobic disorders. Journal of Nervous and Mental Disease, 178:434, 1990.

Butler G, et al. Anxiety management: Developing effective strategies. Behaviour Research and Therapy, 25:517, 1987.

Coleman JC, Butcher JN, Carson RC. Abnormal Psychology and Modern Life (6th ed.). Glenview, IL: Scott Foresman and Company, 1980.

Dohrenwend BP, Dohrenwend BS: Psychiatric disorders in urban settings. In Arieti S (ed). American Handbook of Psychiatry, vol 2. 2nd ed, New York: Basic Books, 1974.

Dubin WR, Weiss KJ. Handbook of Psychiatric Emergencies. Springhouse, PA: Springhouse, 1991.

Ellis A. Reason and Emotion in Psychotherapy. New York: Lyle Stuart, 1962.

Global heart of panic. Science News, 137:334, 1990.

Glod CA. Update Xanax: Pros and cons. Journal of Psychosocial Nursing, 30(6):36, 1992.

Hibbert G. Ideational components of anxiety: Their origin and content. British Journal of Psychiatry, 144:618, 1984.

Hollander A, Liebowitz MR, Gorman JM. Anxiety disorders. In Talbott JA, Hales RE, Yudofsky SC (eds.) Textbook of Psychiatry. Washington, DC: American Psychiatric Press, 1988.

Janoff-Bulman R. Aftermath of victimization: Rebuilding shattered assumptions. In Figley R (ed). Trauma and Its Wake. New York: Bruner-Mazel, 1985.

Kaplan HI, Sadock BJ. Synopsis of Psychiatry, 6th ed. Baltimore: Williams & Wilkins, 1991.

Marchione K, et al. Cognitive behavioral treatment of agoraphobia. Behaviour Research and Therapy, 25:319–328, 1987.

Mattrick R, Peters L. Treatment of severe social phobia. Journal of Consulting and Clinical Psychology, 56:251, 260, 1988.

Maxmen JS. Psychotropic Drugs Fast Facts. New York: Norton, 1991.

Moergen S, et al. Habituation to fear stimuli in a case of obsessive-compulsive disorder. Journal of Behavior Therapy and Experimental Psychiatry, 18:65, 1987.

Ost LG. Coping techniques in the treatment of anxiety disorders: Two controlled case studies. Behavioral Psychotherapy, 13:154–161, 1987.

Post-traumatic stress: Part 1. Harvard Mental Health Letter, 7(8):17, 1991.

Preston J, Johnson J. Clinical Psychopharmacology Made Ridiculously Simple. Miami: MedMaster, 1991.

Rapoport JL. The new biology of obsessive-compulsive disorder. Harvard Mental Health Letter, 5(1):4, 1989.

Rapoport, JL. The Boy Who Couldn't Stop Washing. New York: Plume, 1990.

Saigh P. In vivo flooding of an adolescent's post-traumatic stress disorder. Journal of Clinical Child Psychology, 16:147, 1987.

Schatzberg AF, Cole JO. Manual of Clinical Psychopharmacology, 2nd ed. Washington, DC: American Psychiatric Press, 1991.

Simoni PS. Obsessive-compulsive disorder: The effect of research on nursing care. Journal of Psychosocial Nursing, 29:19, 1991.

Valliant G. Adaptation and ego mechanisms of defense. Harvard Mental Health Letter, 3(7):4, 1986.

Weissman MM, et al. Suicidal ideation and suicide attempts in panic disorder and attacks. New England Journal of Medicine, 321:1210, 1989.

Whitley GG. Ritualistic behavior: Breaking the cycle. Journal of Psychosocial Nursing and Mental Health Services, 29(10):31, 1991.

Further Reading

Andreason N. The Broken Brain. New York: Harper & Row, 1984.

Beck A, Emery G. Anxiety Disorders and Phobias: A Cognitive Perspective. New York: Basic Books, 1985.

Chapman AH, Chapman M. Harry Stack Sullivan's Concepts of Personality Development and Psychiatric Illnesses. New York: Brunner-Mazel, 1980.

Clark DB, Agras WS. The assessment and treatment of performance anxiety in musicians. American Journal of Psychiatry, 148:598, 1991.

Crowe RR, Noyes R, Pauls DL, et al. A family study of panic disorders. Archives of General Psychiatry, 40:1065, 1983.

Dattilio FM. Symptom induction and de-escalation in the treatment of panic attacks. Journal of Mental Health Counseling, 12:416, 1990.

Kidson MA, Jones IH. Psychiatric disorders among aborigines of the Australian western desert. Archives of General Psychiatry, 19(4):413, 1968.

Panic disorder: Part 1. Harvard Mental Health Letter, 7(3):1, 1990.

Panic disorder: Part 2. Harvard Mental Health Letter, 7(4):1, 1990.

Post-traumatic stress: Part 2. Harvard Mental Health Letter, 7(9):1, 1991.

Talbott JA, Hales RE, Yudofsky SC (eds). Textbook of Psychiatry. Washington, DC: American Psychiatric Press, 1988.

Self-study Exercises

Multiple choice

1. Which of the following is one possible etiology of obsessive-compulsive disorder?

   A. Dopamine deficiency
   B. Secondary gain
   C. Faulty learning
   D. Clomipramine excess

2. The plan of care for a client with obsessive-compulsive disorder who has elaborate washing rituals specifies that response prevention is to be used. Which scenario is an example of response prevention?

   A. Not allowing client to wash hands after touching a "dirty" object.
   B. Not allowing client to seek reassurance from staff.
   C. Telling client he must relax whenever he seems tense.
   D. Having client repeatedly touch dirty objects.

3. A client is experiencing a panic attack. The nurse can be most therapeutic by

   A. Telling the client to take slow, deep breaths.
   B. Asking the client what he means when he says, "I'm dying."
   C. Verbalizing mild disapproval of his anxious behavior.
   D. Offering explanations about the sympathetic nervous system's role in symptom production.

4. The nurse caring for a client with panic attacks might anticipate that the psychiatrist would order

   A. Antipsychotic medication
   B. Anticholinergic medication
   C. Antidepressant medication
   D. Antihistamine medication

5. Mr. Thomas is a combat veteran who is being treated for post-traumatic stress disorder. An important nursing task shortly after admission is to

   A. Ascertain how long ago the trauma occurred.
   B. Establish whether the client has chronically elevated blood pressure related to high anxiety.
   C. Set firm limits on acting-out behaviors.
   D. Assess use of chemical substances for anxiety relief.

6. The psychiatrist orders lorazepam, 1 mg by mouth four times a day. The nurse caring for the client should

   A. Question the physician's order, as the dose is excessive.
   B. Teach the client to limit caffeine intake.
   C. Expect to observe mild ataxia and slurred speech.
   D. Explain the long term nature of anxiolytic therapy.

Place a Y before the nursing diagnoses that are commonly seen among clients with anxiety disorders and an N before those that are seldom seen.

7. __N__ *Fluid volume excess*
8. __Y__ *Impaired social interaction*
9. __Y__ *Altered role performance*
10. __Y__ *Risk for infection*
11. __Y__ *Dressing/grooming self-care deficit*
12. __N__ *Body image disturbance*
13. __N__ *Personal identity disturbance*

Match the ego defense mechanism and the anxiety disorder with which it is associated.

14. __B__ Displacement
15. __A__ Isolation
16. __C__ Undoing

   A. Post-traumatic stress disorder
   B. Phobia
   C. Obsessive-compulsive disorder

Place a Y before the interventions that would be helpful in caring for clients with anxiety disorders and an N before those that are not helpful.

17. __N__ Leave anxious clients strictly alone.
18. __N__ Insist that anxious clients sit down.
19. __Y__ Help client link behavior and feelings.
20. __Y__ Provide schedule of daily activities.
21. __N__ Laugh at performance of rituals.
22. __Y__ When a client mentions that his or her obsessive thoughts are "silly," the nurse could respond by saying, "Knowing your unwanted thoughts are irrational and that you are unable to control them seems upsetting to you."

CHAPTER 15

Somatoform and Dissociative Disorders

Helene S. Charron

OUTLINE

Clinical Vignettes
    A Client with Psychogenic
      Amnesia
    A Client with Psychogenic Fugue
    A Client with Depersonalization
      Disorder

    A Client with Multiple Personality
      Disorder
STANDARD VI: EVALUATION
SUMMARY

KEY TERMS AND CONCEPTS ◆ ◆ ◆ ◆ ◆ ◆ ◆ ◆ ◆ ◆ ◆ ◆ ◆ ◆ ◆

The key terms and concepts listed here also appear in bold where they are defined or discussed in this chapter.

ALTERNATE PERSONALITY (SUBPERSON-
    ALITY)
BODY DYSMORPHIC DISORDER
CONVERSION DISORDER
CONTINUOUS AMNESIA
DEPERSONALIZATION DISORDER
DISSOCIATIVE DISORDERS
EGO-SYNTONIC
FACTITIOUS DISORDER (MUNCHAUSEN
    SYNDROME)
GENERALIZED AMNESIA
HYPNOTHERAPY
HYPOCHONDRIASIS
LA BELLE INDIFFERÉNCE

LOCALIZED AMNESIA
MULTIPLE PERSONALITY DISORDER
NARCOTHERAPY
PRIMARY GAIN
PRIMARY PERSONALITY
PSYCHOGENIC AMNESIA
PSYCHOGENIC FUGUE
SECONDARY GAIN
SELECTIVE AMNESIA
SOMATIZATION
SOMATIZATION DISORDER
SOMATOFORM PAIN DISORDER

OBJECTIVES ■

After studying this section on nursing care of clients with somatoform and dissociative disorders, the student will be able to

1. Indicate where somatoform and dissociative disorders fit on the mental health continuum.
2. Discuss psychosocial theories of etiology of somatoform and dissociative disorders.
3. Identify data that should routinely be gathered during the assessment of clients with somatoform disorders and clients with dissociative disorders.
4. Identify three possible nursing diagnoses for the client with a somatoform disorder and for a client with a dissociative disorder.
5. Discuss common reactions health care workers experience when working with clients with somatoform disorders and clients with dissociative disorders.
6. Propose realistic and measurable goals for clients with somatoform disorders and clients with dissociative disorders.
7. Plan interventions for clients employing somatization or dissociation as mechanisms for coping with anxiety.
8. Evaluate effectiveness of care based on established outcome criteria.
9. Identify characteristics of the various somatoform and dissociative disorders according to the *DSM-III-R.*

Anxiety exerts a powerful influence on the lives of individuals. People vary in their ability to cope with anxiety successfully. The ways in which anxiety is manifested dysfunctionally also differ. This chapter will present information about the nursing care of clients who experience somatoform and dissociative disorders. The placement of these disorders on the mental health continuum can be seen in Figure 15–1.

Somatoform Disorders

Somatoform disorders have in common the presence of one or more physical complaints for which adequate physical explanation cannot be found (Kaplan and Saddock 1991). *Soma* is the Greek word for body. **Somatization** can be defined as the expression of psychological stress through physical symptoms. In other words, psychological conflicts are converted into bodily symptoms, and the person reacts with somatic rather than psychic manifestations. **Somatoform disorders** are a group of conditions in which somatization is present. They are characterized by the following:

- Complaints of physical symptoms that cannot be explained by physiological tests
- Existence of a strong possibility that the physical symptoms have been precipitated by psychological factors, such as stress and unmet psychological needs
- Client's inability to voluntarily control the symptom

In these conditions, when anxiety is transformed at an unconscious level into physical symptoms, the primary gain, or purpose for the symptom, is anxiety relief. The physical symptoms are **ego-syntonic,** and the individual believes them to be real. In most somatoform disorders, the individual is worried about the symptom or symptoms and seeks medical assistance. (This characteristic is different from those of clients with obsessions, compulsions, and phobias, whose symptoms are *ego-dystonic*, causing them to view their symptom as "silly.")

An overview of the characteristics of somatoform disorders is shown in Figure 15–2.

Theory

Because no clear etiology exists for somatoform disorders, we will review various theoretical positions.

BIOLOGICAL FACTORS

Studies reported by Kaplan and Sadock (1991) have not shown a conclusive neurophysiologic basis for somatoform disorders. Some researchers suggest that somatoform symptoms arise from faulty perceptions and incorrect assessments of body sensations, caused by attention deficits and cognitive impairments, such as increased distractibility and circumstantial associations.

Some clients may be predisposed to experience severe pain because of abnormalities in brain chemical balance or because of structural abnormalities of the sensory or limbic systems. Pain sensations are probably modulated in the central nervous system; when serotonin and endorphins are deficient, an individual may perceive incoming pain stimuli as being more intense.

Some clinicians believe that **conversion disorder** has an organic basis related to central nervous system– arousal disturbances. The diminished awareness of sensation observed in some clients with conversion disorder could be associated with inhibition of afferent sensorimotor impulses resulting from high arousal.

GENETIC FACTORS

Somatoform disorders have not been identified as being genetically transmitted. Studies have shown that there is an increased likelihood for first-degree relatives of individuals with somatoform pain disorder to be diagnosed with this disorder. Twin studies have shown an increased prevalence of hypochondriasis among identical twins (Kaplan and Sadock 1991).

SOCIOCULTURAL FACTORS

The incidence of *somatoform disorders* is higher among individuals from lower socioeconomic groups, those

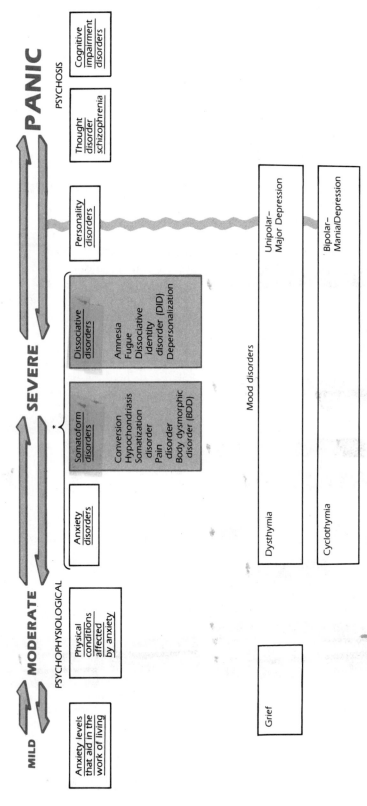

*These disorders are currently classified by presenting clinical symptoms. Previously they were called "neurotic" disorders.

Figure 15–1. *Mental health continuum for somatoform and dissociative disorders.*

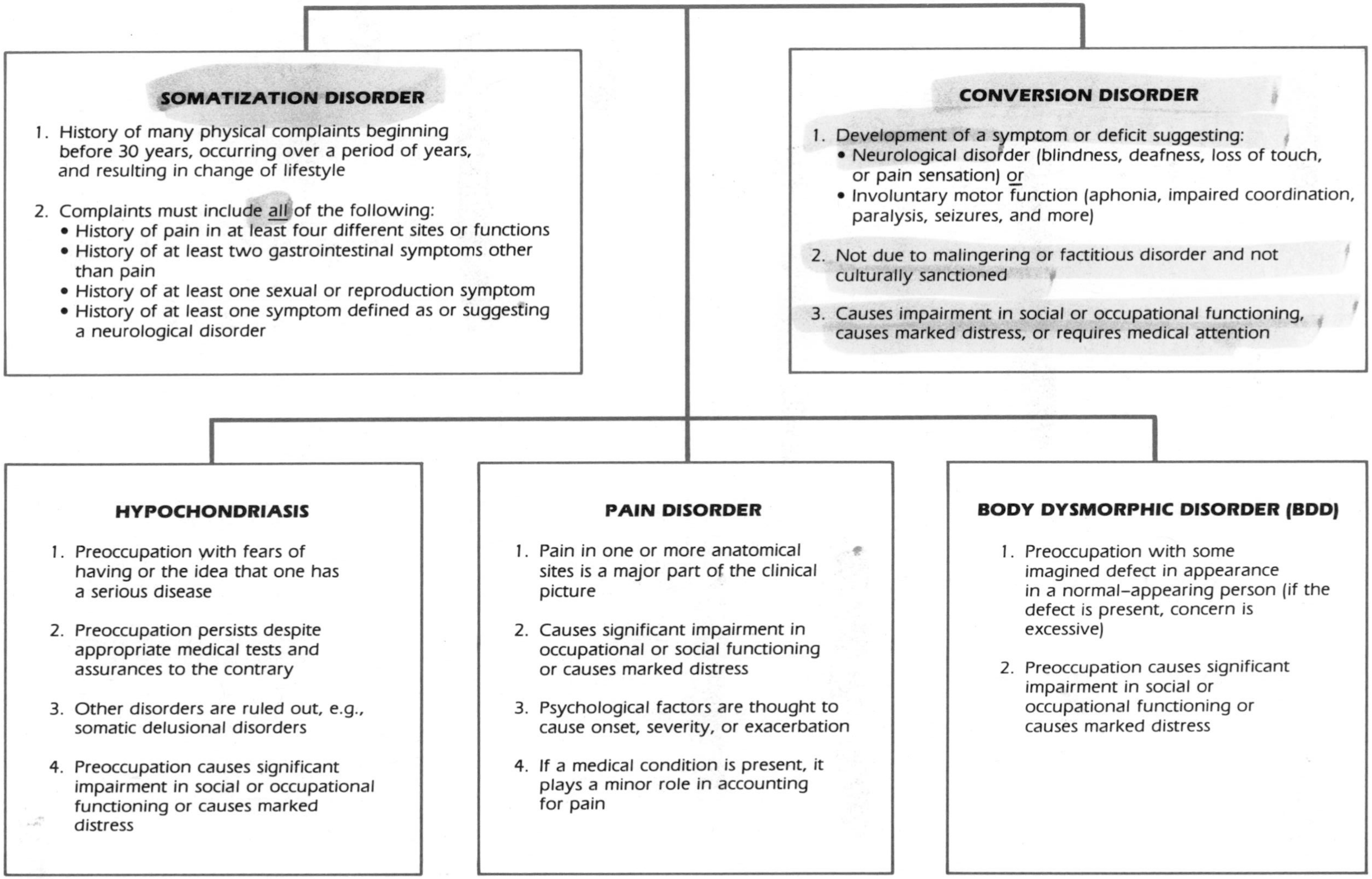

SOMATIZATION DISORDER

1. History of many physical complaints beginning before 30 years, occurring over a period of years, and resulting in change of lifestyle

2. Complaints must include <u>all</u> of the following:
   - History of pain in at least four different sites or functions
   - History of at least two gastrointestinal symptoms other than pain
   - History of at least one sexual or reproduction symptom
   - History of at least one symptom defined as or suggesting a neurological disorder

CONVERSION DISORDER

1. Development of a symptom or deficit suggesting:
   - Neurological disorder (blindness, deafness, loss of touch, or pain sensation) <u>or</u>
   - Involuntary motor function (aphonia, impaired coordination, paralysis, seizures, and more)

2. Not due to malingering or factitious disorder and not culturally sanctioned

3. Causes impairment in social or occupational functioning, causes marked distress, or requires medical attention

HYPOCHONDRIASIS

1. Preoccupation with fears of having or the idea that one has a serious disease

2. Preoccupation persists despite appropriate medical tests and assurances to the contrary

3. Other disorders are ruled out, e.g., somatic delusional disorders

4. Preoccupation causes significant impairment in social or occupational functioning or causes marked distress

PAIN DISORDER

1. Pain in one or more anatomical sites is a major part of the clinical picture

2. Causes significant impairment in occupational or social functioning or causes marked distress

3. Psychological factors are thought to cause onset, severity, or exacerbation

4. If a medical condition is present, it plays a minor role in accounting for pain

BODY DYSMORPHIC DISORDER (BDD)

1. Preoccupation with some imagined defect in appearance in a normal-appearing person (if the defect is present, concern is excessive)

2. Preoccupation causes significant impairment in social or occupational functioning or causes marked distress

Figure 15–2. *Diagnostic criteria for somatoform disorders. (Adapted from American Psychiatric Association. DSM-IV Options Book: Work in Progress. Washington, DC: American Psychiatric Association, 1991.)*

who live in rural rather than in urban settings, and those with little education. Cultural mores may permit certain groups to unconsciously use somatization as an acceptable approach to dealing with life stress.

Conversion disorder was originally thought to be a disorder affecting women exclusively but now is found to occur in men, although to a lesser degree. One reason this disorder may be more prevalent in women is thought to be related to the fact that social mores have not provided women with appropriate ways to express aggression or sexuality.

PSYCHOSOCIAL FACTORS

Freud believed psychogenic complaints of pain, illness, or loss of physical function were related to the repression of a conflict (usually of an aggressive or sexual nature) and the transformation of anxiety into a physical symptom symbolically related to the conflict. In **conversion disorder,** the ego defense mechanisms involved are repression and conversion. According to Freudian theory, in *conversion* symptoms allow a forbidden wish or urge to be partially expressed but sufficiently disguised so that the individual does not have to face the unacceptable wish. Therefore, *the symptom* is said to be *symbolic of the conflict.* The symptom also permits the individual to communicate a need for special treatment or consideration from others. The following is an example of how a symptom can be both symbolic of, and a solution to, a conflict in a conversion disorder:

Anita, aged 18, lives with her mother and stepfather. The stepfather has been physically abusive to Anita for many years. Anita hates him but is dependent on him for financial support. One day, as the family steps off the curb to cross a busy street, the father is hit by a speeding automobile. Anita attempts to shout at her stepfather to warn him, but no sound comes out. She suffers aphonia (loss of voice) that lasts until psychotherapy helps her regain her ability to speak. It is obvious that the conflict is whether to warn her physically abusive and hated stepfather or not to warn him. The loss of her voice solves the problem and makes it impossible to save him.

Behaviorists suggest that conversion disorder symptoms are learned ways of communicating helplessness and that these symptoms allow the individual to manipulate others.

Hypochondriasis is considered by many clinicians to have *psychodynamic* origins. They suggest that anger, aggression, or hostility that had its origins in past losses, rejections, or disappointments is expressed as a need for help and concern from others. The client then rejects the helpers as being ineffective. Other clinicians suggest that hypochondriasis is a defense against guilt or low self-esteem. In this hypothesis, the pain and other somatic symptoms the individual suffers are experienced as deserved punishment. *Cognitive theorists* believe that the client with hypochondriasis focuses on body sensations, misinterprets their meaning, then becomes excessively alarmed by them. Social learning theorists suggest that children who have had medical illnesses are more likely to develop hypochondriasis in adulthood than are children with healthier histories. They also point out that individuals who have survived a severe illness often develop hypochondriacal reactions during convalescence.

Somatoform pain disorder is thought to have a *psychological basis.* According to some theorists, the meaning of pain for the individual may date back to early experiences. Later, the individual's pain may serve an important unconscious function, such as providing atonement for being inadequate or inferior, providing a way to obtain the love and concern of others, or providing punishment for real or imagined wrongdoing. The defense mechanisms responsible are repression and displacement. *Behaviorists* point out that pain symptoms may be learned behaviors and that the symptoms become more intense when they are reinforced by attention from others. In the United States, most individuals are concerned about others who complain of pain, and certainly physicians and nurses are taught to be attentive and responsive to a client's reports of pain. Other reinforcers (secondary gains) are being able to avoid activities the individual considers distasteful, obtaining financial gain from the pain, and being able to gain some advantage in interpersonal relationships as a result of the pain.

In cases of **body dysmorphic disorder,** some theorists believe that the individual invests a part of the body with special meaning that may be traceable to some event occurring at an earlier stage of psychosexual development. The original event is *repressed,* and the attachment of special meaning to a part of the body comes about through *symbolization. Projection* is used when the individual makes statements such as "It makes everyone look at me with horror." or "I know my husband hates it." Refer to Table 15–1 for clinical examples of each of the somatoform disorders and their defenses.

ASSESSMENT

Assessment of clients with somatoform disorders is a complex process, requiring careful and complete documentation.

Table 15-1 ■ SOMATOFORM DISORDERS—DEFENSES AND EXAMPLES

DEFENSE MECHANISMS	EXAMPLE*
Conversion Disorder	
Conversion	Jan, a 28-year-old former secretary, awakes one morning to find that she has a tingling in both hands, and cannot move her fingers. Two days earlier, her husband had told her that he wanted a separation and that she would have to go back to work to support herself.
Somatoform Pain Disorder	
Displacement	Henry, 47, a laborer, "pulled a muscle" in his back a year ago. Two weeks prior to this his wife, a waitress, told him that she wanted to go back to school to get her bachelor's degree. He suffers severe, constant pain, despite negative results from myelograms, computed tomographics scans, magnetic resonance imaging, and neurological exams. He watches television all day and collects disability. His wife, unable now to go to school, waits on him and has assumed his home responsibilities.
Body Dysmorphic Disorder	
Symbolism and projection	Michele, a young, attractive woman, is preoccupied that her nose is too long and "ugly." She is preoccupied and quite distressed over her perception. Two plastic surgeons she consulted are hesitant to reshape her nose but have not altered her thinking that her nose makes her ugly.
Somatization Disorder	
Somatization	Deanna, 27, presents at the doctor's office with excessive, heavy menstruation. She tells the nurse that recently she experienced pain "first in my back and then going to every part of my body." She states that she is often bothered with constipation and frequent vomiting when she "eats the wrong food." She states she had been "unwell" and had suffered from seizures and still has them occasionally. The nurse becomes confused, not knowing what symptoms she wants the doctor to evaluate. Deanna tells the nurse she lives at home with her parents because her poor health makes it hard for her to hold a job.
Hypochondria	
Denial and somatization	Julio, 52 lost his wife to colon cancer 5 months ago, which he "took very well." Recently he saw the sixth physician with the same complaint. He believes that he has liver cancer, despite repeated and extensive diagnostic tests, which are all negative. He has ceased seeing his friends, has dropped his hobbies, and spends much of his time checking his sclera and "resting his liver." His son finally demands that he see a doctor.

*All entail somatization.

Individuals with somatoform disorders resolve conflicts and reduce anxiety with their bodily symptoms. This is considered a **primary gain.** They may also achieve **secondary gains** from their symptoms such as

- Manipulation of relationships
- Avoidance of responsibility through helplessness
- Fulfillment of dependency needs
- Financial gain from insurance, workers' compensation, or sick benefits

During assessment, it is important to determine if the symptoms are under the client's voluntary control. Somatoform symptoms *are not* under the individual's voluntary control; symptoms associated with malingering and factitious disorders are. A client who is **malingering** makes a conscious attempt to deceive others by pretending to have false or exaggerated symptoms, often for financial gain. Low back pain is frequently chosen because it is difficult to disprove. A client with **factitious disorder (Munchausen syndrome)** produces physical signs of illness through voluntary physiological tampering. Such clients may ingest substances that will cause an infection or diarrhea or inject themselves with saliva to cause inflammatory reactions. A prisoner in jail inserted sewing machine needles into his scrotum to gain medical attention. Heating thermometers to give a high reading is common practice among such clients. Individuals who use malingering or who display factitious symptoms deceive others, but not themselves, about the symptoms. By contrast, individuals with somatoform disorders are deceived by their symptoms. They cannot see relationships between symptoms and conflicts that are obvious to others.

Often, clients with *conversion disorder* will report a sudden loss in function of a body part: "I woke up this morning and I couldn't move my arm" or "Suddenly my legs were paralyzed," or "when I tried to speak, I found I had lost my voice." Other common "losses" associated with conversion disorder involve vision and hearing. Some clients with conversion disorder describe their symptoms with an inappropriate lack of concern **(la belle indifférence).** This blandness is found only in a minority of clients. (Pincus and Tucker 1978). Clients with somatization disorder, hypochondriasis, and somatoform pain disorder usually discuss their symptoms dramatically. They often use colorful metaphors and exaggerations: "The pain was searing, like a hot sword drawn across my forehead," or "My symptoms are so rare that I've stumped hundreds of doctors." Individuals with body dysmorphic disorder are concerned about only one part of the body and often seek cosmetic surgery. Their affective display is of disgust with the offending body part.

It may be difficult to differentiate between hypochondriasis and somatization disorder because both may involve multiple somatic complaints. Somatization disorder is usually seen in women and begins before the age of 30. Hypochondriasis begins in the 40s and 50s and extends into old age. It is equally common in men and women (Adler 1981).

Careful diagnostic evaluations must be performed to rule out an organic basis for the symptoms. When somatization disorders are confirmed, laboratory findings and other diagnostic tests will reveal no pathology. Medical histories, however, will show that the client has sought repeated tests and treatments, often from a series of physicians and hospitals. These individuals repeatedly go from doctor to doctor trying to find evidence of illness ("doctor shopping"). When it is suggested that the problem might be psychological and not physical, these clients uniformly resist counseling or therapy.

It is helpful for nurses to assess for (1) presence of secondary gains, (2) cognitive style, (3) ability to communicate emotional needs, and (4) dependence on medication, in addition to collecting data about the nature, location, onset, character, and duration of symptoms.

ASSESSING SECONDARY GAINS

Self-care and role performance may be compromised, depending on the symptoms experienced by the client. Diminished ability to perform usual family, work, and social roles is nearly always present. The physical symptoms may make it difficult, if not impossible, to continue employment. Family roles and processes are altered when one member takes on a sick role. Preoccupation with illness or pain may produce observable emotional and social isolation, inattention to the needs of others, manipulation of others, and excessively demanding behaviors. Powerlessness may be noted as a theme, with clients citing numerous self-care activities and roles they can no longer perform, and responsibilities they have surrendered to others.

Therefore, the nurse might identify a number of *secondary gains* the client may be receiving from the symptoms. These can include (1) getting out of usual responsibilities "legitimately," (2) getting extra attention "legitimately," and (3) manipulating others in the environment. One way to identify the presence of secondary gains is to ask the client questions such as "What can't you do now that you used to be able to do?" or "How has this problem affected your life?"

ASSESSING COGNITIVE STYLE

In general, these clients misinterpret physical stimuli and distort reality regarding their symptoms. For example, sensations a normal individual might interpret as a headache might suggest a brain tumor to a client with somatoform disorder, or indigestion might be interpreted as cancer. Exploring the client's cognitive style may be helpful in distinguishing between hypochondriasis and somatization disorder. The client with *hypochondriasis* exhibits more anxiety and an obsessive attention to detail, along with a preoccupation with the fear of serious illness. The client with *somatization disorder* is often rambling and vague about the details of his or her many symptoms and may give a poor or vague history (Ford 1983).

ASSESSING THE ABILITY TO COMMUNICATE EMOTIONAL NEEDS

Often, clients with somatoform disorders have difficulty communicating their emotional needs. Although able to describe their symptoms, they have difficulty verbalizing feelings, especially those related to anger, guilt, and dependence. The somatic symptom may be the client's chief means of communicating emotional needs. Psychogenic blindness or hearing loss may be saying symbolically, "I can't face this knowledge." Consider the wife who overheard friends discussing her husband's sexual infidelity and developed total deafness.

ASSESSING DEPENDENCE ON MEDICATION

Individuals experiencing many somatic complaints often become dependent on medication to relieve pain or anxiety, or to induce sleep. It is not uncommon for physicians to prescribe diazepam (Valium) or other anxiolytic agents for clients who seem highly anxious and concerned about their symptoms. Clients often return to the physician, seeking prescription renewal. If the client has sought treatment from numerous physicians, the possibility of medication misuse escalates. Dependence on anxiolytics develops quickly; thus, it is important that the nurse assess the types and amounts of medications being used by the client to control pain and anxiety or to promote sleep.

Nursing Diagnosis

Clients with a somatoform disorder present various nursing problems. For example, *ineffective individual coping* may be related to

- Distorted perceptions of body functions and symptoms
- Chronic pain of psychological origin
- Dependence on pain relievers or anxiolytics

Impaired social interaction may be related to preoccupation with illness. When clients focus their psychic and physical energy on somatic symptoms, they have little energy to expend on others or on diversional activities. This tendency to isolate themselves may be due to an unconscious awareness that they may receive little attention in busy social situations or that participating in many social activities might imply wellness rather than illness.

Ineffective family coping related to adoption of the sick role is nearly always present. *Secondary gains* derived by the client nearly always signal the presence of compromised family coping. Adoption of the sick role by a family member causes alterations in family roles; for example, a parent's illness is likely to require children to assume increased responsibility at early ages. The assumption of the illness role by an adolescent may cause the mother to become overinvolved with that child, giving less attention to other siblings or the father.

Self-esteem disturbance may be a useful diagnosis if the client has expressed negative self-evaluation related to losing body function, feeling useless, or not feeling valued by significant others. *Powerlessness* over somatic symptoms of psychogenic origin may be identified if the client has talked about lack of control over his or her life situation.

Self-care deficit might be related to

- Pain associated with somatoform pain disorder
- A specific conversion symptom, such as paralysis, blindness, or loss of voice
- Cognitive impairment: inaccurate belief that client has a life-threatening illness

Planning

CONTENT LEVEL—PLANNING GOALS

Planning client goals and outcomes should be a process in which the client fully participates. Shared decision making can promote goal attainment. It is vital that outcome criteria be realistic and attainable. Setting realistic short term goals helps the client see concrete evidence of progress. Possible goals and outcomes for nursing diagnoses frequently established for clients with somatoform diagnoses follow:

1. *Ineffective individual coping* related to distorted perceptions of bodily functions and symptoms

   By (date), client will cope adaptively, as evidenced by
   - Appropriately interpreting physical symptoms, "The bruises on my leg resulted from bumping the chair, not from leukemia."
   - Verbalizing relationship of conflicts and feelings to somatic symptoms, such as "I was so angry with him but afraid he'd leave me if I showed it. Being sick punished him."
   - Replacing reliance on anxiolytics through the use of alternative coping strategies, such as assertive communication and relaxation techniques.
   - Replacing demanding, manipulative, and attention-seeking behaviors with behaviors that respect others' rights.
   - Expressing feelings verbally rather than acting them out somatically.

2. *Impaired social interaction* related to preoccupation with somatic symptoms or pain

   By (date), client will demonstrate improved social interaction, as evidenced by
   - Establishing and completing a contract to attend a specified number of social and diversional activities daily

- Verbalizing satisfaction with improved level of social interaction
- Sustaining conversations for five or more minutes at a time without mentioning somatic symptoms or their effects

3. *Ineffective family coping* related to the client's adoption of the sick role

By (date), the family will demonstrate interactions that maximize optimal functioning of the client, as evidenced by
- Reports of increased client independence
- Client resumption of preillness roles, including work
- Family reports of absence of manipulative behaviors or excessive dependence

PROCESS LEVEL—NURSES' REACTIONS AND FEELINGS

Nurses and other health care workers often find working with clients with somatoform disorders difficult and unsatisfying. The nurse notes the objective data indicating a lack of physiologic basis for the client's symptoms. The nurse then wonders why this "not sick" client is taking up valuable time that might better be spent on a "sick" client. The tendency, at times, is for nurses to feel resentment or anger toward these clients. These negative feelings occur whether the client is being cared for by medical-surgical staff, who usually prefer to work with clients with physical illnesses, or by psychiatric staff, who often prefer to work with psychotic clients. It is helpful to remember that the symptom the client is experiencing is very real to him or her, even though the objective data do not substantiate a physiologic basis. Anger may also rise when staff find themselves dealing with a client who uses somatic symptoms to manipulate the environment and the people in the environment.

Staff may experience feelings of helplessness over not being able to "make the client realize" that his or her symptom has no organic basis. Clients who use somatization exhibit remarkable resistance to change. They cling to their unrealistic beliefs about the origin of the somatic symptoms, despite objective evidence. Setting goals that have *staged outcomes* (small, attainable steps) can help the nurse avoid feelings of helplessness.

Clients with somatoform disorders should be discussed in clinical conferences to allow staff to ventilate feelings and plan for consistency of care. Being aware of feelings and responses permits effective planning.

Intervention

PSYCHOTHERAPEUTIC INTERVENTIONS

Nursing interventions involve establishing a helping relationship with the client, assisting the client to recognize the somatic symptoms as a coping strategy, and helping the client learn to use more effective coping strategies. To be successful, therapeutic interventions must address ways of helping the client get his or her needs met without resorting to somatization. The *secondary gains* the client has derived from illness behaviors can become less important to the client when underlying needs can be met directly. Collaboration with significant others will be essential for success. Table 15–2 outlines some nursing interventions and rationales for working with clients with somatoform disorders.

HEALTH TEACHING

As previously mentioned, many clients who use somatization as a way of coping with anxiety tend to have little education. Therefore, teaching these clients basic information about body function and health promotion is often warranted. Pictures and charts can be helpful to illustrate the information being taught. It is useful to review with the family the information the client has been given because their information may also be lacking or in error. Teaching assertive communication and stress reduction techniques may help the client control or reduce anxiety and the accompanying somatization.

ACTIVITIES OF DAILY LIVING

When somatization is present, the client's ability to perform activities of daily living (ADLs) may be impaired, and nursing interventions may be necessary. In general, interventions involve using a matter-of-fact approach to support the highest level of self-care of which the client is capable.

For clients manifesting paralysis, blindness, or severe fatigue, an effective nursing approach is to matter-of-factly support clients while expecting them to feed, bathe, or groom themselves. For example, a client who demonstrates paralysis of an arm can be expected to eat using the other arm. The client who is experiencing blindness can be told at what numbers on an imaginary clock the food is located on the plate and encouraged to feed himself or herself. These strategies are effective in reducing secondary gain.

Table 15–2 ■ NURSING INTERVENTIONS AND RATIONALES: SOMATOFORM DISORDERS

INTERVENTION	RATIONALE

Nursing Diagnosis: *Ineffective individual coping* related to inadequate coping skills, as evidenced by total focus on self and physical symptoms

INTERVENTION	RATIONALE
1. Offer explanations and support during diagnostic testing.	1. Reduces anxiety while ruling out organic illness.
2. After physical complaints have been investigated, avoid further reinforcement, e.g., do not take vital signs each time client complains of palpitations.	2. Directs focus away from physical symptoms.
3. Spend time with client at times other than when client summons nurse to offer physical complaint.	3. Rewards non–illness related behaviors and encourages repetition of desired behavior.
4. Observe and record frequency and intensity of somatic symptoms.	4. Establishes a baseline and later evaluation of effectiveness of interventions.
5. Do not imply that symptoms are not real.	5. Psychogenic symptoms are real to the client even though causation is not organic.
6. Shift focus from somatic complaints to feelings or to neutral topics.	6. Conveys interest in client as a person rather than in client's symptoms. Reduces need to gain attention via symptoms.
7. Assess secondary gains that "physical illness" provides for client, e.g., attention, increased dependency, and distraction from another problem.	7. Nurse can work with client to meet these needs in healthier ways and thus minimize secondary gains.
8. Use matter-of-fact approach to clients exhibiting resistance or covert anger.	8. Avoids power struggles. Demonstrates acceptance of anger and permits discussion of angry feelings.
9. Set limits on manipulative behavior that violates rights of others.	9. Protects other clients and significant others.
10. Help client look at result of manipulative behavior on others.	10. Encourages insight. Can help improve intrafamily relationships.
11. Show concern for client and client's anxieties, while avoiding fostering dependency needs.	11. Shows respect for client's feelings while minimizing secondary gains from "illness."
12. Reinforce client's strengths and problem-solving abilities.	12. Contributes to positive self-esteem. Helps client realize that needs can be met without resorting to somatic symptoms.
13. Teach assertive communication.	13. Provides client with a positive means of getting needs met. Reduces feelings of helplessness and the need for manipulation.
14. Teach client stress reduction techniques, such as meditation, relaxation, and mild physical exercise.	14. Can reduce client's need for medication. Provides alternate coping strategies.

Nursing Diagnosis: *Self-care deficit* related to "physical inability," as evidenced by inability to perform usual ADLs

INTERVENTION	RATIONALE
1. Encourage client to perform normal ADLs to highest level of ability.	1. Enhances self-esteem and minimizes secondary gains.
2. Teach client alternative ways to perform ADLs if "physical disability" interferes, assisting only when necessary	2. Gives client support while minimizing secondary gains.
3. Maintain a nonjudgmental approach when assisting client with ADLs.	3. Symptoms are real to client. A person's anxiety level increases when negatively judged; therefore, the need for defense increases.
4. Feed, bathe, and assist with hygiene, if necessary, while encouraging client participation.	4. Client comfort and safety are nursing priorities and may increase client's sense of security.

Nursing Diagnosis: *Diversional activity deficit* related to preoccupation with self and symptoms, as evidenced by complete absorption with self

INTERVENTION	RATIONALE
1. Help client establish a minimum of one daily goal, e.g., attend one activity daily. Gradually increase the number of goals. Expect compliance.	1. Setting initial goals at a low level ensures success and reinforces client's new behaviors.
2. Explore possible uses of community resources for social or diversional activities.	2. Community resources often provide inexpensive opportunities for social interactions. Gives client a sense of control.

ADLs = activities of daily living.

SOMATIC THERAPIES

Clients with somatoform disorders rarely profit from medication. In fact, substance abuse may be a problem for these clients. All medications should be monitored carefully because clients with somatoform disorders tend to use them unreliably.

Clients with somatization disorder and hypochondriasis who display high levels of anxiety may be given short courses of treatment with anxiolytics, and antidepressants may be prescribed for individuals when depression is present. Occasionally, anxiolytics may be prescribed for a short period for a client with a conversion reaction. Clients with somatoform pain disorder rarely benefit from analgesics, sedatives, or anxiolytics; their use often leads to addiction. Recently, antidepressants—amitriptyline (Elavil), imipramine (Tofranil), and doxepin (Sinequan)—have been used with some success to treat somatoform pain. Their mechanism of action in pain relief is still unclear. New studies are being conducted with clomipramine (Anafranil) and fluoxetine (Prozac) to learn if their selective serotonergic action will be effective in treating chronic back pain and body dysmorphic disorder.

THERAPEUTIC ENVIRONMENT

Most clients with somatoform disorders are seen in medical rather than psychiatric settings. Hospitalizations and frequent visits to medical clinics may allow suggestible clients to witness the symptoms of others and later incorporate them into their own symptom repertoires. Because these clients are often rejected by medical-surgical staff, their anxiety levels may rise, causing an intensification of their somatic complaints. The psychiatric setting has the advantages of providing a structured daily routine and activities. Matter-of-fact acceptance by the staff is somewhat easier to achieve.

PSYCHOTHERAPY

Psychoanalytic therapy for clients with somatoform disorders is aimed at helping the client bring the repressed conflict into conscious awareness, connecting the actual feelings associated with the repressed event, and helping the client develop adaptive coping skills.

Behavioral treatment for clients with hypochondriasis, using exposure and response prevention, has seemed moderately effective. In one study (Warwick and Marks 1988), patients showed initial improvement when treated behaviorally, but a five-year follow-up showed

that seven of 17 clients still had concerns about illness.

Salkovskis and Warwick (1986) suggest that a *cognitive-behavioral* approach may also be helpful. They randomly assigned 81 clients with low back pain to one of three groups: an operant-behavioral group, a cognitive-behavioral group, and a control group. The results after one year showed equal improvement among the clients assigned to the two treatment groups.

Family therapy is thought to be an important part of treatment for somatoform disorders by many therapists. The role of family in maintaining somatoform symptoms must be considered. The family's role in bringing about change by collaborating in the treatment of the client cannot be underestimated. At minimum, family therapy can help family members place the client's illness in perspective. Families are taught ways of supporting each other and of minimizing secondary gains. They are also given strategies for coping with predictable problems. The clinical vignettes that follow will discuss both symptoms and treatment. Refer to Figure 15–2 to review the DSM-IV criteria for each.

CLINICAL VIGNETTES

A Client with Somatization Disorder

Susanne Barron, a 26-year-old beautician, is admitted to the hospital following an overdose of sedatives. She states that she is sick of not being able to get help from anyone. In describing herself, she mentions not being well since the age of 14. She describes seizures, fainting spells, and occasional weakness of the left leg. One year ago, she developed abdominal pain, nausea, and diarrhea. Exploratory surgery revealed no significant pathology. The symptoms still recur "sometimes." She mentions experiencing painful menstruation and excessive bleeding over a period of several years. Recently, she has had palpitations and tightness of her chest after emotionally trying events. Ms. Barron lived at home until six months ago, when she married a man 15 years her senior. She states that she is "turned off by sex" because it is painful for her, and she reveals that her husband is upset by her constant illness. He is considering divorce. A short hospitalization is advised.

Although antidepressant medication is considered, Ms. Barron's depression does not warrant its use. In individual therapy, Ms. Barron is able to relate her physical symptoms to her parents' concern with health and illness themes. Her father had been an invalid due to mitral valve disease, and all her mother's attention had been focused on him. Ms. Barron had shared this attention at the times that she, too, was ill. Ms.

Barron's father died when she was 13, and her "illnesses" began soon after. In group therapy, she is able to gain an understanding of how she uses her symptoms to ensure that her emotional needs are met, and how her use of physical symptoms controls others. Her nurse psychotherapist teaches her assertive communication techniques and encourages her to use them to ask directly for what she wants or needs, rather than resort to manipulation. Marital therapy is begun to explore the negative effects of Ms. Barron's coping via somatization. Strategies are devised in which her husband will reinforce "well" behaviors and ignore somatic complaints and helpless behaviors.

By discharge, Ms. Barron's mood is stable, she focuses less on physical symptoms, and she agrees to return to her job and to continue marital counseling.

A Client with Hypochondriasis

Anthony Estada, aged 54, is referred to the mental health center outpatient clinic from the sexually transmitted disease clinic. Mr. Estada has visited the clinic weekly for almost two years, asking for diagnostic tests for various sexually transmitted diseases. He is always told that the tests are negative and that he has no illness. Most recently, his preoccupation has centered on acquired immunodeficiency syndrome (AIDS).

Mr. Estada, a widower whose wife died of uterine cancer three years ago, is a self-employed plumber. Since the onset of his wife's illness and his own preoccupation with illness, his two daughters have visited at least weekly. He has no other social contacts, having given up attendance at an ethnic social club he had once enjoyed.

The client was brought up in a strict religious environment, joined the Navy at 17, and married shortly after discharge. Mr. Estada revealed that despite his religious upbringing, he had several encounters with prostitutes while he was in the Navy. When his wife's illness was diagnosed, he began to wonder if he had acquired a "disease" and passed it on to her. He appears worried as he discusses his concern over having a sexually transmitted disease with the nurse therapist and shares the story of his unsuccessful search for accurate diagnosis and treatment.

Although the nurse therapist is aware that "cure" will be difficult, she decides that a cognitive-behavioral approach might be useful. Cognitive therapy helps him gain an intellectual understanding that his fear of having contracted AIDS over thirty years ago is unrealistic. Mr. Estada is given homework assignments to read literature about AIDS. His daughters are taught to change the subject whenever their father mentions sexually transmitted diseases or AIDS. He contracts with the nurse therapist not to visit the sexually transmitted disease clinic unless he is referred by the therapist. He also agrees to resume attendance at the social club at least once a week. After three months of therapy, Mr. Estada is evaluated as being considerably less preoccupied with the possibility of illness.

A Client with Somatoform Pain Disorder

Robert Priest, aged 36, is referred to the outpatient mental health clinic by his private physician. He has suffered from chronic back pain for two years, during which he has been unable to work as a longshoreman. He leans heavily on a cane and moves slowly and deliberately when he walks. Mr. Priest states that he has had myelograms, computed tomographic scans, and magnetic resonance imaging that showed no cause for his pain. He has used diazepam and various analgesics that afford him little relief. He states that he is never free of severe pain.

His back pain began after playing baseball at a picnic celebrating his wife's graduation from a community college nursing program. She had returned to school against his wishes when their youngest child had entered high school. When she had completed the program, he had grudgingly agreed to her acceptance of a part-time position, but she, instead, chose a full-time position. Now he states, "It's a good thing she went against me, because she's the breadwinner and has to take care of me, now that I can't work."

During therapy, Mr. Priest is withdrawn from medication. He is taught relaxation techniques and self-hypnosis for pain control. He states that being in control of his pain helps him feel like a man, rather than a whimpering baby. His wife and family are taught to reinforce wellness behaviors and ignore comments about pain. Individual counseling gives him support, but he is intensely resistant to uncovering material relevant to the underlying conflict. Job counseling enables him to obtain a position as a dispatcher for a taxi company and resume his former breadwinner role.

A Client with Body Dysmorphic Disorder

Anna Ford, a 32-year-old office worker, is referred to the mental health center clinic by a plastic surgeon. She has experienced preoccupation with the size of her breasts for several years. Initially, she sought breast augmentation from the referring surgeon. After augmentation surgery, she reported seeing another plastic surgeon, hoping to have breast size increased still further. Two years later, she returned to the first surgeon, seeking breast reduction. She was persuaded not to have surgery at that time. Two months ago, she returned to the surgeon expressing dissatisfaction with the size and shape of her breasts.

The nurse psychotherapist begins interventions designed to enhance Ms. Ford's self-esteem and support perceived strengths. Ms. Ford is enrolled in an aerobic exercise program designed to help her feel more comfortable with her body. She is encouraged to consult with a department store fashion consultant for assistance in choosing becoming clothing. Her family are instructed not to reinforce Ms. Ford's expression of dissatisfaction with her body image.

A Client with Conversion Disorder

Pat Norris, a fashion model, is admitted to the neurological unit on the eve of her thirtieth birthday, following a sudden onset of convulsions during a modeling assignment. She is an attractive woman whose manner with female nursing staff is indifferent and with male nursing staff and physicians is coy and flirtatious. The first "seizure" recorded after hospitalization happens during morning rounds. As staff enter her room, Ms. Norris arches her back and begins pelvic thrusting motions while thrashing her arms and legs about on the bed. She does not lose consciousness, is not incontinent, and does not bite her tongue. Afterward, she is alert and well oriented. The second "seizure" occurs in the afternoon during a visit from her mother and father. This episode lasts five minutes. It begins with an outcry that brings nurses running. This time, she exhibits a period of generalized muscle rigidity, followed by pelvic thrusting. Again, there is no biting of the tongue, incontinence, or loss of consciousness. Again, there is an absence of lethargy or confusion after the seizure.

During her hospital stay for a neurological workup, Ms. Norris remains relatively unconcerned about her convulsions *(la belle indifférence)* and their potential impact on her career. She seems to enjoy the attention of the male staff who respond to her attractiveness and vivacious interactions. When she is told that

the results of her electroencephalogram and other tests are negative, she shrugs and agrees to transfer to the mental health unit, "if all the boys [meaning medical staff] could come over" to see her.

On the mental health unit, her seizures continue once or twice daily, but always occur in the presence of others, never with incontinence or self-injury, and always include sensual body movements. Initially, Ms. Norris refuses to come out of her room for fear of "an attack." During this time, helpless, dependent behavior is very noticeable. Visits from her parents seem to support this, as her father calls her his "little girl" or "princess," and her mother frequently pleads with the nurses to take good care of her daughter.

From the early days of admission, the staff discuss having negative feelings about Ms. Norris. Female staff report that Ms. Norris makes them feel as though they are her personal maids. Many of the staff admit wanting to avoid her. Male staff report feeling uncomfortable with her seductiveness, and all staff feel annoyed with her flirtatiousness and dependence.

Her nurse therapist makes a nursing care plan for the staff to follow (Nursing Care Plan 15–1). She also directs all staff to provide a safe environment during "seizures," using as few staff as possible to reduce the attention given. Staff are directed not to discuss seizures with Ms. Norris, but to give positive reinforcement for all appropriate interactions, including discussion of feelings. Limit setting is used to help Ms. Norris become compliant with unit routine. Time with her therapist is directed toward helping Ms. Norris see herself as a capable person with talents and options. The staff learns more about Ms. Norris during the interactions with her, as noted in the evaluation part of the nursing care plan. Ms. Norris is discharged after a two-week hospitalization. She continues in therapy with the nurse psychotherapist for six months and then moves to another city.

Nursing Care Plan 15–1 ■ A PERSON WITH CONVERSION DISORDER: MS. NORRIS

NURSING DIAGNOSIS

Ineffective individual coping (use of conversion symptoms [seizures]) related to repressed anxiety associated with unresolved conflicts

Supporting Data

- Seizures of varying patterns, including limb thrashing, muscle rigidity, and seductive pelvic movements
- No incontinence. No injury. Seizures occur only in presence of others.
- La belle indifférence.

Long Term Goal: Client will cope effectively with life stress without using conversion.

Short Term Goal	Intervention	Rationale	Evaluation
1. Client will adjust to unit routine by (date).	1. Explain routine. Establish expectations regarding unit routines, e.g., do not allow	1. Reduces anxiety. Reduces secondary gain and manipulation.	Goal met Initially refuses to leave room for meals. Misses one

Short Term Goal	Intervention	Rationale	Evaluation
	special privileges. Expect client to eat in dining room, perform ADLs, attend activities.		meal. Goes to dining room thereafter. Performs all ADLs, with special attention to applying make-up.
2. Client will develop trusting relationship with nurse by (date).	2. Be consistent.	2. Enhances trust. Reduces manipulation.	Relationship superficial through day 5, when sincere expression of feelings begins.
3. Client will remain safe.	3. Provide safety measures during seizures but limit attention and discussion about seizures afterwards. Monitor physical condition unobtrusively.	3. Prevent harm. Reduces secondary gain. Minimizes secondary gain while assessing condition.	Client does not sustain injury during seizures. States "I guess my seizures don't interest staff. No one will talk to me about them."
			No seizures after day 6 on psychiatric unit.
4. Client will identify stressor by (date).	4. Encourage client to discuss life, work, significant others, and goals.	4. Uncovers stress, conflict, and strengths.	Repeatedly mentions that 30th birthday means she is over the hill as a model.
5. Client will express feelings about the conflict by (date).	5. Use empathy; encourage exploration of feelings.	5. Conveys understanding.	States that she is scared of losing her glamorous appearance and her job. Demonstrates appropriate affect.
6. Client will identify relationship between stressor, conflict, and symptom by (date).	6. Reflect on anxiety and stress as they relate to use of physical symptoms. Provide opportunity to consider how the relationship might be valid in client's case.	6. Establishes probable causal relationship.	Client notes during session that first seizure occurred on 30th birthday.
7. Client will evaluate possible solutions to the problem by (date).	7. Focus on alternatives available to her to earn a living when modeling is no longer an option.	8. Teaches problem solving.	Client shows fashion sketches to nurse and reveals that she had once thought that she might be a good designer. With encouragement, decides to explore evening classes in illustration and design to prepare for second career.
8. Client will discuss ways to cope with stress in future by (date).	8. Encourage use of alternate anxiety reduction techniques. Encourage client to select and learn such a method.	8. Develops skill in use of a healthy technique.	Client chooses to use jogging and progressive muscle relaxation and attends teaching sessions on each. Thinks each is helpful and plans to continue their use.

NURSING DIAGNOSIS

Chronic low self-esteem related to not seeing self as a capable adult

Supporting Data

- Helpless, dependent behavior
- Seductive, flirtatious behavior
- Manipulative behavior, such as playing one staff member against another and seeking special privileges

Long Term Goal: Client will demonstrate adequate self-esteem by relating in age-appropriate ways.

Short Term Goal	Intervention	Rationale	Evaluation
1. Client will identify maladaptive behaviors of excessive dependence, seductivenss, and manipulation by (date).	1a. Set limits. Use consistent team approach.	1a. Minimizes maladaptive behaviors.	Goal partially met. Client has not named any of the cited interpersonal problems, but incidence of behaviors has decreased to less than one per day.
	1b. Be nonjudgmental and accepting.	1b. When one is accepted by others, self-acceptance is fostered.	
	1c. When negative countertransference occurs, seek supervision.	1c. Supervision helps keep relationship in perspective.	
	1d. Affirm to client that symptoms can improve.	1d. Conveys hope.	

Continued on following page

Nursing Care Plan 15–1 ■ A PERSON WITH CONVERSION DISORDER: MS. NORRIS *(Continued)*

Short Term Goal	Intervention	Rationale	Evaluation
	1e. Express confidence in client's ability to function independently.	1e Reinforces strengths.	Client often states, "If you think I can do it, perhaps I should reconsider and try it."
	1f. Reflect on father's choice of nickname ("princess"). Assist client in assessing role behaviors that might perpetuate the infantile image.	1f. Fosters mature role-taking.	Client admits that it is nice to be pampered by her parents but decides that this might not be congruent with a mature role.
2. Client will try out new adaptive coping strategies by (date).	2a. Encourage client to attend assertiveness training to learn to ask directly for what she needs.	2a. Decreases manipulation.	Client reports that she never realized that people would meet her requests when she asked in an assertive way. Client enjoys using the techniques.
	2b. Encourage client to consider needs of others as an alternative to self-absorption.	2b. Gains satisfaction and increased self-esteem.	Client organizes a makeup class for female clients. Client states that she might start a "make-over" business.

Evaluation

Evaluation is a simple process when measurable behavioral outcomes have been written. For clients with somatoform disorders, nurses often find the goals and outcomes are only partially met rather than totally accomplished. The partial meeting of goals should be considered a positive finding when one considers the remarkable resistance to change these clients often exhibit. Clients are more likely to report the continuing presence of the somatic symptoms but often report that they are less concerned about the symptoms. Families are likely to report relatively high satisfaction with outcomes, even without total eradication of the client's symptoms.

Dissociative Disorders

Theory

Dissociative disorders, like somatoform disorders, are illnesses that provide the individual with a way of avoiding anxiety and at the same time permit certain needs to be met. **Dissociative disorders** involve temporary disturbance or loss of normal ability to integrate the mental processes of consciousness, memory, identity, or motor behavior.

A common dissociative experience is depersonalization, an elusive sensation of being not quite human, not fully alive, or disconnected from parts of one's body. In one study of hospitalized psychiatric patients, 80% said they had had this kind of experience, and 12% said they had a severe or lasting form of it (Harvard Mental Health Letter: Part I 1992).

When the ability to integrate consciousness is impaired, the individual is unable to remember (amnesia). When the ability to integrate identity is affected, fragmented aspects of the self may emerge as distinct personalities (multiple personality). When failure to integrate motor behavior occurs along with identity impairment, the individual wanders from familiar surroundings (fugue). Patients with fugue travel away from their situations and often take on a new identity.

Because the unconscious mind contains learned behaviors, clients with dissociative disorders involving memory loss continue to be able to read, write, and perform certain skills, such as driving a car. This use of automatic behaviors is similar to what goes on in our everyday lives when we say we've been operating on "automatic pilot," that is, performing an act or skill without really concentrating on it.

Mild, fleeting dissociative experiences are relatively common. One study on dissociation (Harvard Mental Health Letter: Part I 1992) suggests that about one third of people have occasionally felt as though they were watching themselves in a movie. Up to 70% of young adults may have brief episodes in which they feel that they are not themselves, or as though the world has a dream-like quality (depersonalization).

The incidence of these experiences declines after age 20. Refer to Figure 15–3 for an overview of the dissociative disorders.

BIOLOGICAL THEORY

The only dissociative disorder to have a reasonably strong biological link is **depersonalization disorder.** Perceiving change in, or loss of the sense of, one's own reality has been associated with neurological diseases, such as epilepsy and brain tumors, and with psychiatric disorders, such as schizophrenia. Thus, any client who presents with depersonalization should have an extensive evaluation to rule out other disease. Depersonalization is also experienced by individuals under the influence of certain drugs, such as alcohol, barbiturates, benzodiazepines, scopolamine, hallucinogens, and beta-adrenergic antagonists, so a careful history of prescription and nonprescription drug use is important. It should be noted that the experience of depersonalization is *ego-dystonic.* The experience of feeling a sense of deadness of one's body, of seeing oneself from a distance, or of perceiving

DISSOCIATIVE AMNESIA

1. One or more episodes of inability to recall important information — usually of a traumatic or stressful nature

2. Other psychological (e.g., DID) and physical (e.g., substance-induced) disorders ruled out.

DISSOCIATIVE FUGUE

1. Sudden, unexpected travel away from home or one's place of work with inability to remember past

2. Confusion about personal identity <u>or</u> assumption of new identity

DISSOCIATIVE IDENTITY DISORDER

1. Existence of two or more distinct subpersonalities, each with its own patterns of relating, perceiving, and thinking

2. At least two of these subpersonalities take control of the person's behavior

3. Inability to recall important personal information too extensive to be explained by ordinary forgetfulness

4. Other causes ruled out

DEPERSONALIZATION DISORDER

1. Persistent or recurrent experience of feeling detached from and outside of one's mental processes or body

2. Reality testing remains intact

3. The experience causes significant impairment in social or occupational functioning, or causes marked distress

Figure 15–3. *Diagnostic criteria for dissociative disorders.* (*Adapted from American Psychiatric Association. Diagnostic and Statistical Manual of Mental Disorders, Fourth Edition (DSM-IV). Washington, DC: American Psychiatric Association, 1994.*)

one's limbs to be larger or smaller than normal is described by clients as being very disturbing.

LEARNING THEORY

Learning theory suggests that dissociative disorders can be explained as learned methods for avoiding stress and anxiety. It is possible to see the pattern of avoidance when an individual deals with an unpleasant event by consciously deciding not to think about it, that is, "tuning out." The more anxiety provoking the event, the greater the need not to think about it. Some individuals practice tuning out and become very good at it. Think about the numbers of times students "tune out" what goes on in lectures, or marriage partners seem unaware of the nagging of the spouse. It seems that the more dissociation is used, the more likely it is to become automatic. When stress is intolerable and ego disintegration is threatened, the individual may unconsciously use dissociation to force offending memory out of awareness. Abused individuals may learn to use dissociation to defend against feeling pain and to avoid remembering. Clients who later remember the event have reported, "It seems as though it happened to someone else."

PSYCHOSOCIAL THEORY

Kopelman (1987) hypothesizes that dissociative disorders involve attempts to use repression to block a traumatic event from awareness and to avoid the anxiety its memory would cause. When complete repression proves impossible because of the strength of the traumatic experience, dissociation of certain mental processes takes place to protect the individual from certain painful memories and accompanying anxiety.

DISSOCIATIVE AMNESIA AND FUGUE

Dissociative amnesia, the most common dissociative disorder, differs from ordinary forgetfulness because the extent of the disturbance is much greater. It has a sudden onset. In **localized amnesia,** the client is unable to remember all events of a circumscribed period of time lasting from a few hours to a few days, such as the hours following the death of a loved one. **Selective amnesia** involves the ability to remember some events during a short period of time but not others. For example, a person can remember an auto accident but not remember the death of someone involved in the accident. **Generalized amnesia** involves the inability to remember one's past lifetime. **Continuous amnesia** is the inability to remember each successive event as it occurs, even though the individual is alert and aware of what is happening at the moment it occurs.

Individuals suffering from **dissociative fugue** physically travel away from their homes and jobs. They are confused about personal identity, or they may even take on new identities and new types of work (APA 1991). In cases in which a new identity is assumed, people tend to lead rather simple lives, rarely calling attention to themselves. Often, after a few weeks to a few months, they suddenly remember their former identities and become unable to remember the time spent in the fugue.

Most theorists agree that spontaneous loss of memory as in dissociative amnesia and dissociative fugue has been preceded by a severely traumatic event. Amnesia or fugue is most likely to occur during a time of great disorganization, such as war or a natural or man-made disaster, in which the threat of physical injury or death is present. Other stressors severe enough to produce psychogenic amnesia or fugue include the loss of a loved one and the stress of having to face the unacceptability of certain acts, such as an extramarital affair.

DISSOCIATIVE IDENTITY DISORDER (DID)

It is believed that severe sexual, physical, or psychological abuse in childhood predisposes an individual to the development of **dissociative identity disorder** (DID), formerly multiple personality disorder. The steps in the development of dissociated personalities are thought to be as follows (Greenberg 1982):

1. A young child is confronted with an intolerable, terror-producing event at a time when defenses are inadequate to handle the intense anxiety.
2. The child dissociates the event and the feelings associated with the event. The dissociated processes are split off from the memory of the primary personality.
3. The dissociated part of the personality takes on an existence of its own, becoming a subpersonality.
4. The subpersonality learns to deal with feelings and emotions that could overwhelm the primary personality.

This process may occur once or several times, creating several subpersonalities. The essential feature of multiple personality is the existence within an individual of two or more distinct subpersonalities, each of whom is dominant at a particular time (APA 1987).

Each **subpersonality** or **alternate personality** (alter) is a fully integrated and complex unit, with its own memories, behavior patterns, and social relationships that dictate how the person will act when that personality is dominant. Often the original or **primary personality** is religious and moralistic, and the subpersonalities are quite different: aggressive, pleasure seeking, nonconforming, or sexually promiscuous. They may think of themselves as being of different sex, race, religion, or sexual orientation. Sometimes, the dominant hand is different, and the voice may sound different; intelligence and electroencephalographic findings may also be different. Subpersonalities may exhibit signs of emotional disturbance. A common alternate personality is a fearful, insecure child. Others may be reckless and promiscuous, acting on forbidden impulses, and may meet DSM-IV criteria for personality disorders. Some subpersonalities have names for themselves; some may be identified by roles they play: Host, who provides the social front for interacting with the world; Protector, who defends against harm; and Persecutor, who attempts to harm or even kill other personalities.

The primary personality is usually not aware of the subpersonalities but may be aware of, and perplexed by, lost time and unexplained events. Experiences such as finding unfamiliar clothing in the closet, being called a different name by a stranger, waking up or coming out of a "blank spell" in strange surroundings, or not having childhood memories are characteristic of MPD. Subpersonalities are often aware of the existence of the others to some degree. Some may even interact with each other. Occasionally, one alternate personality may attempt to harm another. Subpersonalities may "listen in" on whatever personality is dominant at the time. Transition from one personality to another often occurs during times of stress and may be a dramatic or barely noticeable event. Some clients experience the transition when awakening. Shifts from personality to personality last from minutes to months, although shorter periods are more common. Refer to Table 15–3 for clinical examples of dissociative disorders.

Assessment

Collecting objective data includes ruling out the presence of organic or cognitive impairment and intoxication or withdrawal. Electroencephalograms, computed tomographic scans, or magnetic resonance imaging may be ordered. Collecting subjective data focuses primarily on the client identity, memory, and consciousness, but other topics should also be included, such as history, mood, use of alcohol and other substances, impact on client and family, and suicide risk.

ASSESSING IDENTITY AND MEMORY

Initially, the client is asked to identify himself or herself. The nurse will then assess the client's memory. Can the client remember recent and past events? Is memory clear and complete or partial and "fuzzy"? It is also important to get a sense of whether the client may have assumed a new identity, as occurs in some cases of fugue or DID. Clients with amnesia and fugue

Table 15–3 ■ CLINICAL EXAMPLES OF DISSOCIATIVE DISORDERS	
DISORDER	**EXAMPLE**
Depersonalization disorder	Mrs. Terry became highly distressed when she perceived changes in her appearance when she looked in a mirror. She thought her image looked wavy and indistinct. Soon after, she described feeling as though she was floating in a fog with her feet not actually touching the ground. During therapy, it was learned that Mrs. Terry's son had revealed to her his HIV-positive status.
Dissociative amnesia	A young woman was partly dressed and poorly nourished when found by a police road patrol. She had no knowledge of who she was. Her parents identified her when she appeared on a morning news television program. Hospital examination revealed the probability of recent rape. She was able to remember going to a party off-campus but had no recall of the party or events after.
Dissociative identity disorder (DID)	Gertrude, a passive, conservative woman, alternated personalities with Dianna, who was sexy and flirtatious. During therapy, Jane and Evelyn revealed themselves as other distinct personalities.

HIV = human immunodeficiency virus.

may be disoriented to time and place as well as person (identity).

ASSESSING HISTORY OF EVENTS

The nurse will need to gather information about the person's life. For example, has the client sustained a recent injury, such as a concussion? Is there a history of epilepsy, especially temporal lobe epilepsy? Is there a history of early trauma such as physical, mental, or sexual abuse? If DID is suspected, pertinent questions include

- *Have you ever found yourself in a place and didn't know how you got there?*
- *Have you ever found yourself wearing clothes you didn't remember buying, or have you ever found strange clothing in your closet?*
- *Have you ever found new items in your belongings that you can't remember buying?*
- *Have you ever had strange people greet you and talk to you as though they were old friends?*
- *Have you ever found writing or drawings you can't remember doing?*

Does the client have differing sets of memories about his or her childhood? This is often an indicator of DID.

ASSESSING MOOD

Is the individual depressed, anxious, or unconcerned? Many people with DID seek help when the primary personality is depressed. The nurse checks also for mood shifts. When subpersonalities of DID take control, their predominant moods may be very different from that of the principal personality. If the subpersonalities shift frequently, marked mood swings may be noted. Clients with dissociative amnesia or fugue may seem indifferent and unconcerned or may be uneasy or perplexed. A client with depersonalization disorder is likely to exhibit moderate to severe anxiety. This client often seeks help due to fear of "going crazy."

ASSESSING THE USE OF ALCOHOL AND OTHER DRUGS

Specific questions should be asked to identify drug or alcohol use or abuse. Dissociative episodes may be associated with recent use of alcohol. Marijuana is known to produce symptoms of depersonalization. Some clients with dissociative disorders turn to alcohol in an attempt to cope with the disorder itself.

ASSESSING THE IMPACT ON CLIENT AND FAMILY

Has the client's ability to function been impaired? Have disruptions in family functioning occurred? In fugue states, families report being highly distressed over the client's disappearance. Clients with amnesia may be more dysfunctional. Their perplexity and memory loss often render them unable to work and sustain normal family relationships. Families often direct considerable attention and solicitude toward the client but may exhibit concern or resentment at having to assume roles once assigned to the client. Clients with DID often have both work and family problems. Families find it difficult to accept the seemingly erratic behaviors of the client. Employers dislike the lost time that may accompany subpersonalities being in control. Clients with depersonalization disorder are often fearful that others may perceive their appearance as distorted and avoid being seen in public. If they exhibit high levels of anxiety, the family will probably find it difficult to keep relationships stable.

ASSESSING SUICIDE RISK

Whenever a client's life has been substantially disrupted, it is possible for the client to have thoughts of suicide. The nurse gathering data should be alert for expressions of hopelessness, helplessness or worthlessness, and for verbalizations indicating intent to engage in self-destructive or self-mutilating behaviors.

Nursing Diagnosis

Nursing diagnoses for clients with dissociative disorders may include, but are not limited to, those discussed in this section. The nurse will need to know that when dealing with multiple personalities, nursing diagnoses may be required for subpersonalities as well as for the primary personality.

Personal identity disturbance (amnesia or fugue) related to a traumatic event would be an appropriate diagnosis for a client unable to recall his or her identity. This diagnosis would also be appropriate for a client experiencing the symptoms of depersonalization disorder and its feelings of unreality or body image distortions. *Personal identity disturbance* related to childhood abuse could be used when evidence of a traumatic childhood exists.

Ineffective individual coping related to alterations in consciousness, memory, or identity may be the diagnosis if the individual has thought about or attempted suicide or abuses chemicals as a way of dealing with having a dissociative disorder.

Anxiety related to alterations in memory or identity would be an appropriate diagnosis if the client demonstrates symptoms of anxiety attributable to not being in control of his or her behavior, feelings, awareness, or memory. A client with depersonalization disorder would be a likely candidate for this diagnosis.

The diagnoses *altered role performance* related to disturbances in identity or memory and *altered family processes* may be appropriate. Assessment data would include subjective data from the client, such as unexplained absences from work, social inappropriateness, withdrawal from relationships, and other "strange" phenomena.

High risk for violence: self-directed, associated with dissociative disorder or with lack of impulse control with subpersonalities in DID may also be warranted.

Other diagnoses that may be considered include *social isolation, body image disturbance, self-esteem disturbance, powerlessness,* and *sleep-pattern disturbance.*

Planning

CONTENT LEVEL—PLANNING GOALS

Planning involves establishing goals and outcome criteria for each nursing diagnosis. Because each client presents an individual set of circumstances, goals must be individualized and be consistent with each client's assessment. Examples of goals for selected nursing diagnoses follow:

1. *Personal identity disturbance* (amnesia, fugue, multiple personalities)

   By (date), client will demonstrate normal ability to integrate identity, memory, and consciousness, as evidenced by
   - Describing who he or she is
   - Identifying significant others
   - Describing feelings about events in the past
   - Being able to recognize environment
   - Having absence of appearance of subpersonalities
   - Reporting absence of depersonalization episodes

2. *Anxiety* related to alteration in identity or memory associated with severe stress

   By (date), client will demonstrate reduction in anxiety, as evidenced by
   - Verbalizing feelings of comfort and safety
   - Verbalizing ability to control behavior or awareness
   - Using orderly logical thought process

3. *Alteration in role performance* related to loss of memory or presence of multiple personalities

   By (date), client will resume pre-illness roles, as evidenced by
   - Resuming occupation
   - Expressing satisfaction with interactions with family, friends, and coworkers
   - Making decisions about daily living

4. *Social isolation* related to inability to remember, or fear of depersonalization episode

   By (date), client will interact appropriately on a social level with family and peers, as evidenced by
   - Attending a specified number of social or diversional activities weekly
   - Verbalizing satisfaction with ability to interact with others

5. *Ineffective family coping* related to having a family member with a dissociative disorder

   By (date), family will demonstrate interactions that promote optimal functioning of client, as evidenced by
   - Absence of behaviors that promote secondary gain
   - Reports of client's ability to function independently
   - Client's resumption of pre-illness roles

6. *Self-directed violence* related to presence of multiple personalities, one of whom wishes to harm another

   By (date), client will refrain from attempts at self-harm, as evidenced by
   - Reporting wish to live rather than to die
   - Reporting feelings of hope
   - Agreeing to a contract stating that client will not act out against self

PROCESS LEVEL—NURSES' REACTIONS AND FEELINGS

Because nurses see relatively few clients with dissociative disorders, they are often anxious and unsure about the clinical decisions they are called on to make. Nurses may also experience feelings of skepticism while caring for clients with dissociative disorder. Many nurses find it difficult to believe in the authenticity of the symptoms the client is displaying.

The nurse caring for a client with psychogenic amnesia or fugue may experience feelings of frustration in any of the following situations:

- When the client's confusion and bewilderment persist even after identity has been established
- If the client seems helpless and needs assistance with ADLs, such as grooming or nutrition
- If the client seems to be receiving many secondary gains, such as attention, media sensationalism, or avoidance of responsibility

Feeling confused and bewildered by the presence of multiple personalities is not unusual. Anger is commonly experienced as a countertransference reaction toward a subpersonality of a client with DID, if one subpersonality is perceived as immature, challenging, or unpleasant. Some nurses experience feelings of fascination and are caught up in the intrigue of caring for a client with DID. A sense of inadequacy may accompany the need to be ready to interact in a therapeutic way with whatever personality is in control at the moment.

Similarly, the nurse may feel inadequate when the establishment of a trusting relationship occurs very slowly. It is very important to remember that the client with a dissociative disorder has often experienced relationships in which trust was betrayed.

When subpersonalities vie for control and attempt to embarrass or harm each other, crises are common. The nurse must be alert and ready to intervene and always prepared for the unexpected, including the possibility of a client's suicide attempt. Constant hypervigilence by staff can eventually lead to feelings of fatigue. Anxiety may also be experienced by the nurse caring for a client with dissociative disorder in any of the following situations:

- When a client who has regained memory develops panic-level anxiety related to guilt feelings
- When a client becomes assaultive because of extreme confusion and panic levels of anxiety
- When a client attempts to harm himself or herself by acting out against the primary personality or other personalities

If the client manifesting symptoms of a dissociative disorder has been involved in the commission of a crime, the nurse may experience concern over the fact that the medical record is likely to be a court exhibit. Nurses may feel anger in this situation if they believe that the client is faking illness to avoid being found guilty of the crime.

Supervision should always be available for nursing staff caring for a client with dissociative disorder. By discussing feelings as well as the plan for care with a competent peer or peers, nurses can better ensure objective and appropriate care for the client.

Intervention

PSYCHOTHERAPEUTIC INTERVENTIONS

Establishing a Relationship

Hospitalization for clients with dissociative disorders is brief and crisis centered if, indeed, it is required at all. Most therapy is conducted at the outpatient level. Nurses in the inpatient unit will have an opportunity for only a short term relationship. The establishment of a trusting relationship is a primary task. It is likely to be difficult, however, because most clients with dissociative disorders have experienced a lifetime of poor relationships, beginning with childhood abuse. Giving simple explanations of what is expected of the client and being consistent are helpful strategies in establishing the relationship.

Meeting Safety and Security Needs

During the first 24–48 hours of hospitalization, the nurse should be prepared to manage various crises. Suicide attempts are not uncommon. It may be necessary to institute suicide precautions, one-on-one supervision, and a no-suicide contract as safety measures.

Panic-level anxiety may accompany depersonalization episodes or follow memory return in psychogenic amnesia or fugue. In DID, a subpersonality may also appear and become severely anxious. Please refer to Chapter 9, where interventions for severe anxiety are discussed.

The appearance of subpersonalities may be a dramatic occurrence requiring the nurse to obtain as much information as possible about the new personality. The nurse may need to intervene "on the spot," with little opportunity to plan strategies. If a subpersonality has a violent agenda, for example, to destroy another personality or to act out against staff, the nurse may need to institute emergency measures to prevent violence (e.g., seclusion or restraints).

Communicating

Because the appearance of a client with a dissociative disorder is often considered a sensational event, the nurse may be required to deal with reporters seeking information. *The need for confidentiality cannot be overly stressed.* Nurses should not comment to the media but should adhere to agency policy, which usually involves referring all requests for information to the hospital public relations department. Communication among unit staff, however, should be fostered, because knowing the plan of care is essential to reducing chaos and promoting effective care.

Addressing Memory and Identity Alterations

Memory loss deprives the individual of information necessary to solve even simple problems. Absence of family due to distance or estrangement deprives the client of support. The nurse may be the client's chief source of information and guidance, as well as the major support-giving figure. Reality orientation to time, place, and person, if known, may be necessary

and may need to be repeated frequently if the client requests information. However, the nurse should never try to force the client to accept information that he or she is not ready to know. Memory loss and identity disturbance serve protective functions. Table 15–4 offers interventions and rationale for the nursing diagnosis *personal identity disturbance* related to a traumatic event.

ACTIVITIES OF DAILY LIVING

Although a client with dissociative disorder may appear "healthier" than other clients on the inpatient unit, disruptions in ADLs are often noted. The nurse may need to give simple directions to assist the client in completing grooming or ensure nutrition if the client manifests disorientation, confusion, severe anxi-

Table 15–4 ■ NURSING INTERVENTIONS AND RATIONALES: DISSOCIATIVE DISORDERS	
INTERVENTION	**RATIONALE**
Nursing Diagnosis: *Personal identity disturbance* related to a traumatic event, as evidenced by an inability to remember past events	
1. Ensure client safety by providing safe, protected environment and frequent observation.	1. Sense of bewilderment may lead to inattention to safety needs. Some subpersonalities may be thrill seeking, violent, or careless.
2. Provide nondemanding, simple routine.	2. Reduces anxiety.
3. Confirm identity of client and orientation to time and place.	3. Supports reality and promotes ego integrity.
4. Encourage client to do things for himself or herself and make decisions about routine tasks.	4. Builds ego strength, enhances self-esteem by reducing sense of powerlessness, and reduces secondary gain associated with dependence.
5. Assist with other decision making until memory returns.	5. Lowers stress and prevents having to live with the consequences of unwise decisions.
6. Support client during exploration of feelings surrounding the stressful event.	6. Helps lower the defense of dissociation used by the client to block awareness of the stressful event.
7. Do not flood the client with data regarding past events.	7. Memory loss serves the purpose of preventing severe to panic levels of anxiety to overtake and disorganize the individual.
8. Allow client to progress at own pace as memory is recovered.	8. Urging too-rapid progress creates anxiety and resistance.
9. Provide support during disclosure of painful experiences.	9. The concerned presence of others when people are experiencing high levels of anxiety and pain can be healing while minimizing feelings of isolation.
10. Help client see consequences of using dissociation to cope with stress.	10. Increases insight and helps client understand own role in choosing behaviors.
11. Accept client's expression of negative feelings.	11. Conveys permission to have negative or unacceptable feelings.
12. Teach stress reduction methods.	12. Provides alternatives for anxiety relief.
13. If client does not remember significant others, work with involved parties to reestablish relationships.	13. Helps client experience satisfaction and relieves sense of isolation.

ety, or immobilizing grief. Sleep pattern should be observed and documented, as sleep loss and fatigue seem to increase the incidence of depersonalization episodes and may delay memory return.

SOMATIC THERAPIES

Antianxiety medication may be prescribed for very short periods of time to treat severe anxiety states. Antidepressants or psychotropics might be prescribed to treat severe psychiatric symptoms displayed by a DID subpersonality; otherwise, medication does not seem particularly helpful in the treatment of dissociative disorders.

Narcotherapy, or interview under the relaxing influence of sodium amytal or intravenous sodium penthothal, gives the therapist access to the client's repressed memories and conflicts. When the client has experienced psychogenic amnesia or fugue, the therapist may explore dissociated events. When the client being treated has DID, the barbiturate interview may be used to access other personalities. The therapist is often able to learn the names, personalities, and roles played by subpersonalities, as well as how much each knows about the others. The nursing care of the client before and after the interview is similar to that of a client undergoing general anesthesia.

THERAPEUTIC ENVIRONMENT

A quiet, simple, structured, supportive environment is best for a client with a dissociative disorder. Confusion and noise increase anxiety and the potential for depersonalization, delayed memory return, or shifts among subpersonalities.

PSYCHOTHERAPY

For clients with DID, three phases of therapy are described by Coons (1986):

PHASE 1. Phase 1 involves developing trust, followed by establishing communication with all subpersonalities. The therapist must map out the names, roles, attitudes, and behaviors of each personality and should attempt to understand the relationships among the personalities, such as which personalities have alliances and where antagonism exists. The therapist must communicate to each personality that acting out against each other is unacceptable and that each will be held accountable for his or her actions. Contracts with the personalities gaining agreement

not to inflict harm or embarrassment are helpful. This introductory phase usually occurs over several months.

PHASE 2. Phase 2, the working stage, extends over several years. The therapist, the primary personality, and the subpersonalities explore relevant issues, such as anger, sexuality, depression, and dependence, as well as the client's traumatic experiences. Contracting may continue whenever the need arises. If a personality refuses to agree to the terms of the contract, it may be necessary to arrange hospitalization. Compromises among personalities will be negotiated during this phase.

PHASE 3. Phase 3 has as its goal the integration of the personalities. In addition, the therapist works with the newly integrated personality to help with self-acceptance and the use of newly acquired coping strategies.

Hypnotherapy may be used during therapy with clients with dissociative disorder. Like narcotherapy, hypnotherapy allows the conscious mind to relax so that the therapist and client can access material from the unconscious and make contact with subpersonalities.

Individuals with psychogenic amnesia and fugue are usually treated conservatively because spontaneous memory return is common. Supportive therapy to promote feelings of safety and security may facilitate memory return. The therapist may employ gentle leading questions to help the client recall painful events. Whether recall occurs spontaneously or after use of hypnotherapy or narcotherapy, the therapist will help the client fully explore the event and the accompanying feelings.

Because the number of clients with dissociative disorder treated by **behavioral methods** is small, little information is available. However, nonreinforcement of secondary gains and reinforcement of healthy coping strategies should always be part of therapy. Some therapists have used thought-stopping techniques to help clients control depersonalization episodes. The client may be taught to shout "Stop!" or to clap his or her hands when the depersonalization begins.

Because of the relative newness of **cognitive therapy** and the rarity of dissociative disorder, even less information is available about its usefulness to treat this disorder. Cognitive therapists would teach the client about the process of dissociation and how it is used as a protective mechanism. They would explore the cognitive distortions held by the client and foster more accurate perceptions.

Because so many clients with dissociative disorder have a history of abuse as children, and because we know that the pattern of abusive parenting is learned, the nurse therapist must be alert for indications that the client may be involved in abuse of his or her own children.

Family therapy may assist in exploring and reducing role strain and family dysfunction. Often, the family member who has been physically absent due to fugue, mentally absent due to amnesia, or socially absent due to self-imposed isolation associated with depersonalization episodes must be reassimilated into the family. Families with members being treated for DID need support to cope with the client's chaotic behaviors and to accept the integrated personality at the conclusion of therapy.

CLINICAL VIGNETTES

A Client with Dissociative Amnesia

Joan Moore, an office worker, is abducted on her way to work. She is taken to an abandoned house, bound and gagged, and placed in a room with several other women. The captor periodically tortures the other captives. Ms. Moore is left helpless and unable to move for three days. During this time she is terrified that she will be noticed and tortured. When the women are rescued by the police, Ms. Moore appears very tired and extremely hungry, but cheerful and unconcerned. She cannot report what happened during the ordeal, stating that she cannot remember. She is referred to a psychiatrist, who describes her as friendly and casual but showing memory loss about the events of the past three days. A diagnosis of dissociative amnesia is made.

Ms. Moore is given supportive therapy at the hospital for several days. Then, her memory returns spontaneously. She is able to describe feelings of terror and her sense of helplessness. She is left shaken and depressed and decides to enter outpatient therapy. After several months of supportive therapy, her life gradually returns to normal.

A Client with Dissociative Fugue

A middle-aged woman awakens one morning and notices snow outside the window swirling around unfamiliar buildings and streets. The radio tells her it is December. She is perplexed to find herself in a residential hotel in Chicago with no idea of how she has gotten there. She feels confused and shaken. As she leaves the hotel, she is surprised to have strangers recognize her and say, "Good morning, Sally." The name Sally does not seem right, but she cannot remember her true identity. She finds her way to a hospital, where she is admitted to the mental health unit. Eventually, "Sally" is able to remember her true identity, Mary Hunt. She tells her primary nurse tearfully that she now can recall that her husband had

come home one day and "out of the blue" told her that he wanted a divorce to marry a younger woman. Ms. Hunt calls her sister in New York, who returns home with her. Ms. Hunt starts counseling on her return and after three months is adjusting fairly well to the changes in her life.

A Client with Depersonalization Disorder

Tim Smith, aged 14, comes to the mental health clinic with the chief complaint, "I feel like a mechanical boy." He describes "going through the motions" at school but feeling that it is "all unreal." He was an "A" student in middle school but finds high school more difficult. He reports that the depersonalization episodes occur only at school. Because psychological testing and physical evaluation reveal no underlying illness, the diagnosis of depersonalization disorder is made.

During therapy, Tim is able to discuss his need to achieve high grades to compete with his older brother, a mechanical engineering student. Tim reveals that a few weeks before the symptoms began, he had told his brother of an embarrassing incident at school in which a teacher had asked him a question and he did not know the answer. The teacher, who knew his older brother, commented that his brother would never miss an easy question like that. Tim's brother responded to Tim's story by ruffling Tim's hair and saying, "They can't expect someone who's 'out to lunch' to know all the answers." Tim is able to explore the differences between himself and his brother and to see that it is okay to have different abilities and strengths. With this breakthrough, his episodes of depersonalization begin to diminish. He and his therapist work on issues of self-esteem, with the result that as his self-esteem increases, the depersonalization episodes cease altogether.

A Client with Dissociative Identity Disorder

Andrea, a 28-year-old conservative electrical engineer, is the primary personality. Four subpersonalities coexist within Andrea and vie for supremacy.

Michele is a four-year-old who is sometimes playful and sometimes angry. She speaks with a slight lisp and with the facial expressions, voice inflections and vocabulary of a precocious child. She likes to play on swings, draw with a crayon, and eat ice cream. She likes to cuddle a teddy bear and occasionally sucks her thumb. Her favorite outfit is a Mickey Mouse sweatshirt and a pair of jeans.

Lee is a calm, deep-voiced man who says he is 26. He is learning to be a chef and is annoyed when he is not allowed to become dominant and take over Andrea's body to attend his classes. He pleads that he is getting behind in his studies. Lee smokes, and he recently discovered that he needs glasses.

Ann is an accomplished ballet dancer. She is shy but firm about needing time to practice and perform. When she is dominant, she likes to wear white and fixes her hair in a severe, pulled-back style. She does little but dance when she is in control. She reports, "When I'm dancing I don't have to think."

Bridget is near Andrea's age, although she says a lady never tells her age. She dresses seductively in bright colors, wears her hair tousled, and likes to frequent discos and stay out late. She often drinks to excess and has several male admirers. Bridget has many moods. She states that she would like to get rid of Ann and Andrea because they're such goody goodies.

Andrea does not drink, hates ice cream, and sees herself as somewhat awkward in her movements and "not a good dancer." Instead she is a paid soprano soloist in a church choir. Andrea takes public transportation, but Lee and Bridget have driver's licenses. She goes to bed and arises early, but Bridget and Michele like to stay up late. Andrea seeks treatment when she finds herself behind the wheel of a moving car and realizes that she does not know how to drive. She has been concerned for some time because she has found strange clothes in her closet—some of them men's. She has also received phone calls from men who insist that she has flirted with them in bars. She sometimes misses appointments and cannot account for periods of time but does not understand why. Although she goes to bed early, she is often unaccountably tired in the morning.

Because her therapist is familiar with DID, hypnosis is used to confirm the presence of the subpersonalities and to gather data about them. During therapy, Bridget tries to dominate the others. She often speaks about getting rid of the others so she can have fun, so her therapist makes numerous time-limited contracts to prevent self-harm. As a result of hypnosis, the therapist learns that Andrea had been abused by her exacting, perfectionistic mother. Many compromises are made by the personalities during therapy sessions. Michele is the first personality to integrate, followed by Ann. Lee merges with Andrea, lending her calmness and a sense of resolution. Bridget still has not integrated. Therapy has continued for eight years, with Andrea remaining in control more than Bridget.

Evaluation

Treatment is considered successful when outcomes are met. In the final analysis, the evaluation will be positive when

- Client safety has been maintained.
- Anxiety has been alleviated, and the client has returned to a state of comfort.
- Conflicts have been explored.
- New coping strategies permit the client to function at his or her optimal level.
- Stress is handled adaptively without the use of dissociation.

Summary

Somatoform disorders involve client complaints of physical symptoms that closely resemble actual medical conditions. Physical examination and diagnostic testing reveal no organic basis for complaints, however. *Dissociative disorders* make up a group of relatively rare conditions involving a sudden, temporary alteration in consciousness, memory, identity, or motor behavior. The etiology of these disorders is assumed to be psychological: that is, the appearance of symptoms provides relief of anxiety associated with a repressed conflict or a severely traumatic event. Elements of secondary gain are present in many cases of somatoform and dissociative disorders; for example, these illnesses allow a client to avoid responsibilities and to receive attention and sympathy.

Assessment for clients with these disorders involves gathering information about

- The subjective experience of the client
- The presence of physical symptoms
- The presence of alterations in consciousness, memory, identity, or motor behavior
- Safety and security needs
- Prescription and nonprescription drug and alcohol use
- Alterations in coping, role performance, and family function
- The degree of disability

Common nursing diagnoses were explored, among them

- *Ineffective individual coping*
- *Impaired social interaction*
- *Ineffective family coping*
- *Self-esteem disturbance*
- *Self-care deficit*
- *Risk for violence: self-directed*
- *Altered ability to perform ADLs*
- *Anxiety*

Discussions of planning and intervention for clients with somatoform disorders and dissociative disorders included the need to provide for client's safety and security needs, to reduce secondary gain, to encourage performance of ADLs, to promote effective communication, and to provide a therapeutic environment.

Psychotherapy is the treatment of choice for clients with somatoform disorders and dissociative disorders. Anxiolytics and other psychotropics are rarely useful. Hypnosis and interviews under the relaxing influencing of a barbiturate may be useful for gathering data and in the treatment of DID. Cognitive and behavioral therapy techniques are proving useful in the treatment of clients with somatoform disorders and are beginning to be tried in treatment of clients with dissociative disorders.

References

Adler G. The physician and the hypochondriacal patient. New England Journal of Medicine, 304:1394, 1981.

American Psychiatric Association. DSM-IV Options Book: Work in Progress. Washington, DC: American Psychiatric Association, 1991.

American Psychiatric Association. Diagnostic and Statistical Manual of Mental Disorders, 3rd ed, revised (DSM-III-R). Washington, DC: American Psychiatric Association, 1987.

Coons PM. Treatment progress in 20 patients with multiple personality disorder. Journal of Nervous Mental Disease, 174:715, 1986.

Ford CV. The Somatizing Disorders: Illness as a Way of Life. New York: Elsevier, 1983.

Greenberg WC. The multiple personality. Perspectives in Psychiatric Care, 20(3):100, 1982.

Dissociation and dissociative disorders: Part I. Harvard Mental Health Letter, 8(9):1, 1992.

Kaplan HI, Sadock BJ. Modern Synopsis of Comprehensive Textbook of Psychiatry, 3rd ed. Baltimore: Williams & Wilkins, 1991.

Kopelman MD. Amnesia: Organic and psychogenic. British Journal of Psychiatry, 144:293, 1987.

Pincus JH, Tucker GJ. Behavioral Neurology, 3rd ed. New York: Oxford University Press, 1978.

Salkovskis PM, Warwick HMC. Morbid preoccupations, health anxiety and reassurance: A cognitive-behavioral approach to hypochondriasis. Behavior Research and Therapy, 24:597, 1986.

Warwick HMC, Marks IM. Behavioral treatment for phobia and hypochondriasis. British Journal of Psychiatry, 152:239, 1988.

Further Reading

Abrams S. The multiple personality: A legal defense. American Journal of Clinical Hypnosis, 25(4):225, 1983.

Coleman KC, Butcher JN, Carson RC. Abnormal Psychology and Modern Life, 6th ed. Glenview, IL: Scott Foresman & Company.

Dissociation and dissociative disorders: Part II. Harvard Mental Health Letter, 8(10):1, 1992.

Hollender MH. The case of Anna: A reformulation. American Journal of Psychiatry, 137:707, 1980.

Kluft RP. The dissociative disorders. In Talbott JA, Hales RE, Yadofsky SC (eds). Textbook of Psychiatry. Washington, DC: American Psychiatric Press, 1988.

Kluft RP. Psychiatrists debate multiple personality: Discrete entity or just a symptom. Psychiatric News, 23(11):7, 1988.

Satow R. Where has all the hysteria gone? The Psychoanalytic Review, 66:463, 1979.

Stoudenmire GA. Somatoform disorders, factitious disorders and malingering. In Talbott JA, Hales RE, Yadofsky SC (eds). Textbook of Psychiatry. Washington, DC: American Psychiatric Press, 1988.

Self-study Exercises

Multiple choice

1. Somatoform and dissociative disorders fit on the anxiety continuum at the

   A. Mild level
   B. Moderate level
   C. Severe level
   D. Panic level
   E. They do not belong on the continuum, as anxiety has been reduced by ego defense mechanisms.

2. Most theorists agree that the etiology of somatoform and dissociative disorders is

   A. Biological
   B. Psychosocial
   C. Hereditary
   D. Cultural

Place a Y for yes next to necessary data, and an N for nice to know but not essential.

Which data should routinely be gathered during the assessment of a client with a somatoform disorder?

3. _____Y_____ Voluntary control of symptoms
4. _____Y_____ Description of symptoms, including onset

5. ___Y___ Level of self-esteem
6. ___Y___ Results of diagnostic work-ups
7. ___Y___ Dependence on medication
8. ___Y___ ADL limitations

Which data should routinely be gathered during the assessment of a client with a dissociative disorder?

9. ___Y___ Potential for violence
10. ___Y___ Level of confusion
11. ___Y___ History of alcohol or drug abuse
12. ___Y___ Ability to remember
13. ___N___ State of nutrition and fluid balance

Multiple choice

14. Which nursing diagnosis would be appropriate for a client with a somatoform disorder?

   A. *Self-care deficit*
   B. *Personal identity disturbance*
   C. *Fluid volume deficit*
   D. *Altered growth and development*

15. Which nursing diagnosis would be appropriate for a client with a dissociative disorder?

   A. *Altered growth and development*
   B. *Pain*
   C. *Personal identity disturbance*
   D. *Noncompliance*

Identify the helpful interventions with an H and those not helpful with an N.

Which of the following interventions would be helpful for a client with a somatoform disorder?

16. ___N___ Focusing on client's physical symptoms
17. ___N___ Offering sympathy
18. ___H___ Encouraging activity
19. ___N___ Offering advice

Which of the following interventions would be helpful for a client with a dissociative disorder?

20. ___N___ Expose to information about traumatic precipitating event.
21. ___N___ Schedule client for a full range of activities: volleyball, community meeting, unit picnic, and carnival.
22. ___Y___ Develop a no-suicide contract.
23. ___Y___ Observe for mood or behavioral changes.

Multiple choice

24. Which of the following conditions involves assumption of a new identity in a distant locale?

   A. Hypochondriasis
   B. Conversion disorder
   C. Fugue
   D. Depersonalization disorder

25. Which statement about somatoform and dissociative disorders is true?

    A. There is no relationship between these disorders and early childhood trauma or loss.
    B. Clients with these disorders are perceived by nurses as easy to care for.
    C. Clients with these disorders lack awareness of the relationship between symptoms and anxiety and unconscious conflicts.
    D. An organic basis exists for each of these disorders.

CHAPTER 16

Personality Disorders: Antisocial, Paranoid, and Borderline

Kem B. Louie • Antisocial and Paranoid
  Personality Disorders
Suzanne Lego • Borderline Personality
  Disorders

KEY TERMS AND CONCEPTS ♦ ♦ ♦ ♦ ♦ ♦ ♦ ♦ ♦ ♦ ♦ ♦ ♦ ♦

**The key terms and concepts listed here also appear in bold where they are
defined or discussed in this chapter.**

AGGRESSION

ANTISOCIAL, SOCIOPATH,
PSYCHOPATH

DETACHMENT

EGO-SYNTONIC

IMPULSIVENESS

MALADAPTIVE USE OF MANIPULATION
Help Me If You Can
Keep the Ball in the Air

Passive-Aggressor
Seducer

MANIPULATION

MODELING

PROJECTIVE IDENTIFICATION

SIX STEPS IN SETTING LIMITS

SPLITTING

Overview of Personality Disorders

An individual's personality encompasses enduring and
consistent attitudes, beliefs, desires, values, and patterns of behavior. Personality has also been referred
to as an evolving pattern of thinking, perceiving, and
experiencing. Personality patterns determine whether
an individual is liked, how he or she is judged by
others, and what his or her goals and accomplishments are in life. To a certain extent, these patterns
are acquired in early childhood and become lifelong
patterns of behavior.

A personality disorder is "an enduring pattern of
inner experience and behavior that deviates markedly
from the expectations of the individual's culture, is
pervasive and inflexible, has an onset in adolescence
or early adulthood, is stable over time, and leads to
distress or impairment" (APA 1994). The ability to
achieve trust, autonomy, and meaningful relationships
is limited for individuals diagnosed with personality
disorders.

According to the DSM-IV, personality disorders are
grouped into three categories: first, those that appear
odd or *eccentric*: the Paranoid, Schizoid, and Schizotypal
personality disorders; second, those that are *dramatic*
or *emotional*: the Histrionic, Narcissistic, Antisocial, and
Borderline personality disorders; and third, those that

are *anxious* and *fearful*: the Avoidant, Dependent, obsessive-compulsive, and passive-aggressive personality
disorders. Tables 16–1, 16–2, and 16–3 provide characteristics and examples of each of these categories of
personality disorders. In the DSM-IV multiaxial classification system, the disorders are listed and diagnosed under Axis II.

Axis I	Clinical Disorders
	Other Conditions That May Be a Focus of Clinical Attention
Axis II	Personality Disorders
	Mental Retardation
Axis III	General Medical Conditions
Axis IV	Psychosocial and Environmental Problems
Axis V	Global Assessment of Functioning

The personality disorders are conceptualized in Figure 16–1.

Psychiatrists find that people with personality disorders are very difficult to treat. They are most likely
to be clinic dropouts and treatment failures, and they
also make up a large percentage of the jailed population (Perry and Vaillant 1989). Because symptoms of
personality disorders are **ego-syntonic,** i.e., they do
not bother the person, there is no motivation for
change. In relationships, the paranoia, hostility, and
passive-aggressive and manipulative behaviors exhibited by the individual are often viewed as hurtful,
distasteful, deceitful, and infuriating.

Table 16–1 ■ NURSING ASSESSMENT: ("ODD OR ECCENTRIC") PERSONALITY DISORDERS

CHARACTERISTICS	EXAMPLES
Paranoid	
Pervasive and unwarranted suspiciousness—mistrust of people displayed as jealousy, envy, and guardedness. Hypersensitivity to others; feels mistreated or misjudged. Displays restricted affect as lack of humor and lack of tender feelings. Often hypervigilant. May use projection.	Ronald is a successful businessman. He is meticulous and has an intense drive for achievement. He is often described by his business associates as lacking a sense of humor and is perceived as sarcastic, derogatory, and resentful. When his positions or points of view are questioned, he argues and defends them relentlessly, believing others are jealous of him. He has been heard belittling and criticizing others on several occasions. He has no close friends.
Schizoid	
Inability to form social relationships; absence of warm and tender feelings toward others. Indifference to praise, criticism, and feelings of others. Exhibits little or no desire for social involvement. Has few friends. Generally is reserved, withdrawn, and seclusive. Pursues solitary interest or hobbies. Has dull or flat affect; appears cold and aloof.	Juanita is a college graduate who has been working as a librarian for five years. She is very shy and withdrawn but readily assists you when you are looking for a book. When speaking to her, you notice that her speech is monotone, and her appearance very dull. She has no friends, and you've heard her tell a coworker that she is not interested in dating and enjoys her time alone.
Schizotypal	
Exhibits various oddities of thought, perception, speech, and behavior that are not severe enough to be diagnosed as schizophrenia. No dominant characteristic is present. May demonstrate magical thinking, ideas of reference, paranoid ideation, illusions, depersonalization, and speech peculiarities. Socially isolated. Has inappropriate affect.	Wallace lives over a grocery store down the street. Every day you have noticed Wallace going into an empty lot looking for pieces of glass or scraps of metal. He is never seen talking to anyone and is usually alone. Wallace was seen arguing and laughing by himself in front of the store one evening. He was discussing how the voices in the faucet were talking to him. The conversation had lasted ten minutes when the owner asked Wallace to leave.

Data from American Psychiatric Association. Diagnostic and Statistical Manual of Mental Disorders, 3rd ed, revised (DSM-III-R). Washington, DC: American Psychiatric Association, 1987.

All of the personality disorders have four characteristics in common: (1) inflexible and maladaptive response to stress, (2) disability in working and loving, (3) ability to evoke interpersonal conflict, and (4) capacity to "get under the skin" of others.

1. *Inflexible and maladaptive response.* Personality patterns are deeply ingrained in the personality structure and persist, unmodified, over long periods of time. At times, these personality patterns and traits may be compatible with and acceptable within societal norms and are valued by the culture or occupation. For instance, an engineer or administrator needs to possess some compulsive traits, such as the ability to organize complex details and meet deadlines. At other times, these same compulsive traits, when too rigid and limited, may interfere with personal, occupational, or social functioning.
2. *Disability in working and loving, which is generally more serious and pervasive than the similar disability found in*

neurosis. On the mental health continuum, personality disorders fall between neurosis and psychosis (e.g., severe anxiety and panic). Certain characteristics, e.g., withdrawal, grandiosity, and extreme suspiciousness, observed in people with personality disorders are similar to those seen in people with affective and schizophrenic disorders. The difference is that, for the most part, individuals with personality disorders have normal ego functioning and reality testing. There are, however, great disturbances in their ability to find intimate and satisfactory interpersonal relationships or to function at their optimum creative level.

3. *Ability to evoke interpersonal conflict.* In individuals with personality disorders, interpersonal relationships are marked by intense upheavals and hostility within a precarious interpersonal context. People with personality disorders lack the ability to see themselves objectively. Therefore, the need or desire to alter aspects of their behaviors to enrich or

Table 16–2 ■ NURSING ASSESSMENT: ("DRAMATIC OR EMOTIONAL") PERSONALITY DISORDERS

CHARACTERISTICS	EXAMPLES
Histrionic	
Behaviors are dramatic and attention seeking. Prone to exaggeration. Overreacts to situations with irrational, angry outbursts or tantrums. Forms interpersonal friendships quickly but becomes demanding, egocentric, and inconsiderate. Is perceived as shallow and lacking genuineness, although appears charming and appealing. Generally, attractive and seductive; attempts to control the opposite sex or enter into a dependent relationship.	Kelly has many boyfriends. She is attractive, witty, fun to be around, and superficial. She is generally seen and heard with groups of people, often flirting with men. Kelly states she does not have any close girlfriends because "they are jealous of me and that is their problem." She is flamboyant, attention seeking, and very manipulative with others.
Narcissistic	
Exaggerated sense of self-importance as exhibited in extreme self-centeredness and self-involvement. Preoccupied with fantasies of unrealistic goals involving power, wealth, success, beauty, or love. Need for constant admiration and attention, with interpersonal manipulation of others. Inability to empathize with others.	Laura is a junior executive, married, with two children. She prides herself in being able to care for her husband and children and have a career. Her husband complains that she is cold and aloof. Everything done at home must be approved by her, including vacations, social affairs, and school activities. At work, she is competitive with the other executives. She even used her femininity once to obtain a promotion. Because she has potential, she has attracted several offers for a position as vice president.
Antisocial	
History of continuous and chronic antisocial behaviors against society, such as vandalism, fighting, delinquency, thefts, and truancy. Inability to maintain meaningful employment or relationships; impulsive, reckless, lying, or conning others for personal gain. Unable to maintain intimacy with a sexual partner.	Joseph's father died of a drug overdose when he was six weeks old. His mother had difficulty caring for him, so he was placed in foster care. By the age of ten, Joey had had five foster parents and had run away three times. At the age of 11, Joey joined a group of boys much older than he. This is when he began stealing. Being bright and attractive, Joey was able to "talk to the ladies." With older women, he would act lost and ask to use the phone. When their backs were turned, he would take the purse out of their pocketbooks. Staying out late at night and absence from school led Joey to drop out of school. At age 16, he traveled across the country, where he began fighting. He was recently arrested for assault.
Borderline	
Instability is exhibited in interpersonal behavior, where relationships are intense and unstable, marked by impulsive and unpredictable behavior; marked shifts in mood and temper inappropriate at times. Profound disturbance in identity related to self image, gender, values, and future goals.	Rachel was admitted to the hospital for a suicide attempt. She threatened to jump out of a six-story window. When asked how long she felt depressed, she responded "forever." On the unit, Rachel acted helpless—unable to decide what to wear and whether she should continue her medication. At other times, she would demand and threaten to leave the hospital. She was fond of Marvin, her primary nurse, and spent much of her free time with him. For his birthday she even bought him a watch, which he refused to accept. Last night Rachel tried to hang herself in her room.

Data from American Psychiatric Association. Diagnostic and Statistical Manual of Mental Disorders, 3rd ed, revised (DSM-III-R). Washington, DC: American Psychiatric Association, 1987.

maintain important interpersonal relationships is lacking. Thus, annoying and distancing behaviors continue and are usually met with strong negative reactions from others.

4. *Capacity to "get under the skin" of others.* "Getting under the skin" of others refers to the uncanny ability of people with personality disorders to "merge personal boundaries" with others. This merging is

Table 16–3 ■ NURSING ASSESSMENT: ("ANXIOUS AND FEARFUL") PERSONALITY DISORDERS	
CHARACTERISTICS	**EXAMPLES**
Avoidant	
Exhibits hypersensitivity to potential rejection, humiliation, or shame. Socially withdrawn with low self-esteem but desires social relations if given guarantee of uncritical acceptance.	Sal has worked for a public relations firm for three years. He is successful and is liked by his coworkers. His nickname in the office is "Shy Sal." He has made several attempts to date female clients but finds himself unable to ask them out. He is active in a running club and bicycles 20 miles per week. He feels lonely and imprisoned in his body. He is aware of wanting to relate to others but is unable to take the necessary steps.
Dependent	
Passively allows others to take responsibility for individual's own life or some major portion of it. Subordinates own needs to the needs of those whom individual is dependent on. Lacks self-confidence.	Mona is a mother of three children. She enjoys caring for her family. She rarely does anything without approval or permission from her husband. She thought of going back to school, but her husband thought it was a stupid idea. She agreed with him after thinking it over. Once, she bought an expensive outfit to wear to a church affair and social. She later apologized and promised not to buy clothes without his permission.
Obsessive-Compulsive	
Restricted in ability to express warm and tender emotions. Preoccupied with conformity, such as rules, trivial details, and procedures. Exhibits superior attitudes when working with others; work and productivity are valued more than pleasure and relationships; tends toward perfectionism.	Jason worked in the accounting department of a community hospital. He was punctual, neat, and meticulous about his appearance and work. At home he was the same way with his family and hobbies. He was generally in the basement working on projects, and when interrupted, he became furious. His family complained that he was not a warm and emotionally feeling man, but he was able to provide the family with financial security.

Data from American Psychiatric Association. Diagnostic and Statistical Manual of Mental Disorders, 4th ed (DSM-IV). Washington, DC: American Psychiatric Association, 1994.

manifested by the intense effect they have on others (Perry and Vaillant 1989). The process is often unconscious and the results undesirable.

Recent research in the identification of biological markers and biogenetic predispositions for many of the personality disorders has yielded important findings. Evidence that genetic factors contribute to the development of personality disorders comes from a study of 15,000 pairs of twins. Kaplan and Sadock (1991) found that the incidence of personality disorders in monozygotic twins was significantly higher than that in fraternal twins.

Many theorists, however, still believe that the origin of personality disorders is the failure to develop an identity compatible with society. The loss or absence of parents or parental substitutes and limited contact with adults and peers in the early stages of development deprive a child of establishing an ego identity through the process of identification. A defect in personality may also occur as a result of frustration when the child is unable to achieve satisfaction of fundamental needs such as love, security, recognition, respect, and success.

Personality disorders are characterized by their long term nature and repetitive, maladaptive, and often self-defeating behaviors. These behaviors are not experienced as uncomfortable or disorganized by the individual, as are the symptoms experienced by a client with a neurotic disorder. It is important to note that with personality disorders, other areas of personal functioning may be very adequate. The predominant maladaptive behaviors may affect only one aspect of the person's life. Therefore, many individuals with personality disorders do not seek treatment unless a severe crisis or trauma precipitates other symptoms. Nurses and other health professionals should consider the following points when working

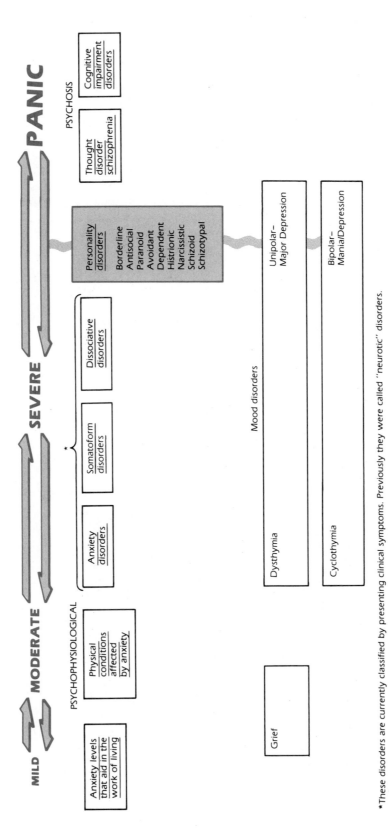

Figure 16–1. *Mental health continuum for personality disorders.*

*These disorders are currently classified by presenting clinical symptoms. Previously they were called "neurotic" disorders.

with any person presenting with a personality disorder (Perry and Vaillant 1989; Kaplan and Sadock 1991):

1. Personality disorders and drug and alcohol abuse often go hand in hand.
2. Personality disorders are often overdiagnosed in clients who are ethnically and culturally different from the diagnostician.
3. Psychoactive drugs should be used only if they are clearly indicated. "Just as there is no pill that will teach Norwegian, it is unlikely that pills will alter character" (Perry and Vaillant 1989). Because of the high incidence of polydrug abuse, sedative-hypnotic drugs should be avoided whenever possible.

Despite cautions about prescribing drugs, antipsychotics may be useful for brief periods to control agitation, rage, and brief psychotic episodes. Pimozide (Orap) has been helpful in reducing paranoid ideation in some clients, and antidepressants may be useful at times, particularly for borderline patients.

The personality disorders seen most often in the health care system are the borderline personality and the antisocial personality. Because the behaviors central to these disorders often cause upheaval and disruption on psychiatric units as well as on medical-surgical wards and clinics, these two disorders will be examined. The paranoid personality will also be discussed because of its prevalence.

Antisocial Personality Disorders

Kem B. Louie

OBJECTIVES ■

After studying this section on antisocial personality disorders, the student will be able to

1. Discuss four characteristics common to all personality disorders.
2. Indicate where personality disorders fit on the mental health continuum.
3. Differentiate between the psychodynamic etiological theory and the family etiological theory for the antisocial personality disorder.
4. For the following areas of assessment, describe the characteristics commonly found in people with antisocial disorders: (a) affect, (b) relationships with others, and (c) behavioral patterns.
5. Identify three possible nursing diagnoses for the antisocial client.
6. Discuss three common reactions health care workers often have toward antisocial clients.
7. Outline nursing interventions for the following client behaviors: (a) manipulation, (b) impulsiveness, (c) aggression, and (d) detachment.
8. Contrast and compare five possible therapies for use with selected antisocial clients.

Prior to the DSM-III, individuals diagnosed as having **antisocial** personalities were referred to as **psychopaths, sociopaths,** or impulsive characters. These terms are often used interchangeably.

One of the earliest studies of antisocial personality disorders was conducted by McCord and McCord (1956). In their classic book *The Psychopath*, the authors delineate six behavioral traits:

- Being antisocial or performing crimes against society.
- Being driven by uncontrollable desires to seek excitement.
- Acting highly impulsively, with no stable goals.
- Acting aggressively and reacting to frustration with fury.
- Feeling little guilt or remorse when committing an amoral act.
- Having a warped capacity for love, i.e., being cold and compassionless.

The authors emphasize that it is the total personality that constitutes this syndrome rather than a single behavior. Modlin (1983) points out that antisocial behaviors alone (e.g., fighting, drinking, stealing, and sexual assaults) do not constitute an antisocial personality disorder. Pathology in antisocial personalities is manifested interpersonally; therefore, the diagnosis is made based on the client's history and on psychological testing.

In his pioneering work with antisocial individuals, Cleckley (1964), a psychiatrist, described the main features of this group in a way that is still relevant today (Box 16–1).

Cleckley asserted that these traits are found not only in criminal personalities but also in society's most respected roles and settings, e.g., businessmen, scientists, physicians, and psychiatrists. Harrington (1972) quotes William Krasner:

> (These people) . . . do well in the more unscrupulous types of sales work, because they take such delight in 'putting it over on them,' getting away with it, and having so little conscience about defrauding their customers. They become private detectives, police, bodyguards, strikebreakers. Many go much higher to become politicians and industrialists where . . . their complete lack of scruples overcomes their more or equally able rivals.

There has been limited progress in understanding and treating antisocial syndromes. Reid (1985) cites four reasons for this:

1. It has been difficult to study syndromes that do not come to medical attention.
2. Because of the frustration and difficulty in treating antisocial syndromes, mental health research funds go to support study in other needed areas (e.g., depression and cancer).
3. Because the success rate of treating these clients has been markedly poor, there is little motivation to inspire interest.
4. Because the clients cause injury, hurt, and loss of property and freedom, there is limited compassion for them.

Box 16–1. MAIN FEATURES OF ANTISOCIAL PERSONALITY DISORDERS

- Superficial charm and good intelligence
- Absence of delusions and other signs of irrational thinking
- Absence of nervousness or neurotic manifestations
- Unreliability
- Untruthfulness and insincerity
- Lack of remorse and shame
- Antisocial behavior without apparent compunction
- Poor judgment and failure to learn from experience
- Extreme self-centeredness and incapability for love
- General poverty in major affective reactions
- Specific loss of insight
- Unresponsiveness in general interpersonal relations
- Fantastic and intrusive behavior with alcohol use and sometimes without
- Suicide rarely carried out
- Sex life impersonal, trivial, and poorly integrated
- Failure to follow any life plan

Data from Cleckley H. The Mask of Sanity, 4th ed. St. Louis: CV Mosby, 1964, pp. 364–400.

However, *some* progress has been made in understanding and treating antisocial syndromes.

Theory

The DSM-IV has identified criteria for the identification of antisocial personality disorder (Box 16–2).

Research that has been conducted on people with antisocial personalities has been limited because they are not confined to one institution or setting. There is, nonetheless, strong evidence supporting four hypotheses regarding the etiology for antisocial disorders: (1) psychodynamic issues, (2) family influences, (3) social and environmental influences, and (4) biological influences.

Note that antisocial behaviors are not a single entity. Recurrently antisocial persons, especially those who are frequently violent, may have multiple influ-

---

Box 16–2. DIAGNOSTIC CRITERIA FOR ANTISOCIAL PERSONALITY DISORDER

- Is unable to sustain consistent work behavior (including similar behavior in academic settings if the person is a student)
- Fails to conform to social norms with respect to lawful behavior (whether arrest record or not), e.g., destroying property, harassing others, stealing, or pursuing an illegal occupation
- Is irritable and aggressive, as indicated by repeated physical fights or assaults (not required by one's job or to defend oneself)
- Is irresponsible and repeatedly fails to honor financial obligations, as indicated by defaulting on debts or failing to provide child support or support for other dependents on a regular basis
- Fails to plan ahead or is impulsive
- Is deceitful and manipulative and has no regard for the truth, as indicated by repeated lying, uses of aliases, or conning others for personal profit or pleasure
- Is reckless regarding his or her own or others' personal safety, as indicated by driving while intoxicated or recurrent speeding
- Is glib or superficial
- Lacks empathy
- Lacks remorse
- Prone to blaming others or offering plausible rationalization for wrongdoing

Reprinted with permission from the DSM-IV Options Book: Work in Progress, 9/1/91. Copyright 1991 American Psychiatric Association.

---

ences and vulnerabilities that predispose them to develop antisocial personality disorders. The following theories identify numerous influences that may cause, in varying degrees and combinations, an individual to develop an antisocial personality.

PSYCHODYNAMIC ISSUES

From a psychodynamic viewpoint, psychopathology is thought to be caused by a fixed disturbance of developmental growth.

A child who has drifted through a series of foster homes, who has been abandoned by his or her par-

ents, or who has suffered severe emotional deprivation may show antisocial traits early in life. Lack of validation, emotional warmth, and physical security interfere with normal ego development. Ego pathology in early life is further compounded during the stage of superego development (3–5 years) and results in disturbances in superego formation. These disturbances are manifested by the individual's failure to develop control over the expression of his or her basic needs. Consequently, personality defenses are designed to gratify impulses and to provide pleasure and immediate relief of tension. The pleasures have a primitive, oral quality and are related to physiological responses, such as those experienced after drinking, drugs, sex, or acquiring property. People with these disorders have a limited capacity to experience pleasure in interpersonal relationships or for warm and sincere relationships. Missing is the ability to love, form friendships, and experience loyalty.

People with personality disorders, like all of us, use various defense mechanisms. When the defense mechanisms of people with personality disorders are effective, anxiety and depression are kept out of awareness. The unwillingness to avow feelings of anxiety and depression is a major reason people with personality disorders avoid treatment. Once defenses are lowered, painful feelings of anxiety and depression often surface, and people with antisocial personalities may employ the other defenses, such as aggression or sexual acting out. Use of alcohol or illicit drugs is also common among people with antisocial personality disorders.

FAMILY INFLUENCES

The family histories of antisocial persons seem to play an important etiological role. Frequently, the antisocial individual was an unwanted child or illegitimate. Often, parents of antisocial individuals are divorced or deserted their families. As children, many antisocial individuals were exposed to violent tempers, physical abuse, cruelty, and sexual abuse by their caretakers. Violent behavior has its origins in early extraordinary physical and sexual abuse. Furthermore, in dysfunctional families, inconsistent and ineffective discipline can teach the child to be deceitful, superficial, and narcissistic. The teaching of moral values and behaviors may also be lacking in these families.

SOCIAL AND ENVIRONMENTAL INFLUENCES

Society and environment influence the family's child-rearing practices. In a longitudinal survey of 411 males aged 8 to 32 years, Farrington (1989) found several indicators of future antisocial behaviors. The best predictors were economic deprivation, family criminality, poor child-rearing practices, school failure, hyperactivity, impulsivity, and attention deficit.

Everyone seems to agree that most of the violent crime in this country is committed by men 18 to 24 years of age. The more males in this age group in a given population, the higher the crime rate.

Antisocial personality disorder can be detected in early adolescence (APA 1994). Predominant characteristics include emotional immaturity and impulsive need for gratification. These preadolescents or adolescents may steal, run away, act destructively, be quarrelsome, demonstrate guiltlessness, and act openly rebellious. This behavior is generally directed toward parents and teachers.

BIOLOGICAL INFLUENCES

Genetic and biological studies concerning the antisocial individual yield interesting data. Conclusions based on studies of antisocial individuals have been summarized by Kaplan and Sadock (1991):

1. There appears to be a genetic predisposition to antisocial behaviors that is also associated with alcoholism.
2. Adopted children of criminal fathers are more likely to become delinquent than adopted children of noncriminal fathers.
3. There is a greater correlation for criminal behavior in monozygotic (identical) than in dizygotic (fraternal) twins.
4. Learning disabilities and mild mental retardation are more prevalent in the criminal population than in the general population.
5. Electroencephalographic changes (slow-wave activity) are common in antisocial and borderline clients.
6. Depletion of serotonin as well as its metabolite, 5-hydroxyindoleacetic acid (5-HIAA), is seen in people who are impulsive and aggressive.
7. Hormonal secretions, such as increased levels of testosterone, 17-estradiol, and estrone, may be linked with impulsive behaviors.

Researchers have also found that psychophysiological measures, such as poor skin conductance conditioning and lower resting heart rate levels, are significant predictors of antisocial behaviors (Raine and Mednick 1989). So, in answer to the question "What is the etiology of antisocial personality disorder," there seems to be no single cause of recurrent, aggressive, antisocial behavior. As more information becomes available, it becomes more apparent that recurrent antisocial aggressive behavior results from biological, psychological, and social interactions.

Assessment

The nurse will encounter individuals with antisocial personality patterns in many settings. These include emergency rooms, prisons, general hospital settings, clinics, and psychiatric units. People brought into clinics and hospital settings are usually brought in against their will. The person with an antisocial personality may appear to health care professionals of the opposite sex as colorful, seductive, and engaging. Health care workers of the same sex often find them manipulative and demanding (Vaillant and Perry 1990).

Antisocial traits are found in everyone (depending on the time or situation, if needs feel urgent, or if inner controls have not been developed or are weakened). *For the person with an antisocial personality, immediate gratification of needs overrides all social or moral dictates.*

Assessment of antisocial individuals should focus on (1) affect, (2) relationships with others, and (3) behavioral patterns.

AFFECT

ANXIETY. People with antisocial personalities can appear charming, self-confident, and verbally glib and can make social contacts easily. Such a person may appear free of anxiety or depression. It has been said that people with antisocial personality structures do not experience anxiety or depression. However, some clinicians believe that the antisocial behavior is a defense against a very low tolerance for anxiety. Indeed, antisocial behavior may be viewed as a defense against painful anxiety and chronic depression (Kaplan and Sadock 1991). The antisocial person may project anxiety by attacking sensitive areas or habits in another, thereby shifting the focus from himself to someone else in the environment.

GUILT. There seems to be a total lack of guilt after an antisocial person participates in a lie, swindle, theft, or murder. If the person does experience remorse, the emotion is fleeting and soon forgotten and in no way alters the person's behavior. The individual explains his actions by denying doing something or denying finding anything wrong in what he or she does. Rationalizations include "everyone else does it" or "no one cares about that anyway . . . it's all built into the system."

SHALLOWNESS. There is a shallow quality to the antisocial person's affective responses. Although the person may be dramatic, engaging, and filled with apparent emotion, the emotions are superficial and aimed at influencing the listener. The listener is often left with feelings of detachment and a lack of connectedness, although the emotions the antisocial person displayed had been intense.

RELATIONSHIPS WITH OTHERS

A person with antisocial character traits is unable to love, cherish, or even care about another person. All emotional energy is focused on the self, and other people exist only to fulfill personal needs. When people are no longer needed, they are discarded and easily replaced by others. People associated with such an individual, especially family and friends, suffer. Relationships with an antisocial individual are punctuated by brutal and irresponsible behavior (Harrington 1972).

A person with an antisocial personality structure is incapable of forming relationships and is often hurtful and deceitful to those close to him or her. However, such a person can often elicit loyalty and adoration. Charles Manson is such an example. Manson inspired blind devotion in his followers who, on command, would kill as a means of social protest, for revenge, for pleasure, at random, and for no reason. Harrington (1972) quotes a speech of Albert Speer's regarding Adolph Hitler:

> . . . Hitler could fascinate, he wallowed in his own charisma, but he could not respond to friendship. Instinctively he repelled it. The normal sympathies men and women enjoyed were just not in him. At the core, in the place where the heart should be, Hitler was a hollow man. He was empty. . . . We who were really close to him, or thought we were, all came to sense this, however slowly. . . . We were all, all of us, simply projections of his own gigantic ego. . . . And yet, Hitler was my destiny. As long as he was alive, he dominated my spirit. . . . The man's drive, his iron will, his daemonism fascinated even while it repelled. . . . It was he who manipulated me. I was enthralled.

BEHAVIORAL PATTERNS

Lying, cheating, swindling, murdering, deceiving others, prostitution, rebelliousness, irresponsibility, and drug addiction are just a few behaviors associated with the antisocial personality. Lying is often pathological, i.e., it is done for no apparent reason. Cheating and swindling family, friends, and business associates is done cleverly and without remorse. Murder

---

Box 16–3. NURSING ASSESSMENT FOR ANTISOCIAL CLIENT

- What is the presenting problem according to the client? What is it according to others (e.g., family and police)?
- Who has identified and defined the problem?
- What functions does the problematic behavior serve for the client at this time?
- What are the client's emotional state and reactions to the problems?
- In what way and to what extent does the client perceive the antisocial behavior as a problem?
- What particular circumstances or stress precipitated the behavior?
- How is the client handling the problem? How has the client handled the problem in the past?
- How would the client like to see the problem resolved?
- What is the client's developmental history?
- Is the client employed? What is the pattern of employment?
- How does the behavior affect the job or role functioning?
- What is the client's physical condition and status?
- What substances (i.e., drugs and alcohol) are abused? How much is taken? When was the last time it was taken?
- Has the client ever been arrested or convicted of a crime?
- Does the client have any meaningful or lasting relationships?

---

may have no motive, give pleasure, or act as revenge for a minor slight. Sex is often used as a tool to manipulate or punish or as a lark. Sex is not within the context of sharing joy and love, as in a normal intimate relationship. Drug addiction is common among people with antisocial personality disorders, as is chronic alcoholism. Physical and verbal aggression is a frequent outlet for frustration. These individuals display a lack of responsibility that is often manifested by an inability to hold a permanent job. Antisocial individuals often engage in illegal occupations, such as selling drugs and stolen goods and engaging in prostitution. Inability to function in the role of parent is often manifested by neglect, sadistic abuse, and desertion. Box 16–3 lists other areas the nurse may assess.

Surprisingly, some people with this disorder are extremely talented or intelligent but never function to their potential. People with antisocial personality disorders do *not* have thought disorders. Even though they choose not to take responsibility for their actions, *they are held responsible in a court of law.*

Nursing Diagnosis

People with antisocial traits are usually admitted to psychiatric institutions for reasons other than their personality disorder, e.g., for substance abuse or by court order.

The data collected from the client provide the nurse with information about the presenting problem or behaviors, emotional state, precipitating situations, and maladaptive coping behaviors. The antisocial client may exhibit any number of problematic behaviors. These behaviors are not in themselves pathological or maladaptive. Behaviors that are repetitive or rigid or those that present an obstacle to meaningful relationships or functioning are considered in the management and care of the client.

Nursing diagnoses must be consistent with the treatment plan agreed on by each member of the interdisciplinary team. In fact, all clinicians involved in the care of the antisocial client must agree to the diagnoses, goals, and plan.

Nursing diagnoses may be numerous. The person with a diagnosis of antisocial personality disorder often presents with gross behavioral problems. These behaviors usually cause a great deal of difficulty in interpersonal relationships. Therefore, *ineffective individual coping* may be diagnosed. *Ineffective coping* may be evidenced by overt hostility, manipulation of others, egocentricity, habitual disregard of social norms, or dependence on drugs, alcohol, or both.

Many people with antisocial personality disorders end up in jail, juvenile courts, and houses of detention because of unlawful behavior and physical aggression toward others. Therefore, the nursing diagnosis of *high risk for violence directed at others* is often applicable. *High risk for violence directed at others* may be evidenced by lack of impulse control, overt aggression and hostility, or emotional immaturity.

Often a person with an antisocial personality may have a parenting role. Because by definition a person with an antisocial personality disorder is unable to empathize, cherish, or support the needs of another human being, children suffer emotionally from such a parent. Therefore, the nursing diagnosis of *altered parenting*, as evidenced by abuse, rejection, inadequate resources, or impaired judgment, is possible.

Planning

Planning nursing interventions for a person with antisocial characteristics is done on the (1) content level —planning goals, and the (2) process level—nurses' reactions and feelings.

CONTENT LEVEL—PLANNING GOALS

Setting goals for people with antisocial personality disorders is not easy. Too often, goals are set that are way beyond the capabilities of the client. Because antisocial behaviors reflect lifelong habits of coping with the world, change comes very slowly, if at all. When goals are too high, health care personnel become frustrated and angry with the client for not meeting the goals. Therefore, it is important that the goals be set interactively with the client. Unfortunately, the client often is not motivated to change, because the client usually sees nothing wrong with his or her behavior.

Building on a person's strengths and offering alternative behaviors can be useful. Telling the person not to do something often meets with resistance from the client and results in frustration on the clinician's part and power struggles between the two.

For the nursing diagnosis *high risk for violence directed at others,* the following goals may be appropriate:

Long Term Goals

- Client will avoid situations that may stimulate aggressive acts by (date).
- Client will demonstrate alternative and acceptable behaviors to deal with aggressive thoughts or feelings by (date).
- Client will show an increase in ability to control unacceptable impulses.

Short Term Goals

- Client will name two situations that trigger aggressive acts by (date).
- By (date) client will verbalize anger and frustration related to one incident that stimulated aggressive behavior.
- Client will develop one alternative behavior to relieve frustration and anger through role-playing and practice by (date).
- Client will demonstrate a decrease in aggressive behaviors by (date).

Ineffective individual coping is always present. Most evident characteristics are projection of blame onto others and manipulation. Often, this manipulation is used to get immediate gratification of some wish or desire. At other times, manipulation is used to keep individuals or groups so confused and distracted that there is little to stop the client from getting his or her way. The aim of intervention is to decrease the unacceptable behaviors. Possible goals follow:

Long Term Goals

- Client will adhere to rules and laws by (date).
- Client will develop healthier relationship with one other individual or group by (date).

Short Term Goals

- Client will acknowledge manipulative behaviors pointed out by staff by (date).
- Client will verbalize awareness of manipulative behaviors by (date).
- Client will state and demonstrate one appropriate method of getting some of his needs met by (date).

PROCESS LEVEL—NURSES' REACTIONS AND FEELINGS

Initially, nurses working with antisocial clients may find them charming and intelligent. After a while, nurses react with frustration and anger when these individuals resist or defy their assistance. As clients continue to test the limits of the treatment program or to manipulate others, including the staff, nurses experience increased anger, disappointment, helplessness, and despair. It is sometimes difficult to understand how a person who is reasonably intelligent repeatedly gets into trouble with family, friends, employers, and the law. Crimes include theft, embezzlement, forgery, robbery, rape, and other acts of violence. Often, the nurse's response when hearing about these crimes is moralistic condemnation and contempt.

Beginning students and practitioners in psychiatric nursing are educated to help clients gain insight into their problems. Antisocial clients do not experience subjective anxiety or guilt that ordinarily motivates people to change, nor do they perceive a need for change. This attitude can elicit feelings of frustration, hopelessness, or anger in the nurse.

Nurses may unwittingly foster the problematic behaviors of their clients. For example, a nurse may admire and be envious of the manner in which a client is able to con or manipulate the system. At other times, a client's rebellious behavior may meet

some unconscious need for vicarious enjoyment or punishment for the nurse. When this occurs, the nurse and client can support a pathological situation. Being aware of these feelings and responses to antisocial clients can help nurses work with them in a more therapeutic manner. Frequent staff meetings and peer supervision are crucial in maintaining objectivity for those working with antisocial individuals.

The goal of treatment with these clients is movement toward behavioral change, particularly those behaviors that are judged by society to be inappropriate and that present an obstacle to developing and maintaining meaningful relationships.

Often, these long term goals focus on bringing about cognitive changes in the client. Specifically, clients are helped to examine and identify their maladaptive behaviors and how these behaviors affect their lives. For some antisocial individuals, this insight can lead to motivation for change. Change is sometimes possible through an integrated comprehensive treatment approach based on individual client assessment and goals. Treatment modalities that have been effective with some individuals are identified subsequently.

Intervention

PSYCHOTHERAPEUTIC INTERVENTIONS

Of the many problematic behaviors exhibited by the antisocial personality, the following predominate and cause the most frustration for nurses and health care professionals: (1) manipulation, (2) impulsiveness, (3) aggression, and (4) detachment.

MANIPULATION. Manipulation by itself is not a maladaptive behavior. It can be purposeful behavior directed at getting needs met. However, the term manipulative behavior often has a negative connotation in the field of psychiatry. **Maladaptive use of manipulation** occurs when (Chitty and Maynard 1986)

1. It is the primary method used to get needs met.
2. The needs, goals, and feelings of others are disregarded.
3. Others are dehumanized and treated as objects to fulfill the needs of the manipulator.

Manipulation of the staff may be achieved by the client by playing various roles:

The Seducer. In the role of **seducer,** the manipulative client is initially extremely responsive to the nurse's therapeutic endeavors. He or she wants only to talk to "his" or "her" nurse. The client appears to share great insights with the nurse early on and always says just what the nurse wants to hear. The seduction may include bringing gifts and doing thoughtful favors for "his" or "her" nurse. Once the groundwork is set, this special relationship or closeness with the nurse is used to gain special favors, e.g., staying out an hour later on pass, making bargains with the nurse (if I do . . . can I then have . . .), and asking for special privileges. If the nurse turns down these requests, the client instills guilt, "I thought you liked me" or "I thought we understood each other." The nurse is now in a no-win situation. If the requests are refused, the nurse loses the "therapeutic" relationship with the client. If the nurse gives in, the manipulative behaviors are reinforced, and the nurse feels controlled and put down by the client.

The Passive-Aggressor. Instead of wooing the nurse, as does the seducer, the **passive-aggressor** manipulates in ways that push the nurse away. People with antisocial personalities have an uncanny ability to detect weak spots in others. The manipulator intuitively knows what will make others anxious and uses this knowledge for exploitation. For example, if the nurse is young and sexually inexperienced, one passive-aggressive approach would be to make sexual overtures or to try to touch the nurse. Or, if the nurse is highly obsessional—and many are—the client can get at the nurse by "exposing" how imperfect the nurse really is. This is done by pointing out the nurse's errors or commenting on the nurse's personal or professional problems in front of other clients and staff.

Keep the Ball in the Air. This is an often-used and highly successful maneuver to get staff so crazy and befuddled that the manipulator can pretty much do as he or she chooses and get what he or she wants with little opposition. The technique **keep the ball in the air** is also used by a person in the manic phase of a bipolar depression (see Chapter 18). Eric Berne (1964) calls this "Let's You and Him Fight." This can be played out in numerous scenarios. One is to tell nurse X, "You really are interested in the patients. I don't at all believe what nurse Y said about you." The manipulator then goes to nurse Y with false tales or half-truths about nurse X. Of course, this is carried out with nurses Z and Q as well. Pretty soon the staff is split and distrustful of one another. Staff energies are soon channeled into squabbling and trying to straighten out who said what to whom. While the staff is thus occupied, the manipulator goes about pretty much as he or she pleases. This same game can be played by telling nurse Z that "nurse X said I could stay out an hour later on pass" after nurse Y told the manipulator that he could not stay out later. Again,

staff becomes confused about the guidelines for treatment.

Help Me If You Can. In **help me if you can,** the manipulator controls by evoking feelings of helplessness in others. All the client has to do is act helpless, cry a lot, and refuse to talk. Soon everyone is trying to find out what the crying is about, stop the crying, and get the client to talk. Staff members are now focused on getting at the "key" to helping this client and are frustrated by their efforts.

An important step in decreasing manipulative behaviors is to set clear and realistic limits on specific behaviors. A manipulative client may overtly react to the limit setting with resentment and resistance; however, some manipulative clients really want some limits placed on their behaviors. **Six steps in setting limits** follow (Chitty and Maynard 1986):

1. Set limits only in those areas in which there is a clear need to protect the client or others.
2. Establish realistic and enforceable consequences of exceeding limits.
3. Make the client aware of the limits and the consequences when limits are not adhered to before incidents occur. The client should be told in a clear, polite, and firm manner what the limits and consequences are and should be given the opportunity to discuss any feelings or reactions to these limits and consequences.
4. All limits should be supported by *all the staff.* The limits should be written in the care plan and communicated verbally as well.
5. When the limits are consistently adhered to, a decision to discontinue the limits should be made by the staff and noted on the nursing care plan. The decision should be based on consistent behavior, not on promises or sporadic efforts.
6. The staff should formulate a plan to address their own difficulty in maintaining consistent limits.

Table 16–4 outlines some goals and interventions aimed at decreasing manipulative behaviors.

IMPULSIVENESS. Antisocial behavior often includes impulsive actions. **Impulsiveness** is an action that is abrupt, unplanned, and directed toward immediate gratification. Thinking things over or considering the effects of the action on others does not occur. These clients have a history of unpredictable and hasty decisions. Frustration is poorly tolerated and often precipitates an impulsive response. A client's impulsive behavior has been described as erratic, self-serving, and thoughtless. In certain situations, the antisocial client's impulsive behavior is able to generate fear and aggression in others. The nurse can work with the client to modify this impulsive behavior. Table 16–5 identifies a goal and possible interventions to aid in decreasing impulsive behavior.

Table 16-4 ■ GOALS AND INTERVENTIONS FOR MANIPULATIVE BEHAVIOR

GOAL	INTERVENTION
Client will demonstrate limiting setting on own for manipulative behavior by (date).	Identify manipulative behaviors by client.
	Set limits on manipulative behaviors by communicating expected behaviors.
	Convey to the team consistency of approach in setting limits.
	Be realistic as to which behaviors can be limited.
	Assist client in developing means of setting limits on own behavior.
	Assess degree of insight into manipulative behavior and motivation to change.
	Avoid getting into power struggles by accusing and arguing with client.
Client will develop two alternative nonmanipulative behaviors by (date).	Discuss client's behaviors in nonjudgmental and non-threatening manner.
	Assist client in identifying personal strengths and effective communication skills.
	Assist client in testing out alternative behaviors for obtaining needs or fulfilling expectations.
	Support client and provide feedback in trying new behaviors.

AGGRESSION. Aggression is a behavior that frequently occurs in antisocial clients. **Aggression** is "any verbal and/or nonverbal, actual or attempted, forceful abuse of the self upon another person or thing." Aggressive behaviors often lead to violence. Aggression is but one expression of anger. Table 16–6 identifies some goals and interventions for decreasing aggressive behavior. See Chapter 22.

DETACHMENT. Detachment refers to interpersonal and intrapersonal dissociation from affective expression. Individuals who manifest these behaviors have been labeled cold, aloof, and distant. This behavior is thought to be learned and is defensive. The individual also dissociates himself or herself from society and does not internalize social standards and values. Right and wrong have little personal meaning for this person. Table 16–7 identifies one goal and several interventions useful for working with a detached client.

PSYCHOTHERAPY

During counseling sessions, the antisocial person will challenge therapists and seek to outwit them. Antisocial clients are known to set up situations to test the therapist's skills, catch inconsistencies, arouse anger, and whenever possible, belittle or humiliate the therapist. The goals of the therapist are to see things from the client's point of view, convey a sense of trust, and create a feeling of alliance. A balance of professional

Table 16-5 ■ GOAL AND INTERVENTIONS FOR IMPULSIVE BEHAVIOR

GOAL	INTERVENTION
Client will identify impulsive acts and give examples of situations in which they occur by (date).	Identify the needs and feelings preceding impulsive acts.
	Discuss current and previous impulsive acts.
	Explore impact of such acts on self and others.
	Recognize cues of impulsive behaviors that may injure others.

Table 16-6 ■ GOALS AND INTERVENTIONS FOR AGGRESSIVE BEHAVIOR

GOAL	INTERVENTION
Client will demonstrate control and responsibility in two situations in which he or she previously used aggressive action by (date).	Encourage client to spend time talking out instead of acting out intense feelings of frustration. Communicate positive expectations to the client. Assist client in developing concrete external controls. Assist client in problem-solving techniques to cope with frustration or tension. Provide feedback on results. Limit choices to those that are safe and appropriate.
Client will cope with stress and aggression in a nonviolent manner most of the time by (date).	Assist client in identifying feelings of anxiety, expectations, anger, frustration, disappointment, or perceived threats. Assist client in verbalizing these feelings. Assist client in describing precipitating events or situations leading to aggressive behavior. Assist client in exploring present situation by discussing situations in the past that have aroused similar feelings. Assist client in identifying previous coping behaviors. Assist client in exploring consequences of behavior on self and others. Assist client in developing more effective coping behaviors and interpersonal skills.

firmness, authority, and tolerance for the client's behaviors must be maintained.

Unfortunately, psychotherapy has proved to be unsuccessful with this personality disorder (McCord 1982; Frosch 1983). Because people with this disorder neither experience subjective anxiety nor view their behavior as a problem, they have no motivation for change. They are also unable to form attachments to others. Without strong interpersonal relationships, a therapeutic alliance cannot evolve, and the therapeutic alliance or relationship is the cornerstone of psychotherapy.

Other therapies have met with somewhat more success in selected clients. For example:

1. *Group therapy* has been successful with some antisocial clients. Often, however, aggressive behaviors have disrupted group functions. Generally these

Table 16-7 ■ GOAL AND INTERVENTIONS FOR DETACHMENT BEHAVIOR

GOAL	INTERVENTION
Client will develop an increased sense of relatedness to others by (date).	Assist client in establishing rapport in interpersonal relationships. (However, nurse may need to supervise relationships to prevent harm to vulnerable clients.) Assist client in identifying patterns of past relationships with significant others. Assist client in describing feelings related to detachment. Assist client in exploring more effective interpersonal skills that increase sense of belonging. Expect client to maintain the rules of the treatment and milieu.

clients are unable to identify with their therapists or even keep appointments. Group therapy is not recommended on an outpatient basis.

2. *Self-help groups* in which clients share and discuss their feelings and behaviors may encourage development of group responsibility and loyalty. This is especially true if the group is composed of other individuals with antisocial personality disorders. When these individuals feel they are among peers, their lack of motivation may change (Kaplan and Sadock 1991).

3. *Therapy based on modeling* also seems successful with the less aggressive antisocial individuals (McCord 1982). **Modeling** is demonstrating the desired behaviors. The client learns to imitate these behaviors in appropriate situations.

4. *Transactional therapy* has had some success with certain antisocial adolescents (McCord 1982). The emphasis of the treatment is on current and future situations in which the individual and therapist develop a contract outlining specific responsibilities and goals for both the therapist and the client. The individual eventually learns to incorporate responsibility when the person's "adult" monitors the "parent" and "child" messages.

5. *Behavior modification* has helped in extinguishing certain problematic behaviors. Positive reinforcement, or conditioning using monetary or other rewards, has been shown to be more successful than using negative reinforcement, i.e., punishment (McCord 1982). Positive reinforcements (e.g., tokens or privileges) are given when desired behaviors occur. For example, positive reinforcement can be used to decrease aggressive behaviors. When a client demonstrates a decrease in aggressive behavior, the client receives a token, which may be exchanged for privileges or other desired rewards.

6. *Family therapy* should begin immediately after the client is admitted to an inpatient unit because the family or spouse may be consciously or unconsciously contributing to and supporting the problematic behaviors (Frosch 1983). Therapy is directed toward assisting each member of the family to understand his or her own role and to deal with the client's behaviors.

Specific changes in social groups, such as families, schools, or entire communities, may benefit the antisocial client. For example, instruction in effective family communication, the use of behavioral contracts, and immediate responses to individual or family crises have decreased the rate of second-time offenders among adolescents (Wade 1977). Academic training, vocational training, and job placement have also been responsible for lower rearrest rates (Quay and Love 1977).

Evaluation

Many of the goals of treatment are long term. Short term goals and interventions need to be realistic. Short term goals are mainly focused on the protection of other patients and the generation of behavioral changes that help the client adjust to the milieu. Equally important is the nurse's awareness of personal feelings and reactions to the client. This awareness can be gained by talking to other nurses and by being supervised by another nurse.

If the goals are not met within a specific time period (while the client is hospitalized), further referrals need to be made to the family, community, or legal system.

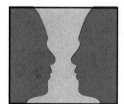

Case Study: Working with a Person Who Has an Antisocial Personality Disorder

Donald Mann, a 32-year-old divorced man, was hospitalized for uncontrollable aggressive impulses. On admission, there was no indication of thought disorders, hallucinations, or depressed affect. He was angry because he felt "forced" to voluntarily admit himself into the hospital. His boss had stated that if he didn't, he would be fired from his job. He had threatened a fellow history teacher and later assaulted him. The client stated, "I was only arguing a historical point, and I got carried away." He smiled and winked his eye as he was relating the course of events to the nurse, Ms. Burke. He stated he was unable to finish writing a book because his third wife had divorced him. When asked about his childhood, he commented, "Fighting is synonymous with being a street kid." He had a history of wife abuse and frequent barroom fights. For the past year, he had been employed as a teacher of history in a private college. He had had numerous teaching positions in various states. Mr. Mann stated that he enjoyed teaching and especially liked the students.

On the unit, Mr. Mann was generally cooperative. However, on two occasions he violated the rules of the unit. Once he was found with a bottle of alcohol ("I was celebrating one of our famous presidents"). The second incident involved threatening to harm another client on the unit. On both occasions, he had responded glibly, "I'm sorry." The female staff usually had no difficulty dealing with him, but the male staff generally complained about him.

On the third day after admission, Mr. Mann threatened another client. The unit coordinator asked Ms. Burke to write a comprehensive care plan on Mr. Mann. His infractions of the rules and aggressiveness were disrupting the unit. Ms. Burke, who had admitted him to the unit, had spent time with him over the past few days. She often felt flattered by his attention. He had told her that he found her "the best nurse on the

unit." That afternoon, his case was to be presented at a staff conference.

During the meeting, each female member stated that Mr. Mann had stated that she was his favorite. He would also "tell tales" to each staff member about the other staff members. The female staff would often do special favors for Mr. Mann, e.g., getting him cigarettes, the paper, or candy. The male members found him argumentative, infuriating, and contemptuous. They tried to avoid him as much as possible. It was clear that almost everyone had strong positive or negative reactions to Mr. Mann. During the meeting, many of the female staff felt annoyed and angry at being manipulated. The staff together decided on goals and a plan of approach.

Assessment

Ms. Burke divided her data into subjective and objective components.

OBJECTIVE DATA

1. Has had two incidents of infractions of the rules
2. Has past history of spouse abuse
3. Assaulted coworker prior to admission
4. Has had three marriages
5. Is argumentative with male staff
6. Rationalizes improper and aggressive behaviors—sees nothing wrong

7. Has difficulty with interpersonal relationships at work
8. Has physically threatened another client
9. Is verbally aggressive with male staff
10. Has made sexual advances toward female staff
11. Manipulates special favors from female staff

SUBJECTIVE DATA

1. Sets one staff member against another, "Nurse Y said this about you . . ."
2. States he was "forced into coming to the hospital"

3. Tells each female nurse that she is his favorite

Nursing Diagnosis

The staff thought two nursing diagnoses were the most important initially.

1. *Ineffective individual coping* related to inadequate psychological resources, as evidenced by verbal manipulation
   - Tells each female nurse that she is his favorite
   - Sets one staff member against another
   - Manipulates "special favors" from female nurses
   - Makes sexual advances toward female staff
   - Is insincere and superficial

2. *High risk for violence directed at others* related to antisocial character, as evidenced by history of overtly aggressive acts
   - Is verbally aggressive with male staff
   - Has threatened physical assault toward another client
   - Has history of spouse abuse
   - Rationalizes violent behavior; does not see behavior as undesirable
   - Has had two episodes of infraction of rules
   - Assaulted a coworker prior to admission

Planning

CONTENT LEVEL—PLANNING GOALS

Ms. Burke and the rest of the staff decided on a number of strategies that would, it was hoped, reduce Mr. Mann's manipulation and aggressiveness. Long term and short term goals were set. The aim of the goals was to

alter Mr. Mann's behavior while he was on the unit and to elicit more appropriate behaviors for meeting needs and responding to frustration.

Continued on following page

Planning
(Continued)

Nursing Diagnosis	Long Term Goals	Short Term Goals
1. *Ineffective individual coping* related to inadequate psychological resources, as evidenced by verbal manipulation	Client will ask directly for basic needs.	1a. Client will state awareness of manipulative behavior by (date). 1b. Client will state awareness of thoughts and expectations surrounding two situations of manipulation by (date).
2. *High risk for violence directed at others* related to antisocial character, as evidenced by history of overt, aggressive acts	Client will demonstrate appropriate behaviors in response to frustration, without violence, most of the time.	2a. Client will talk about his anger and frustration rather than acting out by (date). 2b. By (date) client will develop two appropriate alternative behaviors to relieve frustration.

PROCESS LEVEL—NURSES' REACTIONS AND FEELINGS

During the planning it was decided that Ms. Burke would be the primary nurse during the day, and Ms. Hubb during the evening shift. Ms. Burke was to get supervision from the psychiatric clinical nurse specialist on the unit. The nursing coordinator suggested that communication regarding Mr. Mann be given in some detail during shift reports until modification of his aggressive and manipulative behavior was evident.

Intervention

The nursing care plan involved input from all staff members. It was anticipated that Mr. Mann would become easily frustrated and angry when limits were set on his manipulative and aggressive behavior. Ms. Burke (on days) and Ms. Hubb (on evenings) would be the two staff members primarily working with Mr. Mann. All requests, favors, and sharing of personal information would be channeled through these two nurses. Setting limits was an important aspect of the care plan. Both Ms. Burke and Ms. Hubb were to set the limits on flattery, gifts, and compliments. When such behavior occurred, interaction would be refocused back to Mr. Mann.

Very clear limits were set regarding aggressive behavior. He was told that angry and inappropriate verbal aggressiveness would result in losing a privilege on the unit for that day (e.g., no telephone calls, no television at night). Physical acting out had more severe consequences. For any physical assault, weekend passes would be withheld, and any other appropriate precautions would be taken, such as time in the quiet room or use of medication.

Expected client behaviors were clearly explained, and when elicited, would meet with recognition and positive feedback. The following is an interview between the nurse and Mr. Mann following his threat to strike another client.

Dialogue	Therapeutic Tool/Comment
N: I would like to talk with you about what happened this morning. MR. M: OK, shoot.	Be clear as to the purpose of the interview.
N: Tell me what started the incident.	Use open-ended statements. Maintain a nonjudgmental attitude.
MR. M: Well, as I told you before, I always had to fight to get what I wanted in life. My father and mother abandoned me emotionally when I was a child. N: Yes, but tell me about this morning.	Redirect client to present problem or situation.

MR. M: OK, I never liked Richard since I met him; he has it in for me. I just know it. He doesn't get along with anyone here. Just two days ago he almost had a fight.

N: Donald, what do you mean, Richard has it in for you?

Explore situation.

MR. M: When I'm talking to one of the nurses, he stares and makes comments under his breath.

N: What does he say?

Encourage description.

MR. M: How I'm "in" with the nurses. I'm just trying to do what is expected of me here.

N: You mean that Richard is envious of your relationship with the nurses?

Validate the client's meaning.

MR. M: Right, he really doesn't want to be here. He doesn't care about all that therapeutic junk.

N: You seem to know a lot about how Richard thinks. I wonder how that is?

Assist client to make association to present situation.

MR. M: He reminds me of someone I knew when I was young. His name was Joe Brown. We called him "Bones."

N: Tell me more about Bones.

Explore situation further.

MR. M: We called him Bones because he was skinny as bones. He was into drugs and never ate. He was also called Bones because he was selfish. He never shared anything. He never even had a girl that I knew about.

N: So Richard reminds you of someone who is selfish and lonely?

Make interpretation of information. Note increasing anxiety.

MR. M: That's right. I've had three marriages and girlfriends on the side. No one can take them away from me, just let them try (*angrily*).

N: What makes you so angry now?

Identify feelings and explore threat or anxiety.

MR. M: Richard—I know he wants to be like me, but he can't. I'll hurt him if he makes any more comments about me.

N: Donald, you will not hurt anyone here on the unit.

Set limits on and expectations of client's behavior.

MR. M: I'm sorry. I didn't mean that.

N: It's important that we examine your part in the incident this morning and how to cope without threats or violence.

Focus on client's responsibility and suggesting alternative methods of coping with situation.

MR. M: Listen, I know I've gotten into trouble because I can't control my temper, but that's due to the fact that I won't get any respect until I can show them I don't fear them.

Exhibits rationalization.

N: Who are they?

Clarify pronoun.

MR. M: People like Richard.

N: You've told me that fighting was a way of survival as a child, but as an adult, there are other ways of handling situations that make you angry.

Show empathy and suggest other means of coping.

Continued on following page

Intervention *(Continued)*	MR. M: You're right. I've thought about this. Do you think it would help if you gave me some meds to control my anger?	Exhibits superficial and concrete thinking—possible manipulation.
	N: I wasn't thinking of medications but rather a plan of being aware of your anger and talking it out instead of fighting it out.	Clarify meaning toward behavioral change.
	MR. M: I told you before, I have to fight.	
	N: Have you thought about the consequences of your fighting?	Identify results of impulsive behavior.
	MR. M: I feel bad afterwards. I sometimes wish it hadn't happened.	
	N: Tell me about a time when you felt this way.	Explore previous situations of impulsiveness.
	MR. M: I really loved my third wife, but she made me mad. I didn't want to hurt her, but I couldn't help myself.	
	N: Couldn't help yourself?	Use reflection to get client to further describe situation.
	MR. M: She wanted me to stay home and not go out with the guys, but I didn't want her to tell me what to do.	
	N: And then what happened?	Continue to explore situation.

Evaluation	As expected, Mr. Mann became outraged when limits were set. He started to shout at the doctor and called him names. The staff calmly told him that because of his inappropriate shouting he was unable to use the phone for the rest of the day, as outlined in his plan. Over the next few days, he did some more testing, for example, yelling and throwing a can of soda at one of the evening staff. He was taken to the seclusion room for	an hour. That weekend, he was refused a pass. By the end of the third week, his behavior on the unit showed marked modification. His pitting of staff against staff was thwarted. By discharge, his verbal aggressiveness flared up once in a while, but much less often than on previous occasions. Refer to Mr. Mann's written care plan (Nursing Care Plan 16–1).

Nursing Care Plan 16–1 ■ *A PERSON WITH ANTISOCIAL PERSONALITY DISORDER: Mr. Mann*

NURSING DIAGNOSIS

Ineffective individual coping **related to inadequate psychological resources, as evidenced by verbal manipulation**

Supporting Data

- Sexual advances toward female staff.
- Infraction of rules on unit.
- Attempts to set staff at odds with each other.
- Insincere and superficial.
- Manipulates special favors from nurses.

Long Term Goal: Mr. Mann's manipulative behavior on the unit will be minimal by discharge.

Short Term Goal	*Intervention*	*Rationale*	*Evaluation*
1. Mr. Mann will state awareness of manipulative behavior by (date).	1a. One nurse assigned to Mr. Mann on both evening and day shifts. 1b. One-to-one interaction with primary care staff on a day-to-day basis. 1c. Communicate clear limits on manipulative behavior.	1a–b. Limits chance of mixed communication. Decreases ability to manipulate staff. 1c–f. Clear expectations for behavior and conse-	Goal partially met After two weeks, client acknowledged some manipulative behaviors and stated that he understood the consequences of continuing some of his manipulative behaviors.

	1d. Communicate expected behavior.	quences provide sound framework for intervention.	
	1e. Spell out the consequences of manipulation.		
	1f. Share limits, expected behavior, and consequences of manipulation with all other staff daily at report time and at team conferences.		
	1g. Avoid power struggles; do not be defensive.	1g. Arguments take focus away from client and issue.	
	1h. Offer positive reinforcement and feedback when expected behavior is evident.	1h. Can increase expected behavior.	
2. Mr. Mann will state awareness of thoughts and expectations surrounding two situations of manipulation by (date).	2a. Identify situations in which client is manipulative.	2a–c. Change in behavior facilitated when client is aware of each manipulation.	Goal partially met Client was able to discuss one incident with primary nurse in terms of expectation and thoughts.
	2b. Explore needs or expectations in each manipulative situation.		
	2c. Discuss impact of manipulative behavior on self and others.		

NURSING DIAGNOSIS

High risk for violence directed at others **related to antisocial character, as evidenced by history of overtly aggressive acts**

Supporting Data

- Past history of wife abuse.
- Past history of fighting.
- Assaulted a coworker prior to admission.
- Threatened another client on the unit.
- Rationalizes behavior—does not see anything wrong.
- Two episodes of infraction of rules.
- Verbally aggressive with male staff.

Long Term Goal: Mr. Mann will demonstrate appropriate behaviors in response to frustration, without violence, most of the time.

Short Term Goal	Intervention	Rationale	Evaluation
1. Mr. Mann will verbalize anger and frustration rather than act out by (date).	1a. Identify feelings of anxiety, anger, and frustration. 1b. Encourage appropriate verbalization of these feelings with the nurse. 1c. Discuss events that lead to aggressive behavior.	1a–b. Client learns to talk it out instead of act it out. 1c. Client learns to acknowledge and anticipate feelings of frustration that can lead to aggression.	Goal met Client initiated discussions twice with nurse when he "felt like wasting" another client. Physical acting out had decreased in incidence by end of third week.
2. By (date) Mr. Mann will develop two appropriate alternative behaviors to relieve frustration.	2a. Explore relief felt when aggression is used by client. 2b. Discuss impact or consequences of behavior on self and others. 2c. Explore alternative behaviors in coping with anger or frustration. 2d. Assist client in developing effective communication skills. 2e. Provide feedback to client on behaviors. 2f. Reward client when not using aggressive behaviors.	2a–d. Learning to deal appropriately with aggression allows client to take responsibility for his own behavior. 2e–f. Positive feedback and rewards help elicit desired behaviors.	Goal partially met Initially, the client continued to test staff by throwing things and name calling. On (date), the client sought out nurse two times when angry to discuss thoughts and feelings. By third week, the incidence of verbal and physical acting out had sharply declined.

Summary—Antisocial Personality Disorders

The personality disorders are classified on axis II of the DSM-III-R and DSM-IV. Individuals with personality disorders generally do not seek assistance or intervention because their defense mechanisms are ego-syntonic, that is, the defenses are not at odds with their sense of self. The three major groups of personality disorders are (1) paranoid, schizoid, and schizotypal; (2) histrionic, narcissistic, antisocial, and borderline; and (3) avoidant, dependent, obsessive-compulsive, and passive-aggressive.

Antisocial personality disorders are characterized by acts against society, impulsiveness, aggressiveness, lack of remorse or guilt, shallow affect, and superficial interpersonal relationships. Various biological, cultural-environmental, and psychological theories have been presented to explain the dynamics of this personality disorder.

When hospitalized, clients with antisocial personality disorders evoke strong emotions in nurses. Frustration, anger, disappointment, and despair are usually experienced by health care professionals caring for these clients. Being aware of these feelings and responses to antisocial clients can assist nurses in understanding and caring for them.

Areas to be assessed include (1) affect, (2) relationships with others, and (3) behavioral patterns. Numerous nursing diagnoses may be identified. These include *ineffective individual coping, high risk for violence directed at others,* and *altered parenting.* Goals and interventions are aimed at behavioral change. Most goals are long term in nature. Four specific problematic behaviors (manipulation, impulsiveness, aggression, and detachment) were presented, along with guidelines for intervention. Firm limits need to be set in a nonjudgmental and calm manner. Clear expectations for change in behavior need to be stated. A consistent approach among team members is vital. Other therapies that have been beneficial include behavior modification, group therapy, family therapy, and changes in the social environment.

Paranoid Personality Disorder

Kem B. Louie

OBJECTIVES ■

After studying this section on paranoid personality disorder, the student will be able to

1. Describe seven characteristics of a person with a paranoid personality disorder.
2. Discuss at least two theories of etiology.
3. Identify four common but intense countertransferential feelings experienced by health care professionals.
4. Employ in role-playing with a peer four tools the nurse can use when working with a paranoid individual.

The essential characteristic of persons with paranoid personality disorder (PPD) is the pervasive and unwarranted tendency to interpret the actions of others as deliberately demeaning or threatening (APA 1987). Other characteristics include expecting to be exploited or harmed by others, questioning without justification the loyalty or trustworthiness of friends or coworkers, bearing grudges or acting unforgiving or mistrustful of others, being quick to react with anger, and questioning without justification fidelity of a spouse or sexual partner.

People with PPD include "many of life's least lovable character types—the bigot, the injustice collector, the pathologically jealous spouse, and the fanatic" (Perry and Vaillant 1989).

Individuals diagnosed with PPD can be viewed by

others as capable, ambitious, and energetic, but generally they are often seen as hostile, stubborn, and defensive. They have a great need to control, are inflexible, and avoid intimacy except with those that they absolutely trust. During periods of extreme stress, individuals with PPD may experience transient psychotic symptoms.

There are seven characteristic behaviors typical of the individual with PPD:

1. *Suspiciousness and mistrust.* The paranoid individual is preoccupied with being tricked, maneuvered, or framed. Behaviors of mistrust and suspiciousness include being guarded and secretive, looking for hidden meanings or motives, questioning loyalty of others, and expecting harm.

2. *Rigidity.* People with PPD are steadfast and inflexible in their views of the world. In order to confirm their expectations of others, they are often argumentative and justify their position by excessive rationalization. They make "mountains out of molehills" to prove their points.

3. *Hypervigilance.* Paranoid individuals are hypersensitive to nuances in their interpersonal relationships. They look for hidden motives and scrutinize how things are conducted. These individuals are keen observers and are more attentive to others in their environment than are most individuals.

4. *Distortion of reality.* Cognitively, these individuals distort the facts and give them special meanings. Therefore, they have a distorted perception of reality.

5. *Projection.* Paranoid individuals cope with their anxiety by blaming or attributing unacceptable feelings, desires, and attitudes to others.

6. *Restricted affect.* They are seen as cold, aloof, and humorless, and as lacking tender feelings. They frequently use coping mechanisms, such as intellectualization and rationalization, to avoid any emotional feelings.

7. *The process of exclusion.* Due to their pervasive suspiciousness, relationships with paranoid individuals are strained. They further alienate themselves from others because they perceive others acting according to their expectations.

Theory

PSYCHODYNAMIC ISSUES

Paranoia is theorized as a protective psychological response (Oxman et al. 1982). When the individual ex-periences anxiety, he or she reacts with anger, mistrust, and increased sensitivity. These anxious feelings are too difficult for the person to acknowledge; therefore, his or her feelings are *denied and projected* onto others. Individuals blame or attribute to others their own painful thoughts or feelings. This maladaptive response becomes the basis for the projection process.

Paranoid persons have more intact mental functioning and less personality disorganization than others with mental illness. They are able to use *compensation* for their anxious feelings and thoughts.

Another defense mechanism used by paranoid individuals is *reaction-formation.* They appear strong and independent, but they are truly feeling insecure and powerless.

As tension and anxiety increase, and the denial, projection, intellectualization, rationalization, and reaction-formation fail to decrease the anxiety, other mechanisms may be used, e.g., aggression and psychotic symptoms, such as paranoid delusions and hallucinations.

FAMILY INFLUENCES

Paranoid individuals often come from families who are harsh and strict and demand perfection and high achievement. Children in these families often are the recipients of irrational and overwhelming parental rage (Perry and Vaillant, 1989).

SOCIAL AND ENVIRONMENTAL INFLUENCES

Stress can precipitate paranoid thinking in people with PPD. These individuals may initially seem perfectly normal, but when their stress level increases, greater energy is required to mobilize defenses and maintain control. Paranoid thinking seems to show up more as the individual matures than during younger years. Stresses include increased responsibilities, illness, family loss, divorce, rejection, unemployment, and loneliness.

Numerous researchers have reported that sensory deprivation or defects can lead to paranoid ideas (Cameron 1959; Eisendorfer and Wikie 1972). These researchers found a higher proportion of paranoid symptoms among deaf psychotics than among psychotics with normal hearing. Suspiciousness also has been found in children who are deaf and in patients who temporarily lose their sight due to the wearing of an eye patch (Eisendorfer and Wikie 1972; Kaplan and Sadock 1991).

BIOLOGICAL INFLUENCES

There is not much evidence presently that suggests strong biological links to PPD. However, some adaptation studies show a relationship between PPD and chronic schizophrenia (Perry and Vaillant 1989).

Rockford et al. (1981) found that electroencephalograms (EEGs) differentiate some paranoid patients from individuals in the general population. The electroencephalograms from paranoid patients exhibit a different organization, with a magnitude of variance larger in the left hemisphere. These hemispheric differences tend to return to normal if the paranoid symptoms are treated by medications. The central features of the diagnostic criteria for PPD are found in Box 16–4.

Box 16–4. DIAGNOSTIC CRITERIA FOR PARANOID PERSONALITY DISORDERS

A pervasive distrust and suspiciousness of others such that their motives are interpreted as malevolent, beginning by early adulthood and present in various contexts, as indicated by at least four of the following:

1. Expects, without sufficient basis, to be exploited or harmed by others
2. Questions, without justification, the loyalty or trustworthiness of friends or associates
3. Is reluctant to confide in others because of unwarranted fear that the information will be used against him or her
4. Reads hidden demeaning or threatening meanings into benign remarks or events (e.g., suspects that a neighbor put out trash early to annoy him or her)
5. Tendency to bear grudges persistently, i.e., to be unforgiving of insults, injuries, or slights
6. Perceives attacks on his or her character or reputation that are not apparent to others and is quick to react with anger and counterattack
7. Has recurrent suspicions without justification, e.g., regarding fidelity of spouse or sexual partner

Adapted from American Psychiatric Association. DSM-IV Options Book: Work in Progress. Washington, DC: American Psychiatric Association, 1991.

Box 16–5. NURSING ASSESSMENT OF PARANOID PERSONALITY DISORDER

- Demonstrates behavior that is aggressive, abusive, angry, or hostile
- Demonstrates varying degrees of mistrust and secretiveness
- Blames other individuals or groups when he or she feels insecure or uncomfortable
- Responds to stressful situations with statements that distort and show misunderstanding
- Acts aloof or remains withdrawn in order to maintain superiority
- Makes statements that convey feelings of jealousy, insecurity, fearfulness, and distrust of others

---

Assessment

Assessment of the paranoid thinking process is often difficult because the illness may be hidden behind aggressive behaviors, and initial validation of the client's subjective information may not be available to the nurse. In addition, the individual may appear to be in control, and the personality may appear to be normal.

The nurse can assess clues to paranoid thinking by

- Listening for themes of denial, rationalization, and projection.
- Identifying clusters of behaviors, such as being guarded, suspicious, and aloof, and acting superior.
- Listening to the nurse's own personal feelings when he or she interacts with a paranoid client, such as distancing, lack of emotional contact, superiority, and the urge to engage in power struggles with the client. The nurse may feel attacked or belittled by the client and may wish to retaliate. These feelings should alert the nurse that he or she is experiencing common reactions to a paranoid client's projection process.

Box 16–5 identifies data a nurse may find while assessing a person with PPD.

Nursing Diagnosis

Nursing diagnoses may be numerous; however, *impaired social interactions* and *ineffective individual coping* are nearly always present. *Impaired social interactions* are often related to feelings of mistrust and suspiciousness of others. *Ineffective coping* is manifested by excessive use of projection and blame. *High risk for violence* may also be an appropriate diagnosis if a client feels threatened by others and is fearful of being harmed by others.

Planning

CONTENT LEVEL—PLANNING GOALS

For the nursing diagnosis *impaired social interactions* related to feelings of mistrust, as evidenced by nonparticipation and withdrawal, appropriate goals would include

Short Term Goal

- The client will participate in one to two nonthreatening ward activities by (date).

Long Term Goal

- The client will participate with others in goal-directed activity in relative comfort, as evidenced by the absence of demeaning, angry, or aggressive behaviors.

For the nursing diagnosis *ineffective individual coping* related to increase in anxiety, as evidenced by use of projection and blame, appropriate goals would include

Short Term Goal

- The client will discuss thoughts and feelings regarding situations in which he or she feels threatened.

Long Term Goal

- The client will handle stressful situations in the absence of excessive or prolonged projection or blame.

PROCESS LEVEL—NURSES' REACTIONS AND FEELINGS

As mentioned, the cornerstone of the paranoid defensive structure is the use of projection: a person attributes his or her own unacknowledged and unacceptable feelings to others. Often, a person with PPD will direct angry, demanding, or hurtful statements toward the nursing staff or therapist. At times, these remarks are aimed at real, although minor, truths or vulnerabilities in specific staff members. Staff may feel many common countertransferential reactions in these situations. Perry and Vaillant (1989) state that staff must learn to feel safe in experiencing these reactions and yet must be trained not to act on them. Common reactions are getting angry with the patient, denying the truth, wishing to control the patient, and losing one's concentration. When these countertransferential feelings are acted on, they propagate the "inhumanity found throughout the criminal justice, mental health, and welfare systems" (Perry and Vaillant 1989).

A common emotional reaction by staff to a paranoid person's excessive fault-finding and "injustice collecting" is a defensive and argumentative posture triggered by a need to defend one's innocent and well-meaning position.

Beginning practitioners and nurses as well as experienced therapists need to talk to professional and experienced peers or supervisors when intense negative feelings surface. Staff do best when they can anticipate and understand the situation and disentangle themselves from the patient's intense projections of self-hate, hurt, and rage. The most useful approach staff can take is that of strict honesty, concern for the patient's rights, and a formal, but concerned, distance.

Intervention

Clients with paranoid personality disorders can often appear normal. When their defensive structure is working, they do not view themselves as having a problem. Often, others in their environment, such as family or employers, are traumatized by their behavior and bring them into treatment. Otherwise, these clients are admitted to a hospital for only coexisting psychological or physical problems.

Paranoid individuals are usually extremely sensitive, and they easily misinterpret the words or intentions of others. Therefore, clear and simple messages are often least likely to be misconstrued. Staff should match their verbal message with their nonverbal behaviors. Double messages are confusing to a paranoid person (as, indeed, they are to all of us) and can escalate distrust and further decrease his or her sense of security. For example, if the nurse says she is interested in what the person is thinking and feeling but frequently looks at her watch and appears distracted, the client will doubt the validity of the nurse's statement.

When the nurse is working with a person who is paranoid, courtesy, honesty, and respect are the cardinal rules in treatment. A straightforward approach should be consistently used throughout one's dealings with a person who is paranoid. If staff are accused by the patient of a minor fault (e.g., being late or forgetting to give a message), then a simple apology is more useful to the patient than a defensive explanation (Perry and Vaillant 1989).

A detached, neutral but concerned manner is usually less threatening to a paranoid person. A warm, gushing approach may be interpreted as intrusive, false, and threatening.

Useful tools for a nurse working with a client with a PPD include

- *Focusing on the client's feelings and behavior,* not on the explanation of that behavior. This method can help minimize defensiveness on the part of the client and can increase the nurse's understanding of the client's experience.
- *Providing structure.* Providing structure can increase the client's sense of security, thus helping to minimize acting-out behaviors.
- *Setting limits on destructive behaviors.* However, when limits are set, feelings of anxiety and depression may surface. Staff need to be available to listen to the client and offer appropriate support during this time.
- *Helping the client think through the consequences of actual or intended actions.* This pragmatic approach is much more useful to the client than interpretations of behaviors.

Table 19–11 in Chapter 19 identifies specific therapeutic approaches for nurses to use with a paranoid client.

Evaluation

There are no adequate and systematic long term studies of PPD. In many cases, the paranoid structure is life-long, whereas in others, as the person matures, the paranoid traits give way to reaction-formation, appropriate concern for moral issues, and altruistic concerns. In still others, the paranoid personality structure may be a prodromal indication of subsequent development of schizophrenia (Kaplan and Sadock 1991).

Vignette: Paranoid Personality Disorder

Jason, 40, is admitted to the inpatient unit. His mother reports that he has been hearing voices for the past two months. This is Jason's first admission. On the mental status examination, he denies hearing voices and states that he is voluntarily admitting himself to sort out his problems with his marriage.

Two months ago, he separated from his wife after 10 years of marriage. His mother states that her son has been having marital difficulties for the past five years. He has two daughters, five and six years old. He spends most of his time with his family and on weekends works around the house. He states that he does not like to socialize with others very much. He is an only child, and his father died when Jason was three years old.

He has been employed as a postal worker for 15 years. He is viewed by his coworkers as a diligent, hard worker who gets his work done on time. He is always rated as an excellent employee. Jason admits that he would like to be promoted to supervisor but says others in the company do not like to see him get ahead. When asked why he thinks this, he responds, "They know that I could do a better job. I have my own ideas of how things should be done. They get tired of hearing me, so now I just don't tell them anymore."

The following interview with Jason identifies specific communication skills used by the nurse. Can you identify some of Jason's defenses used during the interview (ideas of reference, denial, rationalization, and reaction-formation)?

JASON: I think there is too much partying around here—all the patients want to do is plan for another social.

NURSE: What seems to be the problem? (*clarifying*)

JASON: I just don't think that all the people here should socialize so much, especially the patients and the doctors. I think that they may be talking about me.

NURSE: Have you actually heard anything said about you? (*seeking validation*)

JASON: No, but I know, I see them whispering and looking at me. They're probably wondering why I'm here—I'm not like them. They can see that I'm smarter than most patients here. You know that I have my degree in political science, but unfortunately I couldn't get a job at the time when I graduated from college.

NURSE: Have you ever felt like this at your job at the Post Office? (*exploring*)

JASON: Listen, I know what you're getting at, but the reason I'm here has nothing to do with my job at the Post Office.

NURSE: I'm wondering what makes you angry about what I've just asked you? (*clarifying*)

JASON: You know that I can't talk about these things because they'd find out, and they have this grudge against me.

NURSE: Who are they? (*clarifying*)

JASON: The patients and doctors.

NURSE: Anyone in particular? (*clarifying*)

JASON: Allen and Dr. Jones.

NURSE: What makes you think Allen and Dr. Jones have a grudge against you? (*exploring*)

JASON: The first day when I arrived on the unit, while the assistant was checking my belongings, I heard Allen and Dr. Jones plotting something in the treatment room. When I got up and walked by they stared at me together. It's the way they look at you, and you know.

NURSE: So the stare made you feel uncomfortable? (*seeking validation*)

JASON: Yes, I mean I had just arrived and there they were just staring at me for no reason. I later found out that Allen lives a block away from the post office and probably recognizes me.

Summary—Paranoid Personality Disorder

The essential characteristic of a person with PPD is the pervasive and unwarranted tendency to interpret the actions of others as deliberately demeaning or threatening. Paranoid individuals have a great need to control, are inflexible, and avoid intimacy. There are no conclusive data to support any one etiology; however, twin studies point to a possible genetic link, although childhood backgrounds are usually tortured and unloving. Some behaviors noted on assessment of clients with PPD include

- Behaving aggressively
- Blaming and accusing others (projection)
- Acting aloof and withdrawn, often accomplished through anger, sarcasm, and demeaning behaviors
- Feeling superior (reaction-formation)
- Demonstrating mistrust and secretiveness

In the hospital, nursing diagnoses often include *impaired social interaction* and *ineffective coping*. *Risk for violence* may also be present. Nursing goals are aimed at making the client feel more comfortable and secure in his or her surroundings.

Nurses, staff, and even experienced therapists may experience intense countertransferential reactions, which have been identified in this section. These reactions need to be discussed and evaluated with a more experienced clinician if inappropriate reactions on the part of personnel are to be avoided. The projections of the paranoid process can attack sensitive and vulnerable aspects in any individual. To provide the most useful treatment for a person with PPD, professional support needs to be available to staff working closely with such a person.

Courtesy, honesty, and respect are the cardinal rules in treatment for a paranoid client. Other tools that are helpful to the client are mentioned in this section, and the reader is referred to Chapter 19 for other specific therapeutic measures for working with paranoid people.

Borderline Personality Disorders

Suzanne Lego

OBJECTIVES ■

After studying this section on borderline personality disorders, the student will be able to

1. Describe a textbook picture of a client with a borderline personality disorder.
2. Discuss three etiological theories of borderline personality disorder.
3. Act out five characteristics of the borderline personality.
4. Discuss five reactions health care workers could experience when working with a borderline client.

5. Identify three possible nursing diagnoses applicable to the borderline client.
6. For the following typical behaviors seen in borderline clients, discuss the nursing interventions and rationale for each: (a) hostility, (b) self-destruction, and (c) demanding behavior.
7. Indicate three possible outcomes of successful interventions when working with a borderline client.

The diagnosis *borderline personality disorder* (BPD) has received a great deal of attention in the past several years. Many papers, books, lectures, and professional presentations have focused on this problem. Clients with BPD are given much attention on inpatient units and in emergency rooms, where they are often branded "troublemakers" or "problem patients." The committee that devised the DSM-III seriously contemplated substituting the term *unstable* for borderline, and others have called clients in this category "the personality disorder who decided not to specialize" (Vaillant and Perry 1985).

Reference was first made in 1938 to the client on the borderline between psychosis and neurosis. Over the years, these clients were labeled "ambulatory schizophrenics," "pseudoneurotic schizophrenics," and "as if" personalities. The last term arose because these clients identified so completely with the person on whom they were dependent and because their own emotional experiences were derived to such a great extent from those of others (Vaillant and Perry 1985). These people are plagued by problems of identity and unstable interpersonal relationships.

In psychiatric settings, clients with BPD are more likely to be female than male. One reason is that males with BPD often end up in jails or prisons. Another reason is that separation problems play a large part in the etiology of BPD and are more pronounced in females in our society than in males (Simmons 1992). Smoyak (1985) observes that "nurses are in an excellent position to observe the rapid mood shifts, the unanticipated lashing out at other patients and staff, the clever and devious games of pitting one staff member against another, the emotional lability, and the covert and overt self-destructive behaviors. Such challenging behaviors require skilled intervention strategies."

Theory

Three theoretical contributions to the study of the etiology and development of the borderline personal-

ity disorders are presented: constitutional theory, Kernberg's contribution, and Masterson's contribution.

CONSTITUTIONAL THEORY

Some authors have hypothesized that borderline clients have inherited an incapacity to tolerate stress. Others believe that they have a constitutional inability to regulate affect, predisposing them to psychic disorganization under certain early adverse environmental conditions (Vaillant and Perry 1985).

KERNBERG'S CONTRIBUTION

Otto Kernberg hypothesizes that in infancy these clients perceive their mothers as strongly nurturing, loving, and protective, as well as hateful, depriving, and punishing without warning. These mothers let needs go unmet for long periods of time and abandon the infants unpredictably. The infant perceives both contradictory views of the mother and becomes highly anxious. To reduce anxiety, the mother is "split" into a "good" and "bad" mother. **Splitting** is a primitive defense in which persons see themselves or others as all good or all bad, unable to integrate the positive and negative qualities of the self or others into an integrated whole. The person may alternately *idealize* and *devalue* the same person (APA 1987). This primitive defense is carried into adult life, and others are experienced either as strongly nurturing and objects of inordinate attachment or as hateful, mean, and sadistic. The "good" person is idealized, and the "bad" person is devalued. The client can feel good only by a flight into *omnipotence*. When the client experiences hate toward another person, along with feelings of extreme dependence, anxiety ensues. The client reduces the anxiety triggered by these conflicting feelings through the use of *projective identification* and *denial*. **Projective identification** occurs when the client infuses the nurse with unwanted parts of the self in a powerfully controlling way (Tansey and Burke 1989). For example, the client feels rage and is able to infuse the nurse with rage toward the client in a very short time. This process is unconscious on the client's part and is often unsettling to the nurse.

MASTERSON'S CONTRIBUTION

James Masterson has described the borderline client's problems as beginning during Mahler's rapprochement subphase of the separation-individuation process of development, between 18 and 36 months of age. At this time, the toddler begins to move away from the mother but returns from time to time for "emotional refueling," and reassurance that the mother will not disappear. The developmental task is to learn that separation is acceptable and rewarding. However, mothers of these clients do not reward separation but rather discourage it by emotionally abandoning the child. That is, the child is punished for autonomous behavior and rewarded for crying, clinging, dependent behavior. This clinging behavior leads to an "emotional reunion" with the mother that comes to be longed for and repeated throughout life. By the same token, moves toward autonomy and independence lead the patient to experience what Masterson calls "abandonment depression" (Masterson 1976). In later life, clients with BPD tend to become depressed each time they experience success or growth, fearing that this will separate them forever from their mothers.

Box 16–6 identifies the DSM-III-R criteria for BPD.

Assessment

The nurse assesses the client for behaviors that are consistent with the diagnosis of borderline personality disorders. On an inpatient unit, some of these behaviors include the following:

- Hostile, demanding behavior
- Splitting—hating some nurses and loving others, or loving a nurse for a period and then suddenly hating her because of a feeling of rejection by the nurse
- Devaluation—constant, biting criticism of staff
- Manipulation—playing staff against one another by lying or distortions
- Clinging, lonely behavior
- Self-mutilation
- Suicide threats or gestures
- Alcohol or drug abuse
- Sexual promiscuity
- Inappropriate overreactions to stress

Box 16–6. DIAGNOSTIC CRITERIA FOR BORDERLINE PERSONALITY DISORDER

A pervasive pattern of instability of mood, interpersonal relationships, self-image, affect, and control over impulses, beginning by early adulthood, and present in various contexts, as indicated by at least *five* of the following:

1. A pattern of unstable and intense interpersonal relationships characterized by alternating between extremes of overidealization and devaluation
2. Impulsiveness in at least two areas that are potentially self-damaging (e.g., spending, sex, substance abuse, shoplifting, reckless driving, or binge eating). (Do not include suicidal or self-mutilating behavior covered in item 5)
3. Affective instability: marked reactivity of mood (e.g., intense episodic dysphoria, irritability, or anxiety lasting a few hours, rarely a few days)
4. Inappropriate, intense anger or lack of control of anger (e.g., frequent displays of temper, constant anger, and recurrent physical fights)
5. Recurrent suicidal threats, gestures, or behavior, or self-mutilating behavior
6. Identity disturbance: persistent and markedly disturbed, distorted, or unstable self-image or sense of self (e.g., feeling that one does not exist or embodies evil)
7. Chronic feelings of emptiness or boredom
8. Frantic efforts to avoid real or imagined abandonment. (Do not include suicidal or self-mutilating behavior covered in item 5)

Reprinted with permission from the DSM-IV Options Book, Work in Progress, 9/1/91. Copyright 1991 American Psychiatric Association.

- Projection of own hostility onto others on whom the client feels dependent
- Occasional psychotic behavior

From the research results of a study of 465 individuals with a DSM-III-R diagnosis of BDP, three core problem areas were identified (Hurt and Clarkin 1990):

1. *Affective cluster*: intense, inappropriate anger, affective lability, and unstable interpersonal relationships.
2. *Identity cluster*: chronic feelings of emptiness and boredom, identity disturbances, and intolerance of being alone.
3. *Impulse cluster*: self-damaging acts and impulsive behaviors.

Past history of many adult female clients with BPD may also include childhood sexual abuse. A study reported by Goldman (1992) supports the hypothesis that a history of sexual and physical abuse is associated with BPD. Shearer et al. (1990) found that female patients with BPD who had a history of childhood abuse were significantly more likely to have a concomitant diagnosis of an eating disorder, substance abuse, or a seizure disorder.

Nursing Diagnosis

The behavior of a person with a borderline personality is punctuated with angry outbursts, impulsive acts, and manipulation. Often, these clients carry out physically self-damaging acts, such as suicidal or self-mutilating behaviors. Because these acts are usually impulsive, hospitalization may be necessary to ensure a safe environment. When this happens, an appropriate nursing diagnosis would be *high risk for violence to self or others*. Violence to self or others may be evidenced by behaviors such as anxiety, self-mutilation, frequent displays of temper, and poor impulse control.

These clients often complain of chronic boredom or emptiness. Uncertainty about such things as gender identity, self-image, and career choice may add to the client's already high anxiety state. Therefore, *severe or panic levels of anxiety* may be related to a number of internal or external factors or conditions.

Borderline persons are often very manipulative. They use manipulative tactics to get their needs met. Similar to the behaviors of the person with an antisocial personality, their manipulations may result in harm to others. At other times, they act out anxiety in the form of impulsive acts. Impulsive acts may include promiscuity, gambling (Selzer 1992), shoplifting, binge eating, excessive spending, and drug use. Therefore, their ability to cope with anxiety is maladaptive. *Ineffective individual coping* may be evidenced by manipulation of others, inability to solve problems, impulsive acts, or chronic use of maladaptive behaviors.

Planning

In planning intervention with borderline clients, the nurse should be aware of the etiology of this condition. The key concepts are, first, the client's extreme, primitive dependency, and second, the client's extreme, primitive anger. Although these feelings began

in very early relationships, they are often triggered in current relationships, including interactions with the nurse. When each of the client's symptoms or problem behaviors is examined, these two issues will exist.

Considering this, the nurse provides a consistent, nurturing environment in which appropriate expression of anger is tolerated. This is easier said than done. To achieve this, the nurse deals directly and openly with the client's manipulation, splitting, devaluation, and other aspects of the neediness and anger.

CONTENT LEVEL—PLANNING GOALS

Many goals formulated in the hospital setting are short term. Usually, hospitalization for a client with a borderline personality is of short duration. Extended hospital stays can result in the client's becoming less functional in daily life. It is important that the client with BPD be directed toward continuing outpatient therapy upon discharge. This plan is articulated the day that the client enters the hospital and continues to be reiterated throughout the stay.

For the nursing diagnosis *high risk for self-directed violence*, the following goals could apply:

Long Term Goals

- Client will report absence of self-destructive thoughts.
- Client will name two people to contact if suicidal thoughts occur in the future.

Short Term Goals

- Client will remain safe while in the hospital.
- By (date) client will discuss desire to hurt self rather than do it.
- Client will express feelings in a nondestructive manner (e.g., talking, physical activity, or writing) by (date).

For the nursing diagnosis *severe-to-panic levels of anxiety*, the following goals may be considered:

Long Term Goals

- Client will state how to lower anxiety using an appropriate outlet by (date).
- Client will express a feeling of being more relaxed than anxious by (date).

Short Term Goals

- By (date), client will state that he or she is relaxed in a situation that usually produces anxiety.
- Client will talk about feeling anxious and identify increases in anxiety by (date).

Goals appropriate for the nursing diagnosis *ineffective individual coping* related to inadequate psychological resources could be the following:

Long Term Goals

- Client will solve most problems in a straightforward manner that injures neither self nor others by (date).
- Client will display ability to seek adaptive and acceptable solutions to problematic life situations by (date).
- Client will name two people available to discuss problems and help with solutions by (date).
- Client will name activities that help to decrease anxiety (e.g., exercise, dancing, talking, singing, or jogging) by (date).

Short Term Goals

- Client will discuss feelings of frustration and deal with them appropriately rather than acting them out by (date).
- Client will name two acceptable alternatives to maladaptive coping skills by (date).
- By (date), client will solve one situation that was usually formerly acted out maladaptively.

PROCESS LEVEL—NURSES' REACTIONS AND FEELINGS

Because borderline clients exhibit such strong anger and dependency, they evoke equally strong feelings in nurses. Their need to split others into "good" and "bad" people extends to the nurse and other staff. In addition, these clients are highly attuned to the vulnerable spots in others and, therefore, can make nurses feel highly anxious. Smith and Lego (1984), in *The American Handbook of Psychiatric Nursing*, compiled the following lists of individual and group reactions of nurses to borderline clients:

INDIVIDUAL REACTIONS

1. Feelings of massive responsibility for the client's welfare
2. Feelings of guilt because of failure to help the client
3. Omnipotent urges to rescue the client from the mishandling of others
4. Feelings of intense love and attachment to the client
5. Promises to keep secrets for the client as a token of trust and esteem
6. Feeling honored that the client "finally opened up"
7. Feeling highly confirmed in professional identity
8. Feeling highly repudiated in professional identity
9. Experiencing a need for excessively firm limits on the amount and quality of attention given to the client
10. Guilt by association with some value or person viewed as hostile by the client
11. Feelings of disappointment in one's work
12. Feelings of being emotionally drained to the extent that one's personal relationships suffer
13. Manifestations of the nurse's latent personality difficulties
14. Hostile acting out toward the clients by discharging them or resigning them from the setting
15. Contempt, jealousy, or envy of the seemingly "normal" client who manages to get considerable attention
16. Feelings of general paranoia and fear of the client's next projection
17. Feeling emotionally exposed and vulnerable because of the client's partly true projections
18. Defensiveness, counterattacking, rejection, and appeasement of the client

GROUP REACTIONS

1. Diagnostic uncertainty, with contradictory evaluations of clients, occurs.
2. Groups of staff members may feel emotionally isolated from one another.
3. Two or more staff members may become suspicious of the motives and behaviors of other staff members toward the client.
4. Lunch hour and coffee break time may be dominated by discussion of specific clients.
5. The nucleus of an "in-group" may believe that they are the only ones who can help the client.
6. Loss of morale and confusion may be seen in the "out-group."
7. Staff cleavage, with excessive clash of opinions, is seen by outside observers.
8. Blurring of staff-client role boundaries is seen in many forms (for example, client and staff discuss another staff member, or staff share personal information with the client).
9. Split in- and out-groups make the following accusations:
   a. "Ins" accuse "outs" of being cold and insensitive.
   b. "Outs" accuse "ins" of being too permissive and gullible and of spoiling the client.
10. Splits within departments in a hospital structure may be seen.
11. Administrative decisions to change client's therapist occur when the therapist is part of the "bad" split.

Table 16–8 ■ INTERVENTIONS FOR TYPICAL BEHAVIORS OF CLIENTS WITH BORDERLINE PERSONALITY DISORDER		
EXAMPLE OF BEHAVIOR	**NURSING INTERVENTION**	**THEORETICAL RATIONALE**
Hostility: "You are the worst nurse on this unit. I'm surprised they let you graduate from nursing school. You're a disgrace to your profession! I'm so mad, I could tear this unit apart. Maybe I will!"	In a calm way, the nurse asks the client to talk about what is causing all this anger, clarifies what has happened, sets limits, and provides safety for all the clients.	The client's rage has been touched off by anxiety about being cared for properly or about separation from caregivers. The nurse provides reassurance that anything can be discussed, that emotional security will not be withheld, and that the environment is safe. The client is helped to see that hostility can be faced and is manageable.
Self-destruction: The client gets angry during a therapeutic community meeting, runs to her room, breaks a lightbulb, and cuts her wrist superficially.	The nurse provides first aid but does not focus inordinate attention on the injury. Rather, attention is paid to the thoughts and feelings that led to the self-mutilation.	Self-destructive acts are unconsciously motivated by self-hatred, anger toward others, and a desire for "reunion" with the mother. The nurse helps the client explore these feelings without reinforcing the clinging, needy feelings.
Demanding Behavior: The client demands a pass even though she has been told she cannot leave for one week because she returned from her last pass drunk. "My doctor is hereby fired! I demand a new doctor and a transfer to another unit!"	The nurse calmly sets limits, pointing out they are a result of the client's inappropriate acting out. "Because you got drunk on pass, you cannot have another pass for a week. You knew the rule before you left on pass. You cannot change doctors or nurses but must stay and deal with what you are thinking and feeling. That is the only way to change."	The client's acting out and demanding behavior cover her need for ego boundaries and control, her anger at earlier deprivation, and her fear of growth and separation. The nurse provides the missing ego, attempts to supply the previously missing emotional attachment, and provides reality testing about separation.

Consistent supervision and peer support for the nurse are necessary to maintain objectivity and avoid staff confusion. Conferences with all members of the health team can be extremely valuable.

Intervention

Health care personnel working with a borderline client must deal with many challenging behaviors. The client's hostility and self-destructive or demanding behaviors are perhaps the most difficult. Table 16–8 shows examples, interventions, and theoretical rationales for borderline clients who display hostile, self-destructive, and demanding behavior. Borderline clients are nearly always treated with individual psychotherapy while in the hospital. The nurse supports the goals of psychotherapy. Team meetings are held often to counteract the effects of the clients' attempts to split staff.

Medications are given to clients with BPD for clinical emergencies only. They are used for targeted symptoms, such as acute anxiety, and are eliminated when those symptoms clear up. "Drugs reinforce the patient's philosophy that life is easy and reinforce the rewarding fantasy, which acts as a resistance to therapy and must be dealt with in treatment" (Masterson 1988).

Long term psychotherapy is the treatment of choice for these clients. The goals are to manage the acting out and to promote insight.

A recent study of 30 borderline clients demonstrated the effectiveness of psychotherapy in a twice-weekly outpatient setting. After 12 months, all clients demonstrated a significant reduction in impulsivity, affective lability, anger, and suicidal behavior. Equally encouraging was that 30% of the clients no longer met the DSM-III-R criteria for BPD, compared with 100% before treatment (Stevenson and Meares 1992).

Evaluation

Short Term Goals

Nurses evaluate their interventions with borderline clients throughout the nursing process. When intervention is successful, the client

- Communicates in a nondefensive way
- Displays less anger
- Displays less neediness
- Displays less acting out

Long Term Goals

- Given enough time, about two of three hospitalized clients with BPD will get better. These clients tend to begin to "mellow" in their 30s

(Stone 1990). The prognosis is less favorable if the client suffers from major depression or abuses alcohol or other drugs.

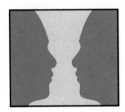

Case Study: Working with a Person Who Has a Borderline Personality Disorder

Mary Drake was a 24-year-old single secretary who lived alone. She had been seen in the emergency room several times for superficial suicide attempts. She was admitted because she had cut her wrists, ankles, and vagina with glass and had lost a lot of blood. This event was precipitated by her graduation from a community college.

Upon admission she was sweet, serene, and grateful to all the nurses, calling them "angels of mercy." Within one week she was angry at half of the nurses, demanding a new primary nurse, saying that the one she had (to whom she had grown attached) hated

her. She had managed to sneak alcohol onto the unit and was found in bed with a young male client. She continually broke unit rules and then pleaded to have this behavior forgiven and forgotten. When angry, she threatened to cut herself again. When asked why she cut herself, Ms. Drake stated, "I was tired." She appeared restless and tense and frequently asked for antianxiety medication. When asked what she was anxious about, she said "Uh . . . I don't know . . . I feel so empty inside." Ms. Drake frequently paced up and down the halls looking both angry and bored.

Assessment

Ms. McCarthy, a recent graduate and Ms. Drake's primary nurse, organized the data into subjective and objective components.

OBJECTIVE DATA

1. Makes frequent, superficial suicide attempts
2. Requests antianxiety medication frequently
3. Paces up and down the hall much of the day

4. Threatens self-mutilation when anxious
5. Brings alcohol onto the unit after pass
6. Is found in bed with male client

SUBJECTIVE DATA

1. Initially "loved" her primary nurse; now "hates" her and wants another nurse
2. States she is restless and tense

3. Complains of feeling empty inside
4. Describes self as angry and bored much of the time

Nursing Diagnosis

Ms. McCarthy formulated three initial nursing diagnoses that had the highest priority during this time.

1. *Moderate to severe anxiety* related to threat to self-concept, as evidenced by inability to relax
   - States she feels "empty"
   - Is restless and tense
   - Requests antianxiety medication frequently
2. *Ineffective individual coping* related to inadequate psychological resources, as evidenced by self-destructive behaviors
   - After stating that she feels frustrated,

client goes on pass and comes back with alcohol
   - After stating that she loves her therapist, client is found in bed with a male client
   - After stating that she hates her primary nurse, client demands a new primary nurse
3. *High risk for self-directed violence* related to anxiety and emptiness, as evidenced by suicidal gestures and poor impulse control
   - Is admitted following self-mutilation
   - Threatens self-mutilation when anxious
   - Threatens self-mutilation on the unit

Continued on following page

Planning

CONTENT LEVEL—PLANNING GOALS

The nurse decided on the following goals:

Nursing Diagnosis	Long Term Goals	Short Term Goals
1. *Moderate to severe anxiety* related to threat to self-concept, as evidenced by inability to relax	Client will state that she feels relaxed more than she feels tense by discharge.	1. By (date) client will state she is relaxed in a situation that usually produces anxiety, e.g., after visiting hours.
2. *Ineffective individual coping* related to inadequate psychological resources, as evidenced by self-destructive behavior	Client will solve problems in a manner that injures neither self nor others by (date).	2. By (date) client will discuss feelings of frustration and deal with them appropriately rather than act them out.
3. *High risk for self-directed violence* related to anxiety and emptiness, as evidenced by suicidal gestures and poor impulse control	Client will state that she will use an alternative coping device when thoughts of self-mutilation occur.	3. By (date), client will discuss desire to mutilate self rather than do so.

PROCESS LEVEL—NURSES' REACTIONS AND FEELINGS

Ms. McCarthy talked to Ms. Drake's therapist twice a week in staff meetings. The therapist impressed upon Ms. McCarthy the difficulty health care workers have in dealing effectively with people with borderline personality disorders. These clients constantly act out their feelings in self-destructive and maladaptive ways. They usually are not aware of their feelings or what triggered their actions.

The most difficult area for many health care workers is dealing with the intense feelings and reactions these clients can instill and provoke in others. Ms. McCarthy set a time twice a week for supervision with Ms. Drake's therapist. At the next meeting, common goals and intervention strategies were discussed.

Intervention

Working with Ms. Drake, the nurse found, was not easy. Many times the nurse felt angry and frustrated with Ms. Drake when acting-out behaviors occurred. With supervision, Ms. McCarthy was better able to deal with her feelings. The nurse became better able to focus on Ms. Drake's actions and work with her to figure out what feelings and events triggered the actions. See Ms. Drake's nursing care plan, including interventions and rationales (Nursing Care Plan 16–2).

Evaluation

Ms. Drake appeared to come a long way in the three weeks she was on the unit. Her acting-out behaviors decreased. She had not threatened or attempted to mutilate herself in two weeks. Although her sessions with her therapist were often stormy, there was more discussion of feelings. Her pacing of the halls had decreased, and she appeared less tense most of the time. She still continued to ask for her antianxiety medication at frequent intervals but was willing to talk about what she thought the anxiety was about with both her primary nurse and the therapist. She agreed to continue therapy with her therapist on a biweekly basis after discharge.

Nursing Care Plan 16–2 ■ A PERSON WITH BORDERLINE PERSONALITY DISORDER: Ms. Drake

NURSING DIAGNOSIS

Moderate to severe anxiety **related to threat to self-concept, as evidenced by inability to relax**

Supporting Data

- States that she feels "empty."
- Is restless and tense.
- Requests antianxiety medication frequently.

Long Term Goal: Ms. Drake will state that she feels relaxed more than she feels tense by discharge.

Short Term Goal	Intervention	Rationale	Evaluation
1. By (date) Ms. Drake will state she is relaxed in a situation that usually produces anxiety (e.g., after visiting hours).	1a. Talk to client prior to event to help her observe and describe what she is expecting from the event.	1a. Understanding expectations that may or may not be met helps to identify source of anxiety and opens the way to more effective problem solving for unmet needs.	Goal met Client was able to discuss situation that was potentially anxiety provoking and appeared relaxed after discussion.
	1b. Engage client in physical activity, such as jogging or aerobics class.	1b. Exercise reduces physical tension and can increase endorphins, thereby increasing feelings of well-being.	Instead of pacing the halls today, she talked pleasantly with other clients after exercise class.

NURSING DIAGNOSIS

Ineffective individual coping **related to inadequate psychological resources, as evidenced by self-destructive behaviors**

Supporting Data

- After stating that she feels "frustrated," client goes on pass and returns with alcohol.
- After stating that she loves her therapist, client is found in bed with another client.
- After stating that she hates her primary nurse, client demands a new primary nurse.

Long Term Goal: Ms. Drake will solve problems in a manner that injures neither self nor others by (date).

Short Term Goal	Intervention	Rationale	Evaluation
1. By (date), Ms. Drake will discuss feelings of frustration and deal with them appropriately rather than act out.	1. Talk with client when she is frustrated regarding her goal, the block to the goal, and ways to either change the goal or reach it in an appropriate way.	1. Discussing and understanding the dynamics of frustration help to reduce the frustration by helping the client take positive action.	Goal met Ms. Drake was able to experience problems and deal with them appropriately. Acting out was minimal or absent. For example, client had an appointment for a job interview. She wanted to stay in bed and avoid the interview. Instead, she talked with the nurse about the fear of "growing up" and was able to get up and go to the interview.
2. By (date), Ms. Drake will discuss transference feelings and deal with them appropriately rather than act out.	2. Talk with client when she is experiencing strong positive or negative transference feelings, helping her to understand and experience all her feelings without acting them out.	2. Discussing and understanding the meaning of transference feelings and splitting help to reduce the potential for acting out.	

NURSING DIAGNOSIS

High risk for self-directed violence **related to anxiety and emptiness, as evidenced by suicidal gestures and poor impulse control**

Supporting Data

- Is admitted following self-mutilation.
- Threatens self-mutilation when anxious.
- Attempts self-mutilation on the unit.

Long Term Goal: Ms. Drake will state that she no longer has the desire to mutilate herself.

Short Term Goal	Intervention	Rationale	Evaluation
1. By (date) Ms. Drake will discuss desire to mutilate self rather than do so.	1a. Assist client in observing potential situations for self-mutilation.	1a–b. Observing, describing, and analyzing thoughts and feelings reduces the	Goal met Ms. Drake was able to experience troubling thoughts and

Continued on following page

Nursing Care Plan 16–2 ■ A PERSON WITH BORDERLINE			
PERSONALITY DISORDER: Ms. Drake *(Continued)*			

Short Term Goal	Intervention	Rationale	Evaluation
	1b. Talk with client about these situations, eliciting thoughts and feelings.	potential for acting them out destructively.	feelings without self-mutila-tion. Stated, "I was mad at my therapist today and de-cided to cut my arms after the session. Instead, I told her I was angry, and together we figured out why."
	1c. Encourage more appropriate ways to deal with these feelings.	1c. Offers alternative behav-iors that can be more satisfying and growth promoting.	
	1d. Take care to safeguard envi-ronment at times when staff is busy and client's anxiety is acute.	1d. Times of increased anxi-ety, frustration, or anger without external controls could increase probabil-ity of client self-mutilat-ing behaviors.	

Summary—Borderline Personality Disorders

Working with people with borderline personality dis-orders is a challenge to nurses and other health care professionals. These clients are recognizable by their highly unstable, angry, manipulative, and self-destruc-tive behaviors, which are derived from primitive de-fenses. These defenses mask extreme neediness, anger, and fear of separation from nurturance. They present unique nursing challenges and stir up irra-tional, uncomfortable feelings in nurses. Intervention is directed toward providing emotional consistency, exploring anger in appropriate ways, and promoting gradual separation-individuation.

References

American Psychiatric Association. Diagnostic and Statistical Manual of Mental Disorders, 3rd ed, revised (DSM-III-R). Washington, DC: American Psychiatric Association, 1987.

American Psychiatric Association. Diagnostic and Statistical Manual of Mental Disorders, 4th ed (DSM-IV). Washington, DC: American Psychiatric Association, 1994.

Berne E. Games People Play: The Psychology of Human Relation-ships. New York: Grove Press, 1964.

Cameron J. Paranoid conditions and paranoia. In Arieti S (ed). American Handbook of Psychiatry. New York: Basic Books, 1959, pp 475–484.

Chitty KK, Maynard CK. Managing manipulation. Journal of Psycho-social Nursing and Mental Health Services, 24(6):9, 1986.

Cleckley H. The Mask of Sanity, 4th ed. St. Louis: CV Mosby, 1964.

Eisendorfer A, Wikie F. Auditory changes in the aged. Journal of the American Geriatric Society, 8:377, 1972.

Farrington D. Early predictors of adolescent aggression and adult violence. Violence and Victims, 4(2):70, 1989.

Frosch JP. The treatment of antisocial and borderline personality disorders. Hospital and Community Psychiatry, 34:243, 1983.

Goldman SJ, Dangelo EG, Demaso DR, Mezzacappa E. Physical and sexual abuse histories among children with borderline personality disorders. American Journal of Psychiatry, 149(12):1723–1726, 1992.

Harrington A. Psychopaths. New York: Simon & Schuster, 1972.

Hurt SW, Clarkin JF. Borderline personality disorder: Prototype ty-pology and development of treatment manual. Psychiatric Annals, 20(1):13, 1990.

Kaplan HI, Sadock BJ. Synopsis of Psychiatry, 6th ed. Baltimore: Williams & Wilkins, 1991.

McCord WM. The Psychopath and Milieu Therapy. New York: Aca-demic Press, 1982.

McCord WM, McCord, J. The Psychopath: An Essay on the Criminal Mind. Princeton: D. Van Nostrand Company, 1956.

Masterson JF. Psychotherapy of the Borderline Adult. New York: Brunner-Mazel, 1976.

Masterson JF. The Search for the Real Self: Unmasking the Person-ality Disorders of Our Age. New York: The Free Press, 1988.

Modlin HC. The antisocial personality. Bulletin of the Menninger Clinic, 47:129, 1983.

Oxman T, Rosenberg S, Tucker G. The language of paranoia. Ameri-can Journal of Psychiatry, 139:257, 1982.

Perry JC, Vaillant GE. Personality disorders. In Kaplan HI, Sadock BJ (eds). Comprehensive Textbook of Psychiatry V, Baltimore: Wil-liams & Wilkins, 1989.

Quay HC, Love CT. The effect of a juvenile diversion program on rearrests. Criminal Justice and Behavior, 5:410, 1977.

Raine A, Mednick S. Biosocial longitudinal research into antisocial behavior. Review in Epidemiology, 37:515, 1989.

Reid WH (ed). The antisocial personality: A review. Hospital and Community Psychiatry, 36(8):831, 1985.

Rockford J, Weinaaple M, Goldstein L. The quantitative hemispheric EEG in adolescent psychiatric patients with depressive or para-noid symptomology. Biological Psychiatry, 16:47, 1981.

Selzer J. Borderline omnipotence in pathological gambling. Archives of Psychiatric Nursing, 6, 1992.

Shearer SL, et al. Frequency and correlation of childhood sexual and physical abuse histories in adult female borderline inpa-tients. American Journal of Psychiatry, 147(2):214, 1990.

Simmons D. Gender issues and borderline personality disorder: Why do females dominate the diagnosis? Archives of Psychiatric Nurs-ing, 6, 1992.

Smith MC, Lego S. The client who has a borderline personality disorder. In Lego S (ed). The American Handbook of Psychiatric Nursing. Philadelphia: JB Lippincott, 1984.

Smoyak SA. Borderline personality disorder (editorial). Journal of Psychosocial Nursing, 23:5, 1985.

Stevenson J, Meares R. An outcome study of psychotherapy for patients with borderline personality disorder. American Journal of Psychiatry, 149(3):358, 1992.

Stone MH. The Fate of the Borderline Patients. Successful Outcome and Psychiatric Practice. New York: Guilford Press, 1990.

Tansey MJ, Burke WF. Understanding Countertransference: From

Projective Identification to Empathy. Hillsdale, NJ: Analytic Press, 1989.

Vaillant GE, Perry JC. Personality disorders. *In* Kaplan HI, Sadock BJ (eds). Comprehensive Textbook of Psychiatry IV. Baltimore: Williams & Wilkins, 1985.

Wade TC. A family crises intervention approach to diversion from the criminal justice system. Juvenile Justice Journal, 7:230, 1977.

Further Reading

Beck CM, Rawlins RP, Williams SR (eds). Mental Health—Psychiatric Nursing. St. Louis: CV Mosby, 1984.

Clack J. Nursing intervention into the aggressive behavior of patients. *In* Burd SF, Marshall MA (eds). Some Clinical Approaches to Psychiatric Nursing. London: Macmillan, 1963.

Closurdo JS. Behavior modification and the nursing process. Perspectives in Psychiatric Care 13:25, 1975.

Epstein L. Countertransference with borderline patients. *In* Epstein L, Feiner AH (eds). Countertransference. New York: Jason Aronson, 1979.

Gerstlev L, Mclellan A, Alterman A, et al. Ability to form an alliance with the therapist: A possible marker of prognosis for patients with antisocial personality disorders. American Journal of Psychiatry, 146:508, 12, 1989.

Houseman C. The paranoid person: A bio-psychosocial perspective. Archives of Psychiatric Nursing, 4(3):176, 1990.

Kernberg OF. Borderline Conditions and Pathological Narcissism. New York: Jason Aronson, 1975.

Kernberg OF. Leadership and organizational functioning: Organization regression. International Journal of Group Psychotherapy, 28:1, 1978.

Kolb LC, Brodie HK. Modern Clinical Psychiatry, 10th ed. Philadelphia: WB Saunders, 1982.

Lanchance R,-Coles. Management of disturbed and aggressive be-havior in psychopaths. Canadian Journal of Psychiatry, 30:13, 1989.

Lewis DO, Bard JS. Multiple personality and forensic issues. Psychiatric Clinics of North America, 14(3):741, 1991.

Loomis ME. Nursing management of acting-out behavior. Perspectives in Psychiatric Care, 8:169, 1970.

MacKinnon RA, Michels R. The psychiatric interview in clinical practice. Philadelphia: WB Saunders, 1971.

Millon T. Disorders of Personality: DSM III: AXIS II. New York: John Wiley & Sons, 1981.

Reid WH (ed). The Treatment of Antisocial Syndromes. New York: Van Nostrand Reinhold Company, 1981.

Sass L. The borderline personality. The New York Times Magazine, 12, August 22, 1982.

Slever LJ, Davis KL. A psychobiological prospective on the personality disorders. American Journal of Psychiatry, 148(12):1647, 1991.

Stringer AY, Josef NC. Methylphenidate in the treatment of aggression in two patients with antisocial personality disorder. American Journal of Psychiatry, 140:1365, 1983.

Toch H. An interdisciplinary approach to criminal violence. Journal of Criminal Law and Criminology, 71:216, 1980.

Tousley M. The paranoid fortress of David J. Journal of Psychosocial Nursing, 22:8, 1984.

Vaillant P, Antonowicz D. Cognitive behavior therapy and social skills training improves personality and cognition in incarcerated offenders. Psychological Reports, 68:27, 1991.

Wilson H, Kneisl C. Psychiatric Nursing, 3rd ed. Menlo Park, CA: Addison-Wesley, 1988.

Winshnie H. The Impulsive Personality. New York: Plenum Press, 1977.

Zamora LC. Anger. *In* Haber J, Leach AM, Schudy SM, et al. (eds). Comprehensive Psychiatric Nursing, 2nd ed. New York: McGraw-Hill, 1982.

Self-study Exercises

ANTISOCIAL PERSONALITY DISORDERS

Place a T (true) or an F (false) next to the possible backgrounds of those children who grow up to have an antisocial personality.

1. _____T_____ They are born to parents who reject them.
2. _____F_____ Parents of antisocial clients have had a fulfilling childhood.
3. _____T_____ As children, antisocial clients were generally exposed to abuse, violent tempers, and cruelty.
4. _____F_____ Authority, goals, and identification of role models were present for these children.

Write a few sentences in answer to the following:

5. Discuss the current thinking regarding the role of anxiety and guilt as they relate to the antisocial personality disorders.

6. Name four behaviors commonly observed in people with antisocial personality disorders.

7. Discuss five steps in setting limits on manipulation.

Multiple choice

8. Choose the characteristic that is *not* common to *all* personality disorders.

    A. Ineffective and maladaptive responses to stress
    B. Difficulty in working and loving
    C. Evokes interpersonal conflict
    D. Always gets into trouble with the law; has no conscience

9. A nurse working with a person diagnosed as antisocial may experience all of the following *except*

    A. Anger
    B. Put-down
    C. Fear
    D. Adoration
    E. True intimacy

10. Choose the least effective therapeutic modality for an antisocial client.

    A. Behavior therapy
    B. Therapy based on modeling
    C. Psychotherapy
    D. Change in social setting

11. The treatment plan for a client with antisocial traits consisted of rewarding him with privileges when he acted appropriately. This is referred to as

    A. Modeling behavior
    B. Cognitive therapy
    C. Civil treatment
    D. Behavior modification

PARANOID PERSONALITY DISORDER

Multiple choice

12. The trait *least* likely observed in a person with a paranoid personality disorder would be

    A. Distortion of reality
    B. Rigidity
    C. Somatic delusions
    D. Hypervigilance

13. The nurse can identify clues to paranoid thinking by *except*:

    A. Listening for themes of denial and projection
    B. Identify specific behaviors, such as suspiciousness and acting superior
    C. Identify personal feelings and reactions to the client
    D. Checking the client medical evaluation

14. When working with a patient with a paranoid defensive structure, the approach that will cause the most difficulty would be a/an

    A. Honest, straightforward approach
    B. Warm, empathetic, and enthusiastic approach

C. Respectful approach
D. Neutral but concerned approach

Place a T (true) or an F (false) next to the possible countertransference reactions a nurse may have to a patient with paranoid personality disorder.

15. __T__ Getting angry with client
16. __T__ Wanting to defend actions
17. __F__ Feeling empathy and concern
18. __T__ Getting into power struggles or arguments
19. __F__ Wanting to rescue the client
20. __T__ Wishing to control the patient

Place a T (true) or an F (false) next to these methods for interviewing a paranoid person.

21. __F__ Avoid setting limits
22. __T__ Provide structure
23. __F__ Interpret the client's behavior to him, i.e., identify what is going on that makes him or her suspicious.
24. __T__ Focus on client's feelings and behaviors.
25. __T__ Help client think through consequences of his or her behavior.

BORDERLINE PERSONALITY DISORDERS

Place a T (true) or an F (false) next to the characteristics of a borderline client according to the DSM-III-R.

26. __T__ Impulsive behavior that is self-damaging, e.g., promiscuity, gambling, overeating, or overspending.
27. __F__ Extreme paranoia, e.g., client thinks people are poisoning or out to hurt him or her.
28. __T__ Relationships intense and very unstable, marked by devaluation and idealization.
29. __F__ Great need to be perfect; very compulsive regarding hygiene and work habits.
30. __T__ Inability to tolerate being alone; chronic feelings of boredom.
31. __F__ Very withdrawn behavior; does not like to call attention to self.
32. __T__ Inappropriate intense anger; problem with impulse control.
33. __T__ Identity disturbances; questions self-image, gender identity, or career goals.
34. __F__ Given to flights of mania when limits are set on impulsive behavior.
35. __T__ Frequent impulsive suicidal gestures or self-mutilation.

Multiple choice

36. Choose the defensive maneuver that is *not* readily used by the borderline client to reduce anxiety or get needs met.

A. Splitting
B. Manipulation
C. Projection
D. Sublimation

Short answer

37. List behavioral outcomes of a successful therapeutic intervention in a borderline personality disorder.

   A. _____
   B. _____
   C. _____

38. Name three nursing diagnoses that could be used with a borderline client.

   A. _____
   B. _____
   C. _____

39. Give the nursing intervention and the rationale for the following behaviors frequently seen in borderline clients:

   A. Hostility_____
   _____

   B. Self-destructive_____
   _____

   C. Demanding_____
   _____

Circle the correct letters

40. Circle *only* the personal reactions nurses and other health care providers may experience when working with a borderline client.

   A. Need to "rescue" client from others.
   B. Feelings of intense love or attachment toward client.
   C. Feeling comfortable soon after establishing a good working relationship.
   D. Contemptuous, jealous, and envious of how client gets attention.
   E. Finding that the client quickly learns appropriate ways to solve problems.
   F. Emotionally exposed and vulnerable related to the client's "partly true" projections.

PEOPLE IN SEVERE TO PANIC LEVELS OF CHRONIC ANXIETY

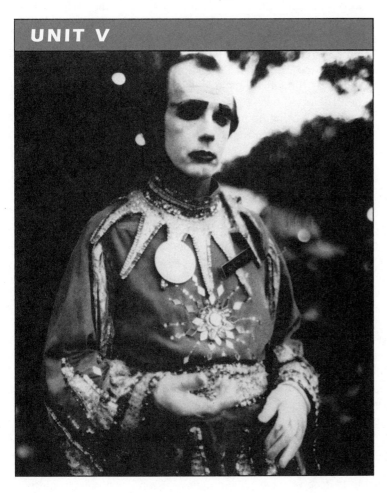

UNIT V

Most of us don't look at things, we look at aspects of things. Our interests are specific. We don't see people, we see clothes or bodies or mirrors of our performance, or we see symptoms of wealth or grace or intellect or sensuality. And slowly we become what we look at most.

HUGH PRATHER, NOTES ON
LOVE AND COURAGE

A Nurse Speaks

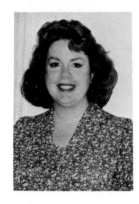

by Anne Cowley Herzog

<u>Danny</u>

I met Danny (not his real name) on a soggy Saturday morning. It doesn't rain often in southern California, but when it does, it can be torrential. Danny was standing on the doorstep of our small psychiatric facility looking like he was about to float away.

He was a short young man, perhaps 5'1" or 5'2". His dirty blond hair was stuck to his very small head. He didn't wear a coat or jacket despite the chilly temperature, and he was coughing and sneezing badly. As he stood there, telling me that the voices in his head were telling him to walk out into the street and in front of a truck, he had an impish grin on his face and big dimples on his grimy cheeks. I didn't know what to make of him.

We brought Danny in and I started to evaluate him for admission. Taking a history was difficult because he often replied to a question with "I don't know." He also seemed quite distracted by the environment. Although Danny seemed tired, he fidgeted in his chair. When I referred back to his statement about the "voices," he didn't seem to know what I was talking about and stated that he hadn't heard any for a long time. Among other things, I learned that he could neither read nor write.

I may have had difficulty gathering a clear history, but on physical examination, Danny had plenty of problems that could easily be noted. His lungs were full of coarse rhonchi bilaterally. His neck, trunk, arms, and legs had multiple bruises and abrasions in various stages of healing. In addition, there was a large, nasty, infected cut on his right shin. He also had copious red-brown, foul-smelling discharge from his left ear. He was extremely thin and rather pale. At no time during the examination did Danny question or object to anything I asked him to do. In fact, he made several little jokes and was very compliant.

As I was finishing the preliminary assessment, Eve (not her real name), a nurse that had been on staff for some time, happened by. She greeted Danny by name. When I seemed surprised that she knew him, she stated, "Danny gets admitted every time it rains." With that, he joined in that he really liked our "place." It was "much better than the others."

An aide took Danny off to the shower, and I went to talk with Eve. She explained the situation to me kindly but with a chuckle because I hadn't recognized what was going on. Danny was moderately developmentally delayed, had some schizophrenic symptomatology, and was homeless. He had been placed in a board and care several times, but he was often the scapegoat of more aggressive residents and would then run away. Danny managed fairly well on the streets, using the local shelter and soup kitchens intermittently. He had a few friends who helped look out for him and protected him from bully attacks when possible. He had no address and was therefore unable to receive most government assistance. Of course, he had no medical insurance. When the weather got bad, competition at the shelters was fierce, and he often could not find room. So, he would arrive at a facility and talk about voices and self-harm. Eve said, "He's learned how to use the system. He's not here to get psychiatric care. He wants three hots and a cot."

Although that seemed to make some sense, I didn't want to believe that we couldn't (read that I couldn't) make a difference in this young man's life. He had restricted cognitive function, no safe environment, and little hope of a better future. Surely *something* could be done.

I phoned the counselor on call that weekend. Margie was fresh from school and enthusiastic. We brainstormed about what could be started immediately and what would have to wait until Monday. When Danny was finished with his shower and was dressed in clean dry clothes from the lost and found, I talked with him about what we would like to do: begin treatment for his various mental and physical needs, have him evaluated for vocational training, get him into a supportive board and care, and so on. He seemed mildly polite about everything but not excited about anything. He really wanted to go watch TV!

In the best of all possible worlds, this story would end with my reporting that Danny now works full-time in a sheltered environment, has improved his problem-solving capabilities, has increased self-esteem, and is a happy member of society. However, it didn't work out quite that way. We were able to help him with some problems during his admission and then found a temporary slot for him in a local board and care. Later, he went back out on the streets. He died a few months later after a beating from an unknown assailant.

CHAPTER 17

Alterations in Mood: Grief and Depression

Elizabeth M. Varcarolis

OUTLINE •

KEY TERMS AND CONCEPTS • • • • • • • • • • • • • • • •

**The key terms and concepts listed here also appear in bold where they are
defined or discussed in this chapter.**

ANERGIA

ANHEDONIA

ANTICIPATORY GRIEF

ATYPICAL ANTIDEPRESSANTS

DELAYED GRIEF

DYSTHYMIA

GRIEF

HYPERSOMNIA

MAJOR DEPRESSION

MONOAMINE OXIDASE INHIBITORS
 (MAOIs)

MOOD

MOURNING

PHENOMENA EXPERIENCED DURING MOURNING

PRIMARY AND SECONDARY DEPRESSIONS

PROLONGED GRIEF

PSYCHOMOTOR AGITATION

PSYCHOMOTOR RETARDATION

SEASONAL AFFECTIVE DISORDER (SAD)

SECONDARY GAINS

TRICYCLIC ANTIDEPRESSANTS (TCAs)

VEGETATIVE SIGNS OF DEPRESSION

Mood refers to a prolonged emotion that colors a person's whole psychic life (APA 1987). *Joy, grief, elation,* and *sadness* are all terms used to describe a particular mood.

Normal moods are universal experiences. Happiness and unhappiness are appropriate responses to life events. When sadness, grief, or elation is extremely intense and the mood is unduly prolonged, a mood disorder results.

Mood disorders, also referred to as affective disorders, are divided into two general categories according to the DSM-III-R and DSM-IV classifications: *bipolar disorders* and *depressive disorders*. This chapter discusses grief and the depressive disorders. Chapter 18 discusses the bipolar disorders.

Grief

OBJECTIVES ■

After studying this section on grief, the student will be able to

1. Discuss the three phases of Engel's acute stage (4–8 weeks) of mourning.
2. Give examples of five phenomena people may experience during the long term stage (1–2 years) of mourning.
3. Describe two pathological grief reactions.
4. Discuss five nursing interventions for a family that is grieving.
5. Identify when the work of mourning has been successful.
6. List six factors that can negatively affect the successful work of mourning.

Change is a part of life, and every change involves loss and gain. People come and go in our lives. As we gain experience, we lose our youth—dreams are realized or hopes abandoned. We are constantly faced with giving up one mode of life for another.

Loss is part of the human experience, and grief is the normal response to loss. The loss may be of a relationship (divorce, separation, death, or abortion), of health (a body function or part, or mental or physical capacity), of status or prestige, of security (occupational, financial, social, or cultural), of self-confidence, of a dream, of self-concept, or symbolic. Other losses include changes in circumstances, such as retirement, promotion, marriage, or aging. All losses affect a person's self-concept. People undergoing therapy may grieve as they give up old, familiar —although maladaptive—ways of viewing the world. A loss can be real or perceived. Athough grief and loss are universal experiences, loss through death is a major life crisis (Davis 1992; Parker 1972).

In this chapter, **grief** refers to the subjective feelings and affect that are precipitated by a loss. The term **mourning** refers to the processes (grief work) by which grief is resolved.

Grief is not a mood disorder, although a depressive syndrome is often part of the grieving process. Grief is the normal response to a significant loss. Although it is a normal phenomenon, it may at times be the focus of treatment.

Zisook and Shuchter's (1992) study of 350 widows and widowers found that

1. A depressive episode, as defined by the DSM-III-R, is common within the first year after the death of a spouse.
2. The depressive episode may occur not only in the early months of bereavement but later as well.
3. Among the individuals at highest risk for depressive episodes 13 months *after* their loss were those:
   • Who were younger widows and widowers
   • Who had past histories of depression
   • Who perceived themselves to be in poor health

Mourning is a distinct psychological process. This process involves disengaging strong emotional ties from a significant relationship and reinvesting those ties in a new and productive direction. This reinvestment of emotional energy into new relationships or creative activities is necessary for a person's mental health and future in society. When the grieving process is successful, the griever is released from one interpersonal relationship and able to form new relationships. The entire process of mourning may take a year or more to complete.

A number of theorists have studied the grief process. Some of the most widely known are George Engel, Colin Parkes, Elizabeth Kübler-Ross, Erich Lindemann, John Bowlby, and Edgar Jackson. Although each theorist uses different terminology, the process outlined by them is basically the same. Each describes commonly experienced psychological and behavioral characteristics. These characteristics follow a pattern of response:

1. Shock and disbelief
2. Sensation of somatic distress
3. Preoccupation with the image of the deceased
4. Guilt
5. Anger
6. Change in conduct behavior (e.g., depression, disorganization, or restlessness)
7. Reorganization of behavior directed toward a new object or activity

A person may demonstrate a different clinical picture at each of the stages of mourning. Each stage of grieving has its own characteristics, and the duration and form of each stage may vary considerably from person to person. People react within their own value and personality structure, as well as within their social environment and cultural patterns. Essentially, people are preprogrammed in their response to death. Distinct characteristics, however, can be identified throughout the grieving process.

The process of mourning is often divided into stages. The stages have been identified by Engel as (1) acute and (2) long term.

Acute Stage

The acute state (4–8 weeks) involves shock and disbelief, developing awareness, and restitution.

SHOCK AND DISBELIEF. The bereaved's first response is that of *denial*. The person is emotionally unable to accept his or her terrible loss. Denial functions as a buffer against intolerable pain and allows the person to acknowledge the reality of death slowly. The mourner may appear to be functioning in a robot-like fashion. Often, the bereaved person feels numb. A death may be "accepted" intellectually during this stage—"It's just as well; she was suffering"—although the emotional responses are still repressed. Denial is an important and needed defense and may last a few hours to a few days. *Denial that persists for longer than a few days could indicate difficulty in progressing through the process of mourning.*

DEVELOPING AWARENESS. As denial fades, painful feelings begin to surface. The finality of the loved one's death becomes more of a reality. Waves of anguish and pain are experienced and may be localized in the chest or epigastric area. *Anger* often surfaces at this time. It is not uncommon for doctors and nurses to be the subject of blame. Awareness by staff that anger is often displaced onto people in the hospital environment may decrease defensive staff behaviors. *Guilt* is often experienced, and the bereaved blames him- or herself for taking or failing to take specific actions. Impulsive and self-destructive acts by the mourner, such as pushing one's hand through a window or beating one's head against the wall, may be seen. *Crying* is a common phenomenon during this stage. "It is during this time that the greatest degree of anguish or despair, within the limits imposed by cultural patterns, is experienced or expressed" (Engel 1964). Crying can afford a welcome release from pent-up anguish and tension. Assessment of cultural patterns is important for making clinical judgments about the appropriateness of the bereaved's behavior. Not crying can be the result of cultural programming or environmental restraints. The person may cry in private. *Inability to cry*, however, may be the result of a high degree of ambivalence toward the deceased. A *person who is unable to cry may have difficulty in successfully completing the work of mourning.*

RESTITUTION. Restitution is the formal ritualistic phase of mourning during the acute stage. It is the institutionalization of mourning: it brings friends and family together in the rites of the funeral service and serves to emphasize the finality of death. The viewing of the body, the lowering of the casket, and the various religious and cultural rituals all help the bereaved shed any residual denial in an atmosphere of support. Every human society has its own moral and cultural standards according to which the rituals of mourning take place. The gathering in ritualistic farewell for the deceased provides support and sustenance for the family.

Long Term Stage

After the acute stage has been completed, the main work of mourning goes on intrapsychically for one to two years. The various **phenomena experienced during mourning** by the bereaved are described in Table 17–1.

Unresolved Grief Reaction

Most bereaved persons resolve their loss over time and resume their lives. However, unresolved grief reactions have been called the hidden disease and may account for many of the physical symptoms seen in doctors' offices and hospital units. The "broken heart syndrome" is supported by statistics that show surviving spouses die within a year of their husbands or wives at a much higher rate than do members of control groups (Carr 1985). In some cases, bereaved persons go to pieces, neglect themselves, do not eat, turn to alcohol or drugs, and become susceptible to physical disease. Often the disease is a direct reaction to an emotional loss. Several studies have shown that the health of widows and close relatives declines within one year of bereavement, and medical and psychiatric problems increase (Bowlby and Parkes 1970; Carr 1985).

Normally, reactions to a loss may occur throughout life. However, two specific atypical reactions to grief have been identified: prolonged grief and delayed grief.

In **prolonged grief,** the bereaved remains intensely preoccupied with the memories of the deceased many years after the person has died.

Mrs. Green has lived by herself since her husband died five years ago. When her nephew comes to visit, he finds everything as it was five years ago. Mr. Green's coat is still on the hook in the front hall, and his slippers are by the day bed where he used to nap. Mrs. Green talks tearfully of how much she misses him and mentions many incidents in their life together.

In **delayed grief,** a person may not experience the pain of loss; however, that pain is modified by chronic depression, intense preoccupation with body functioning (hypochondriasis), phobic reactions, or acute insomnia. Suicidal thinking should always be assessed in a person experiencing a pathological grief response, especially if depression is the presenting symptom. Hallucinations, delusions, or obsessions may be seen. These symptoms may not surface for months or years after the death.

Sidney Bolla's wife died of cancer three years ago. Everyone remarked how well he handled himself and how well he did after the funeral was over. He was always a quiet man and kept to himself. Mr. Bolla starts getting severe anxiety attacks one day while in the supermarket. As time progresses, he becomes fearful of going out and suffers from severe insomnia. A neighbor brings him to the hospital when he develops pneumonia and is too fearful to go outside of the house to seek medical attention.

Reactions And Feelings to Death and Dying

Culture plays an important part in the responses called forth in the face of death and dying. Our capacity to grieve stems from our view of death. In contemporary American society, there is a strong denial of death, growing old, and becoming sick (Benton 1978). Rakoff (1973) states:

America conjured into its superficial stereotype, is a country of the eternal now, of the young, face lifting, good teeth into the seventies, old ladies in Bermuda shorts, hair colored at will, endless euphemisms for chronic disease, affliction and death.

Denial and fear of death are strong in the American culture. This denial and fear affect the behavioral responses of the bereaved, the family, and those who support the family in the face of death. Nurses are affected by cultural myths in the same way as the rest of society. When faced with a person who is dying, nurses remember their own losses. Difficult memories and unresolved feelings are often awakened. When

Table 17-1 ■ NURSING ASSESSMENT: PHENOMENA EXPERIENCED DURING MOURNING

SYMPTOMS	EXAMPLES
Sensation of Somatic Distress	
Tightness in the throat, shortness of breath, sighing, "mental pain," exhaustion. Food tastes like sand; things feel unreal. Pain or discomfort may be identical to the symptoms experienced by the dead person. Normally symptoms are brief.	A woman whose husband died of a stroke complains of weakness and numbness on her left side.
Preoccupation with the Image of the Deceased	
The bereaved brings up and thinks and talks about numerous memories of the deceased. The memories are positive. This process goes on with great sadness. The idealization of the deceased lets the bereaved relive the gratifications associated with the deceased and helps resolve any guilt the bereaved has toward the deceased. The bereaved may also take on many of the mannerisms of the deceased through identification. Identification serves the purpose of holding onto the deceased. Preoccupation with the dead person takes many months before it lessens.	A man whose wife just died states, "I just can't stop thinking about my wife. Everything I see reminds me of her. We picked up this seashell on our honeymoon. I remember every wonderful moment we had together. The pain is so great, but the memories just keep coming." His friends notice that when he talks, his hand gestures and expressions are very like those of his recently deceased wife.
Guilt	
The bereaved reproaches him- or herself for real or fancied acts of negligence or omissions in the relationship with the deceased.	"I should have made him go to the doctor sooner." "I should have paid more attention to her, been more thoughtful."
Anger	
The anger the bereaved experiences may not be toward the object that gives rise to it. Often the anger is displaced on to the medical or nursing staff. Often it is directed toward the deceased. The anger is at its height during the first month but is often intermittent throughout the first year. The overflow of hostility disturbs the bereaved, resulting in the feeling that he or she is going "mad" or "insane."	"The doctor didn't operate in time. If he had, Mary would be alive today." "How could he leave me like this . . . how could he?"
Change in Behavior (Depression, Disorganization, Restlessness)	
A person may exhibit marked restlessness and an inability to organize his or her behavior. Routine activities take a long time to do. Depressive mood is common as the year passes and as the intensity of the grief declines. Absence of depression is more "abnormal" than its presence. Loneliness and aimlessness are most pronounced six to nine months after the death.	Six months after her husband died, Mrs. Faye stated, "I just can't seem to function, I have a hard time doing the simplest tasks. I can't be bothered with socializing." "I feel so down . . . so, so empty."
Reorganization of Behavior Directed Toward a New Object or Activity	
Gradually the person renews his or her interest in people and activities. The grieving thus releases the bereaved from one interpersonal relationship, and new ones are free to take its place.	Twenty months after her husband's death, Mrs. Faye tells a friend, "I'll be away this weekend. I am going fishing with my brother and his friend. This is the first time I've felt like doing anything since Harry died."

Table 17–2 ■ NURSING INTERVENTIONS AND RATIONALES: GRIEVING FAMILIES

INTERVENTION	RATIONALE
Nursing Diagnosis: *Family grieving* **related to loss of family member or significant other**	
1. At the death or imminent death of a family member: ● Communicate the news to the family in an area of privacy. ● If only one family member is available, stay with that member until clergy, a family member, or a friend arrives. ● If the nurse feels unable to handle the situation, the aid of another who can support the family should be enlisted.	● Family members can support each other in an atmosphere in which they can behave naturally. ● The presence and comfort of the nurse during the initial stage of shock can help minimize feelings of acute isolation and anxiety. ● The individual or family will need support, answers to questions, and guidance as to immediate tasks and information.
2. If the family requests to see and take leave of the dying or dead person: ● Always grant this request.	● The need to take leave can be of overwhelming importance for some—to kiss good-bye, ask for forgiveness, or take a lock of hair. This helps people face the reality of death.
3. If angry family members accuse the nurse or doctor of abusing or mismanaging the care of the deceased: ● Continue to provide the best care for the dying or final care to the dead. Avoid becoming involved in angry and painful arguments and power struggles.	● Complaints are not directed toward the nurse personally. The anger may serve the purpose of keeping grieving relatives from falling apart. Projected anger may be an attempt to deal with aggression and guilt toward the dying person.
4. If relatives behave in a grossly disturbed manner (e.g., refuse to acknowledge the truth, collapse, or lose control): ● Show patience and tact, and offer sympathy and warmth. ● Encourage the person to cry. ● Provide a place of privacy for grieving.	● Shock and disbelief are the first responses to the news of death, and people need ways to protect themselves from the overwhelming reality of loss. ● Crying helps provide relief from feelings of acute pain and tension. ● Privacy facilitates the natural expression of grief.
5. If the family requests specific religious, cultural, or social customs strange or unknown to the nurse: ● The nurse helps facilitate steps necessary for the family to carry out the desired arrangements.	● Institutional mourning rituals of various cultures provide important external supports for the grief-stricken person.

Data from Engel GL. Grief and grieving. American Journal of Nursing, 64(9):93, 1964.

staff members have not been able to resolve their own conflicts with death, their ability to help others is minimized. Psychological support needs to be available to help staff better understand the grieving process. When nurses examine their own feelings and their personal experience of loss, verbal and nonverbal clues to the needs of a grieving family member of a dying patient become more apparent (Marks 1976).

Sometimes, nurses grieve with family members at the death of a person they have cared for and become fond of. Sometimes an entire staff may mourn the death of a client.

Helping People Grieve

Prolonged and serious alterations in social adjustment, as well as medical diseases, may develop in the absence of proper management during a grief reaction. The nurse's essential task is sharing the client's grief work.

Most important in handling acute grief are talking and listening. The helping person should keep his or her own talking to a minimum. Banal advice and philosophical statements are useless. Unhelpful responses by others, such as "He's no longer suffering" or "You can always have another child" or "It's better this way," can lead the bereaved to believe that others do not understand his or her acute pain and that the personal impact of the loss is being minimized. Such statements can compound feelings of isolation.

More helpful responses are, "His death will be a terrible loss" or "No one can replace her" or "He will be missed for a long time." Statements such as these validate the bereaved's experience of loss and communicate the message that the bereaved is understood and supported.

Talking by the bereaved can serve the purpose of releasing negative emotions. When a person is faced with an unwanted loss, strong feelings of anger, guilt, and hate are normal reactions that need to be expressed to facilitate the process of mourning. It is important that someone listen and encourage the expression of feelings surrounding the person's loss or anticipated loss.

Psychotherapy over six to ten sessions has been found to be helpful during the crisis period. At a later stage, the use of 15 sessions or more has been found to have a good outcome. More complicated or pathological patterns of grief may require special techniques, such as "regrief work" (Middleton and Raphael 1992).

Nurses frequently encounter people faced with loss. For example, on maternity and pediatric units, parents may be anticipating the loss of a terminally ill child **(anticipatory grief)** or experiencing the loss of a stillborn baby. Here the focus of intervention is facilitating the family's mourning. Specific guidelines the nurse can use in the general hospital setting with families of dying or deceased clients are described in Table 17–2.

Resolution of Grief

The work of mourning is over when the bereaved can remember realistically both the pleasures and the disappointments of the lost loved one.

If, after a normal period of time (12–24 months), a person has not completed the grieving process, reassessment and re-evaluation are indicated.

Some of the factors that can affect the successful completion of the mourning process are

1. *The level of dependency in the relationship.* The more dependent the mourner was on the deceased, the more difficult the resolution of the loss.
2. *The degree of ambivalence in the relationship.* Persistent,

unresolved conflicts interfere with successful grief work.
3. *The age of the deceased.* The death of a child may have a more profound effect than that of an older person.
4. *The bereaved person's support system.* A person with few meaningful relationships will have more difficulty letting go of ties with the deceased.
5. *The number of previous losses.* Present losses can trigger the pain of past losses. Unresolved feelings from past losses can complicate the present grief process.
6. *The physical and psychological health of the person grieving.* These factors greatly affect a person's capacity for grief work.

Summary

The process of mourning is a distinct psychological process and is the normal reaction to a loss. A loss can be real or perceived. Types of losses include the loss of a person, the loss of security, the loss of self-confidence, and the loss of a dream. Essentially, the loss results in the loss of self-concept.

The stage of acute grief may last from four to eight weeks; the complete process of mourning (*long term stage*) may take a year or two, or longer. (see Table 17–1).

Culture greatly affects patterns of response to death and dying in both clients and nurses. Grief can reactivate distressing feelings of previous losses in health care workers. If a nurse has unresolved issues of grief and depression, the nurse's ability to help others is greatly minimized. Staff members need psychological support when they work with people who are grieving. Two specific atypical grief reactions are prolonged grief and delayed grief.

Grief work is successful when specific phenomena identified with the process have been experienced. A person in mourning should be given time to talk and relive memories in the presence of a caring person who can share the pain. Guidelines for nursing interventions in a family that is grieving are outlined in Table 17–2.

The work of mourning is complete when the bereaved can remember realistically both the pleasures and the disappointments of the lost relationship. A number of factors can affect the normal process of mourning.

Self-study exercises 1–21 at the end of this chapter will help the student review material covered in this section.

Depressive Disorders

OBJECTIVES ■

After studying this section on depressive disorders, the student will be able to

1. Compare and contrast major depression and dysthymia.
2. Discuss four theories of the etiology of depression.
3. Identify possible behaviors for each of the following areas when assessing a depressed client: (a) affect, (b) thought processes, (c) feelings, (d) physical behavior, (e) communication, and (f) indications of masked depression.
4. Write five nursing diagnoses for a client who is depressed, and include a long term goal and a short term goal for each diagnosis.
5. Name three unrealistic expectations a nurse may have while working with a depressed person that can result in increased feelings of anxiety in the nurse.
6. Identify at least six principles of communication appropriate for a depressed client.
7. Name three interventions and rationales regarding the physical needs of depressed clients in each of the following categories: nutrition, elimination, rest and sleep, hygiene, and activities and recreation.
8. Discuss nursing considerations in administering tricyclic antidepressants, including (a) common side effects, (b) adverse side effects, and (c) drugs that can trigger an adverse reaction.
9. Name two common side effects of the monoamine oxidase inhibitors, and state one serious adverse reaction and the appropriate medical intervention.
10. Identify five foods and four drugs contraindicated with the use of the monoamine oxidase inhibitors.
11. Discuss four atypical antidepressants, and name one indication for each.
12. Describe the procedure used in electroconvulsive therapy, and state two important nursing actions before, during, and after treatment.

Depression, elation, anger, and anxiety are common examples of universally experienced alterations in mood. A **mood** is a "pervasive and sustained emotion that, in the extreme, markedly colors the perception of the world" (APA 1994).

A depressed mood is the most common presenting problem encountered by mental health professionals. Indeed, about 10% of all people seeking medical advice from their family doctor suffer mild to moderate degrees of depression. Unfortunately, doctors often fail to recognize these conditions (Bech 1992). *Depression* is a term that can be used in many ways. *Depression* can refer to a symptom, a syndrome, or a disorder or illness (Zisook and Shuchter 1992).

A depressive illness is painful and can be debilitating. Many well-known and highly creative people have suffered from severe depressions, such as Sigmund Freud, Winston Churchill, Ernest Hemingway, Marilyn Monroe, and Sylvia Plath, Albert Camus, and William James.

The author William Styron, in his book *Darkness Visible: A Memoir of Madness* (1990), describes his depression as a "howling tempest in the brain." He writes further:

Rational thought was usually absent from my mind at those times, hence trance. I can think of no more opposite word for this state of being, a condition of helpless stupor in which cognition was replaced by that "positive and active anguish" . . . The libido made an early exit . . . Many people lose all appetite . . . My few hours of sleep were usually terminated at three or four in the morning, when I stared up into yawning darkness, wondering and writhing at the devastation taking place in my mind.

Most people experience a normal lowering of mood in response to various stressful life events. However, about 15% of the general population experience a depressive episode during their lifetime. A depressive episode is one that usually warrants some kind of treatment. However, only one of four people actually receive treatment for depression (Abraham et al. 1991). Figure 17–1 identifies depression on a continuum from the clinical depression often experienced in a normal grief reaction to an actual mood disorder, dysthymia or a major depression.

When moods become severe or prolonged or affect a person's occupational or interpersonal functioning, the alteration in mood may constitute a mood disorder. The mood disorders in the DSM-IV include the (1) depressive disorders and (2) bipolar disorders. This chapter discusses the depressive disorders, and Chapter 18 covers bipolar disorders.

A depressive illness can be precipitated by various factors. For example, some environmental events are more likely than others to trigger the onset of depression. Death in the family is the most common precipitator of depression. The anniversary of the death of a loved one can precipitate depression in some. The second most common precipitators are separation and divorce. The third is physical illness, followed by a sexual identity threat, work failures, and disappointment in a child (Goodwin 1982).

Depression and fatigue can be important indications of various *medical disorders*, such as hepatitis, mononucleosis, multiple sclerosis, and cancer. About 10–15% or more of major depressive conditions are caused by general medical illness or other conditions (US Department of Health and Human Services 1993).

A depressive syndrome frequently accompanies other *psychiatric disorders*, such as schizophrenia, psychoactive substance dependence disorder, or eating disorders. Therefore, a depressive syndrome can occur as part of a physical illness, another psychiatric disorder, or an organic mental disorder. When it does occur as part of an organic mental disorder or another nonmood psychiatric disorder, the depression is labeled **secondary depression.**

When depression is not secondary to any other process, it is considered to be **primary depression.** The two main primary depressive disorders are (1) major depression and (2) dysthymia.

MAJOR DEPRESSION. In a **major depression,** there is a history of one or more major depressive episodes and no history of manic or hypomanic episodes. In a major depression, the symptoms often interfere with the person's social or occupational functioning and in some cases may include psychotic features. The emotional, cognitive, and behavioral symptoms an individual exhibits during a major depressive episode represent change in the person's usual functioning. When the symptoms of a major depressive episode have subsided, there is usually complete remission, and people are without significant symptoms of depression for two months or more (APA 1991).

DYSTHYMIA. Dysthymia (depressive neurosis) is mild to moderate in degree and characterized by a chronic depressive syndrome that is usually present for many years. The depressive mood disturbance, because of its chronic nature, cannot be distinguished from the person's usual pattern of functioning (APA 1987). Because the individual has minimal social and occupational impairment, hospitalization is rarely necessary unless the person becomes suicidal. The age of onset varies from the early and middle teens to late in life. These clients are at risk for developing major depressive episodes as well as other psychiatric disorders (Hirschfeld and Goodwin 1988). Figure 17–2 shows the diagnostic criteria for depression.

Differentiating a major depression from dysthymia can be difficult because both disorders have similar symptoms. The main differences are in the duration and severity of the symptoms (APA 1994).

SEASONAL AFFECTIVE DISORDER. Another depressive pattern that has received recent attention is **seasonal affective disorder (SAD).** Seasonal depressions have been recorded by physicians since the time of Hippocrates, around 400 B.C. However, it was not until the 1980s that the study of SAD and the effects of light on humans initiated increased interest and biomedical research. Depression seems to appear with a higher frequency in winter (usually beginning in October and November). Characteristic symptoms of winter depression noted in patients with SAD are hypersomnia, fatigue, weight gain, irritability, interpersonal difficulties, decreased libido, and social withdrawal (Oren and Rosenthal 1992; Hirschfeld and Goodwin 1988). The symptoms are not those of classic depression, and they resemble those of atypical depression. People with SAD winter depressions state that they both crave and consume more carbohydrate-rich foods in the winter. Untreated SAD depressive episodes are generally resolved by springtime. Patients with SAD may experience a reversal of their winter symptoms in summer: elation, increase in libido and social activity, and diminished sleep requirements, appetite, and weight (Oren and Rosenthal 1992). Interestingly, many people among the general population may experience mild seasonal symptoms.

Clients with SAD appear to respond to two to three

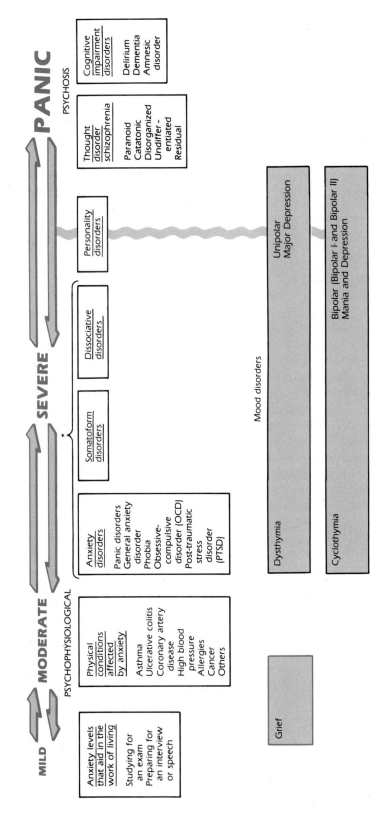

Figure 17–1. *Mental health continuum for grief and depression.*

*These disorders are currently classified by presenting clinical symptoms. Previously they were called "neurotic" disorders.

MAJOR DEPRESSIVE DISORDER

1. Represents a change in previous functions

2. The symptoms cause clinically significant distress or impair social, occupational or other important areas of functioning

3. Five or more of the following occur nearly every day for most waking hours over the same two-week period:

   • Depressed mood

   • Anhedonia

   • Significant weight loss or gain (more than 5% of body weight in one month)

   • Insomnia or hypersomnia

   • Increased or decreased motor activity

   • Anergia (fatigue or loss of energy)

   • Feelings of worthlessness or inappropriate guilt (may be delusional)

   • Decreased concentration or indecisiveness

   • Recurrent thoughts of death or suicidal ideation (with or without plan).

DYSTHYMIA

1. Occurs over a two-year period (one year for children and adolescents), presence of depressed mood

2. Symptoms cause clinically significant distress in social, occupational and other important areas of functioning

3. Presence of two or more of the following:

   • Decreased or increased appetite

   • Insomnia or hypersomnia

   • Anergia or chronic fatigue

   • Anhedonia

   • Decreased self-esteem

   • Poor concentration or difficulty making decisions

   • Perceived inability to cope with routine responsibilities

   • Feelings of hopelessness or despair

   • Pessimistic about the future, brooding over the past, or feeling sorry for self

   • Recurrent thoughts of death or suicide

RELATED PHENOMENA

1. Psychotic features—delusions and hallucinations

2. Seasonal affective disorder (SAD) related to either winter or summer

Figure 17–2. *Diagnostic criteria for depression. (Adapted from American Psychiatric Association. Diagnostic and Statistical Manual of Mental Disorders, 4th ed (DSM-IV). Washington, DC: American Psychiatric Association, 1994.)*

hours of bright light a day (about 200 times brighter than usual indoor lighting). Treatment is provided through the use of "light boxes." Light is thought to have its therapeutic effect through the eyes. Clients report positive results after two to four days of treatment; they also report relapse two to four days after treatment is stopped.

Two newer devices promise more convenience and are hoped to be less time consuming. One is a "dawn-simulator" that will treat patients while they sleep. A second is a head-mounted light visor. The advantage of this device over the light boxes is that it is portable. Both of these newer devices need further study to determine their safety and effectiveness (Oren and Rosenthal 1992).

Theory

Although many theories attempt to explain the cause of depression, there are many psychological, biological, and cultural variables that make identification of any one cause difficult. Four common theories of depression are discussed here: (1) biological, (2) cognitive, (3) psychoanalytical, and (4) learned helplessness.

BIOLOGICAL THEORIES

GENETIC THEORIES. Studies of twins summarized over 50 years consistently show that genetic factors play a role in the development of depressive disorders (Nurnberger and Gershon 1992). Studies of identical twins found that if one twin had a depressive disorder, there was a 72% chance that the other twin would also develop a depressive disorder. However, with fraternal twins, as with siblings, parents, or children of the afflicted person, the risk decreases to 25% (NIMH 1989). There is also an increased incidence of mood disorders among relatives of people diagnosed with mood disorders. Although previous studies supported a possible genetic marker for transmission of mood disorders, the most recent evidence does not indicate this (Nurnberger and Gershon 1992).

BIOCHEMICAL FACTORS. It is currently believed that depression is a biologically heterogeneous disorder: that is, there are probably many central nervous system neurotransmitter abnormalities that can cause clinical depression. These neurotransmitter abnormalities may be the result of inherited or environmental factors or even other medical conditions, such as cerebral infarct, hypothyroidism, acquired immunodeficiency syndrome, drug use, and more (Delgado et al. 1992). Therefore, specific neurotransmitters in the brain are believed to be related to altered mood states. The two main neurotransmitters are *serotonin* and *norepinephrine*, both of which are catecholamines. However, data indicate that dopaminergic activity may be reduced in depression as well (Kaplan and Sadock 1991).

It was long thought that low levels of serotonin and norepinephrine at the synaptic receptor sites in the brain caused depression and that high levels triggered mania. The use of antidepressant drugs supported this biological theory because all antidepressant drugs inhibit the reuptake of serotonin and norepinephrine, increasing the amount of time these neurotransmitters are available to the postsynaptic receptors in the central nervous system. However, it is now considered unlikely that a catecholamine deficiency is the actual cause of depression (Delgado et al. 1992).

Present research is investigating the complex interactions of norepinephrine, serotonin, and acetylcholine, and changes in receptor numbers and sensitivity are being examined (Calarco and Krone 1991). Norepinephrine, serotonin, and acetylcholine also play a role in stress regulation. When these neurotransmitters become overtaxed through stressful events, neurotransmitter depletion may occur. This connection to stress regulation and alteration of mood continues to be evaluated.

At this stage no unitary mechanism of antidepressant action has been found. The relationships between the serotonin, norepinephrine, dopamine, and acetylcholine systems are very complex and need further assessment and research (Delgado et al. 1992).

NEUROENDOCRINE FINDINGS. Although neuroendocrine findings are as yet inconclusive, the most widely studied neuroendocrine symptom in relation to depression has been hyperactivity of the limbic-hypothalamic-pituitary-adrenal axis. Some depressed individuals have a hypersecretion of cortisol. Dexamethasone, an exogenous steroid that suppresses cortisol, is used in the *dexamethasone suppression test* (DST) for depression. Results of the dexamethasone suppression test (DST) are abnormal in about 50% of depressed patients, indicating hyperactivity of the limbic-hypothalamic-pituitary-adrenal axis. However, findings of this test may also be abnormal in people with obsessive-compulsive disorders and other medical conditions (Kaplan and Sadock 1991). Significantly, patients with psychotic major depression are among those with the highest rates of nonsuppression of cortisol on the dexamethasone suppression test (Schatzberg and Rothschild 1992).

SLEEP ABNORMALITIES. Studies show that sleep holds promise as a biological marker. The rapid eye movement (REM) phase of sleep associated with dreaming occurs earlier in two thirds of bipolar and unipolar depressed patients. This sign is referred to as *REM latency*, as Cartwright et al. (1991) reported in a study of people who met the DSM criteria for major depression. Although subjects with REM latency still had the sign a year later, when they were no longer depressed, they had both higher rates of recovery from depression and better life adjustment than did the depressed clients who did not have REM latency. Data also suggest that depressed clients without this sign are not likely to respond to tricyclic antidepressants, which suppress early REM sleep.

COGNITIVE THEORY

Albert Ellis, a well-known cognitive behavior therapist, views emotional disturbance as the product of irrational or illogical thinking. Ellis's rational emotive therapy has had success with people who are shy, are nonassertive in social situations, are experiencing marital problems, or have fears surrounding sexual situations. Expanding on Ellis's work, Aaron T. Beck applied the cognitive behavior theory to depression. Beck proposed that people acquire a psychological predisposition to depression through early life experiences. These experiences contribute to negative, illogical, and irrational thought processes that may remain dormant during most periods but are activated during times of stress (Calarco and Krone 1991). Beck found that depressed persons process information in negative ways, even in the midst of positive factors affecting the person's life. Beck believes three automatic negative thoughts are responsible for people becoming depressed. These three thoughts are called Beck's cognitive triad. They are

1. A negative, self-depreciating view of self
2. A pessimistic view of the world
3. The belief that negative reinforcement or no validation for the self will continue in the future

Automatic negative thoughts refer to thoughts that are repetitive, unintended, and not readily controllable (Haaga and Beck 1992). This cognitive triad holds for all depressions, regardless of clinical subtype.

The goal of cognitive behavior therapy is to change the way clients think and thus relieve the depressive syndrome. This is accomplished by assisting the client in the following:

1. Identifying and testing negative cognitions
2. Developing alternative thinking patterns
3. Rehearsing new cognitive and behavioral responses

PSYCHOANALYTICAL THEORY

Psychoanalytical theory emphasizes unconscious conflicts. This theory proposes that depression is the result of a harsh and punitive superego. Freud believed that through the process of introjection, after the loss of a significant person for whom the individual harbored extreme ambivalence, hostility felt toward this person is then directed toward the self. Therefore, two themes central to the psychoanalytical theory of depression are *loss* and *aggression*. According to psychoanalytical theory, depression is triggered by a loss, and the depressive mood is the result of aggression turned inward toward the self.

LOSS. Freud identified both grief and depression as reactions to a loss, real or symbolic, in his classic *Mourning and Melancholia* (1917). When a person loses a crucial source of security, he or she may become depressed. A sense of helplessness and hopelessness is central to the experience of depression.

When an infant between the ages of six and 36 months experiences the physical or emotional loss of the mothering figure, the biological response is a depressive affect. The loss of the mother's love can be a physical loss (e.g., death or divorce) or an emotional loss (e.g., withdrawal of affection because of depression, alcohol, or narcissism). The loss of the mother disrupts the normal development of the child. This early loss leaves the child extremely vulnerable to losses later in life. The young child interprets the withdrawal of affection (loss) as rejection of his or her self-worth and feels unworthy of love and approval. Numerous early studies supported the relationship

between early loss of a parent (death or divorce) and increased incidence and severity of depressive illness in an individual's later life (Ripley 1977; Bowlby 1961). However, a recent analysis of studies of adult depression as the result of childhood parental loss found little strong or consistent evidence to support a link between parental death and depression (Parker 1992).

AGGRESSION. Psychoanalytical theory states that depression is the result of anger turned inward against the self. The steps in the process of directing anger toward the self are

1. The child experiences emotional rejection, and the child's needs for affection are not met.
2. The child feels hurt and unworthy of love; self-esteem is lowered.
3. Hostility is aroused toward those who have hurt and rejected the child.
4. A state of ambivalence is experienced. The child needs and longs for love from the same people the child rages against for not giving love.
5. The need for acceptance and approval from the parents is so great that the child represses feelings of hostility.
6. Because these feelings of hostility could jeopardize receiving acceptance and approval from the parents, the feelings are pushed out of awareness and turned against the self to maintain acceptance and approval from the parents. Apathy and helplessness are experienced instead.
7. This pattern is set and continues throughout life. Hostility toward others is turned inward against the self in order to maintain the acceptance and approval of others.

Measures aimed at promoting appropriate expressions of anger and activities planned to mobilize aggression are nursing interventions useful for many clients suffering from depression. However, in the last 15 years, the focus of studies of mood disorders has begun to shift from psychoanalytical aspects to inherited biological aspects of these disorders (Mendelson 1992).

LEARNED HELPLESSNESS

One of the most popular theories of the cause of depression is Martin Seligman's theory of learned helplessness. Seligman (1973) states that although anxiety is the initial response to a stressful situation, anxiety is replaced by depression if the person feels that he or she has no control over the outcome of the situation. A person who believes that an undesired event is his or her fault and that nothing can be done to change it is prone to depression.

The theory of learned helplessness has been used to help explain the development of depression in certain social groups, such as the aged, people living in ghettos, and women.

A study by Gulesserian and Warren (1987) found data supporting the theory that "depression is linked with poor adaptational/coping abilities that may lead to learned helplessness, panic and depression." The lack of the following specific coping skills appeared to increase the likelihood of depression: social supports, tension reduction skills, and effective problem-solving skills. The behavioral therapeutic approach includes teaching depressed individuals new and more effective coping skills and ways to increase their self-confidence.

Assessment

Although controversy surrounds the causes of depression, the symptoms of depression seem well accepted. A depressed mood and **anhedonia** (an inability to find meaning or pleasure in existence) are the key symptoms in depression. Almost 97% of people with depression have **anergia** (reduction in or lack of energy). *Anxiety*, a common symptom in depression, is seen in about 90% of patients (Kaplan and Sadock 1991). Thinking is slow, and memory and concentration are usually affected. Depressed people dwell on and exaggerate their perceived faults and failures and are unable to focus on their strengths and successes. A person with major depression may experience delusions of being punished for "doing bad deeds" or "being a terrible person." Feelings of worthlessness, guilt, anger, and helplessness are common. *Psychomotor agitation* may be evidenced by constant pacing and wringing of hands. The slowed movements of *psychomotor retardation*, however, are more common. Somatic complaints (headaches, malaise, backaches) are also common. *Vegetative signs of depression* (change in bowel movements and eating habits, sleep disturbances, and disinterest in sex) are usually present. Dryman and Eaton (1991) reported on a study examining the relationship of depressive symptoms and the subsequent onset of a major depression. Significant symptoms included diminished sexual drive, feelings of worthlessness or excessive guilt, and trouble concentrating or thinking. Sleeping disturbances among women and fatigue among men were also significant symptoms.

Although individual variations in depression occur, commonalities are revealed through the assessment of affect, thought processes, feelings, physical behavior, and communication. Sometimes the symptoms of depression are not so obvious and are masked by other kinds of complaints. Therefore, assessing symptoms that mask depression is useful in all hospital settings.

ASSESSING AFFECT

A person who is depressed sees the world through "gray-colored" glasses. Staff and others often observe that posture is poor; the client may look older than his or her stated age. Facial expressions reflect sadness and dejection, and the person may have frequent bouts of weeping. Conversely, a client may say that he or she is unable to cry. Feelings of hopelessness and despair are readily reflected in the person's affect.

ASSESSING THOUGHT PROCESSES

Identifying the presence of suicidal thoughts and suicide potential has the highest priority in the initial assessment. Approximately two thirds of depressed people contemplate suicide, and 10–15% commit suicide (Kaplan and Sadock 1991). Asking a depressed person openly, "Have you thought about killing yourself?" can encourage the expression of painful pent-up feelings. (Refer to Chapter 21.) The risk of suicide is not necessarily correlated with the severity of the symptoms. Although depressed persons can attempt suicide at any time, the highest mortality occurs within a year of discharge from a psychiatric hospital (Litman 1992), with a decreasing but noticeable suicide rate thereafter.

During the time a person is depressed, the person's ability to solve problems and think clearly is negatively affected. Judgment is poor, and indecisiveness is common. People complain that their mind is slowing down. Memory and concentration are poor. Evidence of delusional thinking may be seen in a major depression. Common examples of delusional thinking are "I have committed unpardonable sins" or "God wants me dead" or "I am wicked and should die."

ASSESSING FEELINGS

Feelings frequently reported by depressed people include (1) anxiety, (2) worthlessness, (3) guilt, (4) helplessness and hopelessness, and (5) anger.

As previously mentioned, *anxiety* is present in about 90% of depressed persons. Feelings of *worthlessness* range from feeling inadequate to having an unrealistic evaluation of self-worth. These feelings reflect the low self-esteem that is a painful partner to depression. Statements such as "I am no good; I'll never amount to anything" are frequent. Themes of one's inadequacy and incompetence are repeated relentlessly.

Guilt is a common accompaniment to depression. Present or past failings are constantly belabored. Extreme guilt can assume psychotic proportions: "I have committed such terrible sins. God is punishing me for my evil ways."

Helplessness is evidenced by the inability to carry out the simplest tasks. Everything is too difficult to accomplish (e.g., grooming, housework, job, and caring for children). With feelings of helplessness come feelings of *hopelessness*. Even though most depressive states are usually time limited, during a depressed period people believe things will never change. This feeling of utter hopelessness can lead people to look at suicide as a way out of constant mental pain. An analysis of the concept of hopelessness by Campbell (1987) cites findings in the literature that have identified hopelessness as one of the core characteristics of depression and suicide, as well as a characteristic of schizophrenia, alcoholism, sociopathy, and physical illness. Campbell identifies the common cognitive and emotional components of hopelessness as having the following attributes:

Negative expectations for the future
Loss of control over future outcomes
Passive acceptance of the futility of planning to achieve goals
Emotional negativism as expressed in despair, despondency, or depression

Anger and irritability are natural outcomes of profound feelings of helplessness. Anger in depression is often expressed inappropriately. For example, anger may be expressed in destruction of property, hurtful verbal attacks, or physical aggression toward others. However, in people who are depressed, anger is most often directed toward the self, resulting in feelings of low self-esteem and worthlessness. An extreme example of turning aggression against the self is suicide. Often the impulse to commit suicide is related to an impulse to murder someone else.

ASSESSING PHYSICAL BEHAVIOR

Complaints of lethargy and fatigue can result in **psychomotor retardation.** Movements are extremely slow, facial expressions are decreased, and the gaze is fixed. The continuum in psychomotor retardation may range from slowed and difficult movements to complete inactivity and incontinence. At other times, the nurse may note **psychomotor agitation.** For example, clients may constantly pace, bite their nails, smoke, tap their fingers, or engage in some other tension-re-

lieving activity. At these times, complaints of feeling "fidgety" and unable to relax are common.

Grooming, dress, and personal hygiene are markedly neglected. A person who usually takes pride in his or her appearance and dress may become sloppy, be poorly groomed, and look shabby and unkempt.

Vegetative signs of depression are universal. Vegetative signs refer to alterations in those activities necessary to support the phenomenon of physical life and growth (eating, sleeping, elimination, and sex). For example, changes in *eating patterns* are common. About 60–70% of people who are depressed report anorexia. Overeating may occur in milder depressions. Changes in *sleep patterns* vary. Often people complain of insomnia, waking at 3:00 A.M. or 4:00 A.M. and staying awake, or only sleeping for short periods. For some, sleep is increased **(hypersomnia)** and provides an escape from painful feelings. In any event, sleep is rarely restful or refreshing. Changes in *bowel habits* are common. Constipation is seen most frequently in psychomotor retardation. Diarrhea occurs less frequently, often in conjunction with psychomotor agitation. *Interest in sex* declines (loss of libido) during depression. Some men experience impotence, which can further complicate marital and social relationships.

ASSESSING COMMUNICATION

A person who is depressed speaks very slowly. Comprehension is slow. The lack of an immediate response by the client to a remark does not mean that the client has not heard or chooses not to reply: the client just needs a little more time to compose a reply. In extreme depression, however, a person may be mute.

ASSESSING INDICATIONS OF MASKED DEPRESSION

Masked depressions are depressions that are not recognized in the familiar form. The manner in which depression is masked depends on the depressed person's (1) cultural background, (2) age and sex, and (3) socioeconomic background, and on (4) heredity factors (Lesse 1983).

In children, truancy, school phobias, underachievement, hyperactivity, learning disorders, and sociopathic behaviors may be the dominant characteristics of underlying depression. In adolescents, underachievement, dropping out of school, compulsive use of drugs and sex, delinquent behavior, and hostile outbursts may indicate masked depression. Adults in the United States may mask depression behind hypo-

Table 17-3 ■ DEPRESSION ON A CONTINUUM

MILD TO MODERATE	SEVERE
Communication	
Slow speech, long pauses before answering; monotone	Slow in extreme; may be mute and not talk at all
Affect	
Crying and weeping, slumping in chair, drooping shoulders, look of gloom and pessimism	May appear without affect; may be experiencing "nothingness"; can sit for hours staring into space
Anxiety may or may not be manifested.	
Anhedonia—inability to experience pleasure	**Anhedonia**
Thinking	
No impairment in reality testing.	*Grasp of reality may be tenuous.*
Thinking is slow, concentration and memory are poor, interest narrows; perspective in situations is lost, e.g.:	Thoughts may indicate delusional thinking, reflecting feelings of:
"Every one always lets me down." "No one cares."	• Low self-esteem • Worthlessness • Helplessness • "I'm no good." • "God is punishing me for my terrible sins." • "My insides are rotting." • "My heart has stopped beating."
Thoughts reflect doubts and indecisions. Thinking is often repetitive in negative cycle, e.g.:	
• "Why was I born? What's life all about?"	
Mild feelings of guilt and worthlessness.	Concentration is extremely poor. Preoccupation with bodily symptoms.
May have suicidal ideation.	**May have suicidal ideation.**
Physical Behavior	
Fatigue and lethargy are hallmark symptoms. They do not prevent the person from working, although the person often works below potential. Initiative and creativity are impaired.	Severe and extreme chronic fatigue and lethargy markedly interfere with occupational functioning, social activities, or relationships with others.
Grooming and hygiene are usually neglected.	Extreme neglect of personal grooming and hygiene.
Vegetative Signs	
Sleep—middle or late insomnia, hypersomnia; EEG studies show shortened REM latency	Sleep—usually insomnia; may have early morning waking at 3:00 or 4:00 A.M.
Energy is often highest in A.M., lowest in P.M.	Energy is often lowest in A.M., highest in P.M.
Eating—may have anorexia or overeat	Eating—usually has anorexia; weight loss of more than 5% in one month
Sexual appetite diminished	Loss of libido
Bowels—constipation if psychomotor retardation; may have diarrhea if psychomotor agitation	Bowels—usually constipation
Psychomotor retardation (slow motor movements)—everything an effort	Psychomotor retardation (most common)
or	*or*
Psychomotor agitation (agitated depression)—pacing up and down halls, wringing hands	Psychomotor agitation

Data from Chapman 1976; APA 1987; Bech 1992.

chondriasis and psychosomatic disorders, as well as compulsive gambling and work habits. Other behavioral patterns associated with underlying depressions include accident proneness, anorexia, bulimia, and substance dependence disorders.

Some adults who present with a masked depression have a characteristic personality profile (Lesse 1983). They are described as intelligent, capable, perfectionistic, hard working, and rigidly inflexible in everyday life. These personality characteristics are thought to be defenses against long-standing feelings of inferiority and inadequacy. Often parents of people who present with masked depressions are also perfectionistic, obsessive-compulsive, highly critical, and domineering.

The symptoms of depression are experienced by people on a continuum from mild to moderate to severe. Table 17–3 organizes the symptoms of depression on a continuum.

Nursing Diagnosis

During the initial assessment, a high priority for the nurse is to identify the presence of suicide potential. Therefore, the nursing diagnosis of *high risk for self-directed violence* should always be considered. The diagnosis of high risk for self-directed violence may be related to a pathophysiological condition (e.g., terminal illness), medical treatment (e.g., dialysis), a situation (e.g., divorce or child abuse), or a maturational issue (e.g., social isolation in the elderly). Suicide rates are high among adolescents, elderly persons, and other specific populations. The risk for self-directed violence needs to be explored when data support this possibility. (See Chapter 21 for significant risk factors.)

Because concentration, judgment, and memory are usually poor and psychotic behavior may be evidenced, *altered thought processes* are often present.

Feelings of worthlessness, guilt, helplessness, anger, and hopelessness all increase feelings of low self-esteem. Therefore, *disturbance in self-esteem, chronic low self-esteem,* or *powerlessness* is often present. Feelings of hopelessness and despair may be viewed as *spiritual distress,* which may be the most appropriate diagnosis.

Many people experiencing a major depressive episode are withdrawn and demonstrate psychomotor retardation, so the focus of care may be *impaired social interaction* or *activity intolerance.*

Most depressed clients exhibit some of the vegetative signs of depression. For example, the nurse may identify *altered nutrition, constipation, diarrhea, and sleep disturbance.*

Disturbance in the ability to function in usual occupational and interpersonal roles suggests *ineffective individual coping. Altered family processes* often surface. The nurse is in a key position to alert other members of the health care team to support the family and to mobilize additional financial and psychological supports.

Planning

The planning of nursing care for a person who is depressed has two levels: (1) the content level—planning long term and short term goals and (2) the process level—nurses' reactions and feelings.

CONTENT LEVEL—PLANNING GOALS

Long term and short term goals are formulated for each nursing diagnosis. Each client is different, and goals are devised according to each person's individual needs. Some possible goals are presented.

When possible, the nurse and client discuss desired outcomes of hospital and health care interventions. Long range goals are identified, and concrete measurable steps are formulated as short term goals. For the following diagnoses, some long term and short term goals are presented.

For the nursing diagnosis *high risk for self-directed violence,* as evidenced by suicidal ideation, the following are possible considerations:

Long Term Goals

- Client will remain safe while in hospital.
- By discharge, the client states that he or she no longer thinks about harming himself or herself.
- By (date), the client will name three places or people he or she can turn to if suicidal thoughts or impulses arise in the future.

Short Term Goals

- Client will make a suicide contract stating that he or she will talk to the nurse or therapist before harming self while in the hospital.
- By (date), the client will discuss with the nurse feelings of anger and frustration.
- By (date), the client will explore with the nurse thoughts, feelings, and circumstances that precede impulses to harm self.
- By (date), the client will demonstrate two alter-

native actions he or she can take when experiencing impulses to harm self.
- Client will name two activities he or she is looking forward to participating in after discharge.

For the nursing diagnosis *altered thought processes*, the following goals might be considered:

Long Term Goals

- By discharge, the client will state that his or her memory has improved.
- By discharge, the client will demonstrate an increased ability to make appropriate decisions.
- By discharge, the client will accurately interpret events happening in the environment.
- By (date), the client will state that he or she was able to participate in an activity that takes moderate concentration (e.g. reading, card games, or Scrabble).

Short Term Goals

- Client will remember to keep appointments, attend activities, and attend to grooming with the aid of medication and nursing interventions while in hospital.
- Client will make two decisions about the future with aid of medications and nursing counseling by (date).
- Client will discuss with nurse three irrational thoughts about self and others by (date).
- Client will demonstrate the ability to concentrate on two five-minute activities (e.g., grooming or recreation) with the aid of medication and nursing interventions by (date).

Goals for a nursing diagnosis of *disturbance in self-esteem* should reflect an increase in the client's sense of self-worth. For example:

- By (date), the client will name two things he or she likes about him- or herself.
- Client will demonstrate an increased interest in personal appearance (grooming, hygiene, and dress) by (date).

Nursing diagnoses concerning *powerlessness* might include the following:

- By (date), the client will discuss one new coping skill he or she has learned.
- By (date), the client will name three alternative solutions to a particular problem.

Often, when people feel hopeless and isolated, they are no longer able to find strength or sustenance from previous religious or spiritual beliefs. General goals for a person in *spiritual distress* are

- Client will state that he or she once again finds strength and meaning in life through personal spiritual beliefs.
- Client will resume usual spiritual activities by (date).

Clients who are depressed are often withdrawn and unwilling or unable to participate in usual activities. General goals for *impaired social interaction* or *activity intolerance* may include the following:

Long Term Goals

- Client will interact freely with at least five other clients throughout the day by (date).
- Client will initiate attending two group activities a day by (date).

Short Term Goals

- By (date), the client will discuss three alternative actions to take when he or she feels the need to withdraw.
- Client will participate in one activity with the nurse by the end of the day.
- By (date), the client will identify two personal behaviors that might push others away.

Goals for any of the vegetative signs of depression should be formulated to show evidence of weight gain, return to normal bowel activity, sleeping six to eight hours per night, or an increase in sexual desire.

For an individual whose work and interpersonal relationships have been negatively affected during the depressive episode, the ability to use previous adaptive coping skills would be a long range goal. For a family in which *altered family processes* have occurred, the long range goal would be resumption of previously satisfying and desired family coping styles.

PROCESS LEVEL—NURSES' REACTIONS AND FEELINGS

The depressed person has enormous needs for recognition and affection; however, he or she may be unable to acknowledge these needs. These intense needs for recognition and affection may be kept unconscious because their recognition could bring up painful feelings of loneliness and rejection. One way a depressed person avoids recognition of painful feelings is by withdrawing. Withdrawal is a defense against perceived hurts and feelings of rejection. During this period of withdrawal, the client has a great need for communication and human company, even though there appears to be a lack of interest in either.

Depressed clients often reject the overtures of the nurses, do not appear to respond to nursing interventions, and appear resistant to change. When this occurs, nurses can experience feelings of frustration, hopelessness, and annoyance. Nurses can alter these problematic responses by (1) recognizing any unrealistic expectations they have of themselves or the client and (2) identifying feelings they have picked up that originate in the client.

Unrealistic Expectations of Self

Nurses new to the hospital setting may have expectations of themselves and their clients that are not realistic, and problems result when these expectations are not met. Unmet expectations usually result in the nurse's feeling anxious, hurt, angry, helpless, or incompetent. Unrealistic expectations of one's self and others may be held by even experienced nurses, and this contributes to staff burnout. Many of the nurse's expectations may not be conscious. However, when these expectations are made conscious and worked through with peers and supervisors, more realistic expectations can be formed and attainable goals can be set. Realistic expectations of one's self and one's client can decrease feelings of helplessness and in-

crease the nurse's self-esteem and therapeutic potential.

Unrealistic expectations are common, especially for nursing students and nurses new to the psychiatric setting. Common expectations and reactions are outlined in Table 17–4.

Client Feelings Picked Up by the Nurse

Intense feelings of anxiety, frustration, annoyance, and helplessness may be experienced by the nurse, although they may originate in the client. These feelings can be important diagnostic clues to the client's experience. Often the nurse senses what the client is feeling through empathy. Sometimes, the client has pushed these feelings out of awareness, and the feelings are manifested behaviorally in psychosomatic complaints, substance abuse, or destructive behaviors. Helping clients recognize these intense negative unconscious feelings is part of the therapeutic process.

When the nurse's feelings of annoyance, hopelessness, and anxiety are the result of empathetic communications with the client, the nurse can discuss these feelings with peers and supervisors in order to separate personal feelings from those originating in

Table 17–4 ■ NURSES' UNREALISTIC EXPECTATIONS OF DEPRESSED CLIENTS		
EXPECTATION	**POSSIBLE RESULTS**	**POSSIBLE OUTCOMES**
Nurse expects to feel needed and helpful to the client.	Client does not respond, shows lack of interest.	Nurse feels useless and ineffectual.
	Client tells the nurse to leave him or her alone and may show hostility.	Nurse feels hurt and avoids the client to avoid arousing these feelings.
Nurse expects to form "therapeutic relationship" with the client.	Client acts aloof and cold.	Nurse feels rejected by client and may withdraw from client to avoid these feelings of rejection.
Nurse expects the client to show signs of improvement after the nurse spends a lot of time with the client.	Client does not improve or slips back to being withdrawn and depressed.	Nurse feels impatient and loses interest in such a "hopeless case."
	Client shows contempt for the nurse after the nurse has worked with the client.	Nurse's self-esteem is lowered. Nurse interprets the client's behavior as a sign of the nurse's incompetence.
	Client's feelings of hopelessness and helplessness are picked up empathetically by the nurse.	Nurse feels helpless and anxious around the client. Nurse withdraws from the client to get away from feeling helpless. *or* Nurse becomes angry at the client: "Why can't you shape up?" or "Stop acting like a baby." Anger may also trigger withdrawal.

the client. If personal feelings are not separated out and examined, withdrawal by the nurse is likely to occur. People naturally stay away from situations and people that arouse feelings of frustration, annoyance, or intimidation. If the nurse has unresolved feelings of anger and depression, the complexity of the situation is bound to be compounded. There is no substitute for competent and supportive supervision to facilitate growth both professionally and personally. Supervision and sharing with peers help minimize feelings of confusion, frustration, and isolation and can increase therapeutic potential and self-esteem in the nurse. The nurse is then free to intervene more directly with the client, and more direct communication can result in increased opportunities for the client to learn new coping skills.

Intervention

The nurse needs to be aware of the secondary gains a client may experience in depression. **Secondary gains** are satisfactions the client derives from the depressive symptoms. As mentioned in Chapter 15, secondary gains may take the form of (1) escaping from responsibilities, (2) getting extra attention from others, or (3) exerting control through manipulation of others in the environment. Secondary gains can be extremely gratifying and can provide rewards an individual was perhaps unable to obtain premorbidly. When the secondary rewards of depression meet previously unmet needs, they can serve to reinforce the symptoms of depression. Therefore, the nurse must minimize any secondary gains. The nurse assists clients in satisfying unmet needs for attention and control in more appropriate and meaningful ways.

PSYCHOTHERAPEUTIC INTERVENTIONS

Nurses often have great difficulty communicating with a client without talking. However, some depressed clients are so withdrawn that they are unwilling or unable to speak. Just sitting with a client in silence may seem like a waste of time to the nurse. Often the nurse becomes uncomfortable not "doing something," and as anxiety increases, the nurse may start daydreaming, feel bored, remember something that "must be done now," and so forth. It is important to be aware that this time spent together can be very meaningful to the depressed person, especially if the nurse has a genuine interest in learning about the depressed individual.

Doris Chan, a senior nursing student, is working with a very depressed, withdrawn woman. The instructor notices the second week that Doris spends a lot of time talking with other students and their clients and little time with her own client. In supervision, Doris acknowledges feeling threatened and useless and says that she wants a client who will interact with her. After reviewing the dynamics of depression, its behavioral manifestations, and the needs of depressed persons, Doris turns her attention back toward her client and spends time rethinking her plan of care. After six weeks of sharing her feelings in postconferences, working with her instructor, and trying a variety of approaches with her client, Doris is rewarded. On her last day, the client tells Doris how important their time together was for the client: "I actually felt someone cared." The staff state that until this time, the client had not responded to anyone.

It is difficult to say when a withdrawn and depressed person is able and ready to respond. However, certain techniques are known to be useful in guiding effective nursing interventions. Some techniques of communication useful with a person who is depressed are listed in Table 17–5.

HEALTH TEACHING

It is important for both clients and their families to understand that depression is a legitimate medical illness over which the client has no voluntary control.

Depressed clients and their families can greatly benefit from learning about the biological symptoms of depression, as well as about the psychosocial and cognitive changes in depression. Review of the medications, side effects, and toxic effects helps families evaluate clinical change and stay alert for reactions that might affect client compliance. Refer to Somatic Therapies for information on the side effects of antidepressants and specific areas to be covered in client and family teaching.

When a client is leaving the hospital, predischarge counseling should be performed with the client and the client's relatives. One purpose of this counseling is to clarify the interpersonal stresses and discuss steps that can alleviate tension for the family system. Predischarge counseling can be done by the psychiatrist, the psychiatric nurse clinician, or the psychiatric social worker.

Buckwalter and Abraham (1987) studied predischarge nursing interventions with depressed clients and their families. Their findings suggest that including families in discharge planning can bring about the following results:

Table 17–5 ■ NURSING INTERVENTIONS AND RATIONALES: WORKING WITH A PERSON WHO IS DEPRESSED

INTERVENTION	RATIONALE
Nursing Diagnosis: *Altered thought process* related to hopelessness, as evidenced by extreme withdrawal and/or verbal statement of low self-worth and hopelessness	
1. Spend short periods of time (5–10 minutes) with the client frequently throughout the day.	1. Frequent short periods minimize anxiety for both nurse and client.
2. Let the client know beforehand when, and for how long, the visits will be.	2. Clear expectations minimize anxiety. Scheduled times bring structure and purpose to empty periods of time.
3. Be on time and stay the full time contracted, even when the client does not acknowledge your presence.	3. Consistency and reliability lay the foundations for trust. The client experiences attention without "having to earn it." When the nurse does not come on time or stay the stated time, a depressed person may personalize the experience: "I'm not worthy of attention."
4. When the client is not speaking, sit with the person in silence for short periods.	4. Even if the client does not acknowledge you, the client knows you are there. Your presence and interest over time can reinforce that you view the client as worthwhile.
5. When a client is mute, make observations of happenings in the environment: "There are many new pictures on the wall" or "You are wearing your new shoes."	5. When a client is not ready to talk, direct questions can raise the client's anxiety level and frustrate the nurse. Pointing to commonalities in the environment draws the client into and reinforces reality.
6. Use simple, concrete words.	6. Slowed thinking and difficulty concentrating impair comprehension.
7. Allow time for the client to respond.	7. Slowed thinking necessitates time to formulate a response.
8. Listen for covert messages and ask about suicide plans.	8. People often experience relief and a decrease in feelings of isolation when they share thoughts of suicide.
9. Spend time listening and sharing feelings.	9. Feeling understood can help diminish feelings of alienation and isolation and facilitate the sharing of painful feelings necessary for healing.
10. *Avoid* laughing, joking, and "acting cheerful."	10. The nurse's cheerful attitude increases feelings of alienation and isolation in the client by contrasting the nurse's "up" feelings with the client's own feelings of low worth.
11. *Avoid* platitudes, such as "Things will look up" or "Everyone gets down once in awhile."	11. Platitudes tend to minimize the client's feelings and can increase feelings of guilt and worthlessness, because the client cannot "look up" or "snap out of it."
12. Accept expressions of anger without becoming defensive. Work at not taking anger personally when it is expressed by the client.	12. Argumentative or self-righteous responses serve to diminish both the client's and the nurse's self-esteem.
13. Encourage the client's verbalization of anger.	13. Sharing difficult feelings can minimize the need to act them out in inappropriate ways.
14. If the client's anger is justified, admit that an error was made.	14. Encourage appropriate expressions of anger and validate that it is all right to have angry feelings.
15. Avoid the use of value judgments: "You look nice this morning." "I like the way you did your hair." Say, instead, "You are wearing a new dress this morning" or "You've changed your hair style."	15. When depressed, a person sees the negative side of everything, for example: <ul><li>Can be interpreted as "I didn't look nice yesterday morning."</li><li>Can be thought of as being done to please the nurse: "If I do my hair another way, maybe he or she will not like it."</li></ul> Neutral comments avoid negative interpretations.

Table continued on following page

Table 17–5 ■ NURSING INTERVENTIONS AND RATIONALES: WORKING WITH A PERSON WHO IS DEPRESSED *Continued*	
INTERVENTION	**RATIONALE**
Nursing Diagnosis: *High risk for self-harm* related to hopelessness and inability to find solution for overwhelming psychic pain, as evidenced by covert or overt clues	
1. Assess the client for overt and covert suicide clues.	1. A high percentage of depressed people have suicidal thoughts.
2. Ask the client directly, "Have you thought of killing yourself?"	2. Often the client is relieved to talk to someone else about these thoughts. Talking about this can minimize painful feelings of isolation and loneliness.
3. Assess the lethality of the suicide plan.	3. If the method is highly lethal (e.g., gun or hanging) and readily available and if the plan is well thought out, the risk is extremely high.
4. Assess high-risk factors.	4. Assessing risk factors can help in determining suicidal risk.
5. Remove all potentially harmful objects from the environment (e.g., belts, straps, ties, sharp objects, glass).	5. Client safety is a nursing priority.
6. If the client is suicidal, place the client on a one-to-one suicide precaution following hospital protocol.	6. Constant one-to-one observation of the suicidal client can maximize client safety. **Always follow hospital protocol.**
7. Form a written no-suicide contract with the client, such as "I will not kill myself during the next eight hours." then renegotiate the contract at that time.	7. Because suicide is often an ambivalent solution, the nurse stresses life-affirming considerations.
8. Secure the promise that the client will seek out a staff member if or when suicidal thoughts emerge or become overpowering.	8. Because people who are suicidal have "tunnel vision," discussing feelings, fears, and any alternatives can lower anxiety and may help the client put events in a more favorable perspective.

1. Increase the family's satisfaction with the depressed family member during the aftercare period
2. Increase the client's use of aftercare facilities in the community
3. Contribute to a high overall adjustment score in the client three months after discharge

Overall, the study findings indicated that the quality of social, family, and community readjustment was positively influenced.

ACTIVITIES OF DAILY LIVING

A depressed person presents with many physical complaints. Because depressed clients may view themselves as worthless, it is often up to the nurse to notice signs and symptoms of physical neglect. Nursing measures for improving physical well-being and promoting adequate self-care are then initiated. Some effective interventions geared to the physical needs of the depressed client are listed in Table 17–6.

SOMATIC THERAPIES

In caring for a person who is depressed, the nurse's main responsibilities associated with somatic therapies are (1) administering medications and (2) applying knowledge of electroconvulsive therapy.

Psychopharmacology

Some readers may find it both interesting and helpful to understand *how* and *why* psychotropic drugs work. Box 17–1 discusses the communication between neurons.

A suicide assessment should be performed with any depressed person. When a depressed person is hospitalized, staff members need to check to make sure all medications are swallowed (not placed in the cheek or under the tongue). Because 10–15 times the prescribed dose of any antidepressant can prove fatal, only a week's supply should be given to a severely

Table 17–6 ■ NURSING INTERVENTIONS AND RATIONALES: PHYSICAL NEEDS OF THE DEPRESSED CLIENT

INTERVENTION	RATIONALE
Nursing Diagnosis: *Activity intolerance* related to poor concentration and motivation, as evidenced by withdrawal from others	
1. While the client is most severely depressed, involve the client in one-to-one activities.	1. Because concentration is impaired, this maximizes the potential for interacting and may minimize anxiety levels.
2. Engage the client in activities involving gross motor activity and calling for minimal concentration, such as taking a walk, making beds with the nurse, setting up chairs, and so forth.	2. Physical activities are thought to help temporarily mobilize aggression and relieve tension.
3. Provide activities that require very little concentration (e.g., walking, playing simple card games, looking through a magazine, drawing, or playing with clay).	3. Concentration and memory are poor in depression. Activities that have no "right" or "wrong" minimize opportunities for the client to put him- or herself down.
4. Eventually bring the client into contact with one other person and then into a group of three.	4. Contact with others distracts the client from self-preoccupations and provides the opportunity for spending more time with people and activities that are based in reality.
5. Eventually involve the client in group activities (e.g., dance therapy, art therapy, or group discussions).	5. Socialization can decrease feelings of isolation. Genuine regard from others can increase feelings of self-worth.
6. In *psychomotor agitation*, provide activities that involve use of the hands and gross motor movements (e.g., ping-pong, volleyball, finger painting, drawing, or working with clay).	6. These activities give the client a more appropriate way of discharging motor tension than pacing and wringing the hands.
Nursing Diagnosis: *Altered nutrition*, less than body requirements related to anorexia, as evidenced by refusal to eat and/or weight loss	
1. Offer small high-caloric and high-protein snacks frequently throughout the day and evening.	1. Low weight and poor nutrition render the client susceptible to illness. Small frequent snacks are more easily tolerated than large plates of food when the client is anorexic.
2. Offer high-protein and high-caloric fluids frequently throughout the day and evening.	2. These fluids prevent dehydration and can minimize constipation.
3. When possible, remain with the client during meals.	3. This reinforces the idea that someone cares, can raise the client's self-esteem, and can serve as an incentive to eat.
4. Ask the client which foods or drinks he or she likes. Offer choices. Involve the dietitian.	4. The client is more likely to eat the foods provided.
5. Weigh the client weekly and observe the client's eating patterns.	5. Monitoring the client's status gives the information needed for revising the intervention.
Nursing Diagnosis: *Sleep-pattern disturbance* related to insomnia, as evidenced by frequent awakenings, difficulty going to sleep, and persistent fatigue	
1. Provide rest periods after activities.	1. Fatigue can intensify feelings of depression.
2. Encourage the client to get up and dress and to stay out of bed during the day.	2. Minimizing sleep during the day increases the likelihood of sleep at night.
3. Provide relaxation measures in the evening (e.g., backrub, tepid bath, or warm milk).	3. These measures induce relaxation and sleep.
4. Reduce environmental and physical stimulants in the evening—provide decaffeinated coffee, soft lights, soft music, and quiet activities.	4. Decreasing caffeine and epinephrine levels increases the possibility of sleep.
5. Spend more time with the client before bedtime.	5. This helps allay anxiety and increases feelings of security.

Table continued on following page

Table 17-6 ■ NURSING INTERVENTIONS AND RATIONALES: PHYSICAL NEEDS OF THE DEPRESSED CLIENT *Continued*

INTERVENTION	RATIONALE
Nursing Diagnosis: *Self-care deficit* **related to poor concentration and lack of motivation, as evidenced by poor grooming and dress**	
1. Encourage the use of toothbrush, washcloth, soap, makeup, shaving equipment, and so forth.	1. Being clean and well groomed can temporarily raise self-esteem.
2. Give step-by-step reminders, such as "Wash the right side of your face, now the left . . . "	2. Slowed thinking and difficulty concentrating make organizing simple tasks difficult.
Nursing Diagnosis: *Constipation* **related to inadequate daily intake**	
1. Monitor intake and output, especially bowel movements.	1. Many depressed clients are constipated. If this condition is not checked, fecal impaction can occur.
2. Offer foods high in fiber and provide periods of exercise.	2. Roughage and exercise stimulate peristalsis and help evacuation of fecal material.
3. Encourage the intake of fluids.	3. Fluids help prevent constipation.
4. Evaluate the need for laxatives and enemas.	4. These prevent the occurrence of fecal impaction.

depressed person when treated on an outpatient basis.

Antidepressant drugs can *positively alter* poor self-concept, degree of withdrawal, the vegetative signs of depression, and activity level. Target symptoms include:

1. Sleep disturbance
   - Early morning awakening
   - Frequent awakening
   - Hypersomnia
2. Appetite disturbance (decreased or increased)
3. Fatigue
4. Decreased sex drive
5. Psychomotor retardation or agitation
6. Diurnal variations in mood (often worse in the morning)
7. Impaired concentration or forgetfulness
8. Anhedonia

However, one main drawback to the use of antidepressant medication is that the client may have to take antidepressant agents from one to three weeks before improvement is noticed. Three major types of antidepressant drugs are the tricyclic antidepressants, the monoamine oxidase inhibitors, and several newer, atypical antidepressants such as the selective serotonin reuptake inhibitors (SSRIs).

TRICYCLIC ANTIDEPRESSANTS. The **tricyclic antidepressants (TCAs)** inhibit the reuptake of norepinephrine and serotonin by the presynaptic neurons in the central nervous system. Therefore, the amount of time that norepinephrine and serotonin are available

to the postsynaptic receptors is increased. This increase in norepinephrine and serotonin in the brain is thought by many to be responsible for mood elevations when TCAs are given to depressed persons.

TCAs benefit about 65–80% of people with nondelusional, unipolar depressions but only about 33% of those with delusional depression (Maxmen 1991). Delusional or psychotic major depression is a severe form of mood disorder characterized by delusions or hallucinations. Some view delusional depression as a distinct disorder (Schwatzburg and Rothchild 1992). Clients with delusional depression respond well to electroconvulsive therapy. Neuroleptic (antipsychotic) agents along with TCAs are also effective for some depressed clients who have psychotic symptoms.

Clients must take therapeutic doses of TCAs for 10–14 days or longer before these agents start to work. The full effects may take from four to eight weeks to be seen. An effect on some symptoms of depression, such as insomnia and anorexia, may be noted earlier. Currently, a person who has had a positive response to TCA therapy will probably be maintained on that medication from six to 12 months in order to prevent an early relapse.

The choice of which TCA to use is based on (1) what has worked for the client or a family member in the past and (2) the drug's side effects. For example, for a client who is very lethargic and fatigued, a more stimulating TCA may be best, such as desipramine (Norpramin) or protriptyline (Vivactil). If a more sedating effect is needed for agitation or restlessness, drugs such as amitriptyline (Elavil) or doxepin (Sine-

Box 17–1. PHYSIOLOGICAL BASIS OF PSYCHOTROPIC DRUG ACTION

Nerve cells communicate by the passage of chemicals (neurotransmitters) from one cell to another. The cell releasing the chemical is called the presynaptic cell, and the cell responding to the chemical, the postsynaptic cell. These terms are used in reference to the synapse, the space separating the two cells. For the neurotransmitter to influence the activity of the postsynaptic cell, it must first combine with a specialized molecule, the postsynaptic receptor. Ultimately, psychotropic drugs exert their effects by increasing or decreasing the activity of the postsynaptic cell.

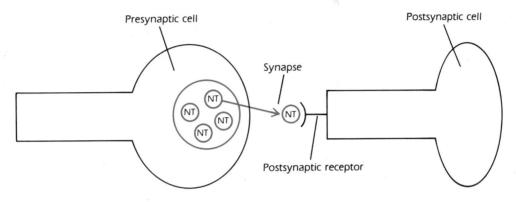

Communication between neurons.

A full explanation of the various ways in which psychotropic drugs alter neuronal activity requires a brief review of the manner in which neurotransmitters are destroyed after attaching to the receptors. As a means of avoiding continuous and prolonged action on the postsynaptic cell, the neurotransmitter is released shortly after attaching to the postsynaptic receptor. Once released, the transmitter is destroyed in one of two ways. One is the immediate inactivation of the transmitter at the postsynaptic membrane. An example of this method of destruction would be the action of the enzyme acetylcholinesterase on the neurotransmitter acetylcholine. Acetylcholinesterase is present at the postsynaptic membrane and destroys acetylcholine shortly after it attaches to nicotinic or muscarinic receptors on the postsynaptic cell.

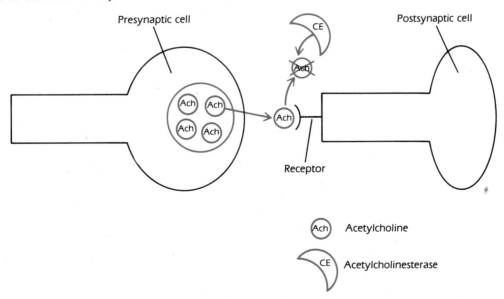

Postsynaptic destruction of neurotransmitter.

Continued

Box 17–1. PHYSIOLOGICAL BASIS OF PSYCHOTROPIC DRUG ACTION (*Continued*)

A second method of neurotransmitter inactivation is a bit more complex. After interacting with the postsynaptic receptor, the transmitter is released and taken back into the presynaptic cell, the cell from which it was released. This process, referred to as the *reuptake* of transmitter, is a common target for drug action. Once inside the presynaptic cell, the transmitter is either recycled or inactivated by an enzyme within the cell. The monoamine transmitters norepinephrine, dopamine, and serotonin are all inactivated in this manner by the enzyme monoamine oxidase.

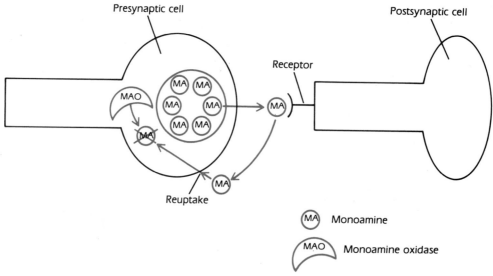

Presynaptic destruction of neurotransmitter.

Looking at this second method, one might naturally ask what prevents the enzyme from destroying the transmitter before its release. The answer is that before release, the transmitter is stored within a membrane and is thus protected from the degradative enzyme. After release and reuptake, the transmitter is either destroyed by the enzyme or re-enters the membrane to be used once again.

(Courtesy of John Raynor.)

quan) may be more appropriate choices. No matter which TCA is given, *the dose should always be low initially and be gradually increased.* Caution should be used, especially in elderly persons, in whom slow drug metabolism may be a problem. Schatzberg and Cole (1991) have found trimipramine (Surmontil) a good choice for the elderly because of its low side effect profile and its rapid effects on promoting sleep. Box 17–2 graphically illustrates how the TCAs are thought to work.

Common Side Effects. The chemical structure of the TCAs is similar to that of the antipsychotic medications. Therefore, the *anticholinergic* actions are similar (e.g., dry mouth, blurred vision, tachycardia, postural hypotension, constipation, urinary retention, and esophageal reflux). These side effects are both more common and more severe in clients taking antidepressants. These side effects are usually not serious and are often transitory, but *urinary retention and severe constipation warrant immediate medical attention.*

Administering the total daily dose of TCA at night is beneficial for two reasons. First, most TCAs have sedative effects, thereby aiding sleep. Second, the minor side effects occur during sleep, thereby increasing compliance with drug therapy because the client experiences fewer side effects during the waking hours. Table 17–7 lists commonly used TCAs, daily dosage ranges, and comments on each, and gives this information for the newer, atypical antidepressants as well.

Serious Side Effects. The most serious side effects of the TCAs are cardiovascular. Arrhythmias, tachycardia, myocardial infarction, and heart block have been reported. Because the cardiac side effects are so serious, the TCAs are considered a risk in clients with cardiac disease and in the elderly. Clients should have

Box 17–2. TRICYCLIC ANTIDEPRESSANT DRUGS: HOW DO THEY WORK?

Whether the original cause of depression is biological, psychological, or social, its symptomatic expression seems to be associated with a deficiency of either or both of the monoamine neurotransmitters norepinephrine and serotonin. The most commonly used pharmacological interventions for the treatment of depression are directed at increasing the activity of these transmitters. Tricyclic antidepressant drugs accomplish this task by blocking the reuptake of norepinephrine and, to a lesser degree, of serotonin into the presynaptic cell, as illustrated. Blocking norepinephrine re-entry into

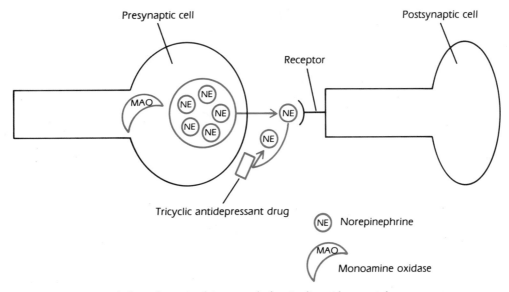

Blockage of norepinephrine reuptake by tricyclic antidepressant drugs.

the presynaptic cell increases the concentration of this transmitter in the synaptic space and, presumably, its action on the postsynaptic cell. This explanation of the beneficial actions of tricyclic drugs is called into question somewhat by the fact that the blockage of transmitter reuptake occurs immediately, whereas the alleviation of depressive symptoms by these drugs usually takes two or three weeks. Although a number of theories attempt to explain this discrepancy, a proven and agreed on explanation is not available at present.

The pharmacological actions of the tricyclic antidepressants are not limited to the blockade of monoamine reuptake and destruction. As is the case with the phenothiazines, these drugs can block muscarinic and alpha$_1$-adrenergic receptors. Many of these agents have quite strong muscarinic blocking ability and can produce the predictable antiparasympathetic responses of blurred vision, constipation, tachycardia, and urinary retention. Alpha$_1$

antagonism blocks the pressor response necessary to avoid orthostatic hypotension.

Although an antidepressant drug might be thought to be somewhat of a stimulant, this is not the case for the tricyclic drugs. In fact, many of these drugs have strong sedating properties. The sedating actions of tricyclic drugs are believed to be due to their ability to block histamine receptors in the brain.

In addition to those untoward effects attributable to known mechanisms of action, most drugs can also have undesirable actions for which there is no clear-cut explanation at present. The most serious toxic and life-threatening effects of tricyclic drugs at high doses are convulsions and the depression of cardiac conductivity and contractility. The therapeutic index (ratio of toxic dose to safe dose) of tricyclic drugs is low, and they are potential agents of accidental and deliberate death.

(Courtesy of John Raynor.)

Table 17–7 ■ DRUG INFORMATION: COMMON ANTIDEPRESSANTS

DRUG	THERAPEUTIC DOSE RANGE (mg/day)	SEDATION	ANTICHOLINERGIC SIDE EFFECTS	COMMENTS
Tricyclic Antidepressants (TCAs)				
Amitriptyline (Elavil)	150–300	High	High	The sedating and anticholinergic effects are difficult for some patients to tolerate. Frequent cause of cardiac arrhythmias.
Protriptyline (Vivactil)	15–60	Low	High	More energizing; useful for lethargy and psychomotor retardation.
Trimipramine (Surmontil)	100–300	High	Mid	Good choice for the elderly: low side effect profile and promotion of sleep.
Doxepin (Sinequan)	75–300	High	Mid	Helps lower anxiety and agitation; sedating.
Imipramine (Tofranil)	75–300	Mid	Mid	Useful in agoraphobia with panic attacks. High incidence of postural hypotension.
Nortriptyline (Aventyl, Pamelor)	40–150	Mid	Mid	Fewest cardiac problems, especially postural hypotension. Useful for the elderly.
Amoxapine (Ascendin)	100–400	Mid	Low	EPS reported—Akathisia, even dyskinesia in some. Drug should be tapered or discontinued when this occurs.
Desipramine (Norpramin)	150–300	Low	Low	More energizing TCA. Also has fewer anticholinergic side effects.
Maprotiline (Ludiomil)	100–225	Mid	Low	Seizures reported at high doses.
Clomipramine (Anafranil)	75–300	High	High	Predominent use for obsessive-compulsive disorders in USA. Also useful in panic disorder.
Atypical Antidepressants (SSRIs)				
Fluoxetine* (Prozac)	20–40	Low	None	Useful in obsessive-compulsive disorder and bulimia; associated with fewer cardiac problems. Wait five to six weeks before changing to an MAOI.
Sertraline* (Zoloft)	50–200	Low	Low	Good side effect profile (similar to that of Prozac) and also useful for obsessive-compulsive disorder.
Parotetine HCL* (Paxil)	20	Low	Low	Most recent SSRI. Initial studies show a beneficial effect on symptoms of anxiety and agitation in depressed clients. The SSRIs have a higher rate of compliance than the TCAs.

DRUG	THERAPEUTIC DOSE RANGE (mg/day)	SEDATION	ANTICHOLINERGIC SIDE EFFECTS	COMMENTS
Trazodone (Desyrel)	150–400	High	None	Fewer cardiac problems than TCAs. Has anti-anxiety properties. Priapism is a rare adverse reaction.
Venlafaxine HCL (Effexor)	75–375	Low	Very low	SSRI-like side effects (anorexia, sexual dysfunction, nervousness). Increases in BP dictate BP monitoring.
Bupropion (Wellbutrin)	200–450	Low	None	Fewer cardiac problems than with TCAs. Seizures reported in 0.4% of patients treated.
Alprazolam** (Xanax)	1.5–4.0	High	High	A benzodiazepine that may treat mild to moderate depressions.

Table 17-7 ■ DRUG INFORMATION: COMMON ANTIDEPRESSANTS *Continued*

Data from Maxmen 1991; Schatzberg and Cole 1991; Preston and Johnson 1991; US Department of Health and Human Services 1993.
*Selective serotonin reuptake inhibitors or blockers.
**Benzodiazepine.
MAOI = monoamine oxidase inhibitor; TCA = tricyclic antidepressant.

a thorough cardiac work-up before beginning TCA therapy.

Adverse Drug Interactions. Individuals taking TCAs can have adverse reactions to a number of other medications. For example, use of a monoamine oxidase inhibitor along with a TCA is often contraindicated. A few of the more common medications usually *not* given while the TCAs are being administered are listed in Box 17–3. Any client who is taking any of these medications along with the TCAs should have medical clearance because some of the reactions can be fatal. Table 17–8 identifies the common and most troublesome side and adverse effects of the TCAs.

Antidepressants may cause a psychotic episode in a person with schizophrenia. In addition, an antidepressant alone can cause a manic episode in a client with bipolar disorder. Depressed clients with bipolar disorder should receive lithium along with the antidepressant.

Contraindications. People who have recently had myocardial infarction (or other cardiovascular problems), those with narrow-angle glaucoma or a history of seizures, and pregnant women should not be treated with TCAs, except with extreme caution and careful monitoring.

Teaching clients and their family members about medications is an expected nursing responsibility. Medication teaching should be started in the hospital.

The client and, whenever possible, one or more family members need to review with the nurse or another qualified health care professional the client's medications, expected side effects, and necessary client precautions. Areas for the nurse to cover in teaching a client receiving TCA therapy are presented in Box 17–4. Clients and family members need to have the infor-

Box 17–3. DRUGS USED WITH CAUTION IN CLIENTS TAKING A TRICYCLIC ANTIDEPRESSANT

- Phenothiazines
- Barbiturates
- Monoamine oxidase inhibitors (MAOIs)
- Disulfiram (Antabuse)
- Oral contraceptives (or other estrogen preparations)
- Anticoagulants
- Some antihypertensives (clonidine, guanethidine, reserpine)
- Benzodiazepines
- Alcohol
- Nicotine (cigarette smoking)

Table 17–8 ■ DRUG INFORMATION: SIDE EFFECTS AND TOXIC EFFECTS OF TRICYCLIC ANTIDEPRESSANTS

PHENOMENA	COMMENTS
Anticholinergic Effects	
Dry mouth, blurred vision, postural hypotension, dry eyes, photophobia, nasal congestion	Most side effects are not serious and are transitory (1–2 weeks). For people with orthostatic hypotension, nortriptyline may be a good alternative.
Urinary retention and *severe constipation.*	Bethanechol, 25–50 mg tid or bid, may help urinary retention. Both urinary retention and severe constipation need immediate medical attention. Check for fecal impaction.
Cardiac Effects	
All patients should be checked for TCA-cardiac interactions before starting a TCA	
1. Low blood pressure (hypotension with dizziness)	1a. Take blood pressure lying and standing. 1b. Instruct the client to rise slowly and hang on to objects. 1c. Instruct the client to use support hose. 1d. Have the doctor change the TCA. 1e. Occurs with greater frequency in patients with cardiac conditions. 1f. Protect the client against falls, especially the elderly client.
2. Tachycardia and arrhythmias	2. Use TCAs with caution in people with cardiac conditions and the elderly.
3. Cardiac ECG changes	3. TCAs are fatal in people with second- and third-degree heart block.
4. Heart failure	4. Use with caution. Monitor the client's vital signs regularly.
Central Nervous System Responses	
1. Sedation (especially during the first 2 weeks)	1. Have doctor prescribe a less sedating TCA and give all at bedtime.
2. Delirium (in high doses)	2. Withhold further doses of the drug and contact the doctor immediately.
3. Memory impairment (especially in elderly clients)	3. Evaluate change in the status of the client's memory.
4. Seizures (with maprotiline)	4. Most seizures reported for maprotiline result from the administration of high doses.
5. "Spaciness," depersonalization	5. Increase the drug dose more slowly or switch the TCA.
6. Tremors	6. Lower the dose. The doctor may prescribe propranolol.
Endocrine and Sexual Effects	
1. Deceased or increased libido	1. Have the doctor evaluate; may change to another TCA.
2. Priapism (trazodone)	2. Medical intervention is crucial within four to six hours to maintain sexual ability.
3. Breast enlargement in women and men	3. Doctor may try an alternate drug if this effect causes embarrassment (men or women).
4. Appetite stimulation–carbohydrate cravings	4. Weight gain can be a problem.

Data from Maxmen 1991; Schatzberg and Cole 1991; Preston and Johnson 1991.
ECG = electrocardiographic; TCA = tricyclic antidepressant.

Box 17–4. TEACHING CLIENTS AND THEIR FAMILIES ABOUT TRICYCLIC ANTIDEPRESSANTS

1. Tell the client and the client's family that mood elevation may take from seven to 28 days. It may take up to 6–8 weeks for the full effect to take place and for major depression symptoms to subside.

2. Have the family reinforce this frequently to the depressed family member because depressed people have trouble remembering and respond to ongoing reassurance.

3. Reassure the client that drowsiness, dizziness, and hypotension usually subside after the first few weeks.

4. When the client starts taking tricyclic antidepressants (TCAs), caution the client to be careful working around machines, driving cars, and crossing streets because of possible altered reflexes, drowsiness, or dizziness.

5. Alcohol can block the effects of antidepressants. Tell the client to refrain from drinking.

6. If possible, the client should take the full dose at bedtime to reduce the experience of side effects during the day.

7. If the client forgets the bedtime dose (or the once-a-day dose), the client should take the dose within three hours; otherwise, the client should wait for the next day. The client should *not* double the dose.

8. Suddenly stopping TCAs can cause nausea, altered heartbeat, nightmares, and cold sweats in two to four days. The client should call the doctor or take one dose of TCA until the physician can be contacted.

---

mation in writing to refer to when at home. Written information should be provided for all medications people will be taking at home.

ATYPICAL ANTIDEPRESSANTS. The atypical **antidepressants** introduced here are trazodone hydrochloride (Desyrel), bupropion hydrochloride (Wellbutrin), fluoxetine hydrochloride (Prozac), and sertraline (Zoloft). These new antidepressant drugs are neither TCAs nor monoamine oxidase inhibitors. The new antidepressant drugs have a lesser incidence of anticholinergic side effects, less cardiotoxicity, and a faster onset of action than the TCAs.

Fluoxetine Hydrochloride (Prozac). Fluoxetine hy-

drochloride is a selective serotonin reuptake inhibitor (SSRI) that has been effective in treating major depressions. Fluoxetine has a much more favorable side effect profile than that of the TCAs. Its major side effects include nausea, tremor, drowsiness, headache, and nervousness. This drug seems to facilitate weight loss and does *not* potentiate seizures. The drug dosage is started at 20 mg per day and can be increased gradually to 40 or 60 mg per day. The maximum recommended daily dose is 80 mg per day, with many clients responding at 60 mg per day or less (Schatzberg and Cole 1991). Fluoxetine has also been found useful for a number of other conditions, such as bulimia nervosa, premenstrual syndrome, and anorexia nervosa (Psychiatry Drug Alerts, 1992; Maxmen 1991).

Timing is important when a client is being switched from one antidepressant to another. For most TCAs, the rule of thumb is that before a person is switched from a TCA to a trial of a monoamine oxidase inhibitor, two weeks should elapse to allow the TCA to leave the person's system. However, in the case of fluoxetine, the time interval should be *five weeks*. This is also true if a depressed individual is to be switched from fluoxetine to a TCA (Psychiatry Drug Alerts 1992).

Sertraline (Zoloft). Sertraline is also an SSRI. This drug has been found effective in depressed persons and in those with obsessive-compulsive disorders. Its side effect profile is similar to that of fluoxetine. The most prominent adverse effects are gastrointestinal (nausea, dyspepsia, and diarrhea). **Paroxetine HCL** (Paxil) and **venlafaxine HCL** (Effexor) are the latest SSRIs. Box 17-5 demonstrates how the serotonin reuptake blockers work. See Appendix A for more information on these drugs.

Trazodone Hydrochloride (Desyrel). Trazodone hydrochloride has been found effective in outpatients who have mild to moderate depression and anxiety, especially those depressed individuals who have difficulty falling asleep (Schatzberg and Cole 1991). The main side effects of this drug appear to be sedation, acute dizziness and fainting (particularly if it is taken on an empty stomach), and priapism. **Priapism** is a persistent erection of the penis due to organic causes, not sexual desire. This condition is serious and may require surgical intervention. If not treated within a few hours, priapism can result in impotence (Schatzberg and Cole 1991).

Bupropion Hydrochloride (Wellbutrin). Bupropion is effective in depressed clients. Bupropion has a favorable side effect profile, although nausea can occur in some clients. It does not induce orthostatic hypotension and stimulate appetite but may cause seizures. For this reason, the drug is contraindicated in people with epilepsy, major head injury, bulimia, and anorexia nervosa (Schatzberg and Cole 1991).

Box 17–5. INHIBITORS OF SEROTONIN REUPTAKE: HOW DO THEY WORK?

Fluoxetine, sertraline, and related selective serotonin reuptake inhibitors (SSRIs) specifically block the reuptake of serotonin (5-hydroxytryptamine) into the presynaptic cell from which it was originally released. As a result of this blockade, in a fashion analogous to the action of tricyclic antide-

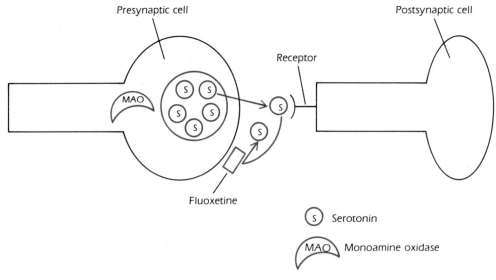

Blockage of serotonin reuptake by fluoxetine.

pressants on norepinephrine, the destruction of the transmitter is reduced and its concentration at the postsynaptic cell is increased. Because these drugs are specific to serotonin and have little or no ability to block muscarinic and other receptors, they tend to have fewer untoward autonomic effects than the tricyclic drugs. In addition, they do not cause as much sedation or have cardiac toxicity. However, to the degree that depression involves norepinephrine deficiency and presents with symptoms of agitation, the serotonin blockers may have less efficacy than the tricyclic antidepressants. Major untoward effects of the serotonin blockers include excessive stimulation and anorexia among susceptible patients.

(Courtesy of John Raynor.)

MONOAMINE OXIDASE INHIBITORS. Monoamine oxidase inhibitors (MAOIs) are not as widely used as TCAs because they have dangerous side effects, the most serious of which is hypertensive crises. The MAOIs are therefore usually contraindicated for people who are debilitated, elderly, or hypertensive; those who have cardiac or cerebrovascular disease; and those who have severe renal and hepatic disease. The MAOIs were traditionally given when the TCAs proved ineffective. At present, MAOI administration is the preferred treatment for "atypical" depression. Atypical depressions that respond well to MAOIs are characterized by clinical features such as:

- Overeating
- Hypersomnia
- Phobic anxiety
- Panic attacks

- Hypochondriasis
- Feeling better in the morning and worse in the evening
- Rejection sensitivity (feeling rejection for the slightest reason or no observable reason at all)
- Chronic pain or hypochondriasis

The most common MAOIs are isocarboxazid (Marplan), phenelzine (Nardil), and tranylcypromine sulfate (Parnate). MAOIs are also effective in some people with (Davidson 1992):

- Panic disorder or anger
- Social phobia
- Generalized anxiety disorder
- Obsessive-compulsive disorder
- Post-traumatic stress disorder
- Bulimia nervosa
- Parkinson's disease

The MAOIs, like the TCAs, block the reuptake of norepinephrine and serotonin in the central nervous system. However, monoamine oxidase is also responsible for the metabolism of tyramine. Therefore, a person taking an MAOI cannot metabolize tyramine. High levels of tyramine in the blood can cause high blood pressure, leading to hypertensive crisis or stroke. Certain foods containing high levels of tyramine are contraindicated for people taking MAOIs (Box 17–6). The MAOIs also interact with various drugs.

On the basis of present evidence, there are no good grounds for the exclusion of reasonable amounts of the following, which are often on lists of foods to avoid (Davidson 1992; Maxmen 1991):

1. Coffee, chocolate, colas, or tea
2. Yogurt and fresh sour cream
3. Soy sauce, tenderized meat, and baker's yeast products (e.g., bread)
4. Avocados, bananas, figs, and raisins

Patients should be carefully selected for MAOI therapy. Periodic reminders of dietary restrictions are advised. Even a clear-thinking person can have difficulty in restaurants and in the homes of friends keeping the list of forbidden foods constantly in mind. It is easy to understand why prescribing an MAOI for someone who is having cognitive difficulty with memory and concentration could be risky. Meperidine hydrochloride (Demerol), epinephrine, and decongestants can be particularly dangerous (Schatzberg and Cole 1991).

Common Side Effects. Some common and troublesome long term side effects of the MAOIs are orthostatic hypotension, weight gain, edema, change in cardiac rate and rhythm, constipation, urinary hesitancy, sexual dysfunction, vertigo, overactivity, muscle twitching, hypomanic and manic behavior, insomnia, weakness, and fatigue (Schatzberg and Cole 1991; Davidson 1992).

Adverse Reactions. The most serious reactions to these agents involve an increase in blood pressure, with the possible development of intracranial hemorrhage, hyperpyrexia, convulsions, coma, and death. Therefore, routine monitoring of blood pressure, especially during the first six weeks of treatment, is advised.

Because so many other drugs, foods, and beverages can have adverse interactions with the MAOIs, increase in blood pressure is a constant concern. The beginning of a hypertensive crisis usually occurs within a few hours after ingestion of the contraindicated substance. The crisis may begin with headaches; a stiff or sore neck; palpitations; an increase or decrease in heart rate, often associated with chest pain; nausea; vomiting; or an increase in temperature (py-

---

Box 17–6. DRUG INFORMATION: FOOD, BEVERAGE, AND DRUG RESTRICTIONS FOR CLIENTS TAKING MONOAMINE OXIDASE INHIBITORS

It is a disservice to patients and promotes noncompliance if depressed individuals are taxed with long lists of substances to avoid.

Foods and Beverages To Avoid

- All cheese, except cream, cottage, and ricotta (80% of all hypertensive crises are secondary to eating aged cheese).
- Red wine, sherry, beer, and liqueurs
- Pickled or smoked fish
- Brewer's yeast products (Marmite, Boveril, some packet soups)
- Fava (broad) beans and Italian green beans
- Chicken or beef liver
- Fermented sausage (bologna, pepperoni, salami, summer sausage)
- Any stale, overripe, or aged foods (pheasant, venison, spoiled fruit, unfresh meats or dairy products)
- Sauerkraut
- Aspartame (the artificial sweetener)

Drug Incompatibilities

- Over-the-counter medications for colds, allergies, or congestion (any product containing ephedrine, phenylephrine hydrochloride, or phenylpropanolamine)
- Tricyclic antidepressants (imipramine, amitriptyline)
- Narcotics
- Antihypertensives (methyldopa, guanethidine, reserpine)
- Amine precursors (L-dopa, L-tryptophan)
- Sedatives (alcohol, barbiturates, benzodiazepines)
- General anesthetics
- Stimulants (amphetamines, cocaine)

Data from Davidson 1992; Maxmen 1991.

---

rexia). When a hypertensive crisis is suspected, immediate medical attention is warranted. Antihypertensive medications, such as phentolamine (Regitine), are slowly administered intravenously. Pyrexia is treated with hypothermia blankets or ice packs. Table 17–9 identifies common side effects and toxic effects. Box 17–7 reviews precautions to go over with clients taking MAOIs and their families.

Table 17-9 ■ DRUG INFORMATION: SIDE EFFECTS AND TOXIC EFFECTS OF MONOAMINE OXIDASE INHIBITORS

Side Effects

- Hypotension
- Sedation, weakness, fatigue
- Insomnia
- Changes in cardiac rhythm
- Muscle cramps
- Anorgasmia or sexual impotence
- Urinary hesitancy or constipation
- Weight gain

Hypotension is the most critical side effect (10%); especially the elderly may sustain injuries from it.

Toxic Effects

Hypertensive crisis

- Severe headache
- Stiff, sore neck
- Flushing, cold, clammy skin
- Tachycardia
- Severe nosebleeds, pupils dilated
- Chest pains, stroke, coma, or death

1. Go to local emergency room immediately—check blood pressure
2. May receive one of the following to lower blood pressure:
   - Intravenous phentolamine (Regitine)

     or
   - Oral chlorpromazine

     or
   - Nifedipine (calcium channel blocker), 10 mg every hour intravenously until relief (one to two doses)

*Related to interaction with foodstuffs and cold medication.

Box 17-7. TEACHING CLIENTS AND THEIR FAMILIES ABOUT MONOAMINE OXIDASE INHIBITORS

- Tell the client and the client's family to avoid certain foods and all medications (especially cold remedies) unless prescribed by and discussed with the client's doctor (see Box 17–6 for specific food and drug restrictions).
- Give the client a wallet card describing the monoamine oxidase inhibitor (MAOI) regimen (Parke-Davis will supply them if contacted at 1-800-223-6432).
- Instruct the client to avoid Chinese restaurants (sherry, brewer's yeast, and other products may be used).
- Tell the client to go to the emergency room right away if he or she develops a severe headache.
- Ideally, blood pressure should be monitored during the first six weeks of treatment (for both hypotensive and hypertensive effects).
- After stopping the MAOI, the client should maintain dietary and drug restrictions for 14 days.

Contraindications. MAOIs may be contraindicated in or with

- Cerebral vascular disease
- Hypertension and congestive heart failure
- Liver disease
- Foods with tyramine, tryptophan, and dopamine (see Box 17–6)
- Medications (see Box 17–6)
- Recurrent or severe headaches
- People having surgery in 10–14 days
- Children under 16 years of age

In summary, some people do not respond to the MAOIs or the TCAs. For others, side effects with these agents prohibit the use of either. The advent of atypical antidepressants, especially the serotonin reuptake inhibitors, has greatly enhanced the ability of the medical profession to decrease the suffering of people with depression. Because of their low side effect profile, the SSRIs are often the first choice, especially for elderly patients.

Electroconvulsive Therapy

Most often, electroconvulsive therapy (ECT) is indicated when antidepressant drugs have no effect. However, in some situations ECT may be considered a

Box 17–8. MONOAMINE OXIDASE INHIBITORS: HOW DO THEY WORK?

As illustrated, inhibitors of the enzyme monoamine oxidase (MAO) act by interfering with the ability of this enzyme to destroy the monoamines norepinephrine, dopamine, and serotonin (5-hydroxytryptamine). Enzyme inhibition eventually leads to an increase in the presynaptic, synaptic, and postsynaptic concentrations of these neurotransmitters. Increased postsynaptic activity of one or more of these transmitters would then account for the beneficial effects of these drugs in certain forms of depression. As with the tricyclic drugs, this explanation still leaves unsolved the problem of the two- to three-week time lag between enzyme inactivation and clinical improvement.

MAO is present in liver cells, as well as in monoamine-releasing neurons. In the liver, this en-

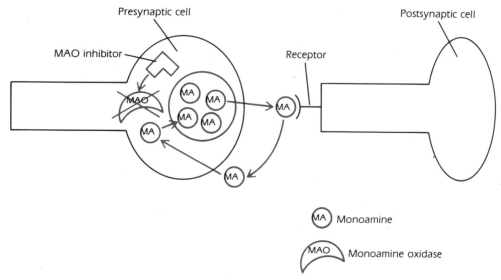

Destruction of monoamine oxidase by an MAO-inhibiting drug.

zyme has the function of destroying circulating endogenous monoamines (e.g., the hormone epinephrine) and exogenous monoamines (e.g., tyramine), which are present in many foods and readily absorbed from the digestive tract. Inactivation of hepatic MAO by MAO-inhibiting drugs can lead to a potentially fatal interaction between these drugs and foods such as aged cheeses, which contain significant amounts of tyramine. This is due to the fact that tyramine can trigger the release of norepinephrine from sympathetic nerve endings. Norepinephrine is a potent vasoconstrictor, and the sudden release of large amounts of norepinephrine in response to tyramine can produce a life-threatening hypertensive crisis. In the absence of MAO-inhibiting drugs, tyramine does not present a problem because it is destroyed by MAO when the absorbed food is brought to the liver by the blood passing through the hepatic portal system. To avoid the possibility of a hypertensive crisis, patients are given a list of proscribed foods that contain large amounts of tyramine.

A large number of pharmacological agents, particularly sympathomimetic drugs, are monoamines and are broken down by hepatic MAO. The plasma level of such drugs resulting from a given dose may be vastly increased in the presence of MAO-inhibiting drugs. Thus, these drugs must be used with great care, if at all, in a patient who is also taking MAO inhibitors. Because many of the monoamine drugs are sold over the counter, patients taking MAO inhibitors must be given a list of drugs as well as foods to be avoided.

(Courtesy of John Raynor.)

primary treatment and be given before a trial of antidepressant medication. ECT is indicated when (APA 1990)

1. There is a need for a rapid, definitive response for either medical or psychiatric reasons (e.g., in acutely suicidal or starving clients)
2. The risks of other treatments outweigh the risks of ECT
3. The client has a history of poor drug response, a history of good ECT response, or both
4. The client prefers it

ECT is very useful in unipolar and bipolar depressive disorders, especially when psychotic symptoms are present (delusions of guilt, somatic delusions, or delusions of infidelity). Clients who have depressions with marked psychomotor retardation and stupor also respond well (Fink 1992). In depressed clients with a major depressive disorder who have responded to medication, there is a 80–90% response rate to bilateral ECT. In depressed medication-resistant clients, the rate is closer to 50% (Devanand et al. 1991).

ECT is also indicated in *manic clients* whose conditions are resistant to lithium and antipsychotic drugs and in *rapid cyclers*. A rapid cycler is a patient with bipolar disorder who has many episodes of mood swings close together (four or more in one year (Grove and Andreasen 1992). (Refer to Chapter 18.) People with *schizophrenia* (especially catatonia), those with *schizoaffective syndromes*, *psychotic patients who are pregnant*, and *patients with Parkinson's disease* can also benefit from ECT.

However, ECT is not necessarily effective in dysthymic depressions or depressed people with character disorders, drug dependence, or depression secondary to situational or social difficulties.

A usual course of ECT for a depressed client is six to 12 treatments given two or three times per week. Although there are no "absolute" contraindications according to Fink (1992), several conditions have special risks demanding special attention and skill, such as clients who have had a recent myocardial infarction, those who have had a cerebrovascular accident, and those with a cerebrovascular malformation or an intracranial mass lesion. These high-risk clients are usually not teated with ECT unless the need is compelling (Fink 1992).

THE PROCEDURE. The procedure is explained to the client, and informed consent must be obtained when voluntary clients are being treated. For involuntary clients, when informed consent cannot be obtained, permission may be obtained from the next of kin.

The client receives nothing by mouth after midnight or at least four hours before treatment is to take place. Vital signs are taken, and the client is re-quested to void. Hairpins, contact lenses, and dentures are removed. Atropine is usually given to reduce tracheobronchial secretions. Table 17–10 describes nursing care with clients undergoing a course of ECT.

POTENTIAL SIDE EFFECTS. The major side effect clients complain of with bilateral treatments is confusion, disorientation, and short term memory loss after treatment. On awakening, the client may be confused and disoriented. The nurse needs to orient the client frequently: "Mr. Taylor, you are in Mercy Hospital. It's 9:00 A.M., and I will take you back to your room, where you will have breakfast." The client will have to be oriented frequently during the course of the treatments. Many people state that they have had memory deficits for the first few weeks before and after the course of treatment. Memory usually recovers completely, although some clients have complained of memory loss lasting up to 6 months (Burns and Stuart 1991). ECT is not a permanent cure for depression, and maintenance treatment with TCAs or lithium decreases the relapse rate.

THERAPEUTIC ENVIRONMENT

When a person is severely depressed, hospitalization is usually indicated. The depressed person needs protection from suicidal acts, a supervised environment for regulating antidepressant medications, and when indicated, a course of ECT. Often, being removed from a stressful interpersonal situation in itself has therapeutic value. Most hospitals have protocols regarding the care and protection of the suicidal client. Chapter 21 covers the nurse's responsibilities in providing a therapeutic environment safe against self-inflicted harm.

PSYCHOTHERAPY

A number of modalities have been applied in the treatment of depression. Studies demonstrate that traditional psychotherapies (e.g., psychoanalytical psychotherapy) are only slightly more effective than placebos in reducing depressive symptoms (Beck and Young 1985).

Most recently, there has been an increased emphasis on short term therapies. Therapies that have received the most attention in outcome research include behavioral therapy, interpersonal psychotherapy, brief psychodynamic therapy, and cognitive therapy.

Interpersonal psychotherapy is a short term psychological treatment of depression. It focuses on the role of the dysfunctional interpersonal relationships in the onset and perpetuation of depression. A study by Elkin (1989) sponsored by the National Institute of

Table 17–10 ■ NURSING CARE IN ELECTROCONVULSIVE THERAPY

1. Provision of emotional and educational support to the patient and family

1a. Encourage the patient to discuss feelings, *including myths* such as:
- Dying from electrocution
- Suffering permanent memory loss
- Suffering impaired intellectual ability

1b. Assess previous knowledge and experience.

1c. Teach the patient and family about what to expect with ECT.

2. Assessment of the pretreatment protocol and the patient's behavior, memory, and functional ability before ECT

2a. Ideally, be present when information for the informed consent is presented to the patient.

2b. Ascertain if the patient and family have received a full explanation, including the option to withdraw the consent at any time.

2c. **Pretreatment care:**
- Withhold food and fluids for six to eight hours before treatment (cardiac medication is given with sips of water).
- Remove dentures, glasses, hearing aids, contact lenses, hairpins, and so on.
- Have patient void before treatment.

2d. **Preoperative medications:**
- Give either glycopyrrolate (Robinul) or atropine to prevent potential for aspiration and to help minimize bradyarrhythmias in response to electrical stimulants.

3. Nursing care during the procedure

3a. Introduce the patient to each member of the treatment team.

3b. Have the client get on a stretcher (padded table) and remove socks and shoes.

3c. Place a blood pressure cuff on one of the client's ankles.

3d. Observe the client's extremities for seizure activity.

3e. As the intravenous line is inserted and EEG and ECG electrodes are attached, give a brief explanation to the patient.

3f. Clip the pulse oximeter to the patient's finger.

3g. Monitor blood pressure throughout treatment.

3h. Medications given:
- Short-acting anesthetic (methohexital sodium [Brevital], thiopental [Pentothal])
- Muscle relaxant (succinylcholine [Anectine])
- 100% oxygen by mask via positive pressure throughout

3i. Check that the bite block is in place to prevent biting of the tongue.

3j. Electrical stimulus given (seizure should last 30–60 seconds).

4. Post-treatment nursing care

4a. Have the patient go to a properly staffed recovery room (with blood pressure cuff and oximeter in place) where oxygen, suction, and other emergency equipment is available.

4b. Once the patient is awake, talk to the patient and check vital signs.

4c. Often the patient is confused; give frequent orientation reassurance; orientation statements are brief, distinct, and simple.

4d. Return the patient to the unit after he or she has maintained a 90% oxygen saturation level, vital signs are stable, and mental status is satisfactory.

4e. Check the gag reflex before giving the patient medicine or breakfast.

Data from Burns CM, Stuart GW. Nursing care in electroconvulsive therapy. Psychiatric Clinics of North America, 14(4):971, 1991.
ECG = electrocardiographic; ECT = electroconvulsive therapy; EEG = electroencephalographic.

Mental Health found interpersonal psychotherapy to be highly effective in reducing depressive symptoms in depressed persons (Luby and Yalom 1992).

Beck's **cognitive therapy** has been gaining momentum. The use of specific cognitive interventions meets with promising success in individual therapy with depressed persons. Cognitive therapy for depression is brief, structured, directive treatment designed to alter dysfunctional beliefs and the negative automatic thoughts typical of depression (Haaga and Beck 1992). Essentially, the depressed person learns

1. The connection between thoughts and feelings
2. The negative thoughts typical of depression
3. How different feelings can emerge when the patient is taught to think differently in the same circumstance (reframing)

A review of several studies (Haaga and Beck 1992) shows apparent prophylactic effects with cognitive therapy in depressed clients, especially those with unipolar depression. That is, people seem to learn something in cognitive therapy that is helpful after the acute phase of treatment, which may help minimize a relapse.

Behavioral therapy has also gained some recognition for success in the treatment of depression. Behavioral therapists attempt to teach depressed people effective coping skills that will increase positive reinforcements from other people and the environment.

The cognitive and behavioral approaches to therapy are thought to be at least as effective as TCA therapy, although pharmacologic treatment remains the standard against which all other treatments are judged (Beck and Young 1985). The National Institute of Mental Health has done research showing that drug therapy and psychotherapy in combination are more effective than either treatment alone.

Group treatment is a widespread modality for the treatment of depression. The treatment of people in groups increases the number of people who can receive treatment at a decreased individual cost. A widely used model for outpatient group treatment is modeled on Beck's cognitive theory of depression (Luby and Yalom 1992).

Another popular group approach is *interactional group therapy*. In this type of therapy, groups consist of clients with different types of disorders. The therapist in this setting focuses on the here-and-now. Maladaptive behaviors displayed within the group are interpreted as the kinds of psychopathology the person displays in his or her outside relationships. Therefore, the target of treatment is not the depression itself but rather the interpersonal manifestations of the disorder (Luby and Yalom 1992).

Evaluation

The short term and long term goals are frequently evaluated. For example, if the client comes into the unit with suicidal thoughts, the nurse evaluates whether suicidal thoughts are still present, whether the depressed person is able to state alternatives to suicidal impulses in the future, whether he or she is able to explore thoughts and feelings that precede suicidal impulses, and so forth. Goals relating to thought processes, self-esteem, and social interactions are frequently formulated because these areas are often problematic in people who are depressed. Physical needs often warrant nursing or medical attention. If a person has lost weight because of anorexia, is the appetite returning? If a person was constipated, are the bowels now functioning normally? If the person was suffering from insomnia, is he or she now getting six to eight hours of sleep per night?

If the goals have not been met, an analysis of the data, nursing diagnoses, goals, and planned nursing interventions is made. The care plan is reassessed and reformulated when necessary.

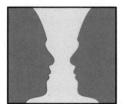

Case Study: Working with a Person Who Is Depressed

June Olston is a 35-year-old executive secretary. She has been divorced for three years and has two sons, 11 and 13 years of age. She was brought into the emergency room by her neighbor. She had tried to kill herself by turning on the gas. The neighbor stated that both of Mrs. Olston's sons were visiting their father for the summer. Mrs. Olston had become more and more despondent after terminating a two-year relationship with a married man four weeks earlier. According to the neighbor, for three years after her divorce, she constantly talked about not being pretty or "good enough" and doubted that anyone could really love her. The neighbor stated that Mrs. Olston had been withdrawn for at least three years. After the relationship with her boyfriend ended, she became even more withdrawn and sullen. Mrs. Olston was about 20 pounds overweight, and her neighbor stated that Mrs. Olston often stayed awake late into the night, drinking by herself and watching TV. She would sleep through most of the day on the weekends.

After receiving treatment in the emergency room, Mrs. Olston was seen by a psychiatrist. The initial diagnosis was dysthymia with suicidal ideation. A decision was made to hospitalize Mrs. Olston for suicide observation and evaluation for appropriate treatment.

The nurse, Ms. Weston, admitted Mrs. Olston to the unit from the emergency room.

NURSE:	Hello Mrs. Olston, I'm Marcia Weston. I will be your primary nurse.
MRS. OLSTON:	Yeah . . . I don't need a nurse, a doctor, or anyone else. I just want to die.
NURSE:	You want to die?
MRS. OLSTON:	I just said that, didn't I? Oh, what's the use. No one understands.
NURSE:	I would like to understand, Mrs. Olston.
MRS. OLSTON:	Look at me. I'm fat . . . ugly . . . and no good to anyone. No one wants me anyway.
NURSE:	Who doesn't want you?
MRS. OLSTON:	My husband didn't want me . . . and now Jerry left me to go back to his wife.
NURSE:	You think that because Jerry went back to his wife that no one else could care for you?
MRS. OLSTON:	Well . . . he doesn't anyway.
NURSE:	Because he doesn't care, you believe that no one else cares about you?
MRS. OLSTON:	Yes . . .
NURSE:	Who do you care about?
MRS. OLSTON:	No one . . . except my sons . . . I do love my sons, even though I don't often show it.
NURSE:	Tell me more about your sons.

The nurse continues to speak with Mrs. Olston. Mrs. Olston talks about her sons with more affect and apparent affection; however, she continues to state that she does not think of herself as worthwhile and that she wants to die.

Assessment

The nurse divides the data into objective and subjective components.

OBJECTIVE DATA

1. Tried to kill herself by inhaling gas fumes
2. Recently broke off with boyfriend
3. Has thought poorly of herself for three years since divorce
4. Has two sons she cares about
5. Twenty pounds overweight
7. Stays awake late at night drinking by herself
8. Withdrawn since divorce

SUBJECTIVE DATA

1. "No one could ever love me."
2. "I'm not good enough."
3. "I just want to die.
4. "I'm fat and ugly . . . no good to anyone."
5. "I do love my sons, although I don't always show it."

Nursing Diagnosis

The nurse evaluated Mrs. Olston's strengths and weaknesses. The nurse decided to concentrate on two initial nursing diagnoses that seemed to have the highest priority.

1. *High risk for self-directed violence* related to separation from two-year relationship, as evidenced by actual suicide attempt
   - Tried to kill herself by inhaling gas fumes
   - Recently broke off with boyfriend
   - Drinks at night by herself
   - Withdrawn for three years, since divorce

2. *Disturbance in self-esteem* related to divorce and recent termination of love relationship, as evidenced by derogatory statements about self
   - "I'm not good enough."
   - "No one could ever love me."
   - "I'm fat and ugly . . . no good to anyone."
   - Works as an executive secretary
   - "I do love my sons, although I don't always show it."

Continued on following page

Planning

CONTENT LEVEL—PLANNING GOALS

Because Mrs. Olston was acutely suicidal, she was put on suicide precautions (see Chapter 21 for suicide precaution protocol). The nurse discussed with Mrs. Olston possible goals related to issues of self-esteem. Although initially Mrs. Olston was very negative about herself, she was able to discuss with the nurse some of her strengths and identify some thoughts, feelings, and behaviors she would like to change about herself. The nurse devised the following long term and short term goals with some input from Mrs. Olston:

Nursing Diagnosis	Long Term Goals	Short Term Goals
1. *High risk for self-directed violence* related to separation from two-year relationship, as evidenced by actual suicide attempt	1. Client will remain safe while in the hospital.	1a. Client will state she has a reason to live by (date).
		1b. Client will state two alternative actions she can take when feeling suicidal in the future.
2. *Disturbance in self-esteem* related to divorce and recent termination of love relationship, as evidenced by derogatory statements about self	2. By discharge, the client will name two things she likes about herself.	2. By (date), the client will name two things she would like to change about herself.

PROCESS LEVEL—NURSES' REACTIONS AND FEELINGS

Ms. Weston is aware that when clients are depressed, they can be very negative, think life is hopeless, and at times be hostile toward those who want to help. At first, when Ms. Weston was new to the unit, she withdrew from depressed clients and sought out clients who appeared more hopeful and appreciative of her efforts. The unit coordinator was very supportive of Ms. Weston when she was first on the unit. Ms. Weston, along with other staff, was sent to in-service education sessions on working with depressed clients, and she was encouraged to speak up in staff meetings about the feelings many of these depressed clients evoked in her. As a primary nurse, she was now assigned a variety of clients. She found that as time went on, with the support of her peers and the opportunity to speak up at staff meetings, she was able to take less personally what clients said and not feel so responsible when clients did not respond as fast as she would like. After two years, she had had the experience of seeing many clients who seemed hopeless and despondent on admission respond well to nursing and medical interventions and go on to lead full and satisfying lives. This also made it easier for Ms. Weston to understand that even though the client may think life is hopeless and believe there is nothing in his or her life to live for, change is always possible.

Intervention

Mrs. Olston was put on 24-hour suicide precautions for the first three days. She appeared to respond positively to the attention from the nurses, as well as to that from some of the other clients on the unit. She told the nurse that since her divorce, she had become more withdrawn and had stopped socializing with others and participating in her usual outside activities. Her married boyfriend never took her out, and together they did not share any social activities. Just being around people who seemed interested in her made her feel better.

Her therapist on the unit used various cognitive therapy approaches with Mrs. Olston. She was encouraged to look at her life and herself differently and evaluate her strengths and those things she valued. The therapist assisted Mrs. Olston in questioning and changing inaccurate thoughts and beliefs she held toward herself and her future. The therapist assisted Mrs. Olston in learning new behaviors to cope with her loneliness, lack of motivation, and negative thinking.

Ms. Weston, the nurse, worked closely with Mrs. Olston's therapist, and together they discussed ways to reinforce what Mrs. Olston was learning in therapy.

For example, the nurse, together with Mrs. Olston, scheduled activities throughout the day, including short rest periods. A record of these activities would be kept by the client and discussed with the therapist. The nurse also role-played with Mrs. Olston some of the new behaviors that Mrs. Olston was learning in her therapy sessions. Refer to Mrs. Olston's nursing care plan (Nursing Care Plan 17–1).

Evaluation

At the end of three days, Mrs. Olston was no longer thought to be suicidal. At the end of the week, she was much less withdrawn: she sought out people on the unit and readily participated in activities. By discharge, she stated that she was anxious to see her children and admitted to missing them terribly when they spent the whole summer away with their father. She was to continue her therapy sessions after discharge and had decided to go to some meetings of Parents Without Partners. She stated that she was looking forward to getting back to work and felt much more hopeful about her life. She had also lost three pounds while in the hospital and was going to attend Weight Watchers once she was discharged. She stated, "I need to get back into the world."

Although Mrs. Olston still had negative thoughts about herself, she admitted to feeling much better about herself. She was no longer suicidal and stated that she was ready to resume previous activities and see old friends.

Nursing Care Plan 17–1 ▪ A PERSON WITH DEPRESSION: Mrs. Olston

NURSING DIAGNOSIS

High risk for self-directed violence **related to separation from two-year relationship, as evidenced by actual suicide attempt**

Supporting Data

- Tried to kill self by inhaling gas fumes.
- Recently broke off with boyfriend.
- Withdrawn for three years since divorce.
- Drinks at night by herself.
- "I just want to die."

Long Term Goal: Client will remain safe while in the hospital.

Short Term Goal	Intervention	Rationale	Evaluation
1. Client will state she has a reason to live by (date).	1a. Staff is to observe the client every 15 minutes while she is suicidal.	1a–b. Ensures client safety. Minimizes impulsive self-harmful behavior.	Goal met By the end of the second day, Mrs. Olston broke down in tears saying how much she loved and missed her children.
	1b. Remove all dangerous objects from the client.		
	1c. Spend regularly scheduled periods of time with the client throughout the day.	1c. Reinforces that she is worthwhile; builds up experience to begin to better relate to nurse on a one-to-one basis.	
	1d. Assist the client in evaluating the positive as well as the negative aspects of her life.	1d. A depressed person is often unable to acknowledge any positive aspects of her life unless they are pointed out by others.	
	1e. Encourage the expression of angry feelings in an appropriate manner.	1e. Providing for expression of pent-up hostility in a safe environment can reinforce more adaptive methods of releasing tension and may minimize the need to act out self-directed anger.	
	1f. Accept the client in her negativism.	1f. Acceptance enhances feelings of self-worth.	

Continued on following page

Nursing Care Plan 17-1 ■ A PERSON WITH DEPRESSION: Mrs. Olston
(Continued)

Short Term Goal	Intervention	Rationale	Evaluation
2. Client will state two alternative actions she can take when feeling suicidal in the future.	2a. Explore usual coping behaviors.	2a. Identifies those behaviors that need reinforcing and new coping skills that need to be introduced.	Goal met By discharge, Mrs. Olston stated that she was definitely going to continue her cognitive-behavioral therapy. She also discussed joining a women's support group that meets once a week in a neighboring town.
	2b. Assist the client in identifying members of her support system.	2b. Evaluate strengths and weaknesses in the support available.	
	2c. Suggest a number of community-based support groups she might wish to discuss or visit (e.g., hotlines, support groups, women's groups, and so forth).	2c. Clients need to be aware of community supports in order to use them.	
	2d. Assist the client in identifying realistic alternatives that she is willing to use.	2d. Unless the client is in agreement with any plan, she will be unable or unwilling to follow through in a crisis.	

NURSING DIAGNOSIS

Disturbance in *self-esteem* related to divorce and recent termination of love relationship, as evidenced by derogatory statements about self

Supporting Data

- "I'm not good enough.
- "No one could ever love me."
- "I'm fat and ugly . . . no good to anyone."
- "I do love my sons, although I don't always show it."

Long Term Goal: By discharge, the client will name two things she likes about herself.

Short Term Goal	Intervention	Rationale	Evaluation
1. By (date), the client will name two things she would like to change about herself.	1a. Assist the client in identifying two realistic things about herself that she would like to change.	1a. Helps the client to problem-solve in two important areas of her life that are amenable to change.	Goal met By the end of the first week, the client stated she (1) wanted to lose weight and (2) wanted to get back to being with some of her friends she had stopped seeing.
	1b. Work with the client to identify the various steps needed to help make these changes come about.	1b. Depressed clients often have difficulty problem solving because of poor concentration and faulty judgment.	
	1c. Identify specific skills the client might need to attain her goals, e.g.: ● Assertiveness training ● More effective communication skills ● Tension-reducing activities	1c. Identifying and teaching more effective coping skills can increase the perception of control and decrease feelings of hopelessness.	
	1d. Work with the therapist to reinforce the skills taught in therapy.	1d. Aids the health team in monitoring client progress and reinforcing positive coping skills.	
	1e. Role-play new coping skills with client.	1e. Aids in incorporating new skills into more automatic behavior.	
	1f. Encourage participation in group activities.	1f. Increases arena in which client can gain positive reinforcement.	

	1g. Assist client in planning a structured daily routine.	1g. Reduces time spent in negative rumination and helps client in thinking more in terms of goal directedness.	
2. Client will identify personal strengths by (date).	2a. Have client list those things she has been told are her strong points.	2a. A depressed person is often unable to see positive aspects in self but is able to identify others' perceptions.	**Goal met**
	2b. Discuss with the client those positive qualities she most admires in herself.	2b. Helps client integrate positive aspects of self.	By discharge, the client was able to admit that (1) even when depressed, she was considered the best secretary in the office, and (2) with the exception of the past weeks, she prides herself on being a good mother to her sons.
	2c. Encourage the client to give the nurse examples of when the client demonstrates these strengths.	2c. Helps to reinforce other more positive aspects of self and abilities.	

Summary

Depression is probably the most commonly seen mental disorder in the health care system. The two primary depressive disorders are major depression and dysthymia. The symptoms in a major depression are usually severe enough to interfere with a person's social or occupational functioning. A person in a major depression may or may not have psychotic symptoms, and the symptoms a person usually exhibits during a major depression are very different from his or her normal premorbid personality.

In dysthymia, the symptoms are often chronic in nature (lasting two or more years) and are considered mild to moderate. Usually a person's social or occupational functioning is not greatly impaired. The symptoms in a dysthymic depression are often congruent with the person's usual pattern of functioning.

There are a number of theories about the cause of depression. Four common theories include psychoanalytical theory, cognitive theory, learned helplessness theory, and psychophysiological theory.

Nursing assessment includes the assessment of (1) affect, (2) thought processes, (3) feelings, (4) physical behavior, and (5) communication. The nurse also needs to be aware of (6) the symptoms that mask depression.

Nursing diagnoses can be numerous. Depressed individuals are always evaluated for *high risk for self-directed violence*. Some other common nursing diagnoses are *altered thought processes, disturbance in self-esteem, altered nutrition, bowel elimination, sleep-pattern disturbance, ineffective individual coping,* and *ineffective family coping.*

Working with people who are depressed can evoke intense feelings of hopelessness and frustration in health care workers. Initially, nurses need support and guidance to clarify realistic expectations of themselves and their clients and to sort out personal feelings from those communicated by the client via empathy. Peer supervision and individual supervision with an experienced nurse clinician or psychiatric social worker or psychologist is useful in increasing therapeutic potential.

Interventions with clients who are depressed involve several approaches. The nurse intervenes therapeutically, using specific principles of communication, planning activities of daily living, administering or participating in somatic therapies, and maintaining a therapeutic environment.

Evaluation is ongoing throughout the nursing process, and the client's outcomes are compared with the stated short term and long term goals. The care plan is revised throughout the client's hospital stay by use of the evaluation process.

Self-study exercises 22–56 will help the student review the material covered in this section.

References

Abraham IL, Neese JB, Westerman PS. Nursing implications of a clinical and social problem. Nursing Clinics of North America, 26(3):527, 1991.

American Psychiatric Association. Diagnostic and Statistical Manual of Mental Disorders, 3rd ed, revised (DSM-III-R). Washington, DC: American Psychiatric Association, 1987.

American Psychiatric Association. DSM-IV Options Book: Work in Progress. Washington, DC: American Psychiatric Association, 1991.

American Psychiatric Association. The Practice of Electroconvulsive Therapy: Recommendations for Treatment, Training and Privileges. Washington, DC: American Psychiatric Press, 1990.

Bech P. Symptoms and assessment of depression. In Paykel ES (ed). Handbook of Affective Disorders, 2nd ed. New York: Guilford Press, 1992.

Beck AT, Young JE. Depression. In Barlow DH (ed). Clinical Handbook of Psychological Disorders. New York: Guilford Press, 1985.

Benton RG. Death and Dying: Principles and Practices in Patient Care. New York: Van Nostrand Company, 1978.

Bowlby J. Separation anxiety: A critical review of the literature. Journal of Child Psychology and Psychiatry, 1:251, 1961.

Bowlby J, Parkes C. Separation and loss within the family. In Anthony E, Koupenik C (eds). New York: John Wiley & Sons, 1970.

Buckwalter KC, Abraham IL. Alleviating the discharge crisis: The effects of cognitive-behavioral nursing intervention for depressed patients and their families. Archives of Psychiatric Nursing, 1(5):350, 1987.

Burns CM, Stuart GW. Nursing care in electroconvulsive therapy. Psychiatric Clinics of North America, 14(4):971, 1991.

Calarco MM, Krone KP. An integrated nursing model of depressive behavior in adults: Theory and implementation. Nursing Clinics of North America, 26(3):573, 1991.

Campbell L. Hopelessness. Journal of Psychosocial Nursing, 25(2):18, 1987.

Carr AL. Grief, mourning, and bereavement. In Kaplan HI, Sadock BJ (eds). Comprehensive Textbook of Psychiatry, (4th ed). Baltimore: Williams & Wilkins, 1985.

Cartwright RD, et al. REM latency and the recovery from depression: Getting over divorce. American Journal of Psychiatry, 148(11):1530, 1991.

Chapman AH. Textbook of Clinical Psychiatry, 2nd ed. Philadelphia: JB Lippincott, 1976.

Davidson JRT. Monoamine oxidase inhibitors. In Paykel ES (ed). Handbook of Affective Disorders, 2nd ed. New York: Guilford Press, 1992.

Davis JM, et al. The effects of a support group on grieving individuals' level of perceived support and stress. Archives of Psychiatric Nursing, 6(1):35, 1992.

Delgado PL, et al. Neurochemistry. In Paykel ES (ed). Handbook of Affective Disorders, 2nd ed. New York: Guilford Press, 1992.

Devanand DP, et al. Electroconvulsive therapy in the treatment-resistant patient. Psychiatric Clinics of North America, 14(4):905, 1991.

Dryman A, Eaton WW. Affective symptoms associated with the onset of major depression in the community: Findings from the US National Institute of Mental Health. Acta Psychiatrica Scandinavica, 84(1):1, 1991.

Elkin I, et al. 1989 National Institute of Mental Health treatment of depression collaborative research program. Archives of General Psychiatry, 46:971, 1989.

Engel GL. Grief and grieving. American Journal of Nursing, 64(9):93, 1964.

Fink M. Electroconvulsive therapy. In Paykel ES (ed). Handbook for Affective Disorders, 2nd ed. New York: Guilford Press, 1992.

Goodwin FK. Depression and manic-depressive illness. Bethesda, MD: US Department of Health and Human Services, National Institute of Mental Health, 1982.

Grove WM, Andreasen NC. Concepts, diagnosis and classification. In Paykel ES (ed). Handbook of Affective Disorders, 2nd ed. New York: Guilford Press, 1992.

Gulesserian B, Warren CJ. Coping resources of depressed patients. Archives of Psychiatric Nursing, 1(6):392, 1987.

Haaga DF, Beck AT. Cognitive therapy. In Paykel ES (ed). Handbook of Affective Disorders, 2nd ed. New York: Guilford Press, 1992.

Hirschfeld RMA, Goodwin FK. Mood disorders. In Talbott JA, Hales RE, Yudofsky SC (eds). Textbook of Psychiatry. Washington, DC: American Psychiatric Press, 1988.

Kaplan HI, Sadock BJ. Synopsis of Psychiatry: Behavioral Sciences and Clinical Psychiatry, 6th ed. Baltimore: Williams & Wilkins, 1991.

Lesse S. The masked depression syndrome—Results of a seventeen year clinical study. American Journal of Psychotherapy, 37:456, 1983.

Lindemann E. Symptomatology and management of acute grief. The American Journal of Psychiatry, 101:141, 1944.

Litman RE. Predicting and preventing hospital suicides. In Maris RW, et al (eds). Assessment and Prediction of Suicide. New York: Guilford Press, 1992.

Luby JL, Yalom ID. Group therapy. In Paykel ES (ed). Handbook of Affective Disorders, 2nd ed. New York: Guilford Press, 1992.

Marks MJ. The grieving patient and family. American Journal of Nursing, 76:1488, 1976.

Maxmen JS. Psychotropic Drugs Fast Facts. New York: WW Norton, 1991.

Mendelson M. Psychodynamics. In Paykel ES (ed). Handbook of Affective Disorders, 2nd ed. New York: Guilford Press, 1992.

Middleton W, Raphael B. Bereavement. In Paykel ES (ed). Handbook of Affective Disorders, 2nd ed. New York: Guilford Press, 1992.

Nurnberger JI Jr, Gershon ES. Genetics. In Paykel ES (ed). Handbook of Affective Disorders, 2nd ed. New York: Guilford Press, 1992.

Oren DA, Rosenthal NE. Seasonal affective disorder. In Paykel ES (ed). Handbook of Affective Disorders, 2nd ed. New York: Guilford Press, 1992.

Parker G. Early environment. In Paykel ES (ed). Handbook of Affective Disorders, 2nd ed. New York: Guilford Press, 1992.

Preston J, Johnson J. Clinical Psychopharmacology Made Ridiculously Simple. Miami, FL: Medmaster, 1991.

Psychiatry Drug Alerts, 2(8):57,59, 1992.

Rakoff VM. Psychiatric aspects of death in America. In Mack A (ed). Death in American Experience. New York: Schocken Books, 1973.

Ripley HS. Depression and the life span epidemiology. In Usdin D (ed). Depression: Clinical, Biological and Psychological Perspectives. New York: Brunner-Mazel, 1977.

Schatzberg AF, Cole JO. Manual of Clinical Psychopharmacology. 2nd ed. Washington, DC: American Psychiatric Press, 1991.

Schatzberg AF, Rothschild AJ. Psychiatric (delusional) major depression: Should it be included as a distinct syndrome in DSM-IV? American Journal of Psychiatry, 149(6):733, 1992.

Schwartz MS, Shockley EL. The Nurse and the Mental Patient: A Study in Interpersonal Relationships. New York: John Wiley & Sons, 1956.

Seligman ME. Fall into hopelessness. Psychology Today, 7:43, 1973.

Styron W. Darkness Visible: A Memoir of Madness. New York: Random House, 1990.

US Department of Health and Human Services, Public Health Service, Agency for Health Care and Research. Depression in primary care: Detection, diagnosis, and treatment. Journal of Psychosocial Nursing, 31(6):19, 1993.

Zisook S. Shuchter. Depression through the first year after the death of a spouse. American Journal of Psychiatry, 148(10):1346, 1992.

Further Reading

Allen MG. Twin studies of affective illness. Archives of General Psychiatry, 33:1476, 1976.

Arieti S. Affective disorders: Manic-depressive psychosis and psychotic depression. In Arieti S (ed). American Handbook of Psychiatry, 2nd ed. New York: Basic Books, 1974.

Beck A. The Diagnosis and Management of Depression. Philadelphia: University of Pennsylvania Press, 1967.

Beck AT. The core problem in depression: The cognitive triad. In Masseman J (ed). Depression: Theories and Therapies. New York: Grune & Stratton, 1970.

Beck MC, Rawlins RP, Williams SR. Mental Health Psychiatric Nursing: A Holistic Life Cycle Approach. St. Louis: CV Mosby, 1984.

Beeber LS. Antidepressant medications. In Lego S (ed). The American Handbook of Psychiatric Nursing. Philadelphia: JB Lippincott, 1984.

Bemporad JR. Psychoanalytically oriented psychotherapy. In Paykel ES (ed). Handbook of Affective Disorders, 2nd ed. New York: Guilford Press, 1992.

Bergersen BS. Pharmacology in Nursing. St. Louis: CV Mosby, 1979.

Bergin AE, Lambert MJ. The evaluation of therapeutic outcomes. In Garfield SI, Bergin AE (eds). Handbook of Psychotherapy and Behavior Change: An Empirical Analysis, 2nd ed. New York: John Wiley & Sons, 1978.

Bunney WE, Murphy DL, Goodwin FK, et al. The switch process from depression to mania: Relationship to drugs that alter brain amines. Lancet, 1:1022, 1970.

Cancro R. Overview of affective disorders. In Kaplan HI, Sadock BJ (eds). Comprehensive Textbook of Psychiatry, 2nd ed. Baltimore: Williams & Wilkins, 1985.

Checkley S. Neuroendocrinology. In Paykel ES (ed). Handbook of Affective Disorders, 2nd ed. New York: Guilford Press, 1992.

Corfman E. Depression, manic depressive illness and biological rhythms. Rockville, MD: US Department of Health and Human Services, National Institute of Mental Health, 1979.

Covi L, Roth D, Lipman RS. Cognitive group therapy of depression: The close-ended group. American Journal of Psychotherapy, 36:459, 1982.

Crary WG, Crary GC. Depression. American Journal of Nursing, 73:472, 1973.

Davison GC, Neale JM. Abnormal Psychology: An Experimental Clinical Approach, 3rd ed. New York: John Wiley & Sons, 1982.

DeGennaro MD, Hymen R, Crannell AM, et al. Antidepressant drug therapy. American Journal of Nursing, 83:1305, 1981.

Dempsey D. The way we die: An investigation of death and dying in America today. New York: Macmillan Publishing Company, 1975.

Donlon PT, Rockwell DA. Psychiatric Disorders: Diagnosis and Treatment. Bowie, MD: Robert J. Brady Company, 1982.

Drake RE, Price JL. Depression: Adaptation to disruption and loss. Perspectives in Psychiatric Care, 13:163, 1975.

Fitzgerald RG, Long I. Seclusion in the treatment and management of disturbed manic and depressed patients. Perspectives in Psychiatric Care, 11:59, 1973.

Freedman AM, Kaplan HI, Sadock BJ. Modern Synopsis of Comprehensive Textbook of Psychiatry, 2nd ed. Baltimore: Williams & Wilkins, 1976.

Gershon ES, Berretini WH, Nurnberger JI, et al. The genetics of affective illness. In Meltzer HY (ed). Psychopharmacology: The Third Generation of Progress. New York: Raven Press, 1987.

Gershon ES, Nurnberger JI, Berretini WH, et al. Affective disorders: Genetics. In Kaplan HI, Sadock BJ (eds). Comprehensive Textbook of Psychiatry, 2nd ed. Baltimore: Williams & Wilkins, 1985.

Gitlin MJ, Jamison KR. Lithium clinics: Theory and practice. Hospital and Community Psychiatry, 35:363, 1984.

Goldstein MJ, Baker BL, Jamison KR. Abnormal Psychology: Experiences, Origins and Interventions. Boston: Little, Brown & Company, 1980.

Goodwin DW, Guze SB. Psychiatric Diagnosis. New York: Oxford University Press, 1984.

Goodwin GM. Tricyclics and newer antidepressants. In Paykel ES (ed). Handbook of Affective Disorders, 2nd ed. New York: Guilford Press, 1992.

Guze SB, Robins E. Suicide and primary affective disorders. British Journal of Psychiatry 117:437, 1970.

Harris E. Lithium. American Journal of Nursing, 81:1310, 1981.

Hart CA, Turner MS, Orfitelli MK, et al. Introduction to Psychotropic Drugs. New York: Medical Examination Publishing Company, 1981.

Hinsie LE, Campbell RJ. Psychiatric Dictionary, 4th ed. New York: Oxford University Press, 1973.

Hirschfeld RMA, Shea MT. Affective disorders: Psychosocial treatment. In Kaplan HI, Sadock BJ (eds). Comprehensive Textbook of Psychiatry, 2nd ed. Baltimore: Williams & Wilkins, 1985.

Hollon SD, Beck AT. Psychotherapy and drug therapy: Comparison and combination. In Garfield SI, Bergin AE (eds). Handbook of Psychotherapy and Behavior Change: An Empirical Analysis, 2nd ed. New York: John Wiley & Sons, 1978.

Jackson EN. Understanding Grief: Its Roots, Dynamics and Treatment. Nashville: Abingdon, 1957.

Jacob M, Frank E, Kupfer DJ, et al. A psychoeducational workshop

for depressed patients, family and friends: Description and evaluation. Hospital and Community Psychiatry, 38(9):968, 1987.

Jacobs LI. Cognitive therapy of postmanic and postdepressive dysphoria in bipolar illness. American Journal of Psychotherapy, 36:450, 1982.

Karb VB, Queener SF, Freeman JB. Handbook of Drugs for Nursing Practice. St. Louis: CV Mosby, 1989.

Klerman GL. Affective disorders. In Nicholi AM Jr (ed). The Harvard Guide to Modern Psychiatry. Cambridge, MA: Belknap Press of Harvard University Press, 1978.

Klerman GL, Weissman MM. Interpersonal Psychotherapy. In Paykel ES (ed). Handbook of Affective Disorders, 2nd ed. New York: Guilford Press, 1992.

Lesse S. The relationship of anxiety to depression. American Journal of Psychotherapy, 36:332, 1982.

Levitt E, Lubin B, Brooks JM. Depression Concepts, Controversies and Some New Facts, 2nd ed. New York: Lawrence Erlbaum Associates, 1983.

Lickey ME, Gordon B. Drugs for Mental Illness: A Revolution in Psychiatry. New York: WH Freeman & Company, 1983.

Major LF. Electroconvulsive therapy in the 1980's. Psychiatry Clinics of North America, 7(3):613, 1984.

Matthysse S, Kidd KK. Evidence of HLA linkage in depressive disorders. New England Journal of Medicine, 305:1340, 1981.

McCoy SM, Garritson S. Seclusion, the process of intervening. Journal of Psychosocial Nursing and Mental Health Services, 21:8, 1983.

Mendelson M. Psychoanalytic Concepts of Depression, 2nd ed. New York: Books Division of Spectrum Publications, 1974.

Merck Manual, 14th ed. Rahway, NJ: Merck & Company, 1982.

Parios R, Taylor CM. Electroconvulsive treatment. In Lego S (ed). The American Handbook of Psychiatric Nursing. Philadelphia: JB Lippincott, 1984.

Parkes CM. Bereavement: Studies of Grief in Adult Life. New York: International Universities Press, 1972.

Pilkonis PA, Frank E. Personality pathology in recurrent depression: Nature, prevalence, and relationship to response. American Journal of Psychiatry, 145(4):435, 1988.

Rees WD, Lutkins S. Morality of bereavement. British Medical Journal, 23:31, 1967.

Scherer JS. Lippincott's Nurses' Drug Manual. Philadelphia: JB Lippincott, 1985.

Schultz JM, Dark SL. Manual of Psychiatric Nursing Care Plans. Boston: Little, Brown & Company, 1982.

Seligman MEP, Abramson LV, Semmell A, et al. Depressive attributal style. Journal of Abnormal Psychology, 88:242, 1979.

Warheit GJ. Life events, coping, stress, and depressive symptomatology. American Journal of Psychiatry, 136(4B):502, 1979.

Weitkamp LR, Stancer HC, Persad E, et al. Depressive disorders and HLA: A gene on chromosome 6 that can affect behavior. New England Journal of Medicine, 305:1301, 1981.

White B, et al. Psychodynamics of depression: Implications for treatment. In Usdin D (ed). Depression: Clinical, Biological and Psychological Perspectives. New York: Brunner-Mazel, 1977.

Whitlock FA. Symptomatic Affective Disorders. New York: Academic Press, 1982.

Self-study Exercises

GRIEF

Identify the phase of grief (shock, developing awareness, restitution) occurring in the acute stage of mourning.

1. _____ A person begins to feel intense feelings of anguish and despair. Anger, guilt, and crying are common at this phase.

2. _____ A person gathers together with family and friends in rituals of saying good-bye and ending the last remnants of denial.

3. _____ A person is not capable of emotionally accepting the intense feelings of pain and may have difficulty accepting the fact of death or may intellectualize feelings instead of feeling them.

True or false

4. _____ Completing the work of mourning takes four to eight weeks.
5. _____ Being with a person who is grieving can bring up one's own feelings of loss and sadness.
6. _____ Nurses have no difficulties dealing with people who are grieving and dying because they are around death so often.

The following are examples of the normal phenomena experienced during the mourning process. Match the example from the left column with the expected phenomenon from the right column.

7. _____ "If his brother had not been so hard on him, he would not have had the heart attack."

8. _____ "There were so many things I wanted to tell him . . . how much he meant to me . . . I should have said more kind things."

9. _____ "It sounds silly, but I am having difficulty swallowing, just the way John did before he died."

10. _____ "I just can't do anything . . . everything is so confusing. I don't even feel like eating or dressing."

11. _____ "Thoughts and memories just keep popping into my head . . . everything I see or do reminds me of the things we used to do together, everything."

12. _____ "I am thinking of resuming typing lessons . . . last night was the first night in a long time that I went to Bingo at church."

A. Sensations of somatic distress

B. Preoccupation with the deceased

C. Guilt

D. Anger

E. Disorganization and depression

F. Reorganization behavior

Evaluate the work of mourning as successful (S) or unsuccessful (U).

13. _____ "She was so strong. Why, I don't even think she cried the whole time—went through the whole process with a 'stiff upper lip.'"

14. _____ "She was a wreck when her sister died. Cried and carried on . . . why, it took her a year or more before she returned to church duties with any zest and started doing things again."

15. _____ "You know, Sid still talks about his mother as if she were alive today—weeps every time he talks about her. Well . . . she's been dead for four years."

16. _____ "I remember the good times we had together, but we had our rough times too before she died."

Multiple choice

17. Regina, a 24-year-old woman whose mother has just died a painful death from cancer, tells the nurse tearfully she does not think she will ever get over her mother's death. Which of the following would be the most appropriate response for the nurse to make?

    A. "Time heals all wounds, and yours will heal in time also."
    B. "It was the best thing that could happen to her; she was in so much pain."
    C. "The loss must be very painful for you."
    D. "The hardest part will be the next couple of months. In a year you will feel fine again."

18. Three of the following are factors that could interfere with Regina's successful resolution of the grief process. Which factor would facilitate the mourning process?

    A. Regina said she loved her mother, but so often their relationship was stormy, and at other times she stated that she hated her mother.
    B. Regina had lost her job two months before, and she and her husband had recently separated.
    C. Regina had always been a good problem solver, and she had many friends whom she counted on as a sounding board and for support.
    D. Regina was always complaining of physical illnesses, and two months ago she was hospitalized with hepatitis.

List three nursing actions that can facilitate a family's grieving process (Table 17–2).

19. _____

20. _____

21. _____

DEPRESSIVE DISORDERS

Indicate whether the following are most likely characteristic of a major depression (MD) or a dysthymic depression (D).

22. _____ May have psychotic symptoms.
23. _____ Usually has a chronic course of two years or more.
24. _____ The symptoms are *not* congruent with the person's premorbid personality.
25. _____ Usually considered mild to moderate in nature. The symptoms do not greatly interfere with the person's occupational or interpersonal functioning.

Identify the corresponding theoretical approach: P (psychoanalytical), C (cognitive), B (biological), L (learned helplessness).

26. _____ The success of the TCAs and the MAOIs helps to support this theory.
27. _____ Thoughts can affect a person's mood.
28. _____ Loss and aggression turned against the self are two of the basic components of this theory.
29. _____ If a person believes he or she has no power to change a situation, and the situation is hopeless, the person can become depressed.

Name two pieces of data one might find with a depressed person on assessment for each of the following:

30. Affect   1. _____   2. _____

31. Thinking   1. _____   2. _____

32. Feelings   1. _____   2. _____

33. Physical Behavior   1. _____   2. _____

34. Communications   1. _____   2. _____

35. Indications of   1. _____   2. _____
     masked depres-
     sion

For each of the following possible nursing diagnoses formulated for the depressed client, write one long term goal and one short term goal:

36. High risk for self-directed violence:
     LTG: _____
     STG: _____

37. Altered thought processes:
     LTG: _____
     STG: _____

38. Social isolation:
     LTG: _____
     STG: _____

Feelings of frustration, anger, and worthlessness may originate in the depressed client and be experienced by the nurse. Which of the following actions by the nurse would be productive (P) and which nonproductive (NP)?

39. _____ Say little and realize that these feelings will go away.
40. _____ Discuss these feelings in team meetings and validate feelings, perceptions, and ways to handle these feelings when with the client.
41. _____ Ask for supervision by an experienced nurse clinician, social worker, or psychologist in order to increase self-awareness and therapeutic skills.

Label the following responses made by a nurse as H (helpful) or NH (not helpful) with a depressed client.

42. _____ "Don't worry, we all get down once in awhile."
43. _____ Don't talk of suicide, the person might get ideas.
44. _____ "Debra, I like your new dress."
45. _____ "I will stay with you for five minutes at 10:00 A.M., 1:00 P.M., and 3:30 P.M. today."
46. _____ Try to cheer the person up with a personal story or joke.
47. _____ If a client says an angry word, help him or her control the anger.

State a common physical problem a depressed person may have for each of the following areas, and offer two suggestions for intervention:

48. *Nutrition*
Problem: _____
Interventions: 1. _____
                 2. _____

49. *Elimination*
Problem: _____
Interventions: 1. _____
                 2. _____

50. *Rest and sleep*
Problem: _____
Interventions: 1. _____
                 2. _____

51. *Physical activity*
Problem: _____
Interventions: 1. _____
                 2. _____

Multiple choice

52. Mr. Smith has been put on amitriptyline (Elavil). The intern asks the nurse how often and when the best time might be to give this drug. Which of the following would be the nurse's best response?

A. Every morning, since it has a stimulant effect.
B. With meals, since it is irritating to the gastric mucosa.
C. At night—the full dose—to aid sleep and minimize side effects when the client is awake.
D. In four divided doses throughout the day.

53. Serious side effects can occur in people with heart conditions when they are given a TCA. Adverse drug reactions can also occur with all the following drugs *except*

A. Insulin
B. MAOIs
C. Alcohol
D. Oral contraceptives, such as estrogen preparations

54. When Mr. Smith did not respond to the TCAs, phenelzine (Nardil), an MAOI, was ordered. Which of the following would *not* be a nursing consideration for Mr. Smith?

A. Wait 10 days after the Elavil has been stopped.
B. Monitor blood pressure closely after the MAOI is started.
C. Stop the medication if the client complains of fatigue and constipation.
D. Carefully teach the client and family about certain foods and drugs that may *not* be taken with an MAOI.

55. Which of the following is an important nursing consideration with ECT?

A. Permanent brain damage occurs with several treatments.
B. ECT has had good results in patients with paranoid schizophrenia and "neurotic" depressions.

C. There are virtually no physical contraindications to ECT.

D. During the course of treatment, a client will need frequent orientation to time, place, and person.

56. Which of the following types of therapy for depressed clients has shown a great deal of promise?

A. Psychoanalytical

B. Cognitive

C. Drug therapy used alone

D. Ego psychology

CHAPTER 18

Alterations in Mood: Elation in Bipolar Disorder

Elizabeth M. Varcarolis

OUTLINE

THEORY

ASSESSMENT
Assessing Mood
Assessing Behavior
Assessing Thought Processes

NURSING DIAGNOSIS

PLANNING
Content Level—Planning Goals
Process Level—Nurses' Reactions and
    Feelings

INTERVENTION
Psychotherapeutic Interventions
Activities of Daily Living
Somatic Therapies
Therapeutic Environment
Psychotherapy

EVALUATION

CASE STUDY: WORKING WITH A
    PERSON WHO IS MANIC

SUMMARY

KEY TERMS AND CONCEPTS

The key terms and concepts listed here also appear in bold where they are
defined or discussed in this chapter.

ANTICONVULSANT DRUGS

BIPOLAR DISORDER

CLANG ASSOCIATIONS

CYCLOTHYMIA

FLIGHT OF IDEAS

HYPOMANIA

LITHIUM CARBONATE

MANIA

PRESSURE OF SPEECH

SCHIZOAFFECTIVE DISORDER

OBJECTIVES

After studying this chapter, the student will be able to

1. Describe characteristics observed during the assessment of a manic client's
   (a) mood, (b) behavior, and (c) thought processes.
2. Formulate three nursing diagnoses appropriate for a manic client, including
   supporting data.
3. Identify one long term and two short term goals for each of the three nursing
   diagnoses.
4. Give examples of unconscious tactics used by a person who is manic to maintain the manic defense.
5. Discuss the rationale for five principles of communication for use with a manic
   client.

465

6. For each of the following areas, identify two interventions a nurse may use when caring for the physical needs of the manic client: nutrition, rest and sleep, elimination, dress and hygiene, and physical activities.
7. Name four (a) expected side effects for a person on lithium therapy, (b) early signs of lithium toxicity, (c) advanced signs of lithium toxicity, and (d) indications of severe toxic effects of lithium.
8. Write a care plan specifying five areas of client teaching regarding lithium carbonate.
9. Indicate two clinical conditions that often respond better to anticonvulsant therapy than to lithium therapy.
10. Describe indications for the use of seclusion with a manic client.

Mood disorders, also referred to as affective disorders, are divided into the bipolar and depressive disorders. The depressive disorders are covered in Chapter 17. This chapter discusses the bipolar disorders. The bipolar disorders include the occurrence of depressive episodes and one or more elated mood episodes.

An elated mood can range from normal elevated mood to hypomania to mania. In extreme mania, thought processes become incoherent, and delusions may be bizarre. Figure 18–1 places hypomania and mania along the mental health continuum.

In **mania,** delusions, poor judgment, and other signs of impaired reality testing are often evident. During a manic episode, a person has marked impairment in his or her social, occupational, and interpersonal functioning.

The symptoms of **hypomania** are less severe than those of mania. A person in hypomania does *not* experience impairment in reality testing, nor do the symptoms markedly impair the person's social, occupational, or interpersonal functioning. Figure 18–2 shows the diagnostic criteria for hypomania and mania.

Mania can be viewed as a reaction-formation to depression. A person in a manic state is thought to be literally running from the psychogenic pain of underlying depression. The frenetic running behavior is evidenced in both the constant physical activity and the racing speech and thought patterns demonstrated by the manic client. Although outwardly the person may act elated, arrogant, and superior, there is almost always a strong depressive force behind the unstable and "upbeat" facade. The elation and hyperactivity seem to help keep feelings of worthlessness and hopelessness at bay. The closer the feelings associated with the depression are to consciousness, the faster the person in mania must run. Mania can escalate to psychotic proportions.

The two major bipolar disorders are (1) bipolar disorder and (2) cyclothymia. Schizoaffective disorder, which is briefly discussed here, consists of both schizophrenic and affective symptoms.

BIPOLAR DISORDER. Bipolar disorder is a mood disorder that includes one or more manic episodes (elevated, expansive, or irritable mood), and usually one or more depressive episodes. Between the elevated and depressed mood episodes, the person may experience long periods of a normal stable mood. The symptoms observed in bipolar disorder are more severe than those seen in cyclothymia.

The manic episode in bipolar disorder may begin suddenly and last a few days to months. Impairment in reality testing may take the form of grandiose or persecutory delusions. There is considerable impairment in social, occupational, and interpersonal functioning. Hospitalization is often warranted to protect the person from the consequences of poor judgment and hyperactivity.

Bipolar disorder has been further divided into two types in the North American literature (Perris 1992, DSM-IV):

1. Bipolar I consists of periods of major depressions plus periods of clear-cut mania.
2. Bipolar II consists of periods of major depression plus periods of hypomania.

CYCLOTHYMIA. Cyclothymia is a chronic mood disturbance of at least two years' duration. Cyclothymia denotes the recurrent experience of some of the symptoms of mania and depression; however, the symptoms do not meet the full DSM-IV criteria for either mania or major depression (American Psychiatric Association 1994). Essentially, the symptoms of cyclothymia consist of alternating periods of dysthymia and hypomania. Periods of normal mood, if present at all, are very short.

The episodes of hypomania or depression are not usually severe enough to warrant hospitalization. Delusions are *never* present, and the person's social, oc-

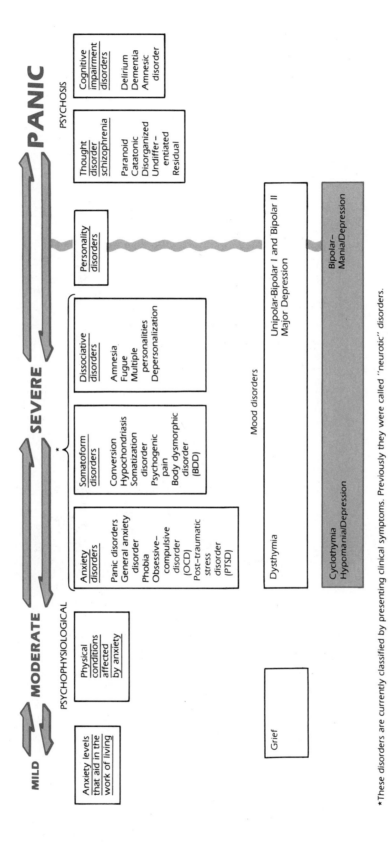

MILD ⟺ MODERATE ⟺ SEVERE ⟺ PANIC

PSYCHOPHYSIOLOGICAL

PSYCHOSIS

Anxiety levels
that aid in the
work of living

Physical
conditions
affected
by anxiety

Anxiety
disorders

Panic disorders
General anxiety
disorder
Phobia
Obsessive–
compulsive
disorder
(OCD)
Post-traumatic
stress
disorder
(PTSD)

Somatoform
disorders

Conversion
Hypochondriasis
Somatization
disorder
Psychogenic
pain
Body dysmorphic
disorder
(BDD)

Dissociative
disorders

Amnesia
Fugue
Multiple
personalities
Depersonalization

Personality
disorders

Thought
disorder
schizophrenia

Paranoid
Catatonic
Disorganized
Undiffer–
entiated
Residual

Cognitive
impairment
disorders

Delirium
Dementia
Amnesic
disorder

*

Mood disorders

Grief

Dysthymia

Unipolar-Bipolar I and Bipolar II
Major Depression

Cyclothymia
Hypomania/Depression

Bipolar-
Mania/Depression

*These disorders are currently classified by presenting clinical symptoms. Previously they were called "neurotic" disorders.

Figure 18–1. *Elation along the mental health continuum.*

1. A distinct period of abnormally and persistently elevated, expansive, or irritable mood for at least 2 weeks

2. During the period of mood disturbance, at least three of the following symptoms have persisted (four if the mood is only irritable) and have been present to a significant degree:

   • Inflated self-esteem or grandiosity

   • Decreased need for sleep (e.g., the person feels rested after only three hours of sleep)

   • Increased talkativeness or pressure to keep talking

   • Flight of ideas or subjective experience that thoughts are racing

   • Distractibility (i.e., the person's attention is too easily drawn to unimportant or irrelevant external stimuli)

   • Increase in goal–directed activity (either socially, at work or school, or sexually) or psychomotor agitation

   • Excessive involvement in pleasurable activities that have a high potential for painful consequences (e.g., the person engages in unrestrained buying sprees, sexual indiscretions, or foolish business investments)

HYPOMANIA

1. Symptoms are less severe than in a manic episode

2. Absence of marked impairment in social or occupational functioning

3. Delusions are never present

4. Hospitalization is not indicated

MANIA

1. Severe enough to cause marked impairment in occupational activities, usual social activities, or relationships

2. Delusions may be present (grandiose, paranoid, or both)

3. Hospitalization is needed to protect client and others from irresponsible or aggressive behavior

Figure 18–2. *Diagnostic criteria for manic symptoms. (Adapted from the American Psychiatric Association. Diagnostic and Statistical Manual of Mental Disorders, 4th ed (DSM-IV). Washington, DC: American Psychiatric Association, 1994.)*

cupational, and interpersonal functioning are not grossly impaired. Hospitalization is rarely necessary unless the person is thought to be suicidal.

SCHIZOAFFECTIVE DISORDER. Schizoaffective disorder was identified and named in 1933. A schizoaffective disorder has the following features (Coryll and Winokur 1992):

• Mixture of schizophrenic and affective symptoms
• Good premorbid adjustment
• Acute onset
• Family history of mood disorder

Schizoaffective disorder has been given many

names, such as schizophreniform psychosis and reactive psychosis (Hirschfeld and Goodwin 1988). When compared with schizophrenic patients, schizoaffective patients have consistently better outcomes. However, when compared with typical affective disorder patients, schizoaffective patients have poorer outcomes (Coryll and Winokur 1992). A relatively good prognosis for a person with a schizoaffective disorder is associated with

• Bipolar features
• Acute onset
• Absence of history of schizophrenia-like symptoms, with no concurrent mood symptoms

Theory

The most accepted hypothesis is that unipolar and bipolar disorders represent two different disorders (Kaplan and Sadock 1991). Table 18–1 lists the differences between bipolar and unipolar disorders.

Bipolar disorders (one or more episodes of both elated and depressed moods) are thought to be distinctly different from nonbipolar depressive disorders, such as major depression or dysthymia (Weissman and Boyd 1985). A vast amount of research is now being conducted to identify causes for the mood disorders. Most of this research is being done in the biological sphere. Some theoretical data pertaining specifically to the etiology of the bipolar disorders are (1) genetic, (2) interactive transmitters system (biogenic amines), (3) social, and (4) psychosocial.

GENETIC. Significant evidence exists to support the theory that bipolar disorders are a result of genetic transmission. For example, there is a higher rate of bipolar disorder and cyclothymia in relatives of patients with bipolar disorders than in those of patients with major depressions or in the general population (Gershon et al. 1985; Weissman and Boyd 1985). A study at National Institutes of Mental Health found that 25% of relatives of bipolar clients had bipolar or unipolar illness. For unipolar clients, 20% of relatives had bipolar or unipolar illness, compared with 7% of relatives of control clients (Nurnberger and Gershon 1992). Twin studies bear out a genetic marker for both the bipolar disorders and the depressive disorders;

however, the incidence of illness is significantly higher in the bipolar disorders. Identical twins are 78–80% more concordant than fraternal twins (14–19%) (Hirschfeld and Goodwin 1988; Nurnberger and Gershon 1992).

BIOGENIC AMINES. The neurotransmitters (norepinephrine, dopamine, and serotonin) have been studied since the 1960s as causal factors in mania and depression. Subsequent research has found that the interrelationships among the neurotransmitter system are very complex. More complex hypotheses have developed since the amine hypotheses were originally proposed. Mood disorders are most likely a result of complex interactions between various chemicals, including neurotransmitters and hormones. Biological research findings support the hypothesis that mood disorders involve pathology of the limbic system, basal ganglia, and hypothalamus (Kaplan and Sadock 1991).

SOCIAL STATUS. Some evidence suggests that the bipolar disorders may be more prevalent in the upper socioeconomic classes. The exact reason for this is unclear; however, people with bipolar disorders appear to achieve higher levels of education and occupational status than nonbipolar depressed individuals. There is, however, no difference in education across various socioeconomic classes with the nonbipolar depressions. Also, a high proportion of bipolar clients has been found among creative writers, highly educated men and women, and professional people.

PSYCHOSOCIAL. Although there is increasing evidence for genetic and biological markers in the etiology of the mood disorders, psychosocial factors are

Table 18–1 ■ DIFFERENCES IN BIPOLAR AND UNIPOLAR DISORDERS

	BIPOLAR	UNIPOLAR
Age of onset	Earlier: 19–30 years (mean, 21 years)	Later: 40–44 years (mean, 40 years)
Sex	Equally frequent in men and women	Twice as frequent in women than in men
Family environment	Higher rate of divorce and marital conflict	Divorce rate same as in general population
Stressful life events	Contributory in the occurrence of both	Contributory in the occurrence of both
Personality traits	"Dominance," "exhibition," and "autonomy" needs higher in bipolar More hypomanic drive toward success and achievement	"Defense of status" and "guilt feeling" higher in unipolar Tendency toward a lack of autonomy
Symptoms in a depressed phase	*More likely to show:* Psychomotor retardation Hypersomnia Fewer somatic complaints Less anxiety	*More likely to show:* Increased motor activity Insomnia Somatic complaints Hypochondriasis
Course and outcome	Higher frequency of relapse than in unipolar	Lower frequency of relapse than in bipolar

Adapted from Perris C. Bipolar-unipolar distinction. *In* Paykel ES (ed). Handbook of Affective Disorders, 2nd ed. New York: Guilford Press, 1992.

still thought to be relevant. For example, manic and hypomanic episodes are viewed by some psychoanalytic theorists as extreme defenses against depression. The manic or hypomanic defense can be viewed as an attempt to avoid inner pain through exhausting activity and an exaggerated, elevated, or expansive mood. In short, the person unconsciously acts out the exact opposite of his or her underlying feelings. Thus, the manic defense can be conceptualized as a reaction-formation to, or denial of, an underlying depression.

Assessment

The three most common initial symptoms in the onset of mania are (1) elated mood, (2) increased activity, and (3) reduced sleep. Not all people in the manic state experience euphoria; some people become extremely irritable, especially when limits are set on their behavior. The nurse evaluates these characteristics when assessing a manic client's (1) mood, (2) behavior, and (3) thought processes.

ASSESSING MOOD

The euphoric mood associated with a bipolar illness is unstable and inconstant. During euphoria, clients may state that they are experiencing an intense feeling of well-being, are "cheerful in a beautiful world," or are becoming "one with God" (Silverstone and Hunt 1992). This mood may change to irritation and quick anger when the elated person does not get his or her way. The irritability and belligerence may be short-lived, or it may become the prominent feature of a person's manic illness. When elated, the person's overjoyous mood may seem out of proportion to what is going on around him or her, and a cheerful mood may be inappropriate to the circumstances.

The person in a manic state may laugh, joke, and talk in a continuous stream, with uninhibited familiarity. Manic people demonstrate boundless enthusiasm, treat everyone with confidential friendliness, and incorporate everyone into their plans and activities. "They know no strangers." Energy and self-confidence seem boundless (Chapman 1976).

Elaborate schemes to get rich and famous and acquire unlimited power are frantically pursued, despite objections and realistic constraints. Excessive phone calls are made, and telegrams are sent to famous and influential people all over the world. The manic is busy all hours of the day and night furthering his or her grandiose plans and wild schemes. To the manic person, there are no limits too high or distances too far. There are no boundaries in reality to curtail the elaborate schemes.

In the manic state, a person often gives away money, prized possessions, and expensive gifts. The manic throws lavish parties, frequents expensive nightclubs and restaurants, and spends money freely on friends and strangers alike. This spending, charging, and high living continue, even in the face of bankruptcy. Intervention is often needed to prevent financial ruin.

As the clinical course progresses, sociability and euphoria are replaced by a stage of hostility, irritability, and paranoia. The high-spirited, jovial, confident, and enthusiastic mood eventually slips, and the forced gaiety and frantic running are revealed as a brittle defense against painful feelings (Klerman 1978). A client describes the painful transition from hypomania to mania (Goldstein et al. 1980):

Hypomania

At first when I'm high, it's tremendous . . . ideas are fast . . . like shooting stars you follow 'til brighter ones appear . . . all shyness disappears, the right words and gestures are suddenly there . . . uninteresting people, things become intensely interesting. Sensuality is pervasive, the desire to seduce and be seduced is irresistible. Your marrow is infused with unbelievable feelings of ease, power, well being, omnipotence, euphoria . . . you can do anything . . . but somewhere this changes. . . .

Mania

The fast ideas become too fast and there are far too many . . . overwhelming confusion replaces clarity . . . you stop keeping up with it—memory goes. Infectious humor ceases to amuse—your friends become frightened . . . everything now is against the grain . . . you are irritable, angry, frightened, uncontrollable, and trapped in the blackest caves of the mind—caves you never knew were there. It will never end. Madness carves its own reality.

Refer to Table 18–2 for the symptoms of mania along a continuum from moderate to panic.

ASSESSING BEHAVIOR

When manic, a person constantly flits from one activity to another, one place to another, one project to another. Many projects may be started, but few, if any, are completed. Inactivity is impossible, even for the

Table 18-2 ■ MANIA ON A CONTINUUM

MODERATE TO SEVERE		PANIC
Hypomanic	**Acute Manic**	**Severe Manic**
Communication		
1. Talks and jokes incessantly, is the "life of the party," gets irritated when not center of attention.	1. May go suddenly from laughing to anger or depression. *Mood is labile.*	1. Totally out of touch with reality.
2. Treats everyone with familiarity and confidentiality; often borders on crude.	2. Becomes inappropriately demanding of people's attention, and intrusive nature repels others.	—
3. Talk is often very sexual in nature—can reach obscene, inappropriate propositions to total strangers.	3. Speech may be marked by profanities and crude sexual remarks to everyone (nursing staff in particular).	—
4. Talk is fresh; flits from one topic to the next. Marked by *pressure of speech.*	4. Speech marked by *flight of ideas,* in which thoughts racing and flying from topic to topic. May have *clang association.*	4. Most likely has *clang associations.*
Affect and Thinking		
1. Full of pep and good humor, feelings of good humor, euphoria, and sociability; may show inappropriate intimacy with strangers.	1. Good humor gives way to increased irritability and hostility, short-lived period of rage, especially when not getting one's way or controls are set on behavior. May have quick shifts of mood from hostility to docility.	1. May become destructive or aggressive—totally out of control.
2. Feels boundless self-confidence and enthusiasm. Has elaborate schemes for becoming rich and famous. Initially, schemes may seem plausible.	2. Grandiose plans are totally out of contact with reality. Thinks one is musician, prominent businessman, great politician, or religious figure, without any basis in fact.	2. May experience undefined hallucinations and delirium.
3. Judgment often poor. Gets involved with schemes in which his job, marriage, or financial status may be destroyed.	3. Judgment extremely poor.	—
4. May get involved with writing large quantities of letters to rich and famous people regarding schemes or may make numerous world-wide telephone calls.	—	—
5. Decreased attention span to both internal and external cues.	5. Decreased attention span and distractibility intensified.	—
Physical Behavior		
1. Overactive, distractible, buoyant, and busily occupied with grandiose plans (not delusions); goes from one action to the next.	1. Extremely restless, disorganized, and chaotic. Physical behavior may be difficult to control. May have outbursts, e.g., throwing things or becoming briefly assaultive when crossed.	1. *Dangerous state.* Incoherent, extremely restless, disoriented, and agitated. Hyperactive. Motor activity is totally aimless (must have physical or chemical restraints to prevent exhaustion and death).
2. Increased sexual appetite; sexually unresponsible and indiscreet. Illegitimate pregnancies in hypomanic female and venereal disease in both male and female are common. Sex used for escape, not for relating to another human being.	2. Too busy—no time for sex. Poor concentration, distractibility, and restlessness too severe.	2. Same as in acute mania but in the extreme.
3. May have voracious appetite, eat on the run, or gobble food during brief periods.	3. No time to eat—too distracted and disorganized.	3. Same as acute mania but in the extreme.
4. May go without sleeping; unaware of fatigue. However, may be able to grab short naps.	4. No time for sleep—psychomotor activity too high; if unchecked can lead to exhaustion and death.	—
5. Financially extravagant, goes on buying sprees, gives money and gifts away freely, can easily go into debt.	5. Same as in hypomania but in the extreme.	5. Too disorganized to do anything.

Data from Chapman 1976; Klerman 1978; Silverstone and Hunt 1992.

shortest period of time. Hyperactivity may range from mild, constant motion to frenetic, wild activity. Writing flowery and lengthy letters and making numerous and excessive long distance telephone calls are common. The spending of large sums of money on frivolous items and giving money away indiscriminately can leave a family in debt.

When a person is *hypomanic*, he or she has a voracious appetite for food as well for indiscriminate sex. Although the constant activity of the hypomanic prevents proper sleep, short periods of sleep are possible. However, a reduced need for sleep is experienced by all manic clients, and some patients may not sleep for several days in a row. The *manic* person is too busy to eat, sleep, or engage in sexual activity. *This nonstop physical activity and the lack of sleep and food can lead to physical exhaustion and even death.*

Modes of dress often reflect the person's grandiose yet tenuous grasp on reality. Dress may be described as outlandish, bizarre, colorful, and noticeably inappropriate. Makeup may be garish or overdone. The manic client is highly distractible. Concentration is poor, and he or she flits from one activity to another without completing anything. Judgment is poor. Impulsive marriages and divorces take place. People often emerge from a manic state startled and confused by the shambles in which their lives are left. The following description conveys one client's experience (Goldstein et al. 1980):

After Mania

Now there are only other's recollections of your behavior—your bizarre, frenetic, aimless behavior—at least mania has the grace to dim memories of itself . . . now it's over, but is it? . . . Incredible feelings to sort through . . . Who is being too polite? Who knows what? What did I do? Why? and most hauntingly, will it, when will it, happen again? Medication to take, to resist, to resent, to forget . . . but always to take. Credit cards revoked . . . explanations at work . . . bad checks and apologies overdue . . . memory flashes of vague men (what did I do?) . . . friendships gone, a marriage ruined.

ASSESSING THOUGHT PROCESSES

Flight of ideas is a nearly continuous flow of speech. The person jumps rapidly from one topic to another. At times, the attentive listener can keep up with the changes, even though direction changes from moment to moment. Speech is rapid, verbose, and circumstantial (including minute and unnecessary details). The goal is to maintain superficiality and escape from

thoughts that would activate the underlying depression. The incessant talking often includes joking, playing on words (puns), and teasing:

How are you doing kid, no kidding around, I'm going home . . . home sweet home . . . home is where the heart is, the heart of the matter is I want out and that ain't hay, . . . hey, Doc . . . get me out of this place. . . .

The content of speech is often sexually explicit and ranges from grossly inappropriate to vulgar. Themes in the communication of the manic may revolve around his or her extraordinary sexual prowess, brilliant business ability, or unparalleled artistic talents (e.g., writing, painting, or dancing). The person may have average ability in these areas, at best.

Some of the manic's tension is drained off by what is termed **pressure of speech.** One can hear the force and energy behind the rapid words. Speech is not only profuse, but loud, bellowing, and even screaming.

As mania escalates, flight of ideas may give way to clang associations. **Clang associations** is the stringing together of words because of their rhyming sounds, without regard to their meaning, such as "Good luck, buck, chuck, duck" or "red, bed, said, ted, led." Pressure of speech is easily detected in the staccato, rapid outpouring of clang associations.

Grandiosity (inflated self-regard) is apparent in either the ideas expressed or the person's behavior. Manic people may exaggerate their achievements or importance, state they know famous people, or believe they have great powers (Silverstone and Hunt 1992). The boast of exceptional powers and status can take delusional proportions in mania. Grandiose persecutory delusions are common. For example, a manic client may think that God is speaking to him or her or that the FBI is out to stop him or her from accomplishing some great feat, such as saving the world. Sensory perceptions may become altered as the mania escalates, and hallucinations may occur. However, in hypomania, there is no evidence of delusions or hallucinations. (See Table 18–2 for an illustration of mania along a continuum from moderate to panic.)

Nursing Diagnosis

Nursing diagnoses can vary for the manic client. When an acutely manic client comes into the hospital, the primary consideration is the prevention of exhaustion and death from cardiac collapse. Because of the client's poor judgment, excessive and constant motor activity, probable dehydration, and difficulty evaluating reality, *high risk for injury* is a likely and appropriate diagnosis if the client's activity level is dangerous to his or her health. Immediate medical and nursing interventions are often vital to prevent physical exhaustion. Bruises or wounds, resulting from falling or bumping into objects, or secondary infections, resulting from lack of nutrition, lack of sleep, and personal neglect, indicate that the client is at risk for injury.

High risk for violence to self or others related to rage reaction, as evidenced by inability to control behavior, occurs frequently when excitation becomes so severe that the client may be destructive, hostile, and aggressive. Aggression is a common feature in mania. At times, intrusive and taunting behavior can induce others to strike out against these clients.

Grandiosity, poor judgment, and giving away of possessions can result in bankruptcy, neglect of family, and impulsive major life changes (e.g., divorce, marriage, or career changes). These behaviors suggest *altered thought processes*. Getting involved in impossible schemes, shady legal deals, and questionable business ventures may be a result of *ineffective individual coping* related to altered affect, caused by changes in body chemistry or inadequate psychological resources.

Defensive coping may be evidenced by the client's manipulative, angry, or hostile verbal and physical behaviors, which are an attempt to gain a sense of control when the manic client is unable to control racing thoughts or erratic behavior.

The client in the acutely manic state may have numerous unmet physical needs. The manic client is too busy to eat and sleep, and is often constipated and poorly groomed. The client's dress may be flamboyant and bizarre. *Fluid volume deficit, altered nutrition* (less than body requirements), *constipation, sleep-pattern disturbance,* and *self-care deficit* are all possible diagnoses.

Because of the manic's rapid speech (flight of ideas), poor attention span, and difficulty concentrating, *altered family process* related to an ill family member should always be assessed. The family as well as the client will need to have questions answered and will need understanding and support.

Planning

Planning interventions for a person who is manic is planned on two levels: (1) the content level—planning goals, and (2) the process level—nurses' reactions and feelings.

CONTENT LEVEL—PLANNING GOALS

After the assessment has been made and the nursing diagnoses placed in order of priority, short term and long term goals are formulated. Goals are made for each nursing diagnosis according to the client's unmet needs. Listed subsequently are possible goals for the following diagnoses:

1. *High risk for injury*:
   - The client's cardiac status will remain stable during hospitalization.
   - While in an acutely manic state, the client will drink 8 ounces of fluid every hour throughout the day.
   - The client will spend time with the nurse in a quiet environment each hour between 7 A.M. and 11 P.M.
   - The client's skin will be free from abrasions and scrapes every day while in the hospital.

2. *High risk for violence directed at others*:
   - By (date) the client will display nonviolent behavior toward others in the hospital, with the aid of medication and nursing interventions.
   - With the aid of seclusion or nursing interventions, the client will refrain from provoking others to physically harm themselves.
   - The client will respond to external controls (medication, seclusion, nursing interventions) when potential or actual loss of control occurs.

3. *Ineffective coping* or *altered thought process*:
   - Client will retain valuables or other possessions while in the hospital.
   - Client will make only one five-minute telephone call per hour.
   - Client will have competent medical assistance and legal protection when signing any legal documents regarding personal or financial matters.

4. *Fluid volume deficit, altered nutrition* (less than body requirements), *constipation, sleep-pattern disturbance,* and *self-care deficit*:
   - Client will have good skin turgor by (time).
   - Client will have normal bowel movements within two days with the aid of high-fiber foods and fluids.
   - Client will take a 10-minute rest period every two hours during the day (8:00 A.M. to 10:00 P.M.), with the aid of the nurse.
   - Client will sleep six hours in 24 hours with the aid of medication and nursing measures within three days.
   - Client will wear appropriate makeup or shave each day while in the hospital.

- Client will wear appropriate attire for age and sex each day while in the hospital.

5. *Altered family process.* Usually, when an episode of mania ceases (a few days to a few months), people return to normal functioning. Often, however, during a manic flight, an individual may unknowingly violently overthrow what was once a "normal" life. People may come out of their manic sprees startled to find themselves broke, without a job, without friends, and without a spouse. Families need to understand what is happening and need support and counseling for themselves. The goals a nurse sets will depend on the complexity of the situation. Often, many members of the health team become involved with supporting the families. For example, social workers, psychologists, psychiatrists, psychiatric nurse clinicians, and staff nurses give important information and realistic reassurances and can make appropriate referrals. Goals may include
   - Family or spouse will meet with the nurse to assess family needs by the end of the week.
   - Family or spouse will discuss prognosis, use of medications, and how to recognize prodromal signs of mania before discharge.

PROCESS LEVEL—NURSES' REACTIONS AND FEELINGS

A nurse working with a manic client for the first time needs guidance and support and needs to become aware of possible client behaviors resulting from the manic defense. The manic client poses problems and requires interventions very different from those of the withdrawn and depressed individual.

First, the manic client, unlike most all other clients on the psychiatric unit, needs to be directed *away* from active environmental stimuli (e.g., upbeat music, activity groups, games, or large meetings) to minimize the escalation of the mania.

A quiet, dimly lit, and calm atmosphere is ideal for the manic. Getting a client to stay in such an environment is a formidable task. The manic needs to be up, to be high, to keep depressive feelings from surfacing. Therefore, the individual rarely stays put for very long. A firm and neutral approach usually works best. *Because the manic client is so distractible, the nurse can use this distractibility to move him or her from potentially problematic situations to more productive activities.* Often, activities that involve motor activity using large muscle groups (e.g., ping-pong or punching bag) as well as writing provide constructive outlets for energy. A few hours of keeping up with a person who is manic can deplete the nurse's energy. Often, nurses take turns monitoring a manic's behavior while the client is still extremely hyperactive.

Second, the manic client can elicit numerous intense emotions from the nurse. A manic client is out of control and fights being controlled. Fear of underlying painful feelings is great. Therefore, the client may use humor, manipulation, power struggles, or demanding behavior to prevent or minimize the staff's ability to set limits on and control dangerous behavior.

When the manic is joking, punning, and being the life of the party, the mood can be infectious. A manic client can be genuinely funny and entertaining. The nurse needs to remain uninvolved or neutral and take measures to prevent further escalation of the mania. Joking with or encouraging the manic's humor is meeting the nurse's needs at the client's expense. The client is running from pain, not to a good time.

Because one motivation of the manic's behavior is to keep painful feelings out of awareness, the behavior of a manic client is often aimed at decreasing the effectiveness of staff control. He or she might accomplish this by getting involved with power plays. For example, the client might taunt the staff by pointing out "faults" or "oversights," drawing negative attention to one or more staff. Usually, this is done in a loud and disruptive manner, which serves to get staff defensive, thereby escalating the environmental tension and the client's degree of mania.

Another unconscious tactic is to divide staff as a ploy to keep the environment unsettled. The manic is very sensitive to the vulnerabilities and conflicts within a group. Often, a manic client will manipulate staff by turning one group of staff against another in an unconscious attempt to discourage outside controls. For example, a client might tell the day shift, "You are the only nurse that listens. On evenings they hardly look at you. You could drop dead, and the nurses wouldn't even know it." To the evening shift the client might say, "Thank God you're here. At last someone who cares. All the day people do is push pills and drink coffee."

In the attempt to ward off painful feelings by maintaining mania, the client can become aggressively demanding, another manic defense. This behavior often triggers frustration and exasperation from the staff. Again, the manic distracts the staff into a defensive position and sets up an environment that allows the manic defense to go unchecked. Setting limits is an important skill for staff to develop.

When the staff start to feel angry at each other and confused, it is often an indication that a client is splitting the staff. Frequent staff meetings dealing with the behaviors of the client and the nurses' responses to these behaviors can help minimize splitting and feelings of anger and isolation by the staff.

The consistent setting of limits is the main theme with a person in mania. *Consistency among staff is imperative* if the limits are to be carried out effectively.

Intervention

PSYCHOTHERAPEUTIC INTERVENTIONS

Table 18–3 suggests basic principles of communication for use with the client who is manic.

ACTIVITIES OF DAILY LIVING

A person in mania has great difficulty meeting personal physical needs. Thus, the nurse finds that much attention is directed toward interventions associated with activities of daily living. Table 18–4 suggests interventions appropriate for safeguarding the physical health of the manic client.

SOMATIC THERAPIES

Lithium Carbonate

Lithium carbonate ($LiCO_3$) is the drug of choice for treating the manic phase of a bipolar disorder. Lithium is a mood stabilizer and is often referred to as an *antimanic* drug. Often, it can calm manic clients, prevent or modify future manic episodes, and protect against future depressive episodes. Lithium is strongly recommended for the treatment of bipolar depression over the tricyclics, which may provoke hypomanic episodes (Abou-Saleh 1992). Lithium aborts 60–80% of acute mania and hypomania in 10–21 days (Maxmen 1991).

Lithium is particularly effective in reducing (Maxmen 1991):

- Elation, grandiosity, and expansiveness
- Flights of ideas
- Irritability and manipulativeness
- Anxiety

To a lesser extent, lithium controls:

- Insomnia
- Psychomotor agitation
- Threatening or assaultive behavior
- Distractibility

Initially when a client comes into the hospital in severe mania, a neuroleptic (antipsychotic) drug is given. Neuroleptics act promptly to slow speech, inhibit aggression, and decrease psychomotor activity. The immediate action of the neuroleptic medication is to prevent exhaustion, coronary collapse, and death. See Chapter 19 for a discussion of the neuroleptic (antipsychotic) drugs. Electroconvulsive therapy may also be used to subdue severe manic behavior, especially in treatment-resistant manic patients and "rapid cyclers," i.e., those who suffer four or more episodes of illness a year. Among bipolar patients, rapid cyclers and those with paranoid-destructive features often respond poorly to lithium therapy (Abou-Saleh 1992).

Lithium must reach therapeutic levels in the client's blood to be effective. This usually takes from seven to 14 days, or longer. As lithium levels become effective in reducing manic behavior, the neuroleptics are usually discontinued. Lithium is 70–80% effective in treating the manic phase of a bipolar disorder; however, it is not a cure. Many clients are on indefinite lithium maintenance and will suffer manic and depressive episodes if the drug is discontinued.

Trade names for lithium carbonate include Lithane, Eskalith, and Lithonate. Initially, 300–600 mg by mouth is given three times a day to reach a *therapeutic* lithium level of 1.0–1.5 mEq/l. Although 0.8–1.2 mEq/l is thought to be an appropriate *maintenance* blood level, 0.8 mEq/l may be too high for some people because each client has individual reactions to lithium. Some patients can avoid a manic or depressive episode on 0.4–0.6 mEq/l (Schatzberg and Cole 1991).

There is a small range between the therapeutic dose and the toxic dose of lithium. Initially, blood levels are drawn weekly or biweekly until the therapeutic level has been reached. After therapeutic levels have been reached, blood levels are drawn every month. After 6 months to a year of stability, blood levels every three months may suffice (Schatzberg and Cole 1991). Blood should be drawn eight to 12 hours after the last dose of lithium.

Many hospital policies state that if blood lithium levels go over 1.5 mEq/l during maintenance therapy, the drug should be withheld for 24 hours and restarted at a lower dose. Toxic effects are usually associated with levels of 2.0 mEq/l or more, although they can occur at much lower levels (even within a therapeutic range).

MAINTENANCE THERAPY. According to Maxmen (1991), the frequency of bipolar relapses in two years is 20–40% of people taking lithium and 65–90% of people not taking lithium. When patients halt lithium, relapse usually occurs within several weeks.

Some suggest that bipolar patients need to be maintained in lithium from nine to 12 months, and some patients may need lifelong lithium maintenance to prevent further relapses. Many patients do well on

Table 18–3 ■ NURSING INTERVENTIONS AND RATIONALES: PSYCHOTHERAPEUTIC NEEDS OF THE CLIENT

INTERVENTION	RATIONALE
Nursing Diagnosis: *Altered thought processes* related to biological changes, as evidenced by hyperactivity and inability to concentrate	
1. Use a firm and calm approach, "John. Come with me. Eat this sandwich."	1. Provides structure and control for a client who is out of control. Can result in feelings of security: "Someone is in control."
2. Use short and concise explanations or statements.	2. Short attention span limits comprehension to small bits of information.
3. Remain neutral; avoid power struggles and value judgments.	3. Client can use inconsistencies and value judgments as justification for arguing and escalating mania.
4. Be consistent in approach and expectations.	4. Consistent limits and expectations minimize potential for client manipulating staff.
5. Avoid getting caught up in joking and repartee. Maintain a calm and neutral manner.	5. Minimizes the manic spiral. Joking and laughing with the manic client is disrespectful of client's needs.
6. Have frequent staff meetings to plan consistent approaches and to set agreed-upon limits.	6 Consistency of all staff is needed to maintain controls and minimize manipulation by client.
7. When limits are decided by staff, they need to be told to the client in simple, concrete terms, including the consequences, e.g., "John, do not yell at or hit Peter. If you cannot control yourself, we will help you." or "The seclusion room will help you feel less out of control and prevent harm to yourself and others."	7. Clear expectations help client experience outside controls, as well as understand reasons for medication, seclusion, or restraints, if he or she is not able to control behaviors.
8. Legitimate complaints should be heard and acted upon.	8. Reduces underlying feelings of helplessness and can raise self-esteem.
9. Accept acting-out behavior (e.g., obscene remarks, crude jokes, and gestures) calmly.	9. Acceptance thwarts the unconscious attempt to trigger anger and get the nurse to act irrationally (out of control), thus maintaining the manic defense.
10. Firmly redirect energy into more appropriate and constructive channels.	10. Distractibility is the nurse's most effective tool with the manic client.
Nursing Diagnosis: *High risk for injury* related to extreme hyperactivity, as evidenced by increased agitation and poor impulse control	
1. Maintain low level of stimuli in client's environment (e.g., away from bright lights, loud noises, and people).	1. Helps decrease escalation of anxiety.
2. Provide structured solitary activities with nurse or aide.	2. Structure provides security and focus.
3. Provide frequent high-calorie fluids.	3. Prevents serious dehydration.
4. Provide frequent rest periods.	4. Prevents exhaustion.
5. Redirect violent behavior.	5. Physical exercise can decrease tension and provide focus.
6. Acute mania may warrant the use of phenothiazines and seclusion to minimize physical harm.	6. Exhaustion and death can result from dehydration, lack of sleep, and constant physical activity.
7. Observe for signs of lithium toxicity.	7. There is a small margin of safety between therapeutic and toxic doses.
8. Protect client from giving away money and possessions. Hold valuables in hospital safe until rational judgment returns.	8. Client's "generosity" is a manic defense consistent with irrational, grandiose thinking.

Table 18–4 ■ NURSING INTERVENTIONS AND RATIONALES: PHYSICAL NEEDS OF THE MANIC CLIENT

INTERVENTION	RATIONALE
Nursing Diagnosis: *Impaired social interaction* related to altered thought processes, as evidenced by intrusive and aggressive social behavior	
1. When possible, provide an environment with minimal stimuli (e.g., quiet, soft music, or dim lighting).	1. Reduced stimuli lessen distractibility.
2. Solitary activities requiring short attention span with mild physical exertion are best initially, e.g., writing, painting (finger painting, murals), woodworking, or walks with staff.	2. Solitary activities minimize stimuli; mild physical activities release tension constructively.
3. When less manic, client may join one or two other clients in quiet, nonstimulating activities (e.g., board games, drawing, cards). *Avoid competitive games.*	3. As mania subsides, involvement in activities that provide a focus and social contact becomes more appropriate. Competitive games can stimulate aggression and increase psychomotor activity.
Nursing Diagnosis: *Altered nutrition* less than body requirements related to excessive physical agitation, as evidenced by inadequate food and fluid intake	
1. Monitor intake, output, and vital signs.	1. Ensures adequate fluid and caloric intake; minimizes dehydration and cardiac collapse.
2. Offer frequent high-calorie protein drinks and finger foods (e.g., sandwiches, fruit, or milk shakes).	2. Constant fluid and calorie replacement are needed. Too active to sit at meals. Finger foods allow "eating on the run."
3. Frequently remind client to eat. "Tom, finish your milkshake." "Sally, eat this banana."	3. The manic client is unaware of bodily needs and is easily distracted. Needs supervision to eat.
Nursing Diagnosis: *Sleep-pattern disturbance* related to biochemical alteration, as evidenced by frequent wakening episodes during the night	
1. Encourage frequent rest periods during the day.	1. Lack of sleep can lead to exhaustion and death.
2. Keep client in areas of low stimulation.	2. Promotes relaxation and minimizes manic behavior.
3. At night, provide warm baths, soothing music, and medication when indicated. Avoid giving client caffeine.	3. Promotes relaxation, rest, and sleep.
Nursing Diagnosis: *Self-care deficit* related to excessive hyperactivity, as evidenced by poor hygiene	
1. Supervise choice of clothes, minimize flamboyant and bizarre dress, e.g., garish stripes, plaids, and loud unmatching colors.	1. Lessens the potential for ridicule, which lowers self-esteem and increases the need for manic defense. Assists client in maintaining dignity.
2. Give simple step-by-step reminders for hygiene and dress. "Here is your razor. Shave the left side . . . now the right side. Here is your toothbrush. Put the toothpaste on the brush."	2. Distractibility and poor concentration are countered by simple, concrete instructions.
Nursing Diagnosis: *Constipation* related to inadequate dietary intake and fluids	
1. Monitor bowel habits; offer fluids and food high in fiber. Evaluate need for laxative. Encourage client to go to the bathroom.	1. Prevent fecal impaction resulting from dehydration and decreased peristalsis.

lower doses during maintenance or "prophylactic" lithium therapy.

Lithium is unquestionably effective in preventing both manic and depressive episodes in bipolar clients. However, complete suppression may occur in only 50% or less, even with compliance to maintenance therapy. Therefore, both the person with a bipolar disorder and his or her spouse need careful instructions about (1) the purpose and requirements of lithium therapy, (2) its side effects, (3) its toxic effects and complications, and (4) when the physician should be contacted. See Box 18–1 for client and family teaching.

INDICATIONS FOR LITHIUM USE. Lithium use

Box 18–1. TEACHING CLIENTS AND THEIR FAMILIES ABOUT LITHIUM

The client and the client's family should be instructed about the following:

1. Lithium can treat your current emotional problem and will also help prevent relapse. So, it is important to continue with the drug after the current episode is resolved.
2. Because therapeutic and toxic dosage ranges are so close, your lithium blood levels must be monitored very closely. More frequently at first, then once every several months after that.
3. Lithium is not addictive.
4. Maintain a normal diet and normal salt and fluid intake (2500–3000 ml/day or six 12-ounce glasses). Lithium decreases sodium reabsorption by the renal tubules, which could cause sodium depletion. A low sodium intake causes a relative increase in lithium retention, which could lead to toxicity.
5. Withhold drug if excessive diarrhea, vomiting, or diaphoresis occurs. Dehydration can raise lithium levels in the blood to toxic levels. Inform your physician if you have any of these problems.
6. Diuretics are contraindicated with lithium.
7. Lithium is irritating to the gastric mucosa. Therefore, take your lithium with meals.
8. Periodic monitoring of renal functioning and thyroid function is indicated with long term use. Discuss your follow-up with your doctor.
9. Avoid taking any over-the-counter medications without checking first with your doctor.
10. If weight gain is significant, you may need to see a physician or nutritionist.
11. Many self-help groups have been developed to provide support for bipolar patients and their families. The local self-help group is (give name and phone number)

You can find out more information by calling (give name and phone number.)

Data from Maxmen 1991; Schatzberg and Cole 1991; Preston and Johnson 1991.

---

2. To attempt to modify milder ongoing or frequent but episodic clinical symptoms, such as chronic depression or episodic irritability
3. To establish a prophylactic maintenance regimen to avert future affective or psychotic episodes
4. To enhance the effect of antidepressants in clients with a major depressive disorder

OTHER INDICATIONS FOR LITHIUM THERAPY. Lithium has been used with success in the following:

Schizoaffective Disorder. Lithium used in combination with neuroleptic therapy can be useful in clients who demonstrate overactivity, insomnia, irritability, or other manic symptoms during an excited episode.

Schizophrenia. For some treatment-resistant clients, a combination of lithium and neuroleptic/antipsychotic drug therapy may prove helpful. It can also be useful in decreasing angry outbursts.

Impulse Control Disorders. Impulse disorders include episodic violence and rage. People who have unpremeditated outbursts of violence, and those in whom rage reactions are seemingly unprovoked by happenings in the environment, often respond well to lithium. Violence that is premeditated, however, is not responsive to lithium.

CONTRAINDICATIONS FOR LITHIUM USE. Before the administration of lithium, a medical evaluation is given to assess a client's ability to tolerate the drug. In particular, baseline physical and laboratory examinations should include renal function; thyroid status, including thyroxine (T_4) and thyroid-stimulating hormone; and evaluation for dementia or neurological disorders, which signal a poor response to lithium (DePaulo 1984).

Other clinical and laboratory assessments, including an electrocardiogram, are done as needed, depending on the individual's physical condition (DePaulo 1984).

Lithium is not given to people who are pregnant, have brain damage, or have cardiovascular, renal, or thyroid disease. Both the fear of and the wish to become pregnant is a major concern among many bipolar women on lithium. Lithium is also contraindicated in mothers who are breast-feeding or have myasthenia gravis and in children under 12 years of age.

EXPECTED SIDE EFFECTS. Mild hand tremors, polyuria, and mild thirst often occur and may persist throughout therapy. Mild nausea and general discomfort may occur initially, and the client can be reassured that these side effects usually subside with treatment. Weight gain is sometimes an undesirable side effect of long term use. Table 18–5 identifies early, advanced, and severe signs of toxic poisoning with lithium. "The major long-term risks of lithium therapy are hypothyroidism and impairment of the kidney's ability to concentrate urine" (Harris 1981).

can be divided into four general clinical situations (Schatzberg and Cole 1991):

1. To control rapidly acute, overt psychopathology, as in mania or psychotic agitation

Table 18–5 ■ DRUG INFORMATION: SIDE EFFECTS AND SIGNS OF LITHIUM TOXICITY

LEVEL	SIGNS*	INTERVENTIONS
Expected Side Effects		
0.8–1.2 mEq/l or less (therapeutic levels)	Fine hand tremors, polyuria, and mild thirst.	Symptoms may persist throughout therapy.
	Mild nausea and general discomfort.	Symptoms often subside during treatment
	Weight gain.	Weight gain may be helped with diet, exercise, and nutritional management.
Early Signs of Toxicity		
Less than 1.5 mEq/l	Nausea, vomiting, diarrhea, thirst, polyuria, slurred speech, muscle weakness.	Medication should be withheld, blood lithium levels drawn, and the dose re-evaluated.
Advanced Signs of Toxicity		
1.5–2 mEq/l	Coarse hand tremor, persistent gastrointestinal upset, mental confusion, muscle hyperirritability, electroencephalographic changes, incoordination.	Use interventions outlined above or below, depending on severity of circumstances.
Severe Toxicity		
2.0–2.5 mEq/l	Ataxia, serious electroencephalographic changes, blurred vision, clonic movements, large output of dilute urine, seizures, stupor, severe hypotension, coma. Fatalities are usually secondary to pulmonary complications.	There is no known antidote for lithium poisoning. The drug is stopped and excretion is hastened. Gastric lavage and treatment with urea, mannitol, and aminophylline all hasten lithium excretion.
Greater than 2.5 mEq/l	Confusion, incontinence of urine or feces, coma, cardiac arrhythmia, peripheral circulatory collapse, abdominal pain, proteinuria, oliguria, hypothyroidism.	Hemodialysis may also be used in severe cases.

Data from Scherer JC. Nurses' Drug Manual. Philadelphia: JB Lippincott, 1985, pp. 631–632.
* Careful monitoring is needed because the toxic levels of lithium are close to the therapeutic levels.

Other Antimanic Drugs

Although lithium is the drug of choice for bipolar clients, 40% of bipolar clients do not respond to or tolerate lithium (Post 1992).

Some subtypes of bipolar clients who often do not respond well to lithium include (Post 1992)

- Those with dysphoric mania (depressive thoughts and feelings during manic episodes)
- Rapid cyclers (four or more episodes a year)
- Those whose initial mood episode was a depression, then mania and then an interval of wellness (D-M-I); they are often nonresponders, compared with those whose initial episode is mania, then depression and then an interval of wellness (M-D-I)

Another possible indication for a positive lithium response occurs in clients who have a family history of bipolar disorder in first-degree relatives. Those with no family history of first-degree relatives with bipolar disorder often have a poorer response to lithium but may respond to the anticonvulsants carbamazepine (Tegretol) or valproic acid (Depakene).

ANTICONVULSANTS AND MILD TRANQUILIZERS. Although many **anticonvulsant drugs** may eventually prove useful in treating mood disorders, carbamazepine and valproic acid have been most frequently studied as long term maintenance therapies (Schatzberg and Cole 1991). According to Maxmen (1991), anticonvulsants have been found to

- Clearly control acute mania (with or without lithium)
- Often prevent mania
- Occasionally treat and prevent unipolar or bipolar depression
- Relieve psychotic symptoms secondary to complex partial seizures
- Infrequently reduce schizophrenia
- Dampen affective swings in schizoaffective patients

- Diminish impulsive and aggressive behavior in some nonpsychotic patients
- Facilitate alcohol and benzodiazepine withdrawal

Clinical benefits include usually being able to control seizures (within hours), mania (within 2 weeks), and depression (within 3 weeks or more).

Carbamazepine. In 25–50% of treatment-resistant bipolar patients, carbamazepine has clear clinical benefits. Some treatment-resistant clients with bipolar disorder improve after taking carbamazepine and lithium or carbamazepine and a neuroleptic. Carbamazepine seems to work better in 60% of rapid cyclers and better in severe paranoid, angry, manic patients than in euphoric, overactive, overfriendly manic patients (Schatzberg and Cole 1991). It is also thought to be more effective in dysphoric manic clients. Table 18–6 gives clinical profiles of lithium and carbamazepine.

For acute mania, lithium and a neuroleptic is more effective than lithium and carbamazepine; however, carbamazepine does not induce tardive dyskinesia and has fewer side effects. Table 18–7 lists side effects and toxic effects of other antimanic (mood-stabilizing) medications. Blood levels of carbamazepine should be monitored at least weekly through the first 8 weeks of treatment because the drug induces liver enzymes, which then speed its own metabolism (Schatzberg and Cole 1991).

Valproic Acid and Divalproex Sodium. Valproic acid (Depakene) and divalproex sodium (Depakote) have been found helpful in initial studies for lithium nonresponders. They can be useful in treating lithium nonresponders who are in acute mania, who are in rapid cycles, who are in dysphoric mania, or who have not responded to carbamazepine. It has also been helpful in preventing future manic episodes.

Clonazepam and Lorazepam. Clonazepam (Klonopin) and lorazepam (Ativan) have been found to be useful in the treatment of acute mania in some treatment-resistant manic clients. Further studies are needed to provide conclusive evidence for its universal use. Table 18–7 lists the major concerns of these other mood stabilizers.

THERAPEUTIC ENVIRONMENT

Hospitalization is indicated for people in the acute manic state. Hospitalization helps the client gain control over extreme hyperactive behavior and allows for medication stabilization. Control of hyperactive behavior almost always includes immediate treatment with a neuroleptic, such as chlorpromazine (Thorazine) or haloperidol (Haldol). However, when a client is dangerously out of control, use of the seclusion room may also be indicated. The seclusion room can provide comfort and relief to many clients who can no longer control their own behavior.

Seclusion serves the following purpose:

1. Reduces overwhelming environmental stimuli
2. Protects a client from injuring self, others, or staff
3. Prevents destruction of personal property or property of others

Seclusion is warranted when documented data by the nursing and medical staff reflect the following points (Roper et al. 1985):

1. Client is unable to control his or her actions.
2. Other measures have failed (e.g., setting limits or using chemical restraints).
3. Behavior has been sustained (continues or escalates despite other measures).
4. Substantial risk of harm to others or self is clear.

The use of seclusion or restraints involves complex therapeutic, ethical, and legal issues. Therefore, most

			BOTH LITHIUM AND
CLINICAL PROFILE	LITHIUM	CARBAMAZEPINE	CARBAMAZEPINE
Mania	+ +	+ +	+ + +
Dysphoria	(+)	+	+ +
Rapid cycling	+	+ +	+ + +
Continuous cycling	(+)	+	+ +
Negative family history	+	+ +	+ + +
Depression	+	+	+ + +
Prophylaxis of Mania and Depression	+ +	+ +	+ + +

Table 18–6 ■ DRUG INFORMATION: CLINICAL PROFILES OF LITHIUM AND CARBAMAZEPINE

Reprinted from PSYCHOTROPIC DRUGS: Fast Facts, by Jerrold S. Maxmen, M.D., by permission of W.W. Norton & Company, Inc. Copyright © 1991 by Jerrold S. Maxmen.

+ = effective; + + = very effective; + + + = possible synergism; (+) = equivocal—may or may not have an effect.

Table 18–7 ■ DRUG INFORMATION: OTHER ANTIMANIC (MOOD-STABILIZING) MEDICATIONS

DRUG	TYPE	MAJOR CONCERNS/SIDE EFFECTS
Carbamazepine (Tegretol)	Anticonvulsant	1. Agranulocytosis or aplastic anemia are most serious side effects.
		2. Blood levels should be monitored through first 8 weeks because drug induces liver enzymes that speed its own metabolism. Dose may need to be adjusted to maintain serum level of 6–8 mg/l.
		3. Sedation is most common problem; tolerance usually develops.
		4. Diplopia, incoordination, and sedation can signal excessive levels.
Valproic acid (Depakene)	Anticonvulsant	1. Baseline liver function tests should be done and monitored at regular intervals. Hepatitis, although rare, has been reported with fatalities in children.
		2. Signs and symptoms to watch for: Fever, chills, right upper quadrant pain, dark-colored urine, malaise, and jaundice.
		3. Common side effects: Tremors, gastrointestinal upset, weight gain, and rarely, alopecia.
Clonazepam (Klonopin)	Benzodiazepine	Same as those of all benzodiazepines, e.g., sedation, ataxia, and incoordination. See Chapter 14, Table 14–9.

hospitals have well-defined protocols for treatment with seclusion. Protocols include a proper reporting procedure through the chain of command when a client is to be secluded. When and what to document and specific nursing responsibilities aimed at safeguarding the client are outlined. For example, a protocol usually specifies who can make the decision for seclusion when a physician is not available, how long a client can be in seclusion without a doctor's written order (e.g., 15–30 minutes), and whom to call if a doctor is not available to write an order (within 15–30 minutes).

Seclusion protocols also identify specific nursing responsibilities. For example, how often the client's behavior is to be observed and documented (e.g., every 15 minutes), how often the client is to be offered food and fluids (e.g., every 30–60 minutes), and how often the client is to be toileted (e.g., every 1–2 hours).

Because phenothiazines are often used with clients in seclusion, vital signs should be taken frequently (every 15 minutes). Refer to Chapter 3 for legal guidelines for seclusion.

When a client does require seclusion to prevent harm to self or others, it is ideal to have one nurse on each shift work with the client on a continuous basis. Communication with a client in seclusion should be concrete and direct, but kind and limited to brief instructions. Clients should be reassured that the seclusion is only a *temporary measure*, and that they will be returned to the unit when they gain control of their behavior (Baradell 1985).

Frequent staff meetings regarding personal feelings about seclusion are necessary to prevent possible dangers. Dangers include the use of seclusion as a form of punishment and leaving a client in seclusion for long periods of time without proper supervision.

PSYCHOTHERAPY

The belief that bipolar clients are not suitable candidates for group therapy has become well accepted among therapists (Luby and Yalom 1992). Bipolar clients have generally been considered poor psychotherapeutic candidates because of their difficult defensive styles. However, two studies have demonstrated that a long term homogeneous group of bipolar clients focusing on interpersonal issues can be successful for this population (Luby and Yalom 1992).

Individual psychotherapy is often useful, especially in conjunction with drug therapy. A survey of lithium clinics revealed that psychotherapy and group psychotherapy were offered in about 84% of clinics (Gitlin and Jamison 1984).

A client describes her feelings about drug therapy and psychotherapy (Jamison and Goodwin 1983):

I cannot imagine leading a normal life without lithium. From startings and stoppings of it, I now know it is an essential part of my sanity. Lithium prevents my seductive but disastrous highs, diminishes my depressions, clears out the weaving of my disordered thinking, slows me, gentles me out, keeps me in my relationships, in my career, out of a hospital, and in psychotherapy. It keeps me alive, too. But psychotherapy heals, it makes some sense of the confusion, it reins in the terrifying thoughts and feelings, it brings back hope, and the possibility of learning from it all. Pills cannot, do not, ease one back into reality. They bring you back headlong, careening, and faster than can be endured at times. Psychotherapy is a sanctuary, it is a battleground, it is where I have come to believe that someday I may be able to contend with all of this. No pill can help me deal with the problem of not wanting to take pills, but no amount of therapy alone can prevent my manias and depressions. I need both.

Evaluation

Depending on the goals the nurse has set, evaluation of goals is done periodically. For example, are the client's vital signs stable, and is he or she well hydrated? Is the client able to control his or her own behavior or respond to external controls? Is the client able to sleep four or five hours per night or take frequent short rest periods during the day? Does the family have a clear understanding of the client's disease and need for medication? Do they know which community agencies may be able to help them?

If goals are not met, the preventing factors are analyzed. Were there incorrect or insufficient data? Were there inappropriate nursing diagnoses or unrealistic goals? Was the intervention poorly planned? After analysis of the goals and care plan are reassessed, the plan is revised, if indicated.

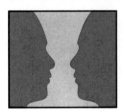

Case Study: Working with a Person Who Is Manic

Mary Horowitz was brought into the emergency room after being found on the highway shortly after her car had broken down. When the police came to her aid, she told them that she was "driving herself to fame and fortune." She appeared overly cheerful, constantly talking, laughing, and making jokes. At the same time, she walked up and down beside the car, sometimes tweaking the cheek of one of the policemen. She was coy and flirtatious with the police, saying at one point, "Boys in blue are fun to do."

She was dressed in a long red dress with a blue and orange scarf around her neck, many long chains of various colors, and a yellow and green turban on her head. When she reached into the car and started drinking from an open bottle of bourbon, the police decided that her behavior and general condition might result in harm to herself or others. When the police explained to Ms. Horowitz that they wanted to take her to the hospital for a general check-up, her jovial mood turned to short-lived anger and rage.

Two minutes after getting into the police car, she was singing "Carry Me Back to Ole Virginia."

On admission to the emergency room, she was seen by a psychiatrist, and her sister was called. The sister stated that Ms. Horowitz had stopped taking her lithium about five weeks before and was becoming more and more agitated and out of control. She stated that Ms. Horowitz had not eaten in two days, had stayed up all night calling friends and strangers all over the country, and had finally fled the house when the sister called the ambulance to take her to the hospital. The psychiatrist contacted Ms. Horowitz's physician, and previous history and medical management were discussed, It was decided to hospitalize her to restart her on lithium. It was hoped that medications and a controlled environment would prevent further escalation of the manic state and prevent possible exhaustion and cardiac collapse.

Assessment

On Ms. Horowitz's admission to the unit, Mr. Atkins was assigned as her primary nurse.. She was unable to sit down. She strode ceaselessly up and down the halls, talking loudly, pointing to other clients, and making loud sexual or hostile comments. Some of the other clients laughed at her actions and her dress.

Mr. Atkins suggested that they go to a quieter part of the unit. Ms. Horowitz turned to him angrily and said, "Let me be . . . set me free, lover . . . I am untouchable . . . I'll get the FBI to set me free."

Mr. Atkins divided the data into subjective and objective components.

OBJECTIVE DATA

1. Little if anything to eat for days.
2. Little if any sleep for days.
3. History of mania.
4. History of lithium maintenance.
5. Constant physical activity—unable to sit.
6. Very loud and distracting to others.
7. Anger when wishes are curtailed.
8. Flight of ideas.
9. Dress loud and inappropriate.
10. Remarks suggestive of sexual themes—called nurse "lover."
11. Some clients found her behavior amusing.
12. Remarks suggested grandiose thinking.
13. Poor judgment.

SUBJECTIVE DATA

1. "Driving myself to fame and fortune."
2. "I'm untouchable . . . I'll get the FBI to set me free."
3. "Let me be . . . set me free, lover."

Nursing Diagnosis

Mr. Atkins discussed Ms. Horowitz's immediate needs with the admitting psychiatrist. The psychiatrist ordered 75 mg of intramuscular chlorpromazine to be given to her immediately. Then he prescribed 75 mg intramuscularly every six hours until she could take the medication by mouth. Thereafter Ms. Horowitz was to receive 100 mg orally three times daily. She was to be observed for behaviors that might indicate harm to herself or others. The medical staff stated that if medication and nursing interventions did not reduce her activity level, the nurses should allow for possible periods of rest and ingestion of fluids and minimize her provocative behavior toward others. Failing that, the use of seclusion would have to be considered. It was agreed that her physical safety was greatly jeopardized.

Mr. Atkins's initial diagnoses reflected the nursing and medical staff's main concern: Ms. Horowitz's physical condition. Although she presented many possible nursing diagnoses and needs at the time, the following two nursing diagnoses were formulated because they focused on her physical safety:

1. *High risk for injury* related to dehydration and faulty judgment, as evidenced by inability to meet own physiological needs and set limits on own behavior
   - Has not slept for days
   - Has not taken in food or fluids for days
   - Constant physical activity—unable to sit

2. *Defensive coping* related to inadequate psychological resources, as evidenced by change in usual communication patterns
   - Very loud and distracting to others.
   - Remarks suggested sexual themes.
   - Some clients found her behavior amusing.
   - Remarks suggested grandiose thinking.
   - Flight of ideas.
   - Loud, hostile, and sexual remarks to other clients.

Planning

CONTENT LEVEL—PLANNING GOALS

Mr. Atkins formulated the following goals:

Nursing Diagnosis	Long Term Goals	Short Term Goals
1. *High risk for injury* related to dehydration and faulty judgment, as evidenced by inability to meet own physiological needs and set limits on own behavior	1. Client's cardiac status will remain stable during manic phase.	1a. Client will be well hydrated, as evidenced by good skin turgor and normal urinary output and specific gravity within 24 hours.
		1b. Client will sleep or rest three hours during the

Planning
(Continued)

		first night in hospital, with the aid of medication and nursing intervention.
		1c. Client's blood pressure and pulse will be within the normal limits within 24 hours, with the aid of medication and nursing measures.
2. *Defensive coping* related to inadequate psychological resources, as evidenced by change in usual communication patterns	2. Within three days, client will respond to verbal external controls when aggression escalates.	2a. Client will engage in safe activities aimed at reducing aggressive energy within 24–48 hours.

PROCESS LEVEL–NURSES' REACTIONS AND FEELINGS

Mr. Atkins had worked on the psychiatric unit for two years. He had learned to deal with many of the challenging behaviors associated with the manic defense. For example, he no longer took most of the verbal insults personally, although many of the remarks could be very cutting and "close to home." He was also better able to recognize and set limits on some of the tactics used by the manic to split the staff. The staff on this unit worked very closely with each other, which made the atmosphere positive and supportive; therefore, communication was good among staff. Frequent and effective communication is needed when working with clients who try to split staff. Clear staff communication is vital to maximize external controls and maintain consistency in nursing care.

The only aspect of Ms. Horowitz's be-havior that Mr. Atkins thought he might have some difficulty with was the sexual assaults and loud sexual comments she might make toward him. He knew that this could make him anxious, and his concern was that his anxiety might be picked up by the client.

When discussing this with the unit coordinator, they both decided that two nurses should provide care for Ms. Horowitz. A female nurse would spend time with her in her room, and Mr. Atkins would spend time with her in quiet areas on the unit. It was decided that neither Mr. Atkins nor any male staff member would be alone with Ms. Horowitz in her room at any time. Mr. Atkins should ask for relief if Ms. Horowitz's sexual remarks and acting-out behaviors were making him anxious.

Intervention

Because the most immediate concerns for Ms. Horowitz upon admission were those of physical safety, 75 mg of intramuscular chlorpromazine was given immediately. Other clients were moved to provide Ms. Horowitz with a single room. She would not allow vital signs to be taken at first; however, eventually vital signs were taken and recorded at regular intervals. After two hours of pacing with Ms. Horowitz and coaxing her into less stimulating areas of the unit, she started taking some fluids. Within five hours, she was drinking 8 ounces of high-caloric fluids per hour, after much reminding and encouragement.

By the next day, Ms. Horowitz's behaviors were much less hyperactive, and although her verbal sexual and aggressive assaults were less intense, she continued to provoke other clients. At this time, Mr. Atkins began to channel some of her physical energy into less disruptive activities. He and Ms. Horowitz did some slow exercises to relaxing music in a quiet part of the unit; he provided writing paper for her, and she spent five to 10 minutes writing furiously. She continued to pace and yell out to other clients, but with continued medication and nursing intervention, Mr. Atkins saw that this behavior was decreasing.

When Ms. Horowitz's sister came to visit, she brought clothes, and Mr. Atkins spent some time with the sister finding out more about Ms. Horowitz. He learned that she was a school teacher, had been depressed for three months prior to her first manic episode two years before, and was recently coming out of her second depressive episode. Although the second depressive episode was less severe than the first, the sister was concerned that Ms. Horowitz would "do something foolish," meaning suicide. Ms. Horowitz was separated from her husband and was having a difficult time adjusting to being back at work.

Mr. Atkins and the female nurse encouraged Ms. Horowitz to dress and groom herself more appropriately because some of the other clients were beginning to laugh at her appearance. Mr. Atkins was aware that ridicule could further lower Ms. Horowitz's self-esteem, thus increasing her anxiety and need for the manic defense.

Ms. Horowitz's behavior was beginning to be controlled by the lithium about 12 days later, and she was being weaned off of the chlorpromazine. At this time, she was able to talk to Mr. Atkins about how upset and depressed she was about her life (job and separation) and the fact that she had to take medication for the "rest of my life." See Nursing Care Plan 18–1.

Mr. Atkins discussed with her some of the side effects that contributed to her noncompliance. He worked with her to reduce and control some of her reactions to lithium. He then reviewed other possible side effects and toxic effects of lithium and dietary and other precautions. At the end of her hospital stay, Ms. Horowitz stated that she was resigned to continuing her lithium. After talking to Mr. Atkins, she decided to re-enter therapy to "help me get back into life."

Evaluation

After two days, the medical staff thought Ms. Horowitz's cardiac status was stable. Her vital signs were within normal limits, she was taking in sufficient fluids, and her urinary output and specific gravity were normal. Although her hyperactivity persisted, it did so to a lesser degree, and she was able to get periods of rest during the day and was sleeping three to four hours during the night.

Ms. Horowitz's hyperactivity continued to be a challenge to the nurses; however, she was able to attend to some activities with the nurse that required gross motor movement and channeled some of her aggressive energy. Shortly after arrival to the unit, Ms. Horowitz started a fight with another client, but seclusion was avoided because she was able to refrain from further violent episodes as a result of medication and nursing interventions. She could be directed toward solitary activities, which drained off some of her energies, at least for short periods of time.

As the effectiveness of the drugs progressed, Ms. Horowitz's activity level decreased, and by discharge she was able to discuss real issues of concern with the nurse and make some useful decisions about her future.

Nursing Care Plan 18–1 ■ A PERSON WITH MANIA: MS. HOROWITZ

NURSING DIAGNOSIS

High risk for injury related to dehydration and faulty judgment, as evidenced by inability to meet own physiological needs and set limits on own behavior

Supporting Data

Has not slept for days
Has not taken in food or fluids for days
Constant physical activity—is unable to sit

Long Term Goal: Client's cardiac status will remain stable during manic phase.

Short Term Goal	*Intervention*	*Rationale*	*Evaluation*
1. Client will be well hydrated, as evidenced by good skin turgor and normal urinary output and specific gravity within 24 hours.	1a. Give chlorpromazine immediately and as needed.	1a. Continuous physical activity and lack of fluids can eventually lead to cardiac collapse and death.	Goal met After three hours Mary took small amounts of fluids (2–4 ounces per hour).
	1b. Check vital signs frequently (every 15 minutes).	1b. Monitor cardiac status—chlorpromazine can lower blood pressure.	
	1c. Place client in private or quiet room (whenever possible).	1c. Reduce environmental stimuli—minimize escalation of mania and distractibility.	

Continued on following page

Nursing Care Plan 18–1 ■ A PERSON WITH MANIA: MS. HOROWITZ *(Continued)*

Short Term Goal	Intervention	Rationale	Evaluation
	1d. Stay with client and divert away from stimulating situations.	1d. Nurse's presence provides support. Ability to interact with others is temporarily impaired.	
	1e. Offer high-calorie, high-protein drink (8 ounces) every hour in quiet area.	1e. Proper hydration is mandatory for maintaining cardiac status.	After five hours, Mary started taking 8 ounces per hour with a lot of reminding and encouragement.
	1f. Frequently remind client to drink: "Take two more sips."	1f. Client's concentration is poor; she is easily distracted.	
	1g. Offer finger food frequently in quiet area.	1g. Client is unable to sit; snacks she can eat while pacing are more likely to be consumed.	
	1h. Maintain record of intake and output.	1h. Enables staff to make accurate nutritional assessment for client's safety.	
	1i. Weigh client daily; take specific gravity at end of each shift as ordered.	1i. Monitoring nutritional status is necessary.	Goal met After 24 hours, specific gravity was within normal limits.
2. Client will sleep or rest three hours during the first night in hospital with aid of medication and nursing intervention.	2a. Continue to direct client to areas of minimal activity.	2a. Lower levels of stimulation can decrease excitability.	Client awake most of first night. Slept for two hours from 4 A.M. to 6 A.M.
	2b. When possible, try to direct energy into productive and calming activities (e.g., pacing to slow, soft music; slow exercise; drawing alone; or writing in quiet area).	2b. Directing client to paced, nonstimulating activities can help minimize excitability.	Was able to rest on second day for short periods and engage in quiet activities for short periods (5–10 minutes).
	2c. Encourage short rest periods throughout the day (e.g., 3–5 minutes every hour) when possible.	2c. Client may be unaware of feelings of fatigue. Can collapse from exhaustion if hyperactivity continues without periods of rest.	
	2d. Client should drink decaffeinated drinks only—decaffeinated coffee, teas, or colas.	2d. Caffeine is a central nervous system stimulant that inhibits needed rest or sleep.	
	2e. Provide nursing measures at bedtime that promote sleep—warm milk, soft music, or backrubs.	2e. Promotes nonstimulating and relaxing mood.	
3. Client's blood pressure (BP) and pulse (P) will be within normal limits within 24 hours with the aid of medication and nursing interventions.	3a. Continue to monitor blood pressure and pulse frequently throughout the day (every 30 minutes).	3a. Physical condition is presently a great strain on client's heart. Chlorpromazine can lower blood pressure. Because client will be getting frequent intramuscular doses of the drug for next 24 hours, close monitoring is needed to maintain client safety.	Baseline on unit not obtained because of hyperactive behavior. Information from family physician stated BP 130/90 and P 88 baselines.
	3b. Keep staff informed by verbal and written reports of baseline vital signs and client progress.	3b. Alerting all staff regarding client status can increase medical intervention if a change in status occurs.	BP at end of 24 hours 130/70; P 80.

Nursing Care Plan 18–1 ■ **A PERSON WITH MANIA: MS. HOROWITZ** *(Continued)*

NURSING DIAGNOSIS

Defensive coping **related to inadequate psychological resources, as evidenced by change in usual communication patterns**

Supporting Data

- Remarks suggest sexual themes.
- Some clients find her behavior amusing.
- Remarks suggest grandiose thinking.
- Has flight of ideas.
- Makes loud hostile and sexual remarks to other clients.

Long Term Goal: Within three days, client will respond to external controls when aggression escalates.

Short Term Goal	Intervention	Rationale	Evaluation
1. Client will engage in safe activities to express hostile and aggressive energy within 24–48 hours with aid of medication and nursing interventions.	1a. Maintain a calm and matter-of-fact (neutral) attitude.	1a. Anxiety can be transmitted from staff to client.	Goal partially met Six hours after admission, client started fight with another client. Staff explained that seclusion might be needed to help her gain control over her behavior.
	1b. Avoid power struggles and defensive postures when client is verbally abusive.	1b. Client does not mean abuse personally; it is part of manic defense. Power struggles and defensive remarks by staff can escalate mania and potentiate violent acting out.	
	1c. Set limits and provide controls when necessary, e.g., "You are not to hit George. Come with me now." or "If you have trouble controlling yourself, we will help you."	1c. When client is out of control, external controls are needed to prevent client from acting out violently.	
	1d. Engage client in solitary activities that use large muscle groups (e.g., punching bag, ping-pong, or pacing with nurse).	1d. Activities client can do alone or with nurse that require large muscle groups can help drain physical tension.	On second day, client was able to participate with nurse in solitary activities using large muscle groups for short periods of time (5–10 minutes).

Summary

Genetic factors appear to play a role in the etiology of the bipolar disorder. There is also little doubt that an excess of, and imbalance in, neurotransmitters are also related to bipolar and unipolar mood swings. The outward gaiety and expansive, self-confident facade of a manic client can be seen as an attempt to keep feelings of depression out of awareness. Mania can be observed on a continuum from hypomania to acute mania.

The three main features of mania are (1) euphoria, (2) hyperactivity, and (3) flight of ideas. The nurse assesses the client's mood, behavior, and thought processes to plan the appropriate nursing interventions.

The analysis of the data helps the nurse choose appropriate nursing diagnoses. Some of the nursing diagnoses appropriate for a client who is manic are *high-risk for violence, defensive coping, ineffective individual coping, altered thought processes,* and *self-esteem disturbance.* Physical needs often take priority and demand nursing interventions. Therefore, *fluid volume deficit* and *altered nutrition* or *elimination,* as well as *sleep-pattern disturbance,* are usually part of the nursing plan. *Altered family process* is also a very important consideration. Support, information, and guidance for the family can greatly affect the client's eventual recovery from his or her manic episode.

Planning nursing care involves setting realistic and measurable short term and long term goals for each of the nursing diagnoses. It is helpful for the nurse to understand that the manic symptoms help keep painful feelings out of awareness. Therefore, the client will go to great lengths to prevent outside controls from limiting manic flight. The manic client has numerous unconscious tactics to keep the nursing staff defensive, divided, and confused. When these tactics are successful, staff are less able to set consistent limits and monitor erratic behaviors. Unconscious tactics include splitting members of the staff against each other through manipulation, loudly and persistently pointing to faults and shortcomings in staff, constantly demanding attention and favors of the staff, and provoking clients as well as staff with profane and lewd remarks. The manic client constantly interrupts activities and distracts groups with his or her continuous physical motion and incessant joking and talking. The feelings aroused in such situations are usually anger and frustration toward the client. When these feelings are not examined and shared, the therapeutic potential of the staff is reduced, and feelings of confusion and helplessness remain.

Working with a manic client can be challenging. Interventions involve using specific principles of therapeutic communication, assisting with activities of daily living and somatic therapies, maintaining a therapeutic environment, and when certified, intervening as a nurse therapist.

Evaluation includes examining the effectiveness of the nursing interventions, changing the goals as needed, and reassessing the nursing diagnoses. Evaluation is an ongoing process and is part of each of the other steps in the nursing process.

References

Abou-Saleh MT. Lithium. In Paykel ES (ed). Handbook of Affective Disorders, 2nd ed. New York: Guilford Press, 1992.

American Psychiatric Association. Diagnostic and Statistical Manual of Mental Disorders, 3rd ed, revised (DSM-III-R). Washington, DC: American Psychiatric Association, 1987.

Baradell JC. Humanistic care of the patient in seclusion. Journal of Psychosocial Nursing, 23(2):9, 1985.

Chapman AH. Textbook of Clinical Psychiatry, 2nd ed. Philadelphia: JB Lippincott, 1976.

Coryll W, Winokur G. Course and outcomes. In Paykel ES (ed). Handbook of Affective Disorders, 2nd ed. New York: Guilford Press, 1992.

DePaulo JR. Lithium. Psychiatric Clinics of North America, 7(3):587, 1984.

Gershon ES, Nurnberger JI, Berretitini WH, et al. Affective disorder genetics. In Kaplan HI, Sadock BJ (eds). Comprehensive Textbook of Psychiatry, 4th ed. Baltimore: Williams & Wilkins, 1985.

Gitlin MJ, Jamison KR. Lithium clinics: Theory and practice. Hospital and Community Psychiatry, 35:363, 1984.

Goldstein MJ, Baker BL, Jamison KR. Abnormal psychology: Experiences, Origins and Interventions. Boston: Little, Brown & Company, 1980.

Harris E. Lithium. American Journal of Nursing, 81:1310, 1981.

Hirschfeld RMA, Goodwin FK. Mood disorders. In Talbott JA, Hales RE, Yudofsky SC (eds). Textbook of Psychiatry. Washington, DC: The American Psychiatric Press, 1988.

Jamison KR, Goodwin FK. Psychotherapeutic treatment of manic-depressive patients on lithium. In Greenhill M, Granlick A (eds). New York: Macmillan Publishing Company, 1983.

Kaplan HI, Sadock BJ. Synopsis of Psychiatry, 6th ed. Baltimore: Williams & Wilkins, 1991.

Klerman GL. Affective disorders. In Nicholi AM Jr (ed). The Harvard Guide to Modern Psychiatry. Cambridge, MA: Belknap Press of Harvard University Press, 1978.

Luby JL, Yalom ID. Group therapy. In Paykel ES (ed). Handbook of Affective Disorders, 2nd ed. New York: Guilford Press, 1992.

Maxmen JS. Psychotropic Drugs Fast Facts. New York: WW Norton, 1991.

Nurnberger JI Jr, Gershon ES. Genetics. In Paykel ES (ed). Handbook of Affective Disorders, 2nd ed. New York: Guilford Press, 1992.

Perris C. Bipolar-unipolar distinction. In Paykel ES (ed). Handbook of Affective Disorders, 2nd ed. New York: Guilford Press, 1992.

Post RM. Anticonvulsants and novel drugs. In Paykel ES (ed). Handbook of Affective Disorders, 2nd ed. New York: Guilford Press, 1992.

Preston J, Johnson J. Clinical Psychopharmacology Made Ridiculously Simple. Miami, FL: Med Master, 1991.

Roper JM, et al. Restraint and seclusion. Journal of Psychosocial Nursing, 23(6):18, 1985.

Schatzberg AF, Cole JO. Manual of Clinical Psychopharmacology. Washington, DC: American Psychiatric Press, 1991.

Scherer JS. Nurses' Drug Manual. Philadelphia: JB Lippincott, 1985.

Silverstone T, Hunt N. Symptoms and assessment of mania. In Paykel ES (ed). Handbook of Affective Disorders, 2nd ed. New York: Guilford Press, 1992.

Weissman MM, Boyd JH. Affective disorders: Epidemiology. In Kaplan HI, Sadock BJ (eds). Comprehensive Textbook of Psychiatry, 4th ed. Baltimore: Williams & Wilkins, 1985.

Further Reading

American Psychiatric Association. DSM-IV Options Book: Work in Progress. Washington, DC: American Psychiatric Association, 1991.

Arieti S. Affective disorders: Manic-depressive psychosis and psychotic depression. In Arieti S (ed). American Handbook of Psychiatry, 2nd ed. New York: Basic Books, 1974.

Bergersen BS. Pharmacology in Nursing. St. Louis: CV Mosby, 1979.

Campbell L. Hopelessness. Journal of Psychosocial Nursing, 25(2): 18, 1987.

Cancro R. Overview of affective disorders. In Kaplan HI, Sadock BJ (eds). Comprehensive Textbook of Psychiatry, 4th ed. Baltimore: Williams & Wilkins, 1985.

Carson R, Butcher JN, Coleman JC. Abnormal Psychology and Modern Life. Glenview, IL: Scott, Foresman & Company, 1988.

Fitzgerald RG, Long I. Seclusion in the treatment and management of disturbed manic and depressed patients. Perspectives in Psychiatric Care, 11:59, 1973.

Goodwin DW, Guze SB. Psychiatric Diagnosis. New York: Oxford University Press, 1984.

Hart CA, Turner MS, Orfitelli MK, et al. Introduction to psychotropic drugs. New York: Medical Examination Publishing Company, 1981.

Hinsie LE, Campbell RJ. Psychiatric Dictionary, 4th ed. New York: Oxford University Press, 1973.

Joyce PR. Prediction of treatment response. In Paykel ES (ed); Handbook of Affective Disorders, 2nd ed. New York: Guilford Press, 1992.

Karb VB, Queener SF, Freeman JB. Handbook of Drugs for Nursing Practice. St. Louis: CV Mosby, 1989.

Lickey ME, Gordon B. Drugs for Mental Illness: A Revolution in Psychiatry. New York: WH Freeman & Company, 1983.

Prien RF. Maintenance treatment. In Paykel ES (ed). Handbook of Affective Disorders, 2nd ed. New York: Guilford Press, 1992.

Self-study Exercises

Choose the most appropriate answer.

1. All of the following may be observed in a person who is manic *except:*

    A. "Hey baby, don't baby me . . . me and you can have some fun, fun and games and sugar and spice . . . "
    B. Quick short periods of anger, quickly changing to another euphoria or depression.
    C. Splitting staff members against each other to prevent control of his or her manic defense.
    D. Although thoughts may be fast, thoughts are never illogical or irrational.

2. Mrs. Jack has been on lithium for months. Her most recent blood level was 2.2 mEq/l. What reactions might the nurse expect to see?

    A. Fine hand tremors, mild thirst, and polyuria.
    B. Diarrhea, vomiting, and slurred speech.
    C. Electroencephalographic changes, ataxia, and seizures.
    D. No untoward effects, because her blood level is within normal limits.

Complete the nursing diagnosis by filling in the related factor(s). For the nursing diagnosis presented, give two pieces of data that would support the diagnosis for a manic client.

3. *High risk for injury* related to _____ as evidenced by:
    Data 1 _____
    Data 2 _____

4. *Impaired verbal communication* related to _____ as evidenced by:
    Data 1 _____
    Data 2 _____

5. *Altered family process* related to _____ as evidenced by:
    Data 1 _____
    Data 2 _____

For each of these nursing diagnoses, state one long term and two short term goals.

6. *High risk for injury:*
    LTG: _____
    STG: _____
    STG: _____

7. *Impaired verbal communication:*
    LTG: _____
    STG: _____
    STG: _____

8. *Altered family process:*
    LTG: _____
    STG: _____
    STG: _____

Identify four unconscious tactics used by a manic client to disrupt the environment and maximize the manic defense.

9. _____

10. _____

11. _____

12. _____

Name two interventions for each of the following areas and give the rationale for the action.

13. Nutrition:
    1. _____
    2. _____
    Rationales: _____

14. Rest and sleep:
    1. _____
    2. _____
    Rationales: _____

15. Dress and hygiene:
    1. _____
    2. _____
    Rationales: _____

16. Activities and recreation:
    1. _____
    2. _____
    Rationales: _____

List at least three cautions a person on lithium should know.

17. _____

18. _____

19. _____

Name three indications for seclusion.

20. _____

21. _____

22. _____

Place an H (helpful) or NH (not helpful) for each of the statements made by the nurse to a manic client.

23. _____ "Tom, come with me to the quiet room."

24. _____ "Comb the left side of your head . . . now the right side."

25. _____ "That's a funny joke, Tom . . . have you heard this one?"

26. _____ "I know the other nurses don't want you to join this group, but I'll let you."

27. _____ "I don't like those remarks. They aren't true, and that kind of behavior is disgusting."

28. _____ "Come away from this group. Let's write instead."

CHAPTER 19

Schizophrenic Disorders

Elizabeth M. Varcarolis

KEY TERMS AND CONCEPTS ♦ ♦ ♦ ♦ ♦ ♦ ♦ ♦ ♦ ♦ ♦ ♦ ♦

The key terms and concepts listed here also appear in bold where they are defined or discussed in this chapter.

ACUTE DYSTONIA

AFFECT

AKATHISIA

AMBIVALENCE

ANERGIA

ANHEDONIA

ASSOCIATIVE LOOSENESS

AUTISM

AUTOMATIC OBEDIENCE

BLOCKING

CLANG ASSOCIATION

CONCRETE THINKING

CONSENSUAL VALIDATION

DECODE

DELUSION

DELUSIONS OF BEING CONTROLLED

DEPERSONALIZATION

DEREALIZATION

DOUBLE-BIND MESSAGE

ECHOLALIA

ECHOPRAXIA

EXTRAPYRAMIDAL SIDE EFFECTS

EXTREME MOTOR AGITATION

FANTASY

HALLUCINATIONS

IDEAS OF REFERENCE

ILLUSIONS

LOOSENESS OF ASSOCIATION

LOSS OF EGO BOUNDARIES

NEGATIVISM

NEOLOGISMS

NEUROLEPTIC (ANTIPSYCHOTIC) MEDICATIONS

NEUROLEPTIC MALIGNANT SYNDROME

PARANOIA

PSEUDOPARKINSONISM

SCAPEGOATING

STEREOTYPED BEHAVIORS

STUPOR

TARDIVE DYSKINESIA

THOUGHT BROADCASTING

THOUGHT INSERTION

THOUGHT WITHDRAWAL

WAXY FLEXIBILITY

WATER INTOXICATION

WORD SALAD

NEGATIVE SYMPTOMS

POSITIVE SYMPTOMS

OBJECTIVES ■

After studying this chapter, the student will be able to

1. Discuss the progression of the disorders known as schizophrenia.
2. Compare four theories that explain the etiology of schizophrenia.
3. Name and briefly define four positive symptoms of schizophrenia.
4. Discuss three behaviors associated with the negative symptoms of schizophrenia.
5. Discuss the onset, premorbid diagnosis, and prognosis of schizophrenia.
6. Formulate three possible nursing diagnoses appropriate for a person with schizophrenia.
7. Describe three countertransference reactions a nurse may experience with a schizophrenic client.
8. Act out interventions for a client who is hallucinating, delusional, and demonstrating looseness of associations.
9. Explain three areas of health teaching appropriate for a family with a schizophrenic member.
10. Discuss four desired effects of the antipsychotic drugs.
11. Assess six side effects of antipsychotic drugs.
12. Identify the kinds of individual, group, and family therapies most useful for schizophrenic clients and their families.
13. Identify six positive outcomes of group work that nurses can do in the hospital setting.
14. Discuss how frequent evaluation of a schizophrenic client's nursing care plan can improve nursing skills and the client's progress.
15. Give the rationale for five specific interventions useful for each of the following: paranoid schizophrenia, catatonic schizophrenia, and disorganized schizophrenia.

Schizophrenia is a major mental disorder with psychotic symptoms marked by a profound withdrawal from interpersonal relationships and cognitive and perceptual disturbances that make dealing with reality difficult. Schizophrenia is a psychotic disorder.

A psychotic disorder differs from other groups of psychiatric disorders in its degree of (1) severity, (2) withdrawal, (3) alteration in affect, (4) impairment of intellect, and (5) regression (Hinsie and Cambell 1981).

SEVERITY. The psychoses, including active forms of schizophrenia, are considered major disorders and involve disruptions in all segments of a person's life. Psychosis may be seen in the major mood disorders, a wide range of organic disorders, and schizophrenia. These disorders are severe, intense, and disruptive. The person with a psychotic disorder suffers greatly, as do those in his or her immediate environment.

WITHDRAWAL. Withdrawal is so severe in psychosis that psychotic individuals are said to be autistic; that is, the person withdraws from reality into a private world. The psychotic individual is more withdrawn than is a person with an anxiety or somatoform disorder, personality disorder, psychophysiological disorder, or any other mental disorder.

AFFECT. The affect, mood, or emotional tone in a person with a psychotic disorder is vastly different from that of "normal" affect. In the mood disorders (see Chapters 17 and 18), one observes the exaggeration of sadness and lightheartedness in the form of depression and mania, respectively. In the schizophrenic disorders, affect may be exaggerated, flat, or inappropriate.

INTELLECT. In psychotic disorders, the intellect is involved in the actual psychotic process; disturbances of language, thought, and judgment result. Therefore, schizophrenia is called a formal thought disorder. Thinking and perceptions of reality are usually severely impaired.

REGRESSION. The most severe and prolonged regressions are seen in the psychoses. There is a falling back to earlier behavioral levels. In schizophrenia, this may include returning to primitive forms of behavior, such as curling up in a fetal position, eating with one's hands, masturbating in public, and so forth.

In 1886, Emil Kraepelin first recognized that a number of clinical syndromes could be seen as one specific disease, which Kraepelin called dementia praecox. Today we call these disorders schizophrenia. Freud viewed schizophrenia as untreatable by psychotherapeutic methods. Sullivan and Fromm-Reichmann, however, engaged in extensive psychoanalytical work with schizophrenic persons. Sullivan believed schizophrenia to be the result of destructive experiences with significant others during the formative years of life. Increased research is being conducted today in the biological, genetic, and neuropathological realms to understand the order and course of schizophrenia.

Data from the National Institute of Mental Health show that 1% of the general population have or will suffer from the symptoms of schizophrenia. People with schizophrenia occupy approximately 50% of the hospital beds for the mentally ill and 25% of all available hospital beds (Berkow et al. 1992).

There seems to be a high prevalence of schizophrenia in the lower socioeconomic classes. This has been attributed to social disorganization and social stresses as well as evidence that some people in a prepsychotic phase drift down the social scale (Berkow et al. 1992).

The symptoms of schizophrenia usually become manifest during adolescence or early adulthood, except for paranoid schizophrenia, which may have a later onset. The process of schizophrenic disorders is often slow, with the exception of catatonia, which may have an abrupt onset.

Theory

Many diverse theories of schizophrenia have been hypothesized by scholars from a variety of disciplines. It is presently thought that schizophrenia is a group of disorders of differing causes. There is no consensus in the literature about what is meant by the classification schizophrenia. Schizophrenia is most reliably classified by a cluster of symptoms and signs, none of which is specific only to schizophrenia. The process of schizophrenia appears complex, and the etiology is perhaps dependent on a variety of factors. Most cases are thought to be a complex interaction between inherited and environmental factors.

The numerous hypotheses relating to the cause of schizophrenia can be divided into two general categories: (1) the biological models which regard schizophrenia as primarily biological in origin, and (2) the environmental models, which suggest that schizophrenia is caused by environmental factors.

BIOLOGICAL MODELS

The most commonly accepted biological models are

1. Neurochemical hypotheses (the dopamine hypothesis and phencyclidine piperidine [PCP] model of schizophrenia)
2. Genetic hypotheses
3. Neuroanatomical findings

Neurochemical Hypotheses

DOPAMINE HYPOTHESIS. Bioamines (brain enzymes) are neurotransmitters to those areas of the brain that mediate emotions, feelings of pleasure and pain, awareness, levels of consciousness, and more. These bioamines are broken down into two categories: catecholamines (epinephrine, dopamine, and norepinephrine) and indolamine (serotonin).

High levels of metabolites (products of metabolism) of the brain bioamines have been found in the urine of clients who are frankly psychotic. When the symptoms worsen, the level of metabolites of catecholamines and indolamine increases in the client's urine.

The dopamine theory of schizophrenia is derived from the study of the action of the neuroleptic (antipsychotic) drugs. Neuroleptics are the drug of choice for treating the symptoms of schizophrenia. The neuroleptics are believed to block the dopamine receptors in the brain, which thereby limits the activity of dopamine and reduces the symptoms of schizophrenia. *Amphetamines*, on the other hand, enhance dopamine transmission. Amphetamines produce an excess of dopamine in the brain and can exacerbate the symptoms of schizophrenia in a psychotic client. In large doses, amphetamines can simulate symptoms of paranoid schizophrenia in a nonschizophrenic person. At least five types of dopamine receptors have been identified (Schizophrenia 1992a).

The dopamine hypothesis, in and by itself, is still not considered conclusive, however. For example, (1) *chronic* schizophrenics show a reduced rather than an increased dopamine turnover, and (2) certain symptoms persist in selected schizophrenics even after they are medicated with these dopamine receptor–blocking antipsychotics (Garza-Trevino et al. 1990). Other neurotransmitters indirectly affecting dopamine pathways must also be involved in schizophrenia (Schizophrenia 1992a).

PHENCYCLIDINE PIPERIDINE HYPOTHESIS. It has long been noted that phencyclidine piperidine (PCP) induces a state that closely resembles schizophrenia. Unlike the amphetamine-induced psychosis in the dopamine hypothesis, PCP psychosis incorporates both the positive symptoms (hallucinations and paranoia) and the negative symptoms (emotional withdrawal and motor retardation) of schizophrenia.

Interest has been renewed in the PCP model of schizophrenia because of growing understanding of mechanisms by which PCP works in affecting behavior at the neuroreceptor level. However, the development of the hypothesis is still in its early stages.

PCP, when ingested, inhibits *N*-methyl-D-aspartate (NMDA) receptor-mediated neurotransmission. Therefore, one possibility is that problems of regulation of receptor-mediated transmission of NMDA might occur in schizophrenia. Thus, PCP-induced psychosis provides a neurochemical hypothesis of schizophrenia different from the dopamine hypothesis (Javitt and Zurkin 1991).

Genetic Hypotheses

Gottesman and Shield (1982) summarized the contribution of genetic studies in the literature to support the genetic hypotheses of schizophrenia. For example:

- Identical twins. Concordance rate (co-twin similarly affected) for schizophrenia is 35–70% greater than that of the general population.
- Identical twin concordance is three times that of fraternal twins.
- Children of schizophrenics placed early for nonfamilial adoption develop schizophrenia as adults at higher rates than the general population does.
- Children of "normal" parents placed in foster homes in which a foster parent later developed schizophrenia do not show an increased rate of schizophrenia.

Although no individual schizophrenic gene has yet been identified, researchers are able to locate markers that are "linked" to a gene that produces vulnerability to schizophrenia (Schizophrenia 1992b).

Neuroanatomical Studies

New technology has been able to support the hypothesis that the symptoms in schizophrenia may be linked to some type of functional or structural brain abnormality. New brain imaging techniques, such as computed tomography, magnetic resonance imaging, and positron emission tomography, provide substantial evidence that some schizophrenics have structural brain abnormalities. Computed tomographic and magnetic resonance imaging studies provide evidence for structural cerebral abnormalities. Findings include (Sandy and Kay 1991)

- Enlargement of the lateral cerebral ventricles
- Cortical atrophy
- Third ventricular dilation
- Ventricular asymmetry
- Cerebellar atrophy

Some schizophrenics may also have changes in the cerebral cortex, the region of the brain that governs higher mental functions. During neurological testing, positron emission tomography scans also show a low rate of blood flow and glucose metabolism in the frontal lobes of the cerebral cortex, which govern planning, abstract thinking, and social adjustment (Schizophrenia 1992a).

ENVIRONMENTAL MODELS

The most prominent theoretical models in this group are the developmental model and the family theory model.

Developmental Model

Harry Stack Sullivan (1953) developed the interpersonal theory for the development of schizophrenia. Sullivan proposed that when an infant grows up in an environment of tenderness, consistent care, warmth, and respect in an atmosphere of minimal anxiety, the child incorporates these values into the sense of self, or ego. Peplau states that when these conditions are met, the child grows to see himself or herself as someone worthy of respect and love. The world is perceived as positive. The child can trust that needs will be met and the environment is safe and secure. This sense of trust stimulates growth.

If hostility, inconsistency of care, ridicule, and rejection are communicated to the infant, trust in the environment is never achieved. The world is perceived as a frightening, hostile, and dangerous place. The child's innate thrust toward growth becomes thwarted.

According to Sullivan, each person maintains contact with reality by consistently checking feelings, thoughts, and actions through interpersonal relationships. The infant initially validates reality with the mother figure. As the child grows, validating perceptions involves more people. This reality checking of thoughts, feelings, and actions with others Sullivan calls **consensual validation**.

If a child grows up in an environment of fear and anxiety, the chances to validate feelings, thoughts, and behaviors are decreased. The child's ability to accurately perceive reality will be greatly impaired. Therefore, a personality deficit or schizophrenia might result. This model is highly theoretical, and there are few data to support it as a model for the development of schizophrenia.

Family Theory Model

Family factors and parental influences are no longer considered a cause of schizophrenia. However, two phenomena observed among some schizophrenic families are presented briefly: double-bind communication and scapegoating.

DOUBLE-BIND COMMUNICATION. The double bind is a form of disturbed communication that takes place within some schizophrenic families. Although the double-bind form of communication probably takes place in all families, it is thought to be excessive among dysfunctional families.

A **double-bind message** contains two contradictory messages given by the same person at the same time, to which the receiver is expected to respond. Most often the receiver is a child. Constant double-bind situations result in feelings of helplessness, fear, and anxiety in the receiver of double-bind messages.

Message	Example
1. An overt message is given, indicating a command or threat to reply.	1. "Come give your mother a kiss."
2. A covert message (posture, gesture, tone of voice) implies the opposite.	2. The mother stiffens and turns her head in disgust as the child approaches.
3. The person is left in a no-win situation. If he or she responds to the verbal message, rejection follows. If he or she responds to the covert message, a reprimand follows.	3. After a period of constant double-bind messages, the child feels paralyzed to act.

SCAPEGOATING. In his work with schizophrenic families, Murray Bowen (1978) revealed profound emotional distance between parents of schizophrenic children. He found that often the parents experienced loneliness, feelings of isolation, and emptiness. Feelings of helplessness, inadequacy, and poor self-esteem can trigger painful levels of anxiety. Many of these parents project personal feelings of pain and anxiety onto an event, situation, or person outside the self. Instead of acknowledging the anxiety-provoking feelings of emptiness and poor self-esteem, the couple projects inner problems onto outward events. For example, the wife projects the cause of her feelings of isolation and loneliness on the "fact" that the husband pays more attention to television and sports than he does to her; the husband defends against his feelings of emptiness and despair by projecting the root of these feelings on the "fact" that his wife appears to care more for her job than for her family.

Scapegoating comes in when the child is the focus of the pain and anxiety within the family. For example, the mother denies her own feelings of inadequacy and helplessness and projects these feelings onto the child. The child then becomes the target of the mother's painful feelings. The *child* is now perceived as inadequate and helpless by the whole family. The mother's projections are then perceived as reality. The feelings that began in the mother become reality in the child (Bowen 1978). Therefore the child becomes the "identified client," or scapegoat for the problems of the parents. The focus of attention onto the child's "problems" relieves the tension between the parents and helps to repress the painful feelings within the parents.

Family studies do suggest that the family life of some schizophrenic persons is disturbed. However, a clear etiological relationship between a pathological family process and schizophrenia has not been established.

Assessment

In 1950, Eugen Bleuler, building on the observations of Emil Kraepelin, coined the term *schizophrenia.* Bleuler's fundamental signs of schizophrenia, referred to as the four As, are still used today for help in the diagnosis of schizophrenia. The four As include

1. **Affect,** the outward manifestation of a person's feelings and emotions. In schizophrenia, one can observe flat, blunted, inappropriate, or bizarre affect.
2. **Associative looseness,** which refers to haphazard and confused thinking that is manifested in jumbled and illogical speech and reasoning. People also use the term **looseness of association.**
3. **Autism,** thinking not bound to reality but reflecting the private perceptual world of the individual. Delusions, hallucinations, and neologisms are examples of autistic thinking in a person with schizophrenia.
4. **Ambivalence,** holding, at the same time, two opposing emotions, attitudes, ideas, or wishes toward the same person, situation, or object. Ambivalence occurs normally in all relationships. Pathological ambivalence is paralyzing.

Sam, a 25-year-old man soon to be discharged from the hospital, constantly tells the social worker he wants his own apartment. When Sam is told that an apartment has been found for him, he states, "But who will take care of me?" Sam is acting out his ambivalence between his desire to be independent and his desire to be taken care of.

In 1959, Kurt Schneider developed a system of diagnosing a person with schizophrenia by ongoing symptoms into first-rank and second-rank symptoms. The World Health Organization in 1975 identified a standard set of symptoms specific to the diagnosis of schizophrenia common to people in a variety of countries. Figure 19–1 lists the different types of schizophrenia based on the DSM-IV *Options Book.*

Renewed interest has been kindled in the study of the positive and negative symptoms of schizophrenia. The positive symptoms (such as hallucinations, delusions, bizarre behavior, and paranoia) are the attention-getting symptoms referred to as *florid psychotic symptoms.* After three decades of analyzing treatment and results of studies, it is indicated that perhaps these florid psychotic symptoms may not be the core deficiency after all. It may actually be the crippling negative symptoms (e.g., apathy, lack of motivation, anhedonia, and poor thought processes) that persist and seem more fundamental (Talbott et al. 1988). This view is supported by the inclusion of greater emphasis on the negative symptoms in the DSM-IV.

Another reason for this interest is that it appears the positive-negative approach may correlate with prognosis as well as biological variables (Grebb and Cancro 1989).

Positive symptoms, such as hallucinations, delusions, bizarre behavior, and paranoia, are associated with

1. Acute onset
2. Normal premorbid functioning
3. Normal social functioning during remissions
4. Normal computed tomographic scan findings
5. Normal neuropsychological test results
6. Favorable response to antipsychotic medication

Negative symptoms, such as apathy, anhedonia, poor social functioning, and poverty of thought, are associated with

1. Insidious onset
2. Premorbid history of emotional problems
3. Chronic deterioration
4. Demonstration of atrophy on computed tomographic scans
5. Abnormalities on neuropsychological testing
6. Poor response to antipsychotic or neuroleptic therapy

Other researchers have not found a clear relationship between positive and negative symptoms (Schizophrenia 1992a); however, in theory, the positive and negative dichotomy is useful for educational purposes (APA 1991). Table 19–1 expands on the discrete attributes of the positive and negative symptoms.

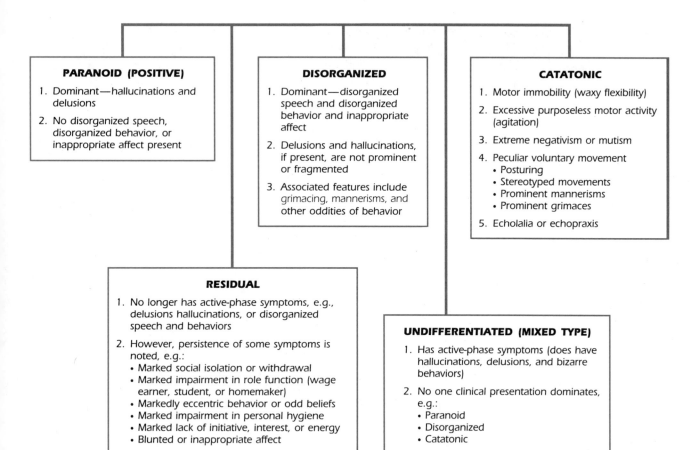

Figure 19–1. *Diagnostic criteria for the subtypes of schizophrenia. (Adapted from the American Psychiatric Association. Diagnostic and Statistical Manual of Mental Disorders, 4th ed (DSM-IV). Washington, DC: American Psychiatric Association, 1994.)*

PRODROMAL SYMPTOMS

Many people who subsequently develop schizophrenia experience prodromal symptoms a month to a year before their first psychotic break. These symptoms represent a clear deterioration in previous functioning. As an adolescent, a person who later develops schizophrenia is often withdrawn from others, lonely, and perhaps depressed. Plans for the future may appear to others as vague or unrealistic (Kolb and Brodie 1982).

There may be a transitional "preschizophrenic" phase a year or two before the disorder is diagnosed. This phase may include such neurotic symptoms as acute or chronic anxiety, phobias, obsessions, and compulsions or may reveal dissociative features. As anxiety mounts, indications of a thought disorder may be present. An adolescent may complain of difficulty with concentration and with the ability to complete school work or job-related work. Eventually there is severe deterioration of work along with the deterioration of the ability to cope with the environment. Such complaints as "mind wandering," inability to concen-

trate, and needing to devote more time to maintaining one's thoughts are heard. Finally, the ability to keep out unwanted intrusions into one's thoughts becomes impossible. Eventually, the person finds that his or her mind becomes so distracted that the ability to have ordinary conversations with others is lost (Kolb and Brodie 1982).

The person may initially feel that something strange or wrong is going on. The person misinterprets things going on in the environment and may give mystical or symbolic meanings to ordinary events. For example, the person may think that certain colors hold special powers or that a thunderstorm is a message from God. The person often mistakes other people's actions or words as signs of hostility or evidence of harmful intent.

As the disease develops, the person suffers from strong feelings of rejection, lack of self-respect, loneliness, and feelings of hopelessness. Emotional and physical withdrawal increase feelings of isolation, as does an inability to trust or relate to others. The withdrawal may become severe, and withdrawal from reality may become evident in hallucinations, delu-

Table 19–1 ■ CORRELATIONS BETWEEN POSITIVE AND NEGATIVE SYMPTOMS

POSITIVE (FLORID)	NEGATIVE (DEFICIT)
Examples	
1. Delusions	1. Apathy
2. Looseness of associations	2. Poverty of speech or content of speech
3. Hallucinations	3. Poor social functioning
4. Bizarre or agitated behaviors	4. Anhedonia
	5. Social withdrawal
Associated Findings	
1. Acute onset	1. Slow onset
2. Least important prognostically	2. Interferes with a person's life
3. History of exacerbations and remissions	3. Positive premorbid history
4. Normal premorbid functioning	4. Chronic deterioration
5. No family history of schizophrenia	5. Family history of schizophrenia
6. Normal computed tomography scan	6. Cerebellar atrophy and lateral and third ventricular enlargement on computed tomography scan
7. Normal neuropsychological testing	7. Abnormalities on neuropsychological testing
8. Good response to antipsychotics	8. Poor response to antipsychotics
Most Useful Interventions	
1. Neuroleptic (antipsychotic) medication	1. Skill training interventions: • Identify areas of skill deficit person is willing to work on • Prioritize skills important to the person
2. Medical assessment to rule out physiological process that may be contributing to symptoms	2. Working with person to identify stressors: • Identify which stressors contribute to maladaptive behaviors • Work with person on increasing appropriate coping skills

sions, and odd mannerisms. Some persons think their thoughts are being controlled by others or that their thoughts are being broadcast to the world. Others may think that people are out to harm them or are spreading rumors about them. Voices are sometimes heard in the form of commands or derogatory statements about their character. The voices may seem to come from outside the room, from electrical appliances, or from other sources.

Early in the disease, there may be preoccupation with religion, matters of mysticism, or metaphysical causes of creations. Speech may be characterized by obscure symbolisms. Later, words and phases may become indecipherable, and these can be understood only as part of the person's private fantasy world. Sometimes the person will make up words. People who have been ill with schizophrenia for a long time often have speech patterns that are incoherent, rambling, and devoid of meaning to the casual observer.

Sexual activity is frequently altered in mental disorders. Preoccupation with homosexual themes may be associated with all psychoses but is most prominent with paranoia. Doubts regarding sexual identity, exaggerated sexual needs, altered sexual performance, and fears of intimacy are prominent in schizophrenia. The process of regression in schizophrenia is accompanied by increased self-preoccupation, isolation, and masturbatory behavior.

Before the 1950s and the advent of antipsychotic drugs, the prognosis for schizophrenia was poor. Today, the outlook is much brighter. With good follow-up therapy and well-controlled maintenance drug treatment, only 10–15% of clients in remission relapse within a year, compared with a 65–70% relapse rate without such treatment (Lehmann and Cancro 1985). The less adherence there is to following a medical maintenance program, the greater the possibility of relapse.

An abrupt onset with good premorbid functioning is usually a favorable prognostic sign. A slow, insidious onset over a period of two or three years is more ominous. Those whose prepsychotic personalities show good social, sexual, and occupational functioning have greater chances for a good remission or a

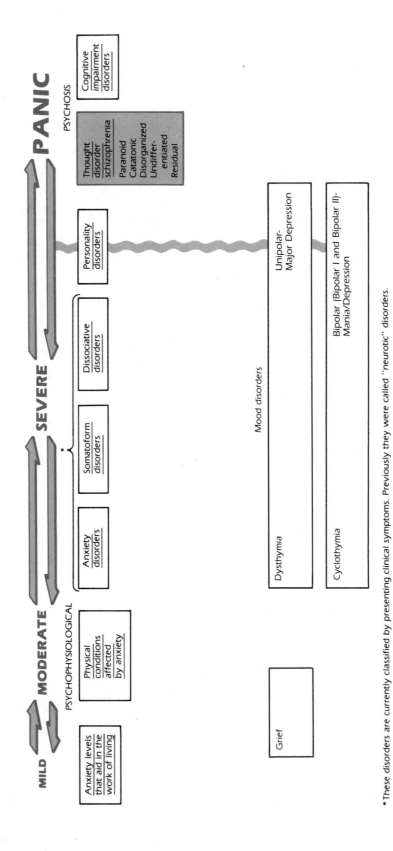

*These disorders are currently classified by presenting clinical symptoms. Previously they were called "neurotic" disorders.

Figure 19–2. *Mental health continuum for schizophrenia.*

complete recovery. Childhood histories of withdrawn, seclusive, eccentric, and tense behavior are unfavorable diagnostic signs. The younger the client is at the onset of schizophrenia, the more discouraging the prognosis. Because schizophrenia is a psychotic disorder, it is placed on the high end of the mental health continuum (Fig. 19–2).

Early psychiatric and medical treatment helps secure a more favorable eventual outcome. A delay of months or years allows the psychotic process to become more entrenched. No single symptom is always present in all cases of schizophrenia or occurs only in schizophrenia alone. The different subtypes of schizophrenia with symptoms are outlined in Figure 19–1. Assessment is organized into assessing positive, negative, and associated symptoms.

ASSESSING POSITIVE SYMPTOMS OF SCHIZOPHRENIA

The positive symptoms appear early in the first phase of the illness. These are the symptoms that get people's attention and often precipitate hospitalization. They are, however, the *least important prognostically* and usually respond to antipsychotic or neuroleptic medication. The positive symptoms are presented in terms of alterations in thinking, perceiving, and behavior.

Alterations in Thinking

Alterations in thinking can take many forms. Delusions, looseness of association, neologisms, concrete thinking, echolalia, clang association, and word salad are considered here.

DELUSIONS. Peplau offers the definition of **delusion** as "an erroneous conclusion drawn from insufficient data." This definition allows for exploring the panic that precedes the conclusion, however faulty, that brings relief to the client (Smoyak 1994). Peplau believes that nurses need to fully understand the operations of anxiety and panic, and how delusions serve to prevent the re-experience of panic episodes (Smoyak 1994).

Most common delusional thinking includes

1. Ideas of reference
2. Delusions of persecution
3. Delusions of grandeur
4. Somatic delusions
5. Delusions of jealousy

Refer to Table 19–2 for definitions and examples of delusions.

About 75% of schizophrenic persons experience delusions at some time during their illness. In schizophrenia, persecutory, grandiose delusions are the

most common, as are those involving religious or hypochondriacal ideas.

In the acute phase of schizophrenia, the person is overwhelmed by panic levels of anxiety and is not able to distinguish what is inside (thoughts) from what is outside (reality). Therefore, a delusion may stimulate behavior for dealing with confusion and the resulting anxiety.

When delusional, a person really believes what he or she thinks to be real *is* real. The person's thinking often reflects feelings of great fear and aloneness. "I know the doctor talks to the CIA about getting rid of me." "Everyone wants me dead." Or delusions may reflect the person's feelings of low self-worth through the use of reaction-formation. "I'm the only one who can save the world, but they won't let me."

It is interesting to note that there may be times that delusions hold a kernel of truth. One patient came into the hospital acutely psychotic. He kept saying the Mafia was out to kill him. Later, the staff learned he had been selling drugs, he had not paid his contacts, and people were out looking to settle the score.

Common delusions observed in schizophrenia are the following (APA 1987):

- **Thought broadcasting,** the belief that one's thoughts can be heard by others (e.g., "My brain is connected to the world mind—I can control all heads of state through my thoughts.").
- **Thought insertion,** the belief that thoughts of others are being inserted into one's mind (e.g., "They make me think bad thoughts and are rotting my brain.").
- **Thought withdrawal,** the belief that thoughts have been removed from one's mind by an outside agency (e.g., "The devil takes my thoughts away and leaves me empty.").
- **Delusions of being controlled,** beliefs that one's body or mind is controlled by an outside agency (e.g., "There is a man from darkness who controls my thoughts with electrical waves.").

LOOSENESS OF ASSOCIATION. Zelda Fitzgerald wrote her husband, the writer F. Scott Fitzgerald, an account of going mad:

Then the world became embryonic in Africa—and there was no need for communication. . . . I have been living in vaporous places peopled with one-dimensional figures and tremulous buildings until I can no longer tell an optical illusion from a reality . . . head and ears incessantly throb and roads disappear (Vidal 1982).

Associations are the threads that tie one thought to another and one concept to another. In schizophrenia, these threads are missing, and connections become

DEFINITION	EXAMPLE
Ideas of Reference	
Misconstruing trivial events and remarks and giving them personal significance	When Maria saw the doctor and nurse talking together, she believed they were talking against her. When she heard on the radio that a hurricane was coming, she believed this to be a message that "bad weather" or harm was going to befall her.
Persecution	
The false belief that one is being singled out for harm by others; this belief often takes the form of a plot by people in power against the person	Sam believed that the secret service was planning to kill him. He became wary of what food he ate because he believed that the secret service was poisoning his food.
Grandeur	
The false belief that one is a powerful and important person	Sally believed she was Mary Magdalene and that Jesus controlled her thoughts and was telling her how to save the world.
Somatic Delusions	
The false belief that the body is changing in an unusual way (e.g., rotting inside)	David kept telling the doctor that his brain was rotting away.
Jealousy	
The false belief that one's mate is unfaithful; may have pieces of so-called proof	Harry kept accusing his girlfriend of going out with other men, even though this was not the case. His "proof" was that she came home from work late twice that week. He persisted in his belief even when the girlfriend's boss explained that everyone had worked late.

*A delusion is a false belief held and maintained as true even with evidence to the contrary. This does not include unrealistic beliefs maintained by one's culture or subculture.

Table 19–2 ■ SUMMARY OF DELUSIONS*

interrupted. In **looseness of association,** thinking becomes haphazard, illogical, and confused:

NURSE: Are you going to the picnic today?
CLIENT: Only five dollars at the top.

This client's response initially seems not to be in keeping with the question asked by the nurse. To the client, however, the response has meaning. This young man always referred to his emotional security in dollars and cents. When he was feeling secure and confident, he spoke of himself as having plenty of money: "I have $500 at the top." At times, the nurse may be able to decipher or **decode** the client's messages and begin to understand the client's feelings and needs. Any exchange in which a person feels understood is useful. Therefore, the nurse might respond to the client in this way:

NURSE: Are you saying, Tony, that you don't feel secure enough to go out with the others today?
CLIENT: Yeah . . . not much at the top today.

If the nurse does not understand what the client is saying, it is important to let the client know this. Clear messages and complete honesty are an important part of the work with schizophrenic persons. Letting the person know *you do not understand* but *would like to understand* or *will try to understand* is honest. If the nurse is confused about the client's message but indicates understanding, this can contribute to increasing this type of message. The client then sees no reason to change his communication.

NEOLOGISMS. Neologisms are words a person makes up that have special meaning for the person. ("I was going to tell him the *mannerologies* of his hospitality won't do." "I want all the *vetchkisses* to leave the room and leave me be.")

Children and creative writers often make up their own words. Their creation of neologisms is imaginative, constructive, and adaptive. Neologisms in the schizophrenic reaction represent regression and disruption in reality functioning.

CONCRETE THINKING. In psychiatry, the term **concrete thinking** usually implies overemphasis on specific details and an impairment in the ability to use abstract concepts. For example, during an assessment, the nurse might ask what brought the client to the hospital. The client might answer "a cab" rather than explaining the need for seeking medical or psychiatric aid. When asked to give the meaning of the proverb "people in glass houses shouldn't throw stones," the person might answer, "Don't throw stones or the windows will break." The answer is literal; the ability to use abstract reasoning is absent.

ECHOLALIA. Echolalia is the pathological repeating of another's word by imitation and is often seen in people with catatonia.

NURSE: Mary, come for your medication.
MARY: Mary, come for your medication.

Echolalia is the counterpart of **echopraxia,** mimicking the *movements* of another, also seen in catatonia.

CLANG ASSOCIATION. Clang association is the meaningless rhyming of words, often in a forceful manner. "They are red, bed, said, fed ned. . . ." This form of speech pattern may be seen in schizophrenia; however, it may also be seen in the manic phase of a bipolar disorder or in an organic condition.

WORD SALAD. Word salad is a term used to identify a mixture of phrases meaningless to the listener and perhaps to the speaker as well. It may include a string of neologisms, as in the following example: "Birds and fishes . . . framewoes . . . mud and stars and thump-bump going."

Alterations in Perceiving

Hallucinations are the major example of alterations in perceiving in schizophrenia, especially auditory hallucinations. The following alterations in perceptions are discussed: hallucinations and loss of ego boundaries (depersonalization and derealization).

HALLUCINATIONS. Hallucinations can be defined as sensory perceptions to which there is no *external stimulus.* The most common types of hallucinations include

- Auditory—hearing voices or sounds
- Visual—seeing persons or things
- Olfactory—smelling odors
- Gustatory—experiencing tastes
- Tactile—feeling body sensations

Refer to Table 19–3 for examples of common hallucinations. Table 19–3 also describes the difference between hallucinations and **illusions.**

Peplau states that hallucinations have three fundamental characteristics (Field 1979):

Table 19–3 ■ SUMMARY OF HALLUCINATIONS*	
DEFINITION	**EXAMPLE**
Auditory	
Hearing voices or sounds that do not exist in the environment but are projections of inner thought or feelings	Anna "hears" the voice of her dead mother call her a whore and a tramp.
Visual	
Seeing a person, object, or animal that does not exist in the environment	Charles, who is experiencing alcohol withdrawal delirium, "sees" hungry rats coming toward him.
Olfactory	
Smelling odors that are not present in the environment	Theresa "smells" her insides rotting.
Gustatory	
Tasting sensations that have no stimulus in reality	Sal will not eat his food because he "tastes" the poison the FBI is putting in his food.
Tactile	
Feeling strange sensations where there are not external objects to stimulate such feelings; common in delirium tremens	A paranoid schizophrenic "feels" electrical impulses controlling his mind. A person experiencing alcohol withdrawal delirium "feels" snakes crawling on his body.

*A hallucination is a false sensory perception for which there is no external stimulus. They are different from illusions in that illusions are misperceptions or misinterpretations of a real experience. For example, a man saw his coat hanging on a coat rack and believed it to be a bear about to attack him. He did see something real but misinterpreted what it was.

1. The perceptions are created within (e.g., voices).
2. The perceptions are then projected onto the real world.
3. The projected perceptions (voices) are then interacted with as if they were real.

It is estimated that 90% of the people with schizophrenia experience hallucinations at some time during their illness. Although manifestations of hallucinations are varied, auditory hallucinations are most common in schizophrenia. These voices may seem to come from outside or inside the person's head. The voices may be familiar or strange, single or multiple. Voices speaking directly to the person or commenting on the person's behavior are most common in schizophrenia. A person may believe the voices are from God, the devil, deceased relatives, or strangers. The auditory hallucinations may occasionally take the form of sounds rather than voices. *Command hallucinations* must be assessed for, because the "voices" may command the person to hurt himself or others. For example, a client might state that "the voices" are telling him to "jump out the window" or "take a knife and kill my child." Command hallucinations are often terrifying for the individual. A person experiencing them is often in panic levels of anxiety, and command hallucinations may signal a psychiatric emergency.

Evidence of possible hallucinatory behavior may be the turning or tilting of the head as if the client is talking to someone or frequent blinking of the eyes and grimacing by the client. Sometimes audible responses are heard.

Visual hallucinations are less often reported in schizophrenia and are more often noted in organic disorders.

Grebb and Cancro (1989) point out that the frequency of hallucinations may vary among cultures. There is some indication that hallucinations are more common in African, West Indian, and Asian cultures than in American and European cultures.

LOSS OF EGO BOUNDARIES. People with schizophrenia often lack a sense of their body in relationship to the rest of the world . . . where they leave off and others begin. For this reason, many schizophrenics are confused over their own sexual identity. A client might say he or she is merging with others or is part of inanimate objects.

1. **Depersonalization** is a nonspecific feeling that a person has lost his or her identity, that he or she is different or unreal. The person may be concerned that body parts do not belong to him or her. Or the person may have an acute sensation that his or her body has drastically changed. For example, people may see their fingers as snakes or their arms as rotting wood. Another may look in a mirror and state his face is that of an animal.

2. **Derealization** is the false perception by a person that the environment has changed. For example, everything seems bigger or smaller, or familiar surroundings have become somehow strange and unfamiliar.

Both depersonalization and derealization can be interpreted as **loss of ego boundaries.**

Alterations in Behavior

Bizarre and agitated behavior is associated with schizophrenia and may take a variety of forms.

BIZARRE BEHAVIOR. Bizarre behaviors may take the form of a stilted rigid demeanor, eccentric dress or grooming, and rituals. The following behaviors are often seen in catatonia.

- **Extreme motor agitation.** Exteme motor agitation is agitated physical behavior, such as running about, in response to inner and outer stimuli. The person may become dangerous to others or suffer exhaustion or collapse and die if not stopped.
- **Stereotyped behaviors.** Stereotyped behaviors are motor patterns that originally had meaning to the person (e.g., sweeping the floor, washing windows) but that have become mechanical and lack purpose.
- **Automatic obedience.** A catatonic client may perform, without hesitation, all simple commands in a robot-like fashion.
- **Waxy flexibility.*** Waxy flexibility consists of excessive maintenance of posture evidenced when a person's arms or legs can be placed in any position and the position is held for long periods of time.
- **Stupor.*** The person who is in a stupor may sit motionless for long periods of time and may be motionless to the point of apparent coma.
- **Negativism.*** Negativism is equivalent to resistance. In *active negativism*, the person does the opposite of what he or she is told to do. When the person does not do things he or she is expected to do (e.g., does not get out of bed, does not dress, does not eat), such behavior is termed *passive negativism.*

AGITATED BEHAVIOR. Clients with schizophrenia may have difficulty with impulse control when they are acutely ill. Because of cognitive deterioration, clients

---

*Waxy flexibility, stupor, and negativism can be considered negative symptoms.

lack social sensitivity and can act out impulsively with others, such as grab another's cigarette, throw food on the floor, and turn television channels abruptly (Grebb and Cancro 1989).

ASSESSING NEGATIVE SYMPTOMS OF SCHIZOPHRENIA

The negative symptoms of schizophrenia develop over a long time. These are the symptoms that most interfere with the individual's adjustment and ability to survive. It is the presence of negative symptoms that *interferes with* the person's ability to

- Initiate and maintain relationships
- Initiate and maintain conversations
- Hold a job
- Make decisions
- Maintain adequate hygiene and grooming

It is the presence of negative symptoms that contributes to the person's poor social functioning and social withdrawal.

On assessment, specific phenomena are noted. During an acute psychotic episode, negative symptoms may be difficult to assess because the positive and more florid symptoms, such as delusions and hallucinations, may dominate. Some of the negative phenomena are outlined in Table 19–4, such as poverty of content of speech, poverty of speech, thought blocking, anergia, anhedonia, affective blunting, and avolition.

Affect is the observable behaviors that express a person's emotions. The affect of a schizophrenic person usually falls into one of three categories: flat or blunted, inappropriate, or bizarre.

A *flat* or *blunted affect* is commonly seen in schizophrenia. In schizophrenia, a person's outward affect may not coincide with his or her inner emotions.

Inappropriate affect refers to an emotional response to a situation that is not congruent with the tone of the situation. For example, a young man, told that his father is ill, breaks out laughing.

Bizarre affect is especially prominent in the disorganized form of schizophrenia. Grimacing, giggling, and mumbling to oneself come under this heading. Bizarre affect is marked when there is inability to relate logically to the environment.

A study suggests that cognitive deficits are more likely to be associated with high negative symptom ratings than with positive. Furthermore, improved cognitive abilities are related to improvement in positive symptoms but not negative symptoms (Addington et al. 1991).

Table 19–4 ■ NEGATIVE PHENOMENA	
PHENOMENON	**EXPLANATION**
Affective blunting	In **affective blunting,** there is severe reduction in the expression, range, and intensity of affects; in **flat affect,** there is no facial expression of emotion
Anergia	Lack of energy: passivity or impersistence at work or school
Anhedonia	Inability to experience any pleasure in activities that usually produce pleasurable feelings; result of profound emotional barrenness
Avolition	Lack of motivation: unable to initiate tasks, such as initiating social contacts, grooming, and other aspects of activities of daily living
Poverty of content of speech	Speech that is adequate in amount but conveys little information because of vagueness, empty repetitions, or use of stereotype or obscure phrases
Poverty of speech	Restriction in the amount of speech—answers range from brief to monosyllabic one-word answers
Thought blocking	A client may stop talking in the middle of a sentence and remain silent
	After a client stopped abruptly: NURSE: "What just happened now?" CLIENT: "I forgot what I was saying. Something took my thoughts away."

ASSESSING ASSOCIATED SYMPTOMS OF SCHIZOPHRENIA

Many other symptoms are associated with schizophrenia. Presented here are (1) withdrawal and fantasy, (2) depression, (3) water intoxication, (4) substance abuse, and (5) violent behavior. These phenomena are not peculiar to schizophrenia but may be found on assessment.

WITHDRAWAL. Withdrawal can be seen as a defense against uncomfortable levels of anxiety. Withdrawal on a continuum may stretch from moderate shyness to stupor. Behaviors become maladaptive in terms of their *frequency, intensity,* and *duration* of use. Most people have personal patterns of withdrawal during stress. For example, a person might sleep late after going to bed early the night before, watch television for long periods and hardly remember what he or she is watching, or read detective stories for escapist pleasure. Or a person can withdraw physically. A man who has had a fight with his wife may go out for a walk with the dog. A student who has been studying for an exam to the point of frustration goes out to a movie. As long as withdrawal activities do not become a substitute for activities in the real world, they may be viewed as adaptive.

Fantasy represents a retreat from reality and an attempt to solve problems in a private world. The difference between most people and a person with schizophrenia, however, is that the schizophrenic person is often not able to tell the difference between distorted perceptions (fantasy) and reality.

A person with schizophrenia withdraws not just from the activities of life but from feelings as well. This often gives the clinical picture of the blunting or flat affect. Where there is no evidence of actual physical withdrawal, there is more often a delusional paranoid structure, which defends against anxiety.

Catatonic stupor is perhaps the most severe form of physical withdrawal. A schizophrenic who responds to his or her own autistic world (fantasy world), and who is unable to interact with the real world, is severely withdrawn from reality.

DEPRESSION. Depression is often seen in people with schizophrenia. The incidence of suicide may be 5–7% higher in schizophrenia than in the general population (see Chapter 21). People with schizophrenia often feel confused, helpless, and isolated and have fewer personal resources for support and comfort.

WATER INTOXICATION. Excessive water consumption by psychiatric clients is receiving much attention. **Water intoxication** is thought to occur in 3–6% of hospitalized psychiatric patients (Bugle et al. 1992). A high percentage of these psychiatric clients are schizo-phrenics. Patients can ingest more than 10–15 liters of fluid per day. When this disorder is not treated, it can lead to cerebral edema, seizures, brain stem herniation, and even death. Water-intoxicated patients might be seen constantly carrying a cup or soda can around, making frequent trips to the water fountain or restroom. Patients have also been observed drinking from toilet, sink, and shower. These patients are often highly agitated and vigorous in their pursuit of fluids (Bugle et al. 1992).

A high percentage of water imbalance in schizophrenic clients is thought to be medication induced. Inappropriate secretion of antidiuretic hormone can be caused by antipsychotics as well as by carbamazepine (Tegretol), lithium, and other drugs. Approaches to the treatment of clients with water intoxication have had positive results (Goldman 1991; Baldwin et al. 1992).

SUBSTANCE ABUSE. A review of the literature by Dixon and associates (1991) found that the incidence of psychoactive drug abuse among schizophrenic patients is considerably higher than in the general population. Their study found that cannabis, alcohol, and cocaine were the drugs used most frequently by people with schizophrenia. These patients reported that all three drugs acutely increased their experience of happiness and decreased feelings of depression. Most patients reported that they used drugs to relieve depression and relax. Others stated that they used drugs to counteract their negative symptoms (to help them increase feelings and emotions, talk more, and increase energy). It has also been reported that drug-abusing schizophrenic patients require more hospitalization, have lower compliance with treatment regimens, and are at a greater risk for suicide. The use of these psychoactive substances appears to have a significant adverse effect on the global outcome of these patients.

VIOLENT BEHAVIOR. Threats of violence and even minor aggressive outbursts are common in acute schizophrenic states and relapses (Berkow et al. 1992). Refer to Chapter 22 for further discussion.

Nursing Diagnosis

As indicated by the assessment, a person with schizophrenia may have a variety of symptoms. Although there may be many clients on a unit with schizophrenia, each may present with different personal needs and defensive behaviors. Each client requires a nursing care plan that reflects individual needs and strategies appropriate to the client's behaviors and level of functioning. Some nursing diagnoses that are appropriate to nurses' work with schizophrenic clients are discussed.

During the course of schizophrenia, a client is likely to experience positive (hallucinations, delusions) and negative (withdrawal, poor social functioning) symptoms. During this time, impairment in thought processes may be evident in the client's ability to reason, problem-solve, make decisions, and concentrate. These distortions alter the client's ability to perceive reality accurately (hallucinations or delusions) and usually impair the client's judgment. A nursing diagnosis of *altered thought process* is appropriate. *Altered thought process* may be related to alteration in biochemical compounds, panic, levels of anxiety, emotional trauma, and so forth.

With alteration in thought process come changes in language and speech. Therefore, *impaired verbal communication* may be a problem to varying degrees. When looseness of associations is severe, the person is unable to communicate needs or feelings. The nurse interacts in a variety of ways to try to understand and help reduce the client's anxiety. Use of neologisms, echolalia, clang associations, and word salad contribute to the client's *impaired verbal communication*.

When a person is unable to interpret the world accurately, his or her ability to cope with the environment is also impaired. Therefore, *ineffective individual coping* is most always present. A person's *ineffective individual coping* may be evidenced by inappropriate use of defense mechanisms and inability to meet role expectations. Symptoms may include withdrawal or excitability, disorganized or regressive behaviors, paranoid or disorganized thinking, and inability to meet basic needs.

A person who is extremely paranoid may have special problems. For example, if the person is refusing to eat because he or she thinks the food is poisoned, then *altered nutrition: less than body requirements* is used.

"Voices" that tell the person to harm others or himself or herself can result in bodily harm or even death to the client or others. *High risk for violence directed at others or self-directed* would take priority (refer to section on paranoia).

During the excited phase of catatonia, a client may be highly agitated and can exhaust himself or herself to a dangerous level if rest and high-calorie fluid replacement are not immediately provided. Extreme hyperactivity can lead to cardiac or respiratory collapse and indicates a nursing diagnosis of *activity intolerance*.

During extreme withdrawal, attention to physical care is vital. Some useful nursing diagnoses might be (1) *constipation/incontinence*, (2) *impaired physical mobility*, or (3) *self-care deficit: feeding, bathing, dressing/grooming, and toileting*.

When the disease becomes chronic, it is not uncommon to note multiple admissions to a unit. Problems with compliance with medications is thought to be a major factor. Families with schizophrenic members may have their own confused patterns of communication and insufficient knowledge of the client's problems or may feel powerless in coping with the client at home. *Ineffective family coping: compromised or disabling* may be an important area for intervention by members of the health care team, especially in relation to discharge planning.

Most people with schizophrenia suffer from a low self-concept. There is often confusion of sexual identity, as well as unrealistic and distorted perception of self. Depersonalization further confuses the person's perception of body image. *Disturbance in self-esteem* is usually present.

Refer to Figure 19–1 for an overview of the criteria for the individual schizophrenic disorders.

Planning

Planning involves more than the identification of measurable and attainable goals. Identification of personal reactions and feelings regarding the client is necessary if the interventions in the nursing care plan are to be carried out effectively. Therefore, planning involves (1) content level—planning goals and (2) process level—nurses' reactions and feelings.

CONTENT LEVEL—PLANNING GOALS

It is important that goals be both meaningful and attainable by nursing action. The goals are usually directed toward the "related to" component of the nursing diagnosis. Therefore, *altered thought process related to isolation* and *altered thought process related to unclear communications* would have different short term and long term goals. The goals listed subsequently are offered as examples and guidelines for nursing actions.

Altered thought process related to panic levels of anxiety, as evidenced by hallucinations or delusions (positive symptoms)

Long and Short Term Goals
- By (date), client will go from panic to severe levels of anxiety with the aid of medication and nursing intervention.
- Client will meet with nurse once a day for 15

minutes in an activity in which the client feels comfortable.

- By (date), client will state that "the voices" or "the thoughts" are less frequent with the aid of medication and nursing intervention.
- By (date), client will engage in one unit activity per day that provides reality testing.
- By (date), client will identify personal interventions that lower hallucinations.
- By (date), client will talk about concrete happenings without talking about delusions or hallucinations for short periods.
- By (date), client will make needs and wants clearer with the aid of medication and nursing interventions.

Ineffective individual coping related to lack of motivation to respond, as evidenced by alteration in social participation (negative symptoms)

Long and Short Term Goals

- By (date), client will meet with nurse for 10 minutes two times a day in an activity in which the client feels safe.
- By (date), client will meet with the nurse and one other client in a simple activity.
- Client will state that he or she feels more comfortable with nurse by (date).
- Client will state that he or she feels more comfortable with one other client or staff member by (date).
- Client will attend one simple group activity each day by (date).

High risk for violence directed at others related to misperceived messages from others, as evidenced by persecutory delusions and hallucinations

Long and Short Term Goals

- By (date), client will state that the voices are less angry, with the aid of medication.
- By (date), client will identify helping behaviors of nurses and staff.
- Client will join the nurse for one activity per day in which he states that he feels safe.
- By (date), client will state that he feels safe on the unit with the staff.

Activity intolerance related to extreme physical activity, as evidenced by constant physical agitation and increased respiration and pulse

Long and Short Term Goals

- Client will decrease high levels of agitation within 20 minutes after intramuscular medication is administered.

- Client will take 8 ounces of a high-calorie fluid every 30 minutes.
- Client will have five-minute rest periods every 30 minutes.

PROCESS LEVEL—NURSES' REACTIONS AND FEELINGS

Working with individuals diagnosed as schizophrenic is bound to bring up strong emotional reactions from health care workers. The psychotic client is intensely anxious, lonely, dependent, and distrustful. The intensity of these emotions can stir up intense, uncomfortable, and frightening emotions in all health care workers. The identification of transference and countertransference phenomena is an important part of the work of the therapeutic process (See Chapter 6).

If personal countertransferential reactions are ignored by the nurse, feelings of helplessness follow. Increased feelings of helplessness escalate anxiety. Without the support, opportunity, and willingness to explore these reactions with more experienced nursing staff, defensive behaviors emerge. Defensive behaviors in the nurse, such as denial, withdrawal, and avoidance, thwart the client's progress and undermine the nurse's self-esteem. These behaviors are associated with staff burnout. Statements such as "These clients are hopeless," "You can't understand these people," and "You waste your time with them" are examples of unexamined or unrecognized emotional reactions to client's behaviors or feelings.

For new nurses introduced into the psychiatric setting, especially for student nurses, the availability of supportive supervision is a *must* if learning is to take place. The student's part in the supervisory process is a willingness to discuss and identify personal feelings as well as to identify problem behaviors. This can be and often is done in group supervision. Experienced psychiatric nurses call this process *peer group supervision.*

Individual supervision provides the greatest opportunity for a better understanding of the interpersonal issues involved in establishing a working relationship with the client. Individual supervision can increase the learner's understanding of the client and the client's situation, competence with therapeutic skills, and self-confidence. Unfortunately, many schools of nursing do not have the time or faculty to provide this learning opportunity for students. Some psychiatric settings encourage the practice of supervision and provide time and personnel for psychiatric nurses and other staff.

Kahn (1984) identifies three strong transferences on the part of schizophrenic clients that can trigger equally strong countertransference reactions among mental health care workers. These three transferences are (1) the dependent transference, (2) the angry transference and (3) the eroticized transference. These issues are best dealt with during supervision. During this time, the transference phenomena are identified, personal reactions of the nurse are explored, and appropriate intervention strategies are suggested and evaluated.

For example, in dealing with *dependency issues*, decisions need to be made about when to gratify modest dependency needs without hindering the development of the client's autonomy. What feelings does the nurse experience in relationship to the client's exhaustive dependency needs? Which responses are rational and which irrational? Do the irrational feelings toward the client block effective therapeutic work?

During supervision of the *angry transference* feelings, the nurse learns to inhibit the urge to act on angry personal responses, to provide alternative experiences for the client to deal with anger, and to understand the function the anger serves for the client (e.g., maintaining distance).

Eroticized transference may be anxiety producing to both the client and the nurse. Supervisors may explore with the nurse-clinician ways for setting clear limits while maintaining effective contact with the client (Kahn 1984).

Menninger (1984) discusses the extreme frustration that staff have with the slow progress of schizophrenic clients. This sense of frustration and feelings of helplessness can lead to burnout. Periodic reassessment of treatment goals and scaling down of expectations can benefit both staff and client.

These are some but by no means all of the kinds of issues that may surface in dealing with a schizophrenic client. Clinical practice with adequate supervision increases the nurse's skills, lowers personal anxiety, increases confidence, and can improve the quality of interpersonal relationships with clients as well as relationships with others.

Intervention

The detrimental effect of stress on a schizophrenic person's environment has been long observed by clinicians. Environmental stress can result in an exacerbation of schizophrenic symptoms. Much of the work with schizophrenic clients involves decreasing taxing levels of environmental stress, thereby lowering the client's level of anxiety and improving the client's perceptions and adaptive responses.

Lowered anxiety levels can decrease the intensity of schizophrenic symptoms and make the client more amenable to engagement in activities and relationships with health professionals, improved family interactions, and involvement in nonthreatening activities. Lowered anxiety levels make it possible for all people, including people with schizophrenia, to define problems and focus on issues.

For planning interventions, it is important not to overlook the adaptive skills of a psychotic client. *Attention should be given to the client's assets and healthy functioning as well as to areas of deficiencies.*

PSYCHOTHERAPEUTIC INTERVENTIONS

Therapeutic strategies for working with schizophrenic clients often involve interventions that address specific behaviors. Psychotherapeutic interventions are aimed at lowering the client's anxiety, decreasing defensive patterns, encouraging participation in the environment and raising the client's level of self-esteem. Refer to the appropriate sections for useful intervention strategies for paranoid, withdrawn, excitable, and regressed behaviors.

All nurses should be familiar with the principles of dealing with phenomena that are certain to arise with most schizophrenic clients. These are the phenomena of (1) hallucination, (2) delusion, and (3) looseness of association.

HALLUCINATION. Understanding the process of hallucinations offers useful guidelines for working with clients who are actively hallucinating. The hallucinatory process starts out in a painfully lonely and isolated person under stress. Hallucinations are a means to allay the terrorizing feelings of alienation and the resulting panic levels of anxiety.

Voices are the most common hallucinatory experience reported by schizophrenic clients. It is important initially to understand what the voices are saying or telling the person to do. The presence of suicidal or homicidal messages indicates priority measures for all members of the health care team.

Peplau believes that an important perspective for nurses to have when working with a client who is hallucinating is to view hallucinations as evidence that loneliness might be a problem. Through hallucinations significant human contact is being sought (Smoyak 1994). The nurse might ask, "What is going on right now?" and follow up with dialogue that "keeps clear that what the person is experiencing can be differentiated from what others see and hear" (Smoyak 1994).

When the client is asked to give up something important, no matter how maladaptive, something more adaptive and useful should be available to take its place, namely, receptive and interested people in the client's environment. Establishing a relationship that minimizes anxiety and is built on honesty, consistency of care, and genuine concern for the client is an important first step. Moller (1989) has outlined 12 steps nurses can take when working with a hallucinating client. These are part of a process that progresses over time and is shared with the hallucinating individual (Table 19–5). Moller cautions that the nurse may become frustrated at times, and that is to be expected.

DELUSIONS. Delusions are a result of misperception of cognitive stimuli. It is useful if the nurse attempts to see the world as it appears through the eyes of the client. In that way, the nurse can better understand the client's delusional experience. For example:

CLIENT: You people are all alike . . . all in on the CIA plot to destroy me.

NURSE: I do not want to hurt you, Tom. Thinking that people are out to destroy you must be very frightening.

First, the nurse clarifies the reality of his or her intent. Second, the nurse empathizes with the client's apparent experience, the feelings of fear. The nurse does not get drawn into the conversation regarding the content of the delusion (CIA and plot to destroy) but looks for the feelings the person may be experi-

---

Table 19–5 ■ MOLLER'S INTERVENTIONS WITH HALLUCINATIONS

STEPS	COMMENTS
1. Establish a trusting interpersonal relationship.	1. Trust can grow when • The nurse is consistent • The nurse asks permission to talk about hallucinations • The nurse is not hurried—the nurse gives the person time to respond and allows the person time to stare into space
2. Look and listen for symptoms of auditory hallucinations.	2. Cues include • Eyes looking around the room • Tilting the head to one side • Mumbling to oneself • Curling up on the bed and withdrawing (experience of hallucinations can be exhausting)
3. Focus on hallucinatory cues and elicit the person's observation and description of the cue.	3. The goal is to empower the person to help them understand their symptoms • "What are you experiencing?" • "I'll be here if you want me." • "I see your eyes moving back and forth. Are you anxious?" Give the person time to answer.
4. Identify whether the hallucination is caused by toxic substances.	4. Ask the client directly whether he or she has taken drugs or alcohol; what was taken; how much, and when? Drugs do not cause schizophrenia but may exacerbate symptoms.
5. If asked, point out simply that you are not experiencing the hallucinations.	5. For the person it is real; the goal is to guide the person through the experience. • "What do you feel you need to do?" • "What are you hearing?"
6. Follow the direction of the individual to help him or her observe and describe present and recent past hallucinations.	6. This may be the first time a person has been allowed to discuss the hallucination. • Gives the person the power to manage hallucinated voices • Provides a quiet environment; gives the person permission to share the content of the hallucinations.
7. Elicit the person's observation and description of the past experience.	7. Encourage the person to discuss when he or she began experiencing hallucinations. It is essential to understand the past in order to manage the present.

Table continued on following page

Table 19–5 ■ MOLLER'S INTERVENTIONS WITH HALLUCINATIONS *Continued*	
STEPS	**COMMENTS**
8. Encourage the person to observe and describe feelings, thoughts, and actions, both present and past, as they relate to hallucination.	8. The goal is to connect the cognitive, emotional, and behavioral components of hallucinations. • Identify what the person was feeling during the hallucination: "Tell me what you think happened." • The person may have developed skill in covering up hallucinations—this frees up energy to manage the symptoms instead.
9. Help the person observe and describe the needs that may underlie the hallucination.	9. Often hallucinations reflect needs for • Power and control • Self-esteem • Anger • Human contact
10. Help the person make the connection between the hallucination and the need it represents.	10. Focus on the loneliness the individual may be feeling. • Encourage the person to identify when hallucinations occur and what triggers them.
11. Suggest and reinforce the person's use of increased interpersonal relationships in meeting persistent needs.	11. The client needs one person who can be trusted to accept him or her. • Persons often are reluctant to "give up" their voices because they have no close friends.
12. Focus on other related aspects of the person's psychopathological behavior.	12. Talk openly and honestly with the client about concerns other than hallucinations. • Eventually, other aspects of the person's life can be explored.

From Moller MD. Understanding and Communicating with an Individual Who Is Hallucinating (videotapes and study guide). Nine Mile Falls, WA: Nurseminars, 1989.

encing. Talking about the client's feeling experience can be useful for the client; talking about delusional material is not.

It is *not* useful to argue with the client regarding the content of the delusion. Doing so can intensify the client's retention of irrational beliefs. Although the nurse does not argue with the client's delusions, clarifying misinterpretations of the environment is useful. For example:

CLIENT: I see the doctor is here, and he is out to get me and destroy me.

NURSE: It is true the doctor wants to see you, but he wants to talk to you about your treatment. Would you feel more comfortable talking to him in the day room?

Interacting with the client on concrete realities in the environment can be useful in minimizing the client's time spent with delusional ruminations. Specific manual tasks within the scope of the client's abilities can often be useful as distractions from delusional thinking. The more time the client spends with reality-based activities or people, the more opportunity the client has to learn to be more comfortable with reality.

LOOSENESS OF ASSOCIATION. Looseness of association often mirrors the client's autistic thoughts. The client's autistic and disorganized ramblings may leave the nurse confused and frustrated. Increase in the client's autistic speech patterns can indicate increased anxiety on the part of the client and reflect his or her difficulty responding to internal and external stimuli.

Decoding is a term used for interpreting the meaning of autistic communications. Decoding is not always possible, but when it is possible, it can help in understanding the client's experience and needs.

The following guidelines may be useful for spending time with a client whose speech is confused and disorganized:

1. Do not pretend you understand the client's communications when you are confused by the client's words or meanings.
2. Tell the client you are having difficulty understanding his or her communications.
3. Place the difficulty in understanding on yourself, *not* the client. For example, say "I am having trouble following what you are saying," *not* "You are not making any sense."

4. Look for recurring topics and themes in the client's communications. For example, "You've mentioned trouble with your brother several times. I guess your relationship with your brother is on your mind."
5. When understanding the client's autistic communications is not possible, just listening to and being accepting of the client can be meaningful.
6. Emphasize what is going on in the client's immediate environment (here-and-now) and involve the client in simple reality-based activities. These measures can help the client better focus his or her thoughts.
7. Tell the client what you do understand and reinforce clear communication and accurate expression of needs, feelings, and thoughts.

HEALTH TEACHING

Teaching methods of health management to clients, families, and other caregivers can be important in stabilization of the schizophrenic person's future adjustment. It is not just the level or source of stress in the client's environment that is crucial; also important is the manner in which people involved deal with the stress, and how effectively stressful issues are resolved.

Psychological strategies aimed at reducing exacerbation of the psychotic symptoms follow (Falloon et al. 1982):

1. Educate the client and the client's family about the illness. Emphasize how stress and medication affect the illness. Such knowledge may increase medication compliance and motivate involvement in psychosocial activities.
2. Assist the client to increase his or her ability to solve problems related to environmental stress.
3. Teach the client coping strategies to deal with the source of symptoms of schizophrenia and the stresses in his or her social environment.
4. Assist family and client to identify sources for ongoing support in dealing with illness.

Studies indicate the importance of the family environment for a schizophrenic client. When a schizophrenic client is returned to a family environment consisting of warmth, concern, and supportive behavior, a relapse is less likely to be suffered. An environment highly critical of the client's behavior, or consisting of intrusive involvement into the client's life, is more likely to correlate with recurrent episodes of schizophrenia (Falloon 1986).

Some of the critical attitudes toward people with schizophrenia result in a lack of understanding of the symptoms of schizophrenia, especially the negative symptoms. For example, the client's apathy, lack of drive, and motivation may be wrongly interpreted as laziness. This erroneous assumption can encourage hostility on the part of family members, caregivers, or people in the community in general. Therefore, further teaching of the disease process of schizophrenia can reduce tensions in families and communities. Educating the client, families, and others is most effective when it is carried out over time. Table 19–6 can be used as a guide for client and family teaching.

ACTIVITIES OF DAILY LIVING

Those clients who have the most difficulty with the rudiments of self-care usually include the disorganized and catatonic schizophrenic in the acute phase of the illness. The paranoid client usually manages basic activities of daily living more competently. Interventions regarding basic activities of daily living and nutritional and sleep factors for paranoid, catatonic, and disorganized clients are discussed later in this chapter.

SOMATIC THERAPIES

Appropriate drugs for psychotic disorders are called **neuroleptic (antipsychotic) medications.** These drugs used to be popularly referred to as the major tranquilizers. There are two groups of neuroleptic (antipsychotic) drugs: standard and atypical. There are also drugs used in conjunction with antipsychotics for treatment-resistant clients.

Clinically active neuroleptic drugs are able to block postsynaptic dopamine receptors in the central nervous system and are equally effective in the treatment of schizophrenia. The choice of drug is often based on

1. Desired side effects (e.g., an agitated client may be given a more sedative antipsychotic)
2. Avoiding adverse side effects (e.g., haloperidol may be used in a person with cardiac problems because of its reduced anticholinergic effects)
3. Client response (what drug works well for a specific individual)

These drugs are effective in most acute exacerbations of schizophrenia and for the prevention or mitigation of relapse. Antipsychotic drugs target the positive symptoms of schizophrenia (such as hallucinations, delusions, disordered thinking, and paranoia) more than the negative symptoms (such as deficits in social interaction, blunted or inappropriate emotional expression, and lack of motivation) (Levinson 1991). Clozapine and Risperidone are exceptions because they can also affect the negative symptoms.

Table 19-6 ■ TEACHING CLIENTS AND THEIR FAMILIES ABOUT SCHIZOPHRENIA

CONTENT	RATIONALE
Medications*	
1. Explain what the medication *can* do to help client. 2. **Needs to be taken regularly.** Schizophrenia is a relapsing disorder. It is extremely important to keep taking the drug even though things seem fine. 3. **Side effects**—what to do to lessen severity if not harmful to client. 4. **Side effects**—are not harmful to client but may cause noncompliance, (e.g., akathisia, impotence): "You may notice inner feelings of restlessness and nervousness" or "You may have difficulty during sex." Do not stop the drug, most side effects can be treated. Call . . . *who to call.* 5. **Toxic effects**—discontinue the medication—*who to call* and appropriate action until medical help is available. 6. **Stopping medications.** Tolerance does not develop, but some clients report a rebound effect if drugs are stopped suddenly (e.g., nausea, vomiting, sleep disturbance, and more). 7. **Risk factors of tardive dyskinesia.** 8. Client should avoid prolonged exposure to the sun; wear sunscreen, sunglasses, long sleeves, and hats. 9. These drugs (neuroleptics) are not addicting.	May help client compliance if 1. Family is supportive and involved 2. Client knows what to expect 3. Client knows medication can be changed to decrease undesirable side effects
Signs of potential relapse	
1. *Client and family* need to be able to identify those symptoms that come before frank psychotic symptoms unique to each client; for example: ● feeling tense ● difficulty concentrating ● trouble sleeping ● increased withdrawal ● increase in bizarre/magical thinking	Early warning signs recognized by both family and client may ward off psychotic relapse if immediate medical attention is sought.
Substances that can exacerbate a psychotic relapse	
1. Marijuana 2. Alcohol 3. Psychomotor stimulants ● Amphetamine ● Crack ● Cocaine	Family support may influence client to minimize intake if involved with substance use.

*Should be written down for client and family.

Essentially, antipsychotic drugs can cause a

1. Reduction in disruptive and violent behavior
2. Increase in activity, speech, and sociability in withdrawn or mute clients
3. Improvement in self-care
4. Improvement in sleep patterns
5. Reduction in the disturbing quality of hallucinations and delusions
6. Improvement in thought processes
7. Decreased resistance to psychotherapy and supportive psychotherapy
8. Reduced rate of relapse (about 2.5 times)
9. Decrease in the intensity of paranoid reactions

Antipsychotic agents are usually effective in three to six weeks. When a client fails to improve after six months of drug therapy, he or she is unlikely to improve at all with that particular medication. The continuation of drug treatment beyond this point increases the client's risk of side effects (e.g., tardive dyskinesia). Only about 10% of schizophrenic clients do not respond to antipsychotic drugs. These clients should not continue to take medication that, for them, holds only risks and no benefit.

Schizophrenia is the most common indication for neuroleptic (antipsychotic) medication. People in acute mania or psychotic depression may respond to a short course of neuroleptics. These agents frequently are effective in the treatment of the behavioral disorders associated with organic brain disease.

STANDARD NEUROLEPTICS. Among the phenothiazine group, the five standard chemical classes of antipsychotic medications are the phenothiazines, thioxanthenes, butyrophenones, dibenzoxazepines, and dihydroindolones. The properties and side effects of these five are similar. The phenothiazines are usually considered the prototype for assessing the action and side effects of these medications.

The choice of specific drugs is often made on the basis of major side effects, which include (1) extrapyramidal side effects, (2) anticholinergic side effects, and (3) sedation. Other side effects include orthostatic hypotension and lowered seizure threshold. For example, chlorpromazine (Thorazine) is the most sedating and has fewer extrapyramidal side effects than do other antipsychotic agents but causes hypotension in large doses. Haloperidol (Haldol) is least sedating and is often used in large doses to reduce assaultive behavior but has a high incidence of extrapyramidal side effects. The value of haloperidol for treating violent behaviors is its effectiveness in controlling hallucinatory phenomena with a low incidence of hypotension. People who are functioning at work or at home may prefer less sedating drugs; clients who are agitated or excitable may do better on a more sedating medication.

The antipsychotics are often divided into *low potency*

Table 19–7 ■ DRUG INFORMATION: SIDE EFFECTS PROFILE OF ANTIPSYCHOTIC DRUGS

DRUG	ANTI-CHOLINERGIC	SEDATION	ORTHOSTATIC HYPOTENSION	LOWERED SEIZURE TRESHOLD	EXTRA-PYRAMIDAL SIDE EFFECTS
Low Potency					
Chlorpromazine (Thorazine)	+ +	+ + +	+ + +	+ + +	+ +
Thioridazine (Mellaril)	+ + +	+ + +	+ + +	+	+
Clozapine (Clozaril)	+ + +	+ +	+ + +	+	0
High Potency					
Trifluoperazine (Stelazine)	+	+	+	+	+ + +
Perphenazine (Trilafon)	+ +	+	+	+	+ + +
Fluphenazine (Prolixin)	+	+	+	+	+ + +
Thiothixene (Navane)	+	+	+	+ +	+ + +
Chlorprothixene (Taractan)	+ +	+ + +	+ + +	+ + +	+ +
Haloperidol (Haldol)	0	+	+	+ +	+ + +
Loxapine (Loxitane)	+	+ +	+	+ +	+ + +
Molindone (Moban)	+ +	+ +	+	0/+	+ +

Adapted from Swonger A and Matejski MP. Nursing Pharmacology: An Integrated Approach to Drug Therapy and Nursing Practice, 2nd ed. Philadelphia: JB Lippincott, 1991.

and *high potency* on the basis of their anticholingeric (ACH) side effects, extrapyramidal side effects (EPS), and sedation:

Low Potency = High Sedation + High ACH + Low EPS
High Potency = Low Sedation + Low ACH + High EPS

Note, however, that all neuroleptics, except clozapine, can cause tardive dyskinesia. For a side effect profile of many commonly used neuroleptics, see Table 19–7.

There are some positive attributes of the phenothiazine-like drugs. It is difficult to take a lethal over-dose. Neither tolerance nor potential for abuse develops. Many of the side effects are minor or temporary. These drugs are used with caution in people with seizure disorders because these neuroleptics can lower the seizure threshold. Table 19–8 identifies some standard antipsychotics for acute symptoms, usual maintenance doses, and some considerations.

Some of the more disturbing side effects caused by the dopamine blockade properties of the neuroleptics are the **extrapyramidal side effects.** Three of the more common extrapyramidal side effects are (1) **acute dystonia** (muscle cramps of the head and neck),

		ACUTE (mg/day)*	**MAINTENANCE (mg/day)***	**SPECIAL**
DRUG	**ROUTES**			**CONSIDERATIONS**
Chlorpromazine (Thorazine)	PO, IM, R	200–1000	50–400	1. Frequently prescribed 2. Increases sensitivity to sun (as with other phenothiazines) 3. Highest sedation and hypotension effects; least potent
Thioridazine (Mellaril)	PO	200–800	50–400	1. Known to cause retinitis pigmentosa in large doses; any diminished vision should be investigated 2. Low incidence of extrapyramidal side effects 3. High incidence of low blood pressure and cardiac effects 4. High incidence of decreased sexuality and retrograde ejaculation in men
Trifluoperazine (Stelazine)	PO, IM	10–60	4–30	1. Low sedation—good for withdrawn or paranoid symptoms 2. High incidence of extrapyramidal side effects 3. Watch for neuroleptic malignant syndrome
Perphenazine (Trilafon)	PO, IM, IV	12–64 30	8–24 15	Can help control severe vomiting and intractable hiccups
Mesoridazine (Serentil)	PO, IM	100–400	25–200	Among the most sedative; severe nausea and vomiting in adults
Fluphenazine (Prolixin)	PO, IM, SC	2.5–60	1–30	Among the least sedative
Thioxanthenes				
Thiothixene (Navane)	PO, IM	10–120	6–30	High incidence of akathisia
Chlorprothixene (Taractan)	PO, IM	50–600	50–400	Weight gain common

Table 19–8 ■ **DRUG INFORMATION: STANDARD ANTIPSYCHOTIC MEDICATIONS**

Table 19-8 ■ DRUG INFORMATION: STANDARD ANTIPSYCHOTIC MEDICATIONS *Continued*

DRUG	ROUTES	ACUTE (mg/day)*	MAINTENANCE (mg/day)*	SPECIAL CONSIDERATIONS
Butyrophenones				
Haloperidol (Haldol)	PO, IM	5–50	1–15	1. Has low sedative properties; is used in large doses for assaultive patients, thus avoiding the severe side effect of hypotension 2. Appropriate for the elderly for the same reason as above; lessens the chance of falls from dizziness or hypotension 3. High incidence of extrapyramidal side effects
Dibenzoxazepines				
Loxapine (Loxitane)	PO, IM	20–160	10–60	Possibly associated with weight reduction
Dihydroindolones				
Molindone (Moban)	PO	40–225	15–100	Possibly associated with weight reduction
Atypical Antipsychotics				
Clozapine (Clozaril)	PO	None	Slow dosage increases to 300–450	1. Used when clients fail to respond to other neuroleptics 2. Target negative and positive symptoms 3. 1–2% incidence of agranulocytosis 4. Weekly white blood cell counts are required 5. Can cause sedation, hypotension, tachycardia, and severe drooling
Risperidone (Risperdal)	PO	None	Slow dosage increases 4–6	1. Improves positive and negative symptoms 2. Can cause orthostatic hypotension, seizures, EPS, dizziness, somnolence, and more
Decanoate: Long-acting				
Haloperidol (Haldol) Decanoate	IM	0	50–100	1. Deep muscle Z-track IM 2. Give every 4 weeks
Fluphenazine (Prolixin) Decanoate	IM	0	25	1. Deep muscle Z-track IM 2. Effective 1–2 weeks
Fluphenazine (Prolixin) Enanthate	IM	0	25–75	1. Deep muscle Z-track IM 2. Effective 3–4 weeks 3. Can cause acute dystonic reactions

Data from Kaplan and Sadock 1991; Maxmen 1991; Berkow 1992.
*Dosages vary with individual responses to antipsychotic agent employed.
IM = intramuscular; PO = oral; R = rectal suppository; SC = subcutaneous.

(2) **akathisia** (restless pacing or fidgeting), and (3) **pseudoparkinsonism** (stiffening of muscular activity in the face, body, arms, and legs). These side effects often appear early in therapy, can be treated, and are reversible. Treatment usually consists of lowering the dosage or prescribing antiparkinsonian drugs, especially centrally acting anticholinergic drugs. Commonly used drugs include trihexyphenidyl (Artane), benztropine mesylate (Cogentin), diphenhydramine hydrochloride (Benadryl), and amantadine hydrochloride (Symmetrel). The first two in this list are antiparkinsonian drugs. Treatment with antiparkinsonian drugs

is not completely benign because the anticholinergic side effects of the antipsychotics may be intensified (e.g., urinary retention, constipation, failure of visual accommodation [blurred vision], cognitive impairment, and delirium) (Berkow et al. 1992).

Table 19–9 identifies common side effects and nursing and medical interventions for these antipsychotic medications. Box 19–1 identifies nursing measures for giving antipsychotic drugs.

Most clients develop tolerance to extrapyramidal symptoms after a few months. Effective nursing and medical management is important during this time to

Table 19–9 ■ DRUG INFORMATION: NURSING MEASURES FOR SIDE EFFECTS OF ANTIPSYCHOTIC MEDICATIONS

SIDE EFFECTS	ONSET	NURSING MEASURES
Anticholinergic Symptoms		
1. **Dry mouth**		1. Frequent sips of water and sugarless candy or gum. If severe, provide Xerolube, a saliva substitute.
2. **Urinary retention and hesitancy**		2. Check patient's voiding; consider catheterization. If severe, bethanechol 10–25 mg two or three times daily may be ordered.
3. **Constipation**		3. Encourage a diet high in fiber; evaluate the need for mild laxative. May need a stool softener. Assess for adequate water intake.
4. **Blurred vision**		4. Usually abates in 1–2 weeks. If patient is on thioridazine, hold and check with physician.
5. **Nasal congestion**		5. Provide nasal decongestants; body will adjust in a few weeks.
6. **Photophobia**		6. Wear sunglasses.
7. **Dry eyes**		7. Artifical tears.
8. **Inhibition of ejaculation or impotence in men**		8. Alert physician; may need alternative medication.
Extrapyramidal Side Effects		
1. **Pseudoparkinsonism:** masklike facies, stiff and stooped posture, shuffling gait, drooling, tremor, "pill-rolling" phenomena	5–30 days	1. Alert medical staff. Physician may lower dosage or switch to another phenothiazine. Try an anticholinergic agent (e.g., trihexyphenidyl [Artane] or benztropine [Cogentin]). Trihexyphenidyl and benztropine are used with caution because a "high" may result; benztropine has become a popular abused drug. Amantadine (Symmetrel) may also be prescribed.
2. **Acute dystonic reactions:** acute contractions of tongue, face, neck, and back (tongue and jaw first) ● **Opisthotonos**—tetanic heightening of entire body, head back and belly up ● **Oculogyric crisis**—eyes locked upward	1–5 days	2. **First choice** Diphenhydramine hydrochloride (Benadryl) 25–50 mg IM/IV. Relief in minutes. **Second choice** Benztropine (Cogentin) 1–2 mg IM/IV. **Prevent further dystonias** with any anticholinergic agent (see Table 19–10). Experience is very frightening. Take patient to quiet area and stay with him or her until medicated.

Table 19–9 ■ DRUG INFORMATION: NURSING MEASURES FOR SIDE EFFECTS OF ANTIPSYCHOTIC MEDICATIONS *Continued*

SIDE EFFECTS	ONSET	NURSING MEASURES
Extrapyramidal Side Effects *Continued*		
3. **Akathisia:** motor inner-driven restlessness (e.g., tapping foot incessantly, rocking forward and backward in chair, shifting weight from side to side)	5–60 days	3. Physician may change antipsychotic or give antiparkinsonian agent. Tolerance doe not develop to akathisia, but akathisia disappears when neuroleptic is discontinued. Propranolol (Inderal), lorazepam (Ativan), or diazepam (Valium) may be used.
4. **Tardive dyskinesia** ● **Facial**—Protruding and rolling tongue, blowing, smacking, licking, spastic facial distortion, smacking movements ● **Limbs** **Choreic**—rapid, purposeless, and irregular movements **Athetoid**—slow, complex, and serpentine movements ● **Trunk**—neck, shoulder, dramatic hip jerks and rocking, twisting pelvic thrusts	6–24 months	4. **No known treatment.** Discontinuing the drug does not always relieve symptoms. Possibly 20% of patients taking the drug for over 2 years may develop tardive dyskinesia. Nurses and doctors should encourage patients to be screened for tardive dyskinesia at least every 3 months.
Cardiovascular Effects		
1. **Hypotension and postural hypotension**		1. Check blood pressure before giving; advise patient to dangle feet before getting out of bed to prevent dizziness and subsequent falls. A systolic pressure of 80 when standing is an indication to hold the current dose. This usually subsides when drug is stabilized in 1–2 weeks. Elastic bandages may prevent pooling. If medically serious, doctor will order volume expanders or pressure agents.
2. **Tachycardia**		2. Patients with existing cardiac problems should *always* be worked up before the antipsychotic drugs are administered. Haloperidol is usually the preferred drug because of its low anticholinergic effects.
Other Side Effects		
1. **Dermatologic changes:** hives, contact dermatitis, photosensitivity; these can reflect hypersensitivity to the drug		1. Notify physician; withdrawal of the drug may be indicated. Teach client to stay out of the sun and to use sunscreen, hat, and sunglasses.
2. **Photosensitivity:** extreme sensitivity in sun; patient is easily sunburned		2. High with chlorpromazine (Thorazine). Advise patient to wear protective clothing and sunscreen when in the sun.
3. **Increased weight:** distressing side effect for many; increase in appetite is attributed to metabolic changes caused by the drug		3. Nurse can work with patient to monitor weight gain and to work with diets; if severe, alternative drugs may be used.
4. **Endocrine changes:** moderate breast enlargement and galactorrhea in women; in both men and women, changes in sexual drive—usually loss of libido; amenorrhea seen occasionally in women		4. Alert physician; may change medication.

Table continued on following page

Table 19–9 ■ DRUG INFORMATION: NURSING MEASURES FOR SIDE EFFECTS OF ANTIPSYCHOTIC MEDICATIONS *Continued*

SIDE EFFECTS	ONSET	NURSING MEASURES
Other Side Effects *Continued*		
5. **Sedation:** this may be a desired effect in early treatment but may become a liability to a person later in treatment or on maintenance therapy.		5. Physician may change to a less sedative neuroleptic (fluphenazine [Prolixin], trifluoperazine [Stelazine]). Give full dose at bedtime. May relieve daytime sedation.
Rare Side Effects		
1. **Agranulocytosis:** usually occurs suddenly and becomes evident during the first 12 weeks; symptoms include sore throat, fever, malaise, and mouth sores; it is a rare occurrence but one the nurse should be aware of; any flulike symptoms should be carefully evaluated.		1. Nurse notifies medical staff STAT. Hold medication. Physician may order blood work done to determine leukopenia or agranulocytosis. If test results are positive, the drug is discontinued, and reverse isolation may be initiated. Mortality is high if the drug is not ceased and treatment initiated.
2. **Cholestatic jaundice:** rare, reversible, and usually benign if caught in time; prodromal symptoms are fever, malaise, nausea, and abdominal pain; jaundice appears 1 week later.		2. Drug is discontinued; bed rest and high-protein, high-carbohydrate diet given. Liver function tests every 6 months should be routine.
3. **Neuroleptic malignant syndrome:** somewhat rare, potentially fatal ● **Severe extrapyramidal**—such as severe muscle rigidity, oculogyric crisis, dysphasia, flexor-extensor posturing, cogwheeling ● **Hyperthermia**—elevated temperature (up to 107° F) ● **Autonomic dysfunction**—such as hypertension, tachycardia, diaphoresis, incontinence	Can occur in first week of drug therapy but often occurs later.	3. ● Stop neuroleptic. ● Transfer STAT to medical unit. ● Bromocriptine can relieve muscle rigidity and reduce fever. ● Dantrolene may reduce muscle spasms. ● Cool body to reduce fever. ● Maintain hydration with oral and IV fluids. ● Correct electrolyte imbalance. ● Arrhythmias should be treated. ● Small doses of heparin may decrease the possibility of pulmonary emboli. ● Early detection increases patient's chance of survival.

Data from Karb et al. 1989; Schatzberg and Cole 1991; Maxmen 1991; Berkow 1992.
IM = intramuscular; IV = intravenous.

encourage compliance with the medications until the disturbing and frightening side effects have been properly managed. Table 19–10 identifies some of the more commonly used drugs for treatment of extrapyramidal side effects.

Perhaps the most troubling side effects for outpatients on neuroleptics are weight gain, impotence, and tardive dyskinesia. Weight gain is most frequently a problem with women and may result in as much as a 100-pound gain in some clients. Discontinuation of the antipsychotic medication may be necessary with the use of an alternative drug. Impotence is occasionally reported by men and may also necessitate switching to alternative drugs.

Tardive dyskinesia, an extrapyramidal side effect that usually appears after prolonged treatment, is more serious and not always reversible. Tardive dyskinesia consists of involuntary tonic muscular spasms typically involving the tongue, fingers, toes, neck, trunk, or pelvis. This potentially serious extrapyramidal side effect most frequently affects women, older clients, and up to 50% of people on long term large-dose therapy. Tardive dyskinesia varies from mild to moderate and can be disfiguring or incapacitating. Early symptoms of tardive dyskinesia are fasciculations of the tongue or constant smacking of the lips. These early oral movements can develop into uncontrollable biting, chewing, sucking motions, keeping the mouth open, and lateral movements of the jaw. In many cases, the early symptoms of tardive dyskinesia disappear when the antipsychotic medication is discontinued. In other cases, however, early symptoms

---

Box 19–1. DRUG INFORMATION: NURSING MEASURES FOR GIVING ANTIPSYCHOTICS

Oral	Dilute with milk, orange juice, or semisolid food to reduce bitter taste Check mouth; make sure medication is not held in cheek or under tongue
Liquid	Protect oral liquid from light
Intramuscular	• Do not hold drug in syringe for more than 15 minutes; may absorb plastic • Give slowly • Give in deltoid (absorbs more rapidly) or buttocks (upper outer quadrant) • Tell patient it may sting • Massage slowly after injection • Alternate sites • Watch for orthostatic hypotension
Decanoate	Long-acting intramuscular injection is oil based and requires a 20- or 21-gauge needle • Use a dry needle at least 20-gauge, 1.5 inches long • Give deep intramuscularly with Z-track method • Do *not* massage

---

are not reversible and may progress. There is no proven cure for advanced tardive dyskinesia.

The National Institute of Mental Health has developed a brief test for the detection of tardive dyskinesia. The test is referred to as AIMES.* The three areas of examination are facial and oral movements, extremity movements, and trunk movement.

Nurses need to know about some rare but serious and potentially fatal side effects of these drugs. Side effects include (1) neuroleptic malignant syndrome, (2) agranulocytosis, and (3) liver involvement.

Neuroleptic malignant syndrome may occur in about 1% of patients exposed to antipsychotics. Neuroleptic malignant syndrome is potentially fatal in about 10% of the cases. It usually occurs early in the course of treatment but has been reported in people after 20 years of exposure (Berkow et al. 1992).

Neuroleptic malignant syndrome is characterized by a decreased level of consciousness, greatly increased muscle tone, autonomic dysfunction including hyperpyrexia, labile hypertension, tachycardia, tachypnea, diaphoresis, and drooling. Treatment includes discontinuation of the antipsychotic and is otherwise pri-

marily supportive symptom relief as noted in Table 19–9.

Agranulocytosis is also a serious side effect and can be fatal. Liver involvement may occur. The nurse needs to be aware of the prodromal signs and symptoms of these side effects and to teach them to their clients and clients' families (see Table 19–9).

ATYPICAL ANTIPSYCHOTICS. In the early 1990s, **clozapine (Clozaril)** was released in this country for use in clients with (1) treatment-resistant schizophrenia and (2) intolerance of the side effects of the standard neuroleptics. Clozapine is credited with dramatic changes in some clients who had not responded to standard neuroleptics. *One* of the advantages of this drug is that both the negative (amotivation, anergia, and impaired judgment) as well as the positive symptoms of schizophrenia (hallucinations, delusion, and aggression) are greatly reduced. Another is that many of the side effects of the standard neuroleptics are absent and do not appear with clozapine. Because clozapine has minimal or no dopamine blockade, there have been no reported pseudoparkinsonism or dystonia and much less akathisia. It also seems unlikely to cause tardive dyskinesia.

However, notable disadvantages include a high incidence of agranulocytosis (1–2% in all clients in the United States). The need to monitor a client's white blood cell count weekly keeps the cost of this drug

---

*A copy of the AIMES test is free. Write to the National Institute of Mental Health, Schizophrenic Disorders Section, Somatic Treatments Branch, Rockville, MD 20857.

Table 19-10 ■ **TREATMENT OF NEUROLEPTIC-INDUCED EXTRAPYRAMIDAL SIDE EFFECTS**

DRUG	ORAL DOSE (mg)	INTRAMUSCULAR OR INTRAVENOUS DOSE (mg)	CHEMICAL GROUP
Amantadine hydrochloride (Symmetrel)	100 bid or tid	0	Dopaminergic agent
Benztropine mesylate* (Cogentin)	1–3 bid	1–2	ACA
Biperiden* (Akineton)	2 bid or qid	2	ACA
Trihexyphenidyl* (Artane)	2–5 tid	0	ACA
Diphenhydramine hydrochloride (Benadryl)	25–50 tid or qid	25–50	Antihistamine
Procyclidine hydrochloride (Kemadrin)	2.5–5 tid	0	ACA

Reprinted from PSYCHOTROPIC DRUGS: Fast Facts, by Jerrold S. Maxmen, M.D., by permission of W.W. Norton & Company © 1991 by Jerrold S. Maxmen.
ACA = anticholinergic drugs, (after one to six months of long term maintenance antipsychotic therapy, most ACAs can be withdrawn); bid = twice a day; tid = three times a day; qid—four times a day.
*Antiparkinsonian drug.

relatively high, and out of reach for many clients. All patients on this drug must be monitored by a patient management system to receive the drug. The incidence of seizures is also high with use of this drug, as high as 15% at doses over 550 mg per day (Schatzberg and Cole 1991). Clozapine can also be sedating, cause hypotension and tachycardia, and, in some, cause severe drooling (Berkow et al. 1992).

Risperidone (Risperdal) is a recent (April 1993) antipsychotic drug. The drug risperidone also targets the negative as well as the positive symptoms of schizophrenia. Risperidone, like clozapine, is also free of the disturbing and disabling neurological side effects of the older phenothiazine-like antipsychotics. Risperidone does not have the risky side effects of Clozaril and can be used as a first-choice drug. Refer to Box 19-2 for antipsychotic drugs and how they work.

ADJUNCTS TO NEUROLEPTIC THERAPY. Other drugs are often used in the treatment of drug-resistant schizophrenia. For example, *lithium* can be useful for suppressing episodic violence in schizophrenia as well as for targeting many of the more disturbing symptoms when it is used along with a more standard antipsychotic. Carbamazepine (Tegretol) has also been found to ameliorate symptoms in some drug-resistant clients with schizophrenia when it is used along with a standard neuroleptic. (See Chapter 18 for more on these drugs).

Benzodiazepines are also being studied as possible adjuncts in the treatment of selected clients with schizophrenia. For example, diazepam (Valium) has been found useful in one study in controlling psychotic symptoms in a small sample of people with

paranoid schizophrenia. Alprazolam (Xanax) has been found useful in several small studies in controlling panic attacks and anxiety symptoms in schizophrenic clients taking antipsychotics (Schatzberg and Cole 1991) (see Chapter 14).

OTHER SOMATIC THERAPIES. Besides antipsychotic medications, the only other recognized somatic treatment for schizophrenia is electroconvulsive therapy in severely catatonic clients. It is indicated when antipsychotic drug therapy fails or is contraindicated. However, electroconvulsive therapy is mostly employed for people with psychotic depression who are violent, suicidal, or participating in self-starvation.

THERAPEUTIC ENVIRONMENT

ACTIVITIES. Effective hospital care involves more than protection of the client from a confusing family, social, or vocational environment. It should also provide healthy substitutes for erecting new identifications, resources for resolving conflicts, and opportunities for learning social and vocational skills.

Group work with schizophrenic patients is oriented toward providing support, an environment in which a patient can develop social skills, and a format to allow friendships to begin (Black et al. 1988). Structured group therapy can target some of the negative symptoms of schizophrenia. For example, participation in activity groups, determined by the client's level of functioning, has been found to decrease withdrawal, promote motivation, modify unacceptable aggression,

Box 19-2. DRUG INFORMATION: HOW THE ANTIPSYCHOTIC DRUGS WORK

It is thought that at least some of the symptoms of psychosis are due to an excess of the neurotransmitter dopamine in those areas of the brain involved in thought and in emotive processes. The majority of antipsychotic drugs, phenothiazines, and related compounds seem to produce many of their beneficial as well as some of their untoward effects by blocking dopamine receptors and thus reducing dopamine-induced responses in the brain.

Although excess dopamine may be released by the presynaptic cells of the psychotic patient, it will not cause a concomitant response in the postsynaptic cell because the receptors to which it must attach are blocked by the antipsychotic drug. Because dopamine is used as a neurotransmitter in many areas of the brain in addition to those involved in thought and emotion, blockage of these receptors can also lead to serious untoward effects. Specifically, dopamine is a neurotransmitter in the basal ganglia, where it is involved in modulating and fine-tuning motor activity. Blockage of dopamine receptors in this area of the brain probably accounts for the extrapyramidal effects, or movement disorders, such as parkinsonian symptoms that often result from the use of antipsychotic drugs. In fact, Parkinson's disease is thought to result from a deficiency of dopamine in the basal ganglia.

Dopamine also plays a normal physiological role as an inhibitor of prolactin release. Blockage of dopamine receptors by the antipsychotic drugs can therefore lead to elevated levels of prolactin in the blood. This abnormally high level of prolactin may induce disturbances like galactorrhea in women and gynecomastia in men.

To more fully understand the pharmacology of the antipsychotic drugs, it is necessary to know that these drugs block other types of receptors in addition to those for dopamine. In particular, they can block the muscarinic receptors for acetylcholine and the alpha$_1$ receptors for norepinephrine. The degree to which individual drugs block these receptors varies to a considerable extent.

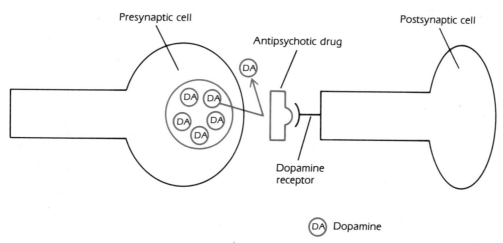

Blockage of dopamine receptors by antipsychotic drugs.

Blockage of Muscarinic Receptors

Because it is the attachment of acetylcholine to muscarinic receptors on smooth muscle, cardiac muscle, and exocrine gland cells that is responsible for the actions of the parasympathetic nervous system, it follows that blockage of these receptors will have antiparasympathetic effects. Included among these antiparasympathetic effects are blurred vision, tachycardia, constipation, and urinary retention.

Blockage of Alpha$_1$ Receptors

Stimulation of alpha$_1$ receptors by norepinephrine is normally responsible for the vasoconstriction necessary to maintain blood pressure in the upright position. Therefore, the consequence of alpha$_1$ receptor blockage is often orthostatic hypotension.

box continued on following page

Box 19–2. DRUG INFORMATION: HOW THE ANTIPSYCHOTIC DRUGS WORK *Continued*

In summary, the blockage of dopamine receptors accounts for the beneficial effects of the antipsychotic drugs. Unfortunately, dopamine blockage accounts for some of the extrapyramidal side effects as well. Other untoward effects result from the blockage of muscarinic and alpha$_1$ receptors. This picture has been somewhat clouded by a novel antipsychotic drug, clozapine. This drug has almost no antidopamine activity and is effective in some pyschotic patients. The mechanism by which clozapine exerts its antipsychotic effects remains uncertain. Although free of many of the untoward effects of the more traditional antipsychotic drugs, clozapine can cause serious and even fatal leukopenia in a small (1–2%) but significant number of patients.

(Courtesy of John Raynor.)

---

and increase social competence. Patients who respond to group therapy while hospitalized may benefit from group therapy on an outpatient basis.

Lancaster (1976) conducted a study that resulted in an increase in self-concept scores of those clients who participated in activity group therapy, in contrast to no increase in the control group. Such activities as drawing pictures, reading poetry, and listening to music were used as a focus of conversation to reduce anxiety and promote socialization. Group functions, such as picnics, reflected growth in social concern for others and the ability to set limits on self and others. Nurses can use activity group therapy in a variety of settings. Lancaster states that "success at tasks and increased involvement with objects and individuals will lead to greater self-esteem in a multiplicity of settings."

In the hospital and outpatient settings, the nurse may participate with other members of the health care team in providing appropriate, structured, and useful activities for the clients. Recreational, occupational, art, and dance therapists are available on many psychiatric units (see Chapter 5).

SAFETY. A client may become physically violent, often in response to hallucinations or delusions. During this time, measures need to be taken to ensure the client's safety as well as the safety of others. If chemical restraints (antipsychotic medication) fail to lessen the person's aggression, such measures as physical restraints and isolation may be indicated. See Chapters 3 and 18 for indications and general guidelines for management of a client in seclusion.

PSYCHOTHERAPY

Medication maintenance has been shown to be the single most important factor in the prevention of relapse in a schizophrenic person. Drugs reduce most of the disturbing, disorganizing, and destructive aspects

of the schizophrenic person's behavior (positive symptoms). Drugs, however, do not improve or affect the underlying apathy, unresponsiveness, and lack of initiative (negative symptoms). Supportive psychotherapy, in addition to drug therapy, results in an even lower rate of relapse than does drug therapy alone. Zahniser and colleagues (1991) identified (1) relationship problems, (2) family concerns, (3) depression, (4) losses, and (5) the role of medication as the most common concerns of schizophrenic clients in therapy. Hilde Bruch (1980) cites a study that identified the elements contributing to successful therapeutic outcomes with schizophrenics, even though the therapists' disciplines were diverse:

> The highest improvement rate was associated with "active participation" with the therapist showing initiative in a sympathetic inquiry, challenging the client's self-deprecatory attitude, and identifying realistic limits as to what is acceptable in the client's behavior.

INDIVIDUAL THERAPY. Intensive insight-oriented psychotherapy is of questionable value with schizophrenic clients. Supportive therapy over long periods, however, has great value and results in helping the person make adjustments to a more useful and satisfactory life. Individual therapy, ideally combined with group therapy, should be made available to the client on an outpatient basis as well as being part of inpatient treatment.

GROUP THERAPY. Group therapy is particularly useful for clients who have had one or more psychotic episodes. It has been shown that groups can benefit the client in the development of *interpersonal skills, resolution of family problems,* and *effective use of community supports.* Groups provide opportunities for socialization in safe settings, the expression of tensions, and sharing problems.

The most useful types of groups for schizophrenics are groups that help the client develop abilities to deal with such issues as day-to-day problems, sharing relevant experiences, learning to listen, asking questions, and keeping topics in focus (Mosher 1982). Groups available on a continuing outpatient basis allow individual growth in these areas.

Some day hospitals and clinics may offer medication groups for clients. Medication groups can help clients (1) deal more effectively with troubling side effects, (2) alert the nurse to potential adverse side effects or toxic effects, (3) minimize isolation among clients receiving antipsychotics, and (4) increase compliance. Refer to Chapter 7 for a discussion of group work with schizophrenic clients.

FAMILY THERAPY. It is unfortunate that more families are not more involved with the therapy of their schizophrenic members because families play such an important role in the course of the illness. Family education and family therapy are known to diminish the negative effects of family life on schizophrenic clients (Hertz 1984).

In family therapy sessions, the family can identify family fears, faulty communications, and distortions. Improved problem-solving skills can be taught, and healthier alternatives to situations of conflict can be explored. Family guilt and anxiety can be lessened, which facilitates change. In some studies, family treatment was even more effective than individual treatment in reducing the severity of symptoms and preventing rehospitalization (Falloon et al. 1982).

The family self-help movement has been an important development in the mental health field. Families of schizophrenics have formed local and national self-help and advocacy organizations. Families with schizophrenic members do have needs. They need to be part of the decision-making process, to have adequate and appropriate help in crises, and to have periodic respite from the hard work of coping with a schizophrenic member (Lamb et al. 1986). Families need help in understanding the disease and the role of medications, setting realistic goals, and developing problem-solving ways for handling tensions and misunderstandings within the family environment. Whether this is in the form of formal family therapy or educational counseling, the family unit needs inclusion and counsel if the schizophrenic member is to become stabilized.

Discharge planning is a vital part of managing schizophrenic clients. Nurses, physicians, and social workers should be aware of the community resources for clients who are to be discharged. Some clients may feel more comfortable with self-help community groups, such as Recovery Inc. and Schizophrenics Anonymous. Information on community resources should be made available to clients and families alike. Examples include community mental health services, home health services, work support programs, and other information sources. Also included should be telephone numbers and addresses of local support groups affiliated with the National Alliance for the Mentally Ill for family and siblings as well as clients.*

Evaluation

Evaluation is always an important step in planning care. Evaluation is especially important in working with people who have chronic psychotic disorders. Modifications may have to be made in the goals set for specific clients. All goals need to be realistic and obtainable. It is not uncommon for the goals set for people with chronic disorders to be too ambitious. A former short term goal often becomes a long term goal. Change is a process that occurs over time. With a person diagnosed as schizophrenic, the time period may be pronounced. Therefore, for preventing both client frustration and staff burnout, short term goals should be realistic and obtainable.

Another advantage to regularly scheduled evaluation with chronically ill clients is that it allows the staff to bring in new data and to reassess the client's problems. Is the client not progressing because a more important need is not being met? Is the staff using the client's strengths and interest to reach identified goals? Are there more appropriate interventions available for this client to facilitate his or her progress?

The active involvement of staff with the client's progress can help sustain interest and prevent feelings of helplessness and burnout. Input from the client can offer valuable data about why a certain desired behavior or situation has not occurred.

Paranoia

Any intense and strongly defended irrational suspicion can be regarded as **paranoia.** Paranoid ideas cannot be corrected by experiences and cannot be modified by facts or reality. *Projection* is the most common defense mechanism used by people who are paranoid. For example, when paranoid individuals feel self-critical, they experience others as being harshly critical

---

*National Alliance for the Mentally Ill, 1901 North Fort Meyers Drive, Suite 500, Arlington, VA, (703) 525-7600. For chapters nearest you, call 1-800-950-NAMI.

toward them. When they feel anger, they experience others as being unjustly angry at them.

Paranoid states may occur in a variety of mental or organic disorders. For example, a person experiencing a psychotic depression or manic episode may display paranoid thinking. Paranoid symptoms can be *secondary* to physical illness, organic brain disease, or drug intoxications.

Paranoid schizophrenia is one of the *primary* paranoid disorders (i.e., those in which the primary symptom is paranoid thinking). The others are paranoid delusional disorder and paranoid personality disorder.

Refer to Chapter 16 for a discussion of paranoid personality disorder.

People with paranoid schizophrenia usually have a later age of onset (e.g., late 20s–30s). It develops rapidly in individuals with good premorbid functioning and tends to be intermittent during the first five years of illness. In some cases, paranoid schizophrenia is associated with a good outcome or recovery (Fenton and McGlashan 1991). The person with a paranoid disorder is usually frightened. Although not always consciously aware of his or her feelings, the paranoid person has deep feelings of loneliness, despair, help-

---

Table 19–11 ■ NURSING INTERVENTIONS AND RATIONALES: PSYCHOTHERAPEUTIC AND PHYSICAL NEEDS OF A CLIENT WHO IS PARANOID

INTERVENTION	RATIONALE
Communications	
Nursing Diagnosis: *Altered thought processes* related to perceptual and cognitive distortions, as evidenced by suspicious thoughts and defensive behavior	
1. Honesty and consistency are imperative. If you say "I'll be back at 11 A.M." or "I'll call your social worker this morning," *always* follow through with what you say you will do.	1. A person who is paranoid will be quick to pick up dishonesty. Honesty and consistency provide an atmosphere in which trust can grow.
2. Avoid a warm and gushing approach. A nonjudgmental, respectful, and consistent approach is most effective.	2. Warmth and gushing can be frightening to a person who needs emotional distance. Matter-of-fact consistency is not threatening.
3. Eliminate physical contact; do *not* touch the client. Ask client's permission if touch is necessary.	3. Touch may be interpreted as a physical or sexual assault.
4. Focus on maintaining ego boundaries; e.g.: • Do not get too physically close • Avoid touching client • Limit time of interaction	4. Perceptions of having personal space invaded can increase client's anxiety.
5. Evaluate themes in hallucinations and delusions.	5. The themes are important to know (e.g., kill self or others), because protective action may have to be taken.
6. Do not argue with the content.	6. Arguing with hallucinations and delusions makes the person defend his or her beliefs more vigorously.
7. When speaking of the client's "voices," note that client hears voices not experienced by you.	7. Increases trust while accepting and acknowledging the client's experience.
8. Resist getting caught up in content; rather, look for the feelings behind the delusions and hallucinations.	8. One cannot logically discuss illogical material, but one *can* discuss feelings, e.g., "I don't know about the FBI trying to harm you, but thinking that must be frightening."
9. Clarify and restate your role. Repeat with patience and understanding.	9. Prevents misinterpretations and minimizes misconstruing the relationship.
10. Use simple and clear language when speaking to client. Explain everything you are going to do before you do it.	10. Prevents misinterpretations and clarifies nurse's intent and actions.
11. Diffuse angry and hostile verbal attacks with a nondefensive stand. Explore with client the origin of his or her angry feelings.	11. The anger a client expresses is often displaced. When staff become defensive, anger of both client and staff escalates. A nondefensive and nonjudgmental attitude provides an atmosphere in which feelings can be explored more easily.

Table 19–11 ■ NURSING INTERVENTIONS AND RATIONALES: PSYCHOTHERAPEUTIC AND PHYSICAL NEEDS OF A CLIENT WHO IS PARANOID *Continued*

INTERVENTION	RATIONALE
Physical Needs	
Nursing Diagnosis: *Altered health maintenance* **related to panic levels of anxiety, as evidenced by refusing to eat or sleep**	
1. Grooming and dress are rarely a problem.	1. Provide the necessary toilet articles and facilities for the client to care for clothes.
2. When client thinks food is poisoned, nurse can provide foods in their own containers, e.g., milk cartons, hard-boiled eggs, or apples.	2. Delusions that food is poisoned are common with paranoid clients. Usually these measures promote adequate nutrition. Tube feeding is instituted as a *last* resort.
3. When the client is unable to sleep, staying with the client for specific time periods can be helpful.	3. Client may feel too vulnerable to sleep. The nurse's presence often helps the client feel more secure, e.g., "I will stay with you 15 minutes" or "I will stay with you until you fall asleep."
4. Use of radio or tape player may decrease anxiety at bedtime.	4. Provides a focus at bedtime other than hallucinations.
Physical Behaviors (Recreation)	
Nursing Diagnosis: *Risk for violence* **related to altered perceptions and cognitive distortion, as evidenced by increased agitation and hostile behaviors**	
1. Maintain low level of stimuli, e.g., avoid groups and provide quiet setting and subdued lighting.	1. Noisy environments may be perceived as threatening.
2. Observe client frequently, e.g., every 15 minutes.	2. Observe for increased agitation and increased motor behavior. Intervene when necessary.
3. Provide verbal and physical limits to client's hostility, e.g., "We won't allow you to hit or hurt anyone here; if you can't control yourself, we will help you."	3. When anxiety is high, the client may feel out of control. Often, firm verbal limits are effective in calming the client. If not, a quiet room or medication may be necessary.
Nursing Diagnosis: *Diversional activity deficit* **related to panic level of anxiety**	
1. Assign solitary, noncompetitive activities that take some concentration (e.g., crossword puzzles, picture puzzles, photography, typing); when client feels less threatened, bridge and chess may be more appropriate, requiring increased concentration.	1. When client is extremely distrustful of others, solitary activities are best. Activities that demand concentration keep the client's attention on reality and minimize hallucinatory and delusional preoccupation.

lessness, and fear of abandonment. The paranoid facade is a defense against painful feelings.

COMMUNICATIONS. Because persons who are paranoid are unable to trust the actions of those around them, they are usually guarded, tense, and reserved. Although the client may keep himself or herself aloof from interpersonal contacts, impairment in functioning may be minimal. To ensure interpersonal distance, he or she may adopt a superior, hostile, and sarcastic attitude. A common defense for maintaining self-esteem used by paranoid individuals is to disparage others and dwell on the shortcomings of others. The client will frequently misinterpret the messages of others or give private meaning to the communications of others **(ideas of reference).** Minor oversights are often interpreted as personal rejection.

During hospitalization, a paranoid client may make offensive yet accurate criticisms of staff and ward policies. It is important that staff not react to these criticisms with anxiety or rejection of the client. Staff conferences, peer group supervision, and working with one's clinical supervisor are effective ways of looking behind the behaviors to the motivations of the client. This provides the opportunity to reduce the client's anxiety and increase staff effectiveness.

PHYSICAL NEEDS. A person with a paranoid schizophrenic disorder usually has stronger ego resources than do individuals with other schizophrenic disorders, particularly with regard to occupational functioning and capacity for independent living (APA 1987). Grooming, dress, and self-care may not be a problem, therefore. In fact, in some cases grooming may be meticulous. Nutrition, however, may pose a problem. A common distortion or delusion is that the food is poisoned. In this case, special foods should be provided in enclosed containers to minimize the suspicion of tampering. If the client thinks that others will harm him when he is sleeping, he may be fearful of going to sleep. Therefore, proper rest may become a problem that warrants nursing interventions.

PHYSICAL BEHAVIORS. A paranoid person may become physically aggressive in response to hallucinations or delusions. Hostile drives are projected on the environment and then acted on. Homosexual urges may be projected onto the environment as well, and fear of sexual advances from others may stimulate aggression or homosexual panic.

An environment that provides the client with a sense of security and safety should minimize anxiety and environmental distortions. Activities that distract the client from ruminating on hallucinations and delusions can also help decrease anxiety. Table 19–11 suggests some basic nursing interventions for clients who are experiencing paranoia.

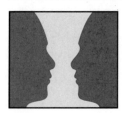

Case Study: Working with a Person Who Is Paranoid

Tom is a 37-year-old man who is currently an inpatient at the Veterans Administration Hospital. He has been separated from his wife and four children for six years. His medical records state that he has been in and out of hospitals frequently for 17 years for his illness, which Tom describes as "hearing voices a lot." Tom is an ex-marine who first "heard voices" at the age of 19 while he was stationed in Okinawa; he subsequently received a medical discharge.

The hospitalization was precipitated by an exacerbation of auditory hallucinations. "I thought people were following me. I hear voices, usually a woman's voice, and she's tormenting me. People say that it happens because I don't take my medications. The medications make me tired and I can't have sex." Tom also admits to using cocaine and marijuana. He is aware that marijuana and cocaine increase his paranoia and that taking drugs usually precedes hospitalization but says that "they make me feel good." Tom

finished 11 years of school but did not graduate from high school. He denies having any close friends. He was in prison for five years for manslaughter and told the nurse, "I was in prison because I did something bad." He was abusing alcohol and drugs at the time, and drug abuse has been related to each subsequent hospitalization.

Ms. Lally is Tom's primary nurse. When Tom meets the nurse, he is dressed in pajamas and bathrobe. His hygiene is intact, and he is well nourished. He tells the nurse that he does not sleep much because "the voices get worse at night." Ms. Lally notes in Tom's medical record that he has had two episodes of suicidal ideation. During those times, the voices were telling him to jump "off rooftops" and "in front of trains."

During the first interview, Tom only occasionally makes eye contact and speaks in a low monotone. At times he glances about the room as if distracted, mumbles to himself, and appears upset.

NURSE:	Tom, my name is Ms. Lally. I will be your nurse while you're in the hospital. We will meet every day for 30 minutes at 10:00 A.M. During that time we can discuss areas of concern to you.
TOM:	Well . . . don't believe what they say about me. I want to start a new . . . are you married?
NURSE:	This time is for you to talk about *your* concerns.
TOM:	Oh . . . (*Looks furtively around the room, then lowers his eyes.*) Someone is trying to kill me, I think . . .
NURSE:	You appear to be focusing on something other than our conversation. Is something making you uncomfortable?
TOM:	The voices tell me things . . . I can't say . . .
NURSE:	I don't hear any voices except yours and mine. I am going to stay with you. Tell me what is happening and I will try to help you.
TOM:	The voices tell me bad things.

Ms. Lally stayed with Tom and encouraged him to communicate with her. As Tom focused more on the nurse, his anxiety appeared to lessen. His thoughts became more connected; he was able to concentrate more on what the nurse was saying, and he mumbled less to himself.

Assessment

After the initial interview, Ms. Lally divides the data into objective and subjective components:

OBJECTIVE DATA

1. Speaks in low monotone voice
2. Poor eye contact
3. Well nourished and hygiene intact
4. Admits to auditory hallucinations
5. Has history of drug abuse—cocaine and marijuana
6. Has no close friends
7. Has been hospitalized since age 19 and has not worked since that time
8. Has had suicidal impulses twice
9. Imprisoned five years for violent acting out (manslaughter)
10. Thoughts scattered when anxious

SUBJECTIVE DATA

1. "Someone is trying to kill me . . . I think."
2. "I don't take my medicine. It makes me tired and I can't have sex."
3. "The voices get worse at night and I can't sleep."
4. Voices have told him to "jump off rooftops" and "in front of trains."

Nursing Diagnosis

Ms. Lally formulates two nursing diagnoses on the basis of her assessment data.

1. *Altered thought processes* related to unclear communication and alteration in biochemical compounds, as evidenced by persecutory hallucinations and intense suspiciousness.
   - Voices have told him to "jump off rooftops" and "in front of trains."
   - "Someone is trying to kill me, I think."
   - Abuses cocaine and marijuana, although paranoia increases, because "it makes me feel good."

2. *Noncompliance with medications* related to side effects of therapy, as evidenced by verbalization of noncompliance and persistence of symptoms.
   - Does not take prescribed medication because "it makes me tired and I can't have sex."
   - Chronic history of relapse of symptoms when out of hospital.

Planning

CONTENT LEVEL—PLANNING GOALS

Ms. Lally decides that initial concentration should be placed on establishing a relationship in which Tom can feel safe with the nurse and comfortable enough to discuss his voices and events that precipitate them. The nurse is also aware that if Tom's anxiety level can be lowered and his suspicions diminished, he will be able to participate more comfortably in reality-based activities and have an increased ability to problem-solve. Because noncompliance with his medications seems to be a major factor in the persistence of Tom's disturbing symptoms, this becomes an important focus for discussion. Ms. Lally plans to evaluate the medication and side effects with the physician and to work with Tom on alternatives to increase his medical compliance.

Nursing Diagnosis	Long Term Goals	Short Term Goals
1. *Altered thought processes* related to unclear communication and alteration in biochemical compounds, as evidenced by persecutory hallucinations and intense suspiciousness	1. Tom will state he is able to function without interference from "his voices" by discharge.	1a. By (date), Tom will state that he feels comfortable with the nurse. 1b. By (date), Tom will name two actions that precipitate the voices and paranoia.

Planning
(Continued)

2. *Noncompliance with medications* related to side effects of therapy, as evidenced by verbalization of noncompliance and persistence of symptoms

2. Tom will adhere to medication regimen by (date).

1c. By (date), Tom will name two actions he can take if the voices start to become upsetting to him.
2a. By (date), Tom will name actions he can take to offset the side effects of medication.
2b. Tom will attend weekly support group for people with schizophrenia.

PROCESS LEVEL—NURSES' REACTIONS AND FEELINGS

On the first day of admission, Tom assaulted another male client, stating that the other client accused him of being a homosexual and touched him on the buttocks. After assessing the incident, the staff agreed that Tom's provocation came more from his own projections (Tom's sexual attraction to the other client) than from anything the other client had done or said.

Tom's difficulty with impulse control frightened Ms. Lally. She had some real concerns regarding Tom's impulse control and the possibility of Tom's striking out at her, especially when Tom was hallucinating and highly delusional. Ms. Lally mentioned her concerns to the nursing coordinator, and it was suggested that Ms. Lally meet with Tom in the day room until he demonstrated more control and less suspicion of others. After five days, Tom was less excitable, and the sessions were held in a room set aside for client interviews. Ms. Lally also spoke with a senior staff nurse regarding her fear. By talking to the senior nurse and understanding more clearly her own fear, Ms. Lally was able to identify interventions to help Tom regain a better sense of control.

Intervention

Ms. Lally made out an initial nursing care plan (Nursing Care Plan 19–1). An important part of her plan was conferring with the physician about the legitimate concerns Tom had regarding his medication. The physician decided to try giving Tom a larger dose of medication at bedtime to minimize his insomnia and a smaller dose during the day to minimize the sedative side effects. The concerns Tom had regarding not being able to sustain an erection were legitimate, and the physician stated that he would try another medication if Tom's complaint of impotence continued. Ms. Lally worked with Tom on continuing his participation in the support group. During team conference, the social worker suggested that if Tom was able to maintain contact with a support group, he might be a good candidate for a group home in the future.

Neuroleptic medications seemed to greatly lower Tom's suspiciousness and his hallucinatory symptoms. This enabled Tom to discuss with the nurse more reality-based concerns and to be more amenable to attending the weekly support group. After the fourth meeting, Tom seemed to view the group more favorably and even spoke of making a friend in the group.

Evaluation

By discharge, Tom said he had a better understanding of his medications and what to do. He knew that marijuana and cocaine would increase his symptoms, but he said sometimes he got lonely and needed to "feel good." He did say he planned to continue with the support group and with outpatient counseling. The reason he gave for deciding to attend outpatient therapy was that he felt Ms. Lally had really cared about him, and that made him feel good. By the time of discharge, he was sleeping much better and said he had more energy during the day.

Nursing Care Plan 19-1 ■ A PERSON WITH PARANOIA: Tom

NURSING DIAGNOSIS

Altered thought processes **related to unclear communication and alteration in biochemical compounds, as evidenced by persecutory hallucinations and intense suspiciousness**

Supporting Data

- Voices have told him to "jump off rooftops" and "in front of trains."
- "Someone is trying the kill me, I think."
- Abuses cocaine and marijuana although paranoia increases: "It makes me feel good."

Long Term Goal: Tom will state that he is able to function without interference from his "voices" by discharge.

Short Term Goals	Intervention	Rationale	Evaluation
1. By (date), Tom will state that he feels comfortable with the nurse.	1a. Meet with Tom each day for 30 minutes. 1b. Use clear, unambiguous statements. 1c. Provide activities that need concentration and are non-competitive.	1a. Short, consistent meetings help establish contact and decrease anxiety. 1b. Minimize potential for mis-construing messages. 1c. Increase time spent in real-ity-based activities and de-crease preoccupation with delusional and hallucina-tory experiences.	Goal met By the end of the first week, Tom said he looked forward to meeting with "my nurse."
2. Tom will name two events that precede the hallucina-tions and delusions by (date).	2a. Investigate content of hallu-cinations with Tom. 2b. Explore those times that voices are most threatening and disturbing.	2a. Identify suicidal or aggres-sive themes. 2b. Identify events that increase anxiety.	Goal met Tom was able to identify that the voices were worse at nighttime. He also stated that after smoking marijuana and taking cocaine, he always thought people were trying to kill him.
3. Tom will name two actions that he can take if the voices start to become upsetting to him by (date).	3. Explore with Tom possible actions that can minimize anxiety.	3. Offer him alternatives while anxiety level is relatively low.	Goal met Tom has the number of a physi-cian he can call when halluci-nations start to escalate.

NURSING DIAGNOSIS

Noncompliance with medications **related to side effects of therapy, as evidenced by verbalization of noncompliance and persistence of symptoms**

Supporting data

- Does not take prescribed medication: "It makes me tired and I can't have sex."
- Chronic history of relapse of symptoms when out of hospital

Long Term Goal: Tom will adhere to medication regimen by (date).

Short Term Goals	Intervention	Rationale	Evaluation
1. By (date), Tom will name ac-tions he can take to offset the side effects of medica-tion.	1a. Evaluate medication re-sponse with physician in hospital. 1b. Educate Tom regarding side effects—how long they last and actions to take.	1a. Identify drugs and dosage that have increased thera-peutic value and decreased side effects. 1b. Can give increased sense of control over symptoms.	Goal met Physician readjusted dose, with the large dose at bedtime to increase sleep and a small dose during the day to de-crease fatigue. Tom stated he slept better at night but still tired during the day.
2. Tom will attend weekly sup-port group for people with schizophrenia by (date).	2. Encourage Tom to join sup-port group for people with schizophrenia.	2. Mutual concerns and prob-lems discussed in an atmos-phere of acceptance—concerns such as housing, expenses, loneliness, and jobs. Group also provides peer support for drug ther-apy maintenance.	Goal met Week 1—Tom attended meet-ing. Week 2—Tom stated that he made a friend. Spoke in the group about "not feeling good" at times. Week 3—Tom said that he might go to group therapy after discharge from hospital.

Table 19–12 ■ NURSING INTERVENTIONS AND RATIONALES: PSYCHOTHERAPEUTIC AND PHYSICAL NEEDS OF A PERSON WHO IS WITHDRAWN

INTERVENTION	RATIONALE

Communications

Nursing Diagnosis: *Impaired verbal communication* related to altered perceptions and cognitive distortions, as evidenced by severe withdrawal and anergia.

INTERVENTION	RATIONALE
1. Stay with the person and sit in silence for short intervals. This is often the first step.	1. Do not demand that the client reply; meet the person at his or her own level. The client may be too anxious or confused to speak.
2. Initiate frequent, short, regular contacts with the withdrawn person.	2. Initially, short intervals are more tolerable for both client and nurse.
3. Before you leave, be specific as to when you will be back, e.g., "I will be back at 1 P.M. for 10 minutes." Always be on time and keep your word.	3. Visit the patient regularly and be back when you say you will. Disappointments caused by you could interfere with forming a relationship. If a delay is unavoidable, explain this to the client.
4. When speaking to the client, use simple, short sentences.	4. The client's thoughts may be confused and attention span short.
5. Make observations about happenings in the environment, e.g., "I see you brought your Bible with you this morning."	5. Focuses attention on common realities in the environment.
6. When the client begins to speak, keep topics neutral and simple.	6. Helps minimize anxiety and frustration.
7. Clarify the client's use of the generalized "they."	7. Clients with weak ego boundaries have difficulty with differentiating others from self. Ask, "Who are *they*?"
8. Meet hostility and rejection with a nonjudgmental and neutral response, e.g., "If you don't want to visit now, I'll be back at 1 P.M. to spend time with you."	8. Often clients are verbally abusive to or rejecting of the nurse; this is rarely personal. When the client can experience acceptance and caring for how he or she is at that moment, feelings of self-worth may increase.
9. Always tell the client you do not understand when you do not.	9. Clients may erroneously think the nurse can "read my mind" or "know" what they are thinking. By correcting this false belief, the nurse clarifies communications and delineates ego boundaries.

Physical Needs

Nursing Diagnosis: *Altered health maintenance* related to biochemical changes, as evidenced by apparent stupor

INTERVENTION	RATIONALE
1. Talk to the client who appears comatose while giving physical care and explain everything that you are doing. Talk as if the client fully understands. Address the client respectfully, e.g., "Mr. Jones, I am going to shave the other side of your face. The water may feel cold."	1. Even though clients may appear comatose, they may be *aware of everything that is going on*. Often clients can remember verbatim the conversations of others around them during the time they were comatose.
2. Monitor intake.	2. Client may be too disorganized to eat or drink.
3. Monitor output.	3. Client may retain urine and feces or be incontinent of urine or feces.
4. Encourage involvement with hygiene and dressing at the client's own level. *Do not do for a client what he or she is able to do.*	4. Sometimes giving short, simple reminders is sufficient for a disorganized client. At other times, the nurse may have to assist the client with grooming and dressing.

Table 19–12 ■ NURSING INTERVENTIONS AND RATIONALES: PSYCHOTHERAPEUTIC AND PHYSICAL NEEDS OF A PERSON WHO IS WITHDRAWN *Continued*	
INTERVENTION	**RATIONALE**
Physical Behaviors (Recreation)	
Nursing Diagnosis: *Impaired social interactions* related to anxiety and inability to concentrate attention outward, as evidenced by poor attention span and withdrawal	

1. Increase participation with others at client's level of tolerance.
  a. Stuporous to very withdrawn: one-to-one simple activities with the nurse, e.g., talking, looking through a magazine, painting, working with clay.
  b. Less withdrawn: simple, concrete activity with nurse and perhaps with one other client, e.g., card games, drawing, Ping-Pong.
  c. Eventually, offer client group activities, e.g., ward meetings, occupational therapy, dance therapy, bingo games.
	a. Those activities that require no verbal response and have no time limit or "right or wrong" are the least threatening.
	  b. Brings the client slowly into contact with others. This provides a greater opportunity for reality orientation and consensual validation.
	  c. Increased participation with others can increase client's ability to validate reality and to experience satisfaction in reality-based activities.

Catatonia

The essential feature of catatonia is abnormal motor behavior. Two extreme motor behaviors are seen in clients with catatonia: extreme motor agitation and extreme psychomotor retardation (even stupor with mutism). Other behaviors identified with catatonia include posturing, waxy flexibility, stereotyped behavior, extreme negativism or automatic obedience, echolalia, and echopraxia. The onset of catatonia is usually abrupt and the prognosis favorable. Severe catatonic symptoms are rarely seen today as a result of chemotherapy and improved individual management.

WITHDRAWN PHASE

COMMUNICATIONS. Clients in the withdrawn phase of catatonia can be so withdrawn that they appear comatose. They can be mute and may remain so for hours, days, weeks, or months. Although such a client may not appear to pay attention to events going on around him or her, the client is acutely aware of the environment and may remember events accurately at a later date.

PHYSICAL NEEDS. When a client is extremely withdrawn, physical needs take priority. A client may need to be hand-fed or tube-fed for adequate nutritional status to be maintained. Normal control over bladder and bowel functions can be interrupted. Assessment of urinary or bowel retention must be made

and acted on when found. Incontinence of urine and feces poses the problem of skin breakdown and potential infection. Because physical movements may be minimal or absent, range-of-motion exercises need to be carried out to prevent muscular atrophy, calcium depletion, and contractures. Dressing and grooming will most likely need direct nursing interventions.

The client with catatonic symptoms may trigger resistance in the staff to nursing interventions because the client refuses to participate in activities or cooperate voluntarily.

PHYSICAL BEHAVIORS. During the withdrawn state, the catatonic person may be on a continuum from decreased spontaneous movements to complete stupor. Waxy flexibility, or the ability to hold distorted postures for extensive periods of time, is often seen. The term *waxy* refers to the holding of any posture that the staff may place the person in. For example, if someone raises the client's arms over his head, the client may maintain that position for hours or longer. This phenomenon is often used as a diagnostic sign. When less withdrawn, a client may demonstrate stereotyped behavior, echopraxia, echolalia, or automatic obedience.

Caution is advised, because even after holding a single posture for long periods, the client may suddenly and without provocation have brief outbursts of gross motor activity in response to inner hallucinations, delusions, and change in neurotransmitters. Table 19–12 suggests specific nursing interventions for a catatonic client who is withdrawn or in a catatonic stupor.

EXCITED PHASE

COMMUNICATIONS. During the excited or hyperactive stage, the person talks or shouts continuously, and the verbalizations may be incoherent.

PHYSICAL NEEDS. A person who is constantly and intensely hyperactive can become completely exhausted and even die if medical attention is not available. Most often a phenothiazine (chlorpromazine) is administered intramuscularly. The client may continue to be agitated, but within limits that are not potentially harmful. During this time of heightened physical activity, the client's body has an increased need for fluids, calories, and rest. During the hyperactive state, a client may be destructive and aggressive to others in response to hallucinations or delusions. Table 19–13 suggests nursing interventions during the excited phase of catatonia. Many of these concerns and interventions are the same as for a bipolar client in a manic phase.

Table 19–13 ■ NURSING INTERVENTIONS AND RATIONALES: PSYCHOTHERAPEUTIC AND PHYSICAL NEEDS OF A PERSON WHO IS HYPERACTIVE

INTERVENTION	RATIONALE
Communications	
Nursing Diagnosis: *Ineffective coping* related to panic level of anxiety, as evidenced by hyperactivity	
1. Use firm, clear statements.	1. Client may be disorganized; needs clear statements. Firmness provides a sense of outside control.
2. Keep patient in quiet area.	2. Helps decrease environmental stimuli and anxiety.
Physical Needs	
Nursing Diagnosis: *Altered health maintenance* related to cognitive disturbances, as evidenced by inability to care for basic needs	
1. Monitor weight and dietary intake.	1. Client may lose calories, fluids, and essential nutrients.
2. Offer high-calorie fluids and "finger foods," e.g., milk, bananas, sandwiches, candy bars, hard-boiled eggs.	2. Foods that a client can carry with him or her when too active to sit during meals help replace and maintain adequate nutrition.
3. Provide rest periods.	3. Minimizes exhaustion and fatigue.
4. Supervise grooming and physical appearance.	4. Client may be too agitated to care for physical appearance.
Physical Behaviors (Recreation)	
Nursing Diagnosis: *Risk for violence* related to biochemical changes, as evidenced by agitation	
1. Watch closely for signs of increased agitation.	1. Client may become increasingly agitated and need a decrease in environmental stimuli or medication. Intervention should be made before anxiety escalates to panic levels, when intervention becomes traumatic for both client and staff.
2. Assess need for intervention if agitation increases (verbal, chemical, or seclusion/restraints)	
Nursing Diagnosis: *Diversional activity deficit* related to cognitive disturbances, as evidenced by hyperactivity and poor concentration	
1. Simple physical activity using large muscle groups may help discharge some physical tension, e.g., pace with the client, Ping-Pong, volleyball.	1. Gross motor activity that requires minimal concentration can reduce anxiety and tension.

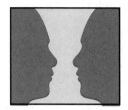

Case Study: Working with a Person Who Is Withdrawn

Mrs. Ling Chou is a 25-year-old woman. She left China for the United States six months ago to join her husband. Before she came to the United States, she lived with her parents and worked in a button factory. In China Mrs. Chou had been educated to speak and understand English. She had always been shy and looked to her parents and now to her husband for guidance and support. Shortly after she arrived in the United States, her mother developed pneumonia and died, and Mrs. Chou was not able to go back to China for the funeral. Mr. Chou states that his wife thought that if she had stayed in China, her mother would not have become ill. She told him recently that evil would come to their one-year-old child because she was unable to take proper care of her mother. Three days before admission, Mrs. Chou became lethargic and spent most of the day staring into space and mumbling to herself. When Mr. Chou asked whom she was talking to, she would answer, "My mother." She had not eaten for two days; at the time of admission, Mrs. Chou sat motionless and mute and appeared stuporous.

The physician noticed that when he took Mrs. Chou's pulse, her arm remained in midair until he replaced it by her side. Mr. Chou said that once his wife became extremely agitated and started to scream and cry while tearing the curtains and knocking over objects. Shortly afterward, she returned to a withdrawn, mute state. Mr. Chou is extremely distraught and confused, and he fears for the safety of their child. Mr. Nolan is assigned to Mrs. Chou as her primary nurse.

Mrs. Chou is sloppily dressed, and her hair and nails are dirty. She is pale, and her skin turgor is poor. She sits motionless and appears unaware of anything going on around her. Mr. Nolan introduces himself and explains what he will be doing beforehand, for example, that he will be taking her blood pressure and pulse and offering her fluids.

While taking her vital signs, he tells Mrs. Chou the date, the time, and where she is. When he is finished taking her vital signs, he offers Mrs. Chou some fluids. She is able to take sips from a straw when the straw is placed in her mouth. Mrs. Chou's intake and output are monitored, and she is placed in a four-bed room next to the nurses' station.

Assessment

Mr. Nolan assesses his data.

OBJECTIVE DATA

1. Motionless and mute for two days
2. Has not taken nourishment for two days
3. Has had one episode of violent and destructive activity
4. Appears to be comatose, eyes not focused, body limp
5. Has had recent shock with mother's death
6. Skin turgor poor
7. Poorly groomed
8. Waxy flexibility

SUBJECTIVE DATA

1. Told husband "evil" would come to the baby because she did not take proper care of her mother

Nursing Diagnosis

Mr. Nolan notes that Mrs. Chou is unable to take care of any basic needs (e.g., nutrition, hygiene, or proper toileting). He identifies *self-care deficit* as the primary initial priority.

Planning

CONTENT LEVEL—PLANNING GOALS

Mr. Nolan formulated the following long term and short term goals:

Planning *(Continued)*	Nursing Diagnosis	Long Term Goals	Short Term Goals
	1. *Self-care deficit* related to immobility, as evidenced by inability to feed, bathe, dress or toilet herself	1. Mrs. Chou will maintain nutritional intake and body weight while in the hospital.	1a. Mrs. Chou will take in 2000 ml of fluid each day.
			1b. Mrs. Chou will eat three meals per day.
		2. Mrs. Chou will maintain normal bladder and bowel function while in the hospital.	2a. Mrs. Chou will void 1000–1500 ml per day.
			2b. Mrs. Chou will have one bowel movement per day.
		3. Mrs. Chou will maintain present muscle tone and flexibility while in the hospital.	3a. Mrs. Chou will participate in passive range-of-motion exercises three times per day for 15 minutes.

PROCESS LEVEL—NURSES' REACTIONS AND FEELINGS

Mr. Nolan found that initially he became impatient with Mrs. Chou. He was used to carrying out nursing procedures quickly and efficiently. Mrs. Chou's morning care demanded a great deal of time. For example, he found himself being impatient with the long periods it took to feed Mrs. Chou. He discussed his impatience with a colleague. During the discussion, it became apparent that it was more Mrs. Chou's total dependency on him that made him anxious. Mr. Nolan sees himself as highly organized and in control, often suppressing many of his own needs and desires to be taken care of. "I guess her total dependency triggers some of my own unmet dependency needs." Once he was able to separate some of his own personal concerns that triggered his reaction, he was able to focus on Mrs. Chou's needs with more patience. He found that the more he talked to Mrs. Chou as if she were able to understand everything he said, the easier it was for him to maintain a certain level of relatedness and interest.

Intervention

Mr. Nolan assigned the psychiatric aide to bathe and dress Mrs. Chou in the mornings. He spent time with Mrs. Chou each morning and afternoon doing range-of-motion exercises, offering her frequent sips of juice or milk, and talking to her—that is, making observations about neutral happenings in the environment. Mr. Chou visited every day, and Mr. Nolan encouraged Mr. Chou to talk to his wife about everyday occurrences in his life and about their future. He also cautioned Mr. Chou that there was a possibility Mrs. Chou could suddenly become agitated and aggressive, and that this was part of the disease.

With the aid of medication therapy and nursing management, Mrs. Chou began to show signs of comprehension. By the end of the seventh day, Mrs. Chou was talking, feeding herself, and able to bathe herself. She appeared to have developed a strong attachment to Mr. Nolan, and told her husband how kind he was to her while she was "away." She even remembered that Mr. Nolan brought in a Chinese music tape during the period when she was stuporous. The psychiatrists thought that Mrs. Chou's catatonic reaction was triggered by her mother's death, and strongly suggested counseling after discharge to facilitate the work of mourning.

Evaluation

Catatonic episodes are generally acute and related to identifiable stressors, and the disorder has a favorable prognosis. Mrs. Chou responded rapidly to medication and Mr. Nolan's nursing intervention. Although much of Mrs. Chou's passivity was culturally determined, the psychiatrists suggested that Mrs. Chou develop more outlets for release of emotional tensions. Mrs. Chou agreed to counseling after discharge.

Disorganized Schizophrenia

The most regressed and socially impaired of all the schizophrenic disorders is the disorganized form. A person diagnosed with disorganized schizophrenia (formally hebephrenia) may have marked looseness of associations, grossly inappropriate affect, bizarre mannerisms, and incoherence of speech and may display extreme social withdrawal (APA 1987). Although delusions and hallucinations are present, they are fragmentary and not well organized. Behavior may be

---

Table 19–14 ■ NURSING INTERVENTIONS AND RATIONALES: PSYCHOTHERAPEUTIC AND PHYSICAL NEEDS OF A PERSON WITH DISORGANIZED SCHIZOPHRENIA

INTERVENTION	RATIONALE
Communications	
Nursing Diagnosis: *Impaired verbal communication* related to perceptual and cognitive distortions, as evidenced by disorganized speech	
1. Speak in short, simple sentences.	1. Thought patterns are disorganized. Simple phrases are best understood.
2. Constantly reinforce reality, e.g., call client by name, state the date, state your name, and so forth.	2. Thinking is often autistic and confused. Stressing common environmental realities provides a tie with reality.
3. Initiate short, frequent contacts.	3. Helps establish a rapport and personal contact in a manner less threatening to client.
4. Allow client time to respond.	4. Because thought process of client is disorganized, time is needed for client to take messages in and compose a response.
Physical Needs	
Nursing Diagnosis: *Altered health maintenance* related to cognitive distortions, as evidenced by difficulty with activities of daily living	
1. Observe for signs and symptoms of physical illness, e.g., cold, thirst, pain.	1. Clients are often disorganized, out of touch with feelings, and unable to assess personal needs or ask for what they need.
2. Check for incontinence and provide fresh clothes when necessary. Use nonpunitive, matter-of-fact approach.	2. Client may be too disorganized to use toilet. Encourage appropriate dress and hygiene.
3. Help clients with hygiene as needed, e.g., set up shaving, give step-by-step instructions; if unable to shave, help with shaving; help with putting on makeup, brushing hair, brushing teeth, and so forth.	3. Can minimize anxiety and help client maintain self-esteem. Meets client at own level. When client is able to do partial care, even though slowly, this type of assistance encourages independent functioning.
4. Lay out clothes that are clean and appropriate. Give simple step-by-step instructions for dress, e.g., "Put in your left arm . . . now right arm . . . pull the sweater over your head."	4. Maintains optimal level of functioning and self-esteem.
5. Encourage appropriate social behaviors, e.g., have clients eat with utensils and cover front with napkin.	5. Increases social interactions. When taking something away, e.g., eating with hands, offer alternatives such as large spoon with which to eat food.
Physical Behaviors (Recreation)	
Nursing Diagnosis: *Diversional activity deficit* related to inability to concentrate, as evidenced by purposeless activity and apathy	
1. Plan and initiate simple, daily routine.	1. Consistent daily routine helps client maintain contact with reality with minimal anxiety.
2. Plan simple, concrete tasks that require minimal concentration and skill, e.g., drawing, walking with nurse, dancing, ward meeting, folding linen.	2. Tasks that match client's concentration and interest can promote socialization, increase contact with reality, provide exercise, and increase self-esteem.

considered "odd," and giggling or grimacing in response to internal stimuli are common. Disorganized schizophrenia has an earlier age of onset (early-middle teens) and often develops insidiously. It is associated with poor premorbid functioning, a significant family history of psychopathological disorders, and a poor prognosis (Fenton and McGlashan 1991).

COMMUNICATIONS. People with disorganized schizophrenia experience persistent and severe perceptual problems. Verbal responses may be marked by looseness of associations or incoherence. Clang associations or word salad may be present. **Blocking,** a sudden cessation in the train of thought, is frequently observed.

PHYSICAL NEEDS. Grooming is neglected. Hair may be dirty and matted, and clothes are inappropriate and stained. There is no awareness of social expectations. A client may be too disorganized to carry out simple activities of daily living.

Basic goals for nursing intervention include encouraging optimal level of functioning, preventing further regression, and offering alternatives for inappropriate behaviors whenever possible. Refer to Table 19–14 for basic nursing considerations.

PHYSICAL BEHAVIORS. Behavior is often described as bizarre. A client may twirl around the room or make strange gestures with his or her hands and face. Social behavior is often primitive or regressed. For example, a client may eat with his or her hands, pick his or her nose, or masturbate in public. Typical behaviors include posturing, grimacing or giggling, and mirror gazing.

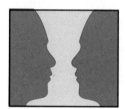

Case Study: Working with a Person with Disorganized Thinking

Martin Taylor, a 36-year-old white unemployed man, has been transferred to an inpatient psychiatric unit for further evaluation. He is accompanied to the unit by his mother and sister. He had been previously hospitalized for three years with the diagnosis of chronic schizophrenia and was doing well at home until two months ago. His only employment was for five months as a janitor after high school graduation. Other significant family history includes a twin brother who died of a cerebral aneurysm in his teens. Martin tells the nurse he has used every street drug available, including LSD and intravenous heroin. His mother states that as a teenager, before his substance abuse, he was an excellent athlete who received average grades. At the age of 17, he had his first psychotic break in the setting of polysubstance abuse. His behavior became markedly bizarre (e.g., eating cat food and swallowing a rubber-soled shoe that required an emergency laparotomy).

Ms. Lamb is Martin's primary nurse. Ms. Lamb meets with Martin after speaking with his mother and sister. Martin is unshaven and his appearance is disheveled. He is wearing a red headband in which he has placed popsicle sticks and scraps of paper. He chain smokes during the interview and frequently gets up and paces back and forth. He tells the nurse that he is Alice from *Alice In the Underground* and that people from space hurt him with needles. His speech pattern is marked by associative looseness and occasional blocking. For example, he often stops in the middle of a phrase and giggles to himself. At one point, when he started to giggle, Ms. Lamb asked him what he was thinking about. He stated, "You interrupted me." At that point, he began to shake his head while repeating in a sing-song voice, "Shake them tigers . . . shake them tigers . . . shake them tigers." He denies suicidal or homicidal ideation. Ms. Lamb notes that Martin has a great deal of difficulty accurately perceiving what is going on around him. He has markedly regressed social behaviors. For example, he eats with his hands and picks his nose in public. He has no apparent insight into his problems; he tells Ms. Lamb that his biggest problem is the people in space.

Assessment

OBJECTIVE DATA

1. Associative looseness
2. Giggles and mumbles to self
3. Poorly and bizarrely dressed
4. Low level of functioning
5. History of bizarre behavior
6. Restless, pacing, and chain smoking
7. Regressed social behaviors
8. Occasional blocking

Assessment
(Continued)

SUBJECTIVE DATA

1. "I am Alice in the Underground."
2. "People from space hurt me with needles."
3. "You interrupted me," in response to being asked what he was thinking.
4. Denies suicidal or homicidal impulses.
5. "My biggest problems are the people from space."

Nursing Diagnosis

Ms. Lamb identifies Martin's deterioration of functioning as one priority for intervention. Ms. Lamb's first diagnosis follows:

1. *Ineffective individual coping* related to confused thought processes and lack of motivation to respond, as evidenced by inability to meet basic needs.
   - Regressed social behaviors
   - Poorly and bizarrely dressed
   - Low level of functioning
   - Frequent looseness of association

Planning

CONTENT LEVEL—PLANNING GOALS

Nursing Diagnosis	Long Term Goals	Short Term Goals
1. *Ineffective individual coping* related to confused thought processes and lack of motivation, as evidenced by inability to meet basic needs	1. Martin will be able to perform three skills in daily living within one month.	1a. Martin will be able to bathe independently in one week. 1b. Martin will make his bed in two weeks. 1c. Martin will be able to make a sandwich with the aid of the nurse in three weeks.

PROCESS LEVEL—NURSES' REACTIONS AND FEELINGS

Working with a client who has limited potential for relating, poorly defined ego boundaries, and limited social skills and who demonstrates regressed bizarre behaviors requires a great deal of skill, patience, and peer support. In the presence of delusions, bizarre behaviors, and regressed social skills, health care workers can experience helplessness, feel overwhelmed, and become anxious. Some anxiety may be caused by empathizing or acknowledging the client's deeply repressed feelings of inferiority, fear, and anger. At times, nurses may have similar repressed feelings that they find difficult to deal with, which may cause them to withdraw from the client in an attempt to minimize their awareness of uncomfortable feelings. Often, the more withdrawn and regressed the client is, the more taxing he or she is to health care workers. Team involvement is necessary to promote success and continued interest in the client. For example, frequent team meetings among the recreational therapist, occupational therapist, nurses, social worker, and psychiatrist can sustain interest in a client's progress, provide mutual support for members of the health care team, and provide new data for reformulating goals and interventions.

Intervention

Ms. Lamb discussed Martin at the weekly health care team conference. Because Martin has a chronic history of deterioration, all members of the health care team agreed to work together on a few concrete goals. A trial daily checklist for activities of daily living was devised for use during the first week and to be reviewed at the next meeting. It included such items as the following:

1. Makes bed
2. Brushes teeth
3. Combs hair
4. Shaves
5. Showers
6. Makes two meals a week
7. Wears clean clothing

Continued on following page

Evaluation

After one month, Martin is able to carry out basic activities of daily living when constant reminders are given. He is able to bathe, shave, comb his hair, and dress more appropriately when given simple instructions and encouragement. The goal of making a sandwich or fixing a simple lunch has not yet been met; Martin starts to eat the food before the task of finishing the sandwich is completed. The social worker is trying to place Martin in a group home where his socialization skills can be increased, his isolation decreased, and his level of functioning maintained.

Undifferentiated Schizophrenia

In the undifferentiated type of schizophrenia, there are *active signs of the disorder* (positive or negative symptoms), but the individual does not meet the criteria for paranoia, catatonia, or disorganized type (APA 1991). Undifferentiated schizophrenia has an early and insidious onset (early-mid teens) like that of disorganized schizophrenia. However, the premorbid state is less predictable, and the disability remains fairly stable, although persistent, over time (Fenton and McGlashan 1991).

Residual Type of Schizophrenia

In the residual type of schizophrenia, there are no longer active phase symptoms, but evidence of two or more residual symptoms continues. Residual symptoms include

- Lack of initiative, interests, or energy
- Marked social withdrawal
- Impairment in role function (wage earner, student, homemaker)
- Marked speech deficits (circumstantial, vague, and poverty of speech or content of speech)
- Odd beliefs, magical thinking, and unusual perceptual experiences

Similar principles of care, as with withdrawn, paranoid, and disorganized schizophrenia, apply to people with undifferentiated and residual schizophrenia as dictated by the client's behavior.

Summary

Psychotic symptoms in schizophrenia are more pronounced and disruptive than symptoms found in other disorders. The basic differences are in degree of severity, withdrawal, alteration in affect, impairment of intellect, and regression.

Hypotheses for explaining the symptoms of schizophrenia are discussed: neurochemical (catecholamines and serotonin), genetic, neuroanatomical, developmental, and family theories. However, no one theory at present can account for all phenomena found in the various schizophrenic disorders.

During the nurse's work with schizophrenic clients, specific symptoms are evident. No one symptom is found in all cases. The positive and negative symptoms of schizophrenia are discussed. The *positive* symptoms are more florid (hallucinations, delusions, looseness of associations) and respond better to antipsychotic drug therapy. The *negative* symptoms of schizophrenia (poor social adjustment, lack of motivation, withdrawal) can be more debilitating and do not respond to neuroleptic (antipsychotic) therapy.

Some nursing diagnoses discussed include *altered thought process, impaired communications,* and *ineffective individual coping.*

Planning on the content level is discussed, and a variety of short term and long term goals are proposed for each of the nursing diagnoses. Planning on the process level involves awareness of personal feelings and reactions to clients' feelings and behaviors. The person with schizophrenia may exhibit strong dependent, angry, and eroticized transferences, among other feelings and reactions, that warrant supervision and peer support for the nurse expected to deal with these issues.

Interventions for people with schizophrenia include therapeutic interventions, health teaching, activities of daily living, somatic therapies, therapeutic environment, and psychotherapy. Each area is discussed, and examples are given.

Paranoid, catatonic (withdrawn and excited), and disorganized schizophrenia are briefly overviewed. Specific nursing interventions are outlined, and a case study for each is presented. Undifferentiated and residual types of schizophrenia are also briefly discussed.

References

Acker C. Drug offers hope to schizophrenia. Philadelphia Inquirer, June 21, 1993.

Addington J, Addington D, Maticka-Tyndale E. Cognitive functioning and positive and negative symptoms in schizophrenia. Schizophrenia Research, 5(2):123, 1991.

American Psychiatric Association. Diagnostic and Statistical Manual of Mental Disorders, 3rd ed, revised (DSM-III-R). Washington, DC: American Psychiatric Association, 1987.

American Psychiatric Association: DSM-IV Options Book: Work in Progress. Washington, DC: American Psychiatric Association, 1991.

Baldwin LJ, et al. Decrease excessive water drinking by chronic mentally ill forensic patients. Hospital and Community Psychiatry, 43(5):507, 1992.

Beard MT, et al. Activity therapy as a reconstructive plan on the social competence of chronic hospitalized patients. Journal of Psychosocial Nursing and Mental Health Services, 16(2):33, 1978.

Berkow R, et al. (eds). Merck Manual, 16th ed. Rahway, NJ: Merck Research Laboratories, 1992.

Black DW, Yates WR, Andreasen NC. Schizophrenia, schizophreniform disorders and delusional paranoid disorders. In Talbott JA, Hales RE, Yudofsky SC (eds). Textbook of Psychiatry. Washington, DC: American Psychiatric Press, 1988.

Bowen M. Family Therapy in Clinical Practice. New York: Jason Aronson, 1978.

Bugle C, Andrew S, Heath. Early detection of water intoxication. Journal of Psychosocial Nursing, 30(11):31, 1992.

Cook JC. Interpreting and decoding autistic communication. Perspectives in Psychiatric Care, 9(1): 1971.

Dixon, et al. Drug abuse in schizophrenic patients: Clinical correlates and reasons for use. The American Journal of Psychiatry, 148(2):224, 1991.

Falloon IRH. Family stress and schizophrenia: theory and practice. Psychiatric Clinics of North America, 9(1):165, 1986.

Falloon IRH, et al. Family management in the prevention of exacerbations of schizophrenia. New England Journal of Medicine, 306:1437, 1982.

Fenton WS, McGlashan TH. Natural history of schizophrenic subtypes. I: Longitudinal study of paranoid, hebephrenic, and undifferentiated schizophrenia. Archives of General Psychiatry, 48(11):969, 1991.

Field WE, Jr. The Psychotherapy of Hildegard E. Peplau. New Braunfels, TX: Atwood Printing, 1979.

Field WE, Ruelke W. Hallucinations and how to deal with them. American Journal of Nursing, 73(4):638, 1973.

Garza-Trevino ES, et al. Neurobiology of schizophrenic syndromes. Hospital and Community Psychiatry, 41(9):971, 1990.

Goldman MB. A rational approach to disorders of water balance in psychiatric patients. Hospital and Community Psychiatry, 42(5):488, 1991.

Gottesman II, Shield S. Schizophrenia, the Epigenetic Puzzle. New York: Cambridge University Press, 1982.

Grebb JA, Cancro R. Schizophrenia: Clinical features. In Kaplan HI, Saddock BJ (eds). Comprehensive Textbook of Psychiatry, vol I. Baltimore: Williams & Wilkins, 1989.

Hertz MI. Recognizing and preventing relapse in patients with schizophrenia. Hospital and Community Psychiatry, 35(4):344, 1984.

Hinsie L, Cambell RJ. Psychiatric Dictionary, 5th ed. New York: Oxford University Press, 1984.

Javitt DC, Zurkin SR. Recent advances in the phencyclidine model of schizophrenia. American Journal of Psychiatry, 148(10):1201, 1991.

Kahn ME. Psychotherapy with chronic schizophrenics: Alliance, transference and countertransference. Journal of Psychosocial Nursing, 22(7):20, 1984.

Kaplan HI, Sadock BJ. Synopsis of Psychiatry, 6th ed. Baltimore: Williams & Wilkins, 1991.

Karb VB, Queener SF, Freeman JB. Handbook of Drugs for Nursing Practice. St. Louis: CV Mosby, 1989.

Kolb LC, Brodie HKH. Modern Clinical Psychiatry, 10th ed. Philadelphia: WB Saunders, 1982.

Lamb RH, et al. Families of schizophrenics: A movement in jeopardy. Hospital and Community Psychiatry, 37(4):353, 1986.

Lancaster J. Schizophrenic patient activity groups as therapy. American Journal of Nursing, 76(6):949, 1976.

Lehmann HE, Cancro R. Schizophrenia: Clinical features. In Kaplan HI, Sadock BJ (eds). Comprehensive Textbook of Psychiatry, 4th ed. Baltimore: Williams & Wilkins, 1985.

Levinson DF. Pharmacologic treatment of schizophrenia. Clinical Therapy, 13(3):326, 1991.

MacKinnon RA, Michels R. The Psychiatric Interview in Clinical Practice. Philadelphia: WB Saunders, 1971.

Maxmen JS. Psychotrophic Drugs Fast Facts. New York: WW Norton, 1991.

Menninger WW. Dealing with staff reactions to perceived lack of progress by chronic mental patients. Hospital and Community Psychiatry, 35(8):805, 1984.

Moller MD. Understanding and Communicating with an Individual Who Is Hallucinating (video). Omaha, NE: NurScience, 1989.

Mosher LR. A psychosocial approach to returning schizophrenia. The Schizophrenic Outpatient, 1:1, 1982.

Preston T, Johnson J. Clinical Psychopharmacology. Miami: Med Master, 1991.

Sandy KR, Kay SR. The relationship of pineal calcification to cortical atrophy in schizophrenia. International Journal of Neuroscience, 57(3–4):179, 1991.

Schatzberg AF, Cole JO. Manual of Clinical Psychopharmacology, 2nd ed. Washington, DC: American Psychiatric Press, 1991.

Schizophrenia: The present state of understanding—Part I. Harvard Mental Health Letter, 8(11):1, 1992.

Schizophrenia: The present state of understanding—Part II. Harvard Mental Health Letter, 8(12):1, 1992.

Smoyak SA, Hildegard E. Peplau awarded honorary doctorate. Journal of Psychosocial Nursing, 32(11):45–46, 1994.

Sullivan HS. The Interpersonal Theory of Psychiatry. New York: WW Norton, 1953.

Swonger A, Matejski. Nursing Pharmacology. Glenview, IL: Scott, Foresman, 1988.

Talbott J, Hales R, Yadofsky SC. Textbook of Psychiatry. Washington, DC: American Psychiatric Press, 1988.

Vidal G. The Second American Revolution and Other Essays (1976–1982). New York: Random House, 1982.

Zahniser JH, Courey RD, Herghbarger K. Individual psychotherapy with schizophrenic outpatients in the public mental health systems. Hospital and Community Psychiatry, 42(9):906, 1991.

Further Reading

Aaronson LS. Paranoia as a behavior alienation. Perspectives in Psychiatric Care, 15(1), 1977.

Arieti S. American Handbook of Psychiatry, vol 3. New York: Basic Books, 1974.

Bruch H. Psychotherapy in schizophrenia: Historical considerations. In Strauss J (ed). The Psychotherapy of Schizophrenia. New York: Plenum Book Company, 1980.

Cancro R. Individual psychotherapy in the treatment of chronic schizophrenic patients. American Journal of Psychotherapy, 37(4):493, 1983.

Chapman AH. Textbook of Clinical Psychiatry: An Interpersonal Approach. Philadelphia: JB Lippincott, 1976.

Crow TJ. Positive and negative schizophrenic symptoms and the rule of dopamine. British Journal of Psychiatry, 137:383, 1980.

Irving S. Basic Psychiatric Nursing, 3rd ed. Philadelphia: WB Saunders, 1983.

Johnson-Soderberg S. Theory and practice of scapegoating. Perspectives in Psychiatric Care, 15(4):153, 1977.

Lickey ME, Gordon B. Drugs for Mental Illness: A Revolution in Psychiatry. New York: WH Freeman, 1983.

Rickelman B. Brain bio-amines and schizophrenia: A summary of research findings and implications for nursing. Journal of Psychosocial Nursing and Mental Health Services, 17(9):28, 1979.

Roy A. Foreword. The Psychiatric Clinics of North America, 9(1):1, 1986.

Scherer JC. Nurses' Drug Manual. Philadelphia: JB Lippincott, 1985.

Schwartz LH, Schwartz JL. The Psychodynamics of Patient Care. Englewood Cliffs, NJ: Prentice Hall, 1972.

Schwartz MS, Schockley EL. The Nurse and the Mental Patient. New York: John Wiley & Sons, 1956.

Scrak BM, Greenstein RA. Tardive dyskinesia evaluation in a nurse managed prolixin program. Journal of Psychosocial Nursing, 24(5):10, 1986.

Spitz HI. Contemporary trends in group psychotherapy: A literature survey. Hospital and Community Psychiatry, 35(2):132, 1984.

Torry ER. Management of chronic schizophrenic outpatients. Psychiatric Clinics of North America, 9(1):143, 1986.

Weich MJ. Transitional language. In Grolnick SA, Barkin L (eds). Between Reality and Fantasy. New York: Jason Aronson, 1978.

Weiner H. Schizophrenia: Etiology. In Kaplan HI, Sadock BJ (eds). Comprehensive Textbook of Psychiatry, 4th ed. Baltimore: Williams & Wilkins, 1985.

White EM, Kahn ME. Use of modification in group psychotherapy with chronic schizophrenic outpatients. Journal of Psychosocial Nursing and Mental Health Services, 20(2), 1982.

Self-study Exercises

Match the theory of schizophrenia (right column) with the concepts central to that theory (left column).

1. ___D___ Catecholamines
2. ___C___ Identical twin 35–60% concordant schizophrenia
3. ___E___ Double bind
4. ___B___ Hostile environment and lack of consensual validation for the infant
5. ___E___ Scapegoating
6. ___G___ Children of normal parents placed for adoption in homes where schizophrenia later develops do not show increased rate of schizophrenia
7. ___A___ Ventricular enlargement

A. Neuroanatomical

B. Developmental

C. Genetic

D. Dopamine hypothesis

E. Family

Place T (true) or F (false) next to each statement.

8. ___F___ It is impossible to understand a person when his speech is characterized by looseness of association.
9. ___T___ Hallucinations, delusions, and neologisms are examples of positive symptoms.
10. ___F___ Ambivalence in relationships is found only in the mentally ill.
11. ___T___ A man hears the stock market is down and takes that as a sign that God will destroy the world. This is an example of an idea of reference.

Write brief responses in answer to the following.

12. Discuss the difference between a hallucination and a delusion and give examples.

13. Depersonalization and derealization are examples of _____.

14. Give an example of

    A. Clang association

B. Neologism

C. Word salad

15. Name two possible short term goals for *altered thought process*.

A. _____

B. _____

Circle all correct answers.

16. Circle possible outcomes of unresolved countertransferential reactions by a nurse.

    A. Denial
    B. Withdrawal from client
    C. Increase in nurse's self-esteem
    D. Burnout

17. Circle all of the possible outcomes of effective health teaching with client and family. Cross out those that are not possible outcomes.

    A. Increase compliance with medication
    B. Increase problem-solving skills
    C. Minimize misunderstanding of the schizophrenic member within the family or community group
    D. Reduce the occurrence of schizophrenic symptoms from the ingestion of certain drugs (e.g., marijuana, amphetamines)
    E. Help the family identify those symptoms that may signal a possible relapse

18. Circle all the possible effects of neuroleptics (antipsychotic medication).

    A. Reduction in intensity of hallucinations and delusions
    B. Improvement in thought processes
    C. Increase in affect and motivation
    D. Decrease in the intensity of paranoid reactions
    E. Increase in ability to function socially

Place H (hallucinations), D (delusions), or HD (hallucinations and delusions) next to the appropriate intervention.

19. __D__ Look for themes in the client's speech patterns.
20. __H__ Tell the client you do not hear the voices he or she hears.
21. _____ Point out reality and attempt to empathize with the client's experience.
22. _____ Discredit the validity of perceptions (e.g., those so-called voices).
23. _____ Do not argue with the client over the validity of this thinking.
24. __B__ Always validate reality.
25. __B__ Clarify misinterpretations of the environment.
26. __B__ Do not pretend to understand the client when you do not.
27. __D__ Place the focus of difficulty in understanding on yourself (e.g., "I am having a difficult time understanding you.").

Place T (true) or F (false) next to each statement.

28. __F__ All the extrapyramidal side effects are reversible.
29. __T__ Specific antipsychotics are often ordered because of their specific side effects.
30. __F__ The only problem with antipsychotics is that tolerance develops.
31. __T__ Tardive dyskinesia, weight gain, and impotence are among the most troubling side effects in outpatient management.
32. __T__ Fatal side effects from the neuroleptics (antipsychotics) are rare.
33. __F__ A person in a catatonic stupor is totally unaware of anything going on around him or her.
34. __T__ Physical needs may take the highest priority when a person is in either extreme catatonic excitement or stupor.

True (T) or false (F). The following can result from frequent team evaluation of the treatment plan for a chronic schizophrenic client.

35. __T__ Reassessment of problems; important needs may have have missed.
36. __T__ Re-evaluation of the client's strengths and identification of alternative interventions.
37. __T__ Reassessment of goals can renew interest in the client.

True (T) or false (F). A person with paranoid schizophrenia

38. __T__ Often has better ego functions than a person with any other schizophrenic disorder
39. __T__ Uses sarcasm and hostility to maintain emotional distance.
40. __F__ Needs help with grooming and dress
41. __T__ Uses projection as a main defense mechanism

Multiple choice

42. Jerry P., a 17-year-old youth, had a paranoid psychotic break after the death of his twin brother. He was sure everyone wanted him dead and that his food was poisoned. He heard the voice of God demanding that he join his brother. He would not bathe or change his clothes because he believed that the warlocks could then take over his body. Of the following possible nursing diagnoses, which has the highest priority?

   A. *Alteration in nutrition: less than body requirements*
   B. *Alteration in health maintenance*
   C. *Potential for self-harm*
   D. *Alteration in thought processes*

43. If Tom thought his food was poisoned, the nurse should first

   A. Discuss nutrition with Tom
   B. Get an order for tube feedings
   C. Offer Tom food in its own containers (e.g., milk, oranges)
   D. Show him how irrational his thinking is

44. When Tom says, "You are wearing a red sweater. That means you are against me today," he is experiencing

   A. Delusion
   B. Hallucination
   C. Idea of reference
   D. Fantasy

45. When speaking to a person who is paranoid, you would consider all of the following *except*

    A. Use simple, clear language.
    B. Refrain from touching the client.
    C. Be warm and enthusiastic.
    D. Clarify and reiterate your role in a patient manner.

46. Which activity would you choose *initially* for a person who was paranoid?

    A. Listening to music alone
    B. Poker with two other people
    C. Team volley ball
    D. Model airplanes, concentrating by self

47. Medication appropriate for a person in extreme psychomotor agitation is

    A. Lithium
    B. Chlorpromazine (Thorazine)
    C. Chlordiazepoxide hydrochloride (Librium)
    D. Trihexyphenidyl hydrochloride (Artane)

CHAPTER 20

Cognitive Impairment Disorders

Brenda Lewis Cleary

OUTLINE •

KEY TERMS AND CONCEPTS • • • • • • • • • • • • • • • •

**The key terms and concepts listed here also appear in bold where they are
defined or discussed in this chapter.**

AGNOSIA

AGRAPHIA

ALZHEIMER'S DISEASE

APHASIA

APRAXIA

COGNITIVE IMPAIRMENT DISORDER

CONFABULATION

DELIRIUM

DEMENTIA

DYSGRAPHIA

HALLUCINATIONS (TACTILE, VISUAL)

HYPERMETAMORPHOSIS

HYPERORALITY

HYPERVIGILANT

ILLUSIONS

MNEMONIC DISTURBANCE

PERSEVERATION

PRIMARY DEMENTIA

PSEUDODEMENTIAS

SECONDARY DEMENTIA

OBJECTIVES ■

After studying this chapter, the student will be able to:

1. Describe the clinical picture of delirium and contrast it with the clinical picture of dementia.
2. Identify three nursing diagnoses useful for a client with delirium, including supportive data.
3. Formulate three realistic and measurable goals for a client with delirium.
4. Summarize the essential somatic and psychotherapeutic interventions for a client with delirium.
5. Discuss three essential features for each of the four stages of Alzheimer's disease.
6. Give an example of the following phenomena assessed during the progression of Alzheimer's disease:
   A. Apraxia
   B. Agnosia
   C. Aphasia
   D. Confabulation
   E. Hyperorality
7. Choose two nursing diagnoses suitable for a client with Alzheimer's disease and formulate two goals for each.
8. Identify at least three specific nursing interventions for a client with Alzheimer's disease in each of the following areas:
   A. Communication
   B. Activities of daily living
   C. Therapeutic environment
   D. Health teaching with families

The term *organic mental disorders* has long been used to alert clinicians to the possibility of an underlying physical disorder as the cause of mental disturbances. However, the DSM-IV has replaced the term with **cognitive impairment disorder.** The organic mental disorders now include (1) Delirium, Dementia, and Amnestic disorder and other cognitive disorders; (2) mental disorders due to General Medical Conditions; and (3) Substance-Related Disorders.

Table 20–1 identifies the three cognitive impairment disorders and gives a brief description of each. This chapter addresses the broad categories of delirium and dementia because these are by far the most common conditions that nurses encounter.

Delirium usually has a sudden onset and is generally reversible with proper treatment of the underlying cause or causes. **Delirium** can be defined as an acute and reversible condition with multiple etiologies (APA 1987).

Dementia most often has a slow and insidious onset and in many cases, an irreversible course. However, the prognosis depends on the underlying cause. Dementias such as those of the Alzheimer type, which involve *primary* encephalopathy, have no precisely known cause or cure; thus, they are considered irreversible. On the other hand, dementias that are *secondary* to other pathological processes (e.g., neoplasms, trauma, infections, or toxic disturbances) may be improved when the underlying cause is eliminated.

In the next section, the delirium that is a relatively common occurrence in an intensive care unit (ICU) (sometimes referred to as ICU psychosis) is discussed. In the section on dementia, Alzheimer's disease is used as an example.

Figure 20–1 identifies the placement of cognitive impairment disorders on the mental health continuum.

		Table 20–1 ■ **SUMMARY OF COGNITIVE IMPAIRMENT DISORDERS**	
SYNDROME	**CHARACTERISTICS**	**IMPAIRMENT IN SOCIAL AND OCCUPATIONAL FUNCTIONING**	**POSSIBLE CAUSES**
Group 1: Cognitive Impairment Is Relatively Global			
Delirium	• Fluctuating levels of awareness during the day • Clouding of consciousness (confused and disoriented) • Perceptual disturbances (illusions and hallucinations) • Memory, especially recent memory, is disturbed • Alteration in sleep-wake cycle • EEG changes • Developed over a short period of time • Reversible when underlying cause has been treated	Severe	Metabolic, nutritional, or toxic disorders, e.g.: • Hypoxia • Hepatic or renal disorders • Postoperative states • Psychoactive substances • Intoxication or withdrawal
Dementia	• Slow, insidious onset • Impaired long and short term memory • Deterioration of cognitive abilities—judgment, abstract thinking • Often irreversible if untreatable • Significant impairment in social and occupational functioning	Severe	• May be primary (e.g., Alzheimer's disease, Pick's disease, or multi-infarct dementia) • May be secondary (e.g., Parkinson's disease, multiple sclerosis, AIDS, hypothyroidism, or Huntington's chorea) • Prolonged or untreatable delirium
Amnestic Syndrome (relatively uncommon)	• Impairment in short and long term memory • Inability to learn new material • Remote memory better than that of recent events • Confabulation • Apathy, lack of initiative • Emotionally bland	Moderate to severe	• Head trauma • Hypoxia • Herpes simplex encephalitis • Thiamine deficiency • Chronic use of alcohol or other substances

AIDS = acquired immunodeficiency syndrome; EEG = electroencephalographic.

Delirium

Nurses frequently encounter delirium on medical and surgical units in the general hospital setting. During specific phases of a hospital stay, *confusion* may be noted—for example, after surgery or after the introduction of a new drug. The second or third hospital day may herald the onset of confusion for older people with difficulty adjusting to an unfamiliar environment.

Delirium is a syndrome caused by transient malfunctioning but with no destruction of brain cells. De-

lirium is *always* secondary to an underlying medical condition or toxic agent. Delirium may be followed by complete recovery; however, if left untreated or if it is untreatable, delirium may progress to a chronic mental syndrome (dementia) or to irreversible coma and death. Delirium is most often seen in children and those over 60 years of age, although it does occur in all age groups.

The DSM-III-R (APA 1987) states that the essential feature of delirium is a *clouded state of consciousness* and

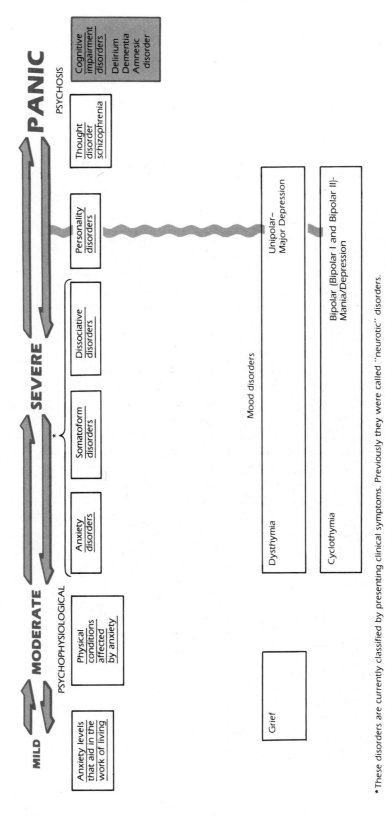

Figure 20–1. Mental health continuum for the cognitive impairment disorders.

*These disorders are currently classified by presenting clinical symptoms. Previously they were called "neurotic" disorders.

that delirium in general is marked by cognitive difficulties. Thinking, memory, attention, and perception are generally disturbed. The clinical manifestations of delirium develop over a short period of time (hours to days) and appear on a continuum from mild to severe.

Delirious states usually *fluctuate in intensity*; consequently, nurses may note varying levels of consciousness and orientation during a short period of time. The condition is often intensified at night. Delirium is characterized by progressive disorientation to time and place. Because delirium increases psychological stress, supportive interventions that lower anxiety and reduce manifestations of the delirium can restore a sense of control (Foreman 1990).

Theory

Delirium can be caused by any number of pathophysiological conditions. Some of the most common causes of delirium include infections, postoperative states, metabolic abnormalities, hypoxic conditions, drug withdrawal states, and drug intoxications. Multiple drug use, or polypharmacy, is frequently implicated in acute organic mental syndromes (Gomez and Gomez 1987). Some drugs commonly responsible for delirium states are digitalis preparations and antihistamines, as well as medications used for treatment of hypertension, depression, and Parkinson's syndrome (Dwyer 1987; Ellison 1984; Lipowski 1983). Other likely offenders include anticholinergics, benzodiazepines, and analgesics, which induce central nervous system depression (Andresen 1992). Box 20–1 lists common causes of delirium.

Assessment

Problems in accurate assessment of delirium or an acute confusional state often arise. First, the degree of reversibility can be determined only retrospectively. Second, the relative acuity of the onset depends on how noxious the stimuli are. Third, a reversible confusional state (delirium) can occur simultaneously with or be superimposed upon an irreversible mental syndrome (dementia), further complicating accurate identification (Foreman 1986).

Generally, the nurse suspects the presence of delirium when a client rather *abruptly develops a clouded state of consciousness. Confusion is a hallmark of delirium.* The person may have difficulty with orientation first to

---

Box 20–1. SUMMARY OF THE ETIOLOGICAL FACTORS OF DELIRIUM

Some major categories that can cause alteration in neural function are outlined below.

A. **Drug intoxications and withdrawals**
   1. Alcohol, anxiolytics, opioids, and central nervous system stimulants (e.g., cocaine and crack)
B. **Infections**
   1. Systemic: pneumonia, typhoid fever, malaria, urinary tract infection, and septicemia
   2. Intracranial: meningitis and encephalitis
C. **Metabolic disorders**
   1. Hypoxia (pulmonary disease, heart disease, and anemia)
   2. Hypoglycemia
   3. Sodium, potassium, calcium, magnesium, and acid-base imbalances
   4. Hepatic encephalopathy or uremic encephalopathy
   5. Thiamine (vitamin B_1) deficiency (Wernicke's encephalopathy)
   6. Endocrine disorders (e.g., thyroidism or parathyroidism)
   7. Hypothermia or hyperthermia
   8. Diabetic acidosis
D. **Neurological diseases**
   1. Seizures
   2. Head trauma
   3. Hypertensive encephalopathy
E. **Drugs**
   1. Digitalis, steroids, lithium, levodopa, anticholinergics, benzodiazepines, central nervous system depressants, or tricyclic antidepressants
F. **Postoperative states**
G. **Psychosocial stressors**
   1. Relocation or other sudden changes
   2. Sensory deprivation or overload
   3. Sleep deprivation
   4. Immobilization

Data from Andresen G. How to assess the older mind. RN, 34, July 1992; Dwyer BJ. Cognitive impairment in the elderly: Delirium, depression, or dementia? Focus on Geriatric Care and Rehabilitation, 1(4):1, 1987; Foreman MD. Acute confusional states in hospitalized elderly: A research dilemma. Nursing Research 35(1):34, 1986; Perry SW, Markowitz J. Organic mental disorders. In Talbott et al. (eds). Textbook of Psychiatry. Washington, DC: American Psychiatric Press, 1988; Seltzer B, Frazier SH. Organic mental disorders. In Nicholi AA (ed). The Harvard Guide to Modern Psychiatry. Cambridge, MA: The Belknap Press of Harvard University, 1980.

time, then to place, and last to person. For example, a client with delirium may think the year is 1972 instead of 1994, that the hospital is home, and that the nurse is his wife. Orientation to person is usually intact to the extent that the person is aware of his or her own identity (Kaplan and Sadock 1991).

Fluctuating levels of consciousness tend to be unpredictable. Disorientation and confusion are usually markedly worse at night and during the early morning. In fact, some clients may be confused or delirious only at night and may remain lucid during the day, a situation referred to as "sundowning."

Data collection should include assessment of (1) cognitive and perceptual disturbances, (2) physical needs, and (3) mood and behavior.

ASSESSING COGNITIVE AND PERCEPTUAL DISTURBANCES

It may be difficult to engage delirious persons in conversation, because they are easily distracted and display marked attention deficits. *Memory* is often impaired. In mild delirium, memory deficits are noted upon careful questioning. In more severe delirium, memory difficulties usually take the form of obvious difficulty in processing and remembering recent events. For example, the person might ask when a son is coming to visit, even though the son has left only an hour before.

Perceptual disturbances are also common. Perception is the processing of information about one's internal and external environment (Dwyer 1987). Various misinterpretations of reality may take the form of illusions or hallucinations.

Illusions are errors in perception of sensory stimuli. For example, a person may mistake folds in the bedclothes for white rats, or the cord of a window blind for a snake. The stimulus is a real object in the environment; however, it is misinterpreted and often becomes the object of the client's projected fear. Illusions, unlike delusions or hallucinations, can be explained and clarified for the individual.

Hallucinations are false sensory stimuli (see Chapter 19). **Visual hallucinations** are a diagnostic symptom of an organic mental syndrome. **Tactile hallucinations** may also be present. For example, delirious people may become terrified when they "see" giant spiders crawling over the bedclothes or "feel" bugs crawling on their bodies. Auditory hallucinations occur more often in other psychiatric disorders, such as schizophrenia and depression.

The delirious individual generally possesses an awareness that something is very wrong. For example, the delirious person may state, "My thoughts are all jumbled." When perceptual disturbances are present, the emotional response is one of fear and anxiety. Verbal and psychomotor signs of agitation should be noted.

Two abilities requiring high cortical functioning may be impaired in delirium: the ability to name an object and the ability to write. **Agnosia** refers to the inability to name objects. Agnosia hampers the person's ability to name objects because it alters perception of stimuli. **Dysgraphia** refers to the inability to write (APA 1987).

ASSESSING PHYSICAL NEEDS

PHYSICAL SAFETY. A person in delirium becomes disoriented and may try to go home. Or, a person may think he or she is home and jump out of a window trying to get away from "invaders." Wandering, pulling out tubes such as intravenous (IV) lines and Foley catheters, and falling out of bed are common dangers that require nursing intervention.

An individual experiencing delirium has difficulty processing stimuli in the environment. Confusion magnifies the inability to recognize reality. The physical environment should be made as concrete and clear as possible. Elevating the head of the bed slightly can maximize orientation to place. Objects such as clocks and calendars can maximize orientation to time. Eyeglasses, hearing aids, and adequate lighting without glare can maximize the person's ability to interpret more accurately what is going on in the environment. Nagley (1986) recommends nurse-client interaction for periods of at least five to 10 minutes, when no other nursing actions are being carried out, to help decrease anxiety and increase awareness of reality.

BACTERIOLOGICAL SAFETY. Self-care deficits may lead to skin breakdown and leave a person prone to infection. Often, this condition is compounded by poor nutrition, forced bedrest, and possible incontinence. These are areas requiring nursing assessment and intervention.

BIOPHYSICAL SAFETY. Autonomic signs, such as tachycardia, sweating, flushed face, dilated pupils, and elevated blood pressure, often occur. These changes must be monitored and documented carefully and may require immediate medical attention.

There are usually changes in the sleep-wake cycle, and the level of consciousness may range from lethargy to stupor or from semicoma to hypervigilance. The **hypervigilant** person is extraordinarily alert and may have difficulty getting to sleep or may be actively disoriented and agitated throughout the night.

ASSESSING MOODS AND PHYSICAL BEHAVIORS

The delirious individual's behavior and mood may change dramatically within a short period of time. Moods may swing back and forth from fear, anger, and anxiety to euphoria, depression, and apathy. These labile moods are often accompanied by physical behaviors associated with feeling states. A person may strike out from fear or anger or may cry, call for help, curse, moan, and tear off clothing one minute and become apathetic or laugh uncontrollably the next. In short, behavior and emotions are erratic and fluctuating. Lack of concentration and disorientation complicate interventions. The following vignette illustrates delirium:

Mrs. Lew, 68, lives with her daughter, Jean, and son-in-law, Ted. Mrs. Lew takes care of the house, does the cooking and cleaning and is active in church activities. She has a number of lady friends and once a week goes to the movies or plays cards "with the girls." One day after work, her daughter Jean comes home to find her mother huddled in a darkened room, terrified. When asked what is wrong, Mrs. Lew states that the house is under siege and she has to hide in the dark, "Can't you hear them?" Outside, the sound of drilling and pounding by construction workers is what Jean hears. Mrs. Lew is experiencing illusions. That night when Jean goes in to check on her mother, she discovers that her mother is gone. Jean finds her wandering in her nightclothes three blocks from the house.

Jean becomes terribly alarmed, even though her husband insists that "it's normal for old people to become confused" and that they have just been fortunate up to now. Mrs. Lew is taken to the emergency room. Upon admission she is oriented to person, but not to time and place. She thinks it is 1942 and that she is back in London during World War II. She keeps shouting, "Get those men out of my house!" She "picks" at things in the air and is so restless, agitated, and incoherent that a mental examination is postponed.

Physical examination of Mrs. Lew reveals bilateral rales in the lower lobes of the lungs, a high white blood cell count, temperature of 101.3° F, and mild dehydration. Diagnosis of bilateral lower lobe pneumonia is made, and within 24 hours of treatment with intravenous fluid, antibiotics, and diligent nursing care, Mrs. Lew becomes oriented to time, place, and person, and her "clouded state of consciousness" disappears.

The doctor explains to the family that Mrs. Lew's temporary delirium had been secondary to the infectious process and that the symptoms of delirium often may appear hours before the signs or symptoms of the underlying disorder.

Nursing Diagnosis

The nurse analyzes the data and considers areas that warrant the highest priority. Delirium is always secondary to some physical disorder or drug toxicity. The priority in medical care is to identify the cause and take appropriate medical or surgical intervention. If the underlying disorder is corrected and reversed, complete recovery is possible. If, however, the underlying disorder is not corrected and persists, sustained neuronal damage can lead to irreversible changes, such as dementia and even death.

Therefore, nursing concerns center on (1) assisting with proper medical management to eradicate the underlying cause, (2) prevention of physical harm due to confusion, aggression, or electrolyte and fluid imbalance, and (3) supportive measures to relieve distress.

Safety needs play a substantial role in nursing care. Clients often perceive the environment as distorted. Objects in the environment are often misperceived (illusions), or imagined (hallucinations), and people and objects may be misinterpreted as threatening or harmful. These misinterpretations are often acted on. For example, feeling threatened or thinking that common medical equipment is harmful, the client may pull off an oxygen mask, pull out an intravenous or nasogastric tube, or try to flee. In such a case, a person demonstrates a *high risk for injury* related to altered cerebral function, as evidenced by sensory deficits or perceptual deficits.

Fever and dehydration may be present; thus, fluid and electrolyte balance may need to be managed. If the underlying cause of the client's delirium results in fever, decreased skin turgor, decreased urinary output or fluid intake, and dry skin or mucous membranes, then the nursing diagnosis of *fluid volume deficit* is appropriate. Fluid volume deficit may be related to fever, electrolyte imbalance, reduced intake, or infection.

Because there may be disruption in the sleep-wake cycle, the client may be less responsive during the day and may become disruptively wakeful during the night. At no time, either during the day or at night, does the client experience a restful sleep; instead, he or she suffers from a fragmented and fluctuating state of consciousness (McHugh and Folstein 1987). Therefore, *sleep pattern disturbance* related to impaired cerebral oxygenation or disruption in consciousness is a likely diagnosis.

Because the delirious person is usually dazed or drowsy, he or she can rarely sustain attention to any mental task. The client may be roused for a moment and coaxed to respond before slipping back to unresponsiveness. Memory is often impaired. Because sustaining communication with a delirious client is difficult, *impaired verbal communication* related to cerebral hypoxia or decreased cerebral blood flow, as evidenced by confusion or clouding of consciousness, may be diagnosed.

Perceptions are disturbed during delirium. Hallucinations, distractibility, illusions, and disorientation are often part of the clinical picture. If any of these symptoms are evident, then *altered thought processes* related to alteration in biochemical compounds, cerebral anoxia, or other disorders must be considered.

Other nursing concerns include *fear, self-care deficits,* and *impaired social interaction. Fear* is most common and may be related to illusions, delusions, or hallucinations, as evidenced by verbal and nonverbal expressions of fearfulness.

Planning

Planning involves (1) the content level—planning goals, and (2) the process level—nurses' reactions and feelings.

CONTENT LEVEL—PLANNING GOALS

The client may present various needs; however, *high risk for injury* is usually present. Appropriate goals might include the following:

- Client will remain safe and free from injury while in the hospital.
- During lucid periods, client will be oriented to time, place, and person with the aid of nursing interventions, such as clocks, calendars, and other orienting information.
- Client will refrain from removing tubes (e.g., intravenous, nasogastric, catheter, or oxygen) while confused, with the aid of frequent orientation by nurse and medications, if necessary.
- Client will remain free from falls and injury while confused, with the aid of nursing safety measures.
- Client will respond to external controls if he or she becomes physically aggressive toward self, other clients, or staff.

Maintaining fluid and electrolyte balance is crucial if the underlying disorder increases the person's metabolic rate and results in increased temperature and decreased circulating fluid volume. Goals for *fluid volume deficit* could include the following:

- Client will be well hydrated within 24 hours.
- Client will take 8 ounces of protein fluid orally once every hour.
- Client's skin turgor or appearance of mucous membranes will be normal within 24 hours.
- Client's specific gravity (urine) will be within normal limits by (time).
- Client's vital signs will become or will remain stable by (time).

Sleep pattern disturbance can cause a problem not only for the delirious client but also for the other clients because it may lead to sleep deprivation and fatigue for all concerned. Creative nursing measures are often necessary. Possible goals follow:

- Client will sleep four to six hours per night within three days.
- Client will state that he or she is comfortable at night with aid of nursing measures (e.g., back rub, light, frequent orientation, or nurse's presence) within (time).
- Client will state accurately where he or she is and what is happening to him or her when awake at night.
- Client's anxiety level will decrease from panic levels to severe or moderate, with aid of medication and nursing interventions.

Because *impaired verbal communication* and *altered thought processes* are usually evident, goals that enhance the client's ability to interpret reality are useful. For example:

- Client will demonstrate accurate perception of the environment by discharge.
- Client will be able to tell nurse where he or she is by (date).
- Client will state that he or she understands that the nurse will provide support when the client is "hearing" or "seeing" frightening things.
- Client will name correct environmental objects or sounds after experiencing an illusion, with aid of nursing interventions.
- Client will be free of hallucinations.

Goals for improving the client's psychosocial status and reducing *fear* and *impaired social interaction* include

- Client will recognize the presence of significant others.
- Verbal ("I am so afraid," "What's happening to me") and nonverbal (e.g., staring, grimacing, or

agitation) expressions of fear will measurably decrease.

PROCESS LEVEL—NURSES' REACTIONS AND FEELINGS

In many cases, delirium is more easily associated with a medical disease. First, delirium is usually treated on a medical or surgical unit, and second, delirium usually responds to specific medical or surgical interventions, depending on the underlying cause. Frequently, this syndrome reverses within a few days or less when the underlying cause is identified and treated. Because the behaviors exhibited by the client can be directly attributed to temporary medical conditions, intense countertransferential reactions are less likely to occur. In fact, intense conflicting emotions are less likely to occur in nurses working with a client in delirium than in those working with a client with dementia, which will be discussed later in this chapter.

However, the nurse may find some behaviors associated with delirium especially "challenging." Because delirium is predictably more severe and incapacitating during the night and early morning hours, night staff often find that a loud, frightened, agitated, and perhaps aggressive, client can take up much of their time. Experienced nurses are aware that even though people in delirium may appear "out of it," they often respond to a calm and caring approach. Maximizing the person's contact with reality during the night can help reduce the anxiety and terror these patients often experience.

However, there are certain instances that may cause staff to have strong negative feelings toward a client in delirium. Such incidents might include withdrawal. For example, nurses working with clients in alcohol withdrawal delirium might think a person "did it to herself" or is "getting what he deserves." Often, nurses exhibit judgmental attitudes toward persons in withdrawal. Unfortunately, negative attitudes by staff serve only to increase the client's anxiety, intensifying feelings of terror, confusion, and defensive behavior.

Interventions

Delirium is seen in all areas of hospital nursing, but most commonly in postoperative, intensive care, and medical units. Whatever the setting, *delirium requires medical intervention.* As mentioned previously, if the underlying cause of delirium is not treated, permanent brain damage may ensue. The nurse is usually charged with meeting many of the physical needs of the delirious person. In addition, lowering the client's anxiety and fear and increasing the client's orientation to reality can help promote comfort, reduce secondary injury, and minimize aberrant behaviors stimulated by fear and misinterpretation of the environment (e.g., climbing out of bed, fighting staff, or pulling out intravenous tubes). Continuous reality orientation is a major goal with a delirious client, although the same information may have to be repeated many times an hour. Table 20–2 suggests basic nursing interventions for use with a delirious client. Suggested interventions address communication and physical needs.

Evaluation

Long term goals for a delirious person include (1) the client will remain safe while in the hospital, and (2) the client will be oriented to time, place, and person by discharge. However, the short term goals need constant assessment.

For example, are the client's pulse and blood pressure within normal limits? Are all intravenous and nasogastric tubes, Foley catheters, and hyperalimentation lines intact? Is the client's urine specific gravity within normal limits? Is the client oriented to time and place? Has the client's anxiety level decreased from panic levels to severe or moderate? Frequent checking of parameters of short term goals helps monitor successful treatment of the client's underlying medical condition, as well as responses to nursing interventions, and helps prevent possible progression to more profound levels of illness or to irreversible neuronal changes.

THE CLINICAL PICTURE OF DELIRIUM

Delirium is relatively common in an intensive care unit (ICU) and is presented here as an example. In the past, the term ICU *psychosis* was used to describe this phenomenon.

A PERSON IN AN INTENSIVE CARE UNIT

The incidence of delirium in an acute care hospital is estimated to be as high as 80% (Roland and Mariche 1992). Nothing quite prepares a person for admission into an ICU. The environment of the ICU is filled with

Table 20–2 ■ NURSING INTERVENTIONS AND RATIONALES: PSYCHOTHERAPEUTIC NEEDS OF A PERSON IN DELIRIUM

INTERVENTION	RATIONALE

Nursing Diagnosis: *Sensory/perceptual alterations* related to transitory neurological dysfunction, as evidenced by fluctuating level of consciousness, perceptual disturbances (illusion or hallucination), and reduced awareness of environment

INTERVENTION	RATIONALE
1. Introduce self and call client by name at the beginning of each contact.	1. With short term memory impairment, person is often confused and needs orienting to time, place, and person.
2. Maintain face-to-face contact.	2. If client is easily distracted, he or she needs help to focus on one stimulus at a time.
3. Use short, simple, concrete phrases.	3. Client may not be able to process complex information.
4. Briefly explain everything you are going to do before doing it.	4. Explanation prevents misinterpretation of action.
5. Encourage the family and friends (one at a time) to take a quiet, supportive role.	5. Familiar presence lowers anxiety and increases orientation.
6. Keep room well lit.	6. Lighting provides accurate environmental stimuli to maintain and increase orientation.
7. Keep head of bed elevated.	7. Helps provide important environmental cues.
8. Provide clocks and calendars.	8. These cues help orient client to time.
9. Encourage family members to bring in meaningful articles from home (e.g., pictures or figurines).	9. Familiar objects provide comfort and support and can aid orientation.
10. Encourage client to wear personal eyeglasses or hearing aid.	10. Helps increase accurate perceptions of visual auditory stimuli.
11. Make an effort to assign the same personnel on each shift to care for client.	11. Familiar faces minimize confusion and enhance nurse-client relationships.
12. When hallucinations are present, clarify reality, e.g., "I know you are frightened, but I do not see spiders on your sheets."	12. Person feels understood and reassured while validating reality.
13. When illusions are present, clarify reality, e.g., "This is a coat rack, not a man with a knife . . . see? You seem frightened. I'll stay with you for a while."	13. Misinterpreted objects or sounds can be clarified, once pointed out.
14. Inform client of progress during lucid intervals.	14. Consciousness fluctuates: client will feel less anxious knowing where he or she is and who you are during lucid periods.
15. Ignore insults and name calling, and acknowledge how upset the person may be feeling. For example:	15. Terror and fear are often projected onto environment. Arguing or becoming defensive only increases client's aggressive behaviors and defenses.

CLIENT: You incompetent jerk, get me a real nurse, someone who knows what they are doing.

NURSE: You are very upset. What you are going through is very difficult. I'll stay with you.

| 16. If client behavior becomes physically abusive, first, set limits on behavior, e.g., "Mr. Jones, you are not to hit me or anyone else. Tell me how you feel." | 16. Clear limits need to be set to protect client, staff, and others. Often client can respond to verbal commands. Use chemical and physical restraints as a last resort, if at all. |

or

"Mr. Jones, if you have difficulty controlling your actions, we will help you gain control." Second, check orders for use of chemical or physical restraints (e.g., posey belt).

Continued on following page

Table 20–2 ▪ NURSING INTERVENTIONS AND RATIONALES: PSYCHOTHERAPEUTIC NEEDS OF A PERSON IN DELIRIUM *Continued*

INTERVENTION	RATIONALE
Nursing Diagnosis: *Risk for injury* related to neurological changes, as evidenced by unstable vital signs, potential for dehydration, skin breakdown, and sleep deprivation	
1. Check pulse periodically, e.g., every hour or every four hours, depending on underlying conditions.	1. Pulse is a good indicator of course of delirium.
2. Check temperature regularly.	2. Hyperthermia may occur.
3. Schedule medications and treatments so that they do not interfere with client's sleep or rest.	3. Fluctuating levels of consciousness prevent adequate rest.
4. Check for skin breakdown and apply appropriate interventions, e.g., turn every two hours; apply lotion for bony prominences; and ensure proper positioning.	4. Breakdown combined with dehydration can develop rapidly when client is on bed rest.
5. Monitor fluid intake and output.	5. Monitor electrolyte balance.
6. Check skin turgor and urine specific gravity. If client appears dehydrated, forcing fluids may be appropriate.	6. Forcing fluids replaces fluid volume.
7. If skin turgor and urine specific gravity are within limits, or if the client is overhydrated, fluids should *not* be forced.	7. Monitoring prevents fluid volume overload.

an air of urgency, danger, and heroism. The aim in the ICU is to maintain life and to resuscitate those clients whose tie to life is tenuous. Strange noises, odors, and bright, fluorescent lights fill the room and add to the confusion of a newly admitted client. Most ICUs are open, with client beds surrounding the core of activity, the nursing station. The client has little privacy and is able to observe life and death situations merely by glancing across the room. Even though a client is in plain view, he or she may be socially isolated. The medical jargon that is the predominant ICU language is totally alien. Isolation is the hallmark of the ICU setting (Cassem and Hackett 1978; Robinson 1974).

Many ICUs are centrally located to give easy access to the operating room, pharmacy, and laboratory. Therefore, they seldom have windows, which adds to disorientation for the client. Equipment that monitors fluid intake and heart rate are huddled around the client's bedside. The client is connected to these life support companions by a series of tubings. For the critically ill client, tubes seem to be connected to every appendage and orifice the client can supply. The ICU environment is terrifying and foreign for most clients. Clients who have had little exposure to the hospital setting are particularly vulnerable.

Being admitted to an ICU denotes a threat to life and evokes predictable psychological and emotional reactions in clients. Fear of death is a common reaction, as is fear of being maimed by the various procedures needed to sustain life. Surrounded by an unfa-

miliar environment and unfamiliar people, the client may become panicked. Nothing else distorts personality quite like panic. Staff are often amazed at the changes in the client's personality when the panic subsides.

ASSESSMENT

Patients in ICUs may develop delirium within two to five days of admission. Initially, the patient may be hypervigilant and then may become disoriented and even belligerent. The development of illusions, hallucinations, delusions, severe agitation, and fluctuating levels of consciousness may ensue. Sleep deprivation is frequently observed and, along with sensory alteration, may be both an outcome as well as an important factor in the etiology of delirium.

Fear and anxiety are bound closely together in the ICU. The technological environment of the ICU coupled with the likelihood of intrusive procedures can bring about an anxious and fearful patient response. Fear of imminent death is always a concern for the patient and family.

Frequent assessments of mental status should be performed on any medicosurgical patient who develops acute cognitive and behavioral changes. The patient must be seen by a registered nurse for the explicit purpose of testing cognitive function (Sullivan and Fogel 1986).

In addition to mental status, the nurse will want to assess communication impairment, sensory depth deficits, threats to safety, and the effects of medication. Richardson (1983) suggested that nursing observations include sensory perceptual abilities, expressive abilities, receptive abilities, and behavioral consequences.

It is also important that the nurse assess all medications every day because a nurse is in a key position to recognize drug reactions before delirium actually occurs. The nurse should also aggressively assess any other potential organic abnormalities because treatment of underlying organic causes is the first order of delirium management (Sullivan et al. 1991). In summary, nursing assessment should detect the following symptoms: disorientation, fluctuating behavior, and disturbances of consciousness, perception, speech, sleep/wake cycle, and psychomotor activity (Morency 1990).

INTERVENTION

Medical management of delirium involves treating the underlying organic causes. Judicious use of neuroleptic or antianxiety agents may also be useful in controlling agitation and psychotic symptomatology (Sullivan et al. 1991).

Nursing care involves encouraging one or two significant others to stay with the delirious patient to avoid the use of physical restraints (Sullivan et al. 1991). The nurse should promote adequate and accurate sensory input through the use of eyeglasses or hearing aids, if appropriate. Communication should occur face to face and should consist of simple, direct statements. Orientation may be aided by maintaining familiar objects in the environment and by using orienting devices, such as calendars and clocks. Although the use of reality orientation is extremely questionable in patients with chronic confusion, it may prove very helpful during lucid periods in patients with acute confusional states, such as delirium. The nurse should allow patients to care for themselves in areas of competency and do only what is necessary for the patient, while providing continuous explanations when physical care is given. Safety may be aided by the use of night lighting and soothing music and by the involvement of significant others in supervising the patient. As with any patient exhibiting psychotic symptoms, a tolerant, calm, matter-of-fact approach by the nurse has proved to be most helpful.

The following vignette highlights the fear and confusion a person may experience when admitted to an ICU.

Clinical Vignette: A Client with Delirium

A 55-year-old married man, Mr. Arnold, is admitted to the ICU after having a three-vessel coronary artery bypass. Mr. Arnold's surgery has taken longer than usual and has necessitated his remaining on a cardiac pump for three hours. He arrives in the ICU without further complications. Upon awakening from the anesthesia, he hears the nurse exclaim, "I need to get a gas." Another nurse answers in a loud voice, "Can you take a large needle for the injection?" During this period of time, Mr. Arnold experiences the need to urinate and asks the nurse very calmly if he can go to the bathroom. Her reply is, "You don't need to go; you have a tube in." He again complains about his discomfort and assures the nurse if she will let him go to the bathroom, he will be fine. The nurse informs Mr. Arnold that he cannot urinate and that he has to keep the "mask" on so that she can get the "gas" and check his "blood levels." Upon hearing this, Mr. Arnold begins to implore louder and states that he sees the bathroom sign "over there." He assures the nurse that he will only take a minute. In reality "the sign" is an exit sign in the unit. To prove to him that a bathroom does not exist in the ICU and that the sign does not indicate a bathroom, the nurse takes off the restraints and leads Mr. Arnold to the sign. He abruptly breaks away from the nurse's grasp and runs toward the entrance to the ICU. He discovers a door, which is the entrance to the nurses' lounge, barricades himself in the room, and pulls out his chest tube, Foley catheter, and intravenous lines. Needless to say, he finds the bathroom that is connected to the lounge. Ten minutes later, the nurses and security personnel break through the barricade and escort Mr. Arnold back to bed. When he becomes fully alert and oriented a day later, he tells the nurses his perception of the previous events. Initially he thought he had been kidnapped and was being held against his will (the restraints had been rather tight). When the nurse had yelled out about blood gas, he had thought she was going to kill him with noxious gas through his face mask (the reason he did not want to wear the face mask). All he could think about was escaping his tormentor and executioner. In this case, the nurse did not assess the alteration in Mr. Arnold's mental status and had allowed him to get out of bed. The medical jargon and loud voices had perpetuated his confusion and distortion of reality. The nurses could have told Mr. Arnold where he was, that the nursing staff were caring for him, and could have better explained the function of his Foley catheter. Furthermore, the staff could have brought in family members to help calm and orient Mr. Arnold.

Dementia

Severe memory loss is *not* a normal part of growing older. Slight forgetfulness is a common phenomenon of the aging process (age-associated memory loss), but not to the extent that it interferes with one's activities of daily living. The majority of people who live to very old age never experience a significant memory loss or any other symptoms of dementia. Most of us know of people in their 80s and 90s who lead active lives, with their intellect intact. Margaret Mead, Pablo Picasso, Duke Ellington, Count Basie, and Ansel Adams are all examples of people who were still active in their careers when they died; all were past 75 years of age (Picasso was 91) (Mace and Rabins 1981). The slow, mild cognitive changes associated with aging should not impede social or occupational functioning.

Dementia, on the other hand, is marked by progressive deterioration in intellectual functioning, memory, and ability to solve problems and learn new skills. Judgment and moral and ethical behaviors decline as personality is altered.

Teusink and Mahler (1984) stress the progressive decline of the demented person in activities of everyday life, the failure of memory and intellect, and the disorganization of the personality. A person's declining intellect often leads to emotional changes, lack of self-care, and finally, to hallucinations and delusions —that is, psychotic symptoms brought on by organic changes.

A person may have progressive dementia from various etiologies; Alzheimer's disease, Pick's disease, Huntington's chorea, multi-infarct dementias, advanced alcoholism (such as in Korsakoff's syndrome), and Creutzfeldt-Jakob's disease are a few examples.

Dementias can be classified as primary or secondary in nature. **Primary dementia** is not reversible, is progressive, and is not secondary to any other disorder. For example, Alzheimer's disease accounts for about 65% of all dementias, and multi-infarct dementia accounts for about 10% of all dementias (Kaplan and Sadock 1991). Both Alzheimer's and multi-infarct dementias are *primary,* progressive, and irreversible.

Secondary dementia occurs as a result of some other pathological process (e.g., metabolic, nutritional, or neurological). Acquired immunodeficiency syndrome (AIDS)–related dementia is an example of a secondary dementia increasingly seen in health care settings. The exact prevalence of AIDS-related dementia is not known, but it may occur in up to 70% of all

---

Box 20–2. SUMMARY OF THE ETIOLOGICAL FACTORS OF DEMENTIA

A. Primary dementias
   1. Alzheimer's disease (senile and presenile dementia)
   2. Multi-infarct dementia
   3. Pick's disease
B. Secondary dementias
   1. Infections
      a. Tuberculosis
      b. Tertiary neurosyphilis
      c. Fungal, bacterial, and viral infections of the brain (Creutzfeldt-Jacob disease)
   2. Trauma; subdural hematoma, hypoxia
   3. Toxic and metabolic disturbances
      a. Korsakoff's syndrome; Wernicke's encephalopathy (thiamine deficiency)
      b. Pernicious anemia (vitamin B_{12} deficiency)
      c. Folic acid deficiency
      d. Thyroid, parathyroid, or adrenal gland dysfunction
      e. Liver or kidney dysfunction
      f. Metal poisoning
      g. Carbon dioxide and some drugs
   4. Neoplasms
   5. Other neurological diseases
      a. Huntington's chorea
      b. Parkinson's disease
      c. Multiple sclerosis
      d. Cerebellar degenerations
   6. Normal pressure hydrocephalus
   7. AIDS-related dementia (HIV encephalopathy)

Data from Mace NL, Rabins PB. The 36 Hour Day. Baltimore: Johns Hopkins University Press, 1981; Seltzer B, Frazier SH. Organic mental disorders. In Nicholi AA (ed). The Harvard Guide to Modern Psychiatry. Cambridge, MA: The Belknap Press of Harvard University, 1980.
AIDS = acquired immunodeficiency syndrome; HIV = human immunodeficiency virus.

AIDS clients. Some clinicians refer to this phenomenon as human immunodeficiency virus (HIV) *encephalopathy* or AIDS dementia complex (Kaplan and Sadock 1991). Refer to Chapter 26 for more information on

Table 20-3 ■ NURSING ASSESSMENT: DELIRIUM VERSUS DEMENTIA

DELIRIUM	DEMENTIA
Onset	
Acute impairment of orientation, memory, intellectual function, judgment, and affect	Slow, insidious deterioration in cognitive functioning
Essential Feature	
Clouded state of consciousness, fluctuating levels of consciousness, and cognitive impairment	Progressive deterioration in memory, orientation, calculation, and judgment; symptoms do not fluctuate
Etiology	
The syndrome is secondary to many underlying disorders that cause temporary, diffuse disturbances of brain function	The syndrome is either *primary* in etiology or *secondary* to other disease states or conditions
Course	
The clinical course is usually brief (hour to days); prolonged delirium may lead to dementia	Progresses over months or years; often irreversible
Speech	
May be slurred; reflects disorganized thinking	Generally normal in early stages; progressive aphasia; confabulation
Memory	
Short term memory impaired	Short term, then long term, memory destroyed
Perception	
Visual or tactile hallucinations; illusions	Hallucinations not prominent
Mood	
Fear, anxiety, and irritability most prominent	Mood labile; previous personality traits become accentuated, e.g., paranoid, depressed, withdrawn, and obsessive-compulsive
EEG	
Pronounced diffuse slowing or fast cycles	Normal or mildly slow

Data from Kaplan HI, Sadock BJ. Synopsis of Psychiatry, 6th ed. Baltimore: Williams & Wilkins, 1991.
EEG = electroencephalogram.

AIDS. Other secondary dementias can result from viral encephalitis, pernicious anemia, folic acid deficiency, and hypothyroidism.

Korsakoff's syndrome is an example of secondary dementia due to thiamine deficiency that may be associated with prolonged, heavy alcohol ingestion. Along with progressive mental deterioration, Korsakoff's syndrome is marked by peripheral neuropathy, cerebellar ataxia, confabulation, and myopathy (APA 1987).

Some secondary dementias are treatable. In about 15% of dementia cases, the symptoms of dementia can be reversed when the underlying cause is eliminated (Cohen 1984; Kaplan and Sadock 1991; Pajik 1984). Refer to Box 20-2 for a summary of illnesses that can cause dementia. At times it is necessary to distinguish delirium from dementia. Some major differences are outlined in Table 20-3.

Because dementia of the Alzheimer's type accounts for 65% of all dementias and is the fourth most prevalent cause of death after heart disease, cancer, and stroke in the adult population (Powell and Courtice 1983), Alzheimer's disease is discussed in detail as an example of dementia.

Alzheimer's Disease

Alzheimer's disease attacks indiscriminately. Its victims are male and female, black and white, rich and poor, all with varying degrees of intelligence. Although the disease can strike at a younger age, most victims are 65 years of age or older. Alzheimer's is "a thief of minds, a destroyer of personalities, wrecker of family finances and filler of nursing homes" (AARP 1986).

Yasmin Aga Khan (the daughter of the famous actress, Rita Hayworth, who was stricken with Alzheimer's disease) once stated that to watch a once proud, beautiful, independent, dignified human being transformed into a dependent, mentally disabled person is terrifying. An estimated 4 million Americans are afflicted with the disease; it affects up to 11% of the population over 65 years of age and 25% or more of the population over 85 years (McHugh and Folstein 1987).

A wide range of problems may masquerade as dementia and be mistaken for Alzheimer's disease. For example, depression in the elderly is often misdiagnosed as dementia (see Table 20–4). Other disorders that often mimic dementia include drug toxicity, metabolic disorders, infections, and nutritional deficiencies. Disorders that mimic dementia are sometimes referred to as **pseudodementias.** That is, although the symptoms may suggest dementia, a careful examination may reveal another diagnosis altogether. Newbern (1991) emphasizes the critical nature of careful evaluation of tractable conditions and that histories of alcohol abuse and affective disorders must be considered. When a cognitive impairment syndrome is suspected, clinical evaluation includes the following (Perry and Markowitz 1988):

1. Confirm the diagnosis
2. Search for underlying causes
3. Identify psychosocial stressors that may exacerbate related emotional and behavioral problems

The diagnosis of Alzheimer's disease includes ruling out other pathophysiological conditions through the history and physical and laboratory tests, such as:

- Chest and skull x-rays
- Electroencephalography
- Electrocardiography
- Urinalysis
- Sequential Multiple Analyzer—12-test serum profile
- Serum triiodothyronine and thyroxine tests
- Complete blood count (CBC)
- Venereal Disease Research Laboratories (VDRL) test
- Serum creatinine assay
- Electrolyte assessment
- Serum vitamin B_{12} assay
- Serum folate assay
- Vision and hearing evaluation

Computed tomography, positron emission tomography, and other developing scanning technology possess diagnostic capabilities by revealing brain atrophy and ruling out other conditions, such as neoplasms. Mental status questionnaires and various other tests to determine mental status deterioration and brain damage are important parts of the assessment.

In addition to a complete physical and neurological exam, the importance of a complete patient history and description of recent symptoms (including questioning significant others) cannot be overestimated (Souder 1992). Gray-Vickrey (1988) recommends a psychiatric history, a dietary evaluation, and a medication evaluation.

Recent studies have revealed that certain clinical diagnostic criteria can substantially improve the diagnostic accuracy in Alzheimer's disease. Four studies using the National Institute of Neurological and Communicative Disorders and Stroke and the Alzheimer's Disease and Related Disorders Association (NINCDS-ADRDA) guidelines found a 91% specificity for diagnosing Alzheimer's Disease (Dewan and Gupta 1992).

Because depression in the elderly is the disorder most often confused with dementia, Table 20–4 identifies features that aid in distinguishing depression from dementia. Medical and nursing personnel should be cautioned, however, because dementia and depression *can* coexist in the same person (Burnside 1988). In fact, studies indicate that as high as 15–30% of people diagnosed with Alzheimer's dementia also meet DSM-IV criteria for a depressive disorder (Alzheimer's Disease Part I 1992).

Theory

Although the cause of Alzheimer's disease is not known, there are numerous hypotheses regarding etiology. These include (1) the genetic model, (2) the toxin model, and (3) other causes. Neurochemical changes and pathological changes are also discussed.

GENETIC MODEL. Family members of Alzheimer's patients have a risk of acquiring the disease that is higher than that of the general population. Recent studies provide evidence that in some *early onset* families, there appears to be a defect on chromosome 21 and chromosome 14. Other studies indicate that *late onset* familial Alzheimer's disease may be linked to alterations on chromosome 19 (Alzheimer's Association 1993). Studies also indicate that the cumulative risk to first-degree relatives approaches or slightly exceeds 50% (Li et al. 1991).

TOXIN MODEL. High levels of aluminum have been found in some people who have died from Alzheimer's disease. Actually, along with the neurofibrillary tangles and senile plaques, increased aluminum concentration is a common finding on autopsy. The question that remains is whether the increased aluminum preceded the disease or was poorly metabolized

Table 20-4 ■ DEPRESSION VERSUS DEMENTIA IN THE ELDERLY

DEMENTIA	DEPRESSION
1. Recent memory is impaired. In early stages, patient attempts to hide cognitive losses; is skillful in covering up.	1. Patient readily admits to memory loss; other cognitive disturbances may or may not be present.
2. Symptoms progress slowly and insidiously; difficult to pinpoint onset.	2. Symptoms are of relatively rapid onset.
3. Approximate or "near-miss" answers are typical; tries to answer.	3. "Don't know" answers are common; patient does not try to recall or answer.
4. Patient struggles to perform well but is frustrated.	4. Little effort to perform; is apathetic; seems helpless and pessimistic.
5. Affect is shallow or labile.	5. Depressive mood is pervasive.
6. Attention and concentration may be impaired.	6. Attention and concentration are usually intact.
7. Changes in "personality," e.g., from cheerful and easygoing to angry and suspicious.	7. Personality remains stable.

as a result of the disease. Aluminum toxicity is known to cause dementia in animals (Wells 1982).

According to the Alzheimer's Association, the link between aluminum and Alzheimer's disease remains questionable. For example, renal dialysis patients who experienced immense increases in aluminum exhibited symptoms of dementia but did not develop the classic plaques and tangles of Alzheimer's disease. This information makes a very strong point against the hypothesis that aluminum toxicity causes Alzheimer's disease.

OTHER CAUSES. Other etiologies under investigation include a slow viral infection, an autoimmune process, head trauma, environmental factors, and decreased blood flow to the brain (Li et al. 1991).

NEUROCHEMICAL CHANGES. Some studies have indicated that people with Alzheimer's dementia have drastically reduced levels of the enzyme acetyltransferase, which is needed to synthesize the neurotransmitter acetylcholine. Some theorists propose that the cognitive defects that occur in Alzheimer's disease, especially memory loss, are a direct result of the reduction in acetylcholine available to the brain.

PATHOLOGICAL CHANGES. Alzheimer's disease results in cerebral atrophy and in neuritic plaques and neurofibrillary tangles that are microscopic abnormalities in brain tissue. Beta-amyloid protein (BAP) is the main component of neuritic plaques, one of the abnormal structures found in the brain of Alzheimer's patients. BAB is now the subject of intense interest in Alzheimer's research (Alzheimer's Research 1994). A more detailed description follows:

1. *Neurofibrillary tangles* form mostly in the hippocampus, the part of the brain responsible for recent (short term) memory as well as emotions. Therefore, memory and emotions are negatively affected.
2. *Senile plaques* are cores of degenerated neuron material lying free of the cell bodies on the ground substances of the brain. The quantity of plaques has been correlated with the degree of mental deterioration.
3. *Granulovascular degeneration* is the filling of brain cells with fluid and granular material. Increased degeneration accounts for increased loss of mental function. Brain atrophy is observable through the use of computed tomography. The definitive diagnosis of Alzheimer's disease can be made only through brain biopsy or autopsy. Soon, however, the diagnosis of Alzheimer's disease may be made with a simple skin test (Alzheimer's 1993).

Assessment

Alzheimer's disease is commonly characterized by progressive deterioration of cognitive functioning. Initially, deterioration may be so subtle and insidious that others may not notice. In the early stages of the disease, the affected person may be able to compensate for loss of memory. Some people may have superior social graces and charm that give them the ability to hide severe deficits in memory, even from experienced health care professionals. This "hiding" is actually a form of *denial*, which is an unconscious protective defense against the terrifying reality of losing one's place in the world. Family members may also unconsciously deny that anything is wrong as a defense against the painful awareness of deterioration of a loved one. As time goes on, symptoms become more obvious and other defensive maneuvers become evident. **Confabulation** (making up stories or answers to maintain self-esteem when the person does not remember) is noticed. For example, the nurse addresses a client who has remained in a hospital bed all weekend:

NURSE: Good morning, Ms. Jones. How was your weekend?

CLIENT: Wonderful. I discussed politics with President Clinton, and he took me out to dinner.

Confabulation is not the same as lying. When a person is lying, he or she is aware of making up an answer; confabulation is an *unconscious* attempt to maintain self-esteem.

Perseveration (the repetition of phrases or behavior) is eventually seen and often is intensified under stress. The *avoidance of answering questions* also is a mechanism by which the client is able to maintain self-esteem unconsciously in the face of severe memory deficits.

Therefore, (1) denial, (2) confabulation, (3) perseveration, and (4) avoidance of questions are four defensive behaviors the nurse might notice during assessment.

The following four signs of Alzheimer's disease have been described (Wolanin and Fraelich-Philips 1981):

1. **Aphasia** (loss of language ability), which progresses with the disease. Initially, the person has difficulty finding the correct word and then is reduced to a few words, then is finally reduced to babbling or becoming mute.
2. **Apraxia** (a loss of purposeful movement in the absence of motor or sensory impairment). The person is unable to perform once-familiar and purposeful tasks. For example, in apraxia of gait, the person loses the ability to walk. In apraxia of dressing, the person is unable to put his or her clothes on properly (may put arms in trousers or put a jacket on upside down).
3. **Agnosia** (loss of sensory ability to recognize objects). For example, the person may lose the ability to recognize familiar sounds (auditory agnosia), such as the ring of the telephone, a car horn, or the door bell. Loss of this ability extends to the inability to recognize familiar objects (visual or tactile agnosia), such as a glass, magazine, pencil, or toothbrush. Eventually the person is unable to recognize people whom he or she loves or even parts of his or her own body.

4. **Mnemonic disturbance** (memory loss). Initially the person has difficulty remembering recent events. Gradually deterioration progresses to include both recent and remote memory.

The degeneration of neurons in the brain is the wasting of working components in the brain. These cells contain memories, receive sights and sounds, and cause hormones to secrete, produce emotions, and command muscles into motion.

Essentially, with Alzheimer's disease one loses a personal history, a place in the world, and the ability to recognize the environment, and eventually, loved ones. Alzheimer's disease robs family and friends, husbands and wives, and sons and daughters of valuable human relatedness and companionship, resulting in a profound grieving process. Alzheimer's disease robs society of productive and active participants. Because of these devastating effects, it challenges mental health professionals and social agencies, the medical and nursing professions, and researchers looking for possible solutions.

Alzheimer's disease has been classified according to the stages of the degenerative process. The number of stages ranges from three to seven, depending on the source. However, four stages, discussed subsequently, are commonly used to categorize the progressive deterioration seen in victims of Alzheimer's disease (Reisberg 1984).

PHASE 1—MILD ALZHEIMER'S DISEASE

The loss of intellectual ability is insidious. The person with mild Alzheimer's disease loses energy, drive, and initiative and has difficulty learning new things. Personality and social behavior remain intact, which often influences others to minimize and underestimate the loss of the individual's abilities. The individual may still continue to work, with the extent of the dementia becoming evident in a new or demanding situation. Depression may occur early in the disease but usually lessens as the disease progresses. Activities such as doing the marketing or managing finances are noticeably impaired during this phase.

Sam Collins, 56, is a lineman for a telephone company. He feels that he is getting old. He keeps forgetting things and writes notes to himself on scraps of paper. One day on the job, he forgets momentarily which wires to connect and connects all the wrong ones, causing mass confusion for a few hours. At home, Sam flies off the handle when his wife, Jean, suggests they invite the new neighbors for dinner. It is hard for him to admit that anything new confuses him, and he often forgets names *(aphasia)* and sometimes loses the thread of conversations. Once he even forgot his address when his car broke down on the highway. He is moody and depressed and becomes indignant when Jean finds three months of unpaid bills stashed in his sock drawer. Jean is bewildered, upset, and fearful that something is terribly wrong.

According to studies quoted by Reisberg (1984), one third of individuals with Alzheimer's disease at this stage decline quickly and may be dead within three years. Another third, although their condition worsens, may still function within the community with support. The final third usually remain at this level for three years or more.

PHASE 2—MODERATE ALZHEIMER'S DISEASE

Deterioration becomes evident during the moderate phase. Often, the person with moderate Alzheimer's disease cannot remember his or her address or the date. There are memory gaps in the person's history that may fluctuate from one moment to another. Hygiene suffers, and ability to dress appropriately is markedly affected. The person may put on clothes backward, button the buttons incorrectly, or not zip zippers (this inability to carry out simple activities is *apraxia).* Often, the person has to be coaxed to bathe.

Mood becomes labile, and the individual may have bursts of paranoia, anger, jealousy, and apathy. Activities such as driving become hazardous; the person may suddenly speed up or slow down for no apparent reason or go through stop signs. Care and supervision become a full-time job for family members. Denial mercifully takes over and protects the person from the realization that he or she is losing control not only of his or her mind but also of his or her life. Along with denial, the person begins to withdraw from activities and people, since he or she often feels overwhelmed and frustrated doing things that were once easy. The person may also have moments of becoming tearful and sad.

For a short period, Sam is transferred to a less complicated work position after his inability to function is recognized. Jean drives him to work and picks him up. Sam often forgets what he is doing and stares blankly. He accuses the supervisor of spying on him. Sometimes he disappears at lunch and is unable to find his way back to work. The transfer lasts only a few months, and Sam is forced to take an early retire-

ment. At home, Sam sleeps in his clothes. He loses interest in reading and watching sports on TV and often breaks into angry outbursts over seemingly nothing. Often he becomes extremely restless and irritable and wanders around the house aimlessly.

PHASE 3—MODERATE TO SEVERE ALZHEIMER'S DISEASE

At this stage, the person is often not able to identify familiar objects or people, even a spouse *(severe agnosia).* The person needs repeated instructions and directions for the simplest tasks *(advanced apraxia):* "Here is the facecloth, pick up the soap . . . now, put water on the facecloth and rub the facecloth with soap . . . ." Often, the individual cannot remember where the toilet is and becomes incontinent. Total care is necessary at this point, and the burden on the families can be emotionally, financially, and physically devastating. The world becomes very frightening to the person with Alzheimer's disease because nothing makes sense any longer. Agitation, violence, paranoia, and delusions are more commonly seen once the mechanisms of denial and withdrawal are no longer effective. Another problem frightening to family members and caregivers is wandering behavior. It is estimated that about 70% of people with Alzheimer's disease may wander and are at risk of becoming lost (Alzheimer's Association 1993).

Institutionalization may be the most appropriate recourse at this time because the level of care is so demanding, and violent outbursts and incontinence may be crises that the family can no longer handle. Some criteria for placement in a nursing home follow:

- The person wanders.
- The person is a danger to himself and others.
- The person is incontinent.
- The person's behavior affects the sleep of others.

Sam is terrified. Memories come and then slip away. People come and go, but they are strangers. Someone is masquerading as his wife, and it is hard to tell what is reality and what is memory. Things never stay in the same place. Sometimes people hide the bathroom where he cannot find it. He in turn has to hide things to keep them safe, but he forgets where he hides them. Buttons and belts are confusing, and he doesn't know what they are doing there, anyway. Sometimes he tries to walk away from the terrifying feelings and the strangers. He tries to find something he has lost long ago . . . if he could only remember what it is.

PHASE 4—LATE ALZHEIMER'S DISEASE

Williams (1986) described what is called a Klüver-Bucy–like syndrome in late Alzheimer's disease, which includes the following symptoms. **Agraphia** (inability to read or write), **hyperorality** (the need to taste, chew, and put everything in one's mouth), blunting of emotions, visual agnosia (loss of ability to recognize familiar objects), and **hypermetamorphosis** (touching everything in sight) are all associated with this syndrome.

At this stage, the ability to talk, and eventually the ability to walk, are lost. If death due to secondary causes (e.g., infection or choking) has not come, the end stage of Alzheimer's disease is characterized by stupor and coma.

Jean and the children kept Sam at home until his outbursts became frightening. Once he was lost for two days after he somehow unlocked the front door. Jean had Sam placed in a Veterans Administration (VA) hospital. When Jean comes to visit, Sam sometimes cries. Sam never talks and is always tied into his chair when she comes to visit. The staff explains to her that although Sam can still walk, he keeps getting into other people's beds and scaring them. They explain that perhaps Sam wants comfort and misses human touch. They encourage her visits, even though Sam does not seem to recognize her. Sam does respond to music. Jean brings a radio, and when she plays the country and western music he has always loved, Sam nods and claps his hands.

Jean is torn between guilt and love, anger and despair. She is confused and depressed. Jean is going through the painful process of mourning the loss of the man she has loved and shared a life with for 34 years.

Three months after admission to the VA hospital, and eight years after the incident of the crossed wires at the telephone company, Sam chokes on some food, develops pneumonia, and dies.

Nursing Diagnosis

Care for a client with dementia, especially Alzheimer's disease, requires a great deal of patience, creativity, and maturity. The needs of such a client can be enormous for nursing staff and for families who care for their loved ones in the home. As the disease progresses, so do the needs of the client and the demands on the caregivers, staff, and family.

One of the most important areas of concern identified by both staff and families is the client's safety. Many people with Alzheimer's disease wander and may be lost for hours or days. Wandering, along with behaviors such as rummaging, may be perceived as purposeful to the Alzheimer's victim. Wandering may result from changes in the physical environment, fear caused by hallucinations/delusions, or lack of exercise (Alzheimer's Newsletter, 1993.)

Seizures are not uncommon in the later stages of this disease. Injuries from falls and accidents can occur during any stage as confusion and disorientation progress. There is a potential for burns if the client is a smoker or is unattended at the stove. Prescription drugs can be taken incorrectly or bottles of noxious fluids can be mistakenly ingested, resulting in a medical crisis. Therefore, *high risk for injury* is always present.

Throughout the course of the disease, the nursing diagnosis may not change (e.g., *high risk for injury*); however, the "related to" and "as evidenced by" components may, and these are the parameters from which meaningful and effective goals are formed. *High risk for injury* can be related to confusion, unsteady gait, faulty judgment, poisons, household hazards, and loss of short term memory. *High risk for injury* can be evidenced by impaired mobility, sensory deficits, history of accidents, and lack of knowledge of safety precautions all of which increase the risks of hospitalization (Hall 1991). Depending on the etiology or evidence, goals are formulated.

Communicating with the client with Alzheimer's disease becomes progressively more difficult. Comprehension diminishes, and the person finds it difficult and then is unable to name objects (*aphasia*). Eventually the inability to recognize objects (*agnosia*) appears. As the person becomes more disoriented, memory diminishes and attention span decreases, and the person is unable to maintain continuity in relationships, events, and the environment. Lowering the person's levels of fear and anxiety, providing a sense of safety, and emphasizing visual and verbal clues are helpful to patients with a diagnosis of *impaired verbal communication*. Impaired verbal communication may be related to many disorders, including aphasia and cerebral impairment. Supporting data include (1) difficulty finding the correct word and (2) inappropriate speech or response.

As time goes on, the person loses the ability to perform tasks that were once familiar and routine (*apraxia*). For example, the person's ability to dress diminishes. At first, supervision or simple directions may be enough; eventually total assistance is needed. This progression applies to bathing, hygiene, grooming, feeding, and toileting—in fact, to all areas of daily living. Therefore, *self-care deficits* involving a variety of functional abilities occur, to varying degrees. Depending on the affected person's disability, goals and interventions are planned. The most effective and respectful goals are those that allow the client to carry out as much of his or her own care as possible.

It may be difficult to view the person with Alzheimer's disease as a once-competent, humorous, and caring person whose life included family and friends. Memory impairment robs people of their continuity and place in life, along with cherished relationships and the joy of living. Unfortunately, the affected person often *is* aware of what is happening to him or her. The loss of one's sense of self causes terror, despair, and isolation. Therefore, *disturbance in self-esteem, role performance,* and *disturbance in personal identity* need to be addressed when planning care. *Powerlessness, hopelessness,* and *grieving* are also important considerations.

Evidence of hallucinations, delusions (usually paranoid), illusions, and memory impairment signals *altered thought processes* related to dementia. The nursing diagnosis of *altered thought processes* is usually part of any care plan for a person with Alzheimer's disease.

Ineffective individual coping is evident among victims of Alzheimer's disease. Besides not being able to function in one's occupational and personal life, as was previously discussed, long-standing personality traits may intensify and manifest in inappropriate behaviors. Common behaviors include hoarding, regression, and being overly demanding. Therefore, nurses and family members often intervene in behaviors that signal ineffective individual coping. Family caregivers may experience compromised or even disabling family coping.

Additional family issues may emerge. Perhaps some of the most crucial aspects of the client's care are support, education, and referrals for the family. The family loses an integral part of its unit. Family members lose the love, the function, the support, the companionship, and the warmth that this person had provided. There are always *altered family processes. Grieving* is an important process for the family to go through; it can make the task ahead somewhat clearer and, at times, less painful.

Mass and Buckwalter (1988) identified four of the most frequently used nursing diagnoses for clients with Alzheimer's disease on a special Alzheimer's unit as

1. Altered thought processes (52%)
2. Self-care deficit (48%)
3. Altered patterns of urinary elimination: incontinence (12%)
4. Altered nutrition: less than body requirements (10%)

Planning

Planning includes (1) the content level—planning goals, and (2) the process level—nurses' reactions and feelings.

CONTENT LEVEL—PLANNING GOALS

For the nursing diagnosis *high risk for injury,* many goals may be appropriate. Some follow:

- Client will remain safe in the hospital or home.
- With the aid of identification bracelet and neighborhood or hospital alert, client will be returned within three hours of wandering.
- Client will remain free of danger during seizures.
- With the aid of nursing interventions, client will not burn self.
- With the aid of nursing guidance and environmental manipulation, client will fall without hurting himself or herself.
- Client will ingest only correct doses of prescribed medications and appropriate food and fluids.

For the nursing diagnosis *impaired communication,* the following goals might be useful:

- Client will communicate needs.
- Client will answer "yes" or "no" to questions.
- Client will state needs in alternative modes when aphasic (e.g., will signal correct word upon hearing it, or will refer to picture or label).
- Client will wear prescribed glasses or hearing aid each day.

For a client with *self-care deficit,* possible goals follow:

- Client will participate in self-care at optimal level.
- Client can follow step-by-step instructions for dressing, bathing, and grooming.
- Client will put on own clothes appropriately, with aid of fastening tape (Velcro) and nursing supervision.
- Client's skin will remain intact, despite incontinence or prolonged pressure.

Disturbance in self-esteem should also be addressed. Often, nurses tend to treat older people or people with cognitive impairments as if they were children. Being treated like a child may very well foster childlike behaviors. Self-esteem is damaged, anxiety increases, and regressive behaviors are fostered. Some goals that might apply follow:

- Client will state both positive and negative comments about his or her personal level of functioning.
- Client will function at his or her highest level within the family.
- Client will state that he or she is aware that people care about him or her.
- Each day, client will participate in simple activities that bring enjoyment (e.g., singing with others, group exercises, or recounting past successes to others).

Altered thought processes, evidenced by hallucinations, delusions, illusions, and severe memory impairment, may play a large role in the care provided by the nurse or families. Some nursing goals that might be appropriate follow:

- Client will acknowledge the reality, after it is pointed out, of an object or sound that was misinterpreted (illusion).
- Client will state that he or she feels safe after experiencing hallucinations.
- Client will remain nonaggressive when experiencing paranoid ideation.
- Client will discuss some aspects of his or her life that hold pleasant memories.

Ineffective individual coping, evidenced by hoarding, regression, and demanding behaviors, can also be a challenge for both nurses and families. Goals include the following:

- Client will retain only hoarded items that do not include potentially dangerous materials, such as glass, metal, or food.
- Client will respond to suggestions by nurse to go to his or her room to masturbate when masturbating in a public area.
- Number and intensity of client's demands on staff or family will decrease with aid of nursing interventions.

Families with a demented member are under tremendous stresses. The stress of caring for an ill family member, who in many ways has become a stranger, can trigger intense feelings of anger, guilt, hopelessness, despair, and grief within the family. If the family is caring for the ill member in the home, the combination of intense emotional conflicts and overwhelming demands to meet the ill family member's multiple physical needs can be tremendous. There are almost always *altered family processes*. Divorces, separations, and other evidence of severe stress may result. Financial drains may leave the family bankrupt. Many supports are needed. Goals for *altered family processes* follow:

- Family members will have the opportunity to express "unacceptable" feelings in a supportive environment.
- Family members will have access to professional counseling.
- Family members will name two organizations within their geographical area that can offer support.
- Family members will participate in ill member's plan of care, with encouragement from staff.
- Family members will state that they have outside help that allows family members to take personal time for themselves (1–7 days) each week or month.
- Family members will have the name of three resources that can help with financial burdens and legal considerations.

In the moderate stages of the illness, nutritional intake may exceed bodily requirements. However, weight gain is not customary, perhaps because of agitation and wandering, which burn up additional calories. As the illness progresses into later stages, *altered nutrition* that is less than body requirements typically ensues. According to Wilson (1990), problems range from patients' forgetting to eat to ingesting nonedible substances. Goals for *altered nutrition* include the following:

- The client will ingest adequate calories, at least 1200 calories per day.
- The client will maintain an adequate fluid intake (1200–1500 ml per day).

The incontinence of Alzheimer's disease may be classified under the nursing diagnosis of *functional incontinence*, i.e., there is no specific physiological problem other than the person with Alzheimer's disease losing the ability to negotiate the environment for adequate toileting. Goals include

- The client will participate in a toileting program.
- As the disease progresses, however, a more realistic goal may be that the client will remain clean and dry.

PROCESS LEVEL—NURSES' REACTIONS AND FEELINGS

Nurses working in any setting with cognitively impaired clients are aware of the tremendous responsibility placed on the caregivers. Severe confusion, psychotic states, and violent and aggressive behaviors can take their toll on staff and family (Burnside 1988). Taking care of clients who are unable to communicate and who have lost the ability to relate and respond to others is extremely difficult, especially for student nurses and nurses who do not understand dementia or Alzheimer's disease.

Nurses working in facilities for clients who are cognitively impaired (e.g., nursing homes and extended care facilities) need special training. Training needs to include education about the process of the disease and effective interventions, as well as knowledge regarding the neuroleptic (antipsychotic) drugs. Support and educational opportunities should be readily available, not just to nurses but to nurse's aides, who are also often directly responsible for administering basic care.

Burnout of staff can be a problem. Burnside (1988) identifies three possible antidotes to burnout:

1. *Revise goals* so that they are realistic. Nurses sometimes set goals that are too high and not realistic. Frustration and discouragement ensue when the goals cannot be met.
2. *Refrain from being swept into a hopeless stance.* Concentrate on finding satisfaction in small accomplishments (e.g., the client is comfortable, is participating in an activity, or is less delusional than previously). Indeed, for this person, such a situation may mark quite an accomplishment.
3. *Research* is a prime factor for eliminating staff burnout. Involving nurses in research helps involve staff in an important activity that can increase nurses' knowledge for caring for the demented client and can add a feeling of purpose to a very demanding job that involves great patience and maturity.

Intervention

Dementia is a progressive global deterioration of mental functioning, with impairment of recent memory and abstract reasoning, and ultimately disorientation. Whether impairments are reversible or irreversible, several nursing interventions can be employed with the cognitively impaired. *The basic principle underlying all care for the cognitively impaired is to facilitate the highest level of functioning a person is capable of in all areas (e.g., self-care and social and family relationships).*

Treatment of dementia is, at present, palliative and supportive in nature. Medical or surgical interventions that attempt to diminish the pathophysiology remain experimental and primarily focus on replenishing neurochemicals in the brain. However, in March of 1993 the FDA approved the drug tacrine (THA, Cognex) for the treatment of mild to moderate symptoms of Alzheimer's disease. Tests showed that tacrine improved functioning and slowed the progress of the disease by about 42% in the patients who took the drug. The most serious side effect is liver damage (Tacrine update 1993).

Low-dose major tranquilizers (neuroleptic or antianxiety agents) may be administered to clients with severe agitation, aggression, or paranoid behavior. Nutrition, hygiene, safety, and elimination needs all should be managed in Alzheimer's patients. There is a strong need for further development of day care programs, respite programs, and special long term Alzheimer's care units.

According to Ninos and Makohon (1985), assisting patients to cope within their environment is the basis for treatment, particularly nursing therapy. Thus, nurses must identify and modify, where possible, specific functional disturbances and assist clients and families in compensating for such disturbances.

Intervention with family members is also critical. The effects of losing a family member to dementia—that is, watching a person who has an important role within the family unit and who is loved and is a vital part of his or her family's history deteriorate—can be devastating. The interventions discussed subsequently are useful.

PSYCHOTHERAPEUTIC INTERVENTIONS

Burnside (1988) suggests the following guidelines for implementing interventions or teaching a severely cognitively impaired person:

1. Do not provide more than one visual clue (object) at one time.
2. Know that the client may lack understanding of the task assigned.
3. Remember that relevant information is remembered longer than irrelevant information.
4. Break tasks into very small steps.
5. Give only one instruction at a time.
6. Report, record, and chart all data.

Table 20–5 gives special guidelines for nurses and family members to use to communicate with a cognitively impaired person.

HEALTH TEACHING

Educating families that have a cognitively impaired member is one of the most important areas for nurses. Families who are caring for a member in the home need to know about strategies for communication (Table 20–5), for activities of daily living (Table

Table 20–5 ■ NURSING INTERVENTIONS AND RATIONALES: COMMUNICATION NEEDS OF A COGNITIVELY IMPAIRED PERSON	
INTERVENTION	**RATIONALE**
Nursing Diagnosis: *Impaired communication* related to cerebral impairment, as evidenced by impairment in memory, judgment, and difficulty defining words and concepts	
1. Always identify yourself and call the person by name at each meeting.	1. Client's short term memory is impaired—requires frequent orientation to time and environment.
2. Speak slowly.	2. Gives client time to process information.
3. Use short, simple words and phrases.	3. Client may not be able to understand complex statements or abstract ideas.
4. Maintain face-to-face contact.	4. Maximizes verbal and nonverbal clues.
5. Be near client when talking, one or two arm-lengths away. Focus on one piece of information at a time.	5. Attention span of client is poor and easily distracted—helps client focus. Too much data can be overwhelming and can increase anxiety.
6. Talk with client about familiar and meaningful things.	6. Allows self-expression and reinforces reality.
7. Encourage reminiscing about happy times in life.	7. Remembering accomplishments and shared joys helps distract client from deficit and gives meaning to existence.
8. When client is delusional, acknowledge client's feelings and reinforce reality. Do not argue or refute delusions.	8. Acknowledging feelings helps client feel understood. Pointing out realities may help client focus on realities. Arguing can enhance adherence to false beliefs.
9. If a client gets into an argument with another client, stop the argument and get them out of each other's way. After a short while (5 minutes), explain to each client matter-of-factly why you had to intervene.	9. Prevents escalation to physical acting out. Shows respect for client's right to know. Explaining in an adult manner helps maintain self-esteem.
10. When client becomes verbally aggressive, acknowledge client's feelings and shift topic to more familiar ground, e.g., "I know this is upsetting for you, since you always cared for others . . . Tell me about your children."	10. Confusion and disorientation easily increase anxiety. Acknowledging feelings makes the client feel more understood and less alone. Topics the client has mastery in can remind him or her of areas of competent functioning and can increase self-esteem.
11. Have client wear prescription eyeglasses or hearing aid.	11. Increases environmental awareness, orientation, and comprehension, which in turn increases awareness of personal needs and the presence of others.
12. Keep client's room well lit.	12. Maximizes environmental clues.
13. Have clocks, calendars, and personal items (e.g., family pictures or Bible) in clear view of client while he or she is in bed.	13. Assists in maintaining personal identity.
14. Reinforce client's pictures, nonverbal gestures, X's on calendars, and other methods used to anchor client in reality.	14. When aphasia starts to hinder communication, alternate methods of communication need to be instituted.

20–6), and for structuring the environment (Table 20–7). Most importantly, they need to know where to get help. Help includes professional counseling and education regarding the process and progression of the disease. Families especially need to know about and be referred to community-based groups that can help shoulder this tremendous burden (e.g., day care centers, senior citizen groups, organizations providing home visits and respite care, and family support groups. The Alzheimer's Association is a national um-

brella agency that provides various forms of assistance to persons with the disease and their families. The Alzheimer's Association recently launched **Safe Return,** the first nationwide program to help locate and return missing people with Alzheimer's disease and other memory impairments (Alzheimer's Association 1993). Information regarding housekeeping, home health aides, and companions should also be available. Such outside resources can help prevent the total emotional and physical fatigue of family mem-

Table 20-6 ■ NURSING INTERVENTIONS AND RATIONALES: ACTIVITIES OF DAILY LIVING FOR A COGNITIVELY IMPAIRED PERSON

INTERVENTION	RATIONALE
Nursing Diagnosis: *Self-care deficit* **related to cognitive impairment as evidenced by deficit in:**	
Dressing and Bathing	
1. Always have client perform all tasks that he or she is capable of	1. Maintains client's self-esteem and uses muscle groups; impedes staff burnout; minimizes further regression.
2. Always have client wear own clothes, even in the hospital	2. Helps maintain client's identity and dignity.
3. Use clothing with elastic, and substitute fastening tape (Velcro) for buttons and zippers	3. Minimizes client's confusion and eases independence of functioning.
4. Label clothing items with client's name and name of item	4. Helps identify client if he or she wanders and gives client additional clues when *aphasia* or *agnosia* occurs.
5. Give step-by-step instructions whenever necessary, e.g., "Take this blouse . . . put in one arm . . . now the next arm . . . pull it together in the front . . . now . . . "	5. Client can focus on small pieces of information more easily; allows client to perform at optimal level.
6. Make sure that water in faucets is not too hot	6. Judgment lacking in client; is unaware of many safety hazards.
7. If client is resistant to doing self-care, come back later and ask again	7. Moods may be labile, and client may forget but often will comply after short interval.
Nutrition	
1. Monitor food and fluid intake	1. Client may have anorexia or be too confused to eat.
2. Offer finger food that client can walk around with	2. Increases input throughout the day; client may eat only small amounts at meals.
3. Weigh client regularly (once a week)	3. Monitors fluid and nutritional status.
4. During period of *hyperorality*, watch that client does not eat non-food items (e.g., ceramic fruit or food-shaped soaps)	4. Client will put everything thought to be food into mouth; may be unable to differentiate inedible objects made in the shape and color of food.
Bowel and Bladder Functions	
1. Begin bowel and bladder program early; start with bladder control	1. Same time of day for bowel movements and toileting—in early morning, after meals and snacks, and before bedtime—can help prevent incontinence.
2. Evaluate use of disposable diapers	2. Prevents embarrassment.
3. Label bathroom door, as well as doors to other rooms	3. Additional environmental clues can maximize independent toileting.
Sleep	
1. Since client may become awake, be frightened, cry out at night, keep area well lit	1. Reinforces orientation, minimizes possible illusions.
2. Maintain a calm atmosphere during the day.	2. Encourage a calming night's sleep.
3. If possible, allow client to sit by desk (in hospital)	3. Increases orientation and feelings of safety and decreases sense of isolation.
4. Nonbarbiturates may be ordered (e.g., chloral hydrate)	4. Barbiturates can have a paradoxical reaction, causing agitation.
5. If medications are indicated, neuroleptics with sedative properties may be the most helpful (e.g., haloperidol [Haldol])	5. Helps clear thinking and sedates.
6. Avoid the use of restraints	6. Can cause client to become more terrified and fight against restraints until exhausted to a dangerous degree.

bers. **Family members can call (800) 272-3900 to locate the nearest Alzheimer's Association.**

Teusink and Mahler (1984) have labeled the processes that the family goes through as (1) denial, (2) overinvolvement, (3) anger, (4) guilt, and (5) resolu-tion. They compare these steps to those of the mourning process, using the model of Kübler-Ross (see Chapters 17 and 26). Scott et al. (1986) confirmed in their research that family support was positively associated with the caregiver's coping effectiveness.

Table 20–7 ■ NURSING INTERVENTIONS AND RATIONALES: MAINTAINING A THERAPEUTIC ENVIRONMENT FOR A COGNITIVELY IMPAIRED PERSON

INTERVENTION	RATIONALE

Nursing Diagnosis: *High risk for injury* related to cognitive impairment

Safe Environment

INTERVENTION	RATIONALE
If client lives with family: 1. Gradually restrict the use of car.	1. As judgment becomes impaired, client may be dangerous to self and others.
2. Remove throw rugs and other objects in person's path.	2. Minimizes tripping and falling.
If client is in hospital or living with family: 3. Minimize sensory stimulation.	3. Decreases sensory overload, which can increase anxiety and confusion.
4. If client becomes verbally upset, listen briefly, give support, then change the topic.	4. Goal is to prevent escalation of anger. When attention span is short, client can be distracted to more productive topics and activities.
5. Label all rooms and drawers. Label often-used objects (e.g., hairbrushes and toothbrushes).	5. May keep client from wandering into other client's rooms. Increases environmental clues to familiar objects.
6. Install safety bars in bathroom.	6. Prevents falls.
7. Supervise client when he or she smokes.	7. Danger of burns is always present.
8. If client has history of seizures, keep padded tongue blades at bedside. Educate family and observe.	8. Seizure activity is common in advanced Alzheimer's disease.
If client wanders: 9. If client wanders during the night, put mattress on the floor.	9. Prevents falls when client is confused.
10. Have client wear Medi-Alert bracelet that cannot be removed (with name, address, and telephone number). Provide police department with recent pictures.	10. Client can be easily identified by police, neighbors, or hospital personnel.
11. Alert local police and neighbors about wanderer.	11. May reduce time necessary to return client to home or hospital.
12. If client is in hospital, have him or her wear brightly colored vest with name, unit, and phone number printed on back.	12. Makes client easily identifiable.
13. Put complex locks on door.	13. Reduces opportunity to wander.
14. Encourage physical activity during the day.	14. Physical activity may decrease wandering at night.
15. Explore the feasibility of installing sensor devices.	15. Provides warning if client wanders.

Nursing Diagnosis: *Impaired social interaction* related to cognitive impairment

Activities

INTERVENTION	RATIONALE
1. Provide picture magazines and children's books when client's reading ability diminishes.	1. Allows continuation of usual activities that the client can still enjoy; provides focus.
2. Provide simple activities that allow exercise of large muscles.	2. Exercise groups, dance groups, and walking provide socialization, as well as increased circulation and maintenance of muscle tone.
3. Encourage group activities that are familiar and simple to perform.	3. Such activities as group singing, dancing, reminiscing, and working with clay and paint all help to increase socialization and minimize feelings of alienation.

Each stage of Alzheimer's disease involves new and different stresses, which can be diminished by professional assistance.

Family members often feel guilty that they did not do or are not doing enough. They may feel frustrated and angry, and they may blame staff, nurses, and doctors. The use of projection helps protect family members from their own feelings of helplessness and hopelessness. It is *vital* that the health care providers understand this phenomenon to minimize defensive responses. Consultation with family members and education about the disease are of enormous benefit.

Family members need to know where and how to place the ill member when this becomes necessary. Eventually the ill person's labile and aggressive behavior, incontinence, wandering, unsafe habits, or disruptive nocturnal activity can no longer be appropriately dealt with in the home. Families need information, support, and legal and financial guidance at this time. When the nurse is unable to provide the relevant information, proper referrals by the social worker are needed. Information regarding advance directives, durable power of attorney, guardianship, and conservatorship should be included (Weiler and Buckwalter 1988).

ACTIVITIES OF DAILY LIVING

Nurses and family members are constantly involved with adequately maintaining the client's self-care, rest, hygiene, and nutrition. Many useful interventions have been devised by health care workers over the years. Neimoller (1990) suggests that prompting activities of daily living among nursing home residents with dementia is more appropriate than other forms of activity therapy. Table 20–6 provides suggestions for nurses and families caring for a victim of Alzheimer's disease.

THERAPEUTIC ENVIRONMENT

Providing a therapeutic environment is another important element of care for a cognitively impaired person. A therapeutic environment can be divided into (1) safety considerations and (2) activities that increase socialization and minimize loneliness. Table 20–7 gives some guidelines for providing a therapeutic environment.

Roper et al. (1991) identify three categories of interventions to reduce agitation in the client with dementia:

- Modifying the environment
- Using interpersonal strategies
- Using physical or chemical restraints

Certainly, the last category is the least preferred and is used only as a last resort.

Evaluation

It is very important that the goals set for clients with cognitive impairment be measurable, within their capabilities, and evaluated frequently. As the person's condition continues to deteriorate, goals should be altered to reflect the person's diminished functioning. Frequent evaluation and reformulation of goals will also help diminish staff frustration, as well as minimize the client's anxiety by ensuring that tasks are not more complicated than the person can accomplish. The overall goals in treatment and nursing care are to promote the client's optimal level of functioning and to retard further regression, whenever possible. Full staff involvement in the evaluation process may increase the likelihood that the goals will be realistic.

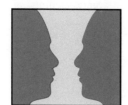

Case Study: Working with a Person Who Is Cognitively Impaired

During the previous four years, Mr. Ludwik had demonstrated rapidly progressive memory impairment, disorientation, and deterioration in his ability to function related to Alzheimer's disease. He is a 67-year-old man who had retired at age 62 to spend some of his remaining "youth" with his wife, Helen, and to travel, garden, visit family, and finally experience the plans they had made over the past forty years. He was diagnosed with Alzheimer's disease at age 63.

Mr. Ludwik had been taken care of at home by his wife and daughter, Daisy. Daisy was divorced and had come home to live with her two young daughters.

The family members found themselves progressively closer to physical and mental exhaustion. Mr. Ludwik had become increasingly incontinent when he could not find the bathroom. He wandered away from home constantly, despite close supervision. The police and neighbors brought him back

Case Study: Working with a Person Who Is Cognitively Impaired *Continued*

home an average of four times a week. Once he was lost for five days, after he had somehow boarded a bus for Pittsburgh, 100 miles from home. He was robbed and beaten before being found by the police and returned home.

He frequently wandered into his granddaughters' rooms at night while they were sleeping and tried to get into bed with them. Too young to understand that their grandfather was lonely and confused, they feared he was going to hurt them. Four times in the past two weeks, he had fallen while getting out of bed at night, thinking he was in a sleeping bag camping out in the mountains.

After a conflicting and painful two months, the family placed him in a nearby nursing home.

Helen Ludwik told the admitting nurse, Mr. Jackson, that her husband wandered almost all of the time. He had difficulty finding the right words for things (*aphasia*) and became frustrated and angry when that happened. Sometimes, he did not seem to recognize the family (*agnosia*). Once he thought Daisy was a thief breaking into the house and attacked her with a broom handle. This caused Daisy to break down into heavy sobs —"What's happened to my father? He was so kind and gentle. Oh God . . . I have lost my father."

Helen Ludwik told Mr. Jackson that Mr. Ludwik could sometimes participate in dressing himself; at other times, when he appeared confused over what went where, he needed total assistance. At this point Mrs. Ludwik began to cry uncontrollably, saying, "I can't bear to part with him . . . but I can't do it any more. I feel like I've betrayed him."

Mr. Jackson then focused his attention on Mrs. Ludwik and her experience. He stated that he knew what a difficult decision this was for her. He said that he believed the nursing home was a proper place for Mr. Ludwik at this time, but that he was also aware that families usually had conflicting and intense emotional reactions of guilt, depression, loss, anger, and other painful feelings. Mr. Jackson suggested that Mrs. Ludwik talk to other families with a cognitively impaired member. "It might help you to know that you are not alone, and having contact with others to share your grief can be healing." One of the groups he suggested was the Alzheimer's Disease and Related Disorders Association (ADRDA), or Alzheimer's Association, for short, a well-known self-help group.

Assessment	Because, indeed, the family was just as much the client as the family member with Alzheimer's disease, Mr. Jackson tried to take the most pressing immediate needs into consideration. He obtained the following data on initial assessment:

OBJECTIVE DATA

1. Wanders away from home about four times a week
2. Was lost for five days and was robbed and beaten
3. Often incontinent when he cannot find the bathroom
4. Has difficulty finding words
5. Has difficulty identifying members of the family at times

6. Has difficulty dressing himself at times
7. Falls out of bed at night
8. Has memory impairment
9. Is disoriented much of the time
10. Gets into bed with granddaughters at night when wandering
11. Family undergoing intense feelings of loss and guilt

SUBJECTIVE DATA

1. "I can't bear to part with him."
2. "I feel I've betrayed him."

3. "I've lost my father."

Nursing Diagnosis	Mr. Jackson evaluated the data. Indeed, many potential nursing diagnoses and several client needs were identified that required intervention by the nursing staff. Mr. Jackson chose four initially; the first one dealt with client safety, two addressed maintaining an optimal level of functioning and preventing further regression, and the fourth dealt with

the very real and immediate needs of a family in crisis. Therefore, Mr. Jackson made the following diagnoses:

1. *High risk for injury* related to altered cerebral functioning, as evidenced by wandering
   - Wanders away from home about four times a week
   - Wanders despite supervision
   - Falls out of bed at night
   - Gets into other people's beds
   - Wanders at night

2. *Altered pattern of urinary elimination: incontinence* related to cerebral impairment or disturbed cognition, as evidenced by inability to find the toilet

   - Incontinent when he cannot find the bathroom

3. *Self-care deficit* (self-dressing deficits) related to impaired cognitive functioning, as evidenced by impaired ability to put on and take off clothing.
   - Sometimes is able to dress with help of wife
   - At other times, is too confused to dress self at all

4. *Family grieving* related to loss and deterioration of family member
   - "I can't bear to part with him."
   - "I feel I've betrayed him."
   - "I've lost my father."
   - Family undergoing intense feelings of loss and guilt

Planning

Mr. Jackson's plan took into account both the content level—planning goals, and the process level—his own emotional reactions to cognitively impaired individuals.

CONTENT LEVEL—PLANNING GOALS

Although Mr. Ludwik had many unmet needs that required nursing interventions, Mr. Jackson decided to focus on the four initial nursing diagnoses previously cited. As other problems arose, they would be addressed.

Nursing Diagnosis	Long Term Goals	Short Term Goals
1. *High risk for injury* related to altered cerebral functioning, as evidenced by wandering	1. Client will remain safe in nursing home.	1a. Client will not fall out of bed at any time. 1b. Client will wander only in protected area. 1c. Client will be returned within two hours if he leaves unit.
2. *Altered pattern of urinary elimination: incontinence* related to disturbed cognition, as evidenced by inability to find the toilet	2. Client will be less incontinent (fewer episodes) by the fourth week of hospitalization.	2a. Client will participate in toilet training. 2b. Client will find the toilet most of the time.
3. *Self-care deficit* (self-dressing) related to impaired cognitive functioning, as evidenced by impaired ability to put on and take off clothes	3. Client will participate in dressing himself most of the time.	3a. Client will follow step-by-step instructions for dressing most of the time. 3b. Client will don own clothes with aid of fastening tape.
4. *Family grieving* related to loss and deterioration of family member	4. All family members will state, in three months' time, that they feel more supported and able to talk about their grieving.	4a. Family members will state that they have opportunity to express "unacceptable" feelings in supportive environment. 4b. Family will state that they have found support from others who have a family member with Alzheimer's disease.

Continued on following page

PROCESS LEVEL—NURSES' REACTIONS AND FEELINGS

Mr. Jackson had worked in this particular unit for a long time. It was a unit especially designed for cognitively impaired individuals, which made nursing care easier than on a regular unit. However, Mr. Jackson would be the first to admit that he had come a long way in the four years he had worked on the unit.

Four years ago, he found himself getting constantly frustrated and angry. He had entered this special unit very enthusiastically and had worked very hard setting goals and trying to implement them. However, he thought no one, especially the clients, cared about what he was doing for them. When the nursing coordinator asked him what made him come to that conclusion, he burst out, "Nothing I do seems to make any difference . . . no one listens to me."

Mr. Jackson had a lot to learn about Alzheimer's disease, and he found that the more he learned, the more he understood about why change took so long or, in some cases, could not take place. He, like everyone before him, learned to become more realistic in formulating goals, thereby lessening his frustration.

He also learned from the other caregivers on the unit many nursing care strategies that increased competent care and decreased frustration. For example, he learned that he could distract certain clients from inappropriate behaviors (e.g., arguing with others or taking things out of other people's rooms) by engaging them in another, enjoyable activity, such as talking about something they were interested in. This reduced Mr. Jackson's initial response of scolding the client, which usually resulted in escalating the client's anxiety, confusion, and sometimes aggression and left Mr. Jackson annoyed and upset.

As time progressed, Mr. Jackson found that he was well suited to this kind of nursing. He had an enthusiastic manner, and his patience, wit, and genuine liking for his clients made him an ideal role model for staff new to the unit. He did a lot of teaching on the unit, both formal and informal. He was compiling a workbook for caregivers of the cognitively impaired.

Intervention

Mr. Jackson gave Mrs. Ludwik the names of two organizations in her community that worked with families of a cognitively impaired member. He emphasized that the Alzheimer's Association support group consisted of other family members who were going through similar circumstances. He gave Mrs. Ludwik the name of the social worker and the nurse clinician assigned to the unit, who could give the family information on the disease, answer questions, and provide support and further referrals. Mr. Jackson asked Mrs. Ludwik to let him know after one week how things were going, and he said that further plans could be made at that time.

Wandering is not an uncommon phenomenon, especially among male clients with Alzheimer's disease. However, because night wandering may be indicative of cardiac decompensation, Mr. Jackson alerted the medical staff. Mr. Ludwik's mattress was placed on the floor to prevent falls, and there was a large area on the unit where he could wander safely. A bright orange vest was made for Mr. Ludwik with his name, unit, and phone number taped on the back, in case he did wander off the unit. A Medic-Alert bracelet was also made up for him, containing the same information. He was en-

couraged to participate in activities that encouraged the exercise of large muscle groups (e.g., exercise and dance groups). He seemed to wander less at night if he had been involved in physical exercise during the day. On the nights that he did wander out of his room, the staff would allow him to wander in the safe area. He was offered snacks, and the room was kept well lit. Sometimes Mr. Ludwik would curl up on the couch and fall asleep.

On the unit, Mr. Jackson and the staff began toilet training Mr. Ludwik; i.e., they took him to the toilet early in the morning, after each meal and snack, and in the evening. On this unit, all the rooms, including the bathrooms, were clearly labeled in large, colorful letters; clocks were placed in every room in clear view, and each room had a large calendar with X's marking off the days.

Mr. Jackson found that, most mornings, Mr. Ludwik was able to follow simple step-by-step instructions for dressing, but that he was much better at this after breakfast than in the early morning hours. Therefore, a schedule was set up that included toileting, breakfast, toileting, and then dressing. When Mr. Ludwik became irritable and refused to dress, Mr. Jackson would involve Mr. Ludwik

Intervention
Continued

in another activity and, after 15 or 20 minutes, suggest dressing. This seemed to work most of the time. Mr. Ludwik always wore his own clothes, unaltered except for the fastening tape that replaced the original buttons and zippers. This seemed to lessen Mr. Ludwik's frustration during dressing.

Mr. Ludwik's love for gardening was sublimated into activities such as finger painting and modeling clay. The activity therapist found that Mr. Ludwik was most content during these times. Refer to Nursing Care Plan 20–1 for more details on Mr. Ludwik's treatment.

Evaluation

At the end of four weeks, Mr. Ludwik was still free from injuries. Placing his mattress on the floor had solved one potential problem. Mr. Ludwik continued to wander at night, but more often he would nap on the couch after having a snack. He did wander off the unit once, when visitors were coming in, but was returned to the unit by the security guard as Mr. Ludwik prepared to leave the hospital. The familiar orange vest had been spotted immediately.

When Mr. Ludwik first came to the unit he had been very disoriented. However, getting used to certain staff members and set routines helped to overcome his disorientation. With the aid of the tape fasteners and constant, short reminders, Mr. Ludwik dressed himself with minimal assistance.

Urinary incontinence showed great improvement over the four-week period. Although Mr. Ludwik was still incontinent, episodes were down to four times a week. He was amenable to the toileting schedule and usually complied without problems.

The family began short term counseling together. Counseling sessions not only gave Helen Ludwik and Daisy an opportunity to express pent-up feelings and receive guidance, but it also gave Mr. Ludwik's granddaughters time to express their own fears and confusion.

Mrs. Ludwik had been to two meetings of an Alzheimer's support group, at which she found great relief. She said she had felt isolated for so long. Her daughter Daisy was planning to go with her to the next meeting.

Nursing Care Plan 20–1 ■ A PERSON WITH COGNITIVE IMPAIRMENT: Mr. Ludwik

NURSING DIAGNOSIS

High risk for injury related to altered cerebral functioning, as evidenced by wandering

Supporting Data

- Wanders despite supervision
- Falls out of bed
- Gets into other people's beds

Long Term Goal: Client will remain safe in nursing home.

Short Term Goal	Intervention	Rationale	Evaluation
1. Client will not fall out of bed at any time.	1a. Spend time with client upon admission.	1a. Lowers anxiety, provides orientation to time and place. Client's confusion will be increased by change.	Goal met
	1b. Label client's room in big, colorful letters.	1b. Offers alternate clues in new surroundings.	
	1c. Remove mattress from bed and place on floor.	1c. Prevents falling out of bed.	Mattress on floor prevented falls out of bed.
	1d. Keep room well lit at all times.	1d. Provides important environmental clues; helps lower possibility of illusions.	
	1e. Show client clock and calendar in room.	1e. Fosters orientation to time.	
	1f. Keep window shade up.	1f. Allows day-night variations.	

Continued on following page

Nursing Care Plan 20–1 ■ **A PERSON WITH COGNITIVE IMPAIRMENT: Mr. Ludwik** *(Continued)*

Short Term Goal	Intervention	Rationale	Evaluation
2. Client will wander only in protected area.	2a. At night take client to large, protected, well-lit room.	2a. Client able to wander safely in protected environment.	Goal met Client continued to wander at night; with supervision, kept out of other clients' rooms most of the time.
	2b. Alert physician to check client for cardiac decompensation.	2b. Possible underlying cause of nocturnal wakefulness and wandering.	By fourth week, client started to nap on couch in large room after snacks during the night.
	2c. Offer snacks when client is up—milk, decaffeinated tea, sandwich.	2c. Helps replace fluid and caloric expenditure.	
	2d. Allow soft music on radio.	2d. Helps induce relaxation.	
	2e. Spend short, frequent intervals with client.	2e. Decreases client's feelings of isolation and increases orientation.	
	2f. Take client to bathroom after snacks.	2f. Helps prevent incontinence.	
	2g. During day, offer activities that include use of large muscle groups.	2g. For some clients, helps decrease wandering.	
3. Client will be returned within two hours if he leaves the unit.	3a. Order Medic-Alert bracelet for client (with name, unit or hospital, phone number).	3a. If client gets out of hospital, he can be identified.	Goal met By fourth week, client wandered off unit only once; was found in lobby and returned by security guard within 45 minutes.
	3b. Place brightly colored vest on client with name, unit, and phone number taped on back.	3b. If client wanders in hospital, he can be identified and returned.	
	3c. Check client's whereabouts periodically during the day and especially at night.	3c. Helps monitor client's activities.	

NURSING DIAGNOSIS

Altered pattern of urinary elimination: **incontinence, related to a cerebral impairment, when client cannot find the toilet**

Supporting Data

● Increasingly incontinent when client cannot find the bathroom

Long Term Goal: Client will be less incontinent by the fourth week of hospitalization.

Short Term Goal	Intervention	Rationale	Evaluation
1. Client will participate in toilet training.	1a. Start toilet training in early morning, after meals and snacks, and before bed.	1. Reduces risk of incontinence.	Goal met For first two weeks, client was very confused in new environment.
	1b. Simplify steps involved in task; present steps one at a time (e.g., "Unbuckle pants, sit down . . . ")	1b. Cueing and task segmentation will increase likelihood of desired behavior.	Client gradually adjusted to toileting.
2. Client will find toilet and be less incontinent by the fourth week.	2a. Frequently identify large sign (or picture) on bathroom.	2a. Frequent orientation to place is helpful to client.	Goat met By fourth week, incontinent episodes decreased from three times a day (rate in first week) to four times a week.
	2b. Simplify clothing. Sweat pants or jogging suits are ideal. Replace any buttons and zippers with fastening tape (*Velcro*).	2b. Modified clothing improves ease of toileting and reduces delay.	
	2c. Evaluate use of incontinence pad.	2c. Can provide dignity and help maintain self-esteem.	

**Nursing Care Plan 20–1 ■ A PERSON WITH COGNITIVE IMPAIRMENT:
Mr. Ludwik** *(Continued)*

NURSING DIAGNOSIS

Self-care deficit **(self-dressing deficit) related to diminished cognitive functioning, as evidenced by impaired ability to put on and take off clothing**

Supporting Data

- Sometimes is able to dress with wife's help
- At other times is too confused to dress self at all

Long Term Goal: Client will participate in dressing himself most of the time.

Short Term Goal	Intervention	Rationale	Evaluation
1. Client will follow step-by-step instructions for dressing.	1a. Refrain from rotating staff.	1a. Minimizes confusion and disorientation.	Goal met By fourth week, client was able to follow instructions for dressing most of the time.
	1b. Always provide client's own clothes.	1b. Maintains client's identity and sense of dignity.	
	1c. Divide tasks into very small steps.	1c. Client can understand one simple comment at a time.	
	1d. Do not hurry client.	1d. Hurrying client can cause increased anxiety, agitation, and disorientation.	
	1e. Calmly give instructions: "Put one leg in trousers . . . now the next leg . . ."	1e. Support and encouragement help lower anxiety and maximize ability to follow instructions.	
2. Client will don own clothes with aid of fastening tape.	2a. Have family replace buttons and zippers with fastening tape.	2a. Fastening shirts and pants is easier.	Goal met Client was able to use fastening tape much of the time to dress self, with close supervision.
	2b. Have client wear pants with elastic in waist.	2b. Lessens need for fastening.	
	2c. Work with client on how to use fastening tape.	2c. Client responds to frequent orientation and step-by-step instruction.	
	2d. When client refuses or is too agitated to follow instructions, come back later.	2d. Client's moods are often labile; forgets easily. Can be redirected later (15 to 20 minutes).	

NURSING DIAGNOSIS

Family grieving **related to deterioration of client's mental status**

Supporting Data

- "I've lost my father."
- "I can't bear to part with him."
- "I feel like I've betrayed him."

Long Term Goal: All family members will state that they feel more supported and able to talk about their grieving in three months' time.

Short Term Goal	Intervention	Rationale	Evaluation
1. Family members will state that they have opportunity to express "unacceptable" feelings in supportive environment.	1a. Make arrangements for family to meet with counselor (e.g., nurse clinician, social worker, or psychologist).	1a. Family is in crisis: family needs to identify feelings and define some plan to regain sense of control and facilitate grief work.	Goal met By the third week, family started attending short term family counseling sessions.
	1b. Encourage spouse's input.	1b. Helps maintain spouse's involvement and may help reduce feelings of guilt.	
	1c. Encourage family members to stay with client and arrange outings (e.g., home visits for holidays, picnics, and weekends).	1c. Increases client's personal identity and aids family members in gradually "letting go."	

Continued on following page

Nursing Care Plan 20–1 ■ A PERSON WITH COGNITIVE IMPAIRMENT: Mr. Ludwik *(Continued)*			
Short Term Goal	*Intervention*	*Rationale*	*Evaluation*
	1d. Encourage family members to express feelings; encourage ongoing sessions with counselor.	1d. Family members need to have a place where they can get support and understanding.	
2. Family will state that they have found support from others who have a family member with Alzheimer's disease.	2a. Offer family written names and phone numbers of available support groups in their vicinity.*	2a. The more support a family has, the better they are able to cope with a complex and painful situation.	Goal met Mrs. Ludwik attended two meetings of an Alzheimer's support group and found it enormously supportive. The daughter planned to attend the next meeting.
	2b. Follow up periodically.	2b. Continue to assess needs and encourage family members to obtain support.	

*A family caring for a client in the home would benefit from, along with the above, (1) companions, (2) other volunteers, (3) home health aides, (4) visiting nurses, (5) day care centers, (6) senior citizen groups, (7) respite care, and (8) financial and legal counseling. Caring for a cognitively impaired family member can quickly lead to physical and emotional exhaustion and can throw the family into crisis.

Summary

Cognitive impairment disorder is the general term that refers to disturbances in orientation, memory, intellect, judgment, and affect due to changes in the brain. Delirium and dementia were discussed in this chapter because they are the cognitive impairment disorders most widely seen by health care workers.

Delirium is marked by acute onset, a clouded state of consciousness, and symptoms of disorientation and confusion that fluctuate by the minute, hour, or time of day. Delirium is always secondary to an underlying condition; therefore, it is temporary, transient, and may last from hours to days once the underlying cause is treated. If the cause is not treated, permanent damage to the neurons could result in dementia or death.

Nursing diagnoses for delirium were suggested, including *high risk for injury, fluid volume deficit, sleep pattern disturbance, impaired verbal communication, fear, self-care deficits,* and *impaired social interaction.* Goals for each of these nursing diagnoses were identified.

The clinical picture of delirium in an intensive care unit was described and medical and nursing intervention were delineated.

Dementia usually has a more insidious onset. Global deterioration of cognitive functioning (e.g., memory, judgment, ability to think abstractly, and orientation) is often progressive and irreversible, depending on the underlying cause. If dementia is primary (e.g., Alzheimer's disease, multi-infarct dementia, or Pick's disease), the course is irreversible. However,

if the underlying cause is treatable, then the progression of the dementia may be halted or reversed.

Alzheimer's disease accounts for 65% of all dementia, and multi-infarct disease, for about 10%; however, these percentages may change with the rising incidence of AIDS-related dementia (HIV encephalopathy).

There are various etiological theories about Alzheimer's disease, none of which is conclusive, although the genetic theory identifies familial tendencies. Signs and symptoms were noted during the progression of the disease through four phases: phase 1 (mild), phase 2 (moderate), phase 3 (moderate to severe) and phase 4 (late). The phenomena of confabulation, perseveration, aphasia, apraxia, agnosia, and hyperorality were explained.

Abraham and Neundorfer (1990) describe a decade of progress related to Alzheimer's disease. There is still no known cause or cure, although the drug tacrine (THA, Cognex) offers some hope for the future. Much research is still needed in unraveling the mysteries of this devastating illness. Duffy et al. (1989) describe a nursing research agenda that includes better care and management of clients with Alzheimer's disease and an emphasis on research-based practice.

People with Alzheimer's disease have many unmet needs and present many nursing problems. There is often a *high risk for injury, impaired verbal communication, self-care deficit, disturbance in self-esteem, altered thought processes, ineffective individual coping,* and always, *altered family processes. Incontinence* and *nutritional deficits* were also discussed.

Goals for each of these nursing diagnoses were identified, and interventions for each were presented, especially in the areas of (1) communication, (2) activities of daily living, (3) health teaching of families and (4) therapeutic environment.

References

Abraham IL, Neundorfer MM. Alzheimer's: A decade of progress, a future of nursing challenges. Geriatric Nursing, May/June:116, 1990.

Alexopoulas GS, Abrams RC. Depression in Alzheimer's disease. Psychiatric Clinics of North America, 14(2):327, 1991.

Alzheimer's Association Newsletter 13(2):4, 1993.

Alzheimer's Disease. Part I. The Harvard Mental Health Letter, 9(3):1, 1992. American Association of Retired Persons (AARP). Coping and caring: Living with Alzheimer's disease. Washington, DC: American Association of Retired Persons, 1986.

Alzheimer's Research Review, 3:1, May/June, 1994.

Alzheimer's in the skin. Discover, 12:26, 1993.

American Psychiatric Association. Diagnostic and Statistical Manual of Mental Disorders 3rd ed, revised (DSM-III-R). Washington, DC: American Psychiatric Association, 1987.

American Psychiatric Association. DSM-IV Options Book: Work in Progress. Washington, DC: American Psychiatric Association, 1991.

Andresen G. How to assess the older mind. RN, 55(7):34, 1992.

Burnside I. Nursing and the Aged, 3rd ed. New York: McGraw-Hill, 1988.

Cassem N, Hackett T. The setting of intensive care. In Hackett T, Cassem N (eds). Massachusetts General Hospital Handbook of General Hospital Psychiatry. St. Louis: CV Mosby, 1978.

Cohen GD. The mental health professional and the Alzheimer patient. Hospital and Community Psychiatry, 35:115, 1984.

Dewan MJ, Gupta S. Toward a definite diagnosis of Alzheimer's disease. Comprehensive Psychiatry, 33(4):282, 1992.

Duffy LM, Hepburn K, Christensen R, et al. A research agenda in care for patients with Alzheimer's disease. Journal of Nursing Scholarship, 21(4):254, 1989.

Dwyer BJ. Cognitive impairment in the elderly: Delirium, depression or dementia? Focus on Geriatric Care and Rehabilitation, 1(4):1, 1987.

Ellison JM. DSM-III and the diagnosis of organic mental disorders. Annals of Emergency Medicine, 13(7):521, 1984.

Foreman MD. Acute confusional states in hospitalized elderly: A research dilemma. Nursing Research, 35(1):34, 1986.

Foreman MD. Complexities of acute confusion. Geriatric Nursing, 11:136, 1990.

Gershon S, Herman S. The differential diagnosis of dementia. Journal of the American Geriatrics Society, 30(11):S58, 1982.

Gomez GE, Gomez EA. Delirium. Geriatric Nursing, 8(6):330, 1987.

Gray-Vickrey P. Evaluating Alzheimer's patients. Nursing 88, 18:34, 1988.

Hall GR. This hospital patient has Alzheimer's. American Journal of Nursing, October 91:45, 1991.

Herst ST, Metcalf BJ. Whys and whats of wandering. Geriatric Nursing, 10:237, 1989.

Heston L, White JA. Dementia: A Practical Guide to Alzheimer's Disease and Related Illnesses. New York: WH Freeman & Company, 1983.

Kaplan HI, Sadock BJ. Synopsis of Psychiatry, 6th ed. Baltimore: Williams & Wilkins, 1991.

Li G, Silverman JM, Mohs KC. Clinical genetic studies of Alzheimer's disease. Psychiatric Clinics of North America, 14(2):267, 1991.

Lipowski ZJ. Transient cognitive disorders (delirium, acute confusional states) in the elderly. American Journal of Psychiatry, 140:1426, 1983.

McHugh PR, Folstein MF. Organic mental disorders. In Michels R, Cavenar JO (eds). Psychiatry, vol I. Philadelphia: JB Lippincott, 1987.

Mace NL, Rabins PB. The 36 Hour Day. Baltimore: Johns Hopkins University Press, 1981.

Mass ML, Buckwalter KC. A special Alzheimer's unit: Phase 1 of baseline data. Applied Nursing Research, 1(1):41, 1988.

Morency CR. Clinical updates. Journal of Professional Nursing, 6(6):356, 1990.

Nagley SJ. Predicting and preventing confusion in your patients. Journal of Gerontological Nursing, 12(3):27, 1986.

Neimoller J. Change of pace for Alzheimer's patients. Geriatric Nursing, 4:86, 1990.

Newbern VB. Is it really Alzheimer's? American Journal of Nursing, 2:51, 1991.

Ninos M, Makohon R. Functional assessment of the patient. Geriatric Nursing, 6:139, 1985.

Pajik M. Alzheimer's disease: Inpatient care. American Journal of Nursing, 84:215, 1984.

Perry SW, Markowitz J. Organic mental disorders. In Talbott JA, Hales RE, Yudofsky SC (eds). Textbook of Psychiatry. Washington, DC: American Psychiatric Press, 1988.

Powell LS, Courtice K. Alzheimer's disease: A guide for families. Reading, MA: Addison-Wesley, 1983.

Reisberg B. Stages of cognitive decline. American Journal of Nursing, 84:225, 1984.

Richardson K. Assessing communication. Geriatric Nursing, July/August 4:237, 1983.

Robinson L. Liaison Nursing: Psychological Approach to Patient Care. Philadelphia: FA Davis, 1974.

Roper JM, Shapira J, Change BL. Agitation in the demented patient: A framework for management. Journal of Gerontological Nursing, 17(3):17, 1991.

Scott JP, Roberto KA, Hutton JT. Families of Alzheimer's victims family support to the caregivers. Journal of American Geriatrics Society, 34:348, 1986.

Seltzer B, Frazier SH. Organic mental disorders. In Nicholi AA (ed). The Harvard Guide to Modern Psychiatry. Cambridge, MA: The Belknap Press of Harvard University, 1980.

Souder E. Diagnosing dementia: Current clinical concepts. Journal of Gerontological Nursing, 18(2):5, 1992.

Spitzer RL, et al. Now is the time to retire the term "organic mental disorders." American Journal of Psychiatry, 149(2):240, 1992.

Sullivan EM, Wanich CK, Kurlowicz LH. Elder care. AORN Journal, 53(3):820, 1991.

Sullivan N, Fogel B. Could this be delirium? American Journal of Nursing, December 86:1359, 1986.

Tacrine update. Alzheimer's Research Review, Summer 1993.

Teusink JP, Mahler S. Helping families cope with Alzheimer's disease. Hospital and Community Psychiatry, 35:152, 1984.

Weiler K, Buckwalter KC. Care of the demented client. Journal of Gerontological Nursing, 14(7):26, 1988.

Wells CE. Chronic brain disease: An update on alcoholism, Parkinson's disease and dementia. Hospital and Community Psychiatry, 33:111, 1982.

Williams L. Alzheimer's: The need for caring. Journal of Gerontological Nursing, 12(2):21, 1986.

Wilson HS. Easing life for the Alzheimer's patient. RN, 53(12):24, 1990.

Wolanin MO, Fraelich-Philips LR. Confusion, Prevention and Cure. St. Louis: CV Mosby, 1981.

Wurtman R. Alzheimer's disease. Scientific American, 252:62, 1985.

Further Reading

Adams M, Hanson R, Norkoal D, et al. Psychological responses in critical care units. American Journal of Nursing, 78:1504, 1978.

Ansbaugh P. Emergency management of intoxicated patients with head injuries. Journal of Emergency Nursing, 3(3):9, 1977.

Burkhalter PK. Nursing Care of the Alcoholic and Drug Abuser. New York: McGraw-Hill, 1975.

Burnside I. Alzheimer's disease: An overview. Journal of Gerontological Nursing, 5(4):14, 1979.

Butz RH. Intoxication and withdrawal. In Estes NJ, Heinemann ME (eds). Alcoholism, 2nd ed. St. Louis: CV Mosby, 1982.

Charles R, Truesdell M, Wood E. Alzheimer's disease: Pathology progression and nursing process. Journal of Gerontological Nursing, 8(2):69, 1982.

Chenitz WC. The nurse's aide and the confused person. Geriatric Nursing, July/August 4:238, 1983.

Chenoweth B, Spencer B. Dementia: The experience of family care-givers. The Gerontologist, 26(3):267, 1986.

Clunn PA, Payne DB. Psychiatric Mental Health Nursing, 4th ed. New York: Medical Examination Publishing Company, 1986.

Cummings JL, Benson DF. Dementia: A Clinical Approach. Boston: Butterworths, 1983.

Davidhizar R, Gunden E, Wehlage D. Recognizing and caring for the delirious patient. Journal of Psychiatric Nursing, 16(5):38, 1978.

Davison GC, Neale JM. Abnormal Psychology and Experimental Clinical Approach, 3rd ed. New York: John Wiley & Sons, 1982.

Dietch JT, Hewett LJ, Jones S. Adverse effects of reality orientation. Journal of American Geriatrics Society, 37:974, 1989.

Fisk A. Alzheimer's disease: A five article symposium (introduction). Postgraduate Medicine, 73:204, 1983.

Folstein MF. Mini-mental state: a practical method for grading the cognitive state of patients for the clinician. Journal of Psychiatric Research, 12:189, 1975.

Frances RJ, Franklin JE. Alcohol and other psychoactive substance use disorders. In Talbott JA, Hales RE, Yudofsky SC (eds). Text-book of Psychiatry. Washington, DC: American Psychiatric Press, 1988.

Gilmore GM. Behavioral management of the acutely intoxicated pa-tient in the emergency department. Journal of Emergency Nurs-ing, 12(1):13, 1986.

Goodwin DW, Guze SB. Psychiatric Diagnosis. New York: Oxford University Press, 1984.

Haber J, Hoskins P, Leach A, et al. Comprehensive Psychiatric Nurs-ing, 3rd ed. New York: McGraw-Hill, 1983.

Inaba-Roland KE, Maricle RA. Assessing delirium in the acute care setting. Heart and Lung, 21(1):48, 1992.

Kelly FM. Caring for the patient in acute alcohol withdrawal. Critical Care Quarterly, 8(4):11, 1986.

Lipkowitz R. Research builds esteem: A model patient/family group program. Generations, 7(1):42, 1982.

Lucas MJ, Steele C, Bognanni. Recognition of psychiatric symptoms in dementia. Journal of Gerontological Nursing, 12(1):11, 1986.

Mackey A. OBS and nursing care. Journal of Gerontological Nursing, 9(2):75, 1983.

McArthur JC. Neurological manifestation of AIDS. Medicine, 66(6):407, 1987.

Ricci M. All-out care for an Alzheimer patient. Geriatric Nursing, April 4:369, 1983.

Schneider E, Emr M. Alzheimer's disease: Research highlights. Geri-atric Nursing, 6:136, 1985.

Smith-DiJulio K. Care of the alcoholic patient during acute episodes. In Estes NJ, Heinemann ME (eds). Alcoholism, 2nd ed. St. Louis: CV Mosby, 1982.

St. George-Hyslop PH, Tanzi RE, Polansky RJ, et al. The genetic defect causing familial Alzheimer's disease on chromosome 21. Science, 235:885, 1987.

Tyler KL, Tyler HR. Differentiating organic dementia. Geriatrics, 39(3):38, 1984.

US Department of Health and Human Services. Q & A: Alzheimer's Disease. Washington, DC: US Department of Health and Human Services, 1985.

Wolanin MO, Halloway J. Relocation confusion: Intervention for pre-vention. Psychosocial nursing care of the aged. In Burnside IM (ed). Nursing and the Aged, 2nd ed. New York: McGraw-Hill, 1980.

Wolanin MO. Scope of the problem and its diagnosis. Geriatric Nursing, July/August 4:227, 1983.

Zabourek RP. Identification of the alcoholic in the acute care set-ting. Critical Care Quarterly, 8(4):1, 1986.

Self-study Exercises

Write DEL (delirium) or DEM (dementia) to categorize each of the following symptoms:

1. _____ Has acute onset.
2. _____ Eventually both short term and long term memory are affected.
3. _____ No or slow changes on electroencephalogram.
4. _____ Fluctuating levels of consciousness.
5. _____ Aphasia and agnosia are commonly observed.
6. _____ Disorientation most severe at night; may be oriented during the day.
7. _____ Confabulation or perseveration commonly observed.
8. _____ Visual tactile hallucinations most common in this syndrome.

Match the terms in the right column with the definitions in the left column.

9. _____ The inability to name objects

10. _____ Difficulty finding the right word—can dete-riorate to muteness

11. _____ Unable to perform once-familiar and simple tasks

12. _____ The need to taste, chew, and put everything in one's mouth

13. _____ Repeating the same word or behavior over and over again.

A. Hypermetamor-phosis

B. Perseveration

C. Hyperorality

D. Apraxia

E. Mnemonic dis-turbance

F. Agnosia

G. Aphasia

H. Confabulation

Short answer

Mark Peters, a Vietnam Veteran, has just been admitted and diagnosed with acute bacterial endocarditis. His temperature is 103°F, his skin turgor is poor, and his urine output is dark amber and scanty. He is agitated and screams in terror when he hears the bleeps from the electrocardiographic monitor. He thinks that he has been captured in Vietnam and that the bleeps are coming from a time bomb, and he is desperate to flee. He thinks it is 1971 and that you are the enemy.

14. Formulate two nursing diagnoses (ND) and identify at least one short term goal (STG) for each diagnosis.
    ND: _____
    related to _____
    as evidenced by _____
    STG: _____

    ND: _____
    related to _____
    as evidenced by _____
    STG: _____

15. Describe the deterioration of a client who is going through the four stages of Alzheimer's disease and identify essential features during each stage.

    A. Phase 1 (mild) _____
    _____

    B. Phase 2 (moderate) _____
    _____

    C. Phase 3 (moderate to severe) _____
    _____

    D. Phase 4 (late) _____
    _____

Mrs. Kendel is a 52-year-old woman who has progressive Alzheimer's disease. She lives with her husband, who has been trying to care for her in the home. Mrs. Kendel often wears evening gowns in the morning, puts her blouse on backward, and sometimes puts her bra on backward outside her blouse.

She often forgets where things are. She makes an effort to cook but often confuses frying pans and pots and sometimes has trouble turning on the stove.

Once in a while she can't find the bathroom in time, often mistaking it for a broom closet. She becomes very frightened of noises and is terrified when the telephone or doorbell rings.

At other times she cries because she is aware that she is losing her sense of her place in the world. She and her husband have always been close, loving companions, and he wants to keep her at home as long as possible.

16. Identify two nursing diagnoses (ND) for Mrs. Kendel as they relate to her being maintained at home.
    ND: _____
    related to _____
    as evidenced by _____

ND: _____

related to _____

as evidenced by_____

17. Help Mr. Kendel by writing out a list of suggestions that he can try at home that might help facilitate (a) communication, (b) activities of daily living, and (c) therapeutic environment.

18. Identify at least seven interventions appropriate to this situation for each of the areas.

19. Identify possible types of resources available for maintaining Mrs. Kendel in the home for as long as possible. Identify the name of one self-help group that you would urge Mr. Kendel to join.

PEOPLE WHO USE SELF-DESTRUCTIVE DEFENSES AGAINST ANXIETY

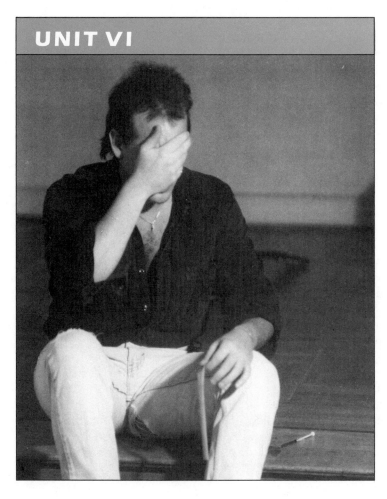

UNIT VI

Many people go throughout life committing partial suicide—destroying their talents, energies, creative qualities. Indeed, to learn how to be good to oneself is often more difficult than to learn how to be good to others.

JOSHUA LIEBMAN

A Nurse Speaks

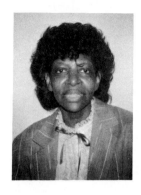

Arnette D. Robinson

The importance of cultural awareness for nurses was made clear to me while I was carrying out field research for my doctoral dissertation, which concerned attitudes toward the elderly held by nursing home aides. In the course of collecting data, I surveyed aides' attitudes and conducted in-service training in cultural awareness.

Since my research was carried out in nursing homes in New York City, the nursing home aides with whom I worked were almost exclusively members of one of three cultural groups: African Americans, English-speaking Caribbean blacks (from Jamaica, Trinidad, Barbados, and Antigua), and Haitians. In all of these cultures, elderly individuals are treated with great respect. Families typically care for older relatives at home, and it is very unusual for an older person to be placed in a nursing home or other institutional setting.

I found that these cultural attitudes had important implications for the way some of the aides viewed the nursing home residents. Some of the aides, especially aides who had been living in the United States for just a short time, tended to assume that the residents must have been placed in the nursing home because they were particularly difficult to get along with or because they had some particular behavioral problem. These aides simply assumed that if the elderly person did not have a problem, he or she would be living at home with the family. It was important that in-service training make these aides aware of the fact that in the United States, nursing home placement is quite common and does not signify that the older individual has any personality or behavioral problem.

A related culturally based issue that arose in my in-service workshops for aides was the feeling of resentment some aides had toward the family members who placed the resident in the nursing home. Coming from cultures in which it would be considered shameful not to take care of a parent at home, some aides felt bitter toward the sons and daughters of the residents. This is a dangerous situation, for two reasons. First, it is important that nursing home staff have good relationships with visiting family members in order to encourage more visits and to exchange information relevant to the resident's well-being. Second, if the aide expresses anger or resentment toward a son or daughter to the resident, the resident may begin to feel misused. This in turn could lead the resident to become angry or depressed.

It was therefore most important to discuss with the aides some of the reasons families place older relatives in nursing homes. These include job transfers or heavy travel requirements, the commonplace occurrence of dual-career families, and the inability to provide required medical care. When the aides recognized the unique pressures placed on families in the context of American culture, they were more understanding of the decision to place the resident in a nursing home.

My experience made it clear to me how important it is for the professional nurse working in a geriatric setting to be aware of cultural differences between staff and patients, as well as cultural differences between different groups of staff members. These differences can have a real impact on patient care.

CHAPTER 21

People Who Contemplate Suicide: Aggression Toward Self

Elizabeth M. Varcarolis

OUTLINE

THEORY
Precipitating Events
Motivating Forces
Theories

ASSESSMENT
Assessing Verbal and Nonverbal Clues
Assessing Lethality of Suicide Plan
Assessing High-Risk Factors

NURSING DIAGNOSIS

PLANNING
Content Level—Planning Goals
Process Level—Nurses' Reactions and
Feelings

INTERVENTION
Psychotherapeutic Interventions
In the Clinic
In the Hospital
On the Telephone Hotlines
Health Teaching
Activities of Daily Living
Somatic Therapies
Therapeutic Environment
Psychotherapy

EVALUATION

CASE STUDY: WORKING WITH A
PERSON WHO IS SUICIDAL

SUMMARY

KEY TERMS AND CONCEPTS

The key terms and concepts listed here also appear in bold where they are
defined or discussed in this chapter.

COMPLETED SUICIDE

NO-SUICIDE CONTRACT

PRIMARY INTERVENTION

SAD PERSONS SCALE

SECONDARY INTERVENTION

SUBINTENTIONED SUICIDE

SUICIDAL IDEATION

SUICIDE

SUICIDE ATTEMPT

TERTIARY INTERVENTION

OBJECTIVES

After studying this chapter, the student will be able to

1. Describe the profile of suicide in the United States, including clues, professions at risk, most common psychopathology, population at risk, and when people may commit suicide.
2. Identify common precipitating events.
3. Act out two verbal and two nonverbal clues that might signal suicidal ideation.

4. Discuss three areas of assessment in determining lethality of plan according to Farberow.
5. Using the SAD PERSONS scale, list the 10 risk factors to consider when assessing for suicide.
6. Describe three expected reactions a nurse may have when beginning work with suicidal clients.
7. Give examples of intervention: primary, secondary, and tertiary (postvention) intervention.
8. Give examples of psychotherapeutic interventions that a nurse may carry out (a) in the clinic, (b) in the hospital, and (c) on a telephone hotline.
9. Write two "no-suicide contracts."
10. Make up a care plan including two nursing diagnoses and four goals for a suicidal client.

Humans are the only creatures that are aware of their own mortality. They are able to contemplate the past as well as the future, to consider their personal end, and to be cognizant of their own death (Mowshowitz 1984).

Whether to live or die is a universal question that has been debated for centuries. Whether a person has the right to suicide is an intensely complex moral, ethical, religious, and legal issue.

People are granted the right to "life, liberty, and the pursuit of happiness." Health care professionals, however, are in frequent contact with people who are following more self-destructive pursuits. Schneidman (1963) has labeled self-destructive behaviors **subintentioned suicide.** Compulsive use of drugs and alcohol, hyperobesity, gambling, self-harmful sexual behaviors, and medical noncompliance are examples of covert, self-destructive behaviors, or subintentioned suicidal acts. By definition, in *subintentioned death*, a person takes part in hastening his or her own death. This participation with one's own death may be on a covert, or unconscious, level. These covert acts of self-destruction, however, are often easier for health care providers to deal with than the overt act of suicide.

Suicide is the ultimate act of self-destruction. In most cases of suicide, crisis precedes the attempt (Clayton 1985). Suicidal risk should always be assessed in any crisis situation. Suicidal thoughts, threats, or attempts are signals of a person or family in high anxiety. Sustained severe to panic levels of anxiety are seen in all crises.

The act of purposeful self-destruction by taking one's own life arouses intense and complex emotions in others. Suicide, which is the act of opting for nonexistence, is an option that some members of our society are adopting at increasing and alarming rates.

In all Western countries, suicide ranks among the fifth to tenth leading causes of death (Roy 1989). This figure does not take into account the many suicides disguised as accidents. Suicide is the second leading cause of death among the 5- to 19-year-old group in this country (Holinger 1990). However, the group that has the highest suicide rate of any other is the elderly (De Leo and Ormskerk 1991).

Among youth who commit suicide, drug use and antisocial personality disorder were found more often in those under 30 years of age. Depression, alcoholism, and illness stressors were found more often among suicide victims over 30 (Roy 1989). However, more important than the degree of depression, *hopelessness about the future* was highly correlated with the seriousness of suicidal intent (Hendin 1992). Box 21–1 provides recent US statistics on suicide.

Although the suicide rate among whites is about two times that of nonwhites, the rate among black women has increased 80% in the last 20 years (Merck Manual 1992). The suicide rate among ghetto youth and certain Native Americans exceeds the national rate, and in some tribes it is five times the national average (Kaplan and Sadock 1991; Merck Manual 1992).

The following summary of statistical findings provides a profile of suicide in America:

- About 75–80% of people who go on to commit suicide give out clues and warnings and often seek help. An estimated 75% of all suicide victims seek help within the four months before they take their lives.
- Of those who commit suicide, 65–70% have made previous attempts. A person who has attempted suicide in the past is at great risk for successful suicide. The risk is highest in the first two years after a suicide attempt, *especially in the first three months.*
- The incidence of suicide is higher in urban areas than in rural areas. It is also higher for those who

Box 21-1. SUMMARY OF SUICIDE STATISTICS

- Suicide is the *eighth* leading cause of death in the United States.
- Suicide is the *second* cause of death among young people 15–19 years.
- The highest suicide rate is for persons over 65 years.
- It is estimated that there are about 10 attempted suicides to one completion.
- 72% of *all* suicides are committed by white males.
- The gender ratio is 4 males to 1 female (4:1).
- Suicide by firearms is the most common method (60% of all suicides).
- Professional persons including lawyers, dentists, military men, and physicians have higher than average suicide rates.
- Suicide is less frequent among practicing members of most religious groups.

Data from National Institute of Mental Health, March 1992; Merck Manual 1992.

are socially mobile or who are migrants. The suicide rate for white Americans is higher than for nonwhites (except young black males). Suicide is more common among the affluent than among the poor. It is also higher in students, the elderly, gifted individuals, immigrants, and Indian-Eskimos.
- The incidence of suicide also seems to be higher in some occupations. Doctors, dentists, lawyers, police officers, and air-traffic controllers have higher suicide rates than does the general population. People who are physically ill are also at higher risk than the general population. The suicide rate is higher for single people than for married people and is higher for divorced males than for divorced females. See Table 21–1 for myths and facts about suicide.
- A significantly greater number of suicide attempters stated that they did not participate in religious activities, according to one study.

Monday is the most frequent day for suicide, morning the most frequent time, and April the most frequent month.

People who have problems with impulse control (drugs or alcohol or use of violence), are depressed, are psychotic, or have a family member who committed suicide are at greater risk than the general public. Up to 75% of clinically depressed people have suicidal ideation or intent (Mullis and Byers 1988).

Figure 21–1 conceptualizes the process of suicide as a self-destructive, problem-solving behavior.

Not all suicides are committed by insane or severely disturbed individuals. Kavenaugh (1972) states that suicide can be a "tortuous ethical decision made by a moral and sane individual." Perhaps a third of those who have attempted suicide unsuccessfully are persons without known psychopathology (Kolb and Brodie 1982), although many of these deaths may have been precipitated by severe stressors including financial loss and illness. When psychopathology does exist, depression and alcoholism are most commonly seen. The one- to three-month period following recovery from a depressive episode is a high-risk period (Roy 1989).

The "right to die" issue is presently controversial. The dilemma is most debated in cases of terminal illness, severe debilitation, intractable pain, and progressive illnesses such as multiple sclerosis. Does someone with a terminal disease and who is in pain have a moral and ethical right to take his or her own life? Is rational suicide in such cases legally and ethically sanctioned?

The questions of whether intentionally ending one's life can ever be rational or praiseworthy, and if so under what circumstances, are presently being hotly

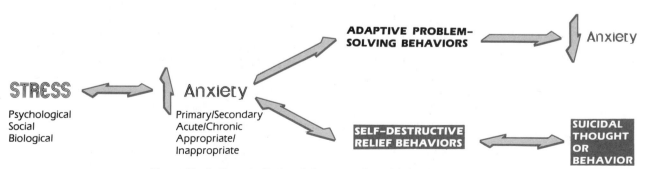

Figure 21–1. *Conceptualization of the process of suicidal thoughts or behaviors.*

Table 21–1 ■ MYTHS VERSUS FACTS: SUICIDE

MYTH	FACT
1. Only people who are mentally ill commit suicide.	1. Suicide can be a decision made by a sane individual.
2. Suicidal persons are fully intent on dying.	2. Most persons who contemplate suicide are highly ambivalent about dying.
3. If a nurse suspects that a person is thinking about suicide, the nurse should not bring up the subject lest the person kill himself.	3. Open dialogue is most often a relief for the suicidal person. Talking can decrease the risk of suicide.
4. Suicide is an impulsive act.	4. The act may be impulsive, but most often suicide has been carefully thought out.
5. The chance of suicide lessens as depression lessens.	5. When depression is lifting, there is more energy to carry out a previously pondered suicide plan.
6. Suicide can be an inherited trait.	6. Alcoholism and depression most likely are genetic, and having a relative who has committed suicide is a risk factor; however, there are no genetic markers for suicide.
7. Most suicidal persons give no warning.	7. About 75% of people who attempt or commit suicide give definite clues to intent.
8. All nonwhites have a lower suicide rate than whites.	8. This is true with the exception of young black males.
9. Professionals such as lawyers, doctors, dentists, police officers, and air-traffic controllers have a low suicide rate.	9. All have higher suicide rates than people in the general population.
10. People who are psychotic have the greatest chance of killing themselves among those with definite psychopathology.	10. People with depression and alcoholism are at greatest risks for suicide among people with psychopathology.
11. Only people with grave problems, mental illness, or physical illness think about suicide.	11. At one time or another, almost everyone contemplates suicide.
12. People who just want attention use suicidal threats as manipulation.	12. Even if a suicide threat is manipulative, the person may actually go on to commit suicide. All *threats should be taken seriously.*
13. Young people who have anti-social and borderline personality disorders never attempt suicide.	13. Both have higher suicide rates than the general population.
14. People who go from "rags to riches" are better protected against suicide than those who go from fortune to poverty.	14. Persons with sudden change in fortune (success, riches, acclaim) are also at risk for suicide.

Data from Harvard Medical School 1986; Kaplan and Sadock 1991; Roy 1989; Simmons 1981.

debated. The Netherlands is used by some as an example of a country with progressive social reforms regarding the practice of euthanasia. However, others strongly disagree.

> Euthanasia in the Netherlands is now an alarming practice that oversteps ethical bounds and administrative controls . . . allowing them (doctors) to become medical killers (Pollard 1991).

Issues such as the right to die with dignity and respect for the wishes of the patient to die in the face of unbearable suffering or progressive disability are presently challenging the health profession in the courts as well as in the ethical arena. We know that 20–40% of all suicide victims have some physical illness (Merck Manual 1992).

Transient thoughts of death and dying are a universal phenomenon. Almost everyone will experience momentary self-destructive thoughts. Obsessive preoccupation with thoughts of suicide, however, is pathological (Kolb and Brodie 1982).

The Center for Study of Suicide Prevention of the United States Public Health Service has classified suicidal behavior into three categories, according to intent: *completed suicide, suicide attempt,* and *suicidal ideation.*

1. **Completed suicide** includes all willful, self-inflicted, life-threatening acts leading to death.
2. **Suicide attempt** includes all willful, self-inflicted, life-threatening attempts that have not led to death. Attempted suicide is most often associated with hysteria, antisocial personality, thought disor-

ders, and various paraphilias (Kaplan and Sadock 1991).

3. **Suicidal ideation** means that the person is thinking about harming himself or herself.

Theory

Because the subject of suicide arouses strong feelings and reactions in all persons, it is wise to examine personal thoughts and ethical beliefs regarding another person's attempt at suicide.

Theoretical considerations and research findings can clarify or modify one's understanding of the phenomena surrounding overt self-destructive behavior. Three areas provide a framework for nurses' work with suicidal persons: (1) precipitating events, (2) motivating forces, and (3) theories.

PRECIPITATING EVENTS

The act of suicide may be precipitated by many internal and external events. Adam (1985) summarized various events from studies in the literature and found that social isolation, severe life events, and sensitivity to loss often precede a suicide attempt.

SOCIAL ISOLATION. Suicidal individuals frequently have difficulty forming and maintaining relationships. Usually there is a high rate of divorce, separation, or single marital status. Norman Cousins maintains that all human history is an endeavor to shatter loneliness. He tells the story of a woman who had recently committed suicide. She had written in her diary every day during the week before her death, "Nobody called today, nobody called today, nobody called today" (Mowshowitz 1984).

SEVERE LIFE EVENTS. Severe life events often precede a suicide attempt. Paykel et al. (1975) found that people who attempted suicide were four times as likely to suffer severe life events (e.g., divorce, death, sickness, blows to self-esteem, legal problems, and interpersonal discord) in the six months prior to their attempts than were people in the general population. Having serious arguments with a spouse, having a new person in the home (baby, elderly parent), and having to appear in court were more frequent occurrences for persons who attempted suicide than for nonsuicidal persons. A study by Parker (1988) found that adolescents attempting suicide experienced more life changes than other adolescents, and had a history of emotional illness in the family.

SENSITIVITY TO LOSS. People who are sensitive to losses may react tragically to separation or loss of a loved one. People who commit suicide after such a loss usually have had insecure or unreliable childhood experiences. Repeated studies demonstrate a significantly higher incidence of broken homes in the childhood of people who commit suicide than in the general population. People from broken homes may be more susceptible to loss of a significant relationship than someone whose background includes more stable or loving relationships.

MOTIVATING FORCES

The suicidal person may be stimulated by numerous motivating forces. The suicide attempt may reflect a desire for reincarnation, a wish-fulfilling fantasy of reunion, or efforts to force love from others. Or, a suicide attempt may be an effort to get away from psychological pain, to atone for past sins, or to escape from severe physical pain or deformity. Another motive could be the wish to instill guilt in a significant other who is perceived as abandoning or rejecting the suicidal person. In this case, suicide can be seen as a means of control and revenge. *All suicidal thoughts and ideas, no matter what the motivation or intent, should be taken seriously.*

THEORIES

Much information has been gathered on suicide from clinical observations, studies, and research. However, no single theory can account for all the data available. Two theoretical models that have influenced suicidologists most are the (1) psychodynamic theories and (2) sociological theories. A more recent area of study is (3) biochemical-genetic theories.

PSYCHODYNAMIC THEORIES. Psychodynamic explanations of suicide focus on the role of aggression and the internalization of hostile or disappointing relationships. Freud described suicide as a murderous attack on an ambivalently loved, internalized significant person. In other words, there would not be a suicide without the repressed desire to kill someone else. This is sometimes referred to as "murder in the 180th degree." Others describe suicide as a wish to be at peace with the internalized significant person.

Other themes besides punishment of inner "objects" and the wish to be reunited with a deceased loved object are the wish for revenge and the wish to get rid of a hated part of the self. Suicide is either a phenomenon of disturbed internalizations of hostile or ambivalent significant persons or an effort to cope with the absence of comforting and deeply loved significant others (Malzberger and Buie 1980). Whatever the introjected or internalized object signifies, *suicide is an attempt to escape from an intolerable situation or intolerable state of mind.*

SOCIOLOGICAL THEORIES. Suicidal crisis involves the unique characteristic of rejecting society, as well as rejecting one's self. The threat of death carries enormous impact for all concerned. No other kind of death leaves family and friends with such long-lasting feelings of shame, guilt, puzzlement, and distress (Van Dongen 1988).

Sociological theory refers to the social and cultural context in which a person lives. "Suicide or dying behaviors do not exist in a vacuum, but are an integral part of the life style of the individual" (Schneidman 1963). Circumstances in a person's cultural and social environment may correlate with a person's opting for death over life. Durkheim is the pioneer of sociological research in the study of suicide. The principal types of suicide found in his studies are the (1) egotistic suicide, (2) anomic suicide, and (3) altruistic suicide.

1. *Egotistic suicide* occurs when a person is insufficiently integrated into society.
2. *Anomic suicide* occurs when a person is isolated from others through abrupt changes in social status or social norms.
3. *Altruistic suicide* occurs as a response to societal demands. The deaths of buddhist monks and of nuns who set themselves on fire to protest the Vietnam War are examples of altruistic suicide.

One extension of Durkheim's theory proposes that the more integrated individuals are in a given society, the lower the risk of suicide. For example, the more meaningful the occupational roles and the higher the status of integration, the lower the risk of suicide (Adam, 1985). Others have established that suicide can be related to sudden change in status more than just to social status alone (Mowshowitz 1984).

BIOCHEMICAL - GENETIC THEORIES. It is difficult to distinguish biochemical or genetic predispositions to suicide from predispositions to depression or alcoholism. Both of these disorders run in families and most likely have a genetic component (Harvard Medical School 1986). However, low levels of the neurotransmitter serotonin are thought to play a part in the decision to commit suicide. Low serotonin levels are related to depressed moods. In a study of people hospitalized for suicide attempts, those with low serotonin levels were more likely to commit suicide than those with normal serotonin levels (Harvard Medical School 1986).

Also, low blood platelet levels of monoamine oxidase have been found in persons with a higher famil-

ial incidence of suicide than in people with normal levels (Kaplan and Sadock 1991). Monoamine oxidase inhibitors are commonly given for the treatment of depression (see Chapter 17).

No theory completely explains why a person will choose to end his or her life. However, a framework for nursing assessment and intervention can borrow from all three theoretical models.

Assessment

Nurses in all areas of work are in contact with people who have a high potential for suicidal behaviors. Patients on the general medical-surgical units often suffer losses in health or losses of function. Many people are hospitalized for alcohol-related medical problems or have alcoholism as a secondary diagnosis. These two groups comprise about 50% of all completed suicides (Kaplan and Sadock 1991).

On maternity wards, women are often undergoing situational crises. These crises may be related to an unwanted newborn or loss of a newborn. On obstetrical units, removal of a breast or uterus can be experienced as traumatic mutilation, resulting in alteration in self-concept and personal identity. In specialized units, such as burn units and intensive care units, nurses are continually dealing with people in physical and emotional crises. Appropriate interventions through referral for a psychiatric consultation or for counseling can prevent a suicide attempt or the actual act of suicide (Kolb and Brodie 1982).

Three areas of assessment will be discussed: (1) verbal and nonverbal suicidal clues, (2) lethality of the suicide plan, and (3) high-risk factors.

ASSESSING VERBAL AND NONVERBAL CLUES

Almost all people considering suicide will send out clues, especially to people they think of as supportive. Nurses often fit this category. Clues may be verbal, behavioral, somatic, or psychodynamic (Reubin 1979).

Verbal Clues	Examples
Overt statements	"I can't take it anymore." "Life isn't worth living anymore." "I wish I were dead." "Everyone would be better off if I died."

Covert statements

"It's OK now, soon everything will be fine."
"Things will never work out."
"I won't be a problem much longer."
"Nothing feels good to me anymore, and probably never will."
"How can I give my body to medical science?"

The nurse should always make overt what is covert. Most often it is a relief for a person contemplating suicide to finally talk to someone about his or her despair and loneliness. Asking someone if he or she is thinking of suicide does *not* "give a person ideas." Self-destructive ideas are a personal decision. Making covert indications of suicide overt *does* make possible a decrease in isolation and can increase problem-solving alternatives for living. Pallikkathayil and McBride (1986) found that suicide attempters were extremely receptive to talking about their suicide crisis, even those that regretted the failure of their attempt. Often these people expressed gratitude for the opportunity to talk to someone. Specific questions to ask include the following (Stevenson et al. 1988):

Are you experiencing thoughts of suicide?
Have you ever had thoughts of suicide in the past?
Have you ever attempted suicide?
Do you have a plan for committing suicide?
If so, what is your plan for suicide?

The following dialogue illustrates how the nurse can make covert messages overt.

NURSE: You haven't eaten or slept well for the past few days, Mary.
MARY: No . . . I feel pretty low lately.
NURSE: How low are you feeling?
MARY: Oh . . . I don't know . . . nothing seems to matter to me anymore . . . it's all so meaningless . . .
NURSE: What is meaningless, Mary?
MARY: Life . . . the whole thing . . . nothingness . . . life is a bad joke.
NURSE: Are you saying that you don't think life is worth living?
MARY: Well . . . yes . . . it's all so hopeless anyway . . .
NURSE: Are you thinking of killing yourself, Mary?
MARY: Yes . . . sometimes I think about it . . . I probably would never go through with it.
NURSE: Let's talk more about what you are thinking and feeling. However, I will need to share your thoughts with other members of the staff.

Be alert for behavioral clues, somatic clues, and emotional clues.

1. **Behavioral Clues** Sudden behavioral changes, especially when depression is lifting and when the person has more energy available to carry out a plan.	1. **Examples** Signs include giving away prized personal possessions, writing farewell notes, making out a will, and putting personal affairs in order.
2. **Somatic Clues** Physiological complaints can mask psychological pain and internalized stress.	2. **Examples** Symptoms associated with chronic stress include headaches, muscle aches, trouble sleeping, irregular bowel habits, unusual appetite, or weight loss.
3. **Emotional Clues** Various emotions can signal possible suicidal ideation.	3. **Examples** Symptoms include social withdrawal, feelings of hopelessness and helplessness, confusion, irritability, and complaints of exhaustion.

ASSESSING LETHALITY OF SUICIDE PLAN

The evaluation of a suicide plan is extremely important in determining the degree of suicidal risk. There are three main elements to be considered when evaluating the lethality of a suicide plan: (1) specificity of details, (2) lethality of proposed method, and (3) availability of means (Farberow 1967). If a person has definite plans for the time, place, and means, he or she is at high risk. Someone who is thinking of suicide but has not thought about when, where, or how is at a lower risk.

The lethality of method also indicates the level of risk, such as how quickly the person would die by that method, thereby lessening the probability of intervention. *Higher-risk* methods, also referred to as "hard" methods, include using a gun, jumping, hanging, carbon monoxide poisoning, and staging a car crash. Example of *lower-risk* methods, also referred to as "soft" methods, include slashing one's wrists, inhaling house gas, and ingesting pills. One study of persons who had attempted suicide showed that those who used hard methods displayed more social disintegration, were more often psychiatrically ill, and had more negative self-esteem (Schmitt and Mundt 1991).

When the means are available, the situation is more serious. For example, a man who states that he will jump from, and has access to, a high building, or that he will shoot himself and has a gun, is a serious risk. When people are psychotic, they are at high risk regardless of the specificity of details, lethality of method, and availability of means, because impulse control, judgment, and thinking are all grossly impaired.

ASSESSING HIGH-RISK FACTORS

Many tools can be used to aid a health care worker in assessing suicidal potential. Patterson et al. (1983) have devised an assessment aid using a brief acronym (**SAD PERSONS scale**) to evaluate 10 major risk factors for suicide potential (Box 21–2). The SAD PERSONS assessment is a simple, clear-cut, and practical guide to gauging suicide potential. Ten categories are described in the assessment tool. The person being evaluated is assigned one point for each applicable category. The person's total points are compared with a scale, which assists health care workers in deter-

mining whether hospital admission is necessary. The decision to admit someone to a hospital unit depends on many variables, such as whether the person lives alone, whether the person has access to a high-risk weapon, and whether the person has attempted suicide previously. The following scale serves as a general guideline:

Points	Guidelines for Intervention
0–2	Home with follow-up care
3–4	Close follow-up and possible hospitalization
5–6	Strongly consider hospitalization
7–10	Hospitalize

Nursing Diagnosis

The nursing diagnoses for a person who is suicidal may address many areas. However, the nursing diagnosis with the highest priority is *high risk for self-harm*.

Box 21–2. NURSING ASSESSMENT: SAD PERSONS SCALE

S	Sex	Men kill themselves three times more than women, although women make attempts three times more often than men.
A	Age	High-risk groups: 19 years or younger 45 years or older, especially the elderly 65 years or over.
D	Depression	Studies report that 35–79% of those who attempt suicide manifested a depressive syndrome.
P	Previous attempts	Of those who commit suicide, 65–70% have made previous attempts.
E	ETOH	ETOH (alcohol) is associated with up to 65% of successful suicides. Estimates are that 15% of alcoholics commit suicide. Heavy drug use is considered to be in this group and is given the same weight as alcohol.
R	Rational thinking loss	People with functional or organic psychoses are more apt to commit suicide than those in the general population.
S	Social supports lacking	A suicidal person often lacks significant others (friends, relatives), meaningful employment, and religious supports. All three of these areas need to be assessed.
O	Organized plan	The presence of a specific plan for suicide (date, place, means) signifies a person at high risk.
N	No spouse	Repeated studies indicate that persons who are widowed, separated, divorced, or single are at greater risk than those who are married.
S	Sickness	Chronic, debilitating, and severe illness is a risk factor.

From Patterson W, et al. Evaluation of suicidal patients: The SAD PERSONS scale. Psychosomatics, 24(4):343, 1983. Other data from Adam 1989; Merck Manual 1992; Stevenson 1988.

High risk for self-harm may be evidenced by various emotional states. Feelings of hopelessness, anger, poor impulse control, frustration, abandonment, and rejection are common among people who are suicidal. Suicide is often related to a loss. The loss of a significant person can leave a person feeling isolated, panicky, and confused. Loss of job, status, money, and sickness can be overwhelming. *High risk for self-harm* can also be related to crises in adolescents, adults, and the elderly. Identity crisis in the adolescent and isolation and loss of spouse in the elderly are situations signaling individuals in trouble.

Ineffective individual coping is also usually present. For example, a person who is clinically depressed, relies heavily on drugs and alcohol, is facing situational or maturational crises, or has chronic mental or physical problems may have impaired problem-solving and coping skills. Therefore, *ineffective individual coping* may be evidenced by the inability to meet role expectations or to meet basic needs related to heavy use of alcohol or drugs, inadequate psychological resources, or unsatisfactory support systems.

Ineffective family coping is often present. A child or teenager may be unable to get the guidance, support, and love he needs from home. Withdrawal of support from other family members can leave a child feeling abandoned, overwhelmed, and confused. This withdrawal of love and support may be related to the parent's own problems with alcohol or drugs, mental disorders, or perceived desertion through divorce or separation. When there are intense feelings of hostility and intolerance between parents, children often get left out or are manipulated and pitted against either or both parents. Therefore, examples of *ineffective family coping* may be evidenced by behavior problems in children, break-up of the family unit, chaotic family communication, or highly ambivalent family relationships.

Suicide is an attempt to end an intolerable life situation or state of mind that people feel helpless or powerless to change. Therefore, feelings of *hopelessness* and *powerlessness* are feelings often described by people who contemplate suicide.

Hopelessness, the belief that nothing can help change an intolerable situation or experience plays a major role in most suicides. Hopelessness can be related to a multitude of physical conditions (e.g., acquired immunodeficiency syndrome or cancer) and situations (e.g., financial or alterations in significant relationships). Hopelessness can be evidenced by verbal statements and cognitive difficulties (e.g., decreased judgment and decreased problem solving).

Powerlessness (thinking one has no control over events) may be related to a lifestyle of helplessness or a current situation that the person perceives as untenable and unalterable. An interpersonal interaction may also be perceived to be unalterably painful or psychologically traumatic. The person may be left feeling powerless or isolated.

People who think of ending their lives often do not feel very good about themselves. Feelings of worthlessness and expressions of shame or guilt are common among some. Therefore, the diagnoses *disturbance in self-esteem* or *chronic low self-esteem* need serious consideration.

Planning

Planning nursing care for a person who is suicidal involves planning on the (1) content level—planning goals and (2) process level—awareness of personal reactions to suicide and the person who is suicidal.

CONTENT LEVEL—PLANNING GOALS

Long term and short term goals are set for each nursing diagnosis. The nurse works with the client to set goals that are consistent with the suicidal person's perceptions and ability to carry out the goals. If a person is thought to be actively suicidal, hospitalization may be appropriate. For the nursing diagnosis *high risk for self harm*, the following goals may apply:

Long Term Goals

- Client will state by (date) that he or she wants to live.
- By (date), client will name two people he or she can call if thoughts of suicide recur.
- Client will name one acceptable alternative to his or her situation by (date).

Short Term Goals

- Client will remain safe while in the hospital.
- Client will make a no-suicide contract with the nurse covering the next 24 hours.
- Client will talk about painful feelings (guilt, anger, loneliness) by (date).

When people are depressed or suicidal, they are often unable to see choices or make decisions that could change their situation. This phenomenon is referred to as "tunnel vision." Clarifying hazards for the client and facilitating the expression of negative feelings are basic interventions. When the client is able to explore alternatives to his or her situation, change in thinking and behavior is possible. When alternatives to suicide are acceptable, feelings of hopelessness diminish. Therefore, goals for *ineffective individual coping*, as evidenced by faulty problem solving, could include the following:

Long Term Goals

- By (date) client will name signs and symptoms that indicate that he or she is starting to feel overwhelmed.
- By (date) client will name two persons that he or she can talk to if suicidal thoughts recur in the future.
- By (date) client will state that he or she has used two new coping mechanisms successfully in a stressful situation.
- By (date) client will state one decision that he or she has made that will improve the situation.

Short Term Goals

- Client will discuss with nurse situations that trigger suicidal thoughts and two feelings about these situations by (date).
- Client will identify three past coping mechanisms and state which were useful and which were not by (date).
- Client will name two effective ways to handle difficult situations in the future by (date).
- Client will state that he or she feels comfortable with one new technique after three sessions of role-playing.

Often a suicidal person is living within a family unit—that is, spouse, children, parent(s), or other significant others. The hopelessness, desperation, irritability, and withdrawal of the suicidal person profoundly affect other members of the family. Feelings of anxiety, denial, guilt, anger, frustration, and hopelessness arise in those close to a suicidal person. In many cases, the suicidal behavior is a reaction to dysfunctional family behavior. If the motive is to instill guilt in a significant person to control and extract revenge, the whole family unit would be in crisis. Therefore, the whole family needs support and counseling. For a diagnosis of *ineffective family coping* related to ineffective patterns of communication, the following goals could be included:

Long Term Goals

- Each family member will state that he or she feels less guilty, angry, or manipulated now (using a scale from 1 to 10), than before working with the nurse.
- Each family member will state that he or she feels better able to communicate with the suicidal member by (date).
- Each family member will state that he or she feels supported (by nurse, counselor, or therapist) and less confused and angry.
- By (date) each family member will state that the communication among all members of the family has improved.

Short Term Goals

- Each family member will state two feelings toward the suicidal member by (date).
- Each family member will state what he or she thinks the problem is by (date).
- Each family member will state three referral sources available for individual or family counseling, support, and guidance during the crises.

Although the motives for suicide may vary and the number of precipitating events may be infinite, all persons with suicidal ideation suffer similar feelings. Intense feelings of deprivation of affection, lack of hope for the future, and profound feelings of worthlessness and low self-esteem are common. The diagnosis of *disturbance in self-esteem* or *chronic low self-esteem* related to feelings of worthlessness may have the following associated goals:

Long Term Goals

- Client will name three things that he or she likes about himself or herself by (date).
- Client will participate in two activities that he or she enjoys and does well by (date).
- Client will state that he or she feels more comfortable around people by (date).
- Client will name one project he or she has completed and feels proud of by (date).
- Client will report feeling better about himself or herself by (date).

Short Term Goals

- Client will state that he or she will continue meeting with the nurse on a regular basis by (date).
- Client will make eye contact with the nurse 50% of the time they are together by (date).
- Client will talk about painful feelings with the nurse by (date).
- Client will begin to look at personal strengths as well as weaknesses by (date).
- Client will participate in his or her treatment plan by (date).

PROCESS LEVEL—NURSES' REACTIONS AND FEELINGS

People who are suicidal present affect and behavior that are difficult for nurses to deal with effectively. All health care professionals who work with people who are suicidal need supervision and guidance by a more experienced health care professional. Most people who are suicidal experience extreme hopelessness and helplessness, are withdrawn and keenly sensitive to rejection, are ambivalent, and may be hostile and angry. Affects such as these can stir up strong negative reactions in others. Birtchnell (1983) has identified numerous reactions in the literature that often arise in health care workers when working with a client who is suicidal. If these and other intense emotional responses are not made known and discussed in supervision, effective intervention will be limited, especially if these feelings are perceived by the suicidal client.

When these feelings are *not* identified, discussed, and resolved, the least that will happen is that the nurse will feel incompetent, experience low self-esteem, and become angry at the client for arousing these feelings. The worst that could happen is escalation or perpetuation of the client's painful feelings. The client may interpret the nurse's anxiety, irritation, and avoidance as validation for his own feelings of poor self-regard and self-hate. When feelings of hopelessness and poor self-esteem escalate, so does the potential for suicide.

The universal reactions of (1) anxiety, (2) irritation, (3) avoidance, and (4) denial by any health care worker caring for a suicidal person are discussed subsequently.

ANXIETY. Anxiety may have numerous sources. However, it is important to recognize that two common sources of anxiety are activated when working with a suicidal client. *First,* Birtchnell (1983) states that there are suicidal inclinations in all of us. A suicidal patient has the capacity to arouse these latent emotions and perhaps bring them out more strongly. *Second,* suicidal behavior or ideations on the part of the client may be interpreted by concerned health care personnel as personal rejection. Both sources of anxiety are usually working at an unconscious level. Nurses must become aware of their anxiety and attempt to identify the source, or the unmet need or expectation. Personal anxiety can then be reduced and not transferred to the client.

IRRITATION. Often people who make repeated suicide attempts are accused by family as well as health care workers of just "trying to get attention" or "looking for sympathy." It is common to hear of friends of family members saying to a suicidal person out of

frustration to "go ahead and get it over with." Such remarks by family and health providers strip the suicidal person of all hope and act as an encouragement for the suicidal person to kill himself or herself (Andriola 1973). No matter how trivial the suicidal attempt may appear, it is a genuine communication that the person is despairing and is unable to find a way out of a desperate situation or state of mind.

AVOIDANCE. People who are suicidal and people who are psychotic are frequently kept at a distance and "handled with kid gloves" by both medical and nursing personnel (Birtchnell 1983). Nurses and physicians may get caught up into taking responsibility for the actions of the suicidal person (rescue fantasy). Then, when things do not go the way the nurse or physician would like them to go, helplessness sets in. Staff then avoid situations or people that stimulate feelings of helplessness and incompetence. When the need to feel in control and responsible for other people's decisions is lessened through experience and supervision, the nurse is better able to refocus energies back to the client.

DENIAL. Denying or minimizing suicidal ideation or gestures is a defense against experiencing the feelings aroused by a suicidal person. Denial can be seen in such statements as, "I can't understand why anyone would want to take his own life." Often, family members and health care professionals are unable to acknowledge suicidal tendencies in someone close to them. Denial also occurs when identification with a suicidal person is strong, such as when a colleague commits suicide or a respected figurehead gives off covert suicidal messages.

PERSONAL STAGES HEALTH CARE WORKERS PASS THROUGH. Hammel-Bissell (1985) documents the "rites of passage" that psychiatric nurses must go through in order to work effectively with a suicidal person. Four stages are presented. Each stage progresses to the next as the nurse works through expected feelings and reactions.

1. The first stage is *naïveté*, in which feelings of shock and denial are prominent.
2. The second stage is termed *recognition*. This stage involves feelings of anxiety, fear, helplessness, and confusion.
3. The third stage, *stage of responsibility*, brings with it a cycle of feeling responsible, guilty, and then angry. This is a very conflicting time for people working with suicidal persons. It is crucial that during this time the nurse is helped by supervision and peer support. The nurse needs to vent these feelings and benefit from the experience of others who have gone beyond this stage. Otherwise, nurses may suffer burnout, may distance themselves from col-

leagues and clients, or may leave the work situation altogether.

4. The fourth and final stage, the *stage of individual choice*, comes through awareness gained through supervision, continuing education, and/or personal therapy. This is the stage when the nurse comes to the realization that the client is the only one in charge of his or her life. This frees the nurse to do whatever is humanly possible to help the client, while realizing that one person cannot ultimately control the decisions of another.

Intervention

Suicide intervention can be divided into three distinct areas: primary, secondary, and tertiary interventions.

Primary intervention includes activities that provide support, information, and education in situations that could otherwise become more serious and even lethal. Primary intervention can be practiced in schools, home, hospitals, and industrial settings.

Secondary intervention is treatment of the actual suicidal crisis. Secondary intervention is practiced in clinics, hospitals, and on telephone hotlines. Most people who are suicidal do not necessarily want to die; they just *don't know how to go on living in an intolerable situation* or state of mind. The client's ambivalence is one of the most important tools a nurse has when working with a suicidal person.

Tertiary intervention (postvention) can refer to (1) interventions with family and friends of a person who has committed suicide or (2) interventions with a person who has recently attempted suicide. Tertiary intervention for the latter is geared toward minimizing the traumatic after-effects of the suicide attempt.

PSYCHOTHERAPEUTIC INTERVENTIONS

Psychotherapeutic skills used by the nurse working with a client who is suicidal are practiced primarily (1) in clinics, (2) in hospitals, and (3) on telephone hotlines. The key element is the establishment of a workable relationship. There is general agreement by workers in this field on the importance of warmth, sensitivity, interest, concern, and consistency on the part of the helping person. Studies indicate that any treatment modality can be effective as long as it (1) includes the establishment of a personal relationship with the suicidal person, (2) encourages more realistic

problem-solving behavior, and (3) reaffirms hope (Evans 1983).

There is no place for hostility, sarcasm, or power struggles in the treatment of a suicidal person. These responses will only enhance poor self-esteem and feelings of hopelessness. Efforts should be geared toward maintaining or raising the suicidal person's self-esteem and self-respect. Cassem (1980) states that "self-esteem or self-respect is the most basic psychic condition to be guarded if life is to continue."

In the Clinic

Usually, people in suicidal crisis are seen in emergency rooms and referred to an outpatient clinic. Indeed, if after initial assessment the person is felt to be at low risk and not in need of hospitalization, referral to a clinic for crisis counseling is always indicated. Hoff (1984) names six techniques that are useful in an outpatient setting:

Technique	Action
1. Relieve isolation.	1. Arrange for person to stay with family or friends. If no one is available and the person is highly suicidal, hospitalization must be considered.
2. Remove all weapons.	2. Weapons and pills are removed by friends, relatives, or nurse.
3. Encourage alternative expression of anger.	3. Have person talk freely about feelings, unmet expectations, and disappointments. Plan with person alternative ways of handling frustration and anger.
4. Avoid final decision of suicide during crisis.	4. Assure the person that the suicidal crisis is a temporary state. Encourage the person to avoid a decision until alternatives can be considered during a noncrisis state (see subsequent discussion of *no-suicide contract*).
5. Re-establish social ties.	5. Contact family members. Arrange for family crisis counseling. Activate links to self-help groups—e.g., Widow-To-Widow, Parents Without Partners, and Al-a-Teen (see Appendix B for referral to self-help groups).

| 6. Relieve extreme anxiety. | 6. After thorough assessment, a tranquilizer may be prescribed to induce sleep and lower anxiety. *Note: only a one-to-three day supply should be given, and only with a return appointment for crisis counseling.* |

All persons receiving crisis counseling for suicidal ideations or actual suicide attempts should be given the opportunity for follow-up counseling or psychotherapy after the immediate crisis is over. **No-suicide contracts** between a counselor and a suicidal client have been used successfully in numerous settings, such as individual therapy, family therapy, group work, and behavioral therapy. The contract is outlined in clear and simple language. The purpose of the no-suicide contract is to give the counselor time to explore alternatives with the client. When the time of the contract is up, the contract is renegotiated. Examples of items in a no-suicide contract include

- "I will talk to my counselor before I harm myself."
- "I will wait until next week before I take any action to harm myself."
- "I will go to the hospital emergency room if I start to have suicidal impulses."
- "I won't kill myself, either on purpose or accidentally, for any reason."

A one-page written contract is signed by the client. Some counselors insert a clause that states that the person will report the importance of the contract to someone (e.g., counselor, friend, or wife) at least once daily. If the client is in the hospital, then the client would talk to the nurse.

Crisis counseling is imperative for a person who is suicidal. A suicidal person may be in an acute crisis situation or may be chronically suicidal. A person who is chronically suicidal usually has the following clinical history (Hatton et al. 1977b):

1. Has eliminated all resources—is isolated and withdrawn from significant others
2. Abuses alcohol, drugs, or both
3. Has recurrent depression
4. Has made several prior suicide threats or attempts over several years' time
5. Has made numerous bids for help, with little or no relief
6. Presents with instability in job performance, interpersonal relationships, or both

Crisis counseling can be effective for the chronically suicidal person; however, it cannot alter personality patterns. More research and clinical study are needed in the area of formulating a treatment plan and intervening successfully with the chronically suicidal person.

In the Hospital

How and when to use hospitalization is somewhat controversial. *"Danger to self or others"* is a general guideline. Legalities are often an important consideration. Either too much or too little restraint may be grounds for liability. Too much restraint may be grounds for abridgment of civil rights, and too little restraint may be grounds for malpractice. Generally, if the primary counselor (e.g., nurse, social worker, or psychologist) determines that the person is highly suicidal, has no immediate supports, and is exhausted and unable to carry out an alternative to suicide, hospitalization is indicated (Hatton et al. 1977b). However, some people are more responsive to treatment when they are not under constant observation. Long term hospitalization may undermine a person's ability to function effectively "on the outside" (Harvard Medical School 1986).

Even when the decision for hospitalization is made, there are no hospitals that are 100% "suicide-proof." Every hospital should have a suicide protocol that attempts to ensure the suicidal client's safety. *Students are advised to become familiar with the suicide protocol in the hospital(s) they are affiliated with.* Box 21–3 lists guidelines for minimizing suicidal behavior on a psychiatric unit (Schultz 1982).

Suicide precautions are meant to provide the client with a sense of security. If the client loses control and makes a suicidal attempt, the staff will step in and assume control. Built into the suicide protocol are frequent interactions between staff and the suicidal client, for example, once every 30 minutes or three times a day for 15 minutes. (See *Therapeutic Environment* for structuring a therapeutic environment while the suicidal person is in the hospital.)

When suicidal adolescents are admitted to a psychiatric unit, further restrictions may be imposed. Phone calls and visitation rights are often limited to the family only; friends, schoolmates, and girlfriends and boyfriends are restricted. This is done to reduce the incidence of *secondary gains* and maintain personal dignity. (Secondary gains are discussed and defined in Chapters 14 and 15.) Positive reinforcement of suicide as a means of receiving attention and sympathy and of temporarily relieving feelings of isolation should be minimized. Better problem-solving techniques and more satisfying ways of achieving attention, affection, and a sense of belonging are explored with the adolescent client.

Box 21–3. GUIDELINES FOR MINIMIZING SUICIDAL BEHAVIOR ON A PSYCHIATRIC UNIT

The Client

1. *Suicide precaution*, include one-on-one monitoring, having client in view *at all times* (one arm's length distance between staff member and client).
   a. *Includes* during toileting
   b. *Includes* during the night

2. *Suicide observation* includes a 15-minute visual check of suicidal client.

3. For each of the above, behavior, mood, and verbatim statements are recorded in the chart every 15 minutes.

The Environment

1. Count silverware and all other sharp objects before and after use by clients.

2. Do not allow clients to spend too much time alone in their rooms, and abolish private rooms altogether.

3. Jump-proof and hang-proof the bathrooms by installing break-away shower rods and recessed shower nozzles.

4. Keep electrical cords to minimum length.

5. Install unbreakable glass in windows. Install tamper-proof screens or partitions too small to pass through. Keep all windows locked.

6. Lock all utility rooms, kitchens, adjacent stairwells, and offices. All nonclinical staff (e.g., housekeepers and maintenance workers) should receive instructions to keep doors locked.

7. Take all potentially harmful gifts (e.g., flowers in glass vases) from visitors before allowing them to see clients.

8. Go through client's belongings with client and remove all potentially harmful objects (e.g., belts, shoelaces, metal nail files, tweezers, matches, and razors).

9. Ensure that visitors do not leave potentially harmful objects in client's room (e.g., matches and nail files).

10. Search clients for harmful objects (e.g., drugs, sharp objects, and cords) on return from pass.

On the Telephone Hotlines

A counselor on a telephone hotline is often a lay person or volunteer who has had special training. At other times, friends, neighbors, relatives, police officers, nurses, and the clergy find themselves at the other end of a telephone cry for help. Guidelines for handling a suicidal phone call are provided here (Hatton et al. 1977a; Neville and Barnes 1985; Frederick 1980). Almost all persons who are suicidal are ambivalent. *Ambivalence is one of the best tools a nurse has when working with a suicidal individual.* Talking with a helping person can help increase the suicidal person's likelihood of staying alive and can provide time to evaluate alternative actions. Essentially, the helping person at-tempts to establish rapport, assess the lethality of the situation, identify the problem, determine appropriate resources, and establish a plan with the caller.

ESTABLISH RAPPORT. Keeping the person on the line as long as possible is the most important thing. As long as the person keeps talking, he or she is not acting out suicidal threats. It is often helpful to acknowledge the person's distress. Although you do not know how the person feels, you can tell the person that you understand that he or she is in distress and is extremely unhappy. This lets the person know that (1) you take his or her concerns seriously, (2) there is no need to complete the suicidal act to make it clear that he or she is in distress, and (3) other alternatives are available; for example (Neville and Barnes 1985),

"The fact that you are considering suicide makes it clear that you are feeling overwhelmed and need some assistance, but there is no need for you to hurt yourself without first talking about what can be done to help you."

Establishing rapport may also be contingent on allowing ventilation of the caller's feelings. The helping person often has to accept angry or manipulative communication. The goal is to keep the caller talking and provide a psychological life-line.

Reinforcing the caller's positive responses is also useful. Any positive responses, thoughts, and actions that the person communicates need to be met with a validation that these were positive and in the person's best interests. For example, if the caller says that he or she was thinking about suicide but decided to call first, this should be reinforced as a positive move (Neville and Barnes 1985): "Your calling me at this time was a very positive move; I am glad you decided to call now."

IDENTIFY THE PROBLEM. The problem needs to be clearly identified. As with all crisis situations, the problem-solving approach is used. The use of reflection and restating are *not* useful in crisis situations (see Chapter 11 for interventions in crisis). The use of problem-solving approaches is helpful. Problem-solving statements help define the problem and explore avenues of action. For example:

Whom have you talked to about your parent's divorce?
How do you think the divorce will change your relationship with your parents?
Have you told them/him/her?
Do you think that they no longer love you?

ASSESS THE LETHALITY OF THE SITUATION

1. If the caller is threatening suicide, evaluate the lethality of the plan (see page 589).
2. If the caller has already taken pills, determine what kind and how many, whether the caller has been drinking, and other relevant medical information.
3. Determine if there is someone nearby—neighbor, bystander, housekeeper, or manager. If the answer is yes, tell the caller that you want to speak to that person right now.
4. If not, try to get the caller's address and explain that you want to get help for him or her.
5. If the caller does not want to give you the address, then instruct the caller on first aid:
   - Taking pills—induce vomiting.
   - Bleeding—apply pressure with bandage.
   - Inhalation poisoning—fresh air, loosen tight clothing.
6. Pass a note to staff member to attempt to have call traced. Notify telephone operator and then the police.

EVALUATE POSITIVE COPING AND ENCOURAGE ALTERNATIVES. Has the caller felt this way in the past? What did he or she do then? What works best? What could the caller do differently in this situation? What does the caller think would help change his or her situation? *Give referrals to appropriate places in the community* that may help alter the situation.

NEGOTIATE A NO-SUICIDE PLAN. As mentioned previously, a clearly worded contract with the caller may give the helping person time to work with the caller on more alternatives. Ideally, the aim is to get the caller into crisis counseling. If that is not possible, a relationship can be attempted over the phone. The wording in the contract should be clear and not conditional. Words such as "try" and "unless" are *not* used.

Not Useful		More Useful
"I will *try* not to kill myself."	→	"When I have thoughts of killing myself, I will go see my counselor."
"I will not kill myself *unless* my wife leaves me."	→	"If my wife does leave me, I will call my counselor right away."
"I will not kill myself *until* I call you."	→	"When I have thoughts of killing myself, I will talk to you."

It is necessary that the person manning the telephone hotline have numerous community resources available for referral. Besides the names and addresses of the resource, telephone numbers and names of contact persons should also be given whenever possible. Dependence is placed on the caller to contact resources for more long term assistance (Hipple and Cimolic 1979).

It is important that the caller is made aware that he or she does have control over his or her own decisions and believes that someone cares about the situation and is available.

Research on the ability of telephone counseling to reduce suicide rates and effect behavioral change is sparse. Severely suicidal people are not thought to make use of life-sustaining avenues such as hotlines. One case study pointed out that only 2% of all suicide victims in Los Angeles County had called the prevention center (Harvard Medical School 1986). However, other studies indicate that telephone counseling may have considerable therapeutic potential (Glatt et al. 1986; Hornblow 1986).

HEALTH TEACHING

Primary intervention in the form of health teaching is an important method of lessening suicidal attempts.

The goal is to reach people before they become so overwhelmed that suicide appears to be a rational alternative. *Primary intervention* relates to the principles of good mental health. The following programs provide support, information, and education:

- Programs on emotional health in the junior and senior high schools
- Drug and alcohol courses that allow "rap sessions" in grade schools and junior and senior high schools
- Special programs in industry for the drug and alcohol abuser
- Seminars for all health care providers on assessment and intervention in suicide, especially for those working in schools, industry, and well-baby clinics
- Seminars and group activities for the elderly that focus on (1) physical concerns such as reactions to medications and physical changes and (2) emotional concerns such as how to cope with loneliness, separations from family, and loss of friends through death

ACTIVITIES OF DAILY LIVING

Because social isolation and withdrawal are often present, active encouragement and advice regarding contacting significant persons and loved ones should be given. Renewing friendships and important relationships can help foster self-esteem. When the crisis pertains to a significant other (e.g., spouse, parent, or child), therapies such as family, couple, or group counseling may be indicated.

Community agencies may be useful in helping a person renew or initiate activities related to work, special interests, hobbies, sports, and other activities that can help enhance self-esteem.

SOMATIC THERAPIES

In cases in which extreme anxiety and lack of sleep occur for several days, the risk of suicide can increase. A tranquilizer will usually take care of both the anxiety and the sleeping problem. If medication is given, the supply should be *for one to three days only*, with a return appointment scheduled for re-evaluation. Tranquilizers, however, should never be given to a highly suicidal individual. Generally, a lethal dose for tranquilizers is 10 times the normal dose. When a drug is combined with alcohol, only half that amount can cause death (Hoff 1984).

When a coexisting psychiatric condition is present in a person who is suicidal, somatic intervention is dictated according to the psychopathology. For example, a person who is suicidal and also holds the diagnosis of schizophrenia may need increased medication. Similar considerations are made for people who are clinically depressed as well as suicidal. Electroconvulsive therapy can save the life of a seriously depressed and highly suicidal person. Refer to Chapter 17 for further information regarding electroconvulsive therapy. It takes one to three weeks of antidepressant therapy before the person experiences an elevation of mood. Electroconvulsive therapy can have more immediate effects.

THERAPEUTIC ENVIRONMENT

Hospitalization is sometimes the most therapeutic intervention. Placing a highly suicidal person in a controlled hospital environment can provide structure and control and can give the person time to evaluate his or her situation with professional staff. During hospitalization, the client's suicidal risk and level of suicidal precaution needed are continually assessed. Table 21–2 lists guidelines for suicide precautions. Repeated monitoring of a person's suicide intent and extent of hopelessness is ongoing. The decision to discontinue suicide precautions is ideally based on clinical observations of nursing staff, physicians, and social workers, as well as on input from the client. Therefore, the decision to continue or discontinue suicide precautions should be based on subjective data and objective clinical observations (Busteen and Johnstone 1983).

PSYCHOTHERAPY

Initial intervention for a suicidal person is crisis intervention. However, all persons should be offered the opportunity for further therapy after the crisis is over. A nurse educated at the master's level may work with suicidal clients in several modalities. Suitable therapies have been mentioned. Couple, individual, family, and group counseling are all useful. This is especially true if a person is chronically suicidal or has coexisting psychopathology, such as depression, borderline symptoms, and schizophrenic disorders.

Tertiary intervention for family and friends ("survivors") of a person who has committed suicide should be initiated as soon after the death as possible (e.g.,

Table 21–2 ■ SUMMARY OF LEVELS OF SUICIDE PRECAUTIONS

POPULATION	EXAMPLES OF CLIENT SYMPTOMS	NURSING CARE
Level I		
Clients who are not verbalizing or suggesting suicidal ideation.	Level I includes all clients admitted to the unit who do not meet the criteria for levels II through IV.	1. Check client's whereabouts at least every hour. 2. Make frequent verbal contact while client is awake
Level II		
Clients who have suicidal ideations and who, after assessment by staff, are assessed to be in minimal danger of activity attempting suicide.	1. The client with vague suicidal ideation but without plan 2. The client who is willing to make a no-suicide contract 3. The client with insight into existing problems	1. Check client's whereabouts every 15 to 30 minutes. 2. Maintain frequent verbal contact while client is awake. 3. Chart client's whereabouts, mood, verbatim statements, and behavior every 15 to 30 minutes. 4. *
Level III		
Clients with suicidal ideations and who, after assessment by unit staff, present clinical symptoms that indicate a higher suicide potential than level II.	1. The client with a concrete suicide plan 2. The client who is ambivalent about making a no-suicide contract 3. The client with minimal insight into existing problems 4. The client with limited impulse control	1. Conduct close observation*—i.e., within visual range of staff while client is awake. Accompany to bathroom. Place client in multiple-client room. Check client every 15 to 30 minutes while client is awake. 2. Chart client's whereabouts, mood, verbatim statements, behavior every 15 to 30 minutes. 3. Ensure that meal trays contain no glass or metal silverware. 4. *
Level IV		
Clients with suicidal ideations or delusions of self-mutilation who, according to assessment by unit staff, present clinical symptoms that suggest a clear intent to follow through with the plan or delusion.	1. The client who is currently verbalizing a clear intent to harm self 2. The client who is unwilling to make a no-suicide contract 3. The client who presents with no insight into existing problems 4. The client with poor impulse control 5. The client who has already attempted suicide in the recent past by a particularly lethal method—e.g., hanging, gun, or carbon monoxide poisoning	1. Conduct one-to-one nursing observation and interaction 24 hours a day (never out of staff's sight). 2. Maintain arm's length at all times. 3. Chart client's whereabouts, mood, and verbatim statements, behavior every 15 to 30 minutes. 4. Ensure that meal trays contain no glass or metal silverware. 5. *

Adapted from Busteen EL, Johnstone C. The development of suicide precautions for an inpatient psychiatric unit. Journal of Psychosocial Nursing and Mental Health Services, 21(5):18, 1983.
*Nurse and physician explain to the client what the nurse will be doing and why. Both nurse and physician document this in chart.

within 72 hours) and continued at least through the first anniversary of the death. Mourning the death of a loved one who has committed suicide is painful at all times. A family of a person who has committed suicide is often faced with the process of mourning without the normal, informal social supports usually provided. Survivors often feel that they are "going crazy." They need to know that these feelings are normal. Survivors need to find outlets for the undercurrent of anger against the deceased, who is responsible for trauma, confusion, and pain inflicted on them. Unfor-

tunately, few survivors of suicide seek out counseling (Van Dongen 1988). Pronounced feelings of anger and guilt are common reactions.

Self-help groups have been found to be extremely beneficial for survivors of a suicidal family member or friend. Many people join self-help groups even if the suicide took place 25–30 years before.

Self-help groups for the survivors of a family member or friend who committed suicide are similar to all other self-help groups. Essentially, self-help groups for family survivors are run by people who have lost someone through suicide. When a professional is involved, it is in the role of facilitator, consultant, or educator—not that of leader. Ideally, lay leaders should have some professional training in group processes and awareness of the limitations of the group experience. Professional therapists (e.g., nurses, social workers, psychiatrists, and psychologists) should be used as a source of referral and should be available for consulting. Referral for individual and family therapy is advised once individual and family problems have been identified.

Likewise, staff and therapists who have been working with a client who successfully commits suicide need support. Staff should have the opportunity to make adequate emotional expression of feelings of self-blame, guilt, and anger. If one of the staff had been closely involved over a long period of time with the client who has committed suicide, the staff member will also pass through a period of grief (Birtchnell 1983). Suicide can be an occupational hazard for a therapist involved in direct client care. Feelings of anger and guilt, experiencing loss of self-esteem, and having intrusive thoughts about the suicide are common. Symptoms similar to those of post-traumatic stress disorder were experienced by a significant percentage of psychiatrists who had a client who committed suicide (Chemtob et al. 1988). Peer support and supervision help work through the loss.

A full-scale psychological postmortem assessment should be carried out among staff. The purpose is to reveal errors in judgment or overlooked clues that could be useful when evaluating future clients. Discussion should center on piecing together the pressures that led up to the client's taking his or her life (Birtchnell 1983).

Tertiary intervention can also be viewed as referring to a person who has survived a suicide attempt. In such a case, efforts to prevent a future attempt (primary intervention) and working with the individual on immediate problems and concerns (secondary intervention) are indicated.

Evaluation

Evaluation of a suicidal client is an ongoing part of the assessment. The nurse must be constantly alert to changes in the suicidal person's mood, thinking, and behavior. As has been mentioned, sudden behavioral changes can signal suicidal intent, especially when the client's depression is lifting and more energy is available to carry out a preconceived plan. A person with a diagnosis of schizophrenia is also at risk when recovering from a psychotic episode. Anniversaries of losses and holiday seasons are particularly difficult times for some people.

Evaluation includes identifying the presence or absence of any clues or thoughts of suicide. The nurse also looks for indications that the person is communicating thoughts and feelings more readily and that his or her social network is widening. For example, if the person is able to talk about his or her feelings and engage in problem solving with the nurse, this would be a positive sign. Is the client increasing his or her social activities and expanding his or her interests? Does the client state that he or she thinks more or fewer suicidal thoughts? Essentially, the nurse evaluates the goals and establishes new ones as different situations arise. Goals for a client who is in a crisis situation may differ from those for a client who is chronically suicidal.

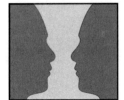

Case Study: Working with a Person Who is Suicidal

Thomas Martin, a 46-year-old social worker, was brought to the hospital for evaluation after an attempted suicide. When he did not show up for work, his coworker called to check on him. His landlady stated that his car was still in the driveway and that she would check his room. She found Mr. Martin lying on the bed, beside an empty bottle of sleeping pills. A strong smell of liquor filled the room and a nearly empty bottle of Scotch was on a table by the bed. An ambulance took Mr. Martin to the emergency room, where his stomach was pumped. He stayed in the emergency room for 16 hours, until he was no longer groggy. He was then seen by a psychiatric nurse, Mrs. Ruiz, for evaluation.

He told Mrs. Ruiz that he had been separated from his wife for two years but had seen his eight-year-old son every week during that time. Three days prior to his suicide attempt, his wife sent him a letter stating that she wanted to remarry and move to Oklahoma with her son and new husband.

Assessment

Mr. Martin's manner was hostile and sarcastic. He told the nurse that it did not matter what anyone did, he would "do it again," and that next time he would succeed. He sat sneering at the nurse saying, "I never liked nurses anyway."

NURSE:	What is it about nurses that you don't like?
MR. MARTIN:	*Mimicking the nurse's tone.* What is it about nurses that you don't like—what dribble. Don't try that therapeutic garbage on me. I don't need help from you or anyone else.
	Silence.
	You're all castrating bitches . . . all women are. I hate all women.
NURSE:	Tell me about one woman who has hurt you.
MR. MARTIN:	*Angrily* . . . Stop prying into my business with your little therapeutic diddies.
	Silence.
	Well . . . my wife . . . she . . . she . . . oh God . . . *At this point Mr. Martin starts sighing deeply, then bursts into tears.*
NURSE:	*Waits a few minutes.* This situation with your wife and son moving away has upset you deeply.
MR. MARTIN:	I don't want to live if I can't see my son. He is all I have left. He is the only thing that ever mattered to me.
NURSE:	You have no friends or family?
MR. MARTIN:	All my family died when I was a kid. As for friends . . . I don't need other people. Anyway, people don't seem to like me much. Look, don't spend time worrying about me. I've got a few more tricks up my sleeve.
NURSE:	Do you mean that you will try to kill yourself again?
MR. MARTIN:	What could it possibly mean to you?
NURSE:	I *am* concerned about you, Mr. Martin.
MR. MARTIN:	Well . . . isn't that the nursie thing to say. . . . Such great understanding.
NURSE:	I do understand that you are very troubled right now and have no one to go to.

Mrs. Ruiz organized her data into objective and subjective components.

OBJECTIVE DATA

1. Male, age 46, no support systems
2. Impending loss of significant relationship with son
3. Possible drinking problem, need more data
4. Suicide attempt
5. Holds responsible job
6. Estranged wife and son moving away from area
7. Appears articulate and bright

SUBJECTIVE DATA

1. "I don't want to live if I can't see my son."
2. "I've got a few more tricks up my sleeve."
3. "He (son) is the only thing that ever mattered to me."
4. "All my family died when I was just a kid."
5. "I don't need other people."
6. "People don't seem to like me much."

Nursing Diagnosis

Mrs. Ruiz analyzed her data and set up her nursing diagnoses in order of priority.

1. *High risk for self-harm* related to suicidal behavior and belief that he has no reason to live
   - Suicide attempt
   - "I don't want to live if I can't see my son."
   - "He is the only thing that ever mattered to me."
   - "I've got a few more tricks up my sleeve."
   - Is holding a responsible job

2. *Impaired social interaction* related to inability to engage in satisfying relationships

Continued on following page

Nursing Diagnosis
(Continued)

- "He (son) is all I have left."
- "All my family died when I was a kid."
- "I don't need other people."
- "People don't seem to like me much."

Mrs. Ruiz discussed the case with the admitting resident. Because Mr. Martin stated that he wanted to kill himself, had no family or friends that could stay with him, and had access to drugs, the decision was made to hospitalize him for further evaluation. Ordinarily, Mrs. Ruiz would follow him in clinic after discharge. In this case, Mrs. Ruiz told the physician that she thought it best for a male psychiatric nurse to work with Mr. Martin after discharge. Mrs. Ruiz explained that she thought that Mr. Martin would have a strong negative transference with a female nurse and, at this time, working with him on alternatives in his life was the main goal. After the immediate crisis was over, working on his interpersonal relationships would take priority.

Planning

Mr. Martin was kept in the hospital for three days. During that time he was placed on suicide precautions, as outlined in Table 21–2. He was discharged to the clinic after the staff thought that he was no longer a suicidal risk.

When asked if he wanted a male nurse instead of a female nurse, he stated, "No . . . I'll talk to the little nursie . . . she's got a thing for me."

CONTENT LEVEL—PLANNING GOALS

The nurse met with Mr. Martin, and both worked out the following goals:

Nursing Diagnosis	Long Term Goals	Short Term Goals
1. *High risk for self-harm* related to loss of a son	1. Mr. Martin will state that he wants to live.	1a. Mr. Martin will make a *no-suicide contract* with the nurse by the end of the first session. 1b. Mr. Martin will talk about painful feelings by (date). 1c. Mr. Martin will look at alternative ways he can keep in touch with his son by (date).
2. *Impaired social interaction* related to social isolation	2. Mr. Martin will state that he feels less isolated and is participating in at least one activity involving other people.	2a. Mr. Martin will discuss feelings of isolation and loneliness by (date). 2b. Mr. Martin will identify three positive aspects of self and job by (date). 2c. Mr. Martin will state that he enjoys one new weekly activity by (date).

PROCESS LEVEL—NURSES' REACTIONS AND FEELINGS

Mrs. Ruiz knew that working with Mr. Martin was going to evoke high anxiety. When talking to her clinical supervisor, it became apparent that the idea of sending Mr. Martin to a male nurse therapist, while logical on the surface, was motivated by Mrs. Ruiz's own anxiety. She was trying to avoid Mr. Martin. "I guess I did try to shove him off. His sarcasm and belittling made me feel put down and angry."

Reviewing that first session with the supervisor clarified a number of important dynamics. First, it became evident that Mr. Martin was experiencing low self-esteem as a result of the impending loss of his son's companionship. The resulting anxiety was turned inward. Mr. Martin's rage at the loss and the inability to change the situation resulted in intense feelings of helplessness. Second, it appeared from the data that Mr. Martin was extremely isolated. It also appeared that most of this isolation was self-imposed. His sarcasm and belittling remarks appeared to be devices to (1) push people away, (2) temporarily lift sagging self-esteem through "one-upmanship," and (3) divert attention from his own fears. The supervisor and Mrs. Ruiz saw the need to relieve Mr.

Martin's isolation without increasing his anxiety to severe levels.

It was important for Mr. Martin to talk about some of his feelings. Identifying and expressing feelings could have a number of benefits. First, talking about pent-up feelings could minimize feelings of isolation. Second, talking about feelings could reduce the need to act them out through self-destructive channels. Third, once identified, these feelings could be more positively discharged and worked through.

Intervention

At first, Mr. Martin was sarcastic, belittling, flirtatious, and hostile. Mrs. Ruiz kept her responses neutral and continued to focus her concern on Mr. Martin's situations and on working with alternatives. She gave him frequent opportunities to talk about his feelings. Initially, Mr. Martin would ridicule the nurse and belittle the idea: "Oh . . . you want to know about my precious painful feelings." Gradually, the testing-out behavior began to diminish. Slowly, and with some reluctance, Mr. Martin began talking about his feelings of loneliness and despair and sense of being a failure as a husband and father. He talked about the pain of his separation from his wife and his feelings of being a failure to his son.

The nurse continued to be neutral, not getting involved with power struggles or becoming defensive. Mrs. Ruiz began to see more clearly how these sarcastic and belittling behaviors helped Mr. Martin to defend against painful feelings of failure and low self-esteem. Refer to Nursing Care Plan 21–1 for specific interventions used with Mr. Martin.

Evaluation

After two months, Mr. Martin stated that although he missed his son desperately, he no longer thought of suicide. He did not want to leave his son that legacy. He was planning his next vacation in Oklahoma, camping with his son for two weeks. His interpersonal relationships were still strained. He was beginning to look at situations that gave rise to his sarcasm and belittling and to relate his actions to feelings that had been unconscious. His sarcasm and belittling toward Mrs. Ruiz had diminished a great deal, although he still resorted to it when he felt threatened. He spent more time on examining his life, feelings, and where he wanted to go, and less on defensive behaviors. Although by this time the crisis was over, Mr. Martin continued counseling with Mrs. Ruiz. He was able to say that at times he felt more comfortable with his coworkers, although he still did not feel at home with others. He had resumed weekly bowling. He stated that he was surprised that he enjoyed it. He had even started talking to a "fellow there who is also divorced and got a rough deal. He's not a bad guy."

Nursing Care Plan 21–1 ■ A SUICIDAL CLIENT AFTER DISCHARGE: Mr. Martin

NURSING DIAGNOSIS

High risk for self-harm related to loss of son.

Supporting Data

- Suicide attempt
- "I don't want to live if I can't see my son."
- "I've got a few more tricks up my sleeve."
- Impending loss of son.

Long Term Goal: Mr. Martin will state that he wants to live.

Short Term Goal	Intervention	Rationale	Evaluation
1. Mr. Martin will make a *no-suicide contract* with nurse by end of first session.	1a. Assess suicide status.	1a. Ongoing periodic check of suicidal status. Higher rate of suicide for those who have attempted suicide.	Goal met Mr. Martin signed contract: "I will not kill myself until I talk to the nurse" (first session).

Continued on following page

Nursing Care Plan 21–1 ■ A SUICIDAL CLIENT AFTER DISCHARGE: Mr. Martin *(Continued)*

Short Term Goal	Intervention	Rationale	Evaluation
	1b. Even if Mr. Martin denies suicide, make a *no-suicide contract.*	1b. Demonstrates concern and offers alternatives if suicidal thoughts return.	
2. Mr. Martin will talk about painful feelings by (date).	2a. Remain neutral in face of hostility and put-downs.	2a. Diminishes power struggles and discourages continuing acting-out behaviors.	Goal met During first to third week, hostile and sarcastic communication was constant.
	2b. Refocus attention back to Mr. Martin.	2b. Arguments and power struggles keep attention focused away from important issues.	By fourth week, Mr. Martin stated, "You really want to know."
	2c. Give frequent opportunities for discussion of feelings through verbal invitation and sated concern.	2c. Aggressive, hostile communications are cover for painful feelings. When client can express feelings in words, there is less need to act them out.	Mr. Martin talked of feeling like a failure as a husband and father.
3. Mr. Martin will look at alternative ways he can keep in touch with his son by (date).	3. Alternative solutions can be problem-solved once feelings and problems are identified.	3. Acceptable alternatives increase a future orientation and decrease hopelessness. Client can experience feelings of control over the situation.	Goal met By fifth week, Mr. Martin talked about taking son on a camping trip during summer recess.

NURSING DIAGNOSIS

Impaired social interaction **related to social isolation.**

Supporting Data

- "He (son) is all I have left."
- "All my family died when I was a kid."
- "I don't need other people."
- "People don't seem to like me much."

Long Term Goal: Mr. Martin will state that he feels less isolated and less frightened of people by (date).

Short Term Goal	Intervention	Rationale	Evaluation
1. Mr. Martin will discuss feelings of isolation and loneliness by (date).	1. Provide opportunities for Mr. Martin to express feelings and thoughts regarding his self-imposed isolation.	1. Before change can take place, clarification of personal feelings and thoughts is necessary.	Goal met By fourth week Mr. Martin spoke of feeling alone—son is only contact to life.
2. Mr. Martin will identify three positive aspects of self and job by (date).	2a. Validate Mr. Martin's strengths.	2a. Positive as well as negative feedback aid in more realistic perception of self.	By fifth week, Mr. Martin stated that he thinks he is a good worker and is respected (if not liked) by his peers.
	2b. Encourage self-evaluation of positive as well as negative aspects of Mr. Martin's life.	2b. Client can begin to see himself more clearly, with increase in self-esteem.	
3. Mr. Martin will state that he enjoys one new weekly activity with at least one other person by (date).	3a. Review previous activities that Mr. Martin enjoyed before his marriage ended.	3a. Change focus from negative present to positive aspects of his past. Can help increase hope and self-esteem.	Goal met By seventh week, Mr. Martin stated that he started bowling again and was surprised that he had a good time.
	3b. Have Mr. Martin choose an activity that he is willing to participate in.	3b. Participating in own problem solving and decision making offers a sense of control and an increase in self-esteem.	

Summary

Suicide is the willful act of ending one's life. A person can also hasten one's death by covert self-destructive behaviors, such as alcoholism, medical noncompliance, hyperobesity, anorexia nervosa, and gambling. Death from such causes is called *subintentioned death*.

Suicidal behavior can be classified into three categories: (1) completed, (2) attempted, and (3) ideation. Statistics surrounding suicide provide a profile that can be useful when assessing a person's suicidal intention. Many complex factors contribute to a person's decision to commit suicide. These factors include psychodynamic, sociological, and biochemical theories.

It is critical for the nurse to assess the client's suicidal intent. The nurse assesses verbal and nonverbal clues, lethality of suicide plan, and high-risk factors. Nursing diagnoses may include a number of problem areas; however, *high risk for self-harm* is the most crucial initially. When planning care, the nurse plans specific goals. Personal reactions to suicide and the suicidal client need to be dealt with. Common and expected reactions were discussed, and supervision with a more experienced health care professional was emphasized.

Intervention in suicide can be on a *primary, secondary,* or *tertiary* level. Various interventions were spelled out. Evaluation is ongoing, especially with a person who has a potential for suicide, because the incidence is often higher when depression is lifting or a person is recovering from a psychotic episode. Goals are evaluated and reset, according to change in the assessment and progress by the client toward mutually agreed-upon goals. A case study was provided to highlight nurses' work with a suicidal client.

References

Adam KS. Attempted suicide. Psychiatric Clinics of North America, 8(2):183, 1985.

Andriola J. A note on the possible iatrogenesis of suicide. Psychiatry, 36:213, 1973.

Birtchnell J. Psychotherapeutic considerations in the management of the suicidal patient. American Journal of Psychotherapy, 37(1):24, 1983.

Busteen EL, Johnstone C. The development of suicide precautions for an inpatient psychiatric unit. Journal of Psychosocial Nursing and Mental Health Services, 21(5):15, 1983.

Cassem NH. Treating the person confronting death. In Nicholi AM (ed). The Harvard Guide to Modern Psychiatry. Cambridge, MA: The Belknap Press of Harvard University Press, 1980.

Chemtob CM, Hamada RS, Baver G, et al. Patient's suicide: Frequency and impact on psychiatrists. American Journal of Psychiatry, 145(2):224, 1988.

Clayton PJ. Suicide. Psychiatric Clinics of North America, 8(2):203, 1985.

Davison GC, Neale JM. Abnormal Psychology. New York: John Wiley & Sons, 1982.

De Leo D, Ormskerk. Suicide in the elderly: General characteristics. Crisis, 12(2):3–17, Sept 1991.

Evans DL. Explaining suicide among the young: An analytic review of the literature. Journal of Psychosocial Nursing and Mental Health Services, 21(5):9, 1983.

Farberow NL. Crisis, disaster and suicide: Theory and therapy. In Schneidman ES (ed). Essays in Self-Destruction. New York: Jason Aronson, 1967.

Frederick CJ. Drug abuse: An indirect self-destructive behavior. In Farberow NL (ed). The Many Faces of Suicide: Indirect Self-Destructive Behaviors. New York: McGraw-Hill, 1980.

Glatt KM, Sherwood DW, Amisson TJ. Telephone hotlines at a suicide site. Hospital and Community Psychiatry, 37(2):178, 1986.

Hammel-Bissell BP. Suicidal casework: assessing nurses' reactions. Journal of Psychosocial Nursing and Mental Health Services, 23(10):20, 1985.

Harvard Medical School Mental Health Letter. Suicide—Part II, 2:1, 1986.

Hatton CL, et al. Intervention. In Hatton CL (ed). Suicide: Assessment and Intervention. New York: Appleton-Century-Crofts, 1977a.

Hatton CL, et al. Theoretical framework. In Hatton CL (ed). Suicide: Assessment and Intervention. New York: Appleton-Century Crofts, 1977b.

Hendrin H. Suicidality and the young. American Journal of Psychiatry, 149(6):850, 1992.

Hipple J, Cimolic P. The use of the telephone in treatment. The Counselor and the Suicidal Crisis: Diagnosis and Prevention. Springfield, MA: Charles C Thomas, 1979.

Hoff LA. People in Crisis: Understanding and Helping, 2nd ed. Menlo Park, CA: Addison-Wesley Publishing Company, 1984.

Holinger PC. The course, impact, and preventability of childhood injuries in the United States. American Journal of Diseases of Children, 144(6):670, 1990.

Hornblow AR. The evolution and effectiveness of telephone counseling services. Hospital and Community Psychiatry, 37(7):731, 1986.

Kaplan HI, Sadock BJ. Synopsis of Psychiatry, 6th ed. Baltimore, MD: Williams & Wilkins, 1991.

Kavenaugh RE. Facing Death. Baltimore: Penguin Books, 1972.

Kolb LC, Brodie HKM. Modern Clinical Psychiatry, 10th ed. Philadelphia: WB Saunders, 1982.

Malzberger JT, Buie D. The devices of suicide. International Review of Psychoanalysis, 7:61, 1980.

Merck Manual of Diagnosis and Therapy. Berkow R, Fletcher AJ (eds). Rahway, NJ: Merck Research Laboratories, 1992.

Mowshowitz I. The special role of the pastoral counselor. In The Will to Live vs. the Will to Die. New York: Human Sciences Press, 1984.

Mullis MR, Byers PH. Social support. Journal of Psychosocial Nursing, 25(4):16, 1988.

Neville D, Barnes S. The suicidal phone call. Journal of Psychosocial Nursing, 23(8):14, 1985.

Pallikkathayil L, McBride AB. Suicide attempts. Journal of Psychosocial Nursing, 24(8):13, 1986.

Parker SD. Accidents or suicide: Do life changed events lead to adolescent suicide? Journal of Psychosocial Nursing, 26(6):15, 1988.

Patterson W, et al. Evaluation of suicidal patients: The SAD PERSONS scale. Psychosomatics, 24(4):343, 1983.

Paykel ES, et al. Suicide attempts and recent life events. Archives of General Psychiatry, 33:327, 1975.

Pollard BJ. Medical aspects of euthanasia. Medical Journal of Australia, 154(9):613, 1991.

Reubin R. Spotting and stopping the suicide patient. Nursing 79, 9(4):83, 1979.

Roche Report: Frontiers of Psychiatry. Suicide support groups: self-help for those left behind. December, 1982.

Roy A. Emergency psychiatry. In Kaplan HI, Sadock BJ (eds). Comprehensive Textbook of Psychiatry V. Baltimore: Williams & Wilkins, 1989.

Schmitt W, Mundt C. Differential typology among patients with hard and soft suicide methods. Nervenarzt, 62(7):440, 1991.

Schneidman ES. Orientation towards death: A vital aspect of the study of lives. In White RW (ed). The study of lives. New York: Atherton Press, 1963.

Schutz BM. Legal Liability in Psychotherapy. San Francisco: Jossey-Bass, 1982.

Simmons S. Suicide potentiality. Washington, DC: U.S. Government Printing Office, U.S. Department of Health and Human Services (NIH Publication No. 82-2308), 1981.

Stevenson JM. Suicide. In Talbott JA, Hale RE, Yudofsky SC. Textbook of Psychiatry. Washington, DC: American Psychiatric Press, 1988.

Van Dongen CJ. The legacy of suicide. Journal of Psychosocial Nursing, 26(1):9, 1988.

Further Reading

Beck AT, et al. Classification and nomenclature. In Resnick H, Hawthorne B (eds). Suicide Prevention in the Seventies. Washington, DC: US Government Printing Office, 1973.

Benton RG. Death and Dying: Principles and Practices in Patient Care. New York: D. Van Nostrand Company, 1978.

Breed W. Occupational mortality and suicide among males. American Sociological Review, 28:179, 1963.

De Leo D, Ormskerk. Suicide in the elderly: General characteristics. Crisis, 12(2):3, 1991.

Donlon PT, Rockwell DA. Psychiatric Disorders: Diagnoses and Treatment. Bowie, MD: Robert J. Brady Company, 1982.

Fitzpatrick JJ. Suicidology and suicide prevention: Historical perspectives from the nursing literature. Journal of Psychosocial Nursing and Mental Health Services, 21(5):9, 1982.

Gibbs J, Martin W. Status integration and suicide: A study in sociology. Eugene, OR: University of Oregon Press, 1964.

Hamlin WT. Adolescent suicide. Journal of the National Medical Association, 74(1):25, 1982.

Hart NA, Keidel GC. The suicidal adolescent. Americal Journal of Nursing, 79(1):80, 1979.

Hipple J, Cimolic P. The Counselor and the Suicidal Crisis: Diagnosis and Prevention. Springfield, MA: Charles C Thomas, 1979.

Hopkins BW. Running away from it all: Suicide among troubled youth. Family Life Developmental Center—Department of Human Developmental Studies, Cornell University, Ithaca, NY, July–August, 1983.

Kenney EM, Karjewski KJ. Hospital treatment of the adolescent suicidal patient. In McIntyre MS, Angle CR (eds). Suicide Attempts in Children and Youth. New York: Harper & Row, 1980.

Kliman AS. Psychological first aid for recovery. In The Will to Live vs. the Will to Die. New York: Human Sciences Press, 1984.

Leggett J. Ross and Tom: Two American Tragedies. New York: Simon & Schuster, 1974.

Menninger K. Man Against Himself. New York: Harcourt, Brace & World, 1938.

Peck ML. Adolescent suicide. In Harron CL, et al (eds). Suicide: Assessment and Intervention. New York: Appleton-Century-Crofts, 1977.

Szasz T. Law, Liberty and Psychiatry. New York: Macmillan, 1963.

Self-study Exercises

Place T (True) or F (False) next to each statement.

1. _____ Attempted suicide is associated with depression and alcoholism.

2. _____ People with antisocial disorders also have a high suicide rate.

3. _____ Once a person is over the suicide crisis, he or she most likely will not attempt suicide in the future.

4. _____ Nonwhites in a low socioeconomic status have the highest rates for suicide.

5. _____ If the nurse thinks that a client may be thinking of suicide, the nurse should not bring up the subject, lest the person get ideas.

6. _____ The suicide rate is higher among gifted individuals, immigrants, police officers, doctors, and the elderly than in the general population.

7. _____ A person who has had a family member commit suicide, is divorced, or has suffered multiple losses is a risk for possible suicide.

Choose the most appropriate response in each case.

8. Choose the type of suicide that is included in Durkheim's theory.

   A. Murder in 180th degree
   B. Low serotonin levels
   C. Anomic
   D. Alcohol abuse or depressed

9. The statement by a suicidal person, "How can I go about giving my body to medical science?" is an example of a(n)

   A. Overt statement.
   B. Behavioral clue.
   C. Emotional clue.
   D. Covert statement.

10. The best response to a client who states, "Things will never work out, but I have an answer now," is

   A. Things have a way of working out in time.
   B. I feel the same sometimes.
   C. I knew you would find a better solution.
   D. What things . . . What kind of answer have you found?

11. Charles Brown, age 52, lost his wife in a car accident four months ago. Since that time, he has been severely depressed and has taken to drinking to "numb the pain." Using the SAD PERSONS assessment scale, how many points does Mr. Brown have?

   A. Three points
   B. Four points
   C. Five points
   D. Six points

12. Which of the following is the *best* way to phrase a *no-suicide contract*?

   A. "I will call my therapist before I harm myself."
   B. "I will not kill myself unless my husband leaves me."
   C. "When I have thoughts of killing myself, I will talk to my counselor."
   D. "I will not try to kill myself until next week."

Next to the intervention, put a P for primary intervention, an S for secondary intervention, or a T for tertiary intervention.

13. _____ Work with the family of a recent suicide victim.
14. _____ Relieve isolation, remove all weapons, and encourage alternative expressions of anger.
15. _____ Place the suicidal person on suicide precautions when he or she is first admitted to the hospital.
16. _____ Work with a teenager who has recently attempted suicide.
17. _____ Provide seminars for the elderly that focus on physical and emotional concerns.
18. _____ Keep the person on the telephone, find out if the person has ingested any drugs, assess the lethality of plan, and work on alternatives.

Name two short term goals for the following nursing diagnoses:

19. *High risk for self-directed violence* related to loss of a loved one

   1. _____
   2. _____

20. *Ineffective family coping* related to lack of sleep and inability to concentrate

   1. _____
   2. _____

For discussion

21. Name and briefly discuss three common and expected emotional reactions that a nurse might have when initially working with people who are suicidal.

CHAPTER 22

People Who Defend Against Anxiety Through Aggression Toward Others

Barbara B. Bauer
Signe S. Hill

OUTLINE

THEORY
Instinctive Theory
Elicited-Drive Theory
Social Learning Theory
Biological Theory

ASSESSMENT
Assessing Factors Related to Aggression
Assessing Verbal and Nonverbal Clues

NURSING DIAGNOSIS

PLANNING
Content Level—Planning Goals
Process Level—Nurses' Reactions and
    Feelings

INTERVENTION
Psychotherapeutic Interventions
Somatic Therapies
Therapeutic Environment
    Therapeutic Environment for the
        Patient
    Therapeutic Environment for Staff

EVALUATION

CASE STUDY: WORKING WITH A
    PERSON WHO IS AGGRESSIVE

SUMMARY

KEY TERMS AND CONCEPTS

**The key terms and concepts listed here also appear in bold where they are
defined or discussed in this chapter.**

AGGRESSION

ANGER

ASSAULTIVE

DE-ESCALATION

EMOTIONAL HONESTY

PARAPHRASAL

SETTING LIMITS

OBJECTIVES

After studying this chapter, the student will be able to

1. Compare four theories that explain the nature of aggression.
2. Identify factors that can precipitate aggressive behavior in clients.
3. Describe the verbal and nonverbal clues that are significant in the assessment of a
   client who is aggressive.
4. Formulate two nursing diagnoses suitable for a client who is aggressive.

5. Develop a long term goal and two short term goals for each of the nursing diagnoses.
6. Give possible reactions in the nurse who is working with a client who is aggressive.
7. Demonstrate two techniques for verbal de-escalation of aggressive behavior.
8. Explain how the use of body language can influence the progress in calming a client who is aggressive.
9. Describe a nonharmful physical intervention technique for a
   A. Wrist grab
   B. Clothing grab
   C. Hair grab
   D. Human bite

Aggressive behavior as a primary means of communication continues to increase in our society, and assaultive behavior in health care settings is a growing problem. Such behavior threatens the welfare of the aggressive clients, other clients, staff, and visitors. The nurse determines what factors contribute to or stimulate an aggressive episode and then what intervention techniques can be used to prevent or decrease this behavior.

It is important to differentiate between aggression and anger. **Aggression** is an action initiated to accomplish a goal that an individual feels cannot be met in any other way. Sometimes this action is triggered by the feeling of anger, frustration, helplessness, low self-esteem, or powerlessness. **Anger** is the *feeling* of rage or hostility, whereas aggression is a verbal or physical response to anger or rage. Figure 22–1 conceptualizes the process of aggression as a destructive problem-solving behavior.

Theory

Various theories concern the nature of human aggression, and some of them have sharply contrasting views. McGuire and Troisi (1989) and Baron (1985) describe a number of frameworks.

INSTINCTIVE THEORY

According to this line of reasoning, human beings are genetically or constitutionally programmed for aggression. The best known supporters of this view were Freud and Lorenz.

Freud initially hypothesized that all human behavior is related to a life instinct that he called Eros. The energy of Eros—libido—exists to enhance or reproduce life. Aggression results from attempts to prevent or block this energy.

After the events of World War I, Freud developed a more pessimistic view. He saw human beings as having a death instinct, Thanatos, that focused on self-destruction. Freud believed that all human behavior was related to the interplay between Eros and Thanatos. The force of Thanatos could lead to self-destruction unless it was neutralized by Eros or redirected through displacement or sublimation. Because displacement or sublimation is never complete, some aggressive energy would be directed toward others.

Lorenz believed aggression that causes harm to others is due to a fighting instinct that human beings

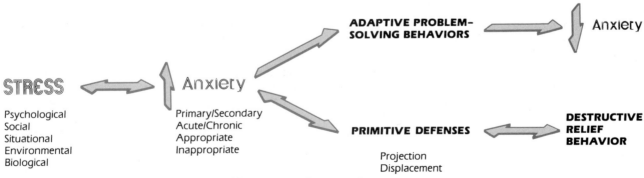

Figure 22–1. *The process of aggression.*

share with many other organisms. His innate-tendency view held that the aggressive energy occurred spontaneously and more or less continuously. The occurrence of aggression related to the amount of stored energy and the presence of aggression-relieving stimuli. Spontaneous eruptions of aggression could occur, however, if enough time had passed since the last aggressive act.

Lorenz saw the possibility of preventing aggressive energy from reaching dangerous levels by the participation in noninjurious aggressive actions. He also believed that feelings of love and friendship for others might prove incompatible with expression of overt aggression toward another.

ELICITED-DRIVE THEORY

The drive theories of aggression assume that aggression is triggered by outside conditions. Examples include past experiences, frustration, specific social situations, loss of face, physical pain, and degree to which needs are being met. These situations could potentially provide strong motivation for harmful assault against others.

Dollard and colleagues (1939) first proposed the frustration-aggression hypothesis. Frustration, which is the blocking of ongoing goal-directed behavior, was viewed as leading to arousal of the aggressive drive. The major goal of this drive was thought to be harm directed at a person or object. This could lead to an attack against persons or objects, especially those considered the cause of the frustration.

SOCIAL LEARNING THEORY

This theory does not accept aggressive drives as being instinctual or biological. In essence, it views aggressive behavior as being part of "you are what you learn." Development of aggressive behavior is thought to be motivated by

1. Acquiring aggressive responses on the basis of past experiences. For example, when adults in a home act aggressively toward each other, babies and children incorporate this behavior as a way of responding to others.
2. Receiving or anticipating rewards for aggressive behavior. For example, soldiers during war receive medals, promotions, and privileges for killing the enemy; gang members receive status and respect for following the gang code; professional athletes reap financial rewards and fame for aggressive be-

havior required in their sport; and organized crime rewards its members through money and privilege.
3. Social or environmental situations that can cause groups to respond aggressively. For example, activists often discover that they receive more attention and media focus in their movements for righting perceived wrongs when they are involved in aggressive acts even though their behavior might result in fines and jail sentences. Their view is "the squeaky wheel gets the oil."

BIOLOGICAL THEORY

A number of biological changes are associated with violence and aggression; for example: brain tumors, temporal lobe epilepsy, and organic brain disorders like Alzheimer's disease and Korsakoff's psychosis. The ingestion of mind-altering drugs can also trigger aggression. Crack cocaine, PCP, alcohol, and even steroids are often closely linked to violent behaviors.

During 1989, the results of independent studies that showed a relationship between impulsive aggression and low levels of the neurotransmitter serotonin were published. The psychiatric diagnoses of the persons involved in one study included major depression and personality disorders. Another study included arsonists and those who attempted or committed murder. Among this group, psychiatric diagnoses included depression, alcohol abuse, antisocial personality, borderline personality, and paranoid personality (Harvard Medical School Mental Health Letter 1989).

Neurotransmitters are chemicals that transmit impulses between nerve cells or neurons. Increasing data show that serotonin may be the most important of the neurotransmitters and potentially affect much of a person's mental life. Unlike other neurotransmitters, serotonin does not seem to have localized receptor sites in a few areas of the brain. "Instead, nerve cells tipped with serotonin-sensitive binding sites cluster deep within the brain stem and send neuronal tentacles snorkeling out through the gray matter. Hence, their uptake and release of serotonin ultimately affects much of our mental life" (Serotonin 1992).

An interesting finding related to aggression is that there are fewer serotonin-releasing neurons in the frontal cortex of persons who experience suicidal thoughts during acute stress. "Some may be born with 'suicidal' brains. Measurement of serotonin debris in the spinal fluid may identify those at risk" (Serotonin 1992).

Research at the National Institute of Mental Health has shown that monoamine oxidase is related to behavior even in newborns. Babies with low levels of monoamine oxidase tend to be more excitable and crankier than are babies with high levels. Levels of monoamine oxidase may be biologically fixed and genetically transmitted in families (Tavris 1989).

The Freedmans along with Brazelton studied the differences in temperament among babies of different cultures. Their work suggested temperamental differences among the human races, but there were also wide variations within racial groups. Work has also been done that indicates there may be a strong hereditary component in some aspects of personality. One aspect of personality studied that is of particular interest in regard to aggressive behavior is emotionality or intensity of reaction. This may appear as a strong temper, a tendency toward fearfulness, violent mood swings, or all of these together. Identical twins with strongly correlated scores were used as partial evidence. No *gene for aggression has been identified, however.* Geneticists think that genes provide humans with a reaction range and that most habits are acquired through learning (Tavris 1989).

The evolutionary biology framework views aggressive behavior as an evolved capacity that can be developed.

> . . . aggressive behavior is not viewed as the result of a specific process, such as a drive, an innate tendency, an eliciting stimulus, or something learned. Rather, like language acquisition, it is an evolved capacity that can be developed, and the development of aggressive behavior (or any other behavior system) generally subserves two ultimate evolutionary functions: Survival and reproduction. Its short-term functions include: Securing preferential or exclusive access to vital resources such as space, shelter, food and mates; and defense of oneself, of those in whom one has direct genetic investment (e.g., offspring, parents), and of selected non-relatives. Proximate mechanisms may be physiological, psychological or contextual (e.g., threat by another) (McGuire and Troisi 1989).

With this view in mind, aggression may be considered adaptive in many situations. Only through careful questioning can it be determined whether the person's aggression should be considered normal or abnormal (McGuire and Troisi 1989).

ASSESSMENT

Assessment of the client with aggressive behavior is a crucial first step in developing a nursing care plan. Areas that need to be considered in an assessment include (1) factors related to aggression and (2) verbal and nonverbal clues.

ASSESSING FACTORS RELATED TO AGGRESSION

When working with a client who is prone to aggression the nurse also needs to be aware of and assess (1) personal, (2) social, (3) situational, and (4) environmental factors (Table 22–1).

ASSESSING VERBAL AND NONVERBAL CLUES

According to Stevenson (1991), violence occurs not as an isolated act but as part of a process. By understanding the cycle of aggression, the nurse can assess the client's potential for violence and intervene early using a proactive approach. The nurse's sensitivity to verbal and nonverbal clues of impending aggression can prevent escalation of behavior. These verbal and nonverbal clues are outlined in Box 22–1.

NURSING DIAGNOSIS

Any person can become violent under certain circumstances. Clients with specific mental disorders have a higher incidence for violent behavior, however. Table 22–2 identifies those mental disorders associated with aggressive events.

In working with clients who are unable to control their behavior, the diagnosis of most concern is *high risk for violence directed at others.*

High risk for violence directed at others can be related to a variety of factors, such as a feeling of loss of control, frequent frustrations, alcohol and other drug ingestion, confusion due to cognitive impairment, or response to stimuli from within. If the client is angry, striking out is a way of demonstrating power and sometimes the only way of communicating with others. Feeling helpless, the client believes that violence is the only way of getting what is perceived as a need.

Ineffective individual coping is an important nursing diagnosis for a client who uses aggressive behavior to deal with anxiety. Such an individual needs to learn to channel angry feelings in constructive ways. Because of illness or environmental factors, the client lacks the necessary problem-solving techniques and coping skills to manage internal or external stresses adequately.

Powerlessness is directly related to aggressive behavior. Because of a perceived feeling of a lack of control

Table 22–1 ■ FACTORS RELATED TO AGGRESSIVE BEHAVIOR

DETERMINANTS	COMMENTS
Personal	

People may be prone to violence if they have
1. A previous history of violence
2. A violent family background: child abuse, spouse abuse
3. Certain mental disorders:
  a. Psychosis—paranoid schizophrenia
  b. Organic—Alzheimer's disease
  c. Antisocial personality disorder
  d. Substance abuse
	Family violence is perhaps the single most treatable phenomenon responsible for violence in our society.
	
	If perception is distorted or there is poor impulse control and confusion because of organic impairment, there is more likelihood of aggressive behavior.

Social	
Frustration	Results in aggression when the frustration is intense or the cause of frustration is seen as undeserved.
Direct provocation from others	Physical abuse and verbal teasing are powerful triggers of aggressive behavior. Once aggression begins, escalation continues to the point at which mild comments may initiate strong reactions.
Exposure to aggressive models • Relationships • Television shows • Films	Attitudes, emotions, and overt behaviors are influenced by exposure to words and acts of others. The link between exposure to TV violence and aggression appears to be that (1) new aggressive techniques are learned, (2) inhibition is reduced, and (3) viewer is desensitized.
Situational	
Heightened physiological arousal	Competitive activities, vigorous exercises, and exposure to arousing films under certain circumstances enhance aggressive behavior if the person has a strong aggressive response tendency.
Pain	May precipitate striking out at any available target, not just those associated with pain.
Sexual arousal	*Mildly erotic material* may reduce aggressive level; *strongly erotic material* may enhance overt aggression.
Environmental	
Air pollution	Exposure to noxious odors (chemical plants, other industries) may increase personal irritability and aggression. Involuntary exposure to cigarette smoke may increase aggression.
Noise	Unpleasant noise may increase overt aggression in those with strong tendency toward aggression.
Crowding	Mixed results—under appropriate conditions, may inhibit or increase aggressive response.
Heat	Does not appear directly related to violence. Reaction to heat is related to combination of factors, although some studies show relationship between weather, mood, and behavior (the Cincinnati Enquirer, 1992).

Data from Baron, RA. Aggression. In Kaplan HI, Sadock BJ (eds). Comprehensive Textbook of Psychiatry, vol 1, 4th ed. Baltimore: Williams & Wilkins, 1985.

Box 22–1. CLUES TO AGGRESSIVE BEHAVIOR

Verbal Clues

- Argumentative
- Shouting profanities
- Repetition of demands, requests, complaints
- Expressing intent to harm others—threatening
- Responding to voices
- False accusations
- Ideas of grandeur
- Disoriented to time, place, person
- Fear of loss of control
- Fear of others

Nonverbal Clues

- Increased motor activity—agitation, pacing, fidgeting
- Irritability
- Rigid posture—clenched fists and jaw
- Angry facial expression
- Responding to voices
- Staring or lack of eye contact
- Excitement
- Extremely quiet—unable to express feelings
- Withdrawal of previously active client

---

over one's life, an individual will act out in an attempt to gain control or power. Human beings become threatened when they begin to lose control over their lives. This is especially noticeable among elderly residents in nursing homes who resent being told when to do things.

Disturbance in self-esteem underlies aggressive behavior, which often consists of accusatory and demeaning remarks that project blame onto others. Demanding, superior, and authoritarian behavior often indicates a de-evaluation of self (Bauer and Hill 1986).

Planning

Planning nursing care for a person who handles anxiety with aggressive behavior involves planning on the (1) content level: planning goals and (2) process level: awareness of personal reactions to aggressive behavior.

CONTENT LEVEL—PLANNING GOALS

It is important to respond to threats of aggression. A client who feels that he or she is not being taken

---

Table 22–2 ■ PSYCHIATRIC DISORDERS ASSOCIATED WITH AGGRESSION

PROBLEM AREA	POSSIBLE CAUSE	STIMULI	BEHAVIOR
Acute psychosis (e.g., paranoid schizophrenia)	Massive disruption in contact with reality	Behavior based primarily on internal rather than environmental stimuli	Less predictable; increased possibility of aggressive behavior
Organic mental disorders (e.g., Alzheimer's disease and Korsakoff's psychosis)	Impaired brain function	Frustration	More limited range or response options available; reacts to frustrating situations with aggressive behavior
Antisocial personality disorder	Internal controls that developed early in the personality structure are rudimentary or lacking	Minor frustration; unable to get immediate satisfaction	Inappropriate aggressive behavior
Borderline personality disorder	Decompensation	Stress-evoking situations	Becomes psychotic; unless the nurse is aware of decompensation, aggressive and unpredictable behavior may come as a surprise
Intoxicated client (e.g., alcohol, crack cocaine)	Reduction of controls; cognitive impairment due to intoxicating substance	Internal: related to physical changes in brain External: related to misinterpretation of environmental stimuli	Abusive and assaultive

seriously may become angrier (Harvard Medical School Mental Health Letter 1991).

Long term and short term goals provide direction in caring and planning for the client. The goals need to be measurable, time limited, and attainable for the individual. When possible, the client needs to participate in the planning of care and the setting of goals. The focus of goals is on the client. Both men and women may use aggressive acting-out behaviors; however, for simplicity the pronoun "his" is used in the following example.

For the nursing diagnosis of *high risk for violence directed at others*, the following goals may apply.

Long Term Goals

- Client will verbalize his needs rather than strike out by (date).
- Client will talk about his feelings without attacking verbally by (date).
- Client will remove himself from situations that provoke aggressiveness by (date).

Short Term Goals

- Client will not harm others while in the hospital.
- Client will identify two positive, alternative ways of dealing with situations that provoke aggressiveness by (date).
- Client will go to his room when he thinks he may be losing control by (date).

Aggression or violence occurs when a person is unable to reach a goal and sees no other option. The individual has only one solution to the problem, and that is to act aggressively. This person can feel helpless and trapped. The nursing diagnosis of *ineffective individual coping* related to a situational crisis may have the following goals.

Long Term Goals

- Client will verbalize the use of three new coping behaviors by (date).
- Client will describe behavioral signs that are an indication of impending aggressiveness by (date).
- Client will list alternative ways of handling his aggressive behavior by (date).

Short Term Goals

- Client, with the help of the nurse, will define his problem by (date).
- Client will discuss with the nurse two situations that trigger his aggressiveness by (date).
- Client will role-play an effective coping technique for dealing with his aggression by (date).

Frustration and anxiety over not having any effect on a particular outcome or situation can result in a feeling of powerlessness. This feeling can trigger an aggressive outburst, which gives a temporary sense of control and power even though it may be destructive. For the nursing diagnosis of *powerlessness*, the following goals may apply.

Long Term Goals

- By (date), the client will state two things that give him some control over his life.
- Client will identify a specific situation in which he feels insecure by (date).
- Client will verbalize the relationship between his aggressive behavior and his sense of powerlessness by (date).
- Client will demonstrate two assertive skills in relating to others by (date).

Short Term Goals

- By (date), the client will talk to the nurse about his feeling of lack of control.
- Client will let the nurse know when he has the feeling that he is losing control by (date).
- Client, with the nurse, will role-play a positive method for gaining control by (date).
- Client will participate in assertiveness training by (date).

The basis of aggressive behavior is usually a feeling of low self-esteem. Underneath all of the defensive and hostile behavior of the aggressive client is a person who is frustrated, bitter, and lonely. Such an individual has a low self-concept and feels that he has to protect himself. In so doing, he drives everyone away. Another nursing diagnosis for a client who is aggressive, therefore, is *disturbance in self-esteem*. In developing goals for this diagnosis, the nurse must remember that self-esteem is earned and not learned (Schmoker 1990).

Long Term Goals

- Client will participate in an activity that makes him feel good about himself by (date).
- Client will state two positive things about himself by (date).
- Client will complete a simple project that he is pleased with by (date).
- By (date), client will state that he feels better about himself.

Short Term Goals

- Client will participate in the planning of his care by (date).

- Client will work with the nurse on emphasizing his strengths by (date).
- Client will use his strengths in selecting a project to work on by (date).
- Client will participate in positive affirmation exercises by (date).

PROCESS LEVEL—NURSES' REACTIONS AND FEELINGS

Aggressive and assaultive behavior in a client can be threatening to health care professionals. This behavior begins to build fear in staff, who often respond by avoiding the client. Avoidance by staff can cause further frustration for the aggressive client.

Staff must be aware of their physical limitations and emotional vulnerability. Through self-understanding, understanding of the client's behavior, and understanding that assaultiveness is a response to a real or perceived situation, many potentially aggressive situations can be prevented.

Bauer and Hill (1986), Miller and Gorski (1981), and Stevenson (1991) emphasize the importance of *self-assessment*. A daily assessment of one's stressors is one way of recognizing and identifying personal stress levels. The nurse should ask himself or herself

- *Are there problems in my home life that are affecting my work?*
- *What are my stresses at work?*
- *Are there certain clients or coworkers who easily upset me?*
- *Are personal issues affecting my interactions with clients? For example, the client may trigger an emotional response because of a similar incident in my personal life.*
- *Am I tired?*
- *Am I afraid of the client? Am I trying to avoid the client?*
- *Do I think the client deserves to be punished?*
- *What is my anxiety level?*

"As arousal increases, judgment decreases" (Stevenson 1991), or as Miller and Gorski (1981) put it, "whenever emotional upset occurs, the brain shuts off." Refrain from reacting solely on an emotional basis so that you do not get caught up in taking care of your own needs and ignoring the needs of the client. For example, if a client calls you names, the verbal attack is usually not toward you personally but toward what you represent (e.g., an authority figure or a reminder of his loss of authority or power). View the situation in a professional, objective way. Talking to colleagues and other professionals often helps staff maintain objectivity.

Other methods that will help maintain self-control include (Miller and Gorski 1981)

1. Breathing deeply to help get oxygen to the brain for meeting the demands of the moment.
2. Having a relaxed posture with your weight balanced evenly on your feet.
3. Focusing thought patterns on optimistic self-talk statements that can increase a sense of self-confidence. For example, "My fear is normal, but I know I can handle the situation." It is most important that you *believe* in what you do!
4. Being alert and intervening in the best way you know how. The nurse's behavior should reflect **emotional honesty,** which means that verbal and nonverbal communication coincide; what is said is reflected in one's body language. If your verbal message does not reflect your body language, the client receives a double message and becomes more confused, anxious, and perhaps agitated.

Intervention

"Every person who becomes violent has, in his own mind, a justifiable reason for the violence and a purpose or goal he believes can be accomplished by violent action" (Miller and Gorski 1981). The client is attempting to meet his personal needs. Therefore, intervention begins with figuring out what the client feels he needs (Stevenson 1991).

PSYCHOTHERAPEUTIC INTERVENTIONS

Psychotherapeutic interventions are aimed at de-escalating anxiety and aggressive verbal or physical behaviors. **De-escalation** means decreasing, at times by degrees, anxiety and aggressive behavior. Constant observations of the client's behavior facilitate early detection of escalating anxiety and agitation. Intervention can ensue in a timely fashion, with avoidance of physical confrontation and physical restraints. Highly structured surroundings with supportive and interpersonal measures can decrease aggressive behavior. Staff members and interveners must calmly state that violence will not be tolerated.

Set limits, because aggression can escalate if a patient senses that others are not in control. **Setting limits,** an important intervention to help clients learn appropriate and desirable behaviors, identifies the rules, guidelines, and standards of acceptable behaviors and defines the consequences of violating those boundaries. The consequences must be clear, consistently enforced, and reasonable. Staff need to speak

Table 22-3 ■ VERBAL AND NONVERBAL INTERVENTION FOR AGGRESSIVE CLIENTS

INTERVENTION	RATIONALE
1. Intervene immediately when the client needs controls or limits. • Separate the client from what is bothering him or her. • If more than one client is involved, go to the one with the *power*; talk *only* to that one.	1. Prevents further escalation of anxiety. • Allows de-escalation of anxiety by removing stimulus. • Focuses on source of disturbance; de-escalates altercation.
2. Approach the client in nonthreatening manner.	2. Prevents further escalation of anxiety.
3. Allow plenty of physical space between yourself and the client.	3. When anxiety is high, people are threatened if their personal space is violated.
4. Maintain a relaxed posture, with hands and arms comfortably at side, and direct eye contact.	4. Threatening postures, such as hands on hips, arms folded on chest, and clenched fists, can encourage defensiveness.
5. Speak slowly and calmly in a "normal" tone of voice. Use person's name and treat the person with respect; for example: • "Mr. Smith, what can I do to help you?" • "Mrs. Brown, its seems as if you are really upset about something." • "George, you appear angry; let's talk about what's bothering you."	5. Slow, calm voice helps minimize client's anxiety, communicate a sense of control. • Calling the person by name in a respectful manner enhances esteem, as in an adult-to-adult exchange. • Acknowledges the client's feelings. • Use of paraphrasal can convert violent impulses into verbal, nondestructive behavior.
6. Refer *only* to yourself (not to policies, rules, supervisors).	6. Referring to policies and rules can decrease the person's sense of personal options and sense of being understood.
7. When setting limits, be firm, understanding, and clear.	7. The purpose of setting limits is to provide a consistent set of expectations, not to control the patient.
8. Give three options: • Two options offer the client a choice. • The third choice is *not* an option and *not* a threat.	8. Giving people choices helps them gain a sense of control. Example: • "I want you to go to your room until you quiet down"; *or* "I want you to help me fold the laundry." • "I cannot allow you to injure yourself, other clients, or me."
9. • If medication is ordered, assess whether other staff need to be present. • Determine in advance the function that each staff person will perform. • Before giving medication, the nurse explains about the medication in a short, simple, and clear manner. • Maintain the same physical level as the client: get up if the client gets up, sit down if the client sits down. • Offer food or drink and offer to talk at regular intervals. • Attempt to identify the cause of the client's disturbance.	9. • Providing external controls can help client maintain control. • Minimizes confusion; provides a sense of security for staff as well as client. • Understanding can decrease anxiety. Patient has a right to know what is being given and the reason for it. • Prevents intimidation and can lessen the perception of a threatening posture. • Provides gratification of basic needs through a constructive outlet. • The reason for client's assaultiveness may be rooted in a legitimate situation.
10. Make an effort to convey acceptance of the client, even though you do not accept his or her behavior.	10. Maintains the client's self-esteem, which can decrease anxiety.
11. Provide diversions that require a short attention span and strenuous physical activity, such as jogging, exercise bike, Ping-Pong.	11. People in high anxiety have scattered thoughts. Physical activity can help reduce muscle tension.
12. Reinforce positive behavior.	12. By focusing on the client's strengths, self-esteem is maintained or increased.
13. Use positive reinforcement whenever possible.	13. Client may be unaware of his or her positive qualities when the emphasis is on the negative aspects of his or her behaviors.

Adapted from Bauer B, Hill S. Essentials of Mental Health Care Planning and Interventions. Philadelphia: WB Saunders, 1986.

slowly and clearly, behave politely, and listen uncritically. Talking softly is useful when clients are loud (Harvard Medical School Mental Health Letter 1991). Box 22-2 lists the steps in limit setting.

An important principle for maintaining safety with a person who is at risk for aggressive behavior is to use the least restrictive means of control. One technique that staff find useful is called **paraphrasal.** Paraphrasal refers to the repeating back to the agitated client in short, clear phrases what you understand the client to be saying. For example, "You are feeling angry at your wife" or "You are angry enough to kill your brother for stealing your car." The purpose is to convert the client's potentially violent impulses into verbal, nondestructive behavior. Clear, respectful, directive statements indicating an interest in understanding the client's immediate feelings are more helpful than open-ended questions. Open-ended questions (e.g., "Tell me more") are *not* helpful with angry individuals in emotionally charged situations (Eichelman 1991).

If the client's anxiety and aggression continue to escalate, chemical restraints may be useful, such as haloperidol (Haldol) or lorazepam (Ativan). If medications do not decrease the threat of harm to a patient or staff member, physical restraint or seclusion is employed. Physical confrontation should always be a last resort. As Stevenson (1991) points out, "The use of force is an encouragement to aggressive behavior and a hindrance to treatment." See Chapter 18 for use of seclusion and restraints.

Verbal and nonverbal intervention skills are used in an attempt to de-escalate the client's aggression. Table 22-3 identifies some useful techniques that staff can use (Bauer and Hill 1986).

SOMATIC THERAPIES

When verbal interventions are not effective in minimizing potential violence, some drugs may be useful in acute situations. Drugs may also be used over time for individuals who are chronically assaultive. Aggression may stem from many sources.

The most useful drugs are neuroleptics (antipsychotics), anxiolytics, lithium, antidepressants, and beta-blockers. These drugs act on neurotransmitter, systems using gamma-aminobutyric acid, norepinephrine, or serotonin. The beta-blocker propranolol acts in the peripheral and central nervous systems to reduce anxiety. Beta-blockers reduce anxiety by suppressing the body's normal fight-or-flight response (Harvard Medical School Mental Health Letter 1991).

Table 22-4 lists psychotropic drugs and the client population for which they are most often used.

Box 22-2. STEPS IN SETTING LIMITS

1. Explain exactly which behavior is inappropriate. Do not assume the individual knows which behavior is inappropriate.
2. Explain why the behavior is inappropriate. Do not assume the individual knows why the behavior is inappropriate.
3. Give the individual reasonable choices or consequences; present them as choices, and always present the positive first.
4. Allow time; if you do not allow time, it may be perceived as an ultimatum.
5. Enforce consequences. Limits do not work unless you follow through with the consequences.

Reprinted from The Art of Setting Limits Participant Manual, p. 8, with permission of the National Crisis Prevention Institute, Inc., © 1991.

THERAPEUTIC ENVIRONMENT

Therapeutic Environment for the Patient

If a client is **assaultive** and it is necessary to intervene physically, the nurse must mentally visualize successful management of the situation for it to be a reality. This concept of mental rehearsal is used in many activities, such as sports and presentations before large groups. It is another way of saying "What you think is what you get." Miller and Gorski (1981) recommend creating common situations in which verbal and physical aggression might occur and then planning all the possible strategies for handling those situations. In this way, possible aggressive situations might be avoided, and those that do occur can be handled more successfully.

Defensive techniques are learned and therefore must be practiced until they become part of the nurse's automatic reaction to assault. This is particularly important because physical assaults sometimes happen quickly. These techniques are often taught to staff through in-service education.

Every situation is different; however, some basic points should be remembered whenever a nurse intervenes with a physically assaultive client (Bauer and Hill 1986).

Table 22-4 ■ DRUG INFORMATION: PSYCHOTROPIC DRUG TREATMENT OF AGGRESSION

DRUG GROUP	INDICATIONS	PRECAUTIONS
Neuroleptics Haloperidol (Haldol) Chlorpromazine (Thorazine)	People with *psychotic ideation*	Oversedation Tardive dyskinesia when used over long periods Other multiple side effects
Anxiolytics Lorazepam (Ativan)	*Acute relief* of violence or aggression	Possible paradoxical rage attacks Oversedation Tolerance and addiction Do not treat with lorazepam for over 6 weeks
Lithium	Aggression or irritability in *manic excitement* Uncontrolled rage attack triggered by "nothing" or minor stimuli May block outbursts in *schizophrenic* clients May diminish hostile outbursts from *organic patients* Does *not* abate premeditated violence	Do lithium work-up (e.g., electrocardiogram, complete blood count with differential) Monitor lithium levels Teach side effects and toxic side effects to patient and family Effective for violence in prisoners and mentally retarded Drug does not affect aggressive behavior until therapeutic blood level is reached

Anticonvulsants
Carbamazepine (Tegretol)
	Aggression from
	   Complex partial seizures
	   Organic mental disorders
		Monitor for bone marrow suppression and blood abnormalities

Beta-blockers Propranolol (Inderol)	Intermittent explosive disorders Psychosis where violence is unrelated to psychotic thought Organic brain disorder	Takes 4–8 weeks Monitor blood pressure and pulse
Nadolol	Chronic paranoid schizophrenia	

1. Do not try to be a hero. Get out of the way and get help, if possible.
2. Maintain a firm base of support for balance if you are suddenly pushed by the client. This can be achieved by placing one foot forward and angling the rear foot to the outside.
3. Keep a proper distance from the client. *Maintain eye contact and relaxed posture with arms loose.* All these factors are less threatening to a client.
4. In a room, do not stand or sit in a corner without a ready exit. At the same time, the client should be able to exit and not feel cornered, because this can be threatening.
5. Always work against the weakest point of any hold (i.e., the area between the thumb and forefinger).
6. Use arms and hands to protect the face and head if a client strikes out; turn the thigh sideways to protect the groin area against a kick.

Some general physical interventions are described. To be effective, however, **these defense techniques must be taught and practiced by staff under qualified supervision.** No technique is a guarantee that injury will be avoided (Bauer and Hill 1986).

WRIST OR ARM GRABS. The weak point of a wrist grab is between the client's thumb and fingers. The wrist can be removed by moving it against the thumb of the attacker's hand in a circular movement. Before implementing the wrist release, evaluate the situation. Sometimes a client grabs a wrist for support or to be close to someone. After a short time, the client may let go. If he does not and the grip is bothersome, kindly ask the client to release his grip before implementing the technique.

CLOTHING GRAB. If a client grabs clothing, place one hand under and close to the grasping hand to keep the clothing against the body. With the heel of the other hand, push the client's grasping hand off in the direction of his knuckles. This technique will protect clothing from being torn.

HAIR GRABS. The best defense is to be careful and not let hair be grabbed.

Hair Grab from Front. When hair is grabbed, prevent pulling of the hair. This can best be done by interlocking the fingers over the attacker's hands and pressing down with the palms of the hands. This alleviates the pain from the grabbing of the hair. Then step back in a crouching position with head pointed toward the ground and elbows pulled in, causing the attacker to release his grip or lose his balance.

Hair Grab from Rear. Placement of the hands should be the same as for the hair grab from the front. Step around as if to face the attacker, moving the upper body down so that the body is bent over at the waist. Facing the attacker, straighten up slowly, keeping the attacker's hand tight to the head.

In both of these interventions after the technique has been applied, squeeze the attacker's hands with the palms of your hands, forcing his grip on the hair to be released.

THE ASSIST (Foster 1979). The assist is used when a coworker is being attacked, usually with hair grabs. The nurse comes up behind the attacker and places one hand over the attacker's eyes. The other hand is placed on the attacker's shoulder. Gently pull the attacker backward and down, using the thigh to guide the attacker to the floor. The attacker, in an effort to regain his balance and vision, will usually release his hands. It is important that the coworker who is being attacked begin to implement the hair grab release; otherwise, the coworker will go backward with the attacker.

CHOKES. The most important thing to remember in a choke is to keep the airway open. Keeping the chin down, but with eyes focused forward, helps relieve pressure on the trachea.

Choke from the Front. Make a fist with both hands. Then, with considerable force, bring the clasped hands up through the attacker's forearms. This will usually release the attacker's grip. It is important then to step back and away from the client.

Choke from the Rear. Keep the chin down and quickly throw hands straight up in the air and pivot around clockwise. This quick action usually breaks the hold.

HUMAN BITES. Human bites are dangerous. Because of the bacteria in the human mouth, broken skin should be treated immediately for prevention of infection. As in the hair grab, do not pull away; instead, move into the attacker's mouth. Release can usually be obtained by placing the forefinger underneath the attacker's nose and pressing upward. The assist can be used to encourage the attack to release the bite.

ESCORTING CLIENTS. For a mildly excited client, or to guide a client down a hallway, the nurse can walk beside the client. The nurse's outside arm is used to hold the client's wrist that is next to the nurse's body. The nurse's other arm, which is next to the client, is placed around the client's waist, grasping the client's forearm. In this way, the nurse can gently guide the client.

To control an excited client when alone, the nurse can grab both of the client's wrists from behind and pull his arms around him. The nurse's left hand grasps the client's right wrist, and vice versa. The client's top arm needs to be tucked under his opposite elbow to decrease movement. This is called the basket hold.

If the person is taller than the nurse, more control can be obtained if the center of gravity is lowered. This can be done by moving the knees into the back of the client's knees and gently lowering the client to the floor.

If two professional staff are working with the client, one staff person should stand on either side of the client. The staff person's outside arm is brought across the staff person's body and clasps the client's wrist. The staff person's other arm, which is next to the client, is brought between the client's arm and chest, clasping the wrist of the staff person's outside arm. Staying close to the client's body decreases the client's movement.

If a client is disturbed, it may be easier to walk him backward. With the client facing backward and two professional staff facing forward, the staff persons hold the client's wrists with their outer hands. The staff persons' inner hands are brought up under the client's armpits, supporting his shoulders. Both staff persons use their feet to push the client's feet out, lowering the client's center of gravity. In this way, the client can be moved backward without any discomfort. *It is important to explain to the client* what is being done and to treat the client with the utmost respect and dignity.

Again, *a word of caution:* Reading about physical management techniques alone is not enough. **They must be properly demonstrated and practiced.** Much of the success in using nonharmful physical intervention techniques is related to spontaneity, surprise, and teamwork. A staff that has been properly trained to intervene with violent and aggressive clients is in an optimal position to (1) increase teamwork and consistency of approach to clients, (2) decrease the rate of injury to clients and staff, and (3) offer staff alternative approaches to aggression (Price-Hoskins 1992). It is hoped that by following the suggested verbal and nonverbal interventions, assaultiveness will be avoided and physical intervention will not be necessary.

Therapeutic Environment for Staff

Recent articles in the literature (Flannery et al. 1991; Lanza 1992; Mahoney 1991) focus on the effect that violence has on staff associated with emergency departments, night shifts, shifts more than eight hours long, and certain patient populations already mentioned (e.g., those who are intoxicated or have dementia).

Therefore, it is extremely important that *all* staff who are working with high-risk groups of patients receive proper training in working with aggressive behavior. If an incident occurs in which a staff member is injured, follow-up should be available to help that individual regain a sense of control and security as well as a sense of effectiveness. A significant factor in providing support as soon as possible is the immediate reporting of all incidents of aggressive behavior. With reporting, events can be reviewed, and more effective techniques for coping can be discussed.

Evaluation

A thorough evaluation of aggressive behavior is significant in preventing further episodes. The nurse needs to be cognizant of factors preceding the client's disruptive behavior. What were the professional staff doing with the client? What was the environment like? What stimuli were present? Are there some staff who work well with the client while other staff elicit a negative reaction?

As mentioned, violence is not an isolated act, so there are clues that precede the act. Most often, the client nonverbally and verbally presents clues of impending changes in behavior. Sometimes these clues are subtle. Impulsive and unpredictable outbursts usually occur when clients have psychiatric problems related to acute psychosis (e.g., schizophrenia or mania), substance abuse, or an organic mental disorder. These clients respond to stimuli from within, so the nurse needs to observe nonverbal behavior, especially eye movements.

After evaluation of the events preceding the aggressive episode, the nurse needs to evaluate the intervention techniques that were used. Was verbal de-escalation successful? For example, "It seems that you are really upset about something," or "Let's sit down and talk about what's bothering you. How about a glass of juice?" In this way, the nurse is evaluating whether the client's goals were realistic and attainable.

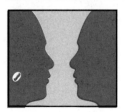

Case Study: Working with a Person Who Is Aggressive

Mr. Richards, 55 years old, was admitted to the local community mental health center this morning by the local police. They received a 911 call from a neighbor who heard Mr. Richards threatening his wife. A frightened Mrs. Richards arrived shortly and gave the following information to the admitting nurse.

My husband works as a plant manager. He's been complaining about his boss since he started working and is suspicious about what is really going on at the plant. It's like the last job he had. The only one he really seems to trust is one of the secretaries. She called me this morning to say he'd walked in as she was making a comment about him in response to what another secretary said, something like "I don't want Mr.

Richards' job." They were joking. He exploded and accused her of plotting to get his job. "My wife's in on this; I'm going to get her," and out he ran. My husband said things like that before, but this time it was different. When he came into the house, he looked different—scary. He began to throw things and shout at me, "I'm going to get you." I ran for the bathroom and locked the door. Thank goodness the neighbor called the police.

When the nurse, Mr. Hall, walked into Mr. Richards' room, Mr. Richards was pacing back and forth. He was frowning, and with a clenched fist he angrily stated, "Get me out of here. I don't belong here. It's my wife's fault."

NURSE:	I can understand why you're angry if you don't know why you're here.
MR. RICHARDS:	You're darn right! My wife should be here. She and the secretary at work are in this together.
NURSE:	Sounds as though you don't trust the secretary or your wife.
MR. RICHARDS:	It's not only them. There's something fishy going on at the plant. Others are plotting to get my job.

Assessment	Mr. Hall divided the data into objective and subjective components.

OBJECTIVE DATA

1. Male, 55 years old
2. Is a plant manager
3. Loud
4. Pacing
5. Clenched fist—frown on face

SUBJECTIVE DATA

1. History of previous suspicious behavior
2. Threatening verbalizations toward others
3. Threw things at home
4. Complains about boss—suspicious about what is going on at the plant
5. Scary look

Nursing Diagnosis	Mr. Hall discussed his assessment of Mr. Richards with the psychiatrist. An antipsychotic medication was ordered, and Mr. Richards was to be observed for behaviors that might indicate a possibility of harm to others. The initial nursing diagnoses for Mr. Richards reflected the staff's concern about his aggressive behavior. The diagnoses of highest priority were: 1. *High risk for violence directed at others* related to suspiciousness of others, as evidenced by hostile, threatening verbalizations

- Thinks something is going on at the plant
- Accusing secretary of plotting to get his job
- Threatening to get his wife

2. *Ineffective individual coping* related to the work environment, as evidenced by aggressive behavior toward others
   - Exploded at work; ran out of the plant
   - Threw things at home
   - Shouted at home

Planning	

CONTENT LEVEL—PLANNING GOALS

Mr. Hall formulated the following goals.

Nursing Diagnosis	Long Term Goals	Short Term Goals
1. *High risk for violence directed at others* related to suspiciousness of others, as evidenced by hostile, threatening verbalizations	1. Mr. Richards will talk about his feelings without attacking verbally by (date).	1a. Mr. Richards will remain nonviolent while in the hospital with aid of medication and nursing interventions. 1b. Mr. Richards will discuss with nurse two situations that trigger his aggressiveness within one week.
2. *Ineffective individual coping* related to the work environment, as evidenced by aggressive behavior toward others	2. Mr. Richards will demonstrate constructive ways of coping with his frustrations by discharge.	2a. Mr. Richards, with the help of the nurse, will define one of his concerns within four days. 2b. Mr. Richards will identify two alternative ways of dealing with situations that provoke aggressiveness within one week.

PROCESS LEVEL—NURSES' REACTIONS AND FEELINGS

The nurse manager on the unit thought it would be best to have a male nurse working with Mr. Richards because he seemed to have difficulty relating to women, especially his wife.

Mr. Hall was comfortable with Mr. Rich-

Evaluation
(Continued)

ards. He realized that his loudness and anger were not directed at him but related to being confined in a hospital. Mr. Hall communicated a relaxed and calming effect and, because of his preparation and experience, felt confident that he could handle an overt aggressive act of Mr. Richards if such behavior occurred.

Intervention

Mr. Hall's focus of care for Mr. Richards was on the prevention of aggressive outbursts. During the team meeting, the staff decided that Mrs. Richards should not visit her husband until he became adjusted to his hospitalization.

While working with Mr. Richards, Mr. Hall was always accepting of Mr. Richards' behavior, allowing him plenty of space. When Mr. Hall went to give Mr. Richards his first dose of prescribed medication, he asked one of the male nursing assistants to go with him. Mr. Hall explained to Mr. Richards in a simple and concise way that the physician had prescribed some liquid medication that would be given in fruit juice. At first, Mr. Richards was not going to take it; but when Mr. Hall explained that the medication would help him so that he could return home quicker, he agreed to try it.

Mr. Hall patiently listened to Mr. Richards' accusations about his work setting without agreeing or disagreeing. As Mr. Hall listened to Mr. Richards, it seemed that there was possibly a legitimate basis for some of his beliefs. After several days of medication, Mr. Richards began to show a trust in Mr. Hall by sharing some of his feelings.

The plant where Mr. Richards worked had been hiring younger men with better qualifications than he had. He was afraid that he would lose his job; some of the supervisors in the plant had been asked to take early retirement. His frustrations at work were being directed at his wife because the home was a safer environment than work.

Mr. Hall found that Mr. Richards loved gardening and was proud of his garden. Mr. Hall reinforced this strength, and he and Mr. Richards discussed more constructive alternatives that Mr. Richards could use to deal with his feelings. By Mr. Hall's emphasizing Mr. Richards' strengths, Mr. Richards began to show more trust in himself and feel more secure.

Mr. Hall was also concerned about Mrs. Richards and discussed with her how to deal with any future outbursts if they should occur.

Evaluation

Assessing the verbal and nonverbal behavior was crucial in preventing Mr. Richards from acting out his aggression. Having the same nurse on each shift work with Mr. Richards on a one-to-one basis over time maximized the potential for trust to develop. Mr. Hall's calm and relaxed manner helped de-escalate Mr. Richards' behavior, especially when he would shout about leaving or object to taking his medication. On discharge, Mr. Richards agreed to continue counseling through the outpatient department. Refer to Nursing Care Plan 22–1.

Nursing Care Plan 22–1 ■ A PERSON WITH AGGRESSIVE BEHAVIOR: Mr. Richards

NURSING DIAGNOSIS

High risk for violence directed at others related to suspiciousness of others, as evidenced by hostile, threatening verbalizations

Supporting Data

- Thinks something is going on at the plant
- Accusing secretary of plotting to get his job
- Threatening to get his wife

Long Term Goal: Mr. Richards will talk about his feelings without attacking verbally by (date).

Short term goals	Intervention	Rationale	Evaluation
1. Mr. Richards will remain nonviolent while in the hospital, with the aid of medication and nursing interventions.	1a. Absorb verbal expressions of anger.	1a. Demonstrates acceptance of Mr. Richards regardless of behavior.	Goal met Verbal and nonverbal interventions were successful in de-escalating Mr. Richards' anxiety.

Nursing Care Plan 22-1 ■ A PERSON WITH AGGRESSIVE BEHAVIOR: Mr. Richards *(Continued)*

Short term goals	Intervention	Rationale	Evaluation
	1b. Give medication as ordered.	1b. Neuroleptics can reduce suspicious behavior that may lead to aggressive outbursts.	
	1c. Listen to complaints and evaluate their validity.	1c. By giving recognition, a sense of trust is developed. When a person feels he or she is taken seriously and is understood, anxiety decreases.	
2. Mr. Richards will discuss with nurse two situations that trigger his aggressiveness within one week.	2a. Identify the precipitating causes of his aggressive behavior.	2a. Knowing the purpose of his behavior helps nurses identify the most useful interventions.	Goal met By the end of the week, Mr. Richards shared with the nurse and appropriate staff things that really irritated him.
	2b. Mr. Richards will share with Mr. Hall his insecurities about his job.	2b. Awareness of underlying reasons for behavior helps in control of that behavior.	
	2c. Isolate specific situations that seem to frustrate him.	2c. Can work with client to cope more effectively in these situations.	

NURSING DIAGNOSIS

Ineffective individual coping **related to the work environment, as evidenced by aggressive behavior toward others**

Supporting Data

- Exploded at work, ran out of the plant
- Threw things at home
- Shouted at wife

Long Term Goal: Mr. Richards will demonstrate three constructive ways of coping with his frustrations by discharge.

Short Term Goals	Intervention	Rationale	Evaluation
1. Mr. Richards, with the help of the nurse, will define one of his problems within four days.	1a. Nurse and client will define the problem and evaluate his response to the situation.	1a. Helps develop an awareness of coping behaviors.	Goal met Mr. Richards was able to talk about his aggressive behavior as being a problem.
	1b. Elicit Mr. Richards' feelings regarding his aggressiveness.	1b. Bringing feelings into awareness helps in dealing with them.	
2. Mr. Richards will identify two alternative ways of dealing with situations that provoke aggressiveness within one week.	2. Explore positive alternative behavior responses (physical activity—working in the garden, jogging, shooting baskets in the gym).	2. Provides opportunity to develop socially acceptable ways of handling frustration.	Goal met By the end of the first week, Mr. Richards would go to the gym and shoot baskets when he was frustrated.

Summary

Violence in our society is a growing problem. The increase in substance abuse, increase in economic and domestic crisis, and increase of confused and disoriented elderly provide some explanation. It is important that health care professionals know how to work with aggressive behavior. Such behavior can be threatening. Nurses need to be aware of their personal feelings, level of anxiety, and physical limitations. Through self-understanding, understanding of the client's behavior, and understanding that assaultiveness is a response to a real or perceived situation that is interfering with achieving a goal, potentially aggressive situations can be prevented.

Factors that might make an individual more prone to aggressive behavior include a previous episode of aggressive behavior; a toxic reaction to medication;

situational, social, or environmental stimuli; and certain psychiatric conditions. The nurse's sensitivity to all clues of impending aggression will lead to a proactive approach rather than a reactive intervention.

The nursing diagnosis of most concern in working with clients who are unable to control their behavior is *high risk for violence directed at others*. Other significant nursing diagnoses include *ineffective individual coping*, *powerlessness*, and *self-esteem disturbance*.

Planning nursing care for a person who handles anxiety with aggressive behavior involves setting realistic, measurable, and time-limited short and long term goals for each of the nursing diagnoses. The verbal and nonverbal interventions by the nurse are crucial in preventing escalation of behavior. Self-confidence, posture, facial expression, tone of voice, and personal space are significant in relating to a disturbed individual. It is important to maintain an emotional honesty; the nurse's verbal and nonverbal communication should give the same message. Double messages lead to further confusion and can escalate anxiety.

Evaluation includes examining effectiveness of verbal and nonverbal intervention techniques. Were they helpful in de-escalating the client's behavior? Were nonharmful physical intervention skills needed? When physical intervention techniques are used, goals need to be reassessed and approaches re-evaluated. Evaluation of aggressive behavior is an ongoing process for ensuring that the least restrictive intervention is always used.

References

Baron RA. Aggression. In Kaplan HI, Sadock BJ (eds). Comprehensive Textbook of Psychiatry, vol I, 4th ed. Baltimore: Williams & Wilkins, 1985.

Bauer B, Hill S. Essentials of mental health care planning and interventions. Philadelphia: WB Saunders, 1986.

Dollard JC, Drok L, Miller N, Mower O, Sears R. Frustration and aggression. New Haven: Yale University Press, 1939.

Eichelman B. Psychiatric mental health nursing with the violent patient. Journal of Psychosocial Nursing and Mental Health Services, 29, 1991.

Flannery RB, et al. A program to help staff cope with psychological sequelae of assaults by patients. Hospital and Community Psychiatry, 42(9):935, 1991.

Foster R. Gentle self defense. Lawrence, KS: Camelot Behavioral Systems Workshop, 1979.

Harvard Medical School Mental Health Letter. Serotonin and aggression: New data, 6(5):6, 1989.

Harvard Medical School Mental Health Letter. Violence, 1(8):1, 1991.

Lanza ML. Nurses as patient assault victims: An update, synthesis and recommendations. Archives of Psychiatric Nursing, 6(3): 163–171, 1992.

Mahoney BS. The extent, nature, and response to victimization of emergency nurses in Pennsylvania. Journal of Emergency Nursing, 17:282, 1991.

Maxmen JS. Psychotropic Drugs Fast Facts. New York: WW Norton, 1991.

McGuire MT, Troisi A. Aggression. In Kaplan HI, Sadock BJ (eds). Comprehensive Textbook of Psychiatry, vol I, 5th ed. Baltimore: Williams & Wilkins, 1989.

Miller M, Gorski T. The management of aggression and violence. Hazel Crest, IL: Human Ecology Systems, 1981.

Price-Hoskins P. Management of aggressive behavior. In Haber et al (eds). Comprehensive Psychiatric Nursing, 4th ed. St. Louis: Mosby–Year Book, 1992.

Schmoker M. Sentimentalizing self-esteem. Education Digest, 55(3):55, 1990.

Serotonin neurotransmitter of the '90s. Psychology Today, 25(5):16, 1992.

Stevenson S. Heading off violence with verbal de-escalation. Journal of Psychosocial Nursing, 29(9):6, 1991.

Tavris C. Anger: The misunderstood emotion. New York: Simon & Schuster, 1989.

The Cincinnati Enquirer. Temperature can heat up emotions. July 11, 1992.

Further Reading

Blair DT, Mew SA. Assaultive behavior: Know the risks. Journal of Psychosocial Nursing, 29(11):25, 1991.

Coccaro EF, et al. Serotonergic studies in patients with affective and personality disorders. Archives of General Psychiatry, 46(7):587, 1989.

Coser LA, et al. Aggressiveness. In Coser LA (ed). Introduction to Sociology, 2nd ed. New York: Harcourt Brace Jovanovich, 1983, p 299.

Coser LA, et al. Kinds-of-people theories. In Coser LA (ed). Introduction to Sociology, 2nd ed. New York: Harcourt Brace Jovanovich, 1983, p 226.

Coser LA, et al. Violence. In Coser LA (ed). Introduction to Sociology, 2nd ed. New York: Harcourt Brace Jovanovich, 1983, p 517.

Gahan K. Everybody gets angry sometime. Journal of Psychosocial Nursing, July-August: 27, 1978.

Gury F, Kavanaugh CK (eds). Psychiatric Mental Health Nursing. Philadelphia: JB Lippincott, 1991.

Hales RE, Yudofsky SC. The American Psychiatric Press Textbook of Neuropsychiatry. Washington, DC: American Psychiatric Press, 1987, p 184.

Harvard Medical School Mental Health Letter. Television violence and children, 1(8):6, 1985.

Iyer PW, et al. Nursing Process and Nursing Diagnosis. Philadelphia: WB Saunders, 1991.

Kerr MM, Nelson MC. Strategies for Managing Behavioral Problems in the Classroom. Columbus, OH: Charles E. Merrill, Publisher of Bell and Howell Company, 1983.

Kreigh HZ, Perko JE. Psychiatric and Mental Health Nursing: Commitment to Care and Concern. Reston, VA: Reston Publishing Company, 1979.

Lathrop V. Aggression as a response. Perspectives in Psychiatric Care, 16(5–6):202, 1978.

Lehmann LS, et al. Training personnel in the prevention and management of violent behavior. Hospital and Community Psychiatry, 34:40, 1983.

Meddaugh DI. Reactance understanding of aggressive behavior in long term care. Journal of Psychosocial Nursing 28(4):28, 1990.

Neville JM. Physical Crisis Intervention: Managing Violent and Assaultive Behavior in the Hospital Setting. East Hanover, NJ: Medical Media Associates Workshop, 1986.

Petrie WM, et al. Violence in geriatric patients. Journal of the American Medical Association, 248(23/30):444, 1982.

Pribula I, Disarming the agitated combative or destructive patient. Free Association, 10(3):5, 1983.

Ryden MB. Moral and perceived control in institutionalized elderly. Nursing Research, 33(3):136, 1984.

Stewart A. Handling the aggressive patient. Perspectives in Psychiatric Care, 16(5–6): 228, 1978.

Taptich BJ, et al. Nursing diagnosis and care planning. Philadelphia: WB Saunders, 1989.

Tupin JP. The violent patient: A strategy for management and diagnosis. Hospital and Community Psychiatry, 34:37, 1983.

Winger J, et al. Aggressive behavior in long term care. Journal of Psychosocial Nursing, 25(4):28, 1987.

Self-study Exercises

The emphasis in learning is on critical thinking. The following questions assist you in this process.

Short Fill-In

Answer each of the following questions in your own words. Clue words are included to facilitate the learning process.

1. What is meant by the *instinctual theory* of aggression? (Clue word: built in.)

2. How did *Freud* view instinct as a basis for aggression? (Clue words: Eros, Thanatos, displacement, innate, inevitable, catharsis.)

3. How did *Lorenz* view instinct as a basis for aggression? (Clue words: fighting instinct, accumulate, release, spontaneously, redirecting, feelings of love and friendship.)

4. What is meant by the elicited-*drive theory* of aggression? (Clue words: situational, frustration, save face, physical pain.)

5. What is the object of the "drive" in the elicited-drive theory? (Clue words: frustration, aggression, harm.)

6. What is meant by the *biological theory* of aggression? (Clue words: impulsive aggression, low levels of serotonin, cultural, hereditary, low monoamine oxidase level, newborns.)

7. What is meant by the *social learning theory* of aggression? (Clue words: past experiences, rewards.)

Match the factors related to aggressive behavior in the right column with the determinants in the left column.

8. _____ TV violence		A. Personal
9. _____ Weather		
10. _____ Crowds		B. Social
11. _____ Erotic material		
12. _____ Family violence		C. Situational
13. _____ Teasing		
14. _____ Competitive activities		D. Environmental
15. _____ Exposure to cigarette smoke		
16. _____ Pain		
17. _____ History of aggressive behavior		
18. _____ Noise		

To prevent escalation of aggressive behavior, the nurse must be sensitive to both verbal and nonverbal clues. In the space provided, *list five verbal* **and** *five nonverbal clues:*

Verbal Clues	*Nonverbal Clues*
19.	24.
20.	25.
21.	26.
22.	27.
23.	28.

In *your own words*, **state** *briefly* **why the following psychiatric problems can increase the possibility of becoming aggressive.**

29. Acute psychosis:

30. Organic mental disorders:

31. Antisocial personality disorder:

32. Borderline personality disorder:

33. Intoxication (alcohol and other drugs):

34. The nursing diagnosis that is of most concern in working with an aggressive client is *high risk for violence directed at others*. In your *own words*, discuss your understanding of factors that may be related to this diagnosis.

35. Briefly explain how *powerlessness* relates to individual aggression, societal aggression, and war.

36. What is the purpose of writing long term goals and related short term goals for the aggressive client? (Clue words: client participation, nursing intervention, continuity.)

37. Because this is a *private* study exercise, consider your own reactions and feelings in response to someone who is aggressive toward you. What do you perceive your own personal feelings to be regarding aggressive clients, your level of anxiety, and your physical limitation? (Clue: Review the list of daily stressors.)

38. Write a personal (short) affirmation that will increase your self-confidence in a fearful situation.

39. Choose four interventions from the list of 13 verbal and nonverbal interventions listed in Table 22–3. Write a *brief* statement of how you might apply each of the four interventions in an actual situation. (Clue: Think of a real client situation. It does not have to be a client on a psychiatric unit.)

    A.

B.

C.

D.

40. In your own words, briefly review four of the basic points for the nurse to remember when interviewing a physically assaultive client.

A.

B.

C.

D.

CHAPTER 23

People Who Depend On Alcohol

Kathleen Smith-DiJulio

OUTLINE •

THEORY
Biological Theories
Psychological Theories
Sociocultural Theories
Definitions

ASSESSMENT
Assessing Levels of Anxiety and Coping
　Styles
Assessing the Level of Alcohol in the
　Body System and Physiological
　Changes
Assessing Psychological Changes
Assessing Social Changes and Available
　Support Systems
Assessing Alcohol Withdrawal and
　Delirium
　　Assessing the Severity of
　　　Withdrawal
　　Assessing for Possible Traumatic
　　　Injuries
　　Assessing for Multiple Withdrawal

NURSING DIAGNOSIS

PLANNING
Content Level—Planning Goals
Process Level—Nurses' Reactions and
　Feelings

INTERVENTION
Psychotherapeutic Interventions
Health Teaching
Somatic Therapies
Therapeutic Environment
Psychotherapy

EVALUATION

**CASE STUDY: WORKING WITH A
　PERSON WHO HAS ALCOHOLISM**

SUMMARY

KEY TERMS AND CONCEPTS • • • • • • • • • • • • • • • • •

**The key terms and concepts listed here also appear in bold where they are
defined or discussed in this chapter.**

ADDICTION

ADULT CHILDREN OF ALCOHOLICS
　(ACoA)

AL - ANON

AL - A - TEEN

ALCOHOL DELIRIUM

ALCOHOL WITHDRAWAL

ALCOHOLICS ANONYMOUS (AA)

ALCOHOLISM

AVERSIVE CONDITIONING

BLOOD ALCOHOL LEVEL (BAL)

CODEPENDENT

DENIAL

DEPENDENCE

DISULFIRAM (ANTABUSE)

DUAL DIAGNOSIS

ENABLER

INTERVENTION PROCESS

PREDICTABLE DEFENSIVE STYLE

TOLERANCE

WITHDRAWAL

OBJECTIVES ■

After studying this chapter, the student will be able to

1. Compare and contrast what is meant by alcohol addiction and alcohol withdrawal.
2. Define alcoholism.
3. Discuss three theories of the cause of alcoholism.
4. Identify significant data found in an alcoholic client, using the five areas of assessment covered in this chapter.
5. Describe the difference in the relationship of blood alcohol levels and behavior between an alcoholic person and a nondrinker.
6. Compare and contrast the symptoms seen in alcohol withdrawal with those in alcohol delirium.
7. Identify four groups of drugs that are given during alcohol delirium and discuss the purpose for each.
8. Formulate six nursing diagnoses that might apply to alcoholic clients, including related etiological factors.
9. Identify two short term goals that might be useful steps in achieving long term sobriety.
10. Write at least four principles of psychotherapeutic intervention that a nurse would use with an alcoholic client.
11. Discuss two issues that a therapist should address when treating alcoholics.
12. Explain three issues that affect the alcoholic during phases of treatment.
13. Discuss five therapeutic modalities used with alcoholic people.
14. Identify four indications that a person is successfully recovering from alcoholism.

Alcohol is the most widely used—and misused—drug in America. It has only been in recent decades that alcoholism has begun to be thought of as a disease rather than a moral weakness. Attitudes change slowly, and moral notions about this disease still prevail; missed diagnoses and lack of treatment for affected individuals are the result. The impact of excessive alcohol use on human health and well-being is substantial, and no one is immune from the gamut of medical-social-emotional-familial-legal-economic problems that uncontrolled alcohol use creates. It is a problem that cannot be ignored.

Two thirds of the nation's adults consume alcohol regularly. One in 10 of these develops problems associated with his or her alcohol use. It has been estimated that one third of hospital admissions are alcohol-related. Alcohol-related traffic accidents continue to be a major problem in our society. Alcohol contributes significantly to the incidence and severity of problems in the home and workplace.

Because of the broad social impact of alcohol use, it is critical that nurses learn to recognize the indicators of a developing alcohol problem. Because alcohol problems in most persons are progressive in nature, early detection is critical for a positive prognosis. There is no arena of nursing practice that can ignore

problems caused by excessive alcohol consumption. People with alcohol problems are seen in clinics, inpatient hospital units, and even schools. Alcohol and drug abuse account for 10% of all emotional problems in the aged (Kaplan and Sadock 1991). Alcohol and substance abuse among adolescents is increasing rapidly and becoming more severe. Substance abuse among women is also on the rise. Women who continue to abuse alcohol during pregnancy run the risk of having an infant born with fetal alcohol syndrome. Health care workers themselves are another population of impaired individuals. A discussion of substance dependence among nurses is found in Chapter 24.

Nurses need to know about alcohol-related problems to care for their clients effectively, wherever they may practice. In addition, the nursing profession is becoming more involved in the treatment of alcoholism, and many nurses are becoming actively involved in all aspects of treatment. This chapter provides fundamental knowledge about alcoholism and focuses on the role of the nurse in both assessment and treatment processes.

Figure 23–1 conceptualizes alcohol abuse as a self-destructive behavior in response to stress.

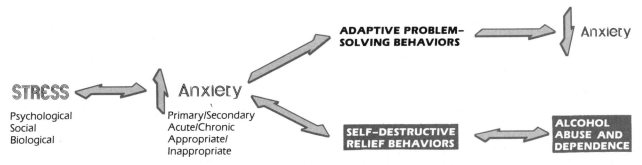

Figure 23−1. *Conceptualization of the process of alcohol abuse and dependence.*

Theory

Alcohol, a psychoactive substance, is used by the majority of the adult population in the United States. Most people who use this central nervous system depressant do so without problems. However, a certain percentage of people develop problems associated with their alcohol use. Alcohol use does occur on a continuum (Fig. 23−2). Movement along this continuum in either direction is a progressive process and takes time.

Alcoholism is the term applied to the end stage of the continuum that includes addiction and dependence. **Addiction** incorporates the concepts of loss of control of alcohol ingestion, drinking despite alcohol-related problems, and a tendency to relapse. **Dependence** can be physical or psychological. Evidence of **tolerance** (increasing amounts of alcohol are required to achieve the desired effect) and **withdrawal** (stopping alcohol use results in specific signs and symptoms) indicates *physical* dependence. *Psychological* dependence involves craving for, and compulsive use of, alcohol. The alcoholic thinks he needs a drink to survive.

The reason one person becomes addicted and another does not seems to depend on a number of factors, including psychosocial and environmental factors as well as genetic predisposition. The difficulty in determining cause and effect is that the diagnosis of alcoholism generally occurs many years after the onset of drinking. Many different factors are involved over the course of those years and probably have an influence on the eventual development of alcoholism in any particular individual. Theories briefly examined here include biological, psychological, and sociocultural theories.

BIOLOGICAL THEORIES

Interest in biological theories was spurred by the observation that alcoholism seemed to run in families. If your ancestors had problems with alcohol, the likelihood seemed to be increased that you would too. The first studies that seemed to indicate a genetic component in the development of alcoholism were by Goodwin et al.(1973, 1974). They studied identical twins of alcoholic and nonalcoholic fathers. All twins studied were adopted at birth; half were placed in alcoholic homes, half in nonalcoholic homes. The children of alcoholic fathers developed alcoholism at a rate significantly higher than that of children of nonalcoholic fathers, even when the children of alcoholic fathers were raised in nonalcoholic homes. Twins raised in alcoholic homes whose biological fathers were not alcoholic did *not* develop alcoholism greater than that of the general population.

Children of alcoholic parents are four times more likely to develop alcoholism than are children of nonalcoholic parents. Sons of alcoholic parents are more

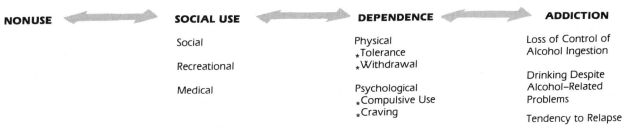

Figure 23−2. A *continuum of alcohol use.*

likely to become alcoholics than are daughters (Kaplan and Sadock 1991).

Current research has largely shifted from looking for an actual gene that causes alcoholism to looking at inherited abnormalities of biochemical factors that predispose to the development of alcoholism. The most promising research in this regard focuses on neuropeptides (also known as endogenous opiates), specifically enkephalins and endorphins. The theory is that a deficiency of these leads to dysphoria. In an attempt to feel better, the affected individual resorts to alcohol use, finds relief, and is thus reinforced for alcohol ingestion. When not drinking, the person again becomes dysphoric, knows that alcohol will improve mood, and so drinks again. Current research involves testing this hypothesis by restoring deficient neuropeptides in those at high risk for developing alcoholism (children of alcoholics) to see whether alcoholism can be prevented. Much change in this area of research is likely to be seen in the next five to 10 years.

It has been demonstrated more recently that alcohol has specific effects on selected neurotransmitter systems, particularly on gamma-aminobutyric acid. This finding helps explain the addictive and cross-tolerance effects that occur when the use of alcohol is combined with barbiturates and benzodiazepines. Both of these drugs also act on gamma-aminobutyric acid (Kaplan and Sadock 1991).

PSYCHOLOGICAL THEORIES

When addiction is conceptualized as a behavioral disorder, one looks to psychological theories for insight into the phenomenon. Knott (1987) described alcoholism as a behavioral impairment due to compulsive alcohol use. The affected individual is overwhelmingly preoccupied with procuring alcohol.

Although there is no addictive personality type, there are psychodynamic factors associated with alcoholism. These include the following (Knott 1987):

1. A *basic depressive personality organization.* Alcoholic persons are frequently described as having a depressed mood; yet they do not always meet the DSM IV criteria for either major depression or dysthymic disorder.
2. An *intolerance for frustration and pain.* This intolerance is exhibited in response to both psychological and physical pain. Much research has centered on the ability of alcohol to reduce tensions.
3. *Lack of success in life.*
4. *Lack of affectionate and meaningful relationships.* Because

of unmet needs, alcoholics require nurturance, which they usually cannot find as adults.
5. *Low self-esteem; lack of self-regard.* Alcoholic people often feel worthless, hopeless, and helpless about themselves and the possibility of their lives ever being any different.
6. *Risk-taking propensity.*

According to psychological theories, a person drinks to feel better. The habit of drinking in response to psychological needs then becomes reinforced, and over time the drinking behavior develops into an addiction.

SOCIOCULTURAL THEORIES

Sociocultural theories attempt to explain differences in the incidence of alcoholism in various groups. Attitudes about alcohol use, which are derived from the society and culture, influence when and how a person drinks. For example, Italians and Jews are thought to have lower alcoholism rates because they have rules about when and how much to drink. In these two cultures, drinking occurs in the context of meals and serves specific social and religious purposes. Drunkenness is frowned upon. The French, in contrast, are said to have high alcoholism rates because it is socially acceptable to drink anywhere and any time, and drunkenness is tolerated.

Another theory correlates alcoholism rates with the degree of cultural stress. This theory is said to explain the higher incidence of alcoholism among black men, especially in urban ghettos. Black women are said to be protected because of their more active involvement in religious groups that promote abstinence.

Women in general are said to have had lower alcoholism rates because of the cultural mores that have prohibited women from public drinking and heavy alcohol intake, although this is changing; alcoholism among women seems to be on the rise.

Theories centering on drinking practices in general place much emphasis on the learning experiences of adolescents. Social practices that encourage drinking as an adult mode of behavior may result in strong pressures to drink. Education about the role of alcohol in one's life and some exposure to it at home (e.g., sampling with meals) may mitigate some of the social pressures toward excessive, frequent alcohol consumption. The higher rates of alcoholism in alcoholic and teetotaling families are thought to derive from this lack of exposure to and thinking about the social role of alcohol.

In summary, *there is no single cause of alcoholism. Multiple factors come to bear to produce this disease in any specific individual.* For example, a child of an alcoholic may have a biochemical deficiency predisposing to alcoholism and may grow up with low self-esteem in a society that has no rituals governing alcohol use. Because of complex biological, psychological, and sociocultural factors, this person is at risk for developing alcoholism.

DEFINITIONS

The lack of consensus on the cause has made precise definition of alcoholism difficult. The *World Health Organization* (1952) defined alcoholics as those excessive drinkers whose dependence on alcohol has attained such a degree that there is an interference with the person's mental, physical, social, and economic well-being or those who show prodromal signs of such development. Put simply, if you have or are developing significant problems in any area of life functioning because of your alcohol intake, then you have an alcohol problem.

In 1977, the Committee on Alcohol Related Disabilities of the World Health Organization endorsed the term *alcohol dependence syndrome* to emphasize the existence of a *recognizable pattern of clinical phenomena.* The essential features of this syndrome include (Mandell 1983)

- Regularity of drinking behavior
- Emphasis on drink-seeking behavior
- Increased tolerance for alcohol
- Repeated withdrawal symptoms that are alleviated by further drinking
- Subjective awareness of a compulsion to drink
- A tendency to relapse

The diagnostic scheme in the DSM-III-R (APA 1987) focuses on the behavioral aspects and the pathological pattern of use, emphasizing the physical symptoms of tolerance and withdrawal. The term alcoholism is replaced by the label alcohol dependence. Also, a distinction is made between alcohol abuse and dependence (alcoholism).

An overview of the diagnostic criteria for alcohol-related disorders is shown in Figure 23–3.

As can be seen, terms describing various patterns of alcohol use have been as confusing as definitions. Definitions of use shown in Figure 23–2 are used throughout this chapter. The terms *addiction* and *alcoholism* are used interchangeably. The most useful definition for assessment purposes is the definition of the World Health Organization, which associates addiction with resultant problems.

Assessment

An objective assessment strategy allows nurses to obtain concrete data useful in diagnosis, planning, referral, and treatment. Most of the information needed for a complete and accurate health assessment is obtained by means of the nursing history. Nurses do basic screening histories on all of their clients. This is the time to begin asking about alcohol use. Because it is relatively recently that alcoholism has been considered a disease, many nurses are not sure of how to ask questions about what was formerly perceived as a "personal matter." The following pointers are helpful in the alcohol history-taking process.

1. Begin by asking the client about the use of *prescribed drugs.* The client is usually honest about these because they are ordered by a physician and thus perceived to be needed. From the answer to this question, an impression can be gained about the person's drug orientation. Some people will express their practice of using medications only when they are absolutely required (e.g., antibiotics for specific infections). Others will begin grumbling that they cannot get the correct prescriptions from any of the doctors they see. "Doctor shopping" and repeated client requests for medications, especially psychotropic medications, are indicators of a possible drug problem. Keep these responses in mind when asking other questions.

2. Next, question the person about *over-the-counter-drugs.* Many do not consider these substances drugs because they are so readily available and advertised. This questioning provides an opportunity for client education about drug effects.

3. Finally, ask the person about commonly used social drugs. The client may be puzzled or bewildered about this category. An explanation that caffeine and nicotine are drugs, followed by an assessment of their use by the client, sets the stage for the drinking history. Emphasize the fact that alcohol is a commonly used drug. Elicit the role that alcohol plays in the everyday functioning of the client.

It is useful at this point to incorporate the *CAGE* questionnaire as part of the assessment protocol. This questionnaire consists of four questions that focus on the main idea of Cutting down alcohol consumption, Annoyance by criticism of drinking, Guilty feelings associated with alcohol use, and Eye-openers, or early morning drinking. The title of the questionnaire was derived by extracting the first letter of the four main ideas, formulating the acronym *CAGE.* The specific questions follow (Mayfield et al. 1974):

ALCOHOL ABUSE

Maladaptive pattern of ETOH use leading to clinically significant impairment or distress, resulting in (within a 12-month period):

1. Inability to fulfill major role obligations at work, school, and home

2. Recurrent legal or interpersonal problems

3. Reduction or absence of important social, occupational, and recreational activities

4. Participation in physically hazardous situations while imparied (driving a car, operating a machine, exacerbation of symptoms, e.g., ulcers)

ALCOHOL DEPENDENCE

Maladaptive pattern of ETOH use leading to clinically significant impairment or distress, manifested by:

1. All criteria for Alcohol Abuse

2. Presence of tolerance to the drug or

3. Presence of ETOH withdrawal syndrome

4. Ingestion to relieve or prevent withdrawal

5. Continuing to use ETOH despite alcohol-related problems

6. Unsuccessful or persistent desire to cut down or control use

7. Increased time spent in getting, taking, and recovering from the substance. May withdraw from family or friends.

ALCOHOL INTOXICATION

1. Recent ingestion sufficient to cause intoxication in most people

2. Maladaptive behavior changes (sexual, aggressive, mood, and judgment)

3. At least one of the following:
   • Slurred speech
   • Incoordination
   • Unsteady gait
   • Nystagmus
   • Flushed face

ALCOHOL WITHDRAWAL

1. Cessation (reduction) of ETOH use that has been heavy or prolonged

2. Two (or more) of the following:
   • Nausea or vomiting
   • Anxiety
   • Transient visual, tactile, or auditory hallucinations or illusions
   • Headache
   • Autonomic activity (sweating, increased pulse over 100)
   • Psychomotor agitation
   • Insomnia
   • Grand mal seizures
   • Increased hand tremor

ALCOHOL-INDUCED DELIRIUM

1. Impaired consciousness (reduced awareness of environment)

2. Changes in cognition (memory, disorientation, language, visual or tactile hallucinations, illusions)

3. Develops over short period of time —hours to days—and fluctuates over a day

4. Evidence of ETOH use (history, physical, laboratory findings) and symptoms developed during withdrawal

Figure 23-3. Diagnostic criteria for alcohol-related disorders. ETOH = ethyl alcohol. (Adapted from American Psychiatric Association. Diagnostic and Statistical Manual of Mental Disorders, 4th ed. (DSM-IV). Washington, DC: American Psychiatric Association, 1994.)

1. Have you ever felt you should *cut down on your drinking*?
2. Have people *annoyed you by criticizing your drinking*?
3. Have you ever felt bad or *guilty about your drinking*?
4. Have you ever had a drink first thing in the morning to steady your nerves or get rid of hangover (**E**ye-opener)?

Two or three yes answers to these questions strongly suggest dependence on alcohol, especially physical dependence in terms of the inability to cut down and the need for an eye-opener (refer to Fig. 23–2). The nurse should also ask how much is drunk on a given occasion. Is it beer, wine, or hard liquor? (See Fig. 23–4 for alcohol equivalents.) What happens when drinking is curtailed? Questioning should not stop until you have asked the client about a whole array of prescribed and nonprescribed drugs. Multidrug use is the norm, and nurses must be on the lookout for it because drugs determine the client's presenting symptoms.

How a person responds to interview questions is a significant factor for assessment purposes. The majority of people give thoughtful, matter-of-fact responses that suggest no alcohol problem. Some will express concern and ask for information and referral. It may have been the first time anyone has asked about their alcohol use! Others will say that they abstain from alcohol. The reasons for abstinence are important. Do they abstain for religious or health reasons? Are they acknowledged alcoholics in recovery? Are they trying to prove to someone else that they can be abstinent? For example: "My husband thinks I drink too much so I'm going to show him. I'm not going to have a drop for two weeks. I can take it or leave it." Such a response indicates possible problems, and further assessment is required. Other responses that serve as "red flag" indicators for the need for further assessment are rationalizations—"You'd drink, too, if . . . "; automatic responses, as if predicted; or slow, prolonged responses, as if the person is being careful about what to say. Last are the practicing alcoholics who admit they have a problem but project an air of hopelessness about ever achieving sobriety (Estes and Heinemann 1986).

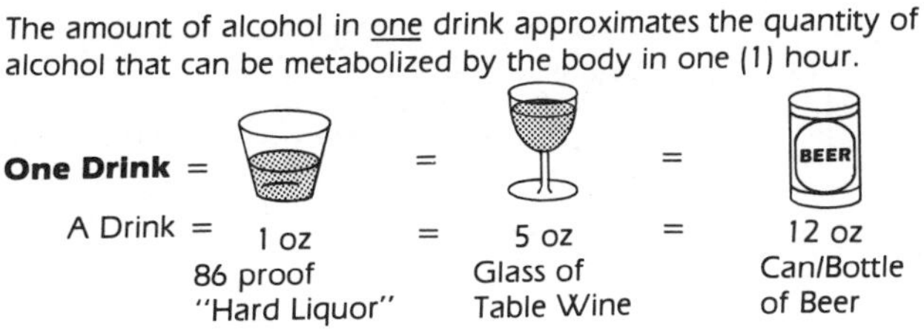

The amount of alcohol in <u>one</u> drink approximates the quantity of alcohol that can be metabolized by the body in one (1) hour.

One Drink =   =   =

A Drink =   1 oz   =   5 oz   =   12 oz
86 proof   Glass of   Can/Bottle
"Hard Liquor"   Table Wine   of Beer

Figure 23–4. *Alcohol equivalents.*

ASSESSING LEVELS OF ANXIETY AND COPING STYLES

Alcoholic people are threatened on a number of different levels in their interactions with nurses. *First*, they are concerned about being rejected. Alcoholic clients are acutely aware that not all nurses are equally willing to care for people with alcoholism, and in fact many clients may have experienced instances of rejection in past encounters with nursing personnel. Therefore, vulnerability is increased each time that they must interact with the health care system.

Second, alcoholic clients may be anxious about recovering because to do so they must give up the substance they think they need to survive—alcohol. *Third*, alcoholics are concerned about failing, not being able to succeed at recovering. Alcoholism is a chronic relapsing condition. In fact, relapse is one of the criteria for diagnosing addiction to alcohol. Most alcoholics have tried recovery at least once before and have relapsed. As a result, many become discouraged about their chances of ever succeeding.

The previously mentioned concerns can threaten the alcoholic person's sense of security and sense of self; thus, anxiety levels are increased. To protect against overwhelming anxiety, the alcoholic establishes a **predictable defensive style** (Wallace 1986). The elements include defense mechanisms, thought processes, and behaviors.

Defense Mechanisms

1. *Denial.* Deliberate denial of certain life difficulties may be a method of coping.
2. *Projection.* The tendency to assume that others are much like oneself and to perceive them as such, as in "It takes one to know one."
3. *Rationalization.* "The alcohol made me do it." "You'd drink too if . . . "

Thought Processes

1. *All-or-none thinking.* Allows structured, restricted choices and highly certain communication.
2. *Selective attention.* Attending only to what can be coped with is an effective way of minimizing anxiety.
3. *Preference for nonanalytical modes of thinking and perceiving.* For example, being influenced more by emotion and what "feels good."
4. *Obsessional focusing.* When the alcoholic spends a lot of energy procuring and ingesting alcohol, there is little left with which to focus on problems that the alcohol may be causing.

Behaviors

1. *Conflict minimization and avoidance.* The alcoholic will go to great lengths to reduce conflict. Conflict, after all, increases anxiety.
2. *Passivity versus assertion.*
3. *Manipulation.* Such as betraying confidences, playing one person against another, requiring special privileges.

The alcoholic is not able to give up these maladaptive coping styles until more positive and functional skills are learned.

ASSESSING THE LEVEL OF ALCOHOL IN THE BODY SYSTEM AND PHYSIOLOGICAL CHANGES

For more thorough assessment of the client addicted to alcohol, it is important to know the person's **blood alcohol level (BAL).** Knowing the BAL assists in determining the level of intoxication, level of tolerance, and whether the person accurately reported recent drinking during the nursing history. These factors are also assessed by means of behavioral cues. The relationship between BAL and behavior in a *nontolerant* individual is shown in Table 23–1.

After tolerance has been built up, there is a discrepancy between the BAL and expected behavior. A person who has developed a tolerance to alcohol may have a high BAL with minimal signs of impairment. For example, a person presented in the emergency department with a BAL of 0.51. He was stuporous and ataxic and had slurred speech. The fact that he was still alive indicated a high tolerance for alcohol. A nursing history conducted when the client sobered up revealed an extensive drinking history. When this is the case, assessing for withdrawal symptoms is important.

The presence of alcohol in the body results in associated physiological problems. A listing of physical problems associated with alcohol use is presented in Box 23–1. A nursing history, physical examination, and laboratory tests are methods used to gather data about alcohol-related physical problems. The extent of impairment depends on individual susceptibility as well as on the amount of heavy drinking.

A thorough nursing history is designed to elicit information about the various physical and psychosocial problems that can occur in people dependent on alcohol.

The drinking history component of the nursing history deserves special mention because it is useful for estimating the degree of addiction as well as the likelihood of withdrawal. Questions are asked to determine how long the client has been drinking, including asking about how long problems with alcohol have been present. Information about the quantity and frequency of drinking is important, and relevant questions include the following:

- *What do you drink?*
- *How much do you drink? Do you ever drink more? How often?*
- *When did you start this drinking bout?*
- *When did you have your last drink?*
- *What have you been drinking? How much per day? (Be certain to ask about beer, wine, and liquor individually. The more you ask, the more information you are likely to obtain.)*
- *What kind of problems has alcohol caused for you? With your family? Friends? Job? Health? Finances? The law?*

With the preceding information, you can make more accurate plans for intervention.

Table 23–1 ■ RELATIONSHIP BETWEEN BLOOD ALCOHOL LEVELS AND BEHAVIOR IN A NONTOLERANT DRINKER		
BLOOD ALCOHOL LEVELS	**BLOOD ALCOHOL ACCUMULATION***	**BEHAVIOR**
0.05 mg%	1–2 drinks	Changes in mood and behavior; judgment is impaired
0.10 mg%	5–6 drinks	Voluntary motor action becomes clumsy; **legal level of intoxication in most states**
0.20 mg%	10–12 drinks	Function of entire motor area of the brain is depressed, causing staggering and ataxia; emotional lability is present
0.30 mg%	15–18 drinks	Confusion; stupor
0.40 mg%	20–24 drinks	Coma
0.50 mg%	25–30 drinks	Death due to respiratory depression

*In excess of alcohol metabolized.

Box 23–1. PHYSIOLOGICAL EFFECTS RELATED TO ALCOHOL USE

Metabolic

Hypoglycemia
Hyperlipidemia
Hyperuricemia

Gastrointestinal System

Increased incidence of cancer of the oral mucosa
Increased acid production
Nausea and vomiting; diarrhea
Esophagitis and varices
Malabsorption of nutrients, especially folic acid, vitamin B$_1$ (thiamine), and vitamin B$_{12}$
Ulcers—gastric and duodenal
Gastritis, enteritis, colitis, hemorrhoids
Fatty liver, alcoholic hepatitis, cirrhosis
Pancreatitis

Neurological System

Sleep disturbance
Peripheral neuropathies
Brain syndromes
Wernicke-Korsakoff syndrome
Cerebellar degeneration

Cardiovascular System

Hypertension, tachycardia due to withdrawal
Decreased mechanical performance of the heart
Cardiomyopathy, after 10 or more years

Respiratory System

Impaired diffusion
Increased incidence of lung infections (e.g., bronchitis, pneumonias)
Smoking effects (e.g., chronic obstructive pulmonary disease)

Genitourinary System

Increased urinary excretion of potassium and magnesium leads to hypomagnesemia and hypokalemia
Hypogonadism, hypoandrogenization, hyperestrogenization in men
Diminished sexual performance
Impotency in males
Decreased menstruation, leading to infertility

Musculoskeletal System

Myopathies

Skin

Infections
Lesions, burns, scars

Hematological System

Anemias
Impaired phagocytosis, which reduces body's response to invasion by bacteria
Leukopenia, which can affect the body's immune system
Hematomas

Data from Smith-DiJulio K. Nursing people experiencing dependence on alcohol and other drugs. In Luckmann J, Sorensen KC (eds). Medical-Surgical Nursing: A Psychophysiologic Approach, 3rd ed. Philadelphia: WB Saunders, 1987, pp 1836–1866.

ASSESSING PSYCHOLOGICAL CHANGES

It is self-evident that alcohol use affects a person's behavior. Certain psychological characteristics are associated frequently with alcohol use, including denial, depression, dependency, hopelessness, low self-esteem, and various psychiatric disorders. It is often difficult to determine which came first, psychological changes or drinking behavior. Some people self-medicate to cope with psychiatric symptoms. For these people, symptoms of psychological difficulty remain even after months of sobriety. In obtaining a nursing history, questions that try to determine whether drinking occurred as an attempt to cope with either a dysphoric or an elated mood can be helpful. Psychological changes that occurred as a result of drinking clear rather quickly with sobriety.

Psychiatric disorders that may be seen concurrently in alcoholics include acute and chronic cognitive impairment disorders, attention deficit disorder, schizophrenia, borderline personality disorder, antisocial personality disorder, anxiety disorders, and disorders of mood (McKelvey et al. 1987; Kaplan and Sadock 1991).

Close attention to mental status will often provide clues to these disorders. If clear-cut alcohol dependency is present along with a well-defined psychiatric disorder, conservative treatment consists of viewing both disorders as primary **(dual diagnosis)** and treating each separately. Because most alcohol dependencies are great "mimickers," a long, well-monitored detoxification period, for observing the appearance or disappearance of mental symptoms, is appropriate.

This often requires skilled psychiatric nursing care when a detoxifying client begins to exhibit the symptoms of major psychiatric problems that must be treated also. Because the majority of psychotropic medications interact adversely with alcohol, trying to treat psychiatric illness in an active alcoholic is discouraged. Alcohol also interferes with medication compliance. Many clinicians are familiar with the well-stabilized bipolar or schizophrenic client who begins to use alcohol, subsequently disrupts or stops taking psychiatric medication, and ends up being rehospitalized for stabilization of his or her disorder.

Denial has become the hallmark psychological characteristic of alcoholism, with the alcoholic person bearing the brunt of the blame for not admitting to having a disease, seeking treatment, and getting cured. **Denial** is a defense mechanism used to avoid the anxiety associated with having to admit something painful or difficult. It is true that the alcoholic person tends to deny having a problem with alcohol, but family and friends often deny the same problem. Also, society denies the problem of alcoholism by failing to allocate funds for alcoholism research, prevention, treatment, and rehabilitation. Nurses and other health care professionals deny the problem by ignoring its existence in their clients. This can result from feelings of hopelessness and helplessness in treating alcoholism owing to gaps in current knowledge of how to do so.

ASSESSING SOCIAL CHANGES AND AVAILABLE SUPPORT SYSTEMS

Deterioration in a person's social status and social relationships often occurs as a result of alcoholism. Job demotion or loss of job, with resultant reduced or nonexistent income, may occur. Meeting basic needs for food, shelter, and clothing is thereby hampered. Marriages and other close relationships deteriorate and fail, and the person often finds him- or herself alone and isolated. This lack of interpersonal and social supports is an important factor in treatment planning for the alcoholic person. These are signs and symptoms of late-stage alcoholism. It is to be hoped that our enhanced assessment skills will allow detection of alcoholism in the early stages before associated problems reach a crisis level.

ASSESSING ALCOHOL WITHDRAWAL AND DELIRIUM

Alcohol withdrawal syndromes occur after the intake of ethyl alcohol (ETOH) has been reduced or has ceased in a person who has had long term exposure to large amounts of alcohol. Alcohol withdrawal reactions range from mild to severe. The severity of the withdrawal reaction depends on the length of the drinking period and the amount of alcohol consumed.

Episodes of *alcohol delirium*, or *delirium tremens*, occur in people with a five- to 15-year history of heavy drinking who often have significant physical illness (Dubin and Weiss 1991). The DSM-III-R (APA 1987) identifies two alcohol withdrawal syndromes: (1) *alcohol withdrawal* and (2) the more severe *alcohol withdrawal delirium*.

Nursing and medical assessment includes (1) assessing the severity of withdrawal, (2) assessing for possible traumatic injuries, and (3) assessing for withdrawal from other drugs.

Assessing the Severity of Withdrawal

ALCOHOL WITHDRAWAL. (6–8 hours after cessation or reduction of ETOH intake). The early signs of withdrawal develop within a few hours after cessation or reduction of ETOH intake; they peak after 24–48 hours and then rapidly and dramatically disappear, unless the withdrawal progresses to alcohol withdrawal delirium.

Early signs of withdrawal include anxiety, anorexia, insomnia, and tremor. The person may appear hyperalert, manifest jerky movements and irritability, startle easily, and experience subjective distress often described as "shaking inside." The person may also report transient, poorly formed hallucinations, illusions, or vivid nightmares. Nausea and vomiting may also occur.

Pulse and blood pressure are usually elevated. Grand mal seizures may also develop. They usually appear in seven to 48 hours after cessation of ETOH intake, particularly in people with a history of seizures.

A client in alcohol withdrawal should be monitored to prevent progression into alcohol withdrawal delirium. Careful assessment followed by appropriate medical and nursing interventions can prevent the more serious withdrawal reactions of delirium. Cross-dependent sedatives are useful on a temporary basis for reducing the symptoms of withdrawal. Cross-dependent sedatives work by controlling the overactivity of the sympathetic nervous system. Drugs frequently used for this purpose include the benzodiazepines, such as diazepam (Valium) and chlordiazepoxide hydrochloride (Librium).

The pulse and blood pressure should be checked hourly for the first eight to 12 hours after admission, at least every four hours during the first 48 hours, and then four times a day thereafter (Smith-DiJulio 1987). *The pulse is a good indication of progress through withdrawal.* Elevation may indicate impending alcohol withdrawal delirium, signaling the need for more rigorous sedation.

ALCOHOL WITHDRAWAL DELIRIUM. (48–72 hours after cessation or reduction of ETOH intake). Alcohol withdrawal delirium is considered a medical emergency and has a 20% mortality rate if left unattended (Kaplan and Sadock 1991). Death is usually due to myocardial infarction, fat emboli, peripheral vascular collapse, hyperthermia, or aspiration pneumonia. The state of delirium usually peaks after three days (72 hours) of abstinence (can occur later) and lasts two to three days.

Along with anxiety, insomnia, anorexia, and delirium, additional features include (Kaplan and Sadock 1991):

1. Autonomic hyperactivity (e.g., tachycardia, diaphoresis, elevated blood pressure)
2. Severe disturbance in sensorium (e.g., disorientation, clouding of consciousness)
3. Perceptual disturbances (e.g., visual or tactile hallucinations)
4. Fluctuating levels of consciousness (e.g., ranging from hyperexcitability to lethargy)

Delusions (paranoid), agitated behaviors, and fever (100–103°F) are usually present.

Whenever possible, an accurate history of *what* the person has been taking (ETOH and other drugs), *when* and *how much* is vital for effective treatment. Such information is a crucial part of the nurse's assessment to be passed on to the medical team. Sometimes family or friends who come in with the indivdual in withdrawal can supply such information.

People experiencing withdrawal are often terrified, confused, and anxious. When the nurse has a kind, warm, and supportive manner, this often can allay anxiety and provide a sense of security. Consistent and frequent orientation to time and place may be necessary. Encouraging the family (one at a time) or close friends to stay with the client in quiet surroundings can also help increase orientation and minimize confusion and anxiety. Pulse and blood pressure need to be monitored frequently. Illusions are usually terrifying for the client. *Illusions* can be clarified, which reduces the client's terror. Interventions are often needed for a client who is hallucinating.

Kaplan and Sadock (1991) warn against the use of physical restraints because a client may struggle against them to the point of exhaustion. Refer to Chapter 20 for interventions appropriate for the client in delirium. Box 23–2 presents a vignette of a person going through alcohol withdrawal delirium.

Box 23–2. CLINICAL VIGNETTE: A CLIENT WITH ALCOHOL WITHDRAWAL DELIRIUM

After her divorce, Mary started having a few drinks after coming home from work. She initially found that these drinks helped her relax and "put me in a good mood." Over time, Mary found that two drinks no longer did the trick and that she required three and then four drinks to achieve the relaxed feeling and mild euphoria she sought. Mary's body was building up a tolerance for the drug, and it took larger and larger doses to get the desired effect. The body is able to adjust to gradually increased doses of certain drugs over time and begins to require a certain level of the drug to function "normally." After 10 years, Mary was drinking a couple of drinks at lunch, before dinner, and during the evening. However, on first glance, the effects of alcohol did not show. Mary was able to "appear normal" with a high blood alcohol level. Mary eventually developed the habit of a taking a drink every morning to settle the "shakes" and prevent tremulousness. She drank in the morning not to feel good but to prevent feeling bad.

In the fall of 1994 after suffering an acute attack of pancreatitis, Mary was hospitalized; she was given intravenous fluids and had a nasogastric tube in place. After three days, Mary became extremely agitated. She screamed that she was being held hostage by Iranian spies. She mistook her water carafe for a time bomb (*illusion*). She became terrified at night, believing she saw giant ants on the walls.

Mary's blood pressure increased from 120/70 on admission to 150/100. Her pulse increased from 88 to 140. She thought it was the winter of 1985, about the time of her divorce.

After alcohol withdrawal delirium was diagnosed, Mary was given 100 mg of chlordiazepoxide hydrochloride (Librium) intramuscularly and then orally every four hours. Her pulse and blood pressure were monitored every hour. She was given 100 mg of thiamine intramuscularly, prophylactically against encephalopathy, as well as magnesium sulfate. Mary had normal skin turgor, and her urine specific gravity was within normal limits; therefore, fluids were not forced.

Her terror at "seeing large ants" was reduced by the nurse's presence and assurances that the nurse did not see the ants. Once the nurse showed her the carafe and poured some of the

Continued

water into a glass, Mary understood that it was not a bomb.

Mary's agitation and aggressiveness became worse at night, and a friend stayed with her, talking in a calm manner and orienting her to her surroundings. When the nurses came to give medication and check vital signs and urinary output, they carefully explained everything they were going to do beforehand to allay misinterpretation of their actions by Mary.

Mary was placed in a private, well-lit room. A minimal amount of environmental stimuli was allowed (e.g., no radios or TV, one visitor at a time). A clock was placed in clear view. The head of her bed was kept elevated to increase environmental orientation, and her bed faced the window to provide further orientation to time of day.

Three days later, Mary was fully oriented although still taking Librium. The episode had frightened her. She agreed to go to an Alcoholics Anonymous meeting and learn about other available avenues to sobriety.

Assessing for Possible Traumatic Injuries

In the emergency department, a person may come in after a fight or accident, with head injuries as well as the noticeable odor of alcohol on his or her breath. Many of these clients have high serum alcohol levels when injuries occur. These high levels of alcohol can greatly interfere with an accurate physical and neurological assessment. Intracranial hematomas, subdural hematomas, and other conditions can go unnoticed if symptoms of acute alcohol intoxication and withdrawal are not distinguished from the symptoms of a brain injury. Therefore, neurological signs (pupil size, equality, and reaction to light) should be assessed, especially with comatose clients suspected of having trauma injuries.

Assessing for Multiple Withdrawal

One danger frequently encountered today is that of multiple drug abuse, or polypharmacy. Multiple drug

and alcohol dependencies are common, and simultaneous withdrawal syndromes are becoming a common phenomenon. The presence of two or more simultaneous withdrawal syndromes can present a bizarre clinical picture and pose problems for safe withdrawal. Again, family and friends may be helpful in gaining important information that can enhance safe withdrawal. Answers to *how much* of *what* was taken and *when* can save people's lives.

Nursing Diagnosis

Appropriate nursing diagnoses depend on an accurate assessment. Whereas the DSM-III-R criteria emphasize patterns of use and physical symptoms, nursing diagnoses identify how dependence on alcohol interferes with a person's ability to meet the activities and demands of daily living.

According to the physical, emotional, and social circumstances of the alcoholic person, nursing diagnoses can be many and varied. Table 23–2 identifies a variety of nursing diagnoses appropriate for use in all hospital settings.

Alcohol impairs health status. When intoxicated, the person is not concerned with being healthy and often does not, or cannot, take responsibility for basic care. Therefore, *altered health maintenance* may be evident.

Alcohol impairs judgment and increases risk-taking behaviors. *Injury* often results. With long term dependence, changes in blood profiles occur. For example, liver function test results are elevated, and hemoglobin and hematocrit are decreased. A multitude of changes occur after long term heavy alcohol use that affect the body's immune system and cardiovascular, gastrointestinal, and genitourinary functioning. Potential for seizures, falls, and accidents is increased; therefore the *high risk for injury* is present.

Disturbance in self-esteem or *chronic low self-esteem* is evidenced by projection of blame/responsibility for problems, denial of problems obvious to others, rationalizations, and expressions of shame or guilt. Low self-esteem is also reflected in the person's self-destructive behaviors and in nonparticipation in health-seeking behaviors.

As with any other disease, alcoholism represents a dysfunction or maladaption to the requirements of everyday life affecting the person's family, social, and occupational functioning. The use of alcohol becomes the main coping device. The disease can progress to the point at which the individual is unable to meet basic needs. Also, related illnesses become prominent and perhaps life-threatening, accidents increase as a

Table 23–2 ■ NURSING DIAGNOSES: PEOPLE WHO ABUSE ALCOHOL

NURSING DIAGNOSIS	COMMENTS
Activity intolerance	Malnutrition Peripheral neuropathies Bacterial endocarditis
Airway clearance, ineffective	Pneumonias
Anxiety	Drug withdrawal Abstinence
Diarrhea	Inflammation, irritation of the bowel due to alcohol ingestion Black, tarry stools from gastrointestinal bleeding
Breathing pattern, ineffective	Alcohol or drug overdose
Cardiac output, decreased	Alcoholic cardiomyopathy
Coping, ineffective family: disabling	Social patterns often become dysfunctional
Coping, ineffective individual	A drug-dependent person has come to see alcohol (drugs) as the solution to every problem; excessive drug-taking is maladaptive, and problem-solving abilities are impaired ● Loses most or all significant others ● Not able to perform on the job ● Usually does not meet basic needs ● Risk of suicide increases ● Denial becomes a major barrier to overcome in effecting change ● Illness rates increase owing to effects of lifestyle as well as drugs ● Accident rate increases owing to intoxication
Fluid volume deficit, potential	Secondary to protracted vomiting or diarrhea
Health maintenance, altered	Choosing to take alcohol and other drugs impairs health status; when intoxicated, the person is not concerned with being healthy and often does not take responsibility for basic care
Injury, high risk for	Alcohol/drugs impair judgment and increase risk-taking behavior; accidents and injury often result; with alcohol dependence, the blood profile becomes abnormal—liver function test results are elevated and hemoglobin and hematocrit are decreased
Knowledge deficit	Ignorance of alcohol/drug effects Ignorance of withdrawal process
Noncompliance	Resumption of alcohol/drug-taking behavior after treatment
Nutrition, altered: less than body requirements	Nutritional deficits are frequent because an intoxicated person is not interested in food; money is spent on alcohol
Oral mucous membrane, altered	Combined with the effects of smoking, leads to an increased incidence of carcinoma of the oropharynx
Parenting, altered: actual or potential	Adults focused exclusively on their own needs to manage drug dependence do not pay attention to the needs of their children Ineffective role-modeling Emotional neglect Increased incidence of physical, sexual abuse
Powerlessness	Central feelings in alcohol- and drug-dependent people
Disturbance in self-esteem **Chronic low self-esteem**	Evidenced by the self-destructive nature of alcohol/drug dependence and by nonparticipation in treatment Not taking responsibility for self

Table continued on following page

Table 23-2 ■ **NURSING DIAGNOSES: PEOPLE WHO ABUSE ALCOHOL** *Continued*	
NURSING DIAGNOSIS	**COMMENTS**
Sensory-perceptual alteration: auditory-visual	Audiovisual hallucinations due to withdrawal
Sexual dysfunction	Alcohol/drug abuse and dependence interfere with sexual arousal and performance: ● Impotence in men ● Decreased vaginal lubrication in women
Sleep pattern disturbance	Central nervous system depressants interfere with rapid eye movement and Stage IV (deep) sleep
Thought processes, altered	Judgment impaired; memory deficits with Wernicke-Korsakoff syndrome; when intoxicated, the alcohol/drug-dependent person is less able to grasp ideas, reason, solve problems, calculate, attend to task
Violence, self-harm, or high risk	Increased risk of suicide; increased incidence of child abuse, domestic violence, including battered woman syndrome

From Smith-DiJulio K. Nursing people experiencing dependence on alcohol and other drugs. In Luckmann J, Sorensen KC (eds). Medical-Surgical Nursing: A Psychophysiologic Approach, 3rd ed. Philadelphia: WB Saunders, 1987, pp 1861–1862.

result of intoxication, and denial becomes a major barrier to change. Sometimes coping becomes impossible, and suicide is attempted. Therefore, *ineffective individual coping* is prominent.

The family goes through many changes as the disease progresses. Family members begin to assume responsibilities for the alcoholic member, communications become dysfunctional, and often the family's activities and energies are organized around the disease and the affected member. Families may go from crisis to crisis, and maladaptions to crises may be evident in the form of spouse abuse or child abuse; thus, *ineffective family coping* may be present.

Planning

On completion of the assessment process, identified problems are assigned priorities, and a plan of care is developed. A plan of care is a guide to action toward improvement or recovery from alcoholism. Planning care is guided by (1) the content level—goals and (2) the process level—nurses' reactions and feelings.

CONTENT LEVEL—PLANNING GOALS

Planning care that may be effective in treating alcoholism requires attention to social status, income, ethnic background, sex, and age because all these contribute to an individual's personality, behavior, and

growth. The goals guide nursing interventions; thus, the goals need to be compatible with the person's personality, desired behaviors, and potential for growth. Therefore, goals for treatment need to be developed *with* the alcoholic person and reflect his or her desires and expectations for the future. Both short term and long term goals must be established.

Long term goals are usually more comprehensive and tend to be viewed as the end product of a hard struggle—for example, sobriety. Gitlow (1988) stated that sobriety or abstinence is not actually the aim of treatment but is a means to an end. The end, or *real purpose of treatment, is to improve function and the person's quality of life.* However, improvement in life cannot take place without sobriety or abstinence for an alcoholic person. Improvement in life is not compatible with the ingestion of alcohol. According to Gitlow (1988), improvement can occur only when there is

1. *Diminishment in psychomotor activity associated with alcohol ingestion.* Use of alcohol results in prolonged and intermittent agitation, enormously uncomfortable for the alcoholic.
2. *Control of organic disease.* Almost every complication of alcoholism requires abstinence for a maximal rate of improvement. Medical therapy in the presence of active drinking fails to achieve a satisfactory recovery.
3. *Potential for change and insight.* It is imposible to develop insight when cognitive functioning is impaired and the brain is sedated. "It's hard to learn to navigate from the deck of a sinking ship."

Therefore, for *ineffective individual coping* related to biochemical changes caused by alcohol ingestion, the goals would be as follows:

Long Term Goals

- Client will maintain sobriety.

Short Term Goals

- Client will attend Alcoholics Anonymous (AA) every night for one month.
- Client will be actively involved with his or her sponsor.
- Client will participate in treatment center after-care group and individual or family counseling.
- Client will name two people to call when experiencing an urge to drink.
- Client will participate in relapse prevention training (identifying the individual's high-risk situations for drinking).
- Client will name two "problem areas" that he or she wants to work on.

Another important area for initial intervention is in the area of self-esteem. Therefore, for the nursing diagnosis *disturbance in self-esteem* or *chronic low self-esteem*, the goals might be as follows:

Long Term Goals

- Client will state that he or she feels good about himself or herself and about the potential for the future.
- Client will demonstrate responsibility in implementing personal treatment goals.
- Client will demonstrate responsibility in implementing personal life goals.

Short Term Goals

- Client will state that AA is assisting him or her to "live one day at a time."
- Client will participate in social skills training.
- Client will role-play assertive communication skills to get needs met and maintain self-esteem.
- Client will demonstrate one new skill learned each week.
- Client will discuss negative aspects of his or her life while keeping the focus on ways to effect positive change.
- Client will state that he or she is more comfortable accepting positive feedback from others regarding personal strengths and positive qualities.

PROCESS LEVEL—NURSES' REACTIONS AND FEELINGS

It is not only within the nursing community but also in the whole medical community that ambivalence, frustration, and confusion operate in the treatment of alcoholism. Gitlow (1988) states, "The special reticence with which the medical community has approached alcoholism demands a greater endeavor for its understanding. Does alcoholism, because of its societal and moral implications, awaken discomfort and fear within the physician? . . . and in the nurse?"

A nurse might want to help but may perceive the alcoholic to be willful, uncooperative, and unworkable.

Alcoholism is a phenomenon of complex etiology involving many factors—mental, physical, genetic, and environmental. Nurses and physicians must be convinced that alcoholism is a disorder, and not a weakness, a nastiness, or someone's "fault" (Block 1988). What do we think alcoholism is?

Are we affected by societal stereotypes—for example, middle-aged, shabby, hedonistic, irresponsible, unemployed, or in some low status job? If alcoholics are viewed as somehow different from ourselves, it will be doubly difficult to recognize alcoholism in our clients, in our colleagues, or in ourselves until it is far advanced (Bissell 1988).

To really come to a personal understanding means that one must examine one's own attitudes, feelings, and beliefs about alcoholism and "alcoholics." It often means that one must examine one's own drinking and that of others, and this is not always pleasant work.

The presence of alcohol in a nurse's own family can overshadow the nurse's interactions with alcoholics. The negative or positive experiences a nurse has had with alcoholics will color all interpersonal interactions with present or future alcoholic clients.

Therefore, it is important to attend to personal feelings that arise in working with alcoholic people. All health care professionals require supervision if they are not experienced in this area. Nurses who do not attend to and work through expected negative feelings that arise during treatment end up in power struggles with the clients, and the therapeutic process becomes generally ineffective.

Intervention

Nurses interact with alcoholics in all areas of nursing practice. General approaches to intervention that apply to all contexts of care are described here.

The aim, in alcoholism treatment, is toward self-responsibility, not compliance. A major challenge is predicting treatment outcome and improving treatment effectiveness by matching subtypes of clients to specific types of treatment. Although alcoholics share some characteristics and dynamics as a group, there are significant differences within the alcoholic population in regard to physiological, psychological, and sociocultural processes. These differences argue against the idea of a single alcoholic personality, and they support the classifying of subtypes of alcoholics. These differences also influence the recovery process, either positively or negatively. Until we can define subtypes, treatment outcomes across types of treatment approaches and programs will remain essentially the same. The choice of inpatient or outpatient care often depends on cost and whether insurance coverage is available. Outpatient programs work best for employed alcoholics with involved social support systems. Those people without support and structure to their day often do better in inpatient programs.

In addition, neuropsychological deficits have been associated with long term drinking. Impairment has been found in abstract reasoning ability, ability to use feedback in learning new concepts, attention and concentration spans, cognitive flexibility, and subtle memory functions. These deficits undoubtedly have an impact on the process of alcoholism treatment (Walker et al. 1986).

Nursing interventions and rationales are presented in Table 23–3. Specific interventions are discussed throughout the rest of the chapter.

PSYCHOTHERAPEUTIC INTERVENTIONS

Principles for psychotherapeutic interventions include the following (Zimberg 1978).

1. Expect sobriety. The distortions, memory loss, and confusion that occur as a result of intoxication make communication and intervention ineffective when the person is intoxicated.
2. Individualize goals and interventions.
3. Set limits on behavior and on conditions under which treatment will continue.
4. Support and redirect defenses rather than attempting to remove them.
5. Recognize that the process of recovery is carried out in stages.
6. Look for therapeutic leverage. Make sobriety worthwhile for the alcoholic (e.g., for keeping one's job, family, friends).

A popular tool for helping the resistant alcoholic person develop a willingness to engage in treatment is the **intervention process** developed by Johnson (1986). This technique can be useful as a response to the first stage of treatment when the alcoholic person has more need for external control. The concept behind the intervention is that alcoholism is a progressive illness and rarely goes into remission without outside help. The strategies for the intervention are outlined in Box 23–3.

HEALTH TEACHING

Nurses must be clear, when communicating with people in all walks of life, in stating that alcohol is a drug and, as such, can have negative consequences. Primary prevention programs aimed at youth must emphasize a "decision about drinking" theme and edu-

Table 23–3 ■ NURSING INTERVENTIONS AND RATIONALES: PEOPLE AFFECTED BY ALCOHOLISM	
NURSING INTERVENTION	**RATIONALE**
1. Support/kindness.	1. Promotes ability to engage in treatment; minimizes anxiety.
2. Reinforce disease concept of addiction.	2. Decreases guilt associated with alcoholic behavior.
3. Effective communication.	3. Establishes trust; role-modeling.
4. Limit setting.	4. Promotes ability to engage in treatment.
5. Maintain consistency.	5. Fosters an objective and nonjudgmental milieu.
6. Education.	6. Client has learning needs related to ● alcoholism as a chronic disease; ● the development of alternative coping skills to deal with stressful or problematic feelings or situations; ● nutrition, hygiene, infection control.
7. Family therapy.	7. Promotes sharing of feelings and identification of destructive patterns that exist within the family system.

Box 23–3. STEPS IN THE INTERVENTION

1. All the people concerned about and affected by the person's drinking are gathered together to present their case. The intervention must be rehearsed before it is actually carried out, usually with the support and guidance of a counselor.
2. Specific evidence related to the drinking is presented by each person, and it is written down so that each person does not have to rely on memory in a tense situation.
3. Timing must be right:
   - There must be current evidence available.
   - It must take place after a crisis is precipitated by alcohol use and *not* when the person is intoxicated or in severe withdrawal.
4. The intervention requires privacy. Hold it in a place where no interruptions can occur.
5. Anticipate the use of defenses. Do not react to them.
6. Demonstrate genuine, but firm, concern.
7. Understand alcoholism as a disease.
8. Present treatment alternatives.
9. Prepare responses to possible outcomes. The goal is to get the affected person treatment. If the alcoholic says yes to treatment, then he or she is taken immediately to a detoxification unit where arrangements have been previously made. If the alcoholic refuses, then family members state his or her decision must force them to make decisions of their own, because they are no longer willing to live with the alcoholic's behavior.

From Johnson VE. Intervention: How to Help Someone Who Doesn't Want Help. Minneapolis: Johnson Institute Books, 1986.

---

cate youngsters about the effect of alcohol on mental processes, physical processes, and mood. Teaching about alcohol's effects on unborn babies should occur in the preteen and teenage years as well as in gynecologists' offices and obstetrics clinics. Nurses can and must play an active role in counteracting the all too prevalent social message that alcohol is a harmless beverage and, in fact, is required for inclusion in many social groups. Such groups as Mothers Against Drunk Drivers (MADD) and Students Against Drunk Drivers (SADD) are natural allies in this effort.

SOMATIC THERAPIES

The predominant somatic therapies for alcoholism treatment are those used for detoxification (management of withdrawal from alcohol) and disulfiram (Antabuse).

ALCOHOL WITHDRAWAL. Not all people who stop drinking require inpatient hospitalization and drug management. This decision depends on the length of time and the amount the client has been drinking, prior history of withdrawal complications, and overall health status. Medication should not be given until the symptoms of withdrawal are seen. Early with-

drawal symptoms are tremors, diaphoresis, rapid pulse (greater than 100), elevated blood pressure (greater than 150/90), and occasional transient tactile or visual hallucinations. Grand mal seizures can occur and are self-limited. The withdrawal process, not the seizure, needs to be treated.

Alcohol delirium need not occur if withdrawal is managed well. However, if the person does develop delirium tremens, immediate medical attention is crucial.

A variety of drugs may be used to prevent or treat alcohol delirium. The best treatment of alcohol delirium is prevention, and adequate sedation is the most important aspect of medical prevention. Sedation can also prevent progression to a deeper and more dangerous level of delirium.

Sedation, in effect, allows safe withdrawal from the drug ETOH; therefore, *a long-acting central nervous system depressant* is substituted for the shorter-acting drug of dependence (ETOH). Although various detoxification procedures may be practiced in different regions of the country, *benzodiazepines* (especially diazepam [Valium] and chlordiazepoxide hydrochloride [Librium]) are the drugs of choice in many areas because of their high therapeutic safety index and anticonvulsant properties. Barbiturates, meprobamate, paraldehyde, and other central nervous system depressants are also safely used in some areas. Clonidine (Catapres), propranolol (Inderal), haloperidol (Haldol), and hydroxyzine hydrochloride (Atarax) have also been used but are not recommended for routine alcohol withdrawal (Dubin and Weiss 1991). In uncomplicated withdrawal, 25–50 mg of chlordiazepoxide hydrochloride may be given every two to four hours. However, once alcohol withdrawal delirium appears, doses of 50–100 mg are given (Kaplan and Sadock 1991). Ten to 20 times the normal doses of these drugs may be needed because cross-tolerance from the drug of dependence often develops. *Danger of an inadvertent overdose is always possible, and close nursing and medical observation is needed, especially during the first 24 hours.*

Thiamine (vitamin B₁) deficiency is often present owing to poor dietary intake and malabsorption. Thiamine replacement is given to prevent Wernicke's syndrome (encephalopathy). Wernicke's syndrome is characterized by nystagmus, ptosis, ataxia, confusion, coma, and possible death (Frances and Franklin 1988).

Hypomagnesemia is another condition found in people with long term drinking problems. *Magnesium sulfate* is often given (1) to increase the body's response to thiamine and (2) to raise the seizure threshold.

Anticonvulsants may or may not be used. Diazepam or phenobarbital may be used on a short term basis to control a client's seizures and prevent status epilepticus. Phenytoin (Dilantin) is less frequently used because seizures usually occur within the first 48 hours of withdrawal and phenytoin takes days to reach an effective blood level; because alcohol withdrawal seizures do *not* represent a primary seizure disorder, a person without such a disorder should not be routinely given phenytoin (Dubin and Weiss 1991). Table 23–4 summarizes drugs used in treatment.

Fluid and electrolyte replacements may be necessary, especially if the client is vomiting, has diarrhea, and is diaphoresing. In these cases, the client may be dehydrated and may need proper fluids and electrolyte replacement (e.g., potassium). However, caution should be taken. Diuresis occurs when blood alcohol levels *rise*, but fluid retention may occur as blood alcohol levels fall; therefore, a person in withdrawal may be *overhydrated*. Rigorous fluid therapy could cause serious complications, such as congestive heart failure.

DISULFIRAM (ANTABUSE). has been used in the treatment of alcoholism for over 30 years. It works on the classical conditioning principle. Disulfiram inhibits *impulsive* drinking because the client tries to avoid the unpleasant physical reaction involved in the alcohol-disulfiram reaction. This reaction consists of facial flushing, sweating, throbbing headache and neck pain,

Table 23–4 ■ DRUG INFORMATION: TREATMENT OF ALCOHOL WITHDRAWAL DELIRIUM

DRUG	DOSE	PURPOSE
Sedatives Benzodiazepines		
Chlordiazepoxide Librium (drug of choice)	25–100 PO every 4 hours (for 5–7 days) in tapering doses	Librium and Valium provide *safe* withdrawal and have *anticonvulsant* effects
Diazepam (Valium)	5–10 mg PO every 2–4 hours in tapering doses	
Phenobarbital/pentobarbital	100 mg PO in tapering doses	Control withdrawal; caution: can depress respiration
Thiamine (vitamin B₁) Given intramuscularly or intravenously before glucose loading	100 mg PO qid	Prevent Wernicke's encephalopathy
Magnesium sulfate (especially if history of seizures)	1 g IM every 6 hours for 2 days	Increases effectiveness of vitamin B₁ Helps reduce status postwithdrawal seizures
Anticonvulsant Phenobarbital		For seizure control
Benzodiazepines		Most effective in short time
Phenytoin (Dilantin)		Takes days to reach therapeutic level
Folic Acid	1 mg PO qid	Malabsorption due to heavy long term alcohol abuse causes deficiencies in many vitamins
Multivitamins	1 daily	

Data from Smith-DiJulio 1987; Frances and Franklin 1988; Dubin and Weiss 1991.

tachycardia, respiratory distress, a potentially serious drop in blood pressure, and nausea and vomiting. The adverse reaction usually begins within minutes to half an hour after drinking and may last 30–120 minutes. These events are usually followed by drowsiness and are gone after the patient has slept. In severe disulfiram reactions, diphenhydramine hydrochloride (Benadryl), 50 mg intramuscularly or intravenously, may help. Hypotension, shock, or arrhythmias are treated symptomatically (Schatzberg and Cole 1991). Consequently, disulfiram should not be prescribed for individuals with a history of serious heart disease, stroke, serious hypertension, or diabetes.

Disulfiram must be taken daily. The action of the drug can last from five days up to two weeks after the last dose (Zuska and Pursch 1988). It is most effectively used early in the recovery process while the individual is making the major life changes associated with long term recovery from alcoholism. Disulfiram should always be prescribed with the full knowledge and consent of the client. The client needs to be told about the side effects and be well aware that any substances that contain alcohol can trigger an adverse reaction. There are three primary sources of "hidden" alcohol—food, medicines, and preparations that are applied to the skin. Foods include:

- All sauces (if made with wine)
- Soups (if made with wine)
- Apple cider
- Anything made with wine vinegar, e.g., pickles, salad dressing
- Flavor extracts (vanilla) used in cooking

Medications include:

- Any elixir (cold medicines, cough medicines)
- Mouthwashes/gargles
- Vitamins/mineral tonics

Skin preparations include:

- Alcohol rubs
- Aftershave lotions/colognes
- Some transdermal patches

People also need to be careful to avoid inhaling fumes from substances that might contain alcohol, such as paints, wood stains, and "stripping" compounds (Guidelines for Antabuse Users 1988). Naltrexone (Trexan, Revia), an opioid antagonist, is now approved for the treatment of alcoholism. Unlike disulfiram, naltrexone decreases the pleasant, reinforcing effects of alcohol without making the user ill. (See page 692 and drug card in glossary.) Unfortunately, voluntary compliance with the disulfiram regimen has often been poor.

THERAPEUTIC ENVIRONMENT

It was formerly thought that you could not help alcoholics until they were ready for help. This is only partially true. It is true that most alcoholics do not present themselves readily for treatment. The motivation of an alcoholic, like that of anyone else who is facing changes in lifestyle, is mixed. Whatever motivation is there can be encouraged. It is part of the nurse's job to help clients become receptive to the possibility of change. *Johnson's intervention*, described earlier in Box 23–3, is useful in this regard.

At all levels of practice, the nurse can play an important role in the intervention process by recognizing the signs of alcohol problems in both client and family and knowing available resources to help with the problem. Table 23–5 identifies important interventions for nurses working with people recovering from alcohol.

The nurse's ability to develop a warm, accepting relationship with the alcoholic can assist the client in feeling safe enough to start looking at problems with some degree of openness and honesty. If the nurse lacks acceptance and empathy, knowledge and skill will not be useful. If the nurse has not worked through strong negative feelings related to alcohol or alcoholism, the nurse should refer the client to another nurse or alcoholism counselor who has dealt with these issues and can begin promoting recovery. The client-counselor relationship is often considered to be more important than the type of treatment pursued (Sanchez-Craig et al. 1991).

Alcoholics often seem indifferent to the destruction they bring on themselves and their families. They also show marked dependency, and they may lean on others, most often loved ones, to solve their problems. This characteristic can give the family and friends an effective means of motivating the alcoholic toward treatment. When family and friends refuse to solve the alcoholic's problems, the alcoholic will be forced to face the consequences of his or her own drinking behavior. Al-Anon teaches family members the three Cs concept. Family members did not *cause* the disease, they cannot *control* it, nor can they *cure* it. They learn that they are not responsible for the disease or for the person affected by it.

A sex difference in willingness to acknowledge alcoholism as a problem has been observed. There are many more barriers for women than for men in acknowledging the need for help with an alcohol problem. Sometimes it is more difficult for women to identify themselves as having alcoholism. This may be due in part to the social stigma against alcoholic behavior in women. Also, many women begin drinking heavily along with an alcoholic partner or spouse, yet

Table 23–5 ■ NURSING INTERVENTIONS AND RATIONALES: PSYCHOTHERAPEUTIC NEEDS OF PEOPLE AFFECTED BY ALCOHOLISM	
INTERVENTION	**RATIONALE**
1. Communicate empathy, focus on feelings. Avoid comments that seem judgmental.	1. Establish a therapeutic alliance based on understanding in an atmosphere of openness and support.
2. Evaluate extent of alcohol use (using a nursing history and standardized test), levels of anxiety, and coping styles as well as support systems.	2. Ascertain strengths and weaknesses, coping skills, available resources, and potential withdrawal reactions.
3. Continually assess • Presence of PDS predictable defensive style • Psychophysiological responses	3. Data collected in initial interview are not complete; assessment is ongoing.
4. Assess for relapse.	4. Alcoholism is a chronic condition; relapse should be addressed.
5. Assess the need for disulfiram (Antabuse).	5. May be an effective adjunct early in treatment.
6. Refer to local resources—always include AA.	6. Behavior change is long term; support, encouragement, and suggestions are needed throughout.
7. Refer to other community agencies as needed.	7. Assistance may be needed in other areas of life functioning (e.g., vocational rehabilitation, socialization, treatment of associated psychiatric disorders).

they do not see their behavior as enough of a problem to warrant seeking help. Those who attempt to get help may find themselves thwarted by actively drinking spouses. Practical problems, such as child care, may also be a barrier to seeking treatment. Given these issues, dealing with alcohol problems in women may be best accomplished at the primary care level (Gearhart et al. 1991).

In terms of treatment goals, it is safest to propose abstinence as a treatment goal for all alcoholics. Abstinence is strongly related to good work adjustments, positive health status, comfortable interpersonal relationships, and general social stability. Treatment must also address the client's major psychological and social problems as well as the drinking behavior. Involvement of appropriate family members is now considered essential by most treatment provides. As previously mentioned Al-Anon and Al-a-Teen are useful support groups for families.

A significant relationship has been noted between a client's feelings of "belongingness" and treatment outcome (Machell 1987). The more a client feels socially involved with peers, the better the chance for successful treatment outcome, continuation of treatment, and lower relapse rates. Nurses should evaluate the feelings of belongingness periodically by questioning clients about how they perceive themselves within their peer group. A client may be immersed in social events but perceive himself or herself as isolated. Clients with an isolated perception stand a

much greater chance of shorter lengths of stay in treatment programs and a higher rate of relapse.

Children of alcoholics deserve special consideration. One of every eight Americans comes from an alcoholic home, and 7 million of these are youngsters facing the daily fear, uncertainty, and problems that result from their parent's alcoholism. School nurses and nurses in pediatric and family practice clinics should assess for alcoholism in the family whenever a child presents for behavioral, mental, or repeated physical complaints that seem to have no basis in fact. A willingness to talk about alcoholism, to respond in a nonjudgmental fashion, and to be a supportive listener allows children relief in knowing that they are not alone and that there is help available. Nurses need to take advantage of their key positions by identifying and providing assistance to children and youth suffering negative consequences of family drinking problems.

PSYCHOTHERAPY

Nurses with advanced training may be involved in psychotherapy with alcoholic clients. Psychotherapy assists clients in identifying and using alternative coping mechanisms to reduce reliance on alcohol. Eventually, psychotherapy can assist recovering alcoholics in becoming comfortable with sobriety.

Psychotherapy with alcoholics takes many forms. It can be individual, group, or family therapy; directive or nondirective therapy; goal-centered or insight-oriented therapy. Whatever type is used, clients need to be informed of what they can expect and cannot expect from the therapy and, likewise, what is expected from them. *No psychotherapy should take place while the client is actively drinking.*

Nurses as therapists may be asked about their own drinking habits. It is best to deal with this issue by exploring the client's underlying concerns about whether the alcoholic client thinks the nurse can understand and help him or her.

Confidentiality must be maintained throughout therapy except when this conflicts with events requiring mandatory reporting (e.g., child abuse).

A number of issues that require addressing occur frequently during the first six months of sobriety. These include the following:

1. Physical changes take place as the body adapts to functioning without alcohol.
2. Numerous signals occur in the client's internal and external world that previously have been cues to drink. Different responses to these cues need to be learned.
3. Emotional responses (feelings that were formerly diluted with alcohol) are now experienced full-strength. Because they are so unfamiliar, they can be anxiety-producing.
4. Responses of family and coworkers to the client's new behavior must be addressed. Sobriety disrupts a system, and everyone in that system needs to adjust to the change.
5. New coping skills must be developed to prevent relapse and to ensure prolonged sobriety. AA makes use of the acronym HALT: "Don't get too Hungry, Angry, Lonely, or Tired." When alcoholics experience these feelings, they are to HALT and implement alternative coping strategies.

Counseling during this early stage of treatment needs to be directive, open and honest, and friendly and caring. Slogans from AA can be helpful in providing initial as well as ongoing motivation for adjusting to life without alcohol. Some examples are "One day at a time," "Easy does it," and "Utilize, don't analyze." These phrases can provide a focus for clients new to recovery. The therapeutic process involves teaching the client to identify the physical and emotional changes that are occurring in the here-and-now. The nurse therapist can then assist in the problem-solving process.

Recovery programs successful in producing abstinence, such as AA, partially owe their success to the intuitive recognition of the fact that in the early stages of recovery the alcoholic protects self-esteem by attempting to minimize the anxiety associated with change and growth. Often the best time for a recovering alcoholic to engage in insight psychotherapy is after two to five years of sobriety—once defenses have been loosened.

Alcoholism therapy must be viewed as a time-dependent process. A particular therapeutic intervention for a recently drinking alcoholic may be entirely inappropriate for one who has managed to achieve several years of sobriety, or vice versa. Besides individual therapy, other specific psychotherapeutic techniques used with alcoholics include behavior therapy and group, family, and marital therapy.

BEHAVIORAL THERAPY. Behavioral therapy is a highly individualized form of treatment. The alcoholic's behavior is carefully assessed before specific intervention strategies are begun. **Aversive conditioning** was the first behavioral technique applied to treatment of alcoholism. In this mode, an aversive event (e.g., emetine-induced nausea and vomiting) is paired with the sight, smell, and taste of alcohol. This aversion needs to be reinforced periodically or it will disappear over time.

A variety of different behavioral techniques are employed for situations the client may face during recovery. Included are skills training (for situations requiring refusal of drinks), assertiveness training, relaxation training, and relapse prevention training, which focuses on interrupting signals to drink (Marlatt 1985). The last approach realistically recognizes that alcoholism is a chronic condition marked by relapses. The possibility of relapse should be discussed, therefore, and options for preventing escalation into a serious drinking episode should be explored. The goal is to help the person learn from those situations so that periods of sobriety can be lengthened over time and so that relapse is not viewed as total failure.

ALCOHOLICS ANONYMOUS. Alcoholics Anonymous (AA) is a self-help group of recovering alcoholics that provides support and encouragement to those involved in continuing recovery. The regular meetings provide role models for recovery as well as guidance from others who have experienced many of the same problems and temptations that the client is facing. AA may also provide a new social group to replace one's old drinking companions. One-to-one-sponsorship allows a person to receive assistance from another AA member on a 24-hour basis as required. The 12-step program (Box 23–4) allows the alcoholic person to "let go" and to take the risks associated with growth and change. There are a variety of groups available in most communities so that a person, by "shopping around," can usually find a compatible group. Meetings may be open to anyone (e.g., friends, or spouses of alcoholics) or closed (restricted to individuals with drinking problems).

Box 23-4. THE TWELVE STEPS OF ALCOHOLICS ANONYMOUS

1. *We admitted we were powerless over alcohol—that our lives had become unmanageable.*
2. *Came to believe that a power greater than ourselves could restore us to sanity.*
3. *Made a decision to turn our will and our lives over to the care of God* **as we understood Him.**
4. *Made a searching and fearless moral inventory of ourselves.*
5. *Admitted to God, to ourselves, and to another human being the exact nature of our wrongs.*
6. *Were entirely ready to have God remove all these defects of character.*
7. *Humbly asked Him to remove our shortcomings.*
8. *Made a list of all persons we had harmed, and became willing to make amends to them all.*
9. *Made direct amends to such people whenever possible, except when to do so would injure them or others.*
10. *Continued to take personal inventory, and when we were wrong, we promptly admitted it.*
11. *Sought through prayer and meditation to improve our conscious contact with God* **as we understood Him,** *praying only for knowledge of His will and the power to carry that out.*
12. *Having had a spiritual awakening as the result of these steps, we tried to carry His message to alcoholics, and to practice these principles in all our affairs.*

Self-help groups formed to help family members of alcoholics deal with many common issues are independent of AA but share many elements of a common belief system structured by the use of AA's 12 steps as their philosophical and operational guide (Ablon 1986).

Al-Anon is a support group for spouses and friends of alcoholics. Al-Anon, like AA, Al-a-Teen, and ACoA (discussed later), works through a combination of educational and operational principles. For example, alcoholism is a disease of the body and the mind, not a moral or perverse whim of the alcoholic (Ablon 1986). This acceptance of the disease concept of alcoholism can remove burdens of guilt, hostility, and shame from family members. Al-Anon also offers pragmatic methods for avoiding "enabling."

Al-a-Teen is a nationwide network for children over 10 years old who have alcoholic parents. It is structured under the guidance of members of Al-Anon. It offers the teenager the chance to exchange feelings and problems with other teenagers going through similar experiences, which can be tremendously therapeutic.

Groups of **Adult Children of Alcoholics (ACoA)** offer support for those who often experience similar difficulties and problems in their adult life as a result of having an alcoholic parent or parents. Adult children of alcoholics were often deprived of a nurturing parent in their formative years.

Self-help groups, like AA and the others described, offer camaraderie and a chance to talk about feelings in a society where that is frowned on (Haaken 1990).

Arising out of the plethora of these groups is the concept of the **codependent** or **enabler.** Not buttressed by any research data, this concept describes a person who is called addicted or sick and is said to benefit from "treatment."

CODEPENDENCY AS A PHENOMENON. Living with an alcoholic is certainly a source of stress and requires family system adjustments. Certain behaviors usually arise when a person attempts to cope with stressful situations. Often these behaviors are those designed to "control" the situation in an attempt to thereby eliminate the source of stress. Whether these behaviors in the case of alcoholism are any different from those present in response to other chronic conditions has yet to be demonstrated (Gomberg 1989). In fact, the behaviors attributed to the codependent (Box 23–5) have come to encompass virtually the entire population of the United States (Gomberg 1989) and are negating skills at which women excel, namely, relationship building and maintenance.

The contemporary codependence literature and the recovery groups that draw on it characterize relationship dilemmas as pathological and vastly oversimplify problems of human dependency and interdependency (Haaken 1990). This has particular appeal now, with social roles in flux and women feeling especially burdened by the combination of traditional caretaking responsibilities and roles introduced by their entry into the work force. New forms of healthy interdependence between people have not been sufficiently realized as the old social contracts have been unraveling. To characterize these symptoms of individual and so-

---

Box 23–5. OVERRESPONSIBLE (CODEPENDENT) BEHAVIORS

Codependent individuals find themselves

1. Attempting to control someone else's drinking
2. Spending inordinate time thinking about the alcoholic person
3. Finding excuses for the person's alcohol abuse
4. Covering up the person's drinking or lying
5. Feeling responsible for the person's alcohol use
6. Feeling guilty for the alcoholic's behavior
7. Avoiding family and social events because of concerns or shame about the alcoholic's behavior
8. Making threats regarding the consequences of the alcoholic's behavior and failing to follow through
9. Eliciting promises for change
10. Feeling like they are "walking on eggshells" on a routine basis to avoid causing problems, especially alcohol use
11. Allowing moods to be influenced by those of the alcoholic
12. Searching for, hiding, and destroying the drinker's alcohol
13. Assuming the alcoholic's duties and responsibilities
14. Feeling forced to increase control over the family's finances
15. Often bailing the alcoholic out of financial or legal problems

---

From Wright DG, Wright B. Dare to Confront. New York: Master Media Ltd, 1990.

---

cial transition as pathological is not helpful to anyone, especially that minority group that already serves as the lightning rod for all sorts of psychological pathology, women. Recent studies seen to support the view that the overresponsible behavior of alcoholic spouses reflect their stressful circumstances more than their disturbed personalities (Montgomery and Johnson 1992). Table 23–6 offers some guidelines for a person in a codependent relationship.

Codependence is overresponsible behavior—doing for others what they could just as well do for themselves. Talking in terms of extremes of over- or underresponsibility points to a need for behavioral change rather than the need for recovery from a "disease" (Krestan and Bepko 1990).

GROUP THERAPY. Group therapy has been helpful for many people recovering from alcoholism. The *advantages of group therapy are*

- Social isolation is decreased.
- Newly recovering alcoholics have models in those with longer histories of sobriety.
- Alcoholics are encouraged to seek support and encouragement from a variety of people.
- The therapist can observe the interpersonal behavior of the clients, without always being directly involved.

Groups can be closed or open, homogeneous or mixed, education- or therapy-oriented. Clients should be screened for admission to the group, and the therapist should maintain good record keeping throughout. *Ground rules* that include commitments to the following points must be developed (Vanicelli 1986):

- Minimal stay in the group
- Expectations of regular attendance or advance notice of absences
- Advance notice to the group if one is considering leaving
- Abstinence and willingness to talk about fears of drinking or actual slips should they occur
- Talk about other difficult issues in the client's life
- Talk about group dynamics
- Confidentiality

Goals for therapy include

- Sobriety
- Motivation to continue to grow and change
- Recognizing and identifying behavior patterns that led to drinking
- Learning new ways to handle old problems
- Developing an emergency plan for high-risk situations that might lead to relapse
- Recognizing and identifying feelings (especially guilt, anger, depression, fear)
- Learning to enjoy life without alcohol

FAMILY THERAPY. Family therapy in alcoholism recognizes that the disease is a "family illness": that is, all members are affected. Alcoholic family members lack trust in each other, lack nurturing closeness, and solve problems in a piecemeal fashion. Children of alcoholics become used to extra and inappropriate responsibilities. Parental role models are distorted. In fact, family equilibrium is established around the alcoholism. Therefore, removal of the drinking behavior becomes a threat!

As with any form of therapy, abstinence from alcohol must be a goal. The family has to begin to learn healthy ways to solve problems. Children of alcoholics are at high risk for developing their own alcoholism. This should be discussed openly at family therapy

Table 23–6 ■ NURSING INTERVENTIONS AND RATIONALES: STRATEGIES FOR CODEPENDENT RELATIONSHIPS

INTERVENTION	RATIONALE
I will not allow myself to	
1. **Argue** when my partner has been drinking or is angry, upset, or strung out because	1a. When I argue, it causes me to become defensive and justify myself.
	1b. Arguments when we are upset accomplish nothing.
	1c. Arguments cause me to become sad or mad.
	1d. During arguments, we say things we regret.
2. **Be put down** and be abused verbally, because	2a. I am human and entitled to make mistakes.
	2b. Putdowns cause me to become defensive. I do not need to defend myself. I am a responsible, caring, and loving individual.
	2c. I *cannot* use putdowns. They do not give me any information about myself or about anything else. However, I *can* use support and guidance if this is a reciprocal process and my support and guidance are listened to.
	2d. Putdowns cause me to become sad, to become mad, and to lose control of myself, and I do not like myself when I lose control, even when my partner provokes it.
3. **Accept more** than my share of responsibility, because	3a. Eventually, I would become resentful and angry.
	3b. I would then feel used and abused.
	3c. It would increase the stress I am feeling.
	3d. I already have more responsibility than I can handle.
	3e. If I accept more than my share of responsibility, I would not have energy and time left for myself first and others second.
4. **Hold in** my emotions, because	4a. I could become physically sick.
	4b. I am entitled to express my feelings provided I do not put anybody else down.
	4c. If I hold in my feelings, they could build up to the point of a blow-up.
	4d. Expressing my feelings lets other people know that my feelings are important, because they are *my* feelings and I am important.
	4e. Feelings are to be shared with those I love and who love me. If people do not care about my feelings, maybe they do not care about me.
	4f. Sharing my feelings with those I love will give them a chance to share their feelings with me.
	4g. Sharing my feelings will help people I love learn to know me better and appreciate me for what I am—an important person.
5. **Let anybody keep me from doing the things I enjoy doing,** because	5a. I deserve some enjoyment out of life.
	5b. My family is part of my life. I enjoy being with them and I should be able to spend time with them without feeling guilty.
	5c. It makes me happy and content to do things I enjoy, including doing absolutely nothing! I am important even when I am doing nothing.

From L'Abate L, Norreson M. Treating codependency. In L'Abate L, Farrar J, Serrilella D (eds). Handbook of Differential Treatments for Addictions. Boston: Allyn & Bacon, 1992, p. 296. Copyright © 1992 by Allyn and Bacon. Reprinted by permission.

sessions. The basic purpose of intervention is to assist the family to motivate a change in their ineffective communication and response patterns. Instilling hope in the family's future is one of the nurse's greatest responsibilities.

When the alcoholic is in inpatient treatment, the family frequently has the opportunity to learn about the disease of alcoholism, family dynamics, communication, and recovery. Structured family therapy may begin at this time. Past behavior, anger, and alcohol use—and the family's role in these—are brought up and dealt with. Plans are made to change behavior as sobriety becomes a part of daily life. The carrying out of these plans must be rehearsed and practiced.

After inpatient treatment of the alcoholic, family members are usually concerned about the alcoholic's returning to drinking. They frequently "walk on eggshells," not thinking or talking about drinking or other problems, in an attempt to prevent a relapse from happening. Ongoing therapy helps them change roles as the need for control is lessened. Spouses frequently are reluctant to give up the position of power they had when the alcoholic drank. Responsibility needs to be renegotiated. Children's roles and changes in behaviors need to be examined as well.

MARITAL THERAPY. For the married couple, issues about time spent at home and about sex are prominent. The alcoholic may not have much libido as he or she begins to recover. Sex is not a paramount urge. Having felt deprived in many areas when the alcoholic was actively drinking, the spouse may want gratification of those unmet needs soon after the alcoholic stops drinking. Couples need further education in the recovery process as they deal with major changes in how they function. For example, the wife may not understand the anger of the newly sober husband. She may balk at his attendance at AA meetings or his kindness to people in AA. She may feel rejected and not needed. These issues predominate in the early months of recovery.

In a study of types of marital therapy with alcoholic couples, it was found that alcohol-focused spouse involvement, as well as behavioral marital therapy, helped alcoholics stay in treatment and that the couples maintained their marital satisfaction better after treatment (McCrady et al. 1986).

Evaluation

Treatment outcome is judged by maintenance of abstinence, decreasing symptomatic denial, acceptable occupational functioning, improving family relationships, and, ultimately, the client's ability to relate normally and comfortably with other human beings.

The ability to use existing supports and skills learned in treatment bodes well for ongoing recovery. For example, recovery is launched if, in response to cues to drink, the client calls his or her sponsor or other recovering alcoholics; increases attendance at AA, aftercare, or other group meetings; or writes feelings in a log and considers alternative action.

In general, the nature and determinants of the alcoholic person's post-treatment functioning are unexplored. In a study of treated alcoholics and their families, it was found that such extra-treatment factors as environmental stressors, coping responses, and social resources had as much influence on the recovery process as did the client's treatment experiences and initial symptoms (Billings and Moos 1983; Estes and Heinemann 1986).

Vaillant and coworkers (1983) concur, stating that alcoholic persons recover not so much because we treat them as because they treat themselves. These authors list *four factors closely associated with remission from alcoholism*:

1. Finding a substitute dependency, such as a compulsive hobby, to replace alcohol
2. Experiencing a consistent aversive event related to drinking, such as use of disulfiram or an obvious adverse health effect
3. Discovering a fresh source of hope and self-esteem
4. Obtaining new social supports, such as new friends or a new job

Awareness and clinical assessment of extra-treatment factors make the evaluation process more meaningful in that the nurse can more adequately understand post-treatment functioning and the process of recovery and relapse. Continuous monitoring and evaluation lead to a better chance for prolonged recovery.

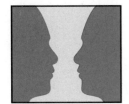

Case Study: Working with a Person Who Has Alcoholism

Mr. Young, aged 49, and his wife arrived in the emergency department one evening, fearful that Mr. Young had had a stroke. His right hand was limp, and he was unable to hyperextend his right wrist. Sensation to fingertips in his right hand was impaired.

Mr. Young looked much *older than his stated age*. He looked to be about 65! His *complexion* was *ruddy* and *flushed*. History taking *was difficult*. Mr. Young answered only what was asked of him, volunteering no additional information. He stated that he had taken a nap that afternoon and that, when he awakened, his right arm was as described.

Mr. Young revealed that he had been unemployed for four years because the company he had worked for had gone bankrupt. He had been unable to find a new job but had an appointment for an interview in 10 days. His wife was now working full time, so the family finances were OK. They had two grown children who no longer lived at home.

Continued on following page

Case Study: Working with a Person Who Has Alcoholism *(Continued)*

He denied any significant medical illness except for *high blood pressure*, just diagnosed last year. His *family history* was negative for illness, with the exception of *alcoholism*. His mother was a recovering alcoholic who had been treated at an inpatient facility and was maintaining her sobriety. Ms. Dee, the admitting nurse, asked Mr. Young questions about his use of alcohol, including quantity, frequency, and withdrawal experiences. In general, he *denied* any significant alcohol involvement. Ms. Dee shared with him the fact that the disease of alcoholism runs in families. Ms. Dee asked Mr. Young whether (1) he knew that and (2) if it concerned him with regard to his own drinking. Mr. Young said he knew and that he did not want to think about it.

Ms. Dee then spoke with Mrs. Young about the events of the day. Ms. Dee stated that she spoke with Mr. Young and that she was concerned that he might have an alcohol problem. Ms. Dee shared the impressions that had led her to that tentative conclusion and asked Mrs. Young to describe her husband's involvement with alcohol. Mrs. Young's shoulders slumped; she sighed and said, "I have spent the entire day talking to a counselor at the local treatment center to see if I can get him in. He won't admit that he has a problem." Mrs. Young then recounted a six-year history of steadily increasing alcohol use. She said that for a while she could not admit to herself that her husband was an excessive drinker. "He tried to hide it, but gradually I knew. I could tell from little changes that he was intoxicated. I couldn't believe it was happening because he had been through the same thing with his mother. And we'd always had such a good relationship. I thought I knew him. Actually, I guess I did, as a working man. Being unemployed and unable to find a job has really floored him. And now he's even going to job interviews intoxicated!"

Mrs. Young recounted how her husband's drinking worsened dramatically with unemployment and how she tried ridding their home of liquor, only to find bottles hidden in their mobile home one day when she went to clean it. She described her feelings, which were like an emotional roller coaster—elated, hopeful when he seemed to be doing OK; dejected and desperate on other occasions, such as the time that she found the alcohol in their mobile home. Mrs. Young hated going to work for fear of what he would do while she was gone. She stated that she was terrified that one day her husband would crack up the car and kill himself, because he often drives when he is intoxicated. Ms. Dee discussed with Mrs. Young her own involvement as part of the family system. Options for Mrs. Young and her husband were discussed.

Meanwhile, the physician in the emergency department had examined Mr. Young. The diagnosis was radial nerve palsy. Mr. Young had most likely passed out and lay on his arm. Because Mr. Young was intoxicated, he had not felt the signals that his nerves sent out to warn him to move (i.e., numbness, tingling). Mr. Young had continued to lie in this position for so long that the resultant cutting off of circulation was sufficient to cause some temporary nerve damage.

Mr. Young's BAL was 0.311 mg%. This is three times the legal limit of intoxication (0.1 mg%). Even though he had a BAL of 0.311, Mr. Young was alert and oriented and not slurring his speech or giving any other outward signs of intoxication. The difference between Mr. Young's BAL and behavior indicated the development of tolerance, a symptom of physical dependence (see Table 23–1).

| **Assessment** | Ms. Dee organized her data into objective and subjective components. |

OBJECTIVE DATA

1. Drives when intoxicated
2. Nerve damage due to passing out while lying on arm
3. Alcohol use has increased during stress of unemployment
4. Alcohol use has impaired his capacity to obtain employment
5. Alcohol use is causing disruption in marital relationship
6. Client unable to see effect of his drinking
7. Family history of alcoholism
8. BAL three times legal limit of intoxication; has developed tolerance

SUBJECTIVE DATA

1. Denies he has an alcohol problem

Nursing Diagnosis

From the data, the nurse formulates the following nursing diagnosis:

Ineffective individual coping related to alcohol use
- Alcohol use has increased during stressful period of unemployment
- Alcohol use has impaired client's capacity to obtain employment
- Alcohol use is causing disruption in marital relationship
- Client unable to see effect of his drinking on his life functioning

Planning

CONTENT LEVEL—PLANNING GOALS

It was decided to allow Mr. Young to sober up in the emergency department because it is difficult to discuss goals when the client is intoxicated. When the client is sober, the nurse establishes goals with the client that are realistic, appropriate, and measurable.

Nursing Diagnosis	Long Term Goals	Short Term Goals
1. *Ineffective individual coping* related to alcohol use	1. Client will abstain from alcohol.	1a. Client will identify the role of alcohol in his life and his risk for alcoholism, given his family history. 1b. Client will agree to remain sober from now to job interview 10 days hence. To assist in this effort, he agrees to • Obtain an appointment at a community alcohol center • Attend at least one AA meeting/day • Call the emergency department nurse to report on the job interview and referral appointments 1c. Client will state two alternative behaviors to engage in when experiencing the urge to drink. 1d. Client will name two ways to begin to rebuild trust in his relationship with his wife.

Continued on following page

Planning *(Continued)*	**PROCESS LEVEL—NURSES' REACTIONS AND FEELINGS** The denial the alcoholic exhibits often results in rejection by nurses, who feel that the alcoholic causes his own problems. Nurses generally feel sympathetic toward spouses and other family members but have a sense of helplessness about being able to effect change. Feelings of rejection, sympathy, and helplessness impair the nurse's ability to facilitate change. True, some alcoholic persons do maintain their denial and effectively resist intervention; but many others welcome the opportunity to begin to learn different ways of coping with life problems. Before dismissing alcoholics as "not wanting help" or being "the only ones that can change things," nurses need to ask themselves if they have done all that they can in an attempt to engage the client in the change process. Ms. Dee had seen many clients with the disease of alcoholism make radical changes in their lives, and she had learned to view alcoholism as a treatable disease. She was aware also that it was the client who made the changes, and she no longer felt responsible when a client was not ready to make that change.
Intervention	Ms. Dee suggested that Mrs. Young attend Al-Anon meetings and gave her information on where she could find groups in her area. She also urged Mrs. Young to discuss what is going on with her grown children and told her about the problems that adult children of alcoholics often experience. She encouraged Mrs. Young to let her children know of support groups they could go to if they felt the need. Ms. Dee also urged Mrs. Young *not* to drive in the car with her husband if he was driving while intoxicated. Ms. Dee stated that she should not protect him from the results of his drinking (e.g., bail him out of jail if he was arrested for driving while intoxicated or make excuses for him). Ms. Dee added that Al-Anon could offer crucial support for her and assist her in minimizing her enabling behaviors, which family members often exhibit. Ms. Dee outlined an initial care plan for Mr. Young (Nursing Care Plan 23–1). Attending AA was a central part of the treatment program, along with a variety of other interventions, like skills training, education, medical intervention, family counseling, and evaluation for disulfiram (Antabuse).
Evaluation	Mr. Young's willingness to become actively involved in planning short term goals is evidence that they were realistic and appropriate. In this case, the main opportunity for evaluating the short term goals is when and if Mr. Young calls back to report on steps he has taken to meet those goals. At that time, he should be supported and applauded for the progress he has made and encouraged to "keep up the good work." Other referrals may be given if indicated. Mr. Young did continue with AA. His denial persists, but he was highly motivated to keep his marriage. He gradually accepted a variety of referrals; as time progressed, he found that the positive feedback and support from others increased his self-esteem, decreased his feelings of isolation, and reinforced his long term goal of sobriety.

Nursing Care Plan 23–1 ■ A PERSON WITH ALCOHOLISM: Mr. Young

NURSING DIAGNOSIS

Ineffective individual coping related to alcohol use

Supporting Data

- Alcohol use increases in response to the stress of job loss, lowered role status
- Alcohol use has impaired client's capacity to obtain employment
- Alcohol use is causing disruptions in relationship with wife
- Family history of alcoholism

Long Term Goal: Client will abstain from alcohol.

Short Term Goal	Intervention	Rationale	Evaluation
1. Client will identify role of alcohol in his life and his risk for alcoholism, given his family history.	1a. Point out relationship between no job and increased alcohol use.	1a. Use assessment data to clarify behavior patterns.	Goal met Client listens to nurse—admitted that going to job interviews intoxicated would lower the chance of getting a job. Stated that he felt so down that he needed alcohol to feel OK.
	1b. Provide information on the disease of alcoholism.	1b. Stressing alcoholism as a disease can lower guilt and help increase self-esteem.	
	1c. Point out the factors placing person at risk for alcoholism.	1c. Children with alcoholic parents are at a greater risk for developing alcoholism themselves.	
	1d. Communicate concern, empathy, nonjudgmental acceptance, warmth.	1d. Helps establish a therapeutic relationship based on understanding and provides an atmosphere of openness and support. Helps client maintain self-esteem.	
2. Client will remain sober from now until job interview (10 days).	2a. Refer to AA. 2b. Refer to local resources for an appointment with alcohol counselor. 2c. List other available supports (e.g., friends, family).	2a–c. Much support and encouragement are needed for making major life changes, such as stopping drinking. A variety of support systems help decrease feelings of alienation and isolation.	Goal met Client calls the emergency department to report on carrying out the plan; states that potential employer wants him back for second interview.
3. Client will state two alternative behaviors that he can exercise when experiencing the urge to drink by (date).	3a. Evaluate client's situation by using a crisis intervention model—that is, assessing precipitating events, support systems, and coping skills.	3a. Identifies high-risk situations and opportunities for change.	Goal met After three weeks, client stated that he attended AA every day. He was learning to identify situations that trigger the urge to drink and was learning new coping behaviors. After five weeks, client had a slip and drank for two days; he decided to try Antabuse.
	3b. Explore alternative coping skills. Skills training may be needed (e.g., assertion, socialization, problem solving).	3b. Behavior change is a learning process. Relapse prevention can be practiced.	
	3c. Encourage participation in AA, group therapy, or other appropriate modalities.	3c. Provide support and minimize feelings of isolation while learning new skills.	

	3d. Referral to a physician for:
	  complete physical examination;
	  possible disulfiram (Antabuse) therapy.
		3d. Antabuse may help provide the external control needed during early months of sobriety; because it can cause physiological crises when taken with alcohol, a physical examination is needed.	

4. Client will name two ways to begin to rebuild trust in his relationship with his wife by (date).	4. Referral to a marital counselor.	4. Alcoholism is a "family illness" adversely affecting those close to the alcoholic.	Goal met Wife has been attending Al-Anon for six weeks, three times per week, after finding a group that she felt comfortable with. Client and wife decided to start couples therapy in two weeks.

Summary

Alcohol use occurs on a continuum, and the development of addiction and dependence is a time-related phenomenon. Various etiological theories attempt to explain why some drinkers develop alcoholism and others do not. Because there is no clear consensus about the nature of alcoholism, notions about treatment are also inconsistent. The more closely clinics are matched to a range of treatment alternatives, the greater the likelihood that sobriety will be achieved and overall life functioning improved.

Nurses encounter alcoholic people in all areas of practice and thus must be prepared for assessing, planning, implementing, and evaluating nursing care of alcoholics. Assessment strategies are outlined in this chapter for determining the severity of the illness, levels of anxiety, and coping styles as well as physiological and psychosocial changes. Some of the nursing diagnoses applicable to alcoholic clients are outlined. Planning nursing care on both process and content levels is discussed. Principles and specific examples of psychotherapeutic intervention are listed. Specific approaches include behavior therapy; individual, group, family, and marital therapy; and Alcoholics Anonymous (AA). Whatever techniques are employed, the nurse must make clear to the client what expectations are reasonable. Issues common in early sobriety are discussed, as are some general approaches to relapse prevention. Factors to be considered in evaluation are described. A case study demonstrates the steps of the nursing process as applied to an alcoholic client.

References

Ablon J. Perspectives on Al-Anon family groups. *In* Estes NJ, Heinemann ME (eds). Alcoholism: Development, Consequences and Interventions. St. Louis: CV Mosby, 1986.

American Psychiatric Association. Diagnostic and Statistical Manual of Mental Disorders, 3rd ed, revised. Washington, DC: American Psychiatric Association, 1987.

American Psychiatric Association. DSM-IV Options Book: Work in Progress. Washington, DC: American Psychiatric Association, 1991.

American Psychiatric Association. Diagnostic and Statistical Manual of Mental Disorders, 4th ed (DSM-IV). Washington, DC: American Psychiatric Association, 1994.

Billings AG, Moos RH. Psychosocial processes of recovery among alcoholics and their families: Implications for clinicians and program evaluators. Addictive Behaviors, 8:205, 1983.

Bissell L. Diagnosis and recognition. *In* Gitlow SE, Peyser HS (eds). Alcoholism: A Practical Treatment Guide, 2nd ed. Philadelphia: Grune & Stratton, 1988.

Block MA. Motivating the alcoholic patient. *In* Gitlow SE, Peyser HS (eds). Alcoholism: A Practical Treatment Guide, 2nd ed. Philadelphia: Grune & Stratton, 1988.

Butz RH. Intoxication and withdrawal. *In* Estes NJ, Heinemann ME (eds). Alcoholism, 2nd ed. St. Louis: CV Mosby, 1982.

Dubin WR, Weiss KJ. Handbook of Psychiatric Emergencies. Springhouse, PA: Springhouse Corporation, 1991.

Estes NJ, Heinemann ME. Alcoholism: Development, Consequences and Interventions. St. Louis: CV Mosby, 1986.

Francis RJ, Franklin JE. Alcohol and other psychoactive substance use disorders. *In* Talbott JA, Hales RE, Yudofsky SC (eds). Textbook of Psychiatry. Washington, DC: American Psychiatric Association, 1988.

Gearhart JG, et al. Alcoholism in women. American Family Physician, 44(3):907, 1991.

Gitlow SE. An overview. *In* Gitlow SE, Peyser HS (eds). Alcoholism: A Practical Treatment Guide, 2nd ed. Philadelphia: Grune & Stratton, 1988.

Gomberg ESL. On terms used and abused: The concept of "codependency." Current Issues in Alcohol/Drug Studies, 3(3/4):113, 1989.

Goodwin DW, Schulsinger F, Hermansen L et al. Alcohol problems in adoptees raised apart from alcoholic biological parents. Archives of General Psychiatry, 28:228, 1973.

Goodwin DW, et al. Drinking problems in adopted and nonadopted sons of alcoholics. Archives of General Psychiatry, 31:164, 1974.

Guidelines for Antabuse Users. Philadelphia: Wyeth-Ayerst Laboratories, 1988.

Haaken J. A critical analysis of the co-dependence construct. Psychiatry, 53:396, 1990.

Harper FD (ed). Alcohol Abuse and Black America. Alexandria, VA: Douglass Publishers, 1976.

Johnson VE. Intervention: How to Help Someone Who Doesn't Want Help. Minneapolis: Johnson Books, 1986.

Kaplan HI, Sadock BJ. Synopsis of Psychiatry, 6th ed. Baltimore: Williams & Wilkins, 1991.

Knott DH. The addictive process. Lecture presented at the University of Utah Summer School on Alcoholism and Other Drug Dependencies, Salt Lake City, June 1987.

Krestan JA, Bepko C. Codependency: The social reconstruction of female experience. Smith College Studies in Social Work, 60(3):216, 1990.

Machell DF. Fellowship as an important factor in alcoholism residential treatment. Journal of Alcohol and Drug Education, 32(2):56, 1987.

Mandell W. Types and phases of alcohol dependence illness. *In* Galanter M (ed). Recent Developments in Alcoholism, vol 1. New York: Plenum Press, 1983, pp 415–447.

Marlatt GA. Relapse Prevention: Maintenance Strategies in the Treatment of Addictive Behaviors. New York: Guilford Press, 1985.

Mayfield D, McLeod G, Hall P. The CAGE questionnaire: Validation of a new alcoholism screening instrument. American Journal of Psychiatry, 131:1121, 1974.

McCrady BS, Noel NE, Abrams DB. Comparative effectiveness of three types of spouse involvement in outpatient behavioral alcoholism treatment. Journal of Studies on Alcohol, 47:459, 1986.

McKelvey MJ, Kane JS, Kellison K. Substance abuse and mental illness: Double trouble. Journal of Psychosocial Nursing, 25(1):20, 1987.

Montgomery P, Johnson B. The stress of marriage to an alcoholic. Journal of Psychosocial Nursing, 30(10):12, 1992.

Sanchez-Craig M, et al. Superior outcome of females over males after brief treatment for the reduction of heavy drinking: Replication and report of therapist effects. British Journal of Addiction, 86:867, 1991.

Schatzberg AF, Cole JO. Manual of Clinical Psychopharmacology, 2nd ed. Washington, DC: American Psychiatric Association, 1991.

Smith-DiJulio K. Nursing people experiencing dependence on alcohol and other drugs. *In* Luckmann J, Sorensen K (eds). Medical-Surgical Nursing. Philadelphia: WB Saunders, 1987, pp 1836–1866.

Vaillant GE, Clark W, Cyrus C, et al. Prospective study of alcoholism treatment: Eight-year follow up. American Journal of Medicine, 75:455, 1983.

Vanicelli M. Group psychotherapy with alcoholics: Special techniques. *In* Estes NJ, Heinemann ME (eds). Alcoholism: Development, Consequences and Interventions. St. Louis: CV Mosby, 1986, pp 374–387.

Walker DR, Donovan DM, Kivlahan DR, Roszell DK. Prediction of alcoholism treatment outcome: Multiple assessment domains. *In* Grant I (ed). Neuropsychiatric Correlates of Alcoholism. Washington, DC: American Psychiatric Press, 1986, pp 109–125.

Wallace J. Alcoholism from the inside out: A phenomenologic analysis. In Estes NJ, Heinemann ME (eds). Alcoholism: Development, Consequences and Interventions. St. Louis: CV Mosby, 1986, pp 3–14.

World Health Organization, Expert Committee on Mental Health. Report on the First Session of the Alcoholism Subcommittee. WHO Organizational and Technical Report Series no. 48, August 1952.

Wright DG, Wright B. Dare to Confront. New York: Master Media Ltd, 1990.

Zimberg S. Principles of alcoholism psychotherapy. In Zimberg S, Wallace J, Blume SB (eds). Practical Approaches to Alcoholism Psychotherapy. New York: Plenum Press, 1978.

Zuska JJ, Pursch JA. Long term management. In Gitlow SE, Peyser HS (eds). Alcoholism: A Practical Treatment Guide, 2nd ed. Philadelphia: Grune & Stratton, 1988.

Further Reading

Brubaker RG, Prue DM, Rychtarik RG. Determinants of disulfiram acceptance among alcohol patients: A test of the theory of reasoned action. Addictive Behaviors, 12:43, 1987.

Edwards G, Gross MM, Keller M. Alcohol related disabilities. Geneva: World Health Organization, 1977. WHO Offset Publication No. 32.

Estes NJ, Smith-DiJulio K, Heinemann ME. Nursing Diagnosis of the Alcoholic Person. St. Louis: CV Mosby, 1980.

Goldberg HI, et al. Alcohol counseling in a general medicine clinic. Medical Care, 29(7):549, 1991.

Hough EE. Alcoholism: Prevention and treatment. Journal of Psychosocial Nursing, 27(1):15, 1989.

Olenick NL, Chalmers DK. Gender-specific drinking styles in alcoholics and nonalcoholics. Journal of Studies on Alcohol, 22(4):325, 1991.

Ross HE. Alcohol and drug abuse in treated alcoholics: A comparison of men and women. Alcoholism: Clinical and Experimental Research, 13(6):810, 1989.

Schaef AW. Co-Dependence: Misunderstood—Mistreated. San Francisco: Harper & Row, 1986.

Self-study Exercises

Match the following.

1. ___F___ Stopping alcohol use results in specific signs and symptoms

2. ___J___ Based on data that alcoholism seems to run in families

3. ___K___ Theory of alcoholism based on observation that different groups have different attitudes and rituals toward alcohol

4. ___H___ A useful definition of alcoholism that associates addiction with resultant problem behaviors

5. ___A___ The number of drinks that would cause a BAL of 0.1 mg% (legally intoxicated)

6. ___D___ BAL level that affects the entire motor area of the brain, causing staggering, ataxia, and emotional lability.

A. 5–6 drinks

B. 10–12 drinks

C. 0.3 mg%

D. 0.2 mg%

E. Psychological theory

F. Withdrawal

G. Dependence

H. World Health Organization definition

I. DSM-III-R criteria

J. Biological theory

K. Sociocultural theory

Identify two possible nursing diagnoses for a person with alcohol problems and formulate two short term goals (STG) (measurable and realistic) for each diagnosis.

7. Nursing Diagnosis 1: _____

STG 1a: _____

STG 1b: _____

8. Nursing Diagnosis 2: _____

   STG 2a: _____

   STG 2b: _____

Multiple choice

9. In intervening with an intoxicated client, it is useful to first

   (A) Let him or her sober up first.

   B. Decide on goals immediately, while the client is still in a good mood.

   C. Gain compliance by sharing your drinking habits with client.

   D. Ask what other drugs client might be taking.

Short answer

10. Name four principles of psychotherapeutic interventions with an alcoholic client.

    A. _____

    B. _____

    C. _____

    D. _____

11. Name two issues a therapist needs to address when treating an alcoholic client.

    A. _____

    B. _____

12. Name and describe five therapeutic modalities used with alcoholic clients.

    A. _____

    B. _____

    C. _____

    D. _____

    E. _____

13. Name four treatment outcomes that indicate effective recovery from alcoholism.

    A. _____   B. _____

    C. _____   D. _____

Match the following for use in treatment of alcohol delirium.

14. __E____ Can prevent Wernicke's encephalopathy   A. Magnesium
15. __B____ Drug of choice for safe withdrawal from   sulfate
            alcohol
16. __A____ Recommended if client has had seizures in   B. Chlordiazepoxide
            the past and to speed the absorption of   hydrochloride
            thiamine
17. __F____ If a client is having seizures during with-   C. Haloperidol
            drawal, this drug is effective and fast-acting

                                                             D. Paraldehyde

                                                             E. Thiamine
                                                                (vitamin B₁)

                                                             F. Diazepam

                                                             G. Phenytoin

Match the following phenomena of an alcoholic with a predictable defensive style.

18. ___G___ Not acknowledging certain life difficulties
19. ___F___ Influenced by emotions—doing what feels good
20. ___E___ Gets others to do things for him, take care of him; instills guilt in others
21. ___C___ Structured, restricted choices
22. ___A___ "It takes one to know one"

A. Projection

B. Rationalization

C. All-or-none thinking

D. Obsessional focusing

E. Manipulation

F. Preference for nonanalytical thinking

G. Denial

23. You know your teaching has been effective when a client states, "I know that as long as I take disulfiram (Antabuse), I need to avoid . . ."

    A. All aged cheeses and meat extracts
    B. Bright sunlight and wear sunscreen
    C. Driving a car and heavy machinery
    D. Cough medicines, mouthwash, and after-shave lotions

24. What do the letters in the acronym HALT stand for?
    "Don't get too . . ."
    H _Hungry_   A _Angry_   L _Lonely_   T _Tired_

CHAPTER 24

People Who Depend On Substances Other Than Alcohol

Mary McAndrew

Psychotomimetics
INTRODUCTION
PCP (Phencyclidine)
    PCP Intoxication
LSD and LSD-like Drugs

Marijuana *(Cannabis sativa)*
CASE STUDY: WORKING WITH A
    PERSON IN PCP INTOXICATION
SUMMARY

KEY TERMS AND CONCEPTS ◆ ◆ ◆ ◆ ◆ ◆ ◆ ◆ ◆ ◆ ◆ ◆ ◆ ◆ ◆

The key terms and concepts listed here also appear in bold where they are defined or discussed in this chapter.

ANTAGONISTIC EFFECT
ANXIOLYTICS
CLONIDINE
EMPLOYEE ASSISTANCE PROGRAMS
FLASHBACKS
LAAM (L-ALPHA ACETYL METHADOL)
METHADONE (DOLOPHINE)
NALOXONE (NARCAN)
NALTREXONE (TREXAN)
PCP (PHENCYCLIDINE) INTOXICATION
POLYDRUG ABUSE

PSYCHOACTIVE SUBSTANCE USE
    DISORDERS
PSYCHOTOMIMETICS
SUBSTANCE ABUSE
SUBSTANCE DEPENDENCE
SYNERGISTIC EFFECT
SYNESTHESIA
THERAPEUTIC COMMUNITIES
TOLERANCE
TOXICOLOGICAL SCREENING
WITHDRAWAL SYMPTOMS

Overview

The history of drugs in the United States begins with European explorers in the fifteenth and sixteenth centuries. Tobacco, cocaine, caffeine, opium, and hallucinogens such as peyote were found in their travels to the New World and Asia and brought back home.

Columbus and other early explorers met Indians who carried rolls of dried leaves that they set on fire—and who then "drank the smoke" that emerged from the rolls. The Indians knew of the strange power of these leaves. They found that nicotine produced a unique combination of effects—both stimulation and tranquilization. People then, as today, found that after they had smoked for a period of time they had to go on smoking or chewing tobacco or taking it as snuff (tobacco ground to a powder and inhaled) for their craving to be satisfied.

Many drugs used by North and South American Indians produced lysergic acid diethylamide (LSD)–

like effects. The effects of these drugs were considered a mystical and religious phenomenon, an experience that would bring humans closer to the gods and nature.

Today, we are perhaps more than ever a drug-oriented society. We use a host of different drugs for various purposes: to restore health, to reduce pain, to reduce anxiety, to increase energy, to create a feeling of euphoria, to induce sleep, and to enhance alertness. Many substances are available to alter mood or state of consciousness. People continue to take drugs today for other than medical reasons. Drugs may make them feel acceptable. Drugs may relieve stress or tension or provide a temporary escape. Peer pressure is also a strong factor in the use of drugs by young people. In many parts of our society, the use of drugs has become a "rite of passage." Sometimes drug use is part of the thrill of taking a risk. From an early age we are "programmed" to accept drugs. The media tell us that drugs are part of the technology that can help make life a little better. They urge us to seek "better living through chemistry" (Resnick 1979).

DRUG ABUSE AND DRUG DEPENDENCE

There is a distinction between use and abuse of drugs. Almost everyone uses a psychoactive substance, even if it is a socially accepted substance, such as coffee or tobacco, but not everyone misuses or abuses drugs. According to the Food, Drug, and Cosmetic Act, *a drug is defined as a substance intended for use in the diagnosis, cure, mitigation, treatment, or prevention of disease.*

The DSM-III-R diagnostic category psychoactive substance use disorders referred to symptoms and maladaptive behavioral changes associated with drugs that affect the central nervous system (APA 1987). The DSM-IV calls this category substance-related disorders. Pathological use of a drug is classified as *substance abuse* and *substance dependence* (Fig. 24–1).

Essentially, substance abuse includes a maladaptive pattern of substance use leading to significant impairment or distress as manifested by

- Inability to fulfill major social, occupational, or school responsibilities
- Recurrent substance-related legal or interpersonal problems
- Recurrent substance use in situations that are physically hazardous (e.g., driving while intoxicated)

Substance dependence includes a maladaptive pattern of substance use leading to clinically significant impairment or distress manifested by

- Impaired control of drug use despite adverse consequences (as described above).
- Development of **tolerance** to the drug (tolerance is a need for higher and higher doses to achieve intoxication or the desired effect).
- **Withdrawal symptoms** occur as a result of continued use (withdrawal symptoms are the negative physiological and psychological reactions that occur when the drug is reduced or no longer taken). Withdrawal symptoms include various physical reactions, such as drowsiness, disorien-

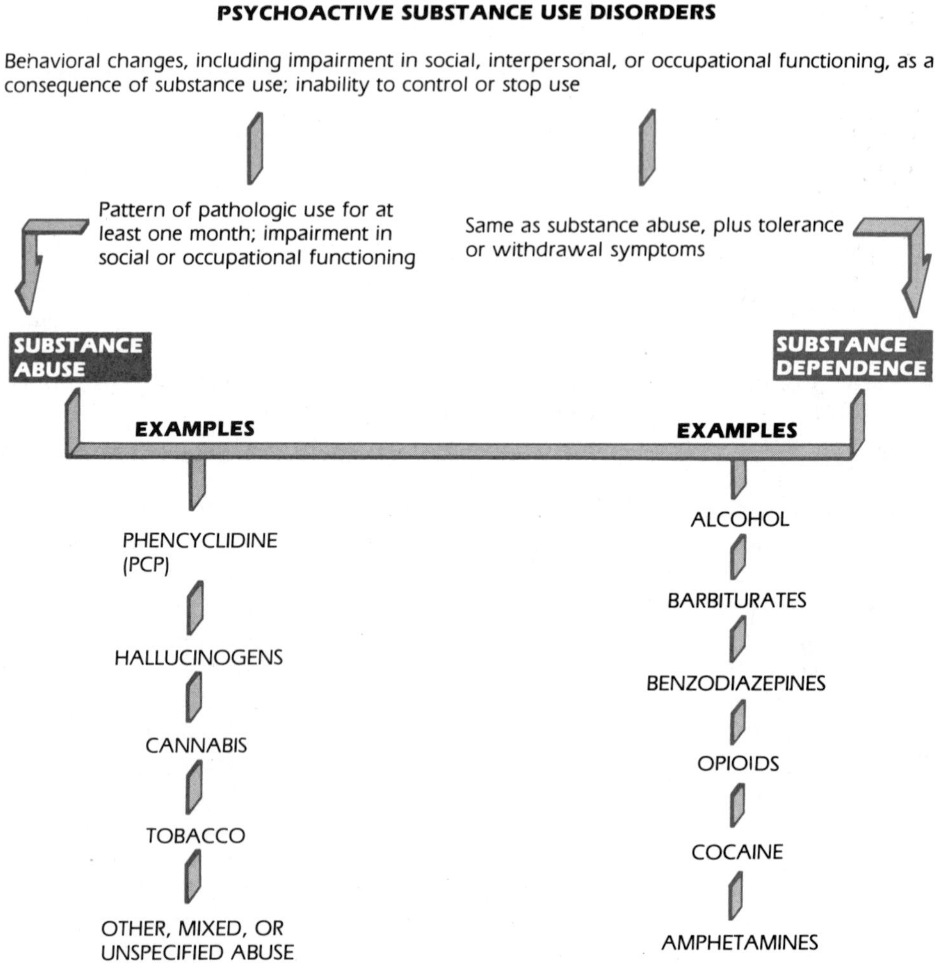

PSYCHOACTIVE SUBSTANCE USE DISORDERS

Behavioral changes, including impairment in social, interpersonal, or occupational functioning, as a consequence of substance use; inability to control or stop use

Pattern of pathologic use for at least one month; impairment in social or occupational functioning

Same as substance abuse, plus tolerance or withdrawal symptoms

SUBSTANCE ABUSE

SUBSTANCE DEPENDENCE

EXAMPLES

EXAMPLES

PHENCYCLIDINE (PCP)

HALLUCINOGENS

CANNABIS

TOBACCO

OTHER, MIXED, OR UNSPECIFIED ABUSE

ALCOHOL

BARBITURATES

BENZODIAZEPINES

OPIOIDS

COCAINE

AMPHETAMINES

Figure 24–1. *Psychoactive substance use disorders.*

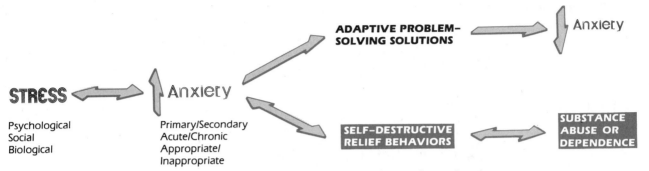

Figure 24–2. *Conceptualization of the process of substance abuse or dependence.*

tation, slurred speech, tremors, abnormal heart rhythms, anxiety, agitation, and insomnia. Refer to Tables 24–2 through 24–5 for more detailed information on signs and symptoms of intoxication and withdrawal.

Other characteristics of drug dependence include a compulsive need to spend more and more time (1) getting the drug in any manner possible (e.g., theft), (2) taking the drug, and (3) recuperating from its effects. Important social, occupational, and recreational activities are given up, leading to such consequences as poor work performance, suspensions or expulsions from school, and neglect of children. Figure 24–2 conceptualizes the process of drug abuse and dependence.

EFFECTS OF POLYDRUG ABUSE (POLYPHARMACY)

The taking of more than one drug at any given time is termed polypharmacy. The pathological use of more than one drug over a period of time is termed **poly-drug abuse.** This is seen in young, adult, and elderly clients. Polydrug abuse poses real hazards to both the individual taking the drugs and the health care worker involved in treating a person who is intoxicated or in withdrawal. Polydrug abuse can have (1) synergistic effects and (2) antagonistic effects.

SYNERGISTIC EFFECT. Some drugs when taken together intensify or prolong the effect of either or both of the drugs. For example, the combination of alcohol plus a benzodiazepine, alcohol plus an opiate, or alcohol plus a barbiturate will all produce a synergistic effect. All these drugs are central nervous system (CNS) depressants. Two of these drugs taken together will result in far greater CNS depression than just the simple sum of the effects of each drug added together. Many unintentional deaths have resulted from lethal combinations of drugs.

ANTAGONISTIC EFFECT. Many people may take a combination of drugs to weaken or inhibit the effect of another drug. For example, cocaine is often mixed with heroin (speedball). The heroin (CNS depressant) is meant to soften the intense letdown of cocaine (CNS stimulant) withdrawal. **Naloxone (Narcan),** an opiate antagonist, is often given to people who have overdosed from an opiate (usually heroin) to reverse respiratory and CNS depression.

DRUG HISTORY. When a person is brought to the emergency room intoxicated or in severe withdrawal, it is vital to know what drug (or drug) the person has taken—and, if possible, the amount, route, and time of each drug. Each drug or category of drugs has unique properties requiring unique measures in case of an overdose or toxic reaction. For example, a person with a history of alcohol and heroin use may be brought into the emergency room stuporous or in a coma. Once the coma is reversed by naloxone, the client may go into alcohol withdrawal tremens 48–72 hours later. It is important for medical teams to know what other drugs the client has ingested. Friends and family members can sometimes supply this information.

DRUG SCREENING. Drug screening can indicate the presence of different drugs in a person's system. After consent for a **toxicological screening** is obtained, 100 ml of urine and 20 ml of blood are taken, and the specimens are collected in the presence of a witness (Bittle et al. 1986). Drug screening should be used in emergency situations and can also be helpful in planning long term treatment.

NEUROLOGICAL EXAMINATION. It must be emphasized that whenever a person is brought into the emergency room in a coma, no matter what the drug history or presence of drugs on or in the body, *a neurological examination should always be completed.* Some people, while intoxicated, get into fights or fall. This could result in a subdural hematoma or other neurological complications. If such complications are not diagnosed early, death may ensue.

CHAPTER ORGANIZATION

This chapter is divided into five sections. The first section, *General Guidelines*, provides guidelines for assessment, diagnosis, planning, and treatment for peo- ple with substance abuse problems. The other four sections discuss antianxiety agents (sedative-hypnotics or anxiolytics), psychostimulants, narcotics, and psychotomimetics.

General Guidelines

OBJECTIVES ■

After studying this section on general guidelines, the student will be able to

1. Compare and contrast the terms "substance abuse" and "substance dependence," as defined by the *DSM-III-R* (APA 1987).
2. Describe tolerance and withdrawal, and give a clinical definition of each.
3. Discuss the synergistic and antagonistic effects of drugs among polydrug abusers and give an example of each.
4. Identify five theories that explain in part the phenomena of substance abuse.
5. Describe four components of the assessment process for working with a person who is chemically dependent.
6. Discuss health teaching on a primary and secondary level as it pertains to drug abuse.
7. Compare and contrast four methods for providing a therapeutic environment for a drug-dependent client, including the indications for each.
8. Identify three psychotherapeutic modalities found useful for substance abusers.
9. State four general goals that will potentiate the client's success at remaining drug-free.

Theory

Hundreds of studies have focused on possible causes of substance abuse. Physical, social, developmental, psychological, cultural, and genetic studies have all failed to identify a single cause or group of causes (Bittle et al. 1986). No matter what the cause, once a person becomes dependent on a chemical agent, the person will continue to take the drug no matter what the physical, social, interpersonal, occupational, or legal consequences. A person will forsake family, friends, and lover and deny his or her own inner potential and talent in favor of the drug. The drug becomes the only thing that matters. The drug is taken initially to induce euphoria, increase feelings of self-esteem, and minimize problems and hurts. As time goes on, the drug is taken to relieve withdrawal symptoms. Therefore, continued use is reinforced by the positive presence of pleasure, by the desire to minimize the effects of withdrawal, or both. As tolerance develops, more and more of the drug is needed to gain the desired effect. More of the person's time revolves around securing the drug, and many people do things they would not do ordinarily, to obtain the drug (e.g., prostitution, stealing, mugging, or even murder).

Because no one theory of drug abuse has been proven, several theories regarding a person's abuse of drugs follow (Cocaine withdrawal step by step 1987; Frances and Franklin 1988).

GENETIC PREDISPOSITION. This theory has gained interest in studies of alcoholics and their children. It is thought by some researchers that alcoholism is caused by a genetically transmitted biochemical defect (see Chapter 23).

NEUROTRANSMITTER DEFECTS. Neurotransmitters are chemicals in the brain that transmit impulses from one cell to another. Certain drugs interfere with the work of neurotransmitters. Most research in this area at present is focused on the drug cocaine. Some researchers think that cocaine dependence is primarily associated with a deficiency in the neurotransmitters dopamine and norepinephrine. It is hoped that by correcting this deficiency, an individual's craving for, and withdrawal symptoms from, cocaine can be reduced.

BIOCHEMICAL ASPECTS. The discovery of endogenous enkephalins and pituitary endorphins (the body's own opiate-like substances) have stimulated interest and information regarding biochemical mechanism underlying opiate actions and effects. The opiate receptors are found in the brain. Under normal conditions, a person's opiate receptors are exposed to certain levels of endorphins and enkephalins. When a person takes certain narcotics, these drugs block the body's opiate receptors, and the body ceases to produce its own natural opiate-like substances, endorphins and enkephalins. When the opiate-like effects of the ingested substance wear off or cease, the body's own endorphin levels remain low, leaving the person dysphoric and in withdrawal.

SOCIOLOGICAL FACTORS. Cultural or peer pressure, especially during adolescence, appears to contribute to drug abuse. Some reasons adolescents give for taking drugs follow:

- For acceptance
- To rebel
- From curiosity
- To relieve boredom

SOCIOECONOMIC CLASS. Being a "drug addict" can give a person a place in a subculture where he or she can be accepted. This is most true in economically deprived and highly stressed and unstable environments, where drugs are taken to numb pervasive feelings of helplessness and to provide a person with a sense of belonging and identity.

SELF-MEDICATION. The myths that "happiness" should be an enduring state, and that anxiety, depression, and loneliness are unnatural and should be avoided at all costs have contributed to the American "pill-popping" phenomenon. Over-the-counter medications are used by a large percentage of our population. Drug abuse, especially polydrug abuse, often is the result of an attempt to treat depression, solve problems, and escape intolerable situations.

Assessment

The assessment of the patient population is becoming more complex because of the increasing number of chemical substances that are used. An additional assessment challenge is the deteriorated physical condition of the increasing number of patients infected with the human immunodeficiency virus (HIV). There is a need to become more sophisticated in assessing patients who abuse drugs. Frequently during the assessment process, questions arise as to whether one is dealing with specific CNS disease—such as dementia, encephalopathy, or an acquired immunodeficiency syndrome (AIDS)–associated opportunistic infection that affects the brain—or a situational depression or the effects of substance abuse. At this point, it is necessary to consider the patient's history, especially if it is corroborated by the family.

Level of consciousness is most important in differentiating between substance abuse effects and HIV-related or other diseases. Even in its advanced state, HIV dementia syndrome, except in its immediate preterminal stage, is not associated with a decreased level of consciousness and orientation. Usually, decreased level of consciousness is the result of the toxic effects of substance abuse.

Selwyn (1990) reports that neurologically HIV-related dementia has been associated with apraxia, particularly, gait apraxia. Gait apraxia is a sort of clumsiness or difficulty negotiating space. Tremors, however, are evidenced by substance abusers.

The importance of a urine toxicology screening on admission and an assessment of current drug abuse cannot be overstressed as part of the evaluation of drug-using, HIV-infected patients or of any drug user who might have an underlying chronic disease, such as hepatitis, tuberculosis, or even a mental disorder. The nurse gathers data about substance abuse from assessing (1) *signs of intoxication or withdrawal*, (2) *level of physiological complications*, (3) *personal history and coping style*, and (4) *drug history*.

ASSESSING SIGNS OF INTOXICATION

Each drug has its own physiological signs and symptoms of intoxication and individual pattern of withdrawal symptoms. Therefore, specific, individualized treatment is necessary when a person is in a coma, intoxicated, or in withdrawal. In the subsequent four sections of this chapter, specific symptoms of intoxications, overdose, and withdrawal are discussed.

Table 24–1 ■ DRUG INFORMATION: PHYSICAL COMPLICATIONS RELATED TO DRUG ABUSE

DRUG	PHYSICAL COMPLICATIONS
Route: Intravenous*	
Narcotics (e.g., heroin) Phencyclidine piperidine (PCP) Cocaine/crack	Acquired immunodeficiency syndrome Hepatitis Bacterial endocarditis Renal failure Cardiac arrest Coma Seizures Respiratory arrest Dermatitis Pulmonary emboli Tetanus Abscesses—osteomyelitis Septicemia ***Note:** The complications listed can result from any drug taken intravenously.
Route: Intravenous, Intranasal	
Cocaine	Perforation of nasal septum (when taken intranasally) Respiratory paralysis Cardiovascular collapse Hyperpyrexia (Note refers to *heading*; complication follow)
Route: Ingestion	
Caffeine	Acid indigestion Peptic ulcer Increased intraocular pressure in unregulated glaucoma Tachycardia Increased plasma glucose and lipid levels
Route: Smoking, Ingestion	
Marijuana	Impaired lung structure Chromosomal mutation—increased incidence of birth defects Micronucleic white blood cells—increased risk of disease due to decreased resistance to infection Possible long term effects on short term memory
Route: Smoking, Chewing	
Nicotine	Heavy *chronic use* associated with Emphysema Cancer of the larynx and esophagus Lung cancer Peripheral vascular diseases
Route: Intravenous	
Heroin	Constipation Dermatitis Malnutrition Hypoglycemia Dental caries Amenorrhea See *Route: Intravenous** for additional complications.
Route: Ingestion	
Phencyclidine piperidine (PCP)	Respiratory arrest See *Route: Intravenous** for additional complications.

ASSESSING THE LEVEL OF PHYSICAL COMPLICATIONS

Drugs of abuse can be lethal. The nurse needs to be aware of the physical side effects of specific drugs of abuse. Common physical complications related to drug abuse are listed in Table 24–1.

ASSESSING PERSONAL HISTORY AND COPING STYLE

The focus of the nursing history is to record the client's perceptions in the area of presenting problems and current lifestyle and to obtain a brief sketch of the client's current life, including family, friends, education, and employment history. The personal history includes having the client identify recent feelings of depression, anxiety, suspiciousness, or hopelessness.

Suicidal ideation is always assessed, especially in the case of toxicity or coma. If the client appears to be suicidal, it should be determined whether there have been previous suicidal attempts. Information regarding suicide history of family members is also elicited. (Refer to Chapter 21 for assessment of suicidal potential.)

ASSESSING DRUG HISTORY

A history of substance abuse includes all drugs taken, amount, length of use, route, and drug preference. It is important to determine how the drugs were used —that is, whether they were taken intravenously, intramuscularly, intradermally ("skin-popped"), or intranasally ("sniffed" or "snorted"); smoked; or taken by mouth. Previous detoxifications and drug-free periods following detoxification also should be included, as well as factors that influenced the client's return to substance abuse.

Essentially, the nurse asks the following questions in a matter-of-fact, nonjudgmental fashion:

- *What drug(s) did you take before coming to the emergency room (hospital, clinic)?*
- *How did you take the drug(s)? (e.g., intravenously, intramuscularly, orally, subcutaneously, smoking, intranasally)*
- *How much of the drug(s) did you take?*
- *When was (were) the last dose(s) taken?*
- *How long have you been using the drug(s)?*
- *How often and how much of the drug(s) do you usually take?*
- *Do you drink alcohol or smoke marijuana? (Often these*

are not considered drugs by some people.) How often? How much?

If the person is not able to provide a drug history, assess for indications of substance abuse, such as dilated or constricted pupils, abnormal vital signs, needle marks, tremors, and history from family and friends (Brauerman and Shook 1987). Check clothing for drug paraphernalia, such as used syringes, crack vials, and evidence of white powder, razor blades, bent spoons, or pipes.

The nurse should also gather data on use or abuse of drugs among family members. Drug abuse by adolescents seems to be related to their parents' use and abuse of drugs, especially alcohol (Brooks 1983). Drug abuse by a family member may also be related to increase in anxiety or conflict within the family (e.g., threatened divorce or separation).

Nursing Diagnosis

Nursing diagnoses for clients with psychoactive substance use disorders are many and varied, owing to the large range of physical and psychological effects of drug abuse or dependence on the user and his or her family. Potential nursing diagnoses for people with psychoactive substance use disorders are as follows:

- *Anxiety*
- *Ineffective individual coping*
- *Altered cardiac output*
- *Impaired communication*
- *Fear*
- *Hopelessness*
- *High risk for infection*
- *Altered parenting*
- *Ineffective breathing patterns*
- *High risk for self-harm*
- *Sexual dysfunction*
- *Sleep-pattern disturbance*
- *Impaired social interaction*
- *Altered thought processes*
- *High risk for violence: self-directed or directed at others*
- *Altered family process*
- *Self-care deficit*
- *Disturbance in personal identity*
- *Diversional activity deficit*
- *Altered nutrition: less than body requirements*
- *Powerlessness*
- *Self-esteem disturbance*
- *Spiritual distress*
- *Impairment of skin integrity*

Planning

CONTENT LEVEL—PLANNING GOALS

Nursing goals will vary widely, depending on whether the client is suicidal, intoxicated, in withdrawal, comatose, in need of learning more effective coping skills, or requiring specific referral information. Specific examples of long term and short term goals will be presented in each of the subsequent sections of this chapter.

PROCESS LEVEL—NURSES' REACTIONS AND FEELINGS

Although nurses may identify with and have sympathy for clients addicted to caffeine or tobacco, their responses to hard-core drug abusers may not be so sympathetic. Substance abusers, particularly repeat substance abusers, are subject to the disdain of many nurses. A client who has overdosed on heroin, LSD, or cocaine may be viewed by health care workers with disapproval, intolerance, and moralistic condemnation and may be considered morally weak. Also, manipulative behaviors that are often seen in these clients lead nurses to feel angry and exploited.

In some areas of the country, the recreational use of cocaine, cannabis, and amphetamine is so common that the nurse may view this occurrence of intoxication or overdose as "rather normal" and may not have much emotional reaction. This attitude is as detrimental as strong emotional disapproval because the nurse may underestimate the importance of supportive measures and client education and the need for follow-up psychotherapeutic intervention.

Perhaps the most detrimental attitude among nurses and other health care workers is that of *enabling. Enabling* is supporting, or denying the seriousness of, the client's physical or psychological substance dependence. Bittle et al. (1986) describe several behaviors that signal enabling by the nurse. The nurse

1. Encourages denial by agreeing that the client only drinks or takes drugs "socially" or when he or she is a little nervous
2. Ignores cues to possible dependency—steers away from drugs to topics more comfortable for the nurse (e.g., anxiety or depression)
3. Demonstrates sympathy for the client's "reasons" (e.g., work, family, or financial problems) for abus-

ing drugs rather than pointing out that these difficulties are often the result of—not the cause of—substance abuse
4. Preaches that the problem can be overcome by will power, thus minimizing the fact that the person is physically or psychologically chemically dependent and has lost control over the use of the drug

Programs for Chemically Impaired Health Care Professionals

A nurse may deny drug abuse or dependence in others in order to reinforce denial of personal drug abuse or dependence. The problem of the chemically impaired health care professional is receiving more recognition and acknowledgement. Nurses and doctors appear to have higher rates of alcohol and prescription drug abuse than people in the general population (Jaffe 1985; Survey 1986).

Alcohol and other drug dependencies in nurses are serious problems for both the nurse and those under his or her care. Descriptive studies of nurses recovering from dependency suggest the following profile: the nurse has a family history of substance abuse, depression, and sexual abuse; is academically and professionally successful; is often divorced; has received professional treatment for substance abuse; and regularly attends recovery self-help groups. Sullivan (1989) reported that 37% of substance-abusing nurses had job-related consequences of drug abuse.

It has also been found that a demanding professional life has an impact on nurses who have experienced stressful family relationships where alcohol or drug use was problematic. Nurses from such backgrounds frequently strive to be "supernurses" and deal with doubts about their feelings of inadequacy by "overachieving" or "overfunctioning."

Drug or alcohol use can become a facilitator for overfunctioning, and it can also set in motion a cycle of drug use. Substance abuse can temporarily help the nurse feel adequate. However, in order to continue the overfunctioning behavior and sustain the temporary feelings of adequacy, the use and abuse of the drug need to continue.

Googins and Kuntz (1981) identify some early indicators that can alert nurse-managers who are sensitive to job performance problems by their staff. These include

- Changing a lifestyle to focus on activities permissive to the use of alcohol or drugs
- Showing inconsistency between statements and actions
- Displaying increasing irritability

- Projecting blame on others
- Isolating one's self from social contacts
- Showing deteriorating physical appearance
- Having frequent episodes of vaguely described illness
- Having frequent tardiness and absenteeism
- Manipulating possession of the narcotic keys for a particular shift
- Having deepening depression

Programs for chemically dependent nurses have been developed in some states in response to a policy statement issued by the American Nurses' Association. The aim of these programs is to protect clients and to keep the nurse in active practice (perhaps with limitations) or to return the nurse to practice after suspension and professional help. Both the medical and nursing professions are formally recognizing this problem, and there is an increased commitment to the rehabilitation of chemically impaired health care professionals, in the form of self-help peer-support groups, hotlines, crisis information, and treatment referral. The section on sedative-hypnotics and anxiolytics in this chapter cites a case study and further discussion of chemically impaired health care professionals.

Intervention

PSYCHOTHERAPEUTIC INTERVENTIONS

Working with a person who is dependent on a psychoactive drug means working with behaviors that almost all substance abusers have in common, including (1) dysfunctional anger, (2) manipulation, (3) impulsiveness, and (4) grandiosity (Zamora 1987). These behaviors and suggested nursing interventions are discussed in Chapter 16. Working with clients who frequently display these behaviors can be challenging and, at times, frustrating. However, supervision, peer support, and team cooperation lessen anxiety and feelings of helplessness among staff and increase the client's opportunity to learn more adaptive coping styles.

Nurses with special training may teach interested clients relaxation techniques or self-hypnosis as an adjunct to other therapies.

Hypnosis can be a useful adjunct to the treatment of chemical dependency because a trance is a natural, nonchemical, and stress-relieving suggestible state. During hypnosis, the client can be given positive sug-

gestions for continued sobriety and for managing day-to-day stress. It can also enhance the person's motivation for continued sobriety, promote nonchemically induced positive feelings, and relieve tension. Attending or speaking at 12-step meetings, coping with anticipated stressful experiences, and preventing a slip back into substance use can all be practiced in a trance state. These experiences can also be coupled with reinforcement of the positive aspects of sobriety. Self-image enhancement can be accomplished as the individual imagines himself or herself chemically free.

Imagery can also be used to help desensitize people to events that they would perceive as threatening or stressful that might elicit relapse or trigger addictive behaviors, and to deal effectively with maintaining recovery. *Imagery* is defined as the internal experience of memories, dreams, fantasies, and visions. Imagery and visualization are compatible with the psychoeducational process necessary for recovery to take place for addicted individuals.

By offering an alternative coping behavior for anxiety reduction, the client may substitute a more adaptive action for lowering anxiety and, as a result, may gain a sense of control and self-esteem.

HEALTH TEACHING

People who abuse or are dependent on psychoactive drugs may develop various physical illnesses (see Table 24–1). A client may need to be hospitalized when a complication is life-threatening (e.g., bacterial endocarditis or pulmonary embolus) or in need of long term care (e.g., hepatitis or severe abscesses).

Health teaching for people who are abusing drugs and plan to continue use includes the following information. The nurse could say something like, "I would rather you seek treatment and not use drugs, but since you are choosing this behavior, here are some ways to minimize your risk." These ways include

1. Instruction on how to administer the drug under antiseptic conditions if the intravenous route is being used (reduces risk for AIDS and hepatitis).
2. Education as to the properties, side effects, and long term physical or emotional effects of the drug.
3. Referral information about community-based clinics, telephone numbers for hotlines, self-help groups, and half-way houses for possible future use.
4. Nutritional information. Many people who use drugs suffer from malnutrition, either because of their lifestyle or because of the properties of the drugs themselves.

Primary Prevention

Primary prevention through health teaching can have an important impact on how youngsters and adolescents choose to solve problems and relate interpersonally. Resnick (1979) offers the following suggestions:

1. Involvement with programs that can strengthen interpersonal and social skills of individuals. An assertiveness training program is an example.
2. More drug education in schools and homes. Peer teaching is often most effective, especially among adolescents.
3. Availability of peer counselors for high school and college students. The normal issues adolescents deal with can be overwhelming for some—e.g., identity problems, occupational goals, heterosexual relationship issues, sexual issues, and drug concerns.
4. Increase in neighborhood recreational and occupational opportunities.
5. Support for families that aims to improve social conditions within the community.
6. Strong community interagency linkage, allowing sharing of resources.

Many communities have youth organizations such as scouting, 4-H clubs, and school clubs. It has been found that the young people who participate in these are at a lower risk for substance abuse. Activities such as these help develop self-confidence and self-esteem in young people.

Part-time job placement can be an important alternative to substance abuse. Earning money on one's own can increase feelings of self-worth and confidence.

Health Teaching For Families

There has been a great deal of research on families with a chemically dependent member. Family intervention is often an important treatment modality in altering maladaptive drug use by one member. Family theorists view a crisis with one member as a signal of a family in distress.

It is believed that some forms of substance abuse may have their roots in the interpersonal context of family relationships (Klagsburn and Davis 1977). Certainly, once substance abuse is integrated into the family experience, the family responds. The response may favor both the abuse pattern and its consequences.

In functional families, there is a coalition between the parents, and the children grow up knowing that the parents will stick together. The parental power is clear, and competing parent-child coalitions are absent (Beavers 1976). In sharp contrast, the marital partners in substance abusing families are typically not in coalition with one another. The power struggle of a spouse to control the substance abuse of the partner leaves its mark, with decreased caring and mutuality.

Conflict between the parents is postulated by Klagsburn and Davis (1977) as a cause of adolescent drug use. The child, by drawing attention to himself or herself, may become a symbolic scapegoat for the unresolved feelings and tensions of the parents.

Clear ego boundaries for each family member are another characteristic of healthy families (Beavers 1976). In the substance-abusing family, there is a pattern of ego enmeshment. A child's fear of separation from the family may be an important dynamic in adolescent drug use, because substance abuse often serves to keep the child within or dependent on the family. To complicate matters, parents themselves often have not emancipated themselves from their families of origin (Weingarten 1980). Often there is no one member who consistently holds the power in a substance-abusing family. In drug-abusing families with adolescents, there is often inconsistent limit setting (Weingarten 1980). The married adult drug abuser often duplicates an earlier conflicted, ambivalent, and immature child-parent relationship with his or her spouse.

As substance abuse is integrated into the family, there may be a pattern of predictable roles for each of the members. Wegscheider (1981) describes six family roles:

1. The chemically dependent person
2. The chief enabler
3. The family hero
4. The scapegoat
5. The lost child
6. The mascot

The *chief enabler* is closest to the substance abuser and, to maintain the norms of family life, becomes increasingly responsible for fulfilling the duties left vacant by the abuser. The *family hero* feels responsible for the family difficulty and attempts to improve the situation. The *scapegoat* acts out of hurt in a defiant manner. The *lost child* withdraws into the self for comfort. The *mascot* uses wit to attract attention and survive in the family system.

Anger, ambivalence, fear, guilt, confusion, and mistrust are frequent feelings in substance-abusing families. Conflict is a norm. Social isolation limits the energy derived from the larger community, and the family is entrapped with its own need to balance relationships. The adequate nourishment required for spontaneous, clear communication is lacking. Victimization caused by immature, impulsive members is frequent.

Counseling and support should be encouraged for all family members. Al-Anon and Al-a-Teen are self-help groups that offer support and guidance for adults and teenagers, respectively, in families with a chemically dependent member.

SOMATIC THERAPIES

Medications are sometimes given in response to withdrawal from drugs. For example, one of the most well-known medical interventions is the methadone maintenance programs developed in the 1960s. This form of treatment for heroin addiction is highly controversial.

Methadone (*Dolophine*) is a synthetic opiate that at certain doses (usually 40 mg) blocks the craving for, and effects of, heroin. However, it is itself highly addicting and when stopped produces withdrawal. *Naltrexone* (*Trexan*) is a nonaddicting narcotic antagonist that has allowed many addicts to live drug free. The use of *clonidine*, initially marketed for high blood pressure, has also proved to be an effective somatic treatment for some chemically dependent individuals when combined with naltrexone (Schloemer and Skidmore 1983; Frances and Franklin 1988). Clonidine is a nonopioid suppressor of opioid withdrawal symptoms. It is also nonaddicting. Other drugs used for clients intoxicated by or withdrawing from certain drugs can include diazepam (Valium) and antipsychotics such as haloperidol (Haldol). (Refer to each section for specific somatic therapies.)

Acupuncture has also been an effective adjunct to treatment for withdrawal from nicotine, caffeine, alcohol, and narcotics for some. The success of acupuncture depends on supplemental lifestyle interventions and client commitment.

THERAPEUTIC ENVIRONMENT

DETOXIFICATION. The first step toward treatment is often detoxification. Each drug has unique properties, and each drug has individual interventions for safe withdrawal (see Tables 24–2 through 24–5). Many individuals do not go further in treatment than detoxification before going back to using heroin.

RESIDENTIAL THERAPEUTIC COMMUNITIES. Many residential therapeutic communities expect the addict to remain for 12–18 months. The goal of treatment is to effect a change in lifestyle, including absti-

nence from drugs. Other anticipated outcomes are the development of social skills and the elimination of antisocial behavior. Follow-up studies suggest that clients who stay 90 days or longer exhibit a significant decrease in illicit drug use and recorded arrests and an increase in legitimate employment (Jaffe 1985). The residential therapeutic community is considered best suited for individuals who have a long history of antisocial behavior (Klein and Miller 1986). Synanon, Phoenix House, and Odyssey House are three of the more familiar names among the more than 300 therapeutic communities in the United States.

OUTPATIENT DRUG-FREE PROGRAMS. Outpatient drug-free programs have the same goals as the therapeutic communities but aim to achieve these goals in an outpatient setting, thus allowing individuals to continue employment and family life. Outpatient drug-free programs are better geared to the polydrug abuser rather than to the heavily addicted heroin client. These centers may offer vocational education and placement, counseling, and individual or group psychotherapy.

Intensive outpatient treatment programs are becoming more popular today. They are also popular with insurance companies because they are viewed as flexible, diverse, cost-effective, and responsive to the specific individual needs of a person.

EMPLOYEE ASSISTANCE PROGRAMS. Employee assistance programs have been developed to provide the delivery of mental health services in occupational settings. Many hospitals and corporations have such programs for their professional staff. Employee assistance programs deal with issues of alcohol and drug abuse and offer employee counseling, information, and referral services (Bittle et al. 1986; Brill et al. 1985).

TWELVE-STEP PROGRAMS. The most effective treatment modalities for all addictions have been the 12-step programs. Alcoholics Anonymous is the prototype of all subsequent 12-step programs developed for any number and types of addictions. Three basic concepts are fundamental to all 12-step programs:

1. Individuals with addictive disorders are powerless over their addiction, and their lives are unmanageable.
2. Although individuals with addictive disorders are not responsible for their disease, they are responsible for their recovery.
3. Individuals can no longer blame people, places, and things for their addiction; they must face their problems and their feelings.

The 12 steps are considered the core of treatment (see Box 23–4 in Chapter 23). Using the 12 steps is often referred to as "working the steps." They are designed to help a person refrain from addictive behaviors as well as to foster individual change and growth. They offer the behavioral, cognitive, and dynamic structure needed in recovery. Besides Alcoholics Anonymous, other 12-step programs include Pills Anonymous, Narcotics Anonymous, Cocaine Anonymous, and Valium Anonymous.

PSYCHOTHERAPY

INDIVIDUAL. Individuals who have abused drugs for a period of time benefit more from analytical or supportive expressive psychotherapy than from standard drug counseling alone (Jaffe 1985). Other approaches that have proven effective for some are cognitive and behaviorally oriented therapies.

GROUP. Groups can help chemically dependent individuals break through denial and rationalization. Group members confront one another regarding drug and antisocial behaviors. Group cohesion fosters growth and commitment toward individual goals. Group interactions increase self-esteem and provide a sense of purpose and belonging. The group modality is especially effective with adolescents because peer relationships are often more acceptable than those of adult authority figures.

FAMILY. Families who have a chemically impaired member need support, information, and guidance. The recovering addict usually has caused disruption, frustration, and confusion among other family members. These and other issues need to be addressed under the guidance of a trained therapist (e.g., nurse, social worker, or psychologist). In fact, some studies suggest that family therapy, in conjunction with regular urinalysis, is superior to standard day counseling in fostering a decrease in illicit drug use (Jaffe 1985).

Evaluation

Evaluation is a continuous process. Short term goals often include the substance abuser's physical safety when the individual's life is threatened, as may be the case in coma, intoxication, and withdrawal. Long term goals involve lifestyle changes, more effective coping methods, improvement in issues involving self-esteem and identity, and improvement in social and interpersonal relationships. Acee and Smith (1987) propose the following goals, which, when met, make possible alternate choices for a more satisfying and productive future.

The client will understand that

1. Chemical dependency is a progressively deteriorating disease if left unchecked.

2. Individuals are not responsible for their disease, but they are responsible for their recovery.
3. Clients cannot blame people, places, or things for their dependency. They must face their problems and their feelings.
4. Rehabilitation and recovery are lifelong enterprises that begin with a commitment to a long term treatment effort.

Summary

Pathological use of drugs is divided into *substance abuse* and *substance dependence*. A person who abuses drugs is one whose social, occupational, psychological, or physical problems are exacerbated by the drug and whose continued use of the drug puts the person in physical danger. Drug dependence includes the preceding characteristics plus *tolerance* or *withdrawal symptoms* when the body is deprived of the drug. The prevalence of polydrug abuse was discussed. The dangers of the *synergistic effect* were mentioned, as well as the *antagonistic effect* that drugs may have on each other. *Toxicological screening* is one way of indicating the presence of different drugs in the body.

Various theories of drug abuse were reviewed. No single theory has been found to explain the reasons for substance dependence and abuse.

Four areas of assessment are (1) signs of intoxication and withdrawal, (2) physical complications, (3) personal history and coping style, and (4) drug history. Because drug use can be precipitated by, or be the cause of, a wide range of psychological and physical problems, possible nursing diagnoses are numerous.

Treatment planning reflects individual needs. Nurses' feelings need to be recognized and discussed with peers because reactions to clients who are chemically dependent are often intense. Some common problematic responses are intolerance, moralistic condemnation, enabling, and denial.

Many treatment modalities were discussed, including detoxification, residential communities, outpatient drug-free programs, and employee assistance programs. Group, family, and individual interventions were addressed under psychotherapy. The greatest emphasis was placed on health teaching and primary prevention. Evaluating whether certain client-centered goals will be met depends in part on the client's being able to meet four basic goals compiled by Acee and Smith (1987).

The problem of drug abuse and dependence among health care professionals was addressed and will be discussed further in the next section.

Sedative-Hypnotics and Anxiolytics

OBJECTIVES ■

After studying this section on sedative-hypnotics and anxiolytics, the student will be able to

1. Name four anxiolytics or antianxiety drugs often abused.
2. Discuss five physical and five psychological signs of sedative-hypnotic or anxiolytic intoxication.
3. Describe emergency medical and nursing treatments for a person who has overdosed, and identify five emergency situations that can occur in anxiolytic intoxication.
4. Discuss treatment for a person who is withdrawing from an anxiolytic CNS depressant.
5. Discuss some of the reactions a nurse might have when working with a chemically impaired nurse.
6. Identify six ways that you as a nurse can help a chemically impaired colleague.

Introduction

BARBITURATES

For centuries, people have sought relief through drugs for anxiety and insomnia. During the nineteenth century, opiates were prescribed to relieve these symptoms. Alcohol was also prescribed as the sedative or hypnotic of choice. Toward the end of the nineteenth century, two German scientists synthesized a new chemical called barbital, a derivative of barbituric acid. This drug was successfully used to facilitate sleep in clients and, given in smaller doses, it would decrease anxiety. In 1903, barbital was introduced into general medical practice under the trade name Veronal, and in 1912, phenobarbital was introduced under the trade name Luminal. Eventually, more than 50 barbiturates were synthesized and accepted for medical use. Long-acting barbiturates were developed for daytime sedation, and short-acting ones were used for prompt sedation and for inducing sleep without delay. These drugs are odorless and tasteless, and precise quantities can be dispensed in capsules or tablets.

During the 1930s and 1940s, it became apparent that these drugs were addictive. A person who be-

comes dependent on barbiturates suffers many of the same withdrawal symptoms as a person withdrawing from alcohol (see Chapter 23). Abrupt withdrawal of these drugs may prove fatal.

Eventually, states began outlawing nonprescription barbiturates. By the end of the 1940s, the United States, which had for decades used barbitures sensibly for anxiety and insomnia, was persuaded that these drugs were "thrill pills." Unfortunately, for some people these warnings served as lures; illicit barbiturate use increased from year to year.

BENZODIAZEPINES

Diazepam (Valium) and chlordiazepoxide (Librium), both benzodiazepines, are known as **anxiolytic,** or antianxiety, medications. These drugs are also called minor tranquilizers. The effects of diazepam, chlordiazepoxide, and other benzodiazepines are similar to those of the barbiturates. The major difference seems to be that a dose of a benzodiazepine that is sufficient to calm anxiety seems to produce a little less sleepiness than does a dose of barbiturates equally effective against anxiety. Benzodiazepines, like all anxiolytic drugs, are CNS depressants. Clients should be advised against the simultaneous ingestion of alcohol

Table 24–2 ▪ DRUG INFORMATION: SEDATIVE-HYPNOTIC OR ANXIOLYTIC AGENTS*

DRUG	INTOXICATION	OVERDOSE		WITHDRAWAL	
		Effects	**Possible Treatments**	**Effects**	**Possible Treatments**

BARBITURATES
Amobarbital
(Amytal)
Pentobarbital
(Nembutal)
Secobarbital
(Seconal)
 	
BENZODIAZEPINES
Diazepam (Valium)
Chlordiazepoxide
(Librium)
Lorazepam (Ativan)
Oxazepam (Serax)
Alprazolam (Xanax)
 	
CHLORAL HYDRATE
 	
GLUTETHIMIDE
(Doriden)
 	
MEPROBAMATE
(Equanil, Miltown)
	PHYSICAL:
	Slurred speech
	Incoordination
	Unsteady gait
	Drowsiness
	Decreased blood
	  pressure
	
	PSYCHOLOGICAL/
	PERCEPTUAL:
	Disinhibition of sex-
	  ual or aggressive
	  drives
	Impaired judgment
	Impaired social or
	  occupational func-
	  tion
	Impaired attention
	  or memory
	Irritability
		Cardiovascular or
		  respiratory de-
		  pression or arrest
		  (mostly with bar-
		  biturates)
		Coma
		Shock
		Convulsions
		Death
			IF AWAKE:
			Keep awake
			Induce vomiting
			Give activated char-
			  coal to aid ab-
			  sorption of drug
			Every 15 minutes
			  check vital signs
			  (VS)
			
			COMA:
			Clear airway—
			  endotracheal tube
			Intravenous (IV)
			  fluids
			Gastric lavage with
			  activated charcoal
			Frequent VS checks
			  after client is
			  stable for shock
			  and cardiac arrest
			Seizure precautions
			Possible hemodialy-
			  sis or peritoneal
			  dialysis
				CESSATION OF
				  PROLONGED/
				  HEAVY USE:
				Nausea/vomiting
				Tachycardia
				Diaphoresis
				Anxiety or irritability
				Tremors in hands,
				  fingers, eyelids
				Marked insomnia
				Grand mal seizures
				
				AFTER 5–15 YEARS'
				  HEAVY USE:
				Delirium
					Carefully titrated de-
					  toxification with
					  similar drug, usu-
					  ally phenobarbital
					**NOTE: Abrupt with-
					  drawal can lead
					  to death.**

Data from Grinspoon and Bakalar 1985; Smith 1984; Bittle et al. 1986; APA 1987.
*DEFINITION: Known as minor tranquilizers, sedatives, hypnotics, and antianxiety agents, these drugs reduce pathological anxiety, tension, and agitation without therapeutic effects on disturbed cognitive or perceptual processes. High potential for dependency; all act differently in the body but produce symptoms of intoxication and withdrawal similar to those of alcohol withdrawal.

and other CNS depressant drugs (Table 24–2). Clients should also be cautioned against engaging in hazardous tasks requiring complete mental alertness, such as operating machinery or driving a motor vehicle. Withdrawal symptoms, similar to those for all sedative-hypnotic or anxiolytic drugs, occur following abrupt discontinuance. These include convulsions, tremors, abdominal and muscle cramps, vomiting, and sweating. Abrupt withdrawal from consistent long term use can prove dangerous, even fatal.

Detoxification should be gradual, because abrupt withdrawal in a person who is physically dependent is dangerous. Supportive measures, including vitamins, restoration of electrolyte imbalance, and prevention of dehydration, are also used. Close observation of the client at this time is also essential (see Table 24–2).

It should be noted that many people obtain these drugs legally, and therefore do not recognize the problem of abuse. The *Physician's Desk Reference* states that many of the benzodiazepines, such as diazepam and chlordiazepoxide, should be used for anxiety on a short term basis only. Yet it is common knowledge that many individuals are given prescriptions for these drugs year after year by their physicians.

SIGNS OF INTOXICATION

Abuse of CNS depressants other than alcohol is determined by three major criteria: (1) a pattern of pathological abuse, (2) impairment in social or occupational functioning caused by the pathological use of the substance, and (3) duration of use, which requires that the disturbance last for at least one month. Use does not have to be continuous throughout a given month but must be frequent enough within a month's time to cause noticeable difficulties in social and occupational functioning.

Symptoms of intoxication include the following (see Table 24–2):

- Mood lability
- Disinhibition of sexual and aggressive impulses
- Irritability
- Loquacity
- Slurred speech
- Incoordination
- Unsteady gait
- Impairment of attention or memory
- Impaired social judgment

Continued misuse of any antianxiety drug has a cumulative toxic effect on the CNS that is life-threatening. In large doses, or in combination with other CNS depressants, antianxiety drugs may cause death.

PHYSICAL COMPLICATIONS

When a client has overdosed on, or is quite intoxicated from, CNS depressants, it is very important for the nurse to observe and record vital signs frequently. These signs include blood pressure, temperature, pulse, respirations, and neurological symptoms. It is also very important to assess respiratory functioning. An intoxicated client should be on seizure precautions; if the client does have a seizure, seizure activity should also be observed and recorded. If a seizure occurs, the client's head and limbs should be protected during the seizure, maintaining a patent airway. A seizure and any periods of apnea should always be timed. Urinary output is often monitored, and specimens are saved for drug screening.

Another possible complication is pulmonary edema. The symptoms of pulmonary edema are anxiety and restlessness, gray complexion, cold, moist hands, cyanotic nail beds, incessant coughing, and noisy and moist breathing.

MEDICAL WITHDRAWAL

Gradual withdrawal from these drugs is the safest method. However, an overdose can constitute a medical emergency (see Table 24–2 for interventions). Recently, a drug has been introduced that is an antagonist to the benzodiazepines and can reverse their effect.

Flumazenil (Mazicon), a benzodiazepine-receptor antagonist, is indicated for a person who has overdosed on benzodiazepines. Because respiratory depression, excessive sedation, and hypotension are among the major adverse effects of a benzodiazepine overdose, prompt intervention is needed to prevent respiratory failure. A code is called immediately while 100% oxygen is administered through a manual ventilation bag. Flumazenil, 0.2 mg, can be given intravenously over 15 seconds. If the level of consciousness does not improve over 45 seconds, a second dose of flumazenil, 0.2 mg, can be given (up to five 0.2-mg doses at 1-minute intervals) (Lammon and Adams 1993).

THE CHEMICALLY IMPAIRED NURSE

Chemical dependence is the number one health problem affecting nurses. Nurses have a 50% higher rate of chemical dependency than the general population. Helping the chemically impaired nurse is difficult but not impossible. The choices for actions are varied, and the only choice that is clearly wrong is to do nothing. Nurses who have worked with chemically impaired nurses state that the majority want to be helped and not protected.

A nurse who demonstrates behaviors consistent with drug abuse or dependence should be reported immediately to the supervisor. This can prevent harm to clients under the nurse's care and save a colleague's professional career or life. By dealing with the problem early on, the supervisor may help stop the process of addiction before more devastating and permanent consequences affect the nurse's life. However, the supervisor's major concern must be with job performance. Clear and accurate documentation is vital, and referral to a drug and alcohol treatment

---

Box 24–1. HOSPITAL PROTOCOL FOR THE CHEMICALLY IMPAIRED NURSE

Step 1. The supervisor contacts the Employee Assistance Counselor (EAC) in the Employee Relations Department to confidentially discuss the problem and review the documentation.

Step 2. The supervisor continues to observe job performance; if it continues to deteriorate, the supervisor arranges a confidential session between the employee and the EAC.

Step 3. The EAC meets with the employee and attempts to get the employee to identify the exact nature of the problem causing a decline in job performance. Often, the employee health nurse is included in this meeting.

Step 4. When alcohol or drug dependency is identified as the problem, the employee is encouraged to take voluntary action. This usually begins with a referral to a local treatment facility, which offers an evaluation and counseling service.

At this point, the problem becomes an employee health problem. After the employee meets with the counselor at the referral agency to discuss treatment needs and possibilities, the

Continued on following page

program should always be an option (Elliot and Williams 1982). Box 24–1 is an example of a hospital protocol for chemically impaired nurses.

However, there are some things that one should definitely *not* do, under any circumstances, when dealing with an alcohol- or a drug-addicted nurse: (Jefferson and Ensur 1982):

1. **Don't** lecture, moralize, scold, blame, threaten, or argue with the person about the problem. Document it and use it to counsel the person about job performance.
2. **Don't** lose your temper.
3. **Don't** "enable" the problem to continue by covering up the consequences, trying to protect the person, making excuses, or doing his or her job.
4. **Don't** give the person an easier work schedule.
5. **Don't** have a holier-than-thou attitude.
6. **Don't** be overly sympathetic. You are not a counselor or big sister or brother.
7. **Don't** accept what you know is a lie. When you know the person is lying, say so. Accepting lies only encourages more lying, and you will lose the person's respect at the same time.
8. **Don't** accept mere promises to "do better," and don't keep switching agreements. When you say that a job is in jeopardy (suspension or termination) if the person's performance does not improve, you must follow through.
9. **Don't** accept the responsibility of letting someone work on your unit or team if impaired by alcohol or drugs. Judgment is the first thing to go.
10. **Don't** put off facing the problem, hoping it will get better with time. It won't.

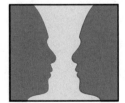

Case Study: Working with a Person Dependent on Diazepam

Elyse, a 34-year-old, recently divorced nurse was brought into the hospital emergency room by two friends who had gone to her apartment after a frantic call from Elyse. When Elyse didn't answer the door, they had the superintendent let them in. They stated that they found Elyse lying on the couch; a half-empty bottle of vodka was open and near the couch. When her friends tried to talk to Elyse, she responded with slurred speech. When she attempted to walk, her gait was unsteady. The friends reported that

when they questioned Elyse about her condition, she became extremely irritable.

Her friends stated that as they sat with Elyse they became increasingly alarmed and phoned Elyse's physician, who encouraged them to take her to the hospital. On the way to the hospital, Elyse abruptly changed her mind and attempted to open the car door. Elyse's friends brought with them an empty bottle of diazepam (Valium) pills, which had recently been prescribed for Elyse.

Assessment

During the assessment, the nurse determined that Elyse displayed some symptoms of intoxication, namely, irritability, slurred speech, incoordination, unsteady gait, and impaired judgment. Because the continued misuse of CNS depressants has a cumulative effect on the CNS that is life-threatening, the staff had to determine immediately how much of the medication Elyse had consumed. Elyse was questioned and drowsily stated that she was not sure how many pills she had taken. The pharmacist was then called. During this time, vital signs were being taken, a gastric lavage was performed, and blood specimens were drawn.

Elyse's blood pressure was 90/60, her pulse was 128, and her respirations were eight to 10 per minute and shallow.

PERSONAL HISTORY AND COPING STYLE

Because Elyse's verbal communication was impaired, the nurse gathered her data from Elyse's two friends and the pharmacist. When it was determined that Elyse's condition was not life-threatening, the nurse continued her assessment. She encouraged Elyse to describe her current problems and also gathered data from Elyse and her two friends about recent stresses in Elyse's life. The nurse learned that Elyse's brother had been killed recently in an automobile accident about a week before Elyse's divorce was finalized. Elyse's friends reported that Elyse had been quite depressed for the past few weeks, and that they had been quite concerned about her.

Elyse had been in charge of the intensive care unit at a nearby hospital. She was bright, ambitious, and respected by her peers. Her friends stated that they knew Elyse was sneaking diazepam from the unit and were concerned, but they had no idea that her abuse of the drug was so serious.

Elyse told her friends that the drug made her feel more relaxed and better able to cope with her problems and her job.

At this time, an accurate history of other substance abuse and length of use, as well as drug preference, could not be made because of Elyse's condition.

Because Elyse's situation could easily have been life-threatening, it was important to assess suicidal ideation and to determine if this was a suicide attempt or gesture. It appeared to the staff that this had been an actual suicidal attempt, because Elyse had taken a substantial amount of diazepam pills with alcohol and had not been expecting visitors.

DRUG HISTORY

Elyse was unable to give any information at this time, and her friends were unaware of her use of any drugs other than diazepam and alcohol.

Nursing Diagnosis

Some nursing diagnoses that pertained to Elyse follow:

1. *High risk for self-directed violence* related to divorce, loss of brother, and drug dependence, as evidenced by drug overdose

2. *Ineffective coping* related to inability to constructively handle losses without alcohol or drugs

Planning

CONTENT LEVEL—PLANNING GOALS

Goals relevant to each of the nursing diagnoses were established.

Nursing Diagnosis	Long Term Goals	Short Term Goals
1. *High risk for self-harm* related to divorce, loss of brother, and drug dependence, as evidenced by drug overdose	1. The client will remain free from self-injury.	1a. The client will make a no-suicide contract with nurse by (date).
		1b. The client will agree to inform the staff of dysphoric feelings she is experiencing by (date).
		1c. The client will discuss with the nurse what she can do to work out feelings by (date).

Continued on following page

Planning
(Continued)

Nursing Diagnosis	Long Term Goals	Short Term Goals
2. *Ineffective coping* related to inability to constructively handle losses without alcohol and drugs	2. Client will name two actions that she can take to improve her self-esteem and quality of life.	2a. Client will discuss with nurse effects of losses (husband and brother) by (date).
		2b. Client will discuss with nurse extent of her substance abuse by (date).
		2c. Client will discuss with nurse and health team members long term treatment plans by (date).
		2d. Client will name three personal strengths by (date).

Some interventions planned to meet three of these short term goals are listed here.

Short Term Goals	Interventions
1a. Client will make a no-suicide contract with nurse by (date).	1. Assess immediate degree of suicidal risk and ask if client is thinking of harming herself.
	2. Discuss with client people she can talk to during the next 24 hours if she feels like harming herself.
	3. Jointly with client work out wording of contract covering the next 24 hours.
	4. Spend time with client for at least 15 minutes twice each day.
2b. Client will discuss with nurse extent of her substance abuse by (date).	1. During scheduled meetings, assist client in connecting the beginning of diazepam and alcohol abuse with feelings surrounding life events.
	2. During scheduled meetings, encourage client to discuss how long she has been abusing alcohol and diazepam, as well as how much and what other drugs she has been taking.
2d. Client will name three personal strengths by (date).	1. Approach client in a positive and open manner.
	2. Assist client to identify personal strengths.
	3. Give positive feedback.

PROCESS LEVEL—NURSES' REACTIONS AND FEELINGS

Word soon spread about a nurse having "overdosed." As accustomed as other nurses were to working with people who were intoxicated or in a coma related to substance abuse, this was different—nurses have strong feelings about "one of their own." Many nurses had a highly moralistic, rigidly judgmental attitude: "She should have known better." "I hope they take her license away." "She's a disgrace." At the other extreme nurses were being enabling: "Poor thing, she had so many tough breaks . . . no wonder she needed something to get over her losses." Both these attitudes toward the chemically impaired nurses are defensive and not objective. Both attitudes can cause problems for the nurses that hold them, and certainly for the chemically impaired nurse-clients who might come under their care.

Because chemical dependency is the number one health problem affecting nurses, and because nurses have a 50% higher rate of chemical dependency than the general population, an in-service education program was set up for the whole nursing staff—this incident reflected concerns that hospital ad-

ministrators had about their own staff. Attitudes, approaches, and resources were covered. It was stressed that a nurse who demonstrated behaviors consistent with drug abuse or dependence should be reported to a supervisor immediately. *First*, this can prevent harm to clients under the nurse's care and, *second*, it may save a colleague's professional career or life.

Guidelines were given to the nursing staff regarding dealing with a chemically impaired colleague.

Intervention

Elyse was placed in the detoxification unit to treat the effects of her diazepam and alcohol abuse. During the initial days of admission, she was on suicide precaution. She was rude and demanding, was contemptuous of the nursing staff, and demanded release from the unit. After several days passed, she became more withdrawn and depressed and started talking more with her primary nurse, Mrs. Brown. Mrs. Brown, who was 51 years old, had many years of nursing experience and had an intelligent and comfortable manner.

Dialogue	Therapeutic Tool/Comment
N: Elyse, I get the impression that life must have been getting very difficult for you lately.	Nurse validates and empathizes.
E: (*Silence*) . . . I don't think you would understand.	
N: I guess sometimes it feels like no one understands, but I would like to try.	Reflecting/empathy.
E: At times . . . I feel I can't go on any more . . . so many losses.	
N: Loss is difficult. Elyse, tell me about your losses.	Encouraging the client to share her painful feelings.
E: My brother's sudden death . . . We were so close . . . I depended on him so much.	
N: It must have been so difficult for you to lose him so suddenly.	Empathy.
E: (*Silence*) . . . No one knows . . . then Harry, he left . . . (*Elyse starts to cry*)	
N: Tell me what you are feeling right now.	Encouraging expression of feelings while feelings are close to the surface.
E: I don't know . . . angry maybe . . . Why does everyone leave me . . . I hate them . . . Oh, I wish I had a Valium now . . .	
N: And what does the Valium do to help you?	Begins to explore the drug dependence in a gently nonthreatening manner.

Elyse became less defensive as time went on and seemed to relate best to Mrs. Brown and the male social worker. He told Elyse about a NA group that was made up of chemically impaired people from the health care professions. He stated that substance abuse disorders among nurses and doctors is a widespread, recognized problem. Elyse still had a tendency to minimize her drug dependence, but she was willing to work on her

Intervention *(Continued)*	feelings about her divorce and her brother's death. By discharge, Elyse had attended two meetings of a Narcotics Anonymous (NA)	group geared toward medical personnel and had started group and individual therapy, which she would continue on an outpatient basis.
Evaluation	On discharge, Elyse was no longer perceived as suicidal. She would continue group and individual therapy on an outpatient basis and agreed to attend NA on a regular basis. Three months after discharge, Elyse wrote to the Director of Nurses to get her old job back. It was agreed that she would work as a staff nurse with the understanding that she would continue therapy and agree to periodic blood and urine testing. For a	probationary period, she was not to give medications or have access to the keys of the medication cabinet. Six months later, Elyse was doing well at work, was attending therapy regularly, and appeared less depressed and more hopeful regarding the future. She was able to admit that drugs had taken control of her life, and she was working hard to turn things around for herself.

Summary

Anxiolytic drugs (barbiturates) have been used since 1903 to induce sleep. Benzodiazepines (e.g., diazepam, alprazolam (Xanax), and chlordiazepoxide) have generally replaced the use of barbiturates because they have fewer sedative qualities and interfere less with motor activities. All these drugs are prescription drugs, are CNS depressants, produce tolerance and withdrawal symptoms, and have a synergistic effect when taken with alcohol. All drugs in this category, although different in action, produce similar withdrawal symptoms. They are all popular and dangerous drugs of abuse. Abrupt withdrawal in a chemically dependent individual can be dangerous, leading to grand mal seizures and death.

The case study highlighted the signs of intoxication and withdrawal of anxiolytic drugs and discussed some nursing responsibilities in the process of assessment, planning, and interventions. The issue of working with a chemically dependent colleague was briefly discussed, and some guidelines were outlined. Behaviors or performances suggesting chemical abuse or dependence need to be reported to a supervisor. Not only will the lives of clients be protected, but the lives and careers of colleagues can be preserved.

Psychostimulants

OBJECTIVES ■

After studying this section on psychostimulants, the student will be able to

1. Identify four psychostimulants and state one unique quality of each.
2. Compare and contrast the signs of intoxication, overdose, and withdrawal symptoms from cocaine and amphetamine use.
3. Discuss three possible nursing interventions for a client addicted to cocaine.

Introduction

AMPHETAMINES

The drug known as amphetamine was first synthesized in 1887; however, its medical uses were not known until 1927. Its effects in enlarging the nasal and bronchial passages and in stimulating the central nervous system were noted, and its effect on elevating blood pressure was discovered (Kramer 1986). This drug was marketed in 1932 under the trade name Benzedrine.

In 1937, researchers found that amphetamines had a paradoxical effect on some children whose functioning is impaired by hyperactivity and an inability to concentrate. It was found that amphetamines, instead of making them even more jittery, had a calming effect on many of these children and notably improved their concentration and performance (see Chapter 27).

By the end of 1971, there were at least 31 amphetamine preparations, including amphetamine-sedative, amphetamine-tranquilizer, and amphetamine-analgesic combinations.

During World War II, the American, British, German, and Japanese armed forces were issuing amphetamines to their men to counteract fatigue, elevate mood, and heighten endurance. After World War II, many physicians prescribed amphetamines routinely for depression and weight loss and as energizers.

After World War II, with the expansion of the legal market for prescribed amphetamines, a modest black market in the drugs also started. Early black market patrons included truck drivers who were trying to maintain schedules that called for long over-the-road hauls without adequate rest periods. Soon, truck stops along the main transcontinental routes were dispensing amphetamines as well as coffee and caffeine tablets to help drivers stay awake. Students were also using amphetamine "pep pills" when cramming for exams.

Stimulants have always been popular drugs of abuse with students, athletes, and entertainers. Now, because of their high potential for abuse and the quickness with which tolerance develops (8–12 weeks) legitimate use of amphetamines is limited to therapy for hyperkinesis in children and for narcolepsy. Amphetamines can be dangerous. Refer to Table 24–3 for the physical and psychological effects of intoxication from abuse of amphetamines and other psychostimulants, possible life-threatening results of overdose, and emergency measures for both overdose and withdrawal.

COCAINE AND CRACK

Cocaine is a naturally occurring stimulant extracted from the leaf of the coca bush. Once the drug of the rich and famous, cocaine use is now spreading to all socioeconomic groups. The drug acts on the CNS and changes the way a person thinks, feels, and behaves. Crack is a cheap, widely available alkalinized form of cocaine. Crack is smoked and takes effect in four to six seconds. Dependence on crack develops rapidly. A popular rock star recovering from crack addiction stated, "If you are on crack, you have three choices: you can get off, you can go crazy, or you can die." The fleeting high obtained from crack (lasting 5–7 minutes) is followed by a period of deep depression that reinforces addictive behavior patterns and guarantees continued use of the drug. With the advent of crack, doctors are seeing a profound increase in the neurological and psychological complications associated with cocaine abuse.

Cocaine has been classified by the federal government as a "schedule II" substance—a drug officially considered to have "high abuse potential with some recognized medical use." Cocaine is consumed in three ways: sniffed intranasally, smoked as freebase or crack, or injected. Various medical problems may develop in the patient, depending on which route is used. Sniffers have problems that relate to deterioration of the nasal passages: sores, hoarseness, and throat infections. Coke smokers can have lung damage, upper gastrointestinal tract problems, and throat damage from the harsh smoke. Intravenous users can develop endocarditis, heart attacks, angina, and needle-related diseases, such as hepatitis and AIDS.

Cocaine exerts two main effects on the body—anesthetic and stimulant—and several related effects. As an anesthetic, it blocks the conduction of electrical impulses within the nerve cells involved in sensory transmissions, primarily pain. It also acts as a stimulant for both sexual arousal and violent behavior.

Cocaine produces an imbalance of neurotransmitters (dopamine and norepinephrine), that may be responsible for many of the physical withdrawal symptoms reported by heavy chronic cocaine users: depression, paranoia, lethargy, anxiety, insomnia, nausea and vomiting, and sweating and chills—all signs of the body struggling to regain its normal chemical balance.

Cocaine's physical effects are virtually identical whether it is snorted, swallowed, smoked, or injected. Differences arise from the speed at which the effects occur, as well as their strength and duration.

Table 24–3 ■ DRUG INFORMATION: PSYCHOSTIMULANTS *

DRUG	INTOXICATION	OVERDOSE		WITHDRAWAL	
		Effects	**Possible Treatments**	**Effects**	**Possible Treatments**
AMPHETAMINES (Long-acting) Dextroamphetamine (Dexedrine) Methamphetamine (Methadrine)	PHYSICAL: Tachycardia Dilated pupils Elevated blood pressure Nausea and vomiting Twitching PSYCHOLOGICAL/ PERCEPTUAL: Assaultive Grandiose Impaired judgment Impaired social and occupational functioning Euphoria Increased energy SEVERE EFFECTS: Resembles paranoid schizophrenia Paranoia with delusions Psychosis Visual, auditory, and tactile hallucinations Severe to panic levels of anxiety Agitated potential for violence NOTE: **Paranoia and ideas of reference may persist for months afterward.**	Respiratory distress Ataxia Hyperpyrexia Convulsions Coma Death associated with hyperpyrexia, convulsions, cardiovascular shock	SUPPORTIVE MEASURES: Acidify urine (ammonium chloride) Phenothiazines to treat psychotic reactions MEDICAL AND NURSING MANAGEMENT FOR: Hyperpyrexia Convulsions Respiratory distress Cardiovascular shock	Depression Agitation Apathy Sleepiness Disorientation	Antidepressants for depression
COCAINE/CRACK (Short-acting) **NOTE:** *High obtained*: Snorted—3 minutes Injected—30 seconds Smoked—4–6 seconds (crack) *Average high lasts*: For cocaine—15–30 minutes For crack—5–7 minutes	PHYSICAL SIGNS: Tachycardia Dilated pupils Elevated blood pressure Insomnia Anorexia PSYCHOLOGICAL/ PERCEPTUAL: Elation Grandiosity Resistance to fatigue Impaired judgment SEVERE EFFECTS (*Chronic Use*): Paranoid thinking Disturbed concentration Psychosis Violent temper outbursts	Seizures Cardiac arrest Respiratory depression/arrest Convulsions Hyperpyrexia Death	MEDICAL AND NURSING LIFE-SAVING MEASURE FOR: Convulsions (prescribe diazepam) Hyperpyrexia (use hypothermia mattress) Respiratory depression/cardiac arrest	Fatigue Depression Apathy Anxiety Chronic users often abuse or are dependent on a narcotic, alcohol, or an anxiolytic to lessen the withdrawal symptoms of cocaine/crack	DETOXIFICATION: Experimental at present: 1. Amino acids (tyrosine and tryptophan) 2. Dopamine agonist 3. Antidepressants (desipramine)

Table 24–3 ■ DRUG INFORMATION: PSYCHOSTIMULANTS * *Continued*

| DRUG | INTOXICATION | OVERDOSE | | WITHDRAWAL | |
		Effects	Possible Treatments	Effects	Possible Treatments
	Formication (tactile hallucinations involving animals or bugs); "cocaine bugs" refer to the sensation some chronic users experience of bugs crawling under their skin CHRONIC USER COMPLAINTS: • Chronic insomnia • Chronic fatigue • Severe headaches • Nasal problems • Poor/decreased sexual performance • Potential toxic cardiovascular effects				
NICOTINE	None known; however, dependence caused by at least several weeks of smoking 10 cigarettes, (0.5 mg nicotine each) per day			Cravings—"nicotine fits" Anxiety Restlessness Difficulty concentrating Disruption in sleep patterns Excessive eating Irritability Constipation Headaches Gastrointestinal disturbances	None known
CAFFEINE	PHYSICAL: Restlessness Excitement Insomnia Flushed face Diuresis Gastrointestinal complaints Cardiac arrhythmias Psychomotor agitation Periods of inexhaustibility Nervousness Rambling flow of thought			None known	

Data from Grinspoon and Bakalar 1985; Smith 1984; Bittle et al. 1986; APA 1987; Gold 1984; Cocaine 1987.
***DEFINITION: Potent central nervous system stimulants with psychoactive and sympathomimetic effects—speeds up body processes.**

The body's peak reaction to the drug occurs about five minutes after it is taken and declines steadily over the following two to five hours. After an initial euphoria, most of cocaine's effects take place between 20–40 minutes after use.

The body reacts to the infusion of cocaine by

- Increased heart rate
- Increased blood pressure
- Increased respirations
- Increased body temperature
- Increased blood sugar levels
- Dilated pupils
- Depressed appetite
- Increased restlessness

Inadequate nutritional intake results from extended cocaine use and can lead to various kinds of infections, seizures, or momentary losses of consciousness. Nasal damage, such as irritation, inflammation, and chronic rhinitis, also may occur when the drug is taken nasally.

Respiratory effects from the use of cocaine can be extremely serious and life-threatening. Serious respiratory symptoms include gasping, rapid or irregular breathing, and lack of oxygen. Anyone suffering from these symptoms should be rushed to a hospital emergency room. Other less serious respiratory effects are bronchitis, hoarseness, coughs, and wheezes.

Taking cocaine by injection is particularly dangerous to the cardiovascular system. It can even bring about a total cardiovascular collapse. Freebasing is the method of use most often leading to heart attacks, but any dose can cause a heart attack. The effects of cocaine on the cardiovascular system can be broken down into three stages:

Stage I:

- Pulse rate increase by 30–50%
- Blood pressure increase of 15–20%
- Irregular heartbeat
- Pounding heart
- Pale skin due to loss of adequate blood flow

Stage II: Anyone experiencing the following cardiovascular reactions to cocaine listed needs to be immediately taken to a hospital emergency room.

- Ventricular contractions
- Extremely high heart rate and blood pressure, possibly resulting in hemorrhage or congestive heart failure
- Rapid falls in blood pressure and irregular heartbeat, resulting in inadequate blood flow
- Rapid, weak, and irregular pulse
- Bluish skin from lack of oxygenated blood supply

Stage III: These symptoms pose danger of rapid death. Anyone experiencing one of these reactions

must receive *immediate emergency medical attention* (Gold 1986).

- Ventricular fibrillation (irregularities of nerve impulses governing heartbeat)
- Overall failure of circulation
- Ashen, gray skin
- Undetectable pulse
- Heart attacks
- Heart stops beating

Some psychological effects from the use of cocaine are extreme mood swings, delusions of extraordinary ability, loss of mental function, and distortion of perception. Cocaine users seek feelings of rapture, exhilaration, confidence, and well-being, as well as sexual excitement.

When the "high" is reached, some common effects are euphoria, talkativeness, contentment, alertness, a need for less sleep, heightened self-awareness, altered sexual feelings, humor, physical neglect, perceptual changes, compulsive behavior, and addiction.

Serious adverse effects include continuous colds, bronchitis, upper respiratory tract infections, asthma, insomnia, anxiety, depression, high blood pressure, circulatory problems, cardiac problems, epilepsy, diabetes, as well as severe digestive disorders, dehydration, anorexia, hallucinations, abscesses, and seizures. Refer to Table 24–3 for the physical, psychological, and withdrawal effects of cocaine abuse.

NICOTINE AND CAFFEINE

Nicotine can act as a stimulant, depressant, or tranquilizer. Because nicotine is one of the most perniciously addicting drugs in common use, most tobacco users are "hooked" and, in effect, locked into the effects of tobacco.

Nicotine (cigarettes, snuff, chewing tobacco) and caffeine (coffee, tea) are common drugs used by people throughout the world. People who smoke over 10 cigarettes a day know how difficult it is to stop smoking once their bodies have become dependent on the drug. It is well known that many medical conditions are associated with and most certainly caused by cigarettes (see Table 24–1). Despite this, many people continue to smoke and use other forms of tobacco because attempting to stop smoking involves enduring severe withdrawal symptoms (see Table 24–3).

Most Americans take caffeine by way of coffee, tea, or cola drinks. People take coffee as a drug—"I've got to have two cups in the morning to function"; for social reasons—"Let's get together for coffee"; or as a reward—"After I finish this job, I'm going to take a coffee break." One cup of coffee contains 100—150 mg of caffeine. Intoxication can result from ingestion of more than 250 mg of caffeine. Restlessness, excitement, cardiac arrhythmias, and nervousness are some of the signs of caffeine intoxication (see Table 24–3).

All stimulants accelerate the normal functioning of the body and affect the CNS. Common signs of stimulant abuse include dilation of the pupils, dryness of the oronasal cavity, and excessive motor activity.

When a person who has ingested a stimulant experiences chest pain, has an irregular pulse, or has a history of heart trouble, the person should be taken to an emergency room immediately.

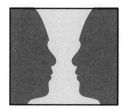

Case Study: Working with a Person Dependent on Cocaine

Fred, aged 17, is an only child of parents who have been separated and divorced for over seven years. Prior to their divorce, the marriage had been described as very chaotic. The parents reportedly had frequent arguments in which they screamed at and occasionally hit each other.

Following the divorce, Fred's parents were awarded joint custody of Fred. Fred would spend two weeks each month with each parent. Fred's father, Mr. F., was an alcoholic whose own father had been distant and rigid. When drunk, Mr. F. would become belligerent and often fight with Fred. The arguments would be heated and occasionally physical.

Fred's mother was a passive-aggressive woman whose father was a belligerent alcoholic. Fred never appeared happy or at ease with either parent. Fred began using cocaine at the age of 15, when he had quite a bit of time on his hands because he had dropped out of school. During this period he usually spent his days "hanging out" at a nearby mall.

During the previous seven months, Fred had been arrested three times for possession of cocaine. When questioned regarding his cocaine abuse, Fred stated that at this point he believes that he has his addiction under control and is not in need of treatment. Mr. and Mrs. F. brought Fred to the hospital, stating that he is unmanageable. Fred was restless and talkative. He stated that he felt great and wanted to leave. His pupils were dilated and nonreactive to light, and his pulse and blood pressure were elevated. His clothes were soaked with sweat. His parents were very vocal, and his mother announced that the next time Fred was arrested, he would be charged as an adult and have a felony conviction.

Assessment

SIGNS OF INTOXICATION AND WITHDRAWAL

In assessing Fred, the nurse observed the following signs of cocaine intoxication:

1. Psychomotor agitation
2. Elation
3. Grandiosity
4. Loquacity
5. Hypervigilance
6. Tachycardia
7. Pupils dilated and nonreactive to light
8. Elevated blood pressure
9. Diaphoresis
10. Nausea and vomiting

PHYSICAL COMPLICATIONS

At present none were noted.

PERSONAL HISTORY AND COPING STYLE

From an interview, the nurse was able to assess Fred's perception of his cocaine use.

Dialogue	Therapeutic Tool/Comment
N: I understand you entered the treatment program yesterday afternoon after your court appearance.	Nurse places the event in time and sequence, validating the precipitating event.
F: Yeah—It was my Dad's idea.	
N: Well, what do you think of the idea?	Encouraging evaluation (actions first, thoughts, then feelings).

Continued on following page

Assessment
(Continued)

Dialogue	Therapeutic Tool/Comment
F: I don't like it. I don't need this place. I'm not a junkie—I just use cocaine, that's all. I can handle it.	
N: From what I've heard, your involvement with cocaine has gotten you into trouble.	Pointing out realities.
F: Yeah, well, I guess I can't deny that . . . but I still don't think I need this place.	
N: Are you saying that you don't think you need a treatment program?	Validating the client's perception.
F: Well, I don't know, I guess maybe I am messed up a bit.	
N: "Messed up."	Restating.
F: Yeah.	
N: What is one thing about you that's messed up?	Nurse encourages client to be specific rather than global.
F: (*Silence*) . . . I guess I feel like I don't belong anywhere.	
N: Talk more about that.	

DRUG HISTORY

Fred told the nurse that he started taking cocaine about two years before at a party. Before that time he drank "with the guys" and "smoked a little pot." He said that now he took alcohol to soften the withdrawal from cocaine when he couldn't get diazepam or methaqualone (Quaaludes). He took the drug intranasally (snorted) and had been tempted to freebase but was frightened. He was presently taking the drug six or seven times a week intranasally. After talking to the nurse and weighing possible future legal complications, Fred agreed to enter the inpatient drug treatment program.

Nursing Diagnosis

Some nursing diagnoses pertaining to Fred follow:

1. *Dysfunctional grieving* related to parental divorce
2. *Knowledge deficit* related to detrimental effects of cocaine
3. *Diversional activity deficit* related to interests or life plan
4. *Ineffective individual coping* related to inadequate psychological resources
5. *Ineffective family coping* related to substance abuse by parents

Planning

CONTENT LEVEL—PLANNING GOALS

Fred and the nurse established goals relevant to each of the nursing diagnoses.

Nursing Diagnosis	Long Term Goals	Short Term Goals
1. *Dysfunctional grieving* related to parental divorce	1. The client will gain an understanding of his underlying feelings regarding his parents' divorce by the time of discharge.	1. The client will meet with his parents in family counseling sessions and discuss his feelings by (date).
2. *Knowledge deficit* related to detrimental effects of cocaine	2. The client will gain knowledge regarding substance abuse and its effects on the body and mind by the time of discharge.	2. The client will attend group educational sessions on substance abuse on four occasions (dates).

3. *Diversional activity deficit* related to lack of interests or life plan

3. The client will have definite plans for his leisure time by the time of discharge.

3. The client will name three activities that interest him and that he would like to get involved in by (date).

4. *Ineffective individual coping* related to inadequate psychological resources

4. The client will state that he feels better able to cope with his feelings by the time of discharge.

4. The client will be able to cope with his painful feelings through participation in group therapy sessions by (date).

5. *Ineffective family coping* related to substance abuse by parents

5. Parents will agree on response (limits) if Fred gets into trouble again by discharge.

5. Client will be able to tell parents how he feels about their divorce.

PROCESS LEVEL—NURSES' REACTIONS AND FEELINGS

The nurse had had to work out many of the personal feelings and reactions she used to have regarding a person dependent on an illicit drug. Her mother had had a serious alcohol problem and had abused diazepam for many years. The nurse had found that going to Al-Anon and other support groups, as well as attending seminars geared toward understanding and working with people dependent on a psychoactive substance, had helped her sort out many of her angry and confused feelings and had altered her initial reactions to people with substance abuse problems. She was aware that most nurses have strong, often negative, reactions to and feelings about people with drug dependence problems. When supervising her colleagues and peers, she encouraged discussion of personal feelings toward drug-dependent clients during staff meetings to maximize the staff's therapeutic value.

Intervention

The inpatient unit combined various appropriate educational programs, family involvement, group therapy with peers, and individual sessions with the primary nurse.

The nurse decided on a set of actions appropriate for reaching each short term goal. These nursing interventions should be seen as guidelines for all nursing staff working with the client to aid in maintaining continuity of care.

Short Term Goals	Interventions
1. The client will meet with his parents in family sessions and discuss his feelings by (date).	1a. Give the client positive support during one-to-one interactions. 1b. Discuss with the client his feelings toward his parents. 1c. Encourage client to participate actively in this phase of treatment.
2. The client will attend group educational sessions on substance abuse every other day, starting on (date).	2a. Discuss with the client the material from the educational sessions on an individual basis. 2b. Answer any questions the client may have. 2c. Reinforce the main points made during the educational sessions.
3. The client will name three activities that interest him and that he would like to get involved in by (date).	3a. Encourage the client to discuss activities that he has enjoyed in the past and that he is good at. 3b. Give client realistic feedback regarding his choices.

Continued on following page

Intervention
(Continued)

Short Term Goals	Interventions
	3c. Provide information regarding additional activities.
4. The client will cope with his painful feelings through participation in group and individual therapy sessions by (date).	4a. Approach the client in an open and positive manner.
	4b. Encourage the client to name painful feelings in a supportive one-to-one session.
	4c. Discuss with the client his support system.

Evaluation

Periodically, Fred and his nurse evaluated the goals.

Short Term Goals	Evaluation
1. The client will meet with his parents in family sessions and discuss his feelings and concerns by (date).	1. As of said date, the client and his mother met, but the father refused to come.
2. The client will attend group educational sessions on substance abuse every other day, starting on (date).	2. As of said date, goal was partially met. The client attended two of the four sessions scheduled.
3. The client will name three activities that interest him and that he would like to get involved in by (date).	3. As of said date, goal was partially met. Fred decided on two activities and has started one—lifting weights in the gym.
4. The client will cope with his painful feelings through participation in group and individual therapy sessions by (date).	4. Goal was partially met. As of said date, client had been verbalizing his feelings in both group and individual sessions.

The family met four times before Fred's dad dropped out. During a session that was evaluating family drug use, Fred's dad left, saying that Fred's problem had nothing to do with him. Fred's mother began to talk to the nurse about her own problems and decided to have individual therapy.

Fred decided to remain with his mother and visit his father periodically when his dad was not drinking. Fred and his mother began to talk a little more about themselves and their feelings. Fred continued his group sessions and was able to listen and share with peers who were experiencing many of the same feelings and were faced with similar problems. He began to feel less isolated and alone and had found one place where he got support and belonged. He still became depressed and often felt lonely, but he told his therapist that he didn't feel so helpless and believed things might get better for him.

Summary

Amphetamines have been around a long time as "diet pills" and "pep pills." They are often abused by students, athletes, and entertainers. Amphetamines are now medically indicated only for hyperkinesis in children and for narcolepsy. Intoxication includes euphoria, impairment in social and occupational functioning, increased energy, impaired judgment, and assaultiveness. Amphetamine psychosis results in symptoms similar to those seen in paranoid schizophrenia (e.g., paranoid delusions; visual, auditory, or tactile hallucinations; high risk for violence; and panic reaction). Overdose of amphetamines and cocaine or crack can lead to hyperpyrexia, convulsions, respiratory depression, and cardiovascular shock. One difference between cocaine or crack and amphetamines is the rate of action. Amphetamines are long-acting and cocaine is short-acting, and dependence develops more rapidly with cocaine and crack.

Nicotine can act as a stimulant and is legal. Consistent use results in dependence on the drug. Despite the harmful effects of nicotine (see Table 24–1), people find it a difficult drug to give up.

The case study highlighted teenage addiction, assessment, planning, and interventions for a young man who was using cocaine.

Narcotics

OBJECTIVES ■

After studying this section on narcotics, the student will be able to

1. Compare and contrast the symptoms of narcotic intoxication with those of narcotic withdrawal.
2. Discuss the pros and cons of the following treatments for narcotic addictions, including which clients are most suited to each type of treatment:
   A. Methadone or LAAM (L-alpha-acetyl methadol) maintenance
   B. Therapeutic communities
   C. Self-help, abstinence-oriented model

Introduction

Opium is derived from the dried juice of the poppy, *Papaver somniferum,* and is an opiate. *Morphine, heroin,* and *codeine* are opiates and belong to the class called narcotics. *Methadone* and *meperidine* (Demerol) are narcotics referred to as opioids rather than opiates. Opium is a raw natural product, and morphine is the chief active ingredient in opium. Each grain of opium contains about one tenth of a grain of morphine. Heroin is produced by heating morphine in the presence of acetic acid (the acid found in vinegar). Heroin is converted back to morphine in the body.

Opium is usually taken orally or "smoked"—that is, it is heated, and its vapors inhaled. Morphine and heroin can also be sniffed, injected under the skin, into a muscle, or, for maximum effect, directly into a vein ("mainlined").

During the nineteenth century, opium was sold legally and was inexpensive. Opiates and countless pharmaceutical preparations containing them were freely accessible.

However, opiate use was frowned on in some circles as immoral. Although deemed immoral, opiate use in the nineteenth century was not subject to the moral sanctions of today—for example, employees were not fired for addiction. Overall, addicts continued to participate fully in the community. Thus, the nineteenth century escaped from one of the most disastrous effects of current narcotics laws and attitudes—the rise of a deviant addict subculture, cut off from respectable society.

During this time, opiates were prescribed for pain as well as for coughs,. diarrhea, dysentery, and many other illnesses. It was not until 1906, when Congress passed the first Pure Food and Drug Act, that a major step forward was taken in control of opiate addiction. This act required that medicines containing opiates be so labeled. In 1914 Congress passed the Harrison Narcotics Act, which cut off altogether the supply of legal opiates to addicts, leading to the production and sale of adulterated, contaminated, and misbranded black-market narcotics.

Codeine is found in small quantities in opium; ordinarily it is taken orally. It is a narcotic and can be addictive if enough is taken. At one time, many cough syrups contained codeine, such as turpin hydrate and codeine elixir, and addicts would buy large quantities. There are tighter controls on codeine cough syrups now.

Methadone is a synthetic narcotic that generally resembles morphine and heroin in its effects but is not derived from opium. It was first synthesized in Germany in 1943, when opiate analgesics were not available because of the war, and was first called Dolophine. Methadone is an effective analgesic, and its physiological effects are the same as those of morphine and heroin. It is a narcotic and produces both psychological and physical dependence. First, tolerance to methadone develops, then physical dependence occurs as repeated doses are taken, and finally withdrawal symptoms take place when the drug is stopped or reduced. One of methadone's most useful properties is its cross-tolerance with other narcotics. When methadone reaches a sufficiently high level in the blood (40 mg), it can block the euphoric effects of heroin. Withdrawal symptoms of people physically dependent on heroin or morphine, including postaddiction craving, can be suppressed by oral administration of methadone. Doses range from 20–80 mg (sometimes up to 120 mg). Refer to Table 24–4 for signs of intoxication, overdose, and withdrawal and treatment.

REVIEW OF ACCEPTED TREATMENTS FOR NARCOTIC ADDICTIONS

Essentially, there are three different models for the treatment of chemical dependency: (1) methadone maintenance, (2) therapeutic communities, and (3) self-help, abstinence-oriented recovery (Klein and Miller 1986).

Methadone Maintenance

During the 1980s, an estimated 70,000–75,000 clients were being treated with methadone. **Methadone** is effective only for approximately 24–36 hours, so the client usually takes methadone every day. A methadone maintenance program is not considered to be an effective treatment in itself. At times, it does keep the client out of the illegal drug subculture, but to be successful, programs have to include counseling and job training sessions.

In the mid-1970s, experimental clinical use began with a longer-acting drug called **L-alpha-acetyl methadol,** or LAAM. **LAAM** is effective for up to three days (72–96 hours), so clients need to come in for their dose only three times a week. This makes it easier for clients to hold down jobs and gives them more freedom than with methadone maintenance. LAAM is also

an addictive narcotic: its therapeutic effects and side effects are the same as those of morphine, including withdrawal symptoms after tolerance has developed (Ling and Blaine 1979). As of July 1993, LAAM has been approved for the treatment of opioid dependence in the United States.

Naltrexone (Trexan) is a relatively pure antagonist that blocks the euphoric effects of opioids. It has low toxicity with few side effects. A single dose provides an effective opiate blockade for up to 72 hours. Taking naltrexone three times a week is sufficient to maintain a fairly high level of opiate blockade. For many clients, long term use results in gradual extinction of drug-seeking behaviors. Naltrexone does *not* produce dependence (Frances and Franklin 1988). In 1971, the United States Congress mandated a large-scale increase in research on narcotic antagonistic drugs. Naltrexone appears to be the best narcotic antagonist that has been developed to date.

As mentioned earlier, **clonidine,** widely used as an antihypertensive, has been found to be a nonopioid suppressor of opioid withdrawal symptoms (Frances and Franklin 1988). Several studies have demonstrated encouraging results using clonidine and naltrexone in treating opiate withdrawal (Charney et al. 1986; Frances and Franklin 1988); however, at this writing, clonidine has not received FDA approval for opioid detoxification.

Therapeutic Communities

Therapeutic communities (TCs), or self-regulating communities, operate on the hypothesis that drug use is a symptom of an underlying character disorder or emotional immaturity. These programs have as a main goal a complete change in lifestyle: abstinence from drugs, elimination of criminal behavior, and development of employable skills, self-reliance, and personal honesty.

There are more than 300 residential TCs in the United States. The TC program includes encounter group therapy, various levels of educational programs, and assigned jobs within the community. TCs use self-government and group pressures, instead of relying on a professional therapeutic staff, to change immature behaviors. Residents of traditional TCs stay for at least 15 months.

Self-help, Abstinence-Oriented Model

Self-help groups patterned after Alcoholics Anonymous—for example, NA, Chemical Dependency Anonymous, and Cocaine Anonymous—help teach in-

Table 24–4 ■ DRUG INFORMATION: NARCOTICS (OPIATES AND OPIOIDS)*

DRUG	INTOXICATION	OVERDOSE Effects	OVERDOSE Possible Treatments	WITHDRAWAL Effects	WITHDRAWAL Possible Treatments

NARCOTICS
Opium (paragenic)
Heroine
Meperidine
  (Demerol)
Morphine
Codeine
Methadone
  (Dolophine)
Hydromorphone
  (Dilaudid)
	PHYSICAL:
	Pupils constricted
	Decreased respiration
	Drowsiness
	Decrease in blood pressure
	Slurred speech
	Psychomotor retardation
	
	PSYCHOLOGICAL/
	  PERCEPTUAL:
	Euphoria
	Dysphoria
	Impairment of attention/memory
	Impaired judgment
		Pupils may be dilated due to anoxia
		Respiratory depression/arrest
		Coma
		Shock
		Convulsions
		Death
			Narcotic antagonist
			—e.g., naloxone (Narcan)
			quickly reverses central nervous system depression
				Yawning
				Anorexia
				Insomnia
				Irritability
				Runny nose (rhinorrhea)
				Panic
				Diaphoresis
				Cramps
				Nausea
				Bone pain
				Chills
				Dilated pupils
					Supportive measures if not life threatening
					
					Short-acting drugs
					—e.g., heroin, morphine
					Peak 48–72 hours
					Course 7–10 days
					
					Long-acting drugs—
					e.g., methadone
					Peak 3–8 days
					Course several weeks

Data from Grinspoon and Bakalar 1985; Smith 1984; Bittle et al. 1986; APA 1987; Jaffe 1985.
*DEFINITION: An opiate derivative or synthetic that affects the CNS and the autonomic nervous system. Medically used primarily as analgesic (pain killer). Consistent use causes tolerance and distressing withdrawal symptoms.

dividuals to face the seriousness of their problem and provide hope and support. Usually, the person first enters the detoxification unit, then may spend some time in the hospital, and finally is referred for outpatient therapy (usually group) and self-help groups.

Klein and Miller (1986) state that generally the *abstinence-oriented model* is best suited for individuals who are somewhat motivated and who are still in the early stage of drug dependence. The *therapeutic community* is best suited for individuals who have a long history of anti-social behavior, especially those ordered there by the court. The *methadone maintenance program* is appropriate for those who have failed at several attempts at abstinence and who are unable to stabilize their lives.

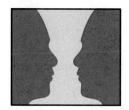

Case Study: Working with a Person Dependent on an Opiate

Bill K., a 20-year-old single man, was brought to the emergency room in a coma. He was accompanied by his mother, with whom Bill lives in a small apartment. Bill had been in his room at home. When his mother was not able to arouse him, she dialed 911 for an ambulance. A syringe and some white powder were found next to Bill.

Bill's breathing was labored, and his pupils were constricted. Vital signs were taken; his blood pressure was 60/40, and his pulse was 132. Bill's situation was determined to be life-threatening.

Bill's mother was extremely distressed, but she was able to report to the staff that Bill had a substance abuse problem and had been taking heroin for six months before entering a methadone maintenance program.

It was determined at this point to administer a narcotic antagonist, and naloxone (Narcan) was given intramuscularly. Following this, Bill's breathing improved, and he responded to verbal stimuli.

Bill's mother later told staff that Bill had been in the methadone maintenance program for the past year but had not attended the program or received his methadone for the past week.

Assessment

SIGNS OF INTOXICATION AND WITHDRAWAL

In an emergency situation, when a patient has overdosed, a history taken from reliable family members, physical examination, and laboratory test (toxicological screening for drugs in blood and urine) as well as analysis of gastric contents provide data for the initial assessment. Bill's physical signs supported the diagnosis of heroin overdose:

Continued on following page

Assessment
(Continued)

1. Constricted pupils (in severe overdose, pupils will be dilated from anoxia)
2. Drowsiness
3. Slurred speech
4. Hypotension
5. Euphoria
6. Dysphoria
7. Apathy
8. Psychomotor retardation
9. Impaired judgment

Other signs and symptoms of intoxication include

PHYSICAL COMPLICATIONS

Bill's mother stated that Bill had problems with constipation; other than that, he appeared healthy to her.

PERSONAL HISTORY AND COPING STYLE

The assessment of psychological status is a part of any nursing assessment, as is an assessment of the client's physical health.

Because Bill's situation was life-threatening, an initial assessment had to be made very quickly. Initially an interview with Bill was not possible; therefore, information had to be gathered from Bill's mother.

DRUG HISTORY

Bill had been attending a methadone maintenance program for the past year, after six months of heroin dependence. His mother stated that he also drank beer and whisky, but she did not know how much.

Nursing Diagnosis

Some nursing diagnoses that pertain to Bill, who had abused heroin, include the following:

1. *Ineffective individual coping* related to failure to develop adequate coping strategies
2. *Noncompliance* related to lack of autonomy in health-seeking behaviors

Planning

CONTENT LEVEL—PLANNING GOALS

Some goals for the client who abuses narcotics follow:

Nursing Diagnosis	Long Term Goals	Short Term Goals
1. *Ineffective individual coping* related to substance abuse—heroin	1. Bill will demonstrate two effective coping skills by discharge.	1. Bill will demonstrate one effective coping skill by (date).
2. *Noncompliance* related to lack of autonomy in health-seeking behaviors	2. Bill will realistically discuss short term goals and available treatment modalities with the nurse and health care team.	2a. Bill will discuss several treatment modalities with the nurse by (date). 2b. Bill will realistically discuss short term goals with the nurse in light of available treatment modalities by (date).

Mr. Samuels, Bill's assigned nurse, identified nursing actions appropriate for reaching each goal. These nursing interventions should be seen as guidelines for all nursing staff working with the client, which maintain continuity of care. Some examples follow:

Short Term Goals	Interventions
1. Bill will demonstrate two effective coping skills by (date).	1a. Approach the client in a positive and open manner. 1b. Provide information about local self-help groups for substance abusers.

1c. Discuss possible alternative behaviors for client to use when anxious or depressed.

1d. Explore with the client coping strategies that used to work for him in the past.

2. Bill will discuss short term goals and available treatment modalities with the nurse by (date).

2a. Obtain a thorough history of substance abuse, including the particular drug(s) taken, length of use, route of administration, and drug preference.

2b. Present history to health care team and evaluate available treatment modalities and community resources.

2c. The health care team will meet with Bill regarding discharge planning.

PROCESS LEVEL—NURSES' REACTIONS AND FEELINGS

Mr. Samuels was a Vietnam veteran. During the war, he had seen many of his friends and colleagues become dependent on opiates. It was during this time that he became familiar with the physical and psychological effects of and long term problems associated with opiate dependence. He had witnessed the disruption and negative changes in the lives of many of his friends.

Intervention

Mr. Samuels knew that Bill's future ultimately rested with Bill. Mr. Samuels talked to Bill regarding his perceptions of his situation, where Bill wanted to go, and what Bill thought he needed to get there.

Dialogue	Therapeutic Tool/Comment
N: Bill, I was in the emergency room Friday afternoon when you were brought in by ambulance.	Placing the event in time and sequence, validating the precipitating event.
B: Were you? I guess a lot of people thought it was over for me.	
N: It certainly looked quite serious.	Emphasizing the reality—*prevents* minimizing situation.
B: Yeah. . . . I should have never left the program. . . . I was doing better, and I just didn't think I needed it anymore.	
N: You said you were doing well.	Reflecting.
B: Yeah. . . . I had a job, and I was beginning to save some money. Wow! I can't believe I blew this whole thing.	
N: I don't know that you really did. Your counselor for the program phoned Dr. L. this morning to find out how you were doing.	Pointing out reality.
B: Do you think they will take me back?	
N: Why don't we talk some more, and after we finish, I'll speak with the other staff about your situation. If you would like to get back into the program, you can call your counselor and we'll support your decision.	Gathering information.

Mr. Samuels met with the other members of the health care team and reviewed the following alternatives for opiate dependent individuals and discussed what might be suitable for Bill.

Evaluation

After reviewing Bill's history, the health care team decided that the self-help, abstinence-oriented recovery treatment might be most helpful. Bill had not been on drugs a long time, he had a job, and he appeared motivated. Naltrexone (Trexan) would be given in conjunction with outpatient therapy and regular attendance at NA meetings.

Three months after discharge, Bill visited Mr. Samuels on the unit. Bill told Mr. Samuels that one of the guys in his neighborhood just died of an overdose, and he was really shaken up. He stated that his job was just OK, but he had made some friends in NA. It was too soon to make any long term plans.

Summary

Opium, morphine, heroin, and codeine are opiates and belong to the class *narcotics*. Methadone and meperidine are nonopiate narcotics referred to as opioids. In 1914, the Harrison Narcotic Act banned the use of narcotics without a prescription.

Signs of intoxication include constricted pupils, drowsiness, decreased blood pressure, psychomotor retardation, and impairment in memory and social functioning. Overdose can lead to respiratory depression, shock, convulsions, and death. Treatment of overdose can be dramatically affected with a narcotic antagonist such as *naloxone* (Narcan). Withdrawal symptoms include yawning, rhinorrhea, insomnia, diaphoresis, muscle cramps, "bone pain," chills, and dilated pupils. Treatment for withdrawal symptoms, which usually are not life-threatening, is mostly supportive.

Treatment modalities vary. Somatic treatment includes *methadone maintenance* (one dose is effective for 24–36 hours) and LAAM (one dose is effective for up to 3 days) as drugs of substitution. These drugs block the craving for, and withdrawal symptoms from, heroin and enable the addicted person to work and carry on a normal social life. One drawback is that these drugs also are addicting and can also produce withdrawal symptoms. *Naltrexone* (Trexan) a narcotic antagonist, is an effective opiate blocker for up to 72 hours and has been a successful treatment modality for many.

Other modalities of treatment include therapeutic communities and self-help, abstinence-oriented therapy. The indication for each form of treatment has been outlined in this section.

P sychotomimetics

OBJECTIVES ■

After studying this section on psychotomimetics, the student will be able to

1. Compare and contrast the signs and symptoms of low-dose, moderate-dose, and high-dose phencyclidine piperidine (PCP) intoxication.
2. Discuss what is meant by *synesthesia* and give two examples.
3. Define *flashback* and give an example.
4. Identify three possible long term results from heavy chronic marijuana use.

Introduction

Psychotomimetics are also known as hallucinogens or mind-altering drugs. People have known and written about hallucinogens for centuries. Our discussion of the psychotomimetics includes phencyclidine piperidine (PCP), LSD and LSD-like drugs, and *Cannabis sativa* (marijuana).

PCP

PCP was first synthesized in 1926, and 30 years later experimental use on human beings began (Shulgin and MacLean 1976). Findings from research studies on humans led to the use of PCP for surgical anesthesia, and PCP was patented under the trade name *Sernyl* in 1960. After five years, it became evident that Sernyl produced many adverse side effects, including acute anxiety, agitation, hallucinations, delirium, muscle rigidity, and seizures (Burns et al. 1975). The acute anxiety experiences responded to brief therapeutic interventions, but acute psychosis caused by PCP resolves slowly (Table 24–5). The severity and frequency of these side effects soon led to the withdrawal of Sernyl from the market for human use.

Since 1967, PCP has been available legally only for use as an anesthetic in veterinary medicine. It was during this same year that its use as a street drug was first reported by Meyers et al. (1967–1968). In various regions of the country, PCP is known as the animal tranquilizer, angel dust, or the **p**eace **p**ill. It can be manufactured from a few readily available chemicals and is relatively simple to synthesize. The illegally produced PCP is manufactured in many forms: powders, pills, capsules, and liquids. It is smoked, sniffed, swallowed, injected, and even used as eye drops.

The route of administration plays a significant role in the severity of PCP intoxication. The onset of symptoms from oral ingestion occurs in about one hour. When taken intravenously, sniffed, or smoked, the onset of symptoms may develop within five minutes (APA 1987). The signs and symptoms of PCP intoxication may range from acute anxiety to acute psychosis. The cardinal signs of both the PCP low-dose experience and the high-toxicity experience include a "blank stare," ataxia, muscle rigidity, vertical and horizontal nystagmus, tendencies toward violence, and generalized anesthesia that lessens the sensations of touch and pain, making staff interventions difficult. *High doses* may lead to hyperthermia, agitated and repetitive movements, chronic jerking of the extremities, hypertension, and kidney failure. Persons with PCP intoxication may become stuporous with their eyes open, may be comatose, or may experience status epilepticus or respiratory arrest (Grinspoon and Bakalar 1985). (see Table 24–5.)

The behavior of a client on PCP often presents difficult management problems for the nursing staff. Client safety is an important issue because the client may fluctuate between immobility and aggressive outbursts. The amount of direct nursing care required varies with the amount of PCP ingested, route of administration, time lapse since last ingestion, and chronicity of use.

PCP Intoxication

LOW DOSE. Clients with **PCP intoxication,** even those requiring minimally restrictive care (those with low-dose toxicity, who have ingested 1–5 mg of PCP), sometimes place themselves in hazardous situations. This possible danger-to-self behavior requires that the client be placed in an environment with minimal, controlled stimuli (Peterson and Stillman 1979). Because of the possibility of paranoia in the client, the environment should be kept as unrestrictive as possible. Seclusion or restraints are indicated only when danger to self or others is present. Limited contact with one staff member should also be maintained with the client. When contact with the client is established, the nurse is careful not to violate the client's personal space.

Please note: Although only one person should interact with the client, no one person should be alone with the client who has ingested PCP. An adequate number of staff members should be present to manage the client if an assaultive situation develops.

The need for monitoring vital signs periodically should be assessed in terms of how agitated the person becomes. Often the physician will order diazepam to reduce agitation and aid sleep. These clients may lose a significant amount of fluids through diaphoresis, and they should be encouraged to drink acidic fruit juices, such as cranberry juice, to replace fluid. Substances such as cranberry juice, ascorbic acid, and ammonium chloride, which acidify the urine, increase the excretion of PCP from the body.

MODERATE DOSE. Clients who have ingested 5–15 mg of PCP (moderate-dose toxicity) present more difficult management problems. Usually these clients are uncommunicative and very stimuli sensitive. They also may exhibit sleep pattern disturbances, varying from continual drowsiness to wakefulness, and can quickly become agitated and combative. This assaul-

Table 24–5 ■ DRUG INFORMATION: PSYCHOTOMIMETICS (HALLUCINOGENS) *

DRUG	INTOXICATION	OVERDOSE		WITHDRAWAL	
		Effects	Possible Treatments	Effects	Possible Treatments
HALLUCINOGENS LSD (lysergic acid diethylamide) Mescaline (peyote) Psilocybin	PHYSICAL: Pupils dilated Tachycardia Diaphoresis Palpitations Tremors Incoordination Elevated temperature, pulse, respiration PSYCHOLOGICAL/ PERCEPTUAL: Fear of going crazy Paranoid ideas Marked anxiety/depression **Synesthesia**—e.g., colors are heard; sounds are seen Depersonalization Hallucinations although sensorium clear Grandiosity—e.g., thinking one can fly	Psychosis Brain damage Death	Keep client in room with low stimuli —minimal light, sound, activity Have one person stay with client— reassure client, "talk down client" Speak slowly and clearly in low voice Diazepam or chloral hydrate for extreme anxiety tension **NOTE:. PCP and LSD-like drugs have different treatments.**	None known	**NOTE: Tolerance develops quickly.**
PCP (phencyclidine piperidine)	PHYSICAL: Vertical or horizontal nystagmus Increased blood pressure, pulse, and temperature Ataxia Muscle rigidity Seizures Blank stare Chronic jerking Agitated, repetitive movements PSYCHOLOGICAL/ PERCEPTUAL: Maladaptive behavior changes Belligerence, assaultiveness, impulsiveness, unpredictability Impaired judgment, social and occupational functioning SEVERE EFFECTS: Hallucinations, paranoia Bizarre behaviors— e.g., barking like a dog, grimacing, repetitive chanting speech	Psychosis Possible hypertensive crisis/cardiovascular accident Respiratory arrest Hyperthermia Seizures	IF ALERT: Caution: If gastric lavage is used, can lead to laryngeal spasms or aspiration Acidify urine (cranberry juice, ascorbic acid); in acute stage, ammonium chloride—may continue for 10 to 14 days Room with minimal stimuli **Do *not* talk down!** Speak slowly, clearly, and in low voice *Diazepam* may be used for agitation *Haloperidol* may be used for severe behavioral disturbance (*not* **a phenothiazine)** MEDICAL INTERVENTION FOR: Hyperthermia High blood pressure Respiratory distress Hypertension	*Tolerance and withdrawal reactions have been reported:* Lethargy Craving Depression **NOTE: Takes 24–48 hours to recover from a high Stays in urine for a week or more Long term effects of chronic PCP abuse may include** ● **Dulled thinking** ● **Lethargy** ● **Loss of memory and impulse control** ● **Depression**	

Table 24-5 ■ DRUG INFORMATION: PSYCHOTOMIMETICS (HALLUCINOGENS) * *Continued*

DRUG	INTOXICATION	OVERDOSE		WITHDRAWAL	
		Effects	Possible Treatments	Effects	Possible Treatments
	Regressive behavior —e.g., public masturbation Violent bizarre behavior, including homicide and suicide Very labile behaviors				
CANNABIS SATIVA (marijuana, hashish)	PHYSICAL: Tachycardia Conjunctional injection Increased appetite Impaired motor ability Talkative PSYCHOLOGICAL/ PERCEPTUAL: Euphoria Intensification of perceptions Apathy Excessive anxiety/paranoia Impaired judgment Slowed perception of time Inappropriate hilarity Impaired memory Heightened sensitivity to external stimuli	Fatigue Paranoia Psychosis—rarely seen			Duration of effects: Smoking: 2–4 hours Ingestion: 5–12 hours **NOTE: Cannabis dependence is associated with such psychological symptoms as** ● **Lethargy** ● **Anhedonia (inability to enjoy life)** ● **Difficulty concentrating** ● **Memory problems**

Data from Grinspoon and Bakalar 1985; Smith 1984; Bittle 1986; APA 1987.

*DEFINITION: Produce abnormal mental phenomena in the cognitive and perceptual spheres. For example, distortion in space and time, hallucinations, delusions (paranoid or grandiose), and synesthesia may occur.

tiveness often is accompanied by periods of amnesia, stupor, and other bizarre behavior (Cohen 1987). Ataxia, generalized twitching, and myoclonic rigidity are seen frequently during the waxing and waning psychotic episodes. Diazepam may be used for its tranquilizing effects and also to reduce severe convulsions. Haloperidol may be used to reduce the aggressive, combative behavior. *Phenothiazines should* NOT *be used because they potentiate the anticholinergic actions of* PCP.

HIGH DOSE. When a client has ingested over 15 mg of PCP (high-dose toxicity), the situation is considered a severe psychiatric emergency, as this is the most life-threatening level of intoxication (Burns et al. 1975; Cohen 1987). This toxic drug state presents a very complex, confusing picture. The person's behavioral, mental, and physical status is unpredictable. Nurses, while maintaining a minimal amount of verbal and tactile stimulation, must resort to the most restrictive forms of physical restraint to

prevent injury or harm to the client or others. Auditory hallucinations, mania, delusions, and severe agitation are typical symptoms (Luisada and Brown 1976). Mental states of disorientation, amnesia, and autistic thought processes also may be noted (Cohen 1987). These clients are also at physical risk because of the possibility of seizures, hyperpyrexia, respiratory distress, and coma. The client may need external respiratory assistance or external cooling to reduce dangerously high body temperatures. Blood pressure may have to be reduced to safe levels and convulsions controlled. After the coma lightens, the patient typically becomes delirious, paranoid, and violently assaultive.

Some chronic PCP users suffer from dulled thinking and reflexes, loss of memory and impulse control, depression, lethargy, and difficulty in concentrating (Grinspoon and Bakalar 1985). Refer to Table 24–5 for physical and psychological signs of PCP intoxication and withdrawal symptoms plus medical treatments. A saying on the street is: "PCP—not an upper or a downer but an insideouter."

LSD AND LSD-LIKE DRUGS

LSD, mescaline (peyote), and psilocybin are hallucinogens. Mescaline and the mushroom *Psilocybe mexicana* (from which psilocybin is isolated) have been used for centuries in their religious rites by Indian peoples living in the southwestern United States and in northern Mexico. A term popular in the 1960s for the psychotomimetic drugs was "psychedelic," which in Greek means "for the soul to be manifest," emphasizing the subjective experience of expansion of consciousness reported by some users (Davison and Neale 1982). LSD was the drug of the 1960s. The hallucinogenic experience was called a "trip." A good trip is characterized by a marked slowing of time, lightheadedness, images in intense colors, and visions in sound **(synesthesia).** People report experiences of spiritual ecstasy or of being united with humankind. During a bad trip, a person may experience severe anxiety, paranoia, and terror compounded by distortions in time and distance. The terrorized person may become violent, unpredictably suicidal, or dangerously grandiose (e.g., thinking he or she can fly). The trip ends when the effects of the drug wear off (8–12 hours for LSD). The best treatment for a person experiencing a bad trip is reassurance, companionship, and protection. Occasionally a tranquilizer (diazepam, chloral hydrate) is indicated (Grinspoon and Bakalar 1985).

Flashbacks are a common effect of hallucinogenic drugs. Flashbacks are the transitory recurrence of psychotomimetic drug experiences when a person is drug-free. Such experiences as visual distortions, time expansion, loss of ego boundaries, and intense emotions are reported. Flashbacks are often mild and perhaps pleasant, but at other times individuals experience repeated recurrences of frightening images or thoughts (Grinspoon and Bakalar 1985). Flashbacks are more likely to occur when a person is fatigued or has smoked marijuana. Prolonged adverse reactions have occurred, lasting 24–48 hours. Reactions have been described as an anxiety attack, depressive reaction, and psychosis.

MARIJUANA (CANNABIS SATIVA)

Cannabis sativa is an Indian hemp plant. Tetrahydrocannabinol (THC) is the active ingredient found in the resin secreted from the flowering tops and leaves of the *Cannabis* plant. THC has mixed depressant and hallucinogenic properties. Marijuana, the leaves of the *Cannabis* plant, is generally smoked ("joint," "reefer," "roach"), but it can be ingested. Some of the many and variable effects of marijuana are listed below (Donlon and Rockwell 1982).

Desired effects:

- Euphoria, detachment, and relaxation.
- Sensations are intensified (e.g., sensory, auditory, visual).
- Time is drawn out.

Concurrent effects:

- Distance perceptions are distorted.
- Tendency toward distractibility, sociability, and hilarity.
- Increases appetite.

Undesirable effects:

- Impairment in ability to drive a car.
- Memory impairment.
- With high doses, hallucinogenic phenomena begin to appear.

Possible effects of heavy chronic use:

- Panic reactions.
- Psychosis.
- Flashbacks.

Individuals with schizophrenia, borderline, or affective disorders may have an exacerbation of symptoms after smoking marijuana. Marijuana users should be aware of the following facts:

1. The effect in the lungs of smoking one marijuana cigarette is equivalent to the effect of smoking twenty tobacco cigarettes. Also, the tar produced by marijuana is considered more carcinogenic than the tar of tobacco (Bittle et al. 1986).
2. Studies suggest that marijuana may be harmful to the reproductive system, although the results as yet are not conclusive. People planning on bearing children might want to exercise caution in marijuana use (Frances and Franklin 1988).
3. People who have abnormal heart function could have difficulty because marijuana increases the heart rate, sometimes dramatically.

Research is still needed, and studies are often conflicting. However, a pilot study found that marijuana-dependent high school students had short term memory defects during the study and after six weeks of abstinence from the drug (McConnell 1988).

Marijuana is often used in conjunction with other drugs of abuse, with which it may have a synergistic effect. For example, marijuana is often used with alcohol and cocaine. *Cannabis* is the most widely used illicit drug in the United States.

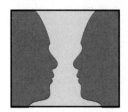

Case Study: Working with a Person in PCP Intoxication

Gina, a 14-year-old teenager, was brought to the emergency room after PCP ingestion. Gina presented with blunted affect. Her speech was incoherent at times, and she was disoriented to date and time.

This was Gina's first visit to the hospital, and she was accompanied by her parents, Mr. and Mrs. Tan.

Gina was described by her parents as having low self-esteem and thinking herself "ugly." They stated that she constantly strove to be accepted by her peers. Mr. and Mrs. Tan explained that recently Gina had been "hanging around" with a group of girls who appeared to them to be very involved in substance abuse. They believed that Gina had become involved with PCP through these girls, even though they had forbidden Gina to socialize with them.

Assessment

SIGNS OF INTOXICATION AND WITHDRAWAL

The nurse noticed

1. Horizontal nystagmus
2. Ataxia
3. Muscle rigidity
4. Agitation
5. Blank facial expression

PHYSICAL COMPLICATIONS

None apparent at present.

PERSONAL HISTORY AND COPING STYLE

According to Gina's parents, this was Gina's first experience with drugs. Gina had been home for over an hour when the symptoms were first noticed. When the nurse asked Mr. and Mrs. Tan about Gina's other friends, Mrs. Tan said, "Well . . . not too many . . . you see we like her to stay home where we can keep an eye on her." The nurse asked both parents what Gina does when she gets upset. Again Mrs. Tan replied rather sharply, "Gina doesn't get upset—why should she?" When the nurse asked Mr. Tan if he could tell the staff anything about Gina's activities or friends, he evaded the nurse's eyes and stated, "I'm away a lot."

DRUG HISTORY

Gina's parents believed that this was Gina's first experience. Further data would be needed from Gina when the drug was out of her system.

Nursing Diagnosis

The nurse in the emergency room discussed her observations with the resident on duty. Both thought that Gina was experiencing low-dose PCP intoxication. The physician suggested that Gina be monitored for an hour or so and then be discharged in the care of her parents. He agreed with the nurse that follow-up care for the family would be advisable, and he would encourage family counseling. The nurse called the social worker and collaborated on plans regarding the following nursing diagnoses:

1. *Disturbance in self-esteem* related to giving into peer pressure in order "to belong"
2. *Altered parental role* related to anxiety over Gina's need to gain independence

---

Planning

CONTENT LEVEL—PLANNING GOALS

Goals relevant to the nursing diagnoses were formulated.

Nursing Diagnosis	Long Term Goals	Short Term Goals
1. *Disturbance in self-esteem* related to giving into peer pressure in order "to belong"	1. Gina will agree to be involved with two school or community activities within six months.	1. Gina will meet with the school counselor within one week and work on developing activities and skills on an ongoing basis.

Continued on following page

Planning
(Continued)

Nursing Diagnosis	Long Term Goals	Short Term Goals
2. *Altered parental role* related to anxiety over Gina's need to gain independence	2. Both parents will state that they feel comfortable encouraging Gina in productive outside activities.	2. Family will meet with family therapist on a regular basis, starting this week, to address family fears, concerns, and frustrations.

PROCESS LEVEL—NURSES' REACTIONS AND FEELINGS

When the nurse first started to care for people with various drug dependent problems, she experienced annoyance and frustration at the behaviors and physical problems resulting from habitual drug abuse. It was through talking to other more experienced staff about her resentments and anger toward substance abusers, and through learning more about substance dependence that she began to feel less overwhelmed. She found that as her experience grew and her ability to interact more effectively increased, her frustration and old feelings of hopelessness regarding people with drug problems began to decrease. She felt especially hopeful for young people who were motivated and had access to community resources.

Intervention

Gina was given diazepam to lower anxiety and agitation. The nurse placed her in a quiet, dimly lit room. Unlike a person who is intoxicated with LSD, mescaline, or other psychedelic drugs, reassurance and verbal support (talking down) is *rarely* useful with a person with PCP intoxication. In fact, increased environmental stimuli can trigger agitation and combativeness in some.

The nurse monitored Gina's vital signs every 15 minutes. Her blood pressure and pulse were moderately elevated (140/90 and 122, respectively) but stable. Because Gina was diaphoretic, the nurse offered her cranberry juice on several occasions.

During this time, the nurse called the social worker and asked him to speak to Gina's parents regarding the observations of the health team and suggested interventions. Initially, Mrs. Tan seemed to bristle at the idea of family therapy but said she would go if it would help keep Gina away from drugs. Mr. Tan looked uncomfortable but also agreed to go. Their caring and concern for Gina appeared genuine.

After several hours, the physician re-examined Gina and said that she could go home in the care of her parents. The social worker would contact the school counselor the following day, and the family had an appointment for family counseling in two days.

Evaluation

Gina was fortunate. She had ingested only 1.5–2.0 mg of PCP, which is considered a low dose, and it had been her first. The nurse was alert to possible contributors to Gina's drug use, such as peer pressure and rebellion through drug use. Other young people are not always so fortunate. People who smoke or ingest PCP more regularly may develop a tolerance to the drug and experience withdrawal symptoms consisting of lethargy, depression, and craving for the drug (Grinspoon and Bakalar 1985).

Three months after the PCP incident, Gina had joined a 4-H club. She seemed to involve herself more easily in outside activities once she had parental encouragement and approval at home. She told the school counselor that her parents were a little more relaxed. She had made a friend in the 4-H club and was finding it easier to talk to her parents since family therapy had begun.

Summary

The psychotomimetics are drugs that produce abnormal mental phenomena in the cognitive and perceptual spheres. For example, there are distortions in space and time, depersonalization; with strong doses, hallucinations, delusions, and synesthesia (the "seeing of sounds" or "hearing of colors") may occur.

PCP intoxication, seen frequently in emergency rooms in the late 1970s, is still seen today. The route of administration plays a large role in the severity of PCP intoxication, as is the case with most drugs. The behaviors and nursing and medical interventions for low-dose, moderate-dose, and high-dose intoxication were discussed.

LSD, mescaline, and psilocybin were popular hallucinogenic drugs of the 1960s. Psychotomimetics have been used for centuries, often in religious rites. PCP, LSD, and LSD-like drugs can cause flashbacks for some users.

There are important differences in the treatment of people with PCP and LSD-like drug intoxication. In particular:

1. Persons with LSD-like drug intoxication respond to verbal support (talking down) if the person is panicky. One does *not* talk down a client with PCP intoxication. The person can become more agitated and assaultive.
2. Phenothiazines may be used at times with LSD-like drugs—but *never* with PCP—although haloperidol may be used.

Other nursing measures for acute intoxication were covered.

Marijuana (*Cannabis sativa*) was discussed under psychotomimetics because they share many of the same properties. For the most part, hallucinations are not experienced with the type of marijuana smoked or ingested in this country. The various effects of marijuana were discussed, and some cautions for use were given. Marijuana is often used in conjunction with other drugs (e.g., alcohol, PCP, and cocaine). *Cannabis* is the most widely used illicit drug in the United States.

References

Acee AM, Smith D. Crack. American Journal of Nursing, 87(5):614, 1987.

American Psychiatric Association. Diagnostic and Statistical Manual of Mental Disorders, 3rd ed, revised (DSM-III-R). Washington, DC: American Psychiatric Association, 1987.

American Psychiatric Association. DSM-IV Options Book: Work in Progress. Washington, DC: American Psychiatric Association, 1991.

Beavers WR. Athenetrial basis for family evaluation. *In* Lewis J, Beaucas WR, Gossit JT, Phillips US (eds). No Single Thread: Psychological Health in Family Systems. New York: Brunner-Mazel, 1976.

Bittle S, Feigenbaum JC, Kneisl CR. Substance abuse. *In* Kneisl CR, Ames SW (eds). Adult Health Nursing: A Biopsychosocial Approach. Menlo Park, CA: Addison-Wesley Publishing Company, 1986.

Brauerman BG, Shook J. Spotting the borderline personality. American Journal of Nursing, 87(2):200, 1987.

Brill P, Herzberg J, Speller JL. Employee assistance programs: An overview and suggested roles for psychiatrists. Hospital and Community Psychiatry, 36(7):727, 1985.

Brooks K. Adult children of alcoholics: Psychosocial stages of development. Focus on Family and Chemical Dependency, 6(5):5, 1983.

Burns R, Lerner S, Gorrado R. Phencyclidine—State of acute intoxication and fatalities. Western Journal of Medicine, 123:348, 1975.

Charney DS, Heninger GR, Kleber HD. The combined use of clonidine and naltrexone as a rapid, safe, and effective treatment of abrupt withdrawal from methadone. American Journal of Psychiatry, 143(7):831, 1986.

Cocaine withdrawal step by step (editorial). Emergency Medicine, April 30:65, 1987.

Cohen S. PCP—New trends in treatment. Drug Abuse and Alcohol News, 7:7, 1987.

Davison GC, Neale JM. Abnormal Psychology. New York: John Wiley & Sons, 1982.

Donlon PT, Rockwell DA. Psychiatric Disorders: Diagnosis and Treatment. Bowie, MD: Robert J. Brady Company, 1982.

Elliot B, Williams E. An employee assistance program. American Journal of Nursing, 82(4):586, 1982.

Frances RJ, Franklin JF. Alcohol and other psychoactive substance use disorders. *In* Talbott JA, Hales RE, Yudofsky SC (eds). Textbook of Psychiatry. Washington, DC: American Psychiatric Press, 1988.

Gold MS. 800-COCAINE. New York: Bantam Books, 1984.

Gold MS. The Facts about Drugs and Alcohol. New York: Bantam Books, 1986.

Googins B, Kuntz N. The role of supervision in occupational alcoholism intervention. Employee Assistance Program Digest, 2:15, 1981.

Grinspoon L, Bakalar JB. Drug dependence: Nonnarcotic agents. *In* Kaplan HI, Sadock BJ (eds). Comprehensive Textbook of Psychiatry, 4th ed. Baltimore: Williams & Wilkins, 1985.

Jaffe JH. Opioid dependence. *In* Kaplan HI, Sadock BJ (eds). Comprehensive Textbook of Psychiatry, 4th ed. Baltimore: Williams & Wilkins, 1985.

Jefferson LV, Ensur BE. Help for the helper: Confronting a chemically-impaired colleague. American Journal of Nursing, 82(4):574, 1982.

Klagsburn M, Davis D. Substance abuse and family interaction. Family Process, 16:149, 1977.

Klein JM, Miller SI. Three approaches to the treatment of drug addiction. Hospital and Community Psychiatry, 37(11):1083, 1986.

Kramer JC. Introduction to amphetamine abuse. Journal of Psychedelic Drugs, II:2, 1986.

Lammon CA, Adams MH. Recognizing benzodiazepine overdose. Nursing 93, 23(1):33, 1993.

Ling W, Blaine JD. The use of LAAM in treatment. *In* DuPont RC, Goldstein A, O'Donnell J (eds). Handbook on Drug Abuse. Washington, DC: National Institute on Drug Abuse, Department of Health, Education, and Welfare, 1979.

Luisada P, Brown B. Clinical management of phencyclidine psychosis. Journal of Clinical Toxicology, 9:539, 1976.

McConnell H. Marijuana update: Heavy use hits short term memory. The Journal, 17(7):9, 1988.

Meyers R, Rose A, Smith D. Incidents involving the Haight-Ashbury population and some uncommonly used drugs. Journal of Psychedelic Drugs, 1 (Winter):139, 1967–1968.

Peterson RC, Stillman RC. Emergency room treatment for phencyclidine (PCP) overdose. Resident Staff Physician, 25:116, 1979.

Resnick HS. It Starts with People: Experiences in Drug Abuse Prevention. Washington, DC: National Institute on Drug Abuse, Department of Health, Education, and Welfare, 1979.

Schloemer NF, Skidmore JW. Opiate withdrawal with clonidine. Journal of Psychosocial Nursing and Mental Health Services, 21(10):8, 1983.

Selwyn P. The role of the chemical depending professional in the management of HIV disease. AIDS Patient Care, 4:34, 1990.

Shulgin A, MacLean D. Illicit synthesis of phencyclidine (PCP) and several of its analogs. Journal of Clinical Toxicology, 9:553, 1976.

Smith MC. The client who is abusing toxic substances other than alcohol. In Lego S (ed). The American Handbook of Psychiatric Nursing. Philadelphia: JB Lippincott, 1984.

Sullivan E. Research update. Addictions Nursing Network, 1(2):18, 1989.

Survey uncovers widespread use of drugs among physicians (editorial). Psychiatric News, 21(20):14, 1986.

Wegscheider S. From the family trap to family freedom. Alcoholism, 1(3):36, 1981.

Weingarten N. Treating adolescent drug abuse as a symptom of dysfunction in the family. In Ellis BG (ed). Drug Abuse from the Family Perspective. Washington, DC: US Government Printing Office, 1980. DHHS Publication No. ADM 80-910.

Zamora LC. Patterns of substance abuse. In Haber J, et al (eds). Comprehensive Psychiatric Nursing. New York: McGraw-Hill, 1987.

Further Reading

Bennett G, Vourahis C (eds). Substance Abuse. New York: John Wiley & Sons, 1983.

Campbell C. Nursing Diagnosis and Intervention in Nursing Practice. New York: John Wiley & Sons, 1984.

Cohen AV. Alternatives to Drug Abuse: Steps Toward Prevention. Washington, DC: National Institute on Drug Abuse, No. 14, Department of Health, Education, and Welfare, 1973.

Count EC. A History of Smoking. London: George G. Harrap and Company, 1931.

Harvard Medical School. Opiate abuse—Part II. The Harvard Medical School Mental Health Letter, 3(8):1, 1987.

Hauschildt E. Addictions in nursing: Reality vs. image. The Journal, 15(12):12, 1986.

Hollister L. Phencyclidine use: Current problems. International Drug Therapy News, 14:5, 1979.

Jaffe JM. Drug addiction and drug abuse. In Goodman LS, Gilman A (eds). The Pharmacological Basis of Therapeutics, 5th ed. New York: MacMillan, 1975.

Kaplan HI, Sadock BJ (eds). Synopsis of psychiatry, 6th ed. Baltimore: Williams & Wilkins, 1991.

Kneisl CR, Ames SW. Adult Health Nursing: A Biopsychosocial Approach. Menlo Park, CA: Addison-Wesley Publishing Company, 1986.

New York State Division of Substance Abuse Services. Report on crack. Albany: The NY State Division of Substance Abuse Services, 1986.

Zamora LC. The client who generates anger. In Haber J, et al (eds). Comprehensive Psychiatric Nursing. New York: McGraw-Hill, 1987.

Zweig C. Drug addicts, acupuncture and retraining. The Journal, 16(3):12, 1987.

Self-study Exercises

GENERAL GUIDELINES

Match the following:

1. _____ G _____ Includes the phenomena of tolerance and withdrawal.
2. _____ D _____ More of the drug is needed to get the desired effect.
3. _____ C _____ The combination of two drugs that enhance the effect of each other to a much greater degree than the sum of the effects of each drug alone.
4. _____ B _____ Naloxone.
5. _____ I _____ Also known as minor tranquilizers or antianxiety agents.
6. _____ A _____ Causes abnormal perceptual and cognitive experiences.

A. Psychotomimetics

B. Opiate antagonist

C. Synergistic

D. Tolerance

E. Withdrawal

F. Substance abuse

G. Substance dependence

H. Synesthesia

I. Anxiolytic

Put P for primary or S for secondary health teaching.

7. _____ P _____ Increase in neighborhood recreational and occupational opportunities.

8. ___S___ Administration of drugs under antiseptic conditions.
9. ___P___ Increase in drug education at home, school—use of peer counselors.

Place T (true) or F (false) next to each statement.

10. ___T___ Therapeutic communities are treatment modalities of choice for individuals who have a long history of antisocial behavior and a poor record in methadone maintenance programs.
11. ___T___ Outpatient drug-free programs are treatment modalities of choice for persons who have a job and have intact family or who are polydrug abusers.

Complete the statement by filling in the appropriate information.

12. _____ Cognitive, analytic, supportive, and psychoanalytic are examples of ___Psychotherapeutic___ intervention strategy.

Short answer

13. List four general goals a drug-dependent (chemically impaired) person should meet in order to begin improving the quality of his or her life.

A. _____
B. _____
C. _____
D. _____

SEDATIVE-HYPNOTIC OR ANXIOLYTIC AGENTS

Indicate withdrawal (W), intoxication (I), or overdose (O).

14. ___I___ Unsteady gait, slurred speech, drowsiness.
15. ___W___ Tachycardia, marked insomnia, diaphoresis, irritability.
16. ___O___ Coma, shock, convulsions, respiratory or cardiovascular depression.
17. ___I___ Impaired social or occupational functioning, impaired judgment or memory.

Short answer

18. Write a paragraph regarding your possible reactions to a drug-dependent client to whom you are assigned.

19. List six actions suggested in this section that you might take if working with a chemically dependent colleague (list in order of priority).

A. _____
B. _____
C. _____
D. _____
E. _____
F. _____

PSYCHOSTIMU-LANTS

Match the following:

20. _____C_____ One of the first psychostimulants used and abused illegally. Medically indicated for hyperkinesis in children and for narcolepsy.

21. _____D_____ A fast-acting drug of the 1980s; expensive, in wide use, and dangerous.

22. _____B_____ An alkalinized form of cocaine acting in four to six seconds; intensely psychologically and perhaps physically addicting.

23. _____A_____ A legal drug of addiction used nationwide since the time of Columbus.

A. Nicotine

B. Crack

C. Amphetamines

D. Cocaine

E. Barbiturates

F. Caffeine

Indicate cocaine (C), amphetamine (A), or both (B).

24. _____B_____ Overdose can result in respiratory depression or arrest, hyperpyrexia, seizures, cardiac shock or arrest, and death.

25. _____C_____ Short-acting; tolerance builds rapidly.

26. _____C_____ Chronic users complain of runny nose due to erosion of nasal septum.

27. _____B_____ Intoxication includes grandiosity, paranoia, impaired judgment, tactile or other hallucinations, and psychosis.

28. _____B_____ Medical management and nursing care are vital in severe overdose.

Choose the answer that most accurately completes the statement.

29. Greta Turk, a highly successful editor, has been taking cocaine intranasally for four years and started freebasing two months ago. For the past week she has been locked in her apartment and has gone through $8000 worth of cocaine. She is unconscious when brought to the hospital. Nursing measures include all of the following *except*:

    A. Monitor vital signs every 15 minutes
    B. Maintain a patent airway; give oxygen when indicated by physician
    C. Observe for seizures and hyperpyrexia
    D. Give ammonium chloride

30. After the drug is out of Greta's system, she will most likely experience

    A. Hyperactivity and diaphoresis
    B. Anxiety and depression
    C. Marked insomnia and coarse, hard hands
    D. Increased sexual impulses and euphoria

31. Greta was admitted to the inpatient treatment unit. As an adjunct to group and individual therapy, the nurse could work with Greta on all of the following *except*:

    A. Educating Greta about the psychological actions of the drug, its dangers, and the latest research
    B. Exploring strengths and activities that Greta enjoyed before becoming involved with the drug
    C. Teaching Greta the indicators for and side effects and action of prescribed medications to ease withdrawal—e.g., antidepressants
    D. Assuming an authoritarian leadership role, because Greta is now so dependent

NARCOTICS

Match the following:

32. _C_ Different from most narcotics because it is synthetic and blocks craving for heroin.
33. _D_ Found in many prescription cough syrups.
34. _B_ Pupils constrict, blood pressure decreases, impaired concentration and judgment.
35. _A_ Yawning, pupils dilated, "bone pain," rhinorrhea.

A. Signs of narcotic withdrawal

B. Signs of narcotic ingestion

C. Methadone or LAAM

D. Codeine

E. Crack cocaine

F. Naloxone

Place T (true) or F (false) next to each statement.

36. _T_ Methadone maintenance at approximately 40 mg can block craving for and withdrawal from heroin; effective for 24–36 hours.
37. _T_ LAAM is effective for up to 3 days and is an addictive narcotic.
38. _T_ Naltrexone is a narcotic antagonist effective for up to 72 hours.

Match the following:

39. _C_ Best suited for motivated individuals in early stages of drug-dependence progression.
40. _A_ Best suited for those with long history of antisocial behavior.
41. _B_ Best suited for those who have had several attempts at abstinence and are unable to stabilize their lives.

A. Therapeutic community

B. Methadone maintenance

C. Self-help, abstinence-oriented model

PSYCHOTO-MIMETICS

Match the following regarding PCP.

42. _B_ Ataxia, "blank stare," muscle rigidity, vertical and horizontal nystagmus, general anesthesia, and tendency toward violence.
43. _D_ May be paranoid or assaultive; give cranberry juice and keep in area of low stimuli and least restrictive environment.
44. _B_ Symptoms vary from drowsiness to agitative and combative; waxing and waning psychotic episodes marked by bizarre behaviors; amnesia and stupor. Diazepam or haloperidol might be given.
45. _C_ Psychiatric emergency—maximum restrictions needed to prevent injury to self and others; physical risks include seizures, hyperpyrexia, and respiratory distress; hallucinations and delusions experienced.

A. Low dose (1–5 mg)

B. Moderate dose (5–15 mg)

C. High dose (15 mg +)

D. Cardinal signs at any dose

Place T (true) or F (false) next to each statement.

46. _____T_____ A flashback is the transitory recurrence, when a person is drug-free, of an experience that a person had while taking a psychotomimetic (LSD-like drug, PCP, marijuana).

47. _____T_____ Synesthesia is perceptual distortion, such as "seeing" sounds or "hearing" colors, triggered by some psychotomimetics.

Short answer

48. If you were counseling a teenager who just started to use marijuana, as part of your health teaching what might be three possible long term physical effects that the teenager should be made aware of?

    A. _____

    B. _____

    C. _____

CHAPTER 25

People Who Defend Against Anxiety Through Eating Disorders

Michelle J. Conant

KEY TERMS AND CONCEPTS ◆ ◆ ◆ ◆ ◆ ◆ ◆ ◆ ◆ ◆ ◆ ◆ ◆ ◆

The key terms and concepts listed here also appear in bold where they are defined or discussed in this chapter.

BINGE-PURGE CYCLE

CRITERIA FOR ADMISSION TO AN
   INPATIENT UNIT FOR PATIENT WITH
Anorexia Nervosa
Bulimia Nervosa
Compulsive Overeating

OBESITY
Developmental Obesity
Reactive Obesity

SYMPTOMS OF ANOREXIA NERVOSA

SYMPTOMS OF BULIMIA NERVOSA

OBJECTIVES ▪

After studying this chapter, the student will be able to:

1. Discuss theories of etiology for eating disorders.
2. Describe five areas of assessment for persons with eating disorders and briefly discuss three aspects of assessment for each area.
3. Compare and contrast the healthy need-satisfaction cycle and the disturbed need-satisfaction cycle.
4. Name at least three settings in which the nurse might encounter persons with eating disorders.
5. Recognize three indications for inpatient treatment for each of the following: anorexia nervosa, bulimia nervosa, and psychogenic obesity.
6. Identify major classifications of drugs used in the treatment of anorexia nervosa and bulimia nervosa.
7. Define anorexia nervosa and describe the "typical" anorexic.
8. Define bulimia nervosa and describe the "typical" bulimic.
9. Discuss obesity due to psychogenic compulsive eating.
10. Formulate nursing diagnoses for a client with anorexia nervosa, bulimia nervosa, and compulsive eating.
11. Construct nursing interventions for clients with each of the following: anorexia nervosa, bulimia nervosa, and compulsive overeating.
12. Identify three problems, apart from problems with eating, that might coexist in a person with an eating disorder.

The eating disorders to be discussed in this chapter are anorexia nervosa, bulimia nervosa, and obesity due to compulsive overeating. The disorders will be discussed as separate entities; it is believed, however, that some common issues are at the core of all these disorders. Eating disorders cannot be placed on a wellness-illness continuum because it has not yet been determined that one is any more pathological than another. Hilde Bruch (1973) was the first to propose that deficits in learning to identify and express needs were present to some degree in all persons with eating disorders. Eating becomes a response of the person when dealing with anxiety.

Victims of anorexia and bulimia are usually white, middle-class adolescent girls and women. However, increasing numbers of young women from all economic, ethnic, and educational backgrounds are seeking treatment for eating disorders.

The incidence of anorexia nervosa has greatly increased since the 1960s, and bulimia has shown a marked increase since the 1970s (Orbach 1985). Currently it is estimated that there is one severe case of anorexia nervosa among every 100–200 adolescent women (Kaplan and Sadock 1991). The onset of anorexia nervosa usually occurs between 13 and 20 years of age, and it is 10–20 times more frequent in women than in men. One extensive search of the literature on male bulimics found the prevalence to be 0.2% of adolescent boys and young men. Male bulimics differ from female bulimics in that males have (Carlat and Camargo 1991):

- Later age of onset
- More premorbid obesity
- Higher incidence of homosexuality and asexuality

Because of the self-destructive and sometimes fatal outcome of these disorders, it is important for nurses to recognize, and have an understanding of, the dynamics of the eating disorders. Studies have shown a mortality rate for anorexia nervosa of 5 to 18% (Kaplan and Sadock 1991).

Some bulimics with vomiting behaviors have suffered fatal complications, such as gastric dilation and gastric rupture (Mitchell et al. 1982). Severe electrolyte imbalances, especially hypokalemia, can lead to cardiac arrhythmias and cardiac arrest. Cardiac failure caused by cardiomyopathy as a result of ipecac (emetine) intoxication is being reported more frequently and often results in death (Halmi 1988).

At this time it is not possible to state the exact cause of eating disorders or to explain why persons exhibit one group of eating behaviors rather than another. For this reason, theories of etiology will be discussed as potentially underlying all three eating disorders.

Because anorexia nervosa and bulimia affect mainly young women, individuals suffering from these syndromes will be referred to with the feminine pronouns. This chapter will address obesity only as it relates to compulsive eating, which is psychogenic in nature. Because the recent literature deals with this type of obesity from a female perspective, the feminine pronouns will be used for this disorder as well.

Figure 25–1 conceptualizes the process of eating disorders as a self-destructive relief behavior.

Theory

This chapter discusses the following theories of etiology: (1) psychodynamic model, (2) sociocultural model, and (3) biological model.

PSYCHODYNAMIC MODEL

The infant develops a healthy ego when the need-response cycle between infant and caregiver, usually the mother, is satisfying (Fig. 25–2). This child will move through the early months of life toward increasing differentiation from the mother, experiencing some separation anxiety and, later, some feelings of helplessness as this separation-individuation process is negotiated. This stage spans approximately six to 30 months of age. With support and encouragement from the mother, the child learns to handle the anxiety of separation. Disturbances in this stage of development occur if the child's need for separation-individuation is responded to with overprotectiveness and anxiety on the part of the mother (Fig. 25–3). Therefore, the child is unable to view the self as separate, with distinct bodily needs and feelings. This nonadjustment is extended even to emotional needs. A distorted body image develops, along with a prevailing sense of ineffectiveness and helplessness in meeting individual needs. As the individual reaches later stages of development requiring increasing separation and independence, such as puberty or leaving the parental home, increased anxiety is experienced.

A child develops the ability to use defense mechanisms and soothe herself to reduce anxieties and protect self-esteem. This is learned through "mirroring" or identifying with these behaviors in the parents (Geist 1982). For the individual who develops eating

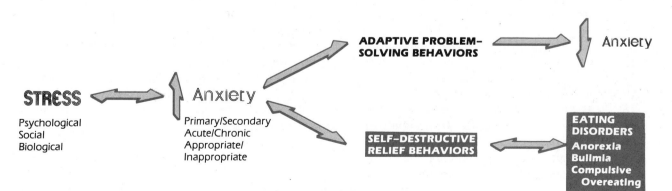

Figure 25–1. *Conceptualization of the process of an eating disorder.*

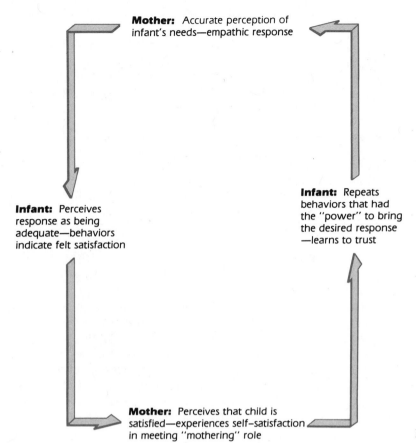

Mother: Accurate perception of infant's needs—empathic response

Infant: Perceives response as being adequate—behaviors indicate felt satisfaction

Infant: Repeats behaviors that had the "power" to bring the desired response —learns to trust

Mother: Perceives that child is satisfied—experiences self–satisfaction in meeting "mothering" role

Figure 25–2. *Healthy need-response cycle.*

disorders, the development of healthy defense mechanisms is disturbed. The child becomes self-critical and is in constant conflict with inner drives and impulses. A sign of self-indulgence is met with self-deprecating thoughts and subsequent feelings of worthlessness. The body becomes the enemy, and it is denied any comfort. Control of the body and its biological needs, such as hunger, becomes a source of constant preoccupation. A break in the self-control arouses fears of a total loss of control, so that often the anorexic or bulimic is viewed as being phobic of food and of body fat. Because the bulimic and anorexic actually experience hunger—although it is suppressed more in the anorexic—they may also exhibit hunger-controlling behaviors, which can be in the form of obsessive thoughts and rituals around eating. This extreme need to control hunger is a response to poor impulse control, as seen in people with addictions.

Mothers of children with eating disorders have been described as being preoccupied with weight and as having given up personal goals for dedication to fulfilling the needs of their families. This life of self-denial engenders anger exhibited through martyrdom, "nagging," or feelings of depression. This conflict is transmitted to the female infant through early feeding experiences that are often mismatched with the

infant's needs. Overfeeding or underfeeding can occur as a response to the mother's feelings rather than the child's needs. Food then becomes the core of the conflict between mother and daughter and is seen as a means of control (Selvina-Palazzoli 1974). There seems to be some correlation with early childhood sexual abuse and bulimia as well (Pribor and Dinwiddle 1992).

SOCIOCULTURAL MODEL

The changing roles of women and the transmission of gender-appropriate role conflict from mother to daughter are believed by some theorists to be at the center of these phenomena. The feminine ideal that society holds for women is that they be compliant and that they subordinate their needs to the needs of others. Open competition is allowed only in the arena of physical beauty. Because "slimness" is the current ideal, the groundwork has been laid for the development of eating disorders. Male infants, on the other hand, repress their feminine identity and fear it, projecting this fear onto all women and attempting to control women through their bodies. Therefore, many women today are faced with conflict. They want to

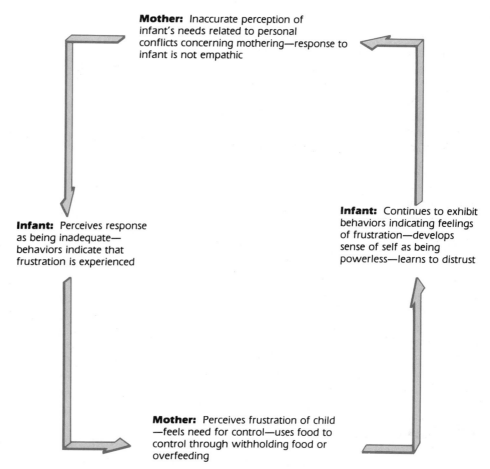

Figure 25–3. *Disturbed need-response cycle.*

compete and achieve in the world but are fearful of rejection by a society that approves and sanctions primarily the roles of wife and mother for women. Achievements outside the home are supported half-heartedly, and they are minimally supported as the primary role for women.

These conflicts can reveal themselves as an eating disorder. Obesity from compulsive eating, for example, can be viewed as a woman's unconscious attempt to rebel against societal pressure to be slim and power-less. This rebellion through obesity exacts a price. Many obese women experience shame and self-hatred and often punish themselves for failing to maintain the feminine ideal. For these women, the rewards for independence and competence do not outweigh the pain of society's judgment (Millman 1980).

BIOLOGICAL MODEL

Although conclusive evidence of biological correlates remains tenuous, some genetic and neurochemical findings warrant further research.

Genetic Factors

In studies of twins with anorexia nervosa, there is evidence of higher concordance rates in monozygotic twins than in dizygotic twins. Also, sisters of anorexic individuals are more likely to be anorexic than are those of controls. Another finding that supports possible genetic factors is that major mood disorders are more common in family members of anorexics than in the general population (Kaplan and Sadock 1991).

Neurochemical Factors

Neurochemical changes in people with anorexia nervosa or bulimia nervosa are more difficult to evaluate. It is hard to know if these chemical changes precede, accompany, or follow the behavioral changes observed in these disorders. Fava et al. (1989) reviewed the literature and found possible evidence of neurochemical factors that might be associated with the patho-genesis of eating disorders. For example, anorexia nervosa appears to be consistently associated with lower concentrations of norepinephrine and 3-methoxy-4-hydroxyphenylglycol (MHPG) in the cerebrospinal fluid. Bulimia nervosa is accompanied by lower-than-normal peripheral noradrenergic functions (norepinephrine). Both of these findings have implications for treatment with psychoactive drugs, especially the tricyclics and monoamine oxidase inhibitors, which directly affect the neurotransmitter systems.

Assessment

When doing a psychiatric nursing assessment (Chapter 8) on a person with an eating disorder, areas such as (1) *weight*, (2) *eating*, (3) *activity*, (4) *family*, (5) *physical signs and symptoms*, and (6) *need for hospitalization* need to be evaluated in depth. Physical signs and symptoms are an important part of the nursing assessment of eating disorders because these disorders are potentially physically debilitating and even fatal. Because depression is often present in eating disorders, the risk for self-harm may be an immediate concern.

ASSESSING WEIGHT

It is important to assess not only the present weight and how much the person has recently lost or gained but also the presence of distorted body image and the influence of mood (anxiety, guilt, depression) or events on weight status.

ASSESSING EATING

The nurse assesses not only the exact eating patterns but also the feelings and behaviors that surround the person's eating. Is there a **binge-purge cycle**? A binge-purge cycle is episodic, uncontrolled, rapid ingestion of large quantities of food over a short period of time often followed by "purging" (vomiting). Are there feelings of anxiety and shame? What is the degree of impulse control? Is the person aware of rigid or compulsive feelings toward eating? Family patterns of eating, attitudes toward food, and eating "in secret" are areas in the nurse's assessment. The nurse also attempts to elicit the function of the bingeing, purging, and fasting behaviors. For the bulimic, the inability to control eating impulses may also suggest an inability to control other impulses as well. According to the DSM-III-R (APA 1987), lying, sexual promiscuity, compulsive drug use, and stealing are often present.

ASSESSING ACTIVITY

The presence of compulsive exercise is determined, and the function the exercise serves, both physically and emotionally, is evaluated.

ASSESSING FAMILY

Although there are similarities in family dynamics for the eating disorders, some researchers hypothesize differences in the styles of interaction between parents of bulimics and parents of anorexics. For example, some researchers state that families of bulimics tend to be more chaotic and disruptive than the families of anorexics. Parents of anorexics are often thought to be more rigid and controlling than those of bulimics. The presence of overt marital conflict in the parents of the client is evaluated, as is presence of poor impulse control (e.g., the use of violence, drugs, or alcohol) in family members. How family members express anger, affection, sadness, and other emotions provides important data. Questions are asked to determine such signs as the presence of competition for parental attention among siblings, the feelings and reactions of other family members to the client's eating behavior, and parental response to emotional needs of children. Table 25–1 identifies some differences that may be found between an anorexic client and a bulimic client. There may be exceptions to these differences in individual cases.

ASSESSING PHYSICAL SIGNS AND SYMPTOMS

Because the eating disorders can be seriously debilitating and in some cases lead to death, careful physical assessment and awareness of specific signs and symptoms are crucial.

Some physical signs and **symptoms of anorexia nervosa** often seen in severe cases include cachexia, hair loss, yellowish skin, cyanosis of the extremities, lanugo, cessation of menses, peripheral edema, and hypotension.

Some physical signs and **symptoms of bulimia nervosa** resulting from frequent vomiting are parotid gland enlargement (called chipmunk facies), chronic hoarseness, sore throat, dental caries from acid regurgitation, electrolyte imbalances (hypokalemia and alkalosis), and dehydration.

The nurse also asks the client about the use of substances for purging (laxatives, diuretics) and evaluates for possible signs of anemia and malnutrition.

Table 25–1 ■ NURSING ASSESSMENT: CONTRASTING CHARACTERISTICS OF ANOREXIA AND BULIMIA

ANOREXIA	BULIMIA
Appearance	
Underweight; 25% below normal weight.	Normal or overweight.
Age	
13–22 years of age; average 18 years. Often younger than bulimics.	20s to 30s; often older than anorexics.
Signs	
Cachexia, hair loss, yellowish skin, lanugo, cyanosis of extremities, peripheral edema, amenorrhea.	Chipmunk facies (enlarged parotid glands), chronic hoarseness, dental caries, dehydration, electrolyte imbalance.
Family Environment	
Rigid and controlled; less overt evidence of marital discord.	More conflicts and overt fighting, chaotic, poor impulse control among family members, e.g., violence, drugs, alcohol.
Clinical Characteristics	
Introverted; more socially isolated than bulimics.	Extroverted, sexually active, high incidence of compulsive behaviors, e.g., promiscuity, drugs, stealing, and suicide attempts.
Awareness of Disorder	
Denies hunger more often than bulimics. More denial of problem than in bulimics.	More aware of own eating disorder than anorexics. More distressed by symptoms than anorexics.

Data from Dickstein 1985; Johnson et al. 1984; Keltner 1984.

Presence or absence of menses, as well as symptoms of premenstrual syndrome, is assessed.

Other forms of mental illness, such as depression, phobias, addictive diseases, and a range of obsessive-compulsive behaviors, are often present in someone with an eating disorder.

A nursing assessment guide (Table 25–2) for a suspected eating disorder can be supplemental to a general psychosocial assessment (refer to Chapter 8). This assessment guide can be adapted for use with anorexia, bulimia, and compulsive eating. The sample questions are a guide and are not necessarily appropriate or complete for all individuals in all settings.

ASSESSING NEED FOR HOSPITALIZATION

Love and Seaton (1991) suggest using Joffe's criteria (Box 25–1) when deciding if patients are candidates for inpatient hospitalization.

Nursing Diagnosis

One of the first concerns a nurse has for someone with an eating disorder is the patient's physical safety. For a severe anorexic, a priority of concern would be *altered nutrition: less than body weight* related to self-starvation. Physical safety for a client who is bulimic may be a priority when severe electrolyte imbalance threatens her life. Therefore, *cardiac output: decreased* related to excessive vomiting and dehydration is a relevant nursing diagnosis. Because depression is often present in people with eating disorders, and because the suicide rate is high for this group, *high risk for self-harm* related to identity crisis must be considered.

Young women with eating disorders usually have distorted self-concepts and low self-esteem. For example, for a person suffering from compulsive overeating, *disturbance in self-esteem* or *chronic low self-esteem* as evidenced by obesity may be an appropriate nursing diagnosis.

Table 25–2 ■ NURSING ASSESSMENT: GUIDE FOR EATING DISORDERS

TO EVALUATE	SAMPLE QUESTIONS
Weight	
1. Presence of distortion or delusions about body image	1a. What do you consider your ideal weight? 1b. Do you often "feel fat"?
2. Influence of moods or events on weight	2a. How do you feel when you gain weight? 2b. What happens just before you decide to lose weight? 2c. (If purging) Would you be able to tolerate gaining 10 pounds if you could stop purging?
3. Feelings about current weight	3. What do you think about your present weight?
4. Fluctuations in weight over time	4a. Have you recently lost weight? 4b. How much? In what period of time?
5. Past treatment history and response to past treatment	5. Have you ever been treated for a weight disorder? Was it successful?
Eating	
1. Exact eating patterns, i.e., amounts and types of food eaten normally and during binges and mealtimes	1a. What do you eat in a typical day? How much? When and where? 1b. What do you eat when you binge? How much? When and where? Why do you terminate binges? 1c. Do you ever induce vomiting after you have eaten? 1d. Do you ever fast? How long? How often?
2. Signs of "secret" eating or shame associated with bingeing	2a. Do you prefer eating alone? 2b. How does your eating change when you are around people?
3. Perception of eating as a problem behavior	3. Do you think your eating pattern is normal?
4. Degree of disabling effects on activities of daily living	4a. How does eating (or not eating) interfere with your life? 4b. Do you find yourself thinking about food and calories often?
5. Anxieties precipitating bingeing and purging	5a. Do you ever fear losing control over your eating? 5b. Do you feel you have any control over purging?
6. Function of the bingeing, purging, and fasting behaviors	6a. How do you feel after your binge? How do you feel after you purge? 6b. How do you feel when you can fast?
Activity	
1. Presence of compulsive exercise as a form of purging	1. Do you exercise? What type and how much each day?
2. Function exercise serves both physically and emotionally	2a. How do you feel physically after exercising? Emotionally? 2b. How do you feel physically if you cannot/do not exercise? Emotionally?
Family (In the context of presenting problem)	
1. Presence of marital conflict in parents' marriage or with spouse if client is married	1a. Do your parents appear to be happy? 1b. How would you describe your marriage?
2. Parental response to emotional needs of children, to separation or independence of children	2a. How do members of your family express anger? 2b. Does your family show affection? How? Sadness? How? 2c. Describe a situation when you brought a problem to your mother or father. What did they do? How did you feel? 2d. How do you feel about expressing opinions that differ from those of your parents? 2e. How did your parents react when you finished high school? Left home for college?

TO EVALUATE	SAMPLE QUESTIONS
Table 25–2 ■ NURSING ASSESSMENT: GUIDE FOR EATING DISORDERS *Continued*	
Family (in the context of presenting problem) *continued*	
3. Feelings and reactions of each family member, spouse, or significant person concerning client's eating behavior and weight	3. What does your mother (father, sibling) do when you refuse meals? Eat too much? Purge?
4. Presence of poor impulse control, i.e., drug or alcohol abuse or excessive tempers in family members	4. Does anyone in your family abuse alcohol? Drugs?
5. Presence of overcontrol of appetites and feelings by family	5. What do your mother, father, siblings do when they are upset, angry, happy, hungry, sad? How do you know when they are angry? Sad? Hungry? Happy?
6. Eating patterns of the family unit	6a. Who plans the family meals? Who does the food shopping? Who pays for the food? 6b. Does your family eat meals together? 6c. Do you speak with each other at these times? 6d. How does it feel for you to eat meals with your family? 6e. How long does it take you to eat a meal?
7. Sexual abuse or incest	7. Do you remember any uncomfortable or frightening physical contact with anyone (e.g., family member, friend of family, babysitter, or teacher)?
Physical Signs and Symptoms	
1. Signs and symptoms often associated with *anorexia nervosa*	1. Is there presence of ● Cachexia or emaciation ● Decreased body temperature ● Peripheral edema ● Cyanosis of the extremities ● Constipation ● Atrophic, dry skin ● Slow pulse ● Yellowish skin ● Amenorrhea ● Hair loss ● Lanugo on skin ● Anemia or malnutrition
2. Signs and symptoms often associated with *bulimia*	2. Is there presence of ● Parotid gland enlargement (chipmunk facies) ● Dehydration ● Chronic hoarseness or sore throat ● Dental caries—loss of enamel on teeth ● Rebound water retention (when purging stops) ● Anemia ● Irregular menses or amenorrhea ● Electrolyte imbalance, i.e., hypokalemia
3. Presence of physical signs of abuse of substances used for "purging," e.g., calluses on knuckles	3a. Do you use laxatives or diuretics to lose weight? How many? How often? 3b. Do you ever take amphetamines, caffeine or diet pills? How many? How often?

Because the issues of control and lack of control are felt to be a central theme, *powerlessness* related to inability to stop the binge-purge cycle, or *ineffective individual coping* related to phobias and rituals surrounding eating could be used.

Often, a person with an eating disorder is consumed with guilt and shame and withdraws from others. Most people who are victims of these disorders are isolated and feel alienated. Building and rebuilding communications with others is an important

---

Box 25–1. CRITERIA FOR INPATIENT ADMISSION OF CLIENTS WITH EATING DISORDERS

Individuals should be admitted who are:

- Suicidal or severely out of control (e.g., self-mutilating or abusing large amounts of laxatives, emetics, diuretics, or street drugs)
- Severely emaciated (30% or more below recommended weight)
- Demonstrating rapid, dramatic weight loss
- Experiencing hypothermia due to loss of subcutaneous tissue (body temperature of less than 36°C)
- Having an imbalance in fluids or electrolytes
- In need of extensive diagnostic work to identify coexisting medical and/or psychiatric problems
- Already medically compromised (e.g., by infections)
- Unable to gain weight repeatedly with outpatient treatment

From Love CC, Seaton H. Eating disorders: Highlights of nursing assessment and therapeutics. Nursing Clinics of North America, 26(3):677, 1991.

---

long term goal. *Social isolation* related to obesity/low self-esteem/shame may be characteristic of some individuals with an eating disorder.

Planning

Planning interventions for people with eating disorders involves planning on the (1) content level and (2) process level. Planning on the *content level* is the actual setting up of client-centered goals and devising specific nursing interventions aimed at meeting those goals. The *process level* is a recognition of the kinds of reactions a client may stimulate in the nurse (countertransference) and awareness of how to deal effectively with these feelings and reactions. Skill and awareness on the part of the nurse to handle personal reactions and feelings help maintain mutual self-esteem and help facilitate the therapeutic process. Inability to recognize strong reactions to the client and deal with them professionally often leads to power struggles and deterioration of the therapeutic relationship.

CONTENT LEVEL—PLANNING GOALS

Interventions planned for clients with eating disorders are derived from the specific goals set and outcomes desired. Some examples of possible short term goals are illustrated here. Specific goals and interventions are discussed under each specific disorder.

An extremely emaciated young girl with anorexia nervosa might have a nursing diagnosis of *altered nutrition: less than body weight* related to self-starvation. Some possible goals follow:

- Client will gain 1 kg per week.
- Client will demonstrate two positive behaviors she can substitute for purging two weeks after treatment starts.

If suicidal thoughts are evident and *high risk for self-harm* is a nursing diagnosis, some possible goals could be

- Client will remain safe with the aid of staff support and supervision.
- By (date), client will be able to name two people she can talk to when thinking of suicide.
- By (date), client will explore feelings of anger and hopelessness with the nurse.

People with eating disorders usually have distortions of body image and a poor self-concept. Negative self-evaluation often takes up much of the person's conscious thought. Therefore, assessing a person's self-concept is important in people with eating disorders. The nursing diagnosis of *disturbance in self-esteem*, as evidenced by obesity, may warrant some of the following short term and long term goals:

- Client will identify two personal strengths by (date).
- By (date), client will name three aspects of her personality that she admires.
- Client will name two personal accomplishments of which she is proud by (date).
- Client will name two important goals she would like to attain in her life.

PROCESS LEVEL—NURSES' REACTIONS AND FEELINGS

Different behaviors often evoke specific reactions in people. Although the nurse may be aware of various reactions and feelings aroused by a client with an eating disorder, some reactions may be expected. These specific countertransferential feelings will be dealt with separately under *Process Level* in the case studies dealing specifically with anorexia, bulimia, and compulsive eating. Health care professionals working with people who have eating disorders should always have supervision available to discuss transference-countertransference issues. Supervision also serves as a guide for validating perceptions and maximizing intervention strategies. Supervision may be informal, as in peer group supervision, or more formal, as with weekly reviews with other members of the health team. Without supervision, nurses may react to clients' behavior emotionally rather than recognize the important underlying issues and intervene accordingly.

Intervention

The nurse may work with a client with an eating disorder in various settings and circumstances. In some settings, the eating disorders may be secondary to other medical disorders. For example, a client with diabetes admitted to a general medical unit for stabilization of insulin may also be obese because of a compulsive eating disorder. A young woman seen in an outpatient clinic because of irregular menses may also be bulimic. Severe cases of anorexia nervosa require hospitalization when malnutrition becomes life threatening. Eating disorders are treated in both inpatient and outpatient settings, depending on the client's priority of needs. The nurse may play various roles when working with a person with an eating disorder.

SOMATIC THERAPIES

To date, there are few specific medications for the treatment of anorexia nervosa or bulimia nervosa. For anorexia clients, perhaps the most promising drug is cyproheptadine (Periactin). Cyproheptadine is an antihistamine and serotonin antagonist that enables anorexia clients to gain weight while exerting an antidepressant effect (Maxmen 1991). Neuroleptics and antidepressants are often prescribed for anorexia. For example, the neuroleptic chlorpromazine (Thorazine) has been useful in the treatment of some severely obsessive-compulsive anorexic clients. Amitriptyline (Elavil), a tricyclic antidepressant and a serotonin-reuptake inhibitor, has also helped some anorexia clients gain weight.

One useful drug in the treatment of bulimia nervosa has been the tricyclic imipramine (Tofranil). Imipramine has been found to reduce the frequency and intensity of binges for some bulimic clients (Pope et al. 1983). Other drugs found useful in some cases of bulimia are fluoxetine (Prozac) at 80 mg per day, lithium, sertraline (Zoloft), phenelzine (Nardil), and naltrexone (an opiate antagonist) (Maxmen 1991).

Symptom relief is of great benefit to the client, but without a change in coping ability, there is little reason to believe that once the medication is stopped the eating behavior will not surface again. Any medication regimen must be monitored carefully, with special attention given to possible side effects or problems that are especially pertinent to this population. One problem is that purging will reduce the actual amount of medication assimilated by the client. For bulimic clients, frequent monitoring of the drug level in the blood is necessary. Another problem is that hypothermia and hypotension, already found in anorexics, are increased by some medications.

THERAPEUTIC ENVIRONMENT

The decision to admit a person with an eating disorder to an inpatient unit, and the type of unit chosen—that is, psychiatric eating disorder unit or medical unit—depend on careful assessment and the client's immediate needs. Because physiological and safety needs must be addressed first, any acute physical distress needing immediate medical attention would warrant admission to a medical unit. Professionals staffing such a unit should have a sound base of knowledge of eating disorders. If the client's physical status is not life threatening, a psychiatric unit staffed by professionals specializing in treating eating disorders is recommended. There has been an increase in these types of units as the number of people suffering from eating disorders has increased. The types of therapeutic approaches used may differ, depending on the theory base used by the professionals in each unit. Indications for in-hospital admission and treatment approaches for anorexia, bulimia, and obesity caused by compulsive eating are discussed subsequently.

Inpatient Treatment for Anorexia Nervosa

The main **criteria for the admission of a person with anorexia nervosa to an inpatient unit** are as follows:

1. Loss of over 15% of minimal normal weight, with signs of extreme resistance to take even a minimum of calories to maintain weight
2. Medical emergencies, regardless of weight, such as serious arrhythmias

3. Severe psychological distress, such as feelings of panic or suicidal ideation, that is persistent and is not relieved by outpatient treatment

Inpatient treatment has a dual focus: nutritional rehabilitation and psychotherapy. A range of weight is set after consulting reliable height and weight charts and considering the person's body frame. This weight range can be set on the low normal end of the chart. The client who is expected to achieve a low normal weight is not as likely to feel that she is being "fattened up."

An individualized diet that achieves a gain of two to three pounds per week will minimize the side effects of refeeding in anorexics (Fig. 25–4). Hyperalimentation and tube feeding may be considered for individuals who do not successfully gain weight. Techniques for forcing clients to eat, for example, using appetite stimulants or using psychotherapy without addressing eating patterns, are inappropriate because they ignore the underlying dynamics of the disorder. Exercise for the purpose of maintaining full range of motion is encouraged, but compulsive exercise to "burn off" calories is discouraged.

Gaining weight is not the only goal. Establishing a normal pattern of eating is necessary so that weight can be maintained on an outpatient basis. Many clients agree to gain weight in order to be discharged but intend to lose the weight after discharge! For this reason, anxiety levels and attitudes during weight gain must be assessed and addressed during the psychotherapy sessions before discharge. One of the most effective methods of treatment for a severe anorexic is based on behavioral therapy. Behavioral therapists who treat clients with anorexia nervosa believe that behavior modification techniques are necessary while the person is suffering from physical starvation. The effects of starvation render the anorexic incapable of benefiting from insight-oriented types of therapy. Some of the effects of starvation are hyperactivity, irritability, and poor concentration and memory. Because of the repression of hunger and distorted body image, there is poor judgment, which makes meeting physical self-care needs difficult, if not impossible.

The following points are important for a behavior modification approach:

1. Weight gain, rather than eating behaviors, is reinforced.
2. A behavioral program must be individually suited to each client.
3. Only an enforceable program is effective, so a means of accurate monitoring must exist, such as regular "weigh-ins."

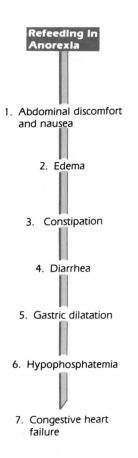

Refeeding in Anorexia

1. Abdominal discomfort and nausea

2. Edema

3. Constipation

4. Diarrhea

5. Gastric dilatation

6. Hypophosphatemia

7. Congestive heart failure

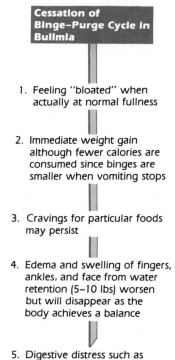

Cessation of Binge–Purge Cycle in Bulimia

1. Feeling "bloated" when actually at normal fullness

2. Immediate weight gain although fewer calories are consumed since binges are smaller when vomiting stops

3. Cravings for particular foods may persist

4. Edema and swelling of fingers, ankles, and face from water retention (5–10 lbs) worsen but will disappear as the body achieves a balance

5. Digestive distress such as "gas" or "heartburn" which results from digesting normal amounts of food rather than purging before digestion is completed

Figure 25–4. *Side effects associated with refeeding in anorexia and with cessation of the binge-purge cycle in bulimia.*

4. Psychotherapy can be integrated with a behavioral program, but the psychotherapist should not be the enforcer of the behavioral program. This helps avoid "power struggles" with the client.
5. Once weight gain commences and eating patterns appear normal, the client is allowed passes to eat in other situations, either alone or with family.

Inpatient Treatment for Bulimia Nervosa

Criteria for the admission of a person with bulimia to an inpatient unit include

1. Inability to interrupt a chronic and frequent binge-purge cycle in spite of outpatient treatment
2. Medical emergencies, such as serious potassium depletion
3. Psychiatric emergencies, such as persistent suicidal ideation

The focus of inpatient treatment for normal-weight bulimics will depend on the problems the individual presents, but generally the focus will be on re-establishment of a normal eating pattern, with avoidance of weight gain and a minimum of the physical side effects caused by the cessation of bingeing and purging (see Fig. 25–4).

Because the bingeing and purging are actually signs of maladaptive coping with severe levels of anxiety and feelings of depression, it is common for these feelings to surface once the behaviors change. It is imperative that more adaptive ways of coping with anxiety are learned. Without the support and teaching by the nurse and other members of the treatment team, the bulimic may develop phobias, experience "anxiety attacks," or abuse drugs or alcohol to deal with anxiety. This work of learning healthier coping skills can begin during inpatient treatment, but long term follow-up consisting of ongoing psychotherapy is necessary to maintain any change.

Four areas of education for bulimics have been identified (Wooley and Wooley 1985). These are (1) physical effects of returning to a normal eating pattern, (2) weight regulation, (3) effects of starvation, and (4) effects of bulimia on health. This information is provided for the client in a structured and intensive program of group and individual sessions.

Inpatient Treatment for Obesity

Obesity due to compulsive eating that is psychogenic in nature is usually treated in an outpatient setting; however, there are some situations in which hospitalization or residential treatment **for compulsive overeating** is recommended:

1. Need for interruption of chronic, uncontrollable eating
2. Presence of potentially dangerous medical conditions that are aggravated by compulsive eating, e.g., diabetes or cardiac problems
3. Need for rapid, supervised weight loss to relieve conditions such as heart disease or to prepare for major surgery
4. Treatment for obesity requiring surgery or drastic dieting
5. Any psychiatric condition that requires inpatient treatment and exists concurrently with compulsive eating

Regardless of whether the inpatient setting is medical or psychiatric, the nurse must maintain a holistic focus in his or her nursing practice. Addressing the "weight problem" and avoiding the client's emotional needs will reinforce for the client that her body is the "problem," and she will continue to deny her feelings. The client with compulsive eating behaviors must be viewed in the context of her need to cope with a poor self-image.

There has been a trend toward assessing each person's eating patterns and needs and formulating individualized plans that can be lifelong rather than focusing on quick weight loss diets. An exercise program may also be prescribed, but careful monitoring is necessary for those who have been leading sedentary lifestyles or who are extremely obese. Identifying the meaning food has in the person's emotional life and the function that compulsive eating serves is an important part of altering compulsive eating patterns. The advantage of a residential setting is that the client can begin working through all aspects of her problem in an intensive program and with the support of others who share her problem. This can be achieved through structured individual and group activities. A program such as this may last from one week to as long as a few months. As with other eating disorders, follow-up focuses on reinforcing and maintaining any progress made.

PSYCHOTHERAPY

There are several psychotherapeutic approaches that may be used, and the choice will determine the types of sessions, the number of sessions, and the length of treatment. Two general issues are addressed, regardless of the specific approach used:

- Body image as it relates to self-image
- Identification and effective expression of needs

A nurse who is educated or certified in specific therapeutic modalities, usually at the master's level, may work with clients who have eating disorders in an outpatient unit, community mental health center, or private practice. Three specific modalities are briefly discussed: (1) individual therapy, (2) group therapy, and (3) family therapy.

Individual Therapy

Numerous theoretical models have been used effectively to treat individuals with eating disorders. Table 25-3 presents an overview of three theoretical

models. The basic therapeutic approaches used in these models are also included.

Group Therapy

Group therapy for persons with eating disorders can be either time-limited, closed groups or long term, open groups. Closed groups do not admit new members once the groups begin meeting, and open groups do. The ideal size of therapy groups is from six to 10 persons.

Analytic or intensive group therapy is long term and open. The dynamics underlying the eating behaviors

Table 25-3 ■ THEORETICAL MODELS FOR EATING DISORDERS

PREMISE	THERAPEUTIC APPROACH
Self-psychology	
Person has a poorly developed sense of self and identity. When threatened, attempts to control anxiety, and "gaining control" takes the form of "controlling" food intake and weight. Anxiety is often stimulated when separation occurs, such as times of increased independence.	1. Explore situational crises (e.g., leaving home, divorcing, or being successful in career). 2. Explore meaning of the crisis. 3. Explore feelings when eating behaviors are used (e.g., fasting, bingeing, purging, or compulsive exercise). 4. Assist connection between feelings and eating behaviors, e.g., "You seem to feel much better about yourself when you can avoid a binge."
Feminist Psychoanalytical Psychology	
The person is very ambivalent about her body. Messages transmitted by the mother that the body is to be feared and controlled and yet is the greatest source of approval from others. Messages hold that issues dealing with one's body (sexuality, power) are "taboo" or "wrong." The daughter learns to (1) withhold information about her problems and (2) deny her needs.	1. Establish a nonjudgmental alliance with client. Encourage the perception that the nurse is on the client's side. 2. Introduce consistency and reliability in scheduling sessions to establish trust. 3. Address the defensive behaviors of withholding or sullenness in a nonthreatening manner, e.g., "It must be difficult to talk about private matters to someone you just met." 4. Avoid power struggles. Do not become invested in whether or not the client gains weight. Refer client to physician to monitor client's weight and assess physical health.
Cognitive Theory	
The concept that people are motivated out of a belief system that is designed to increase feelings of self-esteem. People with eating disorders have faulty belief systems, e.g., food is all "good" or all "bad." This translates into all areas of the person's life, e.g., mistakes mean failure. *Faulty Beliefs* Anorexics—Being thin will solve problems. Bulimics—Food = comfort and removal of food = control. *Compulsive eaters*—"Fat" will protect one from intimacy and independence.	1. Establish a trusting relationship with client. 2. Explore client's belief system. 3. Introduce doubts about beliefs that lead to maladaptive behaviors, e.g., "Being thin doesn't seem to solve your problems, since you are thin now and still unhappy." 4. Explore functions the behavior serves, e.g., eating decreases anxiety. 5. Assist client in modifying false beliefs, e.g., "Being obese may pose some problems in relationships, but intimacy requires more than being thin."

Data from Garner and Bemis 1985; Geist 1982; Goodsitt 1985; Orbach 1985.

are the main focus, and the group leader is generally a facilitator. Group members are encouraged to seek support and meet social needs outside the group membership by using skills learned in group sessions with friends and family. Group sessions are unstructured, with few rules, and group members have primary responsibility for their use of group time and growth. For the person with eating disorders, this personal responsibility and reaching out to others in mutual support are difficult to achieve, yet they are vital lessons to be learned.

Group experiences are invaluable for the client with an eating disorder because social isolation is a common feature for many. Group therapy for women with eating disorders can facilitate communication about sex role socialization experience; choices and conflicts about school, work, and lifestyles; body image misperceptions; and eating patterns and defenses (Dickstein 1985). In the group setting, a person can learn that to be separate and autonomous, with personal needs and desires, is not only possible but encouraged.

Family Therapy

Findings from a recent study supported the theory that certain family relationships contribute to certain psychological and behavioral traits observed in people with eating disorders (Larson 1991). Family therapy is perhaps one way to support family members to make positive changes in their lives.

The overall goal of family therapy is to effect system changes. The focus is off of the person with the eating disorder and on the family as a whole. The family is seen as a system whose parts are in constant interaction with each other. For these troubled families, there has been an ineffectiveness in meeting needs—their own and each other's. This can be a result of faulty communication patterns, difficulties in boundaries and roles, and societal pressure when family norms are challenged. Family life is where separation and identity are learned and, in the case of families that include an anorexic or bulimic person, there seems to be little individuality. The person gets lost in the family system. This dysfunction in the family takes the form of an eating disorder. The functional family, on the other hand, teaches its members to be unique and yet able to cooperate collectively with each other.

The family therapist functions as a participant-observer in the family process and treats the family in an understanding, empathetic, and nonjudgmental manner. It is important to enable the family members to become more differentiated. Using concepts of change theory as a guide, the family must be educated and encouraged to see differentiation as rewarding. Once differentiation has begun, there will be discomfort within the system until these changes become integrated. Positive feedback is important, along with compassion for any feelings of loss or separation anxiety experienced by the family members. Often, anger is expressed during this process, which presents an opportunity to assist the family in learning how to resolve conflict. The eating behavior will often change as this process unfolds. It is important to assist the family in making connections between changes in family patterns and the subsequent changes in the person's eating behaviors. This linking will reinforce that the disorder is a symptom of the dysfunctional family pattern. It is also important to point out that each individual is responsible for his or her own behavior. This will reduce the guilt experienced by parents and siblings and increase feelings of personal power in the person with the disorder by expecting her to "own" her own behavior.

Evaluation

The nurse evaluates the effectiveness of the interventions by determining whether the client-centered goals have been reached by the date set. Specific criteria for evaluating short term goals for clients will be discussed in each of the separate sections on anorexia, bulimia, and obesity due to compulsive eating.

Anorexia Nervosa

The medical term *anorexia* usually applies to a condition in which there is a loss of appetite. In the client with anorexia nervosa, there may *not* be any loss of appetite or disinterest in food, and often the opposite is true. The anorexic is usually preoccupied with food and eating but will suppress her desire for food in order to control her eating. This preoccupation is seen in the anorexic's spending time in planning family menus, choosing restaurants where the family will eat, counting every calorie she ingests, and talking incessantly about food and weight-related issues. A preoccupation with exercise is often present, with the anorexic pushing herself beyond normal limits or needs in order to "work off" every calorie she might have ingested or to "allow" herself to eat a morsel of food.

Ninety-five percent of anorexics are women, and one in 250 teenagers becomes anorexic. Most develop the disorder between the ages of 13 and 22, with the most frequent age being 18. For most, weight was never an issue growing up, although some were slightly overweight. The typical anorexic comes from a white, middle- or upper middle–class family in which divorce or separation is rare. They are usually attractive and intelligent girls who are described as "never being any problem" as children. They tend to over-

achieve in studies and careers and spend a great deal of time in these pursuits. It is no wonder that the anorexic brings out feelings of confusion, anger, and helplessness in parents, friends, and professionals who must stand by and watch a gifted person starve herself "for no reason." In spite of pleas and even threats by concerned people, the anorexic maintains

---

Table 25–4 ■ NURSING INTERVENTIONS AND RATIONALES: PSYCHOTHERAPEUTIC NEEDS OF A PERSON WITH ANOREXIA NERVOSA

INTERVENTION	RATIONALE
Nursing Diagnosis: *Cardiac output decreased* related to binge-purge behaviors, as evidenced by possible fluid and electrolyte imbalance	
1. Monitoring temperature, respiration, and pulse (apical and radial) every day.	1. Increased risk of arrhythmias, bradycardia, and hypotension exists. Hypothermia is often present; therefore, a slight elevation of body temperature above 98.6° F may be a high fever.
2. Observe for tetany or complaint of muscle cramping. Be aware of current electrolyte status.	2. Electrolyte imbalances are common. Subjective complaints of muscle cramping or observation of muscle stiffness in body movement is significant. Frequent electrolyte measures are necessary because of life-threatening complications of hypokalemia.
3. Observe caloric intake closely: (1) amount client eats voluntarily and (2) rituals that decrease amount eaten.	3–7. Because of client's severe anxiety concerning eating and weight in controlled setting, some deception is to be expected. Therefore, objective as well as subjective data collection is essential.
4. Observe closely after eating for signs of purging.	
5. Observe activity level.	
6. Measure urine and fecal output.	
7. Weigh daily at the same time in light clothing.	
Nursing Diagnosis: *Alteration in nutrition* less than body requirements related to distorted body image, as evidenced by body weight 20% or more under ideal weight for height and frame	
1. Make contract for minimal safe weight range, which is a contingency for discharge.	1–2. Participation in planning care increases feelings of control and compliance with treatment. A controlled diet can allay fears of too rapid a weight gain.
2. Give assurance that quick weight gain is not desirable, and that slow, controlled weight gain is the goal.	
3. Meet the client's nutritionist and physician on planning a diet to meet client's physical needs. Allow increasing control over types of food eaten after normal pattern is exhibited.	3. A team approach to planning diet ensures that physical and emotional needs are being met.
4. Respond to signs of distrust and anxiety by acknowledging these feelings in an empathetic manner—avoid interpretation or confrontation in initial stages of relationship.	4. Feelings of worthlessness and anxiety increase as weight increases. Client responds best to support and understanding of fears. To client, gaining weight may mean a threat to survival.
5. Understand that behaviors of deception are expected. Avoid labels such as "bad client" or "liar."	5. Deceptive behaviors are a means of increasing self-esteem and control. Power struggles and negative judgments are to be avoided.

rigid control over her eating, and her only conscious goal is "not to eat." She avoids eating as though phobic of food and experiences anxiety approaching panic when her control is threatened. When she does relinquish control, even slightly, she subjects herself to harsh self-criticism for being "weak" and may experience feelings of hopelessness. In extreme cases, this can lead to suicide. Showing an anorexic the objective facts, such as her actual weight on a scale, her mirror image, or her calorie expenditure as compared with her calorie intake, only increases her need for control.

What would induce a young girl or woman with so many strengths to starve herself, sometimes to death, for the sake of a slim body? It is reported that 5–18% of anorexics die from self-starvation (Kaplan and Sadock 1991). The answer may lie in the possibility that the anorexic is controlling potentially disabling anxiety by controlling her eating. The exact source of this anxiety is different for each individual, but the conflicts most commonly encountered are ones of identity, separation, and autonomy.

Table 25–4 identifies helpful approaches for working with individuals with anorexia nervosa.

DSM-IV CLASSIFICATION

The function of anorexia nervosa as a means of dealing with anxiety rooted in conflict is addressed in the DSM-IV (Diagnostic statistical manuals of the APA 1987). This connection is seen in the following example, in which the character disorder that underlies the eating disorder is placed on axis II. The axis II diagnosis indicates a personality or developmental disorder, whereas axis I indicates a more acute problem. An example is

> Axis I: Anorexia Nervosa
> Axis II: Compulsive Personality Disorder

In the absence of a character disorder, a specific trait may be mentioned on axis II. For example

> Axis I: Anorexia Nervosa
> Axis II: Histrionic Personality Features

The criteria for a diagnosis of anorexia nervosa are specifically stated in Box 25–2.

Box 25–2. DIAGNOSTIC CRITERIA FOR ANOREXIA NERVOSA

A. Refusal to maintain body weight over a minimal normal weight for age and height, e.g., weight loss leading to maintenance of body weight 15% below that expected, or failure to make expected weight gain during period of growth, leading to body weight 15% below that expected.

B. Intense fear of gaining weight or becoming fat, even though underweight.

C. Disturbance in the way in which one's body weight, size, or shape is experienced, e.g., the person claims to "feel fat" even when emaciated or denies the seriousness of the current low body weight.

D. In females, the absence of at least three consecutive menstrual cycles when otherwise expected to occur (primary or secondary amenorrhea). (A woman is considered to have amenorrhea if her periods occur only following hormone, e.g., estrogen, administration.)

Binge-eating/purging type: During the episode of anorexia nervosa, the person engages in recurrent episodes of binge eating.

Restricting type: During the episode of anorexia nervosa, the person does *not* engage in recurrent episodes of binge eating.

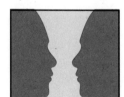

Case Study: Working with a Person Who Has Anorexia Nervosa

Jill is a 16-year-old high school student who was admitted to an eating disorder unit of a local general hospital for anorexia nervosa. She was 5'7" and weighed 90 pounds. Her parents reported a usual weight of 125 pounds and said that she had lost 35 pounds in the previous five weeks. They reported that she refused to eat even her favorite foods. She was taken to the emergency room by her parents, who physically carried her from their home, against her protests. Jill was literally kicking and screaming, protesting that she would "be forced to eat" and would "blow up like a blimp." During her

Continued on following page

Case Study: Working with a Person Who Has Anorexia Nervosa *(Continued)*

initial assessment by her primary nurse, Ms. Heart, Jill was mute and avoided eye contact while maintaining a sullen look on her face. She fidgeted in her seat whenever a question was asked but offered no verbal response. Ms. Heart noted that Jill's nail beds were blue and that she was shivering, although she wore clothing that was heavier than necessary for the well-heated room. Her hair was dull and limp, with some apparent bald patches, and her skin appeared dry, with a yellowish tinge.

Assessment

Ms. Heart divided the data obtained during the initial interview with Jill into objective and subjective components.

OBJECTIVE DATA

1. Rapid weight loss
2. Emaciated appearance
3. Mute
4. Avoids eye contact
5. Sullen facial expression
6. Fidgety
7. Cyanosis of nail beds
8. Dry skin with yellow tinge
9. Shivering with heavy clothing
10. Dull, limp hair with bald patches
11. Physically carried to emergency room

SUBJECTIVE DATA (from parents, as client was mute)

1. "I'll blow up like a blimp."
2. "They'll force me to eat."
3. She was "kicking and screaming" (reported by parents).

Nursing Diagnosis

Ms. Heart reviewed her data and formulated two nursing diagnoses in order of priority.

1. *Altered nutrition: less than body requirements* related to self-starvation
   - Emaciated
   - Rapid weight loss
   - Cyanosis of nail beds
   - Dry skin, yellow tinge
   - Limp hair with bald spot

2. *Ineffective individual coping* related to anxiety over losing control and inability to trust
   - "They'll force me to eat"
   - Physically carried into emergency room
   - Mute
   - Avoids eye contact
   - Sullen facial expression

Planning

CONTENT LEVEL—PLANNING GOALS

Ideally, when planning care, short and long term goals are discussed and set with input from the client. Because Jill's physical starvation had altered her judgment and perception of her physical condition, Ms. Heart set down the short term goals, with input from other members of the health team, and discussed them with Jill. Because Jill's self-starvation was life threatening, attention to gradual weight gain was given priority.

Nursing Diagnosis	Goals
1. *Altered nutrition: less than body requirements* related to self-starvation	1a. Client will gain 0.5–1.5 kg per week. 1b. Client will exhibit a minimum of adverse physical effects from refeeding and starvation during hospital stay (see Figure 25–4).
2. *Ineffective individual coping* related to inability to trust and anxiety over losing control	2a. Client will state that she feels more in control within three weeks. 2b. Client will state that she feels more comfortable with nurse and views nurse as a helping person by four weeks.

PROCESS LEVEL—NURSES' REACTIONS AND FEELINGS

Anorexic clients who exhibit such behaviors as muteness, withdrawal, and sullenness may engender feelings of helplessness and subsequent anger in the nurse. The nurse can use insight into her feelings as a valuable tool in her nursing practice. A lack of self-awareness can interfere with the accepting and nonjudgmental attitude that is especially important in working with the anorexic client. This frightened young woman might be labeled "uncooperative" because of her defenses. Some nurse behaviors that would indicate anger and need for supervision follow:

1. An avoidance of the client
2. An increased attempt to control through arbitrary limit setting

3. Any power struggles or argumentative interactions with the client
4. Infantilizing the client or not providing appropriate limits to compensate for angry feelings

Ms. Heart had been working with clients with eating disorders for two years and had become aware of the signs of her own covert anger in reaction to the clients' behaviors. She continued to be alert to her feelings and actions as clues to what was going on with her clients. Ms. Heart was in weekly supervision with the psychiatric nurse specialist assigned to her unit.

Interventions

Ms. Heart drew her nursing interventions from those outlined in Table 25–4. From these guidelines and input from the health team, Ms. Heart created an individualized plan of care for Jill (Nursing Care Plan 25–1).

Evaluation

Ms. Heart continuously evaluated Jill's progress. She reviewed the short term goals to determine whether they were realistic and to ensure that the planned interventions were appropriate for meeting the goals. See Nursing Care Plan 25–1 for the frequent evaluation and outcome of Ms. Heart's nursing care.

Nursing Care Plan 25–1 ■ A PERSON WITH ANOREXIA NERVOSA: Jill

NURSING DIAGNOSIS

Altered nutrition **related to self-starvation**

Supporting Data

- Emaciated
- Rapid weight loss
- Cyanosis of nail beds
- Dry skin with yellow tinge
- Limp hair with bald spot

Long Term Goal: Client's weight will be within safe limits by discharge.

Short Term Goals	Interventions	Rationale	Evaluation
1. Client will gain 0.5–1.5 kg per week.	1a. Observe caloric intake closely (amount eaten). 1b. Note rituals while eating. 1c. Observe after eating for signs of purging. 1d. Observe activity level. 1e. Measure urine and fecal output. 1f. Weigh daily at the same time in light clothing.	1a–f. Because of client's anxiety regarding eating and weight gain and being hospitalized against client's will, some deception is to be expected. For this reason, objective as well as subjective data collection is essential.	Goal met Week 1—0.5 kg. Week 2—0.7 kg. Week 3—0.9 kg. Week 4—1.1 kg. Week 6—0.8 kg, (after two-pound ankle weight found in pants) Week 7—1.2 kg. Goal is being met, with a slow but steady weight gain.

Continued on following page

Nursing Care Plan 25-1 ■ **A PERSON WITH ANOREXIA NERVOSA: Jill**

(Continued)

Short Term Goals	Interventions	Rationale	Evaluation
	1g. Make contract with client for a minimal safe weight range, as a contingency for discharge.	1g. Involvement in decision making increases sense of control and chances of compliance.	
2. Client will exhibit a minimum of adverse physical effects from refeeding and self-starvation during hospitalization.	2a. Daily monitoring of temperature, respiration, and pulse (apical and radial).	2a. Effects of starvation increase risk of arrythmias, bradycardia, and hypotension. Hypotension is often present.	Goal met Week 1—Within normal limits. Week 2—Within normal limits. Week 3—Within normal limits. Week 4—Within normal limits. Week 5—Within normal limits. Week 6—Within normal limits. Week 7—Within normal limits.
	2b. Observe for muscle twitching, facial twitching, wrist or ankle twitching, and cramping. Check current electrolyte status daily.	2b. Electrolyte imbalances can be life threatening.	Goal met Week 1—Within normal limits. Week 2—Complained of leg cramping, physician notified, and potassium serum levels measured. Week 3—Within normal limits. Week 4—Within normal limits. Week 5—Within normal limits. Week 6—Within normal limits. Week 7—Within normal limits.
	2c. Observe for adverse side effects of refeeding: ● Abdominal discomfort ● Nausea ● Edema ● Constipation or diarrhea ● Gastric dilation ● Hypophosphatemia ● Congestive heart failure	2c. Adverse and possibly fatal effects can occur with overfeeding and too-rapid weight gain.	Goal met Week 1—None. Week 2—complained of abdominal cramping (date). Week 3—complained of nausea, ankle edema (date). Week 4—None. Week 6—complained of constipation (date). Week 7—None.

Bulimia Nervosa

Bulimia nervosa is a clinical entity distinct from anorexia nervosa and compulsive eating. Bulimics can be divided into three different groups. The first are anorexics who have lost their rigid control over eating and who binge. Purging is an attempt to regain control. About 50% of anorexics engage in this behavior (Bruch 1985). The second group consists of anorexics who developed the syndrome of bulimia prior to the onset of anorexia nervosa (Kassett et al. 1988). The third group are persons who are of normal weight or are only slightly overweight who binge and then purge to maintain or lose weight and who report never having had an anorexic episode. There has been an increase in this last type in recent years, or at least an increase in the numbers seeking treatment. It is esti-

mated to occur in as many as 40% of college women (Kaplan and Sadock 1991).

The binge-purge cycle is compulsive in nature and may interfere with the individual's level of daily functioning to the extent that all of her waking time is spent or arranged around these behaviors. Jobs and relationships may be severely affected as the person becomes increasingly more preoccupied with bingeing and purging while simultaneously becoming more isolated. Binges may begin with thousands of calories consumed in a matter of minutes and end because of abdominal distress, sleep, or social interruption. In extreme cases, the person may eat until unconscious. Binge-purge behaviors may affect the lives of bulimics and their families in the same way that alcoholism or drug abuse affects other families. Bulimic behaviors commonly surface in recovering alcoholics, and bulimia and substance abuse sometimes exist simultaneously. Substance abuse and other forms of poor

Table 25–5 ■ NURSING INTERVENTIONS AND RATIONALES: PSYCHOTHERAPEUTIC NEEDS OF A PERSON WITH BULIMIA NERVOSA

INTERVENTION	RATIONALE
Nursing Diagnosis: *Ineffective individual coping* related to disturbance in impulse control, as evidenced by compulsive binge-purge behavior	
1. Communicate empathy; focus on feelings. Avoid comments that seem judgmental.	1. A therapeutic alliance must be based on understanding in an atmosphere of openness and support.
2. Evaluate situation using a crisis intervention model, e.g., assess precipitating events, support system, and coping skills.	2. Strengths and weaknesses, coping skills, available resources, and potential crisis situations need to be ascertained.
3. Continuously assess the presence of purging and the family system.	3. Data collected in initial interview is not complete. Assessment is ongoing.
4. Assess for depression and risk for suicide.	4. Clinical depression is common. Presence of anxiety and feelings of hopelessness indicate high-risk factors.
5. Assess for any immediate physical distress or potential health problems.	5. Immediate physical problem may warrant emergency treatment. Potential health problems warrant some immediate health teaching concerning effects of bingeing and purging.
6. Refer client to physician of her choice for a complete physical examination.	6. An examination is warranted when bingeing and purging are frequent.
7. Refer to a psychiatrist for evaluation for possible pharmacotherapy.	7. Anxiety and possible depression may be relieved by medication, thus making outpatient treatment more manageable.

impulse control are frequently reported in family members of bulimics. This poor impulse control in the bulimic family is similar to the "uncontrollable" nature of the binge-purge cycle.

There is no clearly identified personality type among bulimics, but an underlying depression has been proposed to occur in many. Signs and symptoms of depression, as well as reported suicide attempts and self-mutilation, are often present. The depression may be directly related to the loss of control the bulimic experiences over her eating, or it may remain unchanged regardless of her improvement. A range of personality disorders has been identified in bulimics. Problems with interpersonal relationships, self-concept, and impulsive behaviors are common (Halmi 1988). Forms of poor impulse control include sexual promiscuity, kleptomania, compulsive spending, shoplifting, gambling, and compulsive lying. Other bulimics might guard against these impulses by exhibiting obsessive-compulsive behaviors such as "filling up every minute" to avoid temptation. Any slight deviation from their routine results in feelings of "emptiness" and anxiety. Bulimia may be used as a socially ac-

ceptable substitute for alcoholism and drug addition (Bulik 1987).

Forms of purging may include self-induced vomiting, which can become spontaneous as the behavior persists. Food might simply be chewed and spit out without swallowing, and laxative abuse is common. A minority of bulimics may use diuretics for weight control.

It is thought that the bulimic has a "deficit in the sense of responsibility." The bulimic blames external events or other persons for her behavior. This belief may account for the "assumed helplessness" that bulimics exhibit. The power of others renders her powerless and unable to take charge of her own life (Bruch 1985).

Table 25–5 outlines helpful approaches to use with people with bulimia.

DSM-IV CLASSIFICATION

The DSM-IV criteria for bulimia nervosa (Box 25–3) are very specific, but bulimics may vary greatly in their ability to adjust, so a diagnosis of bulimia nervosa

---

Box 25–3. DIAGNOSTIC CRITERIA FOR BULIMIA NERVOSA

A. Recurrent episodes of binge eating (rapid consumption of a large amount of food in a discrete period of time).

B. A feeling of lack of control over eating behaviors during the eating binges.

C. The person regularly engages in either self-induced vomiting, use of laxatives or diuretics, strict dieting or fasting, or vigorous exercise in order to prevent weight gain.

D. A minimum average of two binge eating episodes a week for at least three months.

E. Persistent overconcern with body shape and weight.

Purging type: Regularly engages in self-induced vomiting or the use of laxatives or diuretics

Nonpurging type: Use of strict diet, fasting, or vigorous exercise, but does not regularly engage in purging.

Reprinted with permission from the DSM-IV Options Book: Work in Progress (9/1/91). Copyright 1991 American Psychiatric Association.

---

alone may be misleading. There may be other, more serious, simultaneous diagnoses. The DSM-IV classifications allow for this need to individualize the bulimic's treatment by using the following system. For example

> Axis I: Bulimia
> Axis II: Borderline Personality Disorder with Depressive Features

A person with this diagnosis might present the binge-purge syndrome along with intense feelings of abandonment and depression that seem related to separation or loss. The treatment plan would need to address bulimia and depression and consider the dynamics of the borderline personality (see Chapter 16).

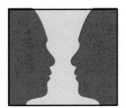

Case Study: Working with a Person Who Has Bulimia Nervosa

Ms. Hunt is a well-groomed 23-year-old woman who was a recent college graduate living at home with her parents and 19-year-old sister. An older sister was married and lived nearby. Ms. Hunt came to the Community Mental Health Center seeking counseling for "anxiety attacks." During the initial assessment by Mr. Hope, the psychiatric nurse clinical specialist, Ms. Hunt reported "feeling panic before leaving home, even to go to work." She would manage to get to work only after "bingeing" but would purge once she

arrived at her job. So far, she had been able to conceal this from her family and her employer but had received numerous warnings about her lateness. She had also experienced "sluggishness and irritability" after bingeing and purging. Ms. Hunt worked as a dietitian in a college cafeteria, which further complicated her situation, as she "sneaked binges and purges" at least twice each workday. She reported "not being able to stop" this cycle and was tearful and speaking rapidly as she was interviewed.

Assessment

Mr. Hope observed that Ms. Hunt was experiencing anxiety during the interview as she related her distress over the emotionally and physically stressful binge-purge cycle. From the assessment, the nurse noted two important strengths: (1) Ms. Hunt had achieved

success in her education, and (2) she had remained employed in spite of a debilitating degree of anxiety. Ms. Hunt's health status and employment status were threatened, but she had some degree of good judgment in seeking assistance at this time.

Assessment
(Continued)

OBJECTIVE DATA

1. Tearful with rapid speech
2. Employed at food-related job
3. Living at home with family of origin
4. Well groomed
5. College graduate
6. Behaviors affect job
7. Behaviors kept secret from family and employer
8. Seems to be seeking help voluntarily

SUBJECTIVE DATA

1. "Panic" before leaving home
2. Reports binge-purge cycle that feels "uncontrollable"
3. "Sluggishness" and "irritability" after bingeing and purging

Nursing Diagnosis

From the data, Mr. Hope formulated the following nursing diagnosis:

Anxiety (severe to panic) related to separation issues
- "Panic" before leaving home
- "Uncontrollable" binge-purge cycle when under stress
- Tearful with rapid speech

Planning

CONTENT LEVEL—PLANNING GOALS

Mr. Hope spent time with Ms. Hunt establishing long term and short term goals that were realistic, appropriate, and measurable.

Nursing Diagnosis	Long Term Goal	Short Term Goals
1. *Anxiety (severe to panic)* related to separation issues	1. Client will demonstrate use of two ways of coping with anxiety by (date).	1a. Within two weeks client will identify specific events that increase her anxiety. 1b. Client will name two alternative coping skills for handling anxiety (other than bingeing and purging) within three weeks.

PROCESS LEVEL—NURSES' REACTIONS AND FEELINGS

The client with bulimia often has extreme anxiety because she feels she is out of control. Once the compulsive binge-purge cycle is in motion, there is a feeling of helplessness to control food. The helpless client may look to the nurse to solve her problems and may exhibit anger when this expectation is not met. Feelings aroused in the nurse from the client's helplessness and extreme dependency might set in motion the need to "take over" or "rescue" the client. These responses on the part of the nurse stem from a "need to be needed" or to "control" this person who feels unable to control her own life. Cues that signal that the nurse has a need to "rescue" the client are listed subsequently. These behaviors signal the need for supervision and can inhibit client progress.

1. Giving the client a diet to follow, believing that poor eating habits are "the problem"
2. Corroborating the client's belief that "food controls her" by telling her to avoid situations in which she might binge rather than focusing on the anxiety that is related to her behaviors
3. Attempting to give the bulimic solutions or "pat answers" rather than using a problem-solving approach

Intervention

Mr. Hope planned individual care for Ms. Hunt, drawing from nursing interventions useful for a person with bulimia (see Table 25–5). Drawing from intervention guidelines and Ms. Hunt's individual situation, Mr. Hope devised Nursing Care Plan 25–2.

Continued on following page

Evaluation

Mr. Hope continuously evaluated the short term goals set for Ms. Hunt. (1) He evaluated her ability to identify situations that produced anxiety and make connections between perceptions, anxiety, and behaviors. (2) He evaluated alterations in her present coping skills and her use of alternative ways of handling stress. Refer to Nursing Care Plan 25–2 for specific observations in the evaluation of Ms. Hunt on a weekly basis. During his interactions with Ms. Hunt, the nurse was watchful for any side effects resulting from the cessation of the binge-purge cycle (see Figure 25–4).

Nursing Care Plan 25–2 ■ A PERSON WITH BULIMIA NERVOSA: Ms. Hunt

NURSING DIAGNOSIS

*Anxiety (**severe to panic**)* **related to separation issues**

Supporting Data

- Panic before leaving home
- "Uncontrollable" binge-purge cycle when under stress
- Tearful with rapid speech

Long Term Goal: Client will demonstrate two ways of coping with anxiety by (date).

Short Term Goals	Interventions	Rationale	Evaluation
1. Within two weeks, client will identify precipitating events that increase her levels of anxiety.	1a. Assess for suicidal risk immediately.	1a. Underlying depression common. High anxiety and feelings of helplessness indicate possible suicidal ideation.	Goal met Week 1—Not at risk at present.
	1b. Work with client on a one-to-one basis two times per week.	1b. Establish therapeutic relationship and evaluate for group participation with others who have eating disorders.	Week 2— Client states she is beginning to see a connection between anxiety and family issues that involve separation, i.e., "growing up," "being different," "leaving home."
	1c. Communicate empathy; focus on feelings of anxiety. 1d. Avoid any comments that may seem judgmental.	1c–d. Establish therapeutic alliance based on understanding. Provide an atmosphere of openness and support. Help maintain self-esteem.	Week 3—Since the client started group, validation from group and support have increased socialization. States she has two new friends with group encouragement.
2. Within four weeks, client will name two alternative coping skills to use when she feels increased anxiety.	2a. Evaluate client's situation using a crisis intervention model, e.g., assessing precipitating events, support system, and coping skills.	2a. To identify anxiety-provoking issues, adaptive and nonadaptive defenses, and possible resources for changes.	Goal met Plans to start back to school in fall for master's degree to fulfill dream of teaching dietitians. To date has three new supports:
	2b. Explore alternative coping skills—relation techniques, talking with friend, activities, problem solving.	2b. Help minimize need to use binge-purge cycle.	1. Group 2. Increase in socialization (friends) 3. Plans for future
	2c. Encourage participation in and provide referred group therapy for eating disorders.	2c. Provide support and reduce feeling of isolation while learning new coping skills.	
	2d. Refer client to a physician for ● Complete exam ● Possible pharmacotherapy	2d. Treat or prevent physical damage from binge-purge behavior. Client's anxiety or depression may be relieved by medication, thus making outpatient treatment more manageable.	

Obesity Due to Compulsive Eating

Obesity is a physical condition that can have several possible etiologies. It can be the result of (1) a medical condition, (2) a lack of an adequate variety of foods, as seen in lower socioeconomic groups whose diets consist mainly of carbohydrates, (3) a side effect of pharmacotherapy such as steroid treatment, or (4) compulsive eating that is psychogenic in its origins. The last type of obesity is discussed here and can be subdivided into two broad categories of either "developmental" or "reactive" obesity (Bruch 1985).

Developmental obesity is the type seen in persons who have been obese since childhood and is the result of overfeeding, beginning as early as infancy. **Reactive obesity** occurs later in life, when compulsive eating becomes a maladaptive coping style at a time of stress. In either case, Hilde Bruch proposed that compulsive eating and obesity are defenses against feelings of depression or more unacceptable acting-out behaviors and that the premature removal of the eating behaviors and subsequent weight loss may allow these feared feelings and behaviors to surface.

If viewed in this way, compulsive eating and "being fat" may serve a similar function for the obese person that fasting and "being thin" serve for the anorexic. For example, a woman, when in an obese state is withdrawn and isolated, blames her lack of close relationships on "being fat." If she were slim, she feels, she would be more physically attractive and would become outgoing. Although this change is desirable, it is also feared because obesity is, for her, a protection from the risks of intimacy. She feels that her "fat" is controlling her fate and, subsequently, denies responsibility for her own isolation. Like the anorexic, she believes that "if I were thin, all my problems would be solved." By holding onto this belief, she avoids the painful process of examining her own participation in her problems.

Like the anorexic and the bulimic, a person who uses food to maintain obesity may be experiencing conflicts about independence, autonomy, separation, and intimacy. Although there are many obese men, the current literature seems to focus on obese women, children, and adolescents. The reason for this is that these populations seek professional counseling for weight-related problems more often than adult males. Although there is a social stigma placed on "fat people" in general, obese women, children, and

---

Table 25–6 ■ NURSING INTERVENTIONS AND RATIONALES: PSYCHOTHERAPEUTIC NEEDS OF A PERSON WHO COMPULSIVELY EATS

INTERVENTION	RATIONALE
Nursing Diagnosis: *Ineffective individual coping* related to low self-esteem and unmet emotional needs, as evidenced by compulsive overeating	
1. Assess suicidal risk.	1. Feelings of hopelessness and poor self-concept indicate high-risk factors.
2. Assess for depression.	2. Compulsive eating can be a way of handling depression and internalizing aggression.
3. Provide structured one-on-one sessions.	3. Frequent opportunities to verbalize feelings can diminish acting out through compulsive eating.
4. Provide structured activities.	4. Structured activities help use empty time and control compulsive eating.
5. Provide group activities, both formal (therapy) and informal (dance, art) ones.	5. Group activities provide feedback, aid development of a more realistic self-image, and allow outlets to relieve tension and aggression.
6. Encourage physical evaluation by physician.	6. Medical abnormalities resulting from obesity need to be evaluated.
7. Encourage consultation by psychiatrist.	7. Need for psychopharmacology, i.e., antianxiety or antidepression medication, must be evaluated
8. Evaluate personal strengths and significant supports with client.	8. Present situation needs to be assessed realistically—strengths must be emphasized and need for support evaluated.

adolescents feel society's disapproval more acutely. Self-esteem is more dependent on body image among these populations. Feelings of shame and guilt, with subsequent depression, are frequent complaints. These feelings may be suppressed through an escalation of the compulsive eating and denial of the obesity. Obesity is denied when an obese person sees only her "better" parts in a mirror or avoids the mirror altogether.

Table 25–6 outlines useful approaches for the nurse to use when working with a compulsive eater.

DSM-III-R CLASSIFICATION

Specific diagnostic criteria for obesity due to compulsive eating are not found in the DSM-III-R. It is possible, however, to use one of two DSM-III-R categories for diagnosis: (1) atypical eating disorders or (2) psychological factor affecting physical condition. An example of the former is:

Axis I: Atypical Eating Disorder
Axis II: Mixed Personality Disorder

and an example of the latter is:

Axis I: Psychological Factor Affecting Physical Condition
Axis II: Dependent Personality Disorder
Axis III: Obesity

Axis III is used, in this case, not only to identify obesity as a medical condition but also to emphasize that it is a result of a psychological condition.

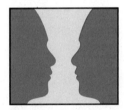

Case Study: Working with a Person Whose Obesity Is Caused by Compulsive Eating

Ms. Robbins is a 45-year-old woman who was admitted to an inpatient mental health unit for depression. Her husband reported that she had not gone to her job for two weeks. Her reasons were vague, and physical complaints were general. She spent most of her days in bed but was awake most of the night. Her husband also reported an apparent increase in her eating, although she denied feeling hungry. The decision to hospitalize Ms. Robbins was made after she verbalized suicidal ideation: "I really don't care what happens to me anymore," "I feel like dying."

Mrs. Worth, a staff nurse on the unit, saw Ms. Robbins for the initial interview. Ms. Robbins was despondent and became tearful when describing her feelings of "worthlessness." She stated, "I can't stand myself—I hate the way I look, but I can't do anything. I feel too ashamed to go to work and have people see me."

Mrs. Worth also noted that Ms. Robbins appeared disheveled and wore tight-fitting clothing. Ms. Robbins stated that she could no longer fit into her clothes. She had gained 40 pounds in the previous two months and at 5'3" weighed 175 pounds. She had no previous history of obesity but reported eating for comfort at times of stress. Ms. Robbins had begun eating compulsively shortly after her father died following a long battle with cancer.

Assessment

Mrs. Worth divided her data into objective and subjective components.

OBJECTIVE DATA

1. Seclusive at home for two weeks
2. Forty-pound weight gain in two months
3. Recent death of father
4. Appeared despondent and became tearful
5. Appeared disheveled
6. 5'3" and 175 pounds
7. Erratic sleep pattern
8. Increased eating without hunger

SUBJECTIVE DATA

1. "I really don't care what happens to me anymore."
2. Feelings of "worthlessness" and "self-loathing"
3. "Ashamed to have people see me."

Nursing Diagnosis

Based on her data, Mrs. Worth formulated the following nursing diagnoses:

1. *Dysfunctional grieving* related to father's death, as evidenced by suicidal thoughts and feelings of worthlessness
   - Forty-pound weight gain in two months (after father's death)
   - Seclusion and social isolation
   - Passive suicidal ideation
   - Feelings of worthlessness and self-loathing

2. *Disturbance in self-esteem* related to obesity, as evidenced by withdrawal and change in usual pattern of responsibility
   - Ashamed to be seen
   - Feeling worthless and expresses self-loathing
   - Disheveled appearance
   - Appears despondent and tearful
   - 5'3" tall and 175 pounds

Planning

CONTENT LEVEL—PLANNING GOALS

After spending time with Ms. Robbins, Mrs. Worth developed goals for her nursing diagnosis. Because Ms. Robbins' physical safety was of utmost importance, priority of interventions was based on the data received from a thorough assessment of suicidal risk and intent (refer to Chapter 21).

Nursing Diagnosis	Long Term Goal	Short Term Goals
1. *Dysfunctional grieving* related to father's death, as evidenced by suicidal thoughts and feelings of worthlessness	1. Within one year's time, client will comfortably state that she remembers the good times and difficult times with her dad.	1a. Client will verbalize feelings about her father's death by the end of four days. 1b. Client will state that she feels better about herself and name two specific strengths by (date).

PROCESS LEVEL—NURSES' REACTIONS AND FEELINGS

Clients who are obese and depressed are often suffering from low self-esteem and shame. When the nurse is confronted with a client who makes self-loathing and self-deprecating statements, there is always a temptation to ease this pain or "take it away." This often indicates a need of the nurse to escape these feelings because they are almost as uncomfortable for the nurse as they are for the client. Some nursing behaviors that can interfere with the development of self-esteem in the client are listed subsequently. Evidence of these behaviors signals the nurse's need for supervision in order to maximize therapeutic intervention.

1. Telling the client that she is wrong about her evaluation of herself rather than exploring her strengths and weaknesses
2. Giving the client compliments that are not genuine
3. Telling the client "not to worry"
4. Focusing on her obesity as the main problem rather than on her feelings about herself. This reinforces her belief that her obese body is "shameful"

Intervention

There are numerous areas and levels of intervention that the nurse can use when working with a client who is obese. This chapter deals with obesity related to maladaptive coping responses. Therefore, the interventions focus on the underlying causes, such as depression, rather than on the physical manifestations, such as diets and exercise. Table 25–6 outlines nursing interventions useful for a client who is a compulsive eater.

Mrs. Worth planned individualized care for Ms. Robbins (Nursing Care Plan 25–3) by using some of the nursing guidelines but tailoring the plan to Ms. Robbins' needs.

Evaluation

Mrs. Worth evaluated her goals during Ms. Robbins' hospital stay. Evidence that appropriate grieving response had been activated would have been seen in Ms. Robbins' ability to talk more completely about her feelings about her father's death. Mrs. Worth noted Ms. Robbins' ability to share painful memories and feelings with her and significant others, and she evaluated appropriate affects regarding the grief reaction. A decrease in

Continued on following page

Evaluation
(Continued)

Ms. Robbins' thoughts about suicide and evidence of more spontaneous socialization were other indicators that the grieving process had been reactivated.

Signs of a more realistic self-concept and rise in self-esteem would have been seen in statements to that effect from Ms.

Robbins' and in specific observations. Was she able to identify specific strengths? Did she speak less frequently about feeling worthless? Did she show an increase in control over eating behaviors? Did her hygiene and grooming improve? Evaluation of goals is noted on Ms. Robbins' care plan.

Nursing Care Plan 25–3 ■ A PERSON WITH PSYCHOGENIC OBESITY: Ms. Robbins

NURSING DIAGNOSIS

***Dysfunctional grieving* related to father's death, as evidenced by suicidal thoughts and feelings of worthlessness**

Supporting Data

- Forty-pound weight gain in two months (after father's death)
- Seclusion and social isolation
- Passive suicidal ideation
- Feelings of "worthlessness" and "self-loathing"

Long Term Goal: Client will start and continue to work through the grieving process by (date).

Short Term Goal	Interventions	Rationale	Evaluation
1. Client will verbalize feelings about her father's death by the end of four days.	1a. Provide structure in client's day through one-to-one sessions with primary nurse.	1a. Gives client opportunity to verbalize feelings of grief, loss, and separation.	Goal met Week 1—Client's affect more appropriate; talking more freely of missing father.
	1b. Provide structured activities throughout the day.	1b. Helps to control compulsive eating.	Week 2—Client continues to express feelings of sadness.
			Week 3—Client was able to express anger over father's leaving her—pounding fist on table. Grief process appears activated.

NURSING DIAGNOSIS

***Disturbance in self-esteem* related to obesity, as evidenced by withdrawal and change in usual patterns of responsibility**

Supporting Data

- Ashamed to be seen
- Disheveled appearance
- Feels worthless and expresses self-loathing
- 5'3" and 175 pounds
- Appears despondent and tearful.

Long Term Goal: Client will resume usual socialization and role-related responsibilities by (date).

Short Term Goal	Interventions	Rationale	Evaluation
1. Client will state that she feels better about her situation and will name two strengths or supports in three weeks.	1a. Evaluate suicide risk.	1a. Suicidal ideation and hopelessness result in high risk for self-destructive behavior.	Goal met Week 1—Vague thoughts of "wanting to die"; suicide risk low.
	1b. Provide group activities, both formal (therapy) and informal (dance, art) ones.	1b. Group activities provide feedback. Aid development of more realistic self-image.	Week 2—More spontaneous participation in group meetings. Hair clean and well groomed.

Short Term Goal	Interventions	Rationale	Evaluation
	1c. Evaluate with client number of personal strengths and supportive significant others.	1c. Potentially more realistic view of situation: ● Actual strengths ● Actual supports available	Week 3—Appearance greatly improved—neatly dressed, nail care, and loss of three pounds. States that she feels better about self. States that she looks forward to going back to work and spending time with husband.

Summary

The eating disorders discussed in this chapter are (1) anorexia nervosa, (2) bulimia nervosa, and (3) obesity due to compulsive eating. There have been various theories to explain the etiology of the eating disorders, including psychodynamic, sociocultural, and biological. A psychiatric nursing assessment for a person with an eating disorder includes the evaluation of specific areas: *weight, eating, activity, family,* and *physical signs and symptoms.*

Nursing diagnoses for a person with an eating disorder can cover a wide range of problem areas. General diagnoses often include *altered nutrition (less or more than body weight), disturbance in self-esteem, ineffective individual coping,* and *social isolation.*

Effective nursing intervention usually entails various therapeutic modes. For example, medications may be used to treat an underlying depression. Inpatient treatment is often indicated when the physical status is life threatening. Examples include a person with anorexia nervosa whose low weight threatens her life and an obese person whose cardiac status is critical. Behavior modification has been found to be an effective approach for some people with eating disorders. Individual, group, and family therapy approaches are also important treatment modalities. Specific profiles of people with anorexia nervosa, bulimia nervosa, and psychogenic obesity were discussed. Specific interventions for each of these three eating disorders were outlined. The case studies demonstrated each eating disorder and nursing involvement within the framework of the nursing process.

References

American Psychiatric Association. Diagnostic and Statistical Manual of Mental Disorders, 3rd ed, revised (DSM-III-R). Washington, DC: American Psychiatric Association; 1987.

American Psychiatric Association. DSM-IV Options Book: Work in Progress. Washington, DC: American Psychiatric Association, 1991.

Bruch H. Eating Disorders: Obesity, Anorexia Nervosa and the Person Within. New York: Basic Books, 1973.

Bruch H. Four decades of eating disorders. In Garner DM, Garfinkel PE (eds). Handbook of Psychotherapy for Anorexia Nervosa and Bulimia. New York: Guilford Press, 1985.

Bulik C. Drug and alcohol abuse by bulimic women and their families. American Journal of Psychiatry, 144(12):1987.

Carlat DJ, Camargo CA. Review of bulimia nervosa in males. American Journal of Psychiatry, 148(7):831, 1991.

Dickstein LJ. Anorexia and bulimia: A review of clinical issues. Hospital and Community Psychiatry, 36:1086, 1985.

Fava M, et al. Neurochemical abnormalities of anorexia nervosa and bulimia nervosa. American Journal of Psychiatry, 146(8):963; 1989.

Garner DM, Bemis K. Cognitive therapy for anorexia nervosa. In Garner DM, Garfinkel PE (eds). Handbook of Psychotherapy for Anorexia Nervosa and Bulimia. New York: Guilford Press, 1985.

Geist RA. Therapeutic dilemmas in the treatment of anorexia nervosa. (Available from Children's Hospital Medical Center.) Boston, 1982.

Goodsitt A. Self-psychology and the treatment of anorexia nervosa. In Garner DM, Garfinkel PE (eds). Handbook of Psychotherapy for Anorexia Nervosa and Bulimia. New York: Guilford Press, 1985.

Halmi KA. Eating disorders. In Talbott JA, Hales RE, Yudofsky SC (eds). Textbook of Psychiatry. Washington, DC: American Psychiatric Press, 1988.

Johnson C, et al. The syndrome of bulimia: Review and synthesis. Psychiatric Clinics of North America, 7:247, 1984.

Kaplan HI, Sadock BJ. Synopsis of Psychiatry, 6th ed. Baltimore: Williams & Wilkins, 1991.

Kasset J, et al. Pattern of onset of bulimic symptoms in anorexia nervosa. American Journal of Psychiatry, 145(10): 1988.

Keltner NJ. Bulimia: Controlling compulsive eating. Journal of Psychosocial Nursing and Mental Health Services, 22:24, 1984.

Larson BJ. Relationship of family communication patterns to eating disorder inventory scores in adolescent girls. Journal of American Dietary Association, 91(9):1065, 1991.

Love, CC, Seaton H. Eating disorders: Highlights of nursing assessment and therapeutics. Nursing Clinics of North America, 26(3):677, 1991.

Maxmen JS. Psychotropic Drugs Fast Facts. New York: WW Norton, 1991.

Millman M. Such a Pretty Face: Being Fat in America. New York: Berkely Books, 1980.

Minuchin S. Psychosomatic Families—Anorexia Nervosa in Context. Cambridge, MA: Harvard University Press, 1978.

Mitchell J, et al. Gastric dilation as a complication of bulimia. Psychosomatics, 23:93, 1982.

Orbach S. Accepting the symptom: Feminist psychoanalytic treatment of anorexia nervosa. In Garner DM, Garfinkel PE (eds). Handbook of Psychotherapy for Anorexia Nervosa and Bulimia. New York: Guilford Press, 1985.

Pope, et al. Bulimia treated with imipramine: A placebo-controlled, double-blind study. American Journal of Psychiatry, 140:554, 1983.

Pribor EF, Dinwiddle SH. Psychiatric correlates of incest in childhood. The American Journal of Psychiatry, 145(1):52, 1992.

Selvina-Palazzoli M. Self-starvation. London: Human Context Books, Chaucer Publishing Company, 1974.

Wooley S, Wooley W. Intensive outpatient group treatment for bulimia. In Garner DM, Garfinkel PE (eds). Handbook of Psychotherapy for Anorexia Nervosa and Bulimia. New York: Guilford Press, 1985.

Further Reading

American Nurses' Association. Standards of Psychiatric and Mental Health Nursing Practice. Kansas City, MO: American Nurses' Association, 1982.

Boskind-White M, White W Jr. Bulimarexia: The binge-purge cycle. Baltimore: Johns Hopkins University Press, 1985.

Chernin K. The Hungry Self: Women Eating and Identity. New York: Time Books, 1985.

Fairburn C. Cognitive-behavioral treatment for bulimia. In Garner DM, Garfinkel PE (eds). Handbook of Psychotherapy for Anorexia Nervosa and Bulimia. New York: Guilford Press, 1985.

Garfinkel PE, Garner DM. Anorexia Nervosa: A Multidimensional Perspective. New York: Brunner-Mazel, 1982.

Garner DM, Garfinkel PE (eds). Handbook of Psychotherapy for Anorexia Nervosa and Bulimia. New York: Guilford Press, 1985.

Haber J, et al. (eds). Comprehensive Psychiatric Nursing, 2nd ed. New York: McGraw Hill, 1982.

Halmi KA, et al. Binge eating and vomiting: A survey of college population. Psychosomatic Medicine, 11:697, 1981.

Lego S. Group-psychotherapy. In Haber J, et al. (eds). Comprehensive Psychiatric Nursing, 2nd ed. New York: McGraw Hill, 1982.

Lucas AR. Pigging out. Journal of the American Medical Association, 82:247, 1982.

Mitchell J, et al. Intensive outpatient group treatment for bulimia. In Garner DM, Garfinkel PE (eds). Handbook of Psychotherapy for Anorexia Nervosa and Bulimia. New York: Guilford Press, 1985.

Orbach S. Fat Is a Feminist Issue. New York: Berkely Publishing Group, 1978.

Pyle R, et al. Bulimia: A report of 34 cases. American Journal of Clinical Psychiatry, 42:60, 1981.

Swift WJ, et al. The relationship between affective disorder and eating disorder: A review of the literature. American Journal of Psychiatry, 143:290, 1986.

Vandereycken W, Meerman R. Anorexia Nervosa: A Clinician's Guide to Treatment. New York: de Gruyter, 1984.

Walsh BT, et al. Bulimia and depression. Psychosomatic Medicine, 47:123, 1985.

Webb LJ. DSM-III Training Manual. New York: Brunner-Mazel, 1981.

Wilson CP, Mintz I. Abstaining and bulimic anorexics: Two sides of the same coin. Primary Care, 9:517, 1982.

Winstead-Fry P. Family therapy and application. In Haber J, et al. (eds). Comprehensive Psychiatric Nursing, 2nd ed. New York: McGraw Hill Book Company, 1982.

Wolman BB. Psychological Aspects of Obesity. New York: Van Nostrand Reinhold, 1982.

Self-study Exercises

Choose the answer that most accurately completes the statement.

1. If the need-satisfaction cycle in early feeding experiences is healthy, the infant will develop

   A. Feelings of frustration
   B. Feelings of loss of control
   C. Feelings of trust
   D. Separation anxiety

2. Some factors in the development of eating disorders may be

   A. A disturbed family system
   B. Inadequate socialization by the mother
   C. Societal expectation
   D. A faulty belief system regarding weight and appearance
   E. All of the above

3. The most important goal for clients with eating disorders is

   A. Achieving a normal weight
   B. The absence of maladaptive eating patterns
   C. The ability to identify and express their own feelings and needs
   D. The ability to have a sexual relationship

4. The typical anorexic or bulimic tends to deal with her imperfections

   A. By taking personal responsibility for her actions
   B. By harsh self-criticism and increasing efforts to be "perfect"
   C. By forgiving her shortcomings
   D. By objectively putting them in perspective

5. Family therapy for anorexics and bulimics would best focus on

    A. The problem of the eating disorder
    B. The fact that the parents are to blame
    C. Separation-individuation of the family members
    D. Better nutrition for the family

Refer to the case study Working with a Person Who Has Anorexia Nervosa *when answering* questions 6–10.

At mealtime, Ms. Heart observes Jill leaving her tray untouched for 30 minutes. Jill then begins cutting her food into tiny pieces and separating them into several piles on her plate. She then takes one piece at a time and chews it several times before swallowing. After a long pause, she drinks a glass of water and begins the process again.

6. Ms. Heart recognizes that Jill

    A. Is using rituals to control her calorie intake
    B. Is anxious about eating
    C. Is trying to deny the hunger she feels
    D. Is exerting control over the only area she feels she can control
    E. All of the above

7. Ms. Heart's most empathic intervention would be

    A. To spoon-feed Jill
    B. To set a time limit for meals
    C. To acknowledge that this is a difficult situation for Jill
    D. To consult with the physician about ordering tube feedings

8. Ms. Heart is aware that Jill may engage in the following behaviors after eating:

    A. Rapidly pacing the halls
    B. Vomiting
    C. Sneaking a laxative
    D. Weighing herself
    E. All of the above

9. The following physical signs are sometimes seen once eating is reestablished:

    A. Edema
    B. Hypothermia
    C. Lanugo
    D. Abdominal distention

10. Once Jill has begun gaining weight, Ms. Heart's priority regarding Jill's mental status is

    A. Assessing for hallucinations
    B. Assessing for hyperactivity
    C. Assessing for purging
    D. Assessing for signs of depression

Refer to the case study Working with a Person Who Has Bulimia Nervosa *when answering* questions 11–15.

11. Before Ms. Hunt will be able to give up her bingeing and purging behaviors without substituting other symptoms, she must

    A. Be given a diet to follow
    B. Learn and practice alternate ways of dealing with anxiety
    C. Take antianxiety medication
    D. Quit her job as a dietitian

12. Ms. Hunt missed her first appointment after her initial interview. She tells Mr. Hope the following week that she was "too anxious to come in and binged and purged instead." The most helpful response from Mr. Hope would be

    A. "You must keep your appointments to be responsible."
    B. "That must have been an uncomfortable feeling. Let's see if we can figure out what you were anxious about."
    C. "How much did you eat when you binged?"
    D. "There's no need to feel anxious about coming here."

13. During a session with Mr. Hope, Ms. Hunt relates a situation in which she is "afraid to be around" a coworker she feels is "lazy" because she fears "losing control." The best response Mr. Hope could use would be

    A. "It's OK—you won't lose control."
    B. "You can't do that or you'll lose your job."
    C. "Tell me more about how you feel when you're around him."
    D. "You can call me if you are afraid of losing control."

14. The following physical complaint, if offered by Ms. Hunt, could warrant *immediate* medical intervention:

    A. Swollen glands
    B. Cramping and weakness of extremities with dizziness
    C. A "bloated feeling" after bingeing
    D. Constipation

15. Mr. Hope realizes that he is feeling the temptation to placate Ms. Hunt when she exhibits anxiety or anger during their session. This could indicate that

    A. He is a good role model
    B. He shares her fear that she is helpless
    C. He wants to help her
    D. He should medicate her

Refer to the case study Working with a Person Whose Obesity Is Caused by Compulsive Eating *when answering questions* 16–18.

16. Considering Ms. Robbins' signs of depression, Mrs. Worth's priority is to

    A. Start Ms. Robbins' in group therapy
    B. Start her on a 1500-calorie diet
    C. Place her on close observation with suicidal precaution
    D. Start her in a hygiene group

17. When Ms. Robbins verbalizes that she feels "too ashamed" to be seen at work, Mrs. Worth's best response would be

    A. "You have nothing to be ashamed of."
    B. "Work will help you keep your mind off your problems."
    C. "Tell me more about your feelings of shame."
    D. "You have a good husband and family to think about."

18. In a group therapy session, Ms. Robbins verbalizes that she feels comfortable talking about her feelings to the group. Group therapy can provide all the following *except*

    A. Opportunities to verbalize feelings
    B. Aids in developing more realistic self-image
    C. Feedback
    D. Physiological safety

19. Ms. Duncan is an obese woman of 30 whose family pattern indicates a history of overeating in response to stress. She is 5'2" tall and has never weighed within a "normal" range for her size. Her obesity is probably

   A. Reactive
   B. Developmental
   C. Organic
   D. All of the above

20. Compulsive eating may serve the function of

   A. Reducing stress
   B. Dealing with conflict
   C. Punishment for guilt
   D. All of the above

PART THREE

MENTAL HEALTH ISSUES: SPECIAL POPULATIONS

POPULATIONS DEALING WITH UNIQUE ISSUES

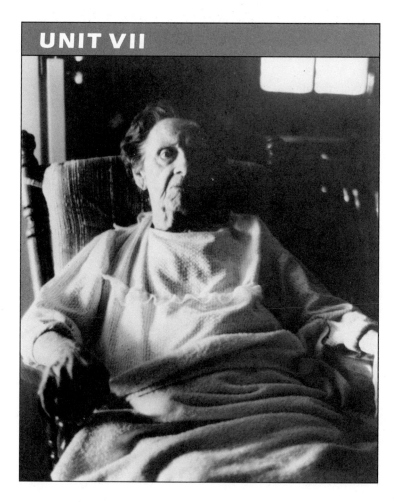

UNIT VII

After all, it is those who have a deep and real inner life who are best able to deal with the "irritating details of outer life."

EVELYN UNDERHILL
THE LETTERS OF
EVELYN UNDERHILL

A Nurse Speaks

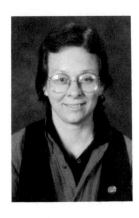

by Carla E. Randall

How do I, as an educator, a nurse, a woman, a lesbian, a risk taker, let it be known that I understand the pain of being hated? I am hated for who others perceive me to be. There is always concern about being negated, overlooked, or denied basic human rights. I evaluate constantly the possibility of being disenfranchised from the students whom I teach and the faculty with whom I share the responsibilities of educating future generations of nurses. I also consider the consequences that might occur if clients had more knowledge of who they are interacting with. Would clients, students, or faculty behave differently if they knew that the nurse, educator, and woman who they are dealing with identifies herself as a lesbian?

There are thousands of us, even hundreds of thousands of us who may be somewhat different than the norm and feel oppressed and marginalized. We feel oppressed and marginalized by mainstream white American culture. Our behaviors and definitions of ourselves do not fit neatly into someone else's definition of normalcy. As students, nurses, and educators, all of us will come into contact with individuals who feel that they are outside the mainstream, that they will not be understood, and that they will be rejected, and who consequently fear that they will receive inadequate health care, especially if differences of any kind are identified or discussed.

As I ponder the task of making my point in a page or two of text, I search for an example that will capture the experience of what it is like to be a lesbian and interact with the health care system. When I go for my yearly physical exam and am asked the routine questions that are commonly asked, I feel invisible and silenced.

You know the questions . . . the routine, inevitable questions . . .

"Are you married?"

"Are you sexually active?"

"What contraception are you presently using?"

"Do you want to become pregnant?"

I'm anxious as the interview begins. I'm cautious, trying to feel out the interviewer. What is safe to say, how open and honest do I dare to be with this person? Do I feel safe enough in this situation to disclose information about myself? How do I know that this person will accept me and provide me with safe and comfortable health care? These questions may seem routine to the interviewer, but to me, no matter how I answer them, they represent a risk. A huge risk.

If I answer the questions simply, without disclosing much of who I am, I leave myself wide open to another whole list of assumptions that leads the interviewer to incorrect conclusions about me, about my life.

"Are you married?" No.

"Are you sexually active?" Yes.

"What contraception are you presently using?" None.

"Do you want to become pregnant?" No.

What conclusion is now drawn about me? I may be viewed as an irresponsible woman who is at risk for an unwanted pregnancy. How much farther from the truth could the interviewer be? I have no fears of possible pregnancy; for that matter, I have no need of contraception. The interviewer is asking questions that may actually compromise my health care because they do not invite me to disclose much about myself.

The frustration that exists is exhausting: the questions imply that the only sexual activity is heterosexual. The assumption has already been made that I am straight. Can't you see me loving a woman? For me to be sexually active, must there be the fear of possible pregnancy? My partner is a woman. How do I say that? Can't you see me as separate from a man? Can't you see that the person I love, the person I have sex with, the person I make my dreams with, is a woman? For me to be myself, to be sexual, and to love someone—means loving a woman.

I look again at this person asking the questions. The questions seem reasonable on the surface. But they all miss providing me an honest interaction with the health care provider. The questions miss seeing me for who I am, and they all avoid discussion of acceptance and honest dialogue.

I'm left trying to second-guess the health care provider. Trying to avoid uncomfortable situations or disclosing more than the health care provider can deal with. What does this person think is sexual? Can this person fathom two women engaged in sexual activity? Is this too shocking? If I answer the questions honestly, will the interviewer be full of disgust, refuse to care for me, treat me in compromising ways, or overlook vital information for my health care because this person does not understand my needs as a lesbian?

How sensitive have these "traditional" questions, these assumptions, been to my dignity . . . to my mental health? Has there been any attempt to see me as anything other than heterosexual? As anything other than needing protection from pregnancy? As anything other than being just like everyone else?

Within our changing roles in society as nurses, as educators, as students, as women or as men, we are challenged to address issues of diversity, of difference, of stretching boundaries, and of learning to accept others while valuing our own uniqueness.

Truly, this decade is about learning to live with and accepting others—be it the single parent creating child care options in a neighborhood . . . the lesbian wanting to be visible in her interactions with the world at large . . . the differently abled man who loudly complains of not having access to downtown shopping areas . . . the psychiatric client who wants to live in a community housing project . . . or you, struggling through nursing school.

Wilma Scott Heidi, a revolutionary nursing leader, in *Feminism for the Health of It,* has suggested that it is not a matter of *if* these things will happen but *when.* I ask each of you to read her book and, when you practice the art of nursing, to ask yourself if your actions include honoring and celebrating the uniqueness of others under your care.

CHAPTER 26

The Hospitalized Person

Jane Bryant Neese

KEY TERMS AND CONCEPTS

The key terms and concepts listed here also appear in bold where they are defined or discussed in this chapter.

CHRONIC PAIN

COPING

HIV ENCEPHALOPATHY

PAIN

PSYCHIATRIC LIAISON NURSE

STAGES IN THE PROCESS OF DYING:
Denial and Isolation
Anger
Bargaining
Depression
Acceptance

OBJECTIVES

After studying this chapter, the student will be able to

1. Discuss areas of stress encountered by a hospitalized person during the process of hospitalization.
2. Identify four positive coping strategies and four negative coping strategies that may be used by a hospitalized person.
3. Describe the role of the psychiatric liaison nurse.
4. Compare and contrast assessment of acute pain and assessment of chronic pain.

5. Explain five nursing interventions effective for reducing pain.
6. In a teaching plan, outline how a nurse can intervene with a person with acquired immunodeficiency syndrome (AIDS).
7. Summarize staff needs and possible staff interventions needed when caring for people who are infected with the human immunodeficiency virus (HIV).
8. Identify nursing interventions that may be useful to a dying person or his or her family during each of Kübler-Ross's five stages.
9. Differentiate between psychophysiological disorders and somatization disorders.
10. Explain how the nurse would implement three of the suggested nursing interventions for a person with a psychophysiological disorder.

Physical and emotional crises occur every day in the medical setting. The stress of being physically ill greatly influences a person's psychological state and emotional reactions. An individual's particular personality structure as well as the nature of his or her illness plays a large part in the coping strategies a person employs to decrease stress. At times, a nurse working in the hospital environment may find that the client's anxiety or coping strategies negatively affect (1) an individual's health and (2) the nurse's ability to administer effective care. Understanding the stresses experienced and strategies used by the hospitalized person can greatly enhance the nurse's effectiveness.

This chapter looks at (1) possible sources of stress for the hospitalized person, (2) various coping strategies used by the hospitalized person, and (3) specific phenomena and possible emotional reactions to each. Four medical conditions that elicit unique emotional needs in a hospitalized person are presented here. The emotional needs of a person (1) in chronic pain, (2) with AIDS, (3) dying of terminal illness, and (4) with a psychophysiological disorder are presented. The role of the psychiatric liaison nurse is discussed because the liaison nurse is an important resource for staff when emotional difficulties arise with a medically ill client.

The Role of the Nurse

When the medically ill person experiences increased levels of anxiety, staff may need assistance in planning care. Most nurses possess sound psychosocial nursing communication skills. However, nurses working on medical or surgical units often become more task oriented and less comfortable with the socioemotional aspects of a client's needs. When this happens, a client's emotional needs may become ignored when the nurse plans care. The client's emotional reaction to his or her situation might, however, trigger frustration and confusion in the staff. Therefore, situations arise in which a hospitalized client's behavior or emotional experience is beyond the skills of the nurse and the health care team. In the general hospital, there are several resources that nurses can contact to help in an emotional crisis. *First*, the psychiatrist diagnoses the psychiatric problem and recommends treatment; however, psychiatrists are accessible only by a physician's order. *Second*, the social worker is often aware of the family's history. The social worker is a useful resource regarding family dynamics and the family's financial situation. However, most social workers are unfamiliar with nursing interventions and lack knowledge of medical diseases. A *third* resource, who knows about medical illnesses, psychiatric illnesses, family dynamics, and the nursing process, is the psychiatric liaison nurse.

PSYCHIATRIC LIAISON NURSE

Psychiatric liaison nursing is a relatively new subspecialty of psychiatric nursing, initiated in the early 1960s (Johnson 1963; Lewis and Levy 1982; Robinson 1974). Usually, the **psychiatric liaison nurse** is a master's-prepared nurse with a background in psychiatric and medical-surgical nursing (ANA 1990). A psychiatric liaison nurse functions as a nursing consultant in the management of psychosocial concerns, and as a clinician in helping the client deal more effectively with physical and emotional problems. Throughout the five steps of the nursing process (assessing, diagnosing, planning, intervening, and evaluating), a psychiatric liaison nurse assists the nursing and medical staff in caring for hospitalized, medically ill clients who are management problems or who have problems that impede client care (Fife 1983; Fife and Lemler 1983; Lewis and Levy 1982). Therefore, the psychiatric liaison nurse is a resource for the nursing staff who feel, for one reason or another, unable to intervene therapeutically with a client.

The psychiatric liaison nurse first meets with the nurse who initiated the consultation. The liaison nurse then reviews the medical records, talks with the physicians, and interviews the client. After interviewing the client, the liaison nurse discusses his or her assessment and suggestions with the referring nurse. If a psychiatric consultation is warranted, the psychiatric liaison nurse will generate the consultation by contacting the client's medical doctor. A case conference is sometimes needed to enhance communication and consistency in the care of a particular client.

Unique Assessment Strategies

Admission into the hospital often signifies that a medical condition is too complex to be treated in an outpatient setting. In emergencies, the client is immediately rushed to the hospital via ambulance and is prepared for entrance into the hospital environment. Numerous stressors will increase anxiety in a person new to the hospital environment. On entering the hospital, the client begins to experience a loss of control and depersonalization. In the admitting office, the person is first asked his or her name and the name of his or her insurance company prior to any discussion of the presenting problem. The client is given a hospital number and an admitting diagnosis as methods of identification. Later, he may no longer be identified as "Mr. Smith," but as the man with acquired immunodeficiency syndrome (AIDS) in room 622.

After being admitted to a room, the client is given a hospital gown and requested to change. Indirectly, the client is beginning to understand that his or her role as provider, father, mother, or boss is changing to the "sick role." The sick role denotes giving up some independent functioning and assuming a more dependent position. A person rarely has time to comfortably adjust to the sick role. Usually within the first few days of hospitalization, the client has given up some identity and independent functioning.

ASSESSING STRESS AND ANXIETY RELATED TO HOSPITALIZATION

The reason for hospitalization generally is illness. The onset of an illness means loss of a previous health state. For some, hospitalization means that the preexisting illness is worsening. For others, hospitalization is their first encounter with a serious illness. Loss of health affects how clients view themselves. If the illness requires surgery or any other mutilating procedure, the client's reaction may be a change in his or her body image and grief over his or her loss. An amputation severely affects a person's self-esteem and body image, especially if the amputation means loss of a job.

If the diagnosis has not been confirmed prior to admission, fear of the unknown can escalate anxiety to severe levels. In some cases, the diagnosis is made, yet the course of treatment is questionable, e.g., chemotherapy in oncology clients. The ultimate fear is the fear of death, especially if surgery is indicated.

Most clients are concerned about their insurance coverage on admission to the hospital. For prolonged hospitalizations, financial concerns become a primary focus and are a major source of stress for the family. The terminally ill client may worry about leaving his or her family with a financial burden after death.

Hospitalization is a stressful period for the client and family and usually precipitates anxiety and confusion. The client's focus shifts from health to illness and from independence to dependence. One is separated from family and support systems. If the illness is terminal, grieving over the loss of health, role, and life is stimulated. Fear of the unknown and financial worries may become the client's major concerns.

The nurse's assessment includes the stressors triggered by the process of hospitalization. When areas of client concern are identified, appropriate supports can be mobilized. Another important area to assess is the way the person copes with stress and anxiety.

ASSESSING COPING STRATEGIES

Coping differs from defense mechanisms in that *defense mechanisms are primarily an unconscious means of regulating internal emotional tension.* **Coping,** however, is a problem-solving behavior that is directed toward influencing, changing, or bringing about equilibrium to a threatening situation (Monat and Lazarus 1991; Weisman 1984). Generally, *coping is seen as a conscious means of altering a stressful event.* The ways people cope are a complicated mixture of how they initially perceive stress, how they respond behaviorally, and how they re-evaluate the stress and correct their response over a period of time (Weisman 1978). Lazarus (1982) defines coping as "not a single act but a constellation of many acts and thoughts engendered by a complex set of demands that may stretch over time." Coping as a constellation is a helpful conceptual model because individuals use various methods of coping in different situations at different times in their lives and with different people. Coping is the client's intervention with a stressor such as illness.

The action of coping has several synonyms, e.g., coping skills, coping strategies, coping modes, coping patterns, and coping mechanisms. For clarity, this chapter uses coping strategies to identify different techniques that physically ill clients use to deal with their illness. Clients are the best source in determining whether their coping has decreased their anxiety. Nurses can help by assessing the client's adaptive coping strategies and strengthening them by positive reinforcement. Open and honest communication helps facilitate positive coping abilities. Supportive, dependable relationships help clients better adapt to their illness.

There are many factors that can influence one's ability to cope. For example, *interpersonal factors* include age, personality, intelligence, values, cultural beliefs, emotional state, and cognitive ability. *Disease-related factors* are type of illness, rate of onset, progression, functional impairment, and whether the disease or impairment is reversible. If a person's illness is a fast-growing malignancy with metastasis to the brain that renders him or her delirious, ability to cope would be seriously compromised. *Environmental factors* include the person's support system (family, friends, or community) and financial stability. Each of these three determinants influences a person's choice of coping strategies.

Seeking information and obtaining guidance is the most commonly reported coping strategy. Nursing staff and physicians tend to reinforce this strategy and are more comfortable when the client does ask questions regarding his or her illness and treatment. The second coping strategy is even more adaptive, that of *sharing concern and finding consolation*. The third coping strategy, *changing emotional tone*, can be helpful or hurtful depending on whether the client is laughing with someone or laughing at someone. Humor and laughter can defuse a tense situation or can escalate anxiety, depending on how it is used. *Suppression* is the fourth coping strategy. Not only is suppression useful at times, it is necessary for clients if they are to continue to deal with their illness. This is especially true with cancer clients or terminally ill clients.

Keeping busy and distracting oneself is also a common strategy. Usually this type of coping only postpones dealing with a difficult situation. Many times, problems of self-worth are at the bottom of postponing dealing with the illness. The sixth coping strategy, *confrontation*, is the cornerstone of many coping strategies because without confrontation, clients avoid the reality of their illnesses. Confrontation is not to be misconstrued as challenging in an angry manner. Confrontation in this case means to address the situ-

ation in a straightforward manner. *Redefinition* means to make virtue out of necessity or transform a deficit into a gain. A person redefines the situation to optimize the problem without compromising the truth. *Resignation* is the eighth coping strategy. Resignation entails acknowledging that the situation is beyond one's control. This is not the same as submitting to defeat but is the ability to recognize one's limitations. Many people, however, take an *impulsive action*. An example of an impulsive action would be abuse of alcohol or attempted suicide. *Reviewing alternatives* suggests that the client is taking the time to reflect on what has happened and is re-evaluating the situation. "Now what are we going to do and where are we going?" is a question frequently asked. Another coping strategy, *escape*, is probably contemplated by more clients than has been reported. No matter how well one copes, it is not surprising that the question "What if . . . ?" is asked and left unanswered. Many clients have stated that they just want to get away from it all. However, few can escape their illness. *Conforming and complying* suggests a more passive stance. Most clients will comply just because compliance with the physician's suggestions is expected.

Another strategy, *blaming someone else*, is not necessarily adaptive but is frequently seen. Crying or raving is an example of *giving vent* or *releasing emotions*. Even though the problem is not solved or altered by releasing emotions, the client may experience a reduction in tension. The last coping strategy is *denying as much as possible* and is the direct opposite of seeking information and sharing concern. Even though health professionals strongly oppose denial, denying as much as possible may have temporary strategic value.

Box 26–1 reviews these coping strategies and identifies those seen in both effective and poor copers. "Effective copers" have a good relationship with the health care team and are optimistic and resourceful. "Poor copers" have higher emotional distress and do not recognize their psychosocial problems.

Intervention strategies for selected hospitalized persons will be presented subsequently.

However, many issues and concerns are experienced by all hospitalized clients. The generalist is often an expert at identifying nursing diagnoses for the physically ill, yet it is vital that the nurse not limit the focus of care to the physical components of the client's condition. In doing so, crucial emotional needs may go unmet. This can result in prolonging recuperation or halting the process of recovery. The medical conditions discussed in this chapter are traumatic, extremely disruptive to the client and his or her family, and may involve a great deal of pain or even death. A competent assessment includes the client's acute concerns, coping strategies, and support sys-

---

Box 26-1. COMMON COPING STRATEGIES USED BY THE HOSPITALIZED PERSON

*   1. Seek information; get guidance.

*   2. Share concern; find consolation.

    3. Laugh it off; change emotional tone.

    4. Forget it happened; put it out of your mind.

*   5. Keep busy; distract yourself.

*   6. Confront the issue; act accordingly.

*   7. Redefine; take a more sanguine view.

    8. Resign yourself; make the best of what can not be changed.

    9. Do something, anything, perhaps exceeding good judgment.

  10. Review alternatives; examine consequences.

† 11. Get away from it all; find an escape, somehow.

* 12. Conform, comply; do what is expected or advised.

† 13. Blame or shame someone, something.

  14. Give vent; feel emotional release.

† 15. Deny as much as possible.

Data from Weisman A. *The Coping Capacity: On the Nature of Being Mortal.* New York: Human Sciences Press, 1984, pp. 36–37.

* Seen most in "effective copers"

† Seen most in "poor copers"

---

tems. Assessing the person's perception of his or her situation and the perception of his or her future is crucial in formulating nursing diagnoses concerning emotional needs, thereby identifying major areas for intervention. For example, a person who is dying may experience the anguish of *spiritual distress.* Grieving in this case may be imminent, and the process of dying may need to be facilitated and supported. A person who has had a myocardial infarction may have overriding concerns regarding *self-esteem* in relationship to self-concept, role performance, or personal identity. If these issues are not addressed, defensive maneuvers such as denial may have a direct impact on the person's medical compliance and could result in premature death. A person who has AIDS may experience extreme *social isolation* or *altered thought process* compounded by a lack of, or distorted, environmental stimuli. *Potential for self-directed violence* should always be evaluated in a person who appears to feel hopeless. Suicide is not an uncommon phenomenon in a hospitalized person who feels overwhelmed, alone, fearful,

and hopeless. *Powerlessness* is experienced to some degree by most all clients. If a sense of powerlessness is experienced by a person who has a high need to feel in control, nursing interventions need to be considered. All levels of *anxiety* will be seen in clients hospitalized for physical conditions. When levels of anxiety result in maladaptive or disorganizing behaviors, swift medical and nursing attention should be made available. Helping the client lower anxiety to more comfortable levels helps maximize the person's ability to participate in his or her care, to problem solve, and to relate more productively to staff, family, and others. *Ineffective family coping* related to a hospitalized family member is also an area that may require specific nursing interventions.

Issues That Affect the Mental Health of Some Hospitalized Persons

A PERSON IN CHRONIC PAIN

Pain is an individual experience, which makes assessment and treatment complicated. Associated with the experience of pain are psychological, physiological, and cultural factors. Health professionals often attempt to define pain as purely physical or psychological (psychogenic) in nature. This view leads to confusion and frustration for both the staff and the client. Zborowski's (1969) classic study described several cultural groups' responses to pain. Stoicism with little verbal and behavioral expression of pain was seen in the old American (descendants of early settlers to the United States), and Irish populations. People from Jewish and Italian backgrounds were more likely to be verbally expressive of their pain. A person's expression of pain often depends on his or her cultural background.

Pain is an ancient warning system of the body, indicating that tissue damage has occurred. In some cases, tissue damage can occur without the person experiencing pain. Conversely, in some cases, even after tissues have healed, pain may continue to be felt by the client.

Pain can be classified into five categories: acute, subacute, recurrent acute, continuous, and chronic. In most cases, *acute pain* is the result of recent tissue damage and lasts up to a few days. *Subacute pain* lasts a few days to a few weeks. In *recurrent acute pain,* the client suffers from a disease that has exacerbations of pain followed by brief periods of remission, as seen in rheumatoid arthritis, migraines, and sickle cell disorders. An underlying malignant disease, such as cancer, is usually the cause of *continuous pain*. **Chronic pain** is characterized by continuous or intermittent pain for more than six months. Neck and back injuries, pancreatitis, and cancer are examples of conditions that can result in chronic pain. This section will focus on management of chronic pain.

For the nurse and the physician, assessment of chronic pain is difficult because most pain models are based on the concept of acute pain. *Acute pain differs from chronic pain in several ways.* In acute pain, the client exhibits more behavioral responses, including motor responses (writhing), vocal responses (crying), and social responses (withdrawal from others). A person in acute pain gives the appearance of being in distress. Often nurses look for the behavioral responses to acute pain when assessing intensity of pain. Physiologically, a client in acute pain has an increase in pulse and blood pressure.

In contrast, a client in chronic pain does not manifest the same behavioral and physiological responses as the client in acute pain. Because of the chronic persistence of pain, a client may slowly adapt to the presence of pain without realizing it. Eventually, the client learns to accommodate to the pain and continues with his or her life while still experiencing pain. In addition, the body begins to adapt to chronic pain. Physiological responses are no longer inclusive data in determining intensity or presence of chronic pain. Often it is the person's adaptation to chronic pain that is his or her undoing. The staff may conclude that the client is not in pain if they are unable to adequately assess the symptoms for chronic pain. How does one measure chronic pain if a person does not behaviorally or physiologically manifest symptoms? The client is the key. Chronic pain is an individual experience. Therefore, the nurse needs to ask the client.

Myths Regarding Pain Control

Many nurses and other health professionals are hesitant to use narcotics for people with chronic pain. This hesitancy stems from fear of "addicting" the client to the narcotic. However, fewer than 1% of clients with chronic pain become physically dependent on medications.

Common myths regarding narcotic and analgesic usage follow (McGuire 1983; Rogers 1984):

1. The use of a potent narcotic can cause drug abuse or "addiction."
2. Withholding narcotics prevents drug abuse.
3. Drug tolerance and physical dependence are the same as drug abuse.

4. The client who "withdraws" is "addicted" or drug dependent.
5. Administering narcotics and analgesics only when needed is the best way to prevent drug abuse and subsequent addiction.
6. A client who asks regularly for medication is "addicted."
7. A client who needs more medication is becoming "addicted" or drug dependent.
8. Demerol is the best injectable narcotic for pain relief.
9. If a client is asleep the client isn't in pain.

There are also other misconceptions about pain control that influence nursing interventions—the misconception, for example, that pain caused by anxiety does not need to be treated. Keep in mind that the physically ill person's perception of pain is influenced by several factors. The *physiological* warning of tissue damage, *psychological* response, and *cultural* influences all contribute to a person's perception of pain. Most people become anxious when they are in pain. Waiting for medication to relieve the pain, especially when the medication schedule is rigid, tends to increase anxiety and thereby increase pain. Anxiety and pain are closely entwined, and both need to be treated. When the client in pain is anxious, the pain still needs to be alleviated through proper medical treatment.

Another misconception is that a nurse is able to judge the "authenticity" of another person's pain. Some nurses have even stated that they can "tell" when a client is in "real" pain because they have worked with "so many" clients in pain. This erroneous belief may come from the nurse's fear of "addicting" a client, fear of being fooled, or personal need for control. This attitude only creates more distrust between nurses and the people under their care.

Another misconception comes from giving a placebo in order to "test" whether the client is "faking" pain. Approximately one third of the hospitalized people with chronic pain will experience pain relief if given a placebo. Some possible reasons for this occurrence are that placebos work if the client trusts the staff. The client becomes less anxious after the placebo is taken. Also, placebos stimulate the body to produce endorphins, which are morphine-like brain chemicals. A placebo trial indicates only that the client can respond positively to a placebo; it *does not* separate psychogenic pain from organic pain. If clients discover that placebos are being used (and they generally do), clients feel tricked and begin to distrust staff. Placebo trials without the person's input can lead to destruction of the nurse-client relationship (Hackett 1978; McGuire 1983; Rogers 1984).

Assessment of Chronic Pain

Assessment of the pain is the first step in management of chronic pain. The nurse needs to find out the site, character, and duration of the pain. Is there anything that makes the pain worse or better? Does the client experience a change in mood because of the pain? Also, is the client newly diagnosed with a malignant disorder or is this a recurrent disease? Differentiate what type of pain the client is experiencing (i.e., acute, subacute, recurrent, continuous, or chronic). A thorough history of analgesic and narcotic usage needs to be taken. The history should include the drug, dosage, route, time interval, length of time on each drug, the effectiveness of each medication, and the side effects. Does one route work better than another route? Because these questions take a considerable amount of time, the nurse may ask the client to write a log documenting pain, type, medication, and route. The nurse can photocopy the log and return the original to the client. If the client does compile a log, the nurse can sit down, discuss the pain, and ask pertinent questions (Foley 1983; Hackett 1978; Rogers 1984).

In discussing the client's pain and previous interventions, the nurse must always accept the client's perception of pain and never think of the pain as imaginary. To alleviate the client's fear of abandonment, the nurse can assure the client that he or she will continue to assist in managing the pain even though there may not be any immediate results. It is also important to stress to the client that different methods of treating pain may not have instant results. In the treatment of chronic pain, the goal should be a decrease in the degree of pain. Some clients, such as those with chronic pancreatitis, will always have some degree of pain. Lessening the pain so that the client can continue functioning is the key to pain management.

Treatment of Chronic Pain

Biofeedback is useful in dealing with headache and chronic back pain by relaxing different muscle groups, thus releasing the tension that causes or aggravates the pain (Greenspan 1981; Hendler and Fernandez 1980; Schuman 1982). Even though biofeedback helps reduce pain, the nurse does not usually have easy access to the equipment to use with clients. The nurse needs to be aware of the availability of biofeedback for the client with chronic pain.

Teaching *relaxation techniques* is another intervention nurses can choose for their clients in chronic pain. Progressive muscle relaxation, rhythmic breathing, and guided imagery are three relaxation techniques that can induce the "relaxation response." Guided imagery is an effective means of deepening relaxation and desensitizing a person to a painful situation or experience. The client is taught to visualize a calm, beautiful place where he or she experiences peace and joy. When a deep sense of relaxation is reached, the client is taught to use images to reduce stress, promote healing, or reduce pain. Before teaching any relaxation technique, the nurse confers with the physician, then evaluates the client's readiness and past experiences with relaxation techniques.

Hypnosis has also frequently helped reduce pain. "Hypnosis depends almost entirely on the client. Only one in four subjects is able to achieve a state of concentration effective enough to control their pain" (Zahourek 1985). Even though hypnosis is more helpful in acute pain, some practitioners have taught autohypnosis (self-hypnosis) to clients who are suggestible. These clients are in a state of resting alertness and are able to block out painful sensations (Wain 1986).

Psychotherapy helps demoralized and desperate clients deal with the terror that pain comes to hold. Behavioral therapy and antianxiety and antidepressant drugs have proved useful. They do not eliminate the pain, but they make it easier to bear by relieving tension, fatigue, anxiety, and insomnia (Kleinman 1989).

When assisting the client with chronic pain, the nurse should accept the client's perception and experience of pain. Each client presents symptoms of pain differently. Promoting a trusting relationship with the client and openly discussing past attempts to control pain are helpful in determining a new approach to pain management. Medications are the most frequently used treatment intervention. Biofeedback and relaxation techniques, such as guided imagery, rhythmic breathing, hypnosis, and progressive muscle relaxation, are other avenues that can help reduce the client's pain.

A 47-year-old single man, Jeff Tide, is admitted to the hospital for weight loss in addition to abdominal and back pain. Past history revealed that Mr. Tide had been shot in the abdomen by a student whom he had taught at a local technical college. As a result of the gunshot wound, Mr. Tide had a pancreatectomy, a colostomy, and an ileostomy. He had several hospitalizations to reverse the colostomy and ileostomy, as well as to correct some abdominal adhesions. After the initial hospitalizations, he attempted to return to work as a professor but was unable to because of pain, nausea, vomiting, and weakness. Three years after the shooting, Mr. Tide was involved in a motor vehicle accident that injured his back. This present hospitalization focuses on Mr. Tide's weight loss secondary to his inability to digest food without compatible pancreatic enzymes, and management of his chronic pain.

Initially Mr. Tide is placed on Percodan (oxycodone hydrochloride, oxycodone terephthalate, and aspirin compound) by mouth for pain, then changed to Tylenol #3 (acetaminophen with codeine) by mouth, and again to Demerol (meperidine), 50 mg by mouth, all to no avail. He continually asks for his pain medication every four hours and requests that the medication and schedule be changed. Soon Mr. Tide becomes frustrated and angry with the nursing staff. He constantly complains about his pain and the staff's poor quality of care. The nurses perceive Mr. Tide as demanding and manipulative. Several times, the nursing staff enter his room to administer the pain medication and find him asleep. Exasperated, the nurses request the psychiatric liaison nurse to assist them in dealing with this "demanding client."

During the interview, the psychiatric liaison nurse assesses that Mr. Tide has had chronic pain for more than five years *(assess the duration of pain)*. The client says that his pain is worse at night and after meals *(assess when the pain occurs)*. He states that at home, he takes one to two Percodan tablets before meals and usually takes two tablets before he goes to bed *(assess previous medication schedule)*. He says that he is in pain most of the day (continuous), which periodically is intolerable. Normally, he rates his pain as a 4 on a 10-point scale *(assess the client's perception of the pain)*. If he misses taking his pain medication, his pain increases to the point where he lies in bed the entire day. Mr. Tide states that he is discouraged about controlling the pain and frustrated that no one is listening to his complaints.

After gathering all the data regarding the client's history, the psychiatric liaison nurse, the nursing staff, and the physician discuss the case and decide to implement the following. The client is to assess his pain on a 10-point scale every time he receives pain medication *(to continually assess pain and changes in pain)*. The pain medication is changed to what he uses at home, incorporating his usual routine. Therefore, the client does not have to ask for pain medication. He can refuse if needed. Mr. Tide will be encouraged to participate in physical therapy and to gradually increase his physical activity. The psychiatric liaison nurse will teach him progressive muscle relaxation, as well as guided imagery. Guided imagery is used to increase his sense of control and potentiate the effectiveness of the medications. The nursing staff are to check on the client every hour to see how he is doing in order to decrease staff avoidance and lessen Mr. Tide's sense of abandonment.

With the use of guided imagery, the client is able to decrease his use of Percodan to one tablet in the morning and two tablets at night. He also begins talking more with the nursing staff. After compatible pancreatic enzymes are established, the client is able to eat without nausea, vomiting, and pain, which previously accompanied eating. He begins ambulating more and is viewed by several nursing staff as an "enjoyable person." Possible discontinuation of his pain medication is discussed with the client but is decided against at this time. The client is discharged with a 5-pound weight gain, an effective pain control plan, and a positive relationship with the staff. This staff learned from Mr. Tide that a pain history and assessment are essential prior to the treatment of chronic pain.

A PERSON WHO HAS ACQUIRED IMMUNODEFICIENCY SYNDROME (AIDS)

What AIDS Is and How It Is Detected

Human immunodeficiency virus (HIV) is a slow retrovirus that is thought to be the causative agent in AIDS. Previously the virus was known as human T-cell lymphotropic virus III (HTLV-III) in the United States and as lymphadenopathy-associated virus (LAV) in Europe.

The virus invades and eventually destroys helper T lymphocytes, thus disrupting the body's immune response. Once the virus has invaded a helper T lymphocyte, it may take from six weeks to 12 months or longer before the presence of HIV antibodies can be detected by testing.

HIV also directly attacks the central nervous system, resulting in various neuropsychiatric symptoms. **HIV encephalopathy** (also called AIDS-related dementia), myelopathy, and neuropathy are possible sequelae. Personality changes include depression, psychosis, and inability to control aggressive impulses. The virus has been identified in blood, semen, tears, saliva, cerebrospinal fluid, and breast milk.

In December 1991, the prevalence of AIDS cases had risen to 199,516 in the United States (Centers for Disease Control [CDC] 1992). Previously, AIDS in the United States was thought to be a disease associated only with homosexual men and intravenous drug abusers; however, a surge in the numbers of infected heterosexual men and women, as well as children, has occurred. Heterosexual contact contributed to a 6% increase in AIDS cases from 1990–1991 (CDC 1992). By 1991, 203,392 pediatric HIV-infected patients had been reported. Therefore, the infection rate of HIV and the subsequent development of AIDS have no boundaries. Every nurse has already, or will, come in contact with someone who is HIV positive or an AIDS victim during his or her early professional career. It is imperative that the nurse's relationship with the HIV or AIDS client remain compassionate and nonjudgmental in order to offer comfort during this anxiety-provoking time.

Psychiatric and Neuropsychiatric Symptoms

Often, nurses work with people who have AIDS in a general hospital setting, although AIDS clients are frequently admitted into the psychiatric units as well. In either case, nurses want to know the kinds of behaviors they might see resulting, either directly or indirectly, from AIDS.

As in no other patient population, the person with AIDS faces the most dramatic changes in self-esteem, daily living habits, and general lifestyle as a result of the illness. People with HIV infection at any of its stages are faced with multiple concerns and existential dilemmas; loss of life, threat of pain, loss of function, social isolation, stigmatization, potential dementia, and economic ruin are at the fore.

There is a segment of the population who are the "worried well," or individuals who believe that their past or current behavior has put them at risk for contracting AIDS. As one homosexual man asked (Bell 1992), "When will I get it? Am I next? Is this cold more than a cold? What is that spot on my leg?" For these individuals, the psychological task is to make a decision about whether to be tested. During this process, the client may become anxious and guilt ridden. It is important that the client consult with sources that give accurate information about the symptoms, treatment, and transmission of AIDS. Guilt may occur from fear of infecting others and of causing undue worry to loved ones. Verbalizing concerns to trusted friends, family, or health professionals can help alleviate some anxiety and guilt (Marcil and Tigges 1992).

Therefore, it is not surprising that feelings of hopelessness and uncertainty can occur. Compounding these feelings of hopelessness is the awareness of negative societal attitudes toward homosexual and bisexual practices, intravenous drug use, and AIDS itself. It is not surprising then that *suicide and suicide ideation* are clinical commonplaces.

Anxiety symptoms take the form of panic attacks, anorexia, tachycardia, insomnia, and agitation. *Intense anger* is frequently experienced and directed toward perceived public discrimination, dissatisfaction with governmental responses, and ineffective medical care (Faulstich 1987). Psychosis and paranoid behaviors may also be exhibited by some clients.

Psychiatric diagnoses include *depression* (reactive and major), the most common diagnosis, *adjustment disorder with depressed mood, dementia, panic disorder, paranoid reactions,* and *psychosis.*

Complicating the diagnosis of depression is the possibility of AIDS-related dementia, also known as **HIV-encephalopathy.** HIV encephalopathy seems to cluster into two broad categories (Perry and Markowitz 1986). One category mimics the signs and symptoms of depression, for example, forgetfulness, poor concentration, loss of libido, apathy, affective blunting, psychomotor retardation, anorexia, fatigue, and social withdrawal. The second category presents with subtle cognitive difficulties and acute psychotic presentation (e.g., delusions, hallucinations, psychomotor agitation, mania, and grandiosity). Approximately 40–70% of people with AIDS will develop some neurological symptoms (Sadovsky 1991), and in about 10% of cases, the neurological symptoms are the first indicators of HIV infection (AIDS Update 1988). Some neuropsychiatric symptoms of AIDS are listed in Box 26–2.

Box 26–2. NEUROPSYCHIATRIC SYMPTOMS IN PEOPLE WITH AIDS

Decrease in sleep
Decrease in appetite
Depressed mood
Withdrawal
Increased somatic complaints
Unkempt physical appearance
Disorientation
Difficulty with verbal expression
Feelings of hopelessness
Decreased feeling of self-worth
Feelings of helplessness
Decreased concentration
Suicidal thoughts
Decreased short term memory
Feelings of punishment
Slow verbal responses
Hallucinations
Delusions

Table 26-1 ■ NURSING DIAGNOSES: A PERSON WITH AIDS	
POSSIBLE NURSING DIAGNOSIS	**RELATED FACTORS**
Ineffective breathing pattern	Pneumocystis carinii pneumonia
Ineffective airway clearance	Respiratory and other opportunistic infections
	Anxiety
Altered nutrition: less than body requirements	Chronic diarrhea
Diarrhea	Lesions of the mouth and esophagus
Fluid volume deficit	Kaposi's sarcoma of the gastrointestinal tract
	Nausea and vomiting induced by medications
	Increased metabolic rate with fevers
Ineffective individual coping	Depression of chronic illness
Sensory-perceptual alterations	Social and physical isolation
High risk for self-harm	Psychological response to catastrophic illness
Spiritual distress	Infections or malignancies of the central nervous system
Social isolation	Imposed isolation requirements
Hopelessness/powerlessness	Community, family, or health care personnel's attitudes
Disturbance in self-esteem	Physical dependency
Anxiety/fear	Poor prognosis
	Symptoms of acute infection
Impaired home maintenance management	Lack of community support services
Grieving	Inadequate home-care information
	Lack of people to assist with care
	Confusion or withdrawal of friends or family

Data from Gong V, Rudnick N (eds). AIDS Facts and Issues. New Brunswick, NJ: Rutgers University Press, 1986.

Table 26-1 identifies frequent nursing diagnoses for clients with AIDS.

Interventions for a Person with AIDS

The HIV-infected individual of course needs intervention. Often, however, care is compromised if health care professionals, family, and friends are not properly educated and are without sufficient peer and outside support. Therefore, staff, the person with AIDS or the HIV-positive client, and family and friends all need attention.

STAFF. The risk for health care workers of becoming HIV positive is stated as being low. Of those who have been punctured from contaminated needles, only 1% have become HIV positive (Breault and Polifroni 1992). Staff have significant concerns regarding their own safety. The present shortage of nursing staff, compounded with the increasing number of AIDS clients needing intensive physical as well as psychological care, raises many valid issues. Many of the following issues can contribute to staff burnout:

- Fear of contagion
- Young age of the afflicted
- Frequent deaths of clients
- Deterioration of the client's physical condition and, often, the psychological state
- Need for extra precautions
- Being the target of the client's anger

Many health care facilities are making an effort to deal with these staff issues and offer support. One psychiatric unit that cared for AIDS and AIDS-related complex clients found that staff significantly benefited from general meetings, small group meetings, individual supervision sessions, educational sessions, and opportunities to ventilate. Box 26-3 identifies some methods nurses can use to prevent burnout.

Education must include housekeeping and dietary staff because auxiliary staff often refuse to enter the room of an HIV-infected individual for fear of contagion. Weekly staff discussion with the Department of Infection Control can decrease misperceptions among all staff.

Knowledge of, and competence in, implementing the hospital's infection control guidelines are crucial.

Box 26-3. SUGGESTIONS FOR PREVENTING STAFF BURNOUT

1. Remember, rewarding and mutually beneficial relationships can be established with your AIDS patients.
2. Use AIDS network groups as a professional reference group to give *you* support.
3. Become familiar with the literature on death and dying and suicide.
4. Discuss and share and become aware of your own feelings about AIDS, persons with AIDS (PWAs), and death.
5. Expect to move through a process in which you feel deep despair before you gain a more balanced sense of reality.
6. Use a voluntary system of rotation with different types of patients.
7. Share feelings and maintain personal relationships with members of a specific nonprofessional community support and socialization group.

Data from Leukefeld C, Fimbres M. Introduction. In Leukefeld C, Fimbres M (eds). Responding to AIDS: Psychosocial Initiatives. Silver Spring, MD: National Association of Social Workers, 1987, as found in Leukefeld CG. Psychosocial initiatives in dealing with AIDS. Hospital and Community Psychiatry, 40(5):454, 1989.

Precautions usually include wearing gloves for contact with blood and body fluids, following special precautions for reusable equipment and supplies, and disposing of used syringes in specially designated impermeable containers. **Each nurse should be very familiar with the disease control protocol practiced in his or her hospital.**

HIV-INFECTED CLIENT. A complicating factor in providing services is the dwindling support system of an HIV client. For example, a person whose support system consists of others in a high-risk group may have witnessed many of his or her peers die of the disease already. Reactions of family and friends might be such that they are unable to support the individual because of their own fears and experiences. Therefore, for the same reason that an individual has an increased need for abundant family support and love, little or none might be available.

The client's ability to trust is perhaps the most basic social psychological process that will determine how the client responds to AIDS (Getty and Stern 1990). Therefore, the nurse's response and attitude toward the client must be nonjudgmental to foster a trusting relationship and to affirm the patient's feelings of self-worth. To help the patient accept his or her illness, the nursing interventions include providing supportive care, which allows the client to maintain maximal competency and control (Sadovsky 1991). The relationship between the patient and nurse should be a partnership, in which the nurse gives accurate information for the patient to make informed decisions. In times of emotional distress, the nurse is available to listen, assess the severity of the distress (e.g., if the patient is suicidal), and offer support. It is important the client knows that he or she will not be abandoned by the staff, especially during the terminal stages of the illness (Sadovsky 1991).

Support groups for people with AIDS are designed to reduce isolation and personal rejection, and are able to provide educational, psychotherapeutic, and social interaction. Support groups can enhance self-esteem by allowing the person to manage his or her life by controlling personal attitudes and decisions in dealing with the disease (Menenberg 1987).

The homosexual community has been very responsive to the needs of AIDS victims; it has been active in fund-raising, legislation, and research and development of community resources (Menenberg 1987). In many areas of the country, there are AIDS therapy groups, which offer emotional and physical support. In addition, there are care partners' groups and parents' support groups that offer assistance to lovers and families of HIV-infected individuals.

Individual and group therapy are often useful in helping the HIV-infected client work through depression and handle the many emotions that arise. Some issues concern drug abuse, possible social isolation, and associated fears or anger that arise over acknowledgment of the disease. Instructions in stress management and problem-solving techniques can be beneficial. As mentioned, antidepressants may be given at times, and benzodiazepines are sometimes useful in reducing extreme anxiety and anxiety reactions. Psychiatric interventions for AIDS-related dementia are similar to the general management of the cognitive impairment disorders. (See Chapter 20.)

Pastoral services can offer spiritual help and can provide a great deal of comfort. Social services provide discharge planning and any necessary referrals. Referrals include information on community re-

INTERVENTION	RATIONALE
Nursing Diagnosis: *Social isolation* related to AIDS as evidenced by feelings of rejection	
1. Assess social supports: Who are the individuals in the client's network? Are they reliable and available? Does the client feel they are supportive?	1. Social support can buffer the effects of physical and psychological stress.
2. Determine which local agencies and resources would be useful and available to the client. For example, • National AIDS Hotline (1-800-342-AIDS) • People with AIDS Coalition Hotline (1-800-828-3280)	2. Clients are often unaware of where they can get specific help and emotional support.
3. Encourage and facilitate verbal expressions of client's concerns, questions, and fears.	3. When others show genuine concern for the client's experience, his or her anxiety may decrease along with feelings of alienation.
Nursing Diagnosis: *Decisional conflict* related to sharing diagnosis with others, as evidenced by fear of rejection	
1. Assist and support client in sharing information with significant others regarding his or her diagnosis of AIDS. For example, role-play what client wants to say to family, lover, and close friends.	1. Many PWAs want their family and close friends to know. Role-playing helps client become more comfortable in disclosing diagnosis.
2. Assess if PWA wants others, such as employer and casual friends, to know diagnosis.	2. Dentist and general practitioner need to know HIV status. Telling employer and casual friends may be risky. Potential for losing job is real.
Nursing Diagnosis: *Moderate to severe anxiety* related to feelings of helplessness, as evidenced by feeling loss of control of one's life	
1. Encourage PWA to participate in determining goals and decision making regarding his or her care.	1. Promotes a sense of control and may reduce anxiety.
2a. Provide accurate information about procedures, tests, transmission, and hospital routines. If nurse is unsure, he or she should contact the Infectious Disease Department in hospital or the local Health Department for up-to-date information.	2a. People often misinterpret the rationale or the reason for procedures and tests. Up-to-date information can reduce anxiety.
2b. Continue to discuss transmission and ways to avoid infecting others.	2b. When anxiety is high, retention of information is diminished.
3. Clarify misperceptions.	3. Helps reduce anxiety, thereby facilitating retention of information.
4. Maintain continuity of nursing care throughout each phase of hospitalization.	4. Continuity helps the PWA maintain trust with the nurse and his or her environment.
Nursing Diagnosis: *Ineffective coping* related to crisis of AIDS, as evidenced by anger and denial	
1. Assess for maladaptive coping strategies, e.g., prolonged denial.	1. Prolonged denial interferes with client's accepting diagnosis and obtaining treatment.
2. Avoid false reassurances, e.g., implying that the cure for AIDS may be at hand.	2. Stories of PWAs who have adjusted to their diagnoses successfully encourage realistic hope.
3. Help the PWA deal with his or her anger. The nurse can • Assess reason for client's anger • Avoid personalizing client's verbal abuse • Encourage realizations that will assist the PWA in resolving some of his or her angry feelings • Use peers to discuss personal feelings and frustrations and to give a clear perspective.	3. Anger is an expected response; however, excess hostility that alienates all support networks is maladaptive. The client's anger often comes from lack of control over situation, fear of isolation, or fear of losing employment.

Data from McGrough KN. Assessing social support of people with AIDS. Oncology Nursing Forum, 17(1):31, 1990; Nyamathi A, Van Servellen G. Maladaptive coping in critically ill patients with acquired immunodeficiency syndrome: Nursing assessment and treatment. Heart and Lung, 18(2):113, 1989.
AIDS = acquired immunodeficiency syndrome; HIV = human immunodeficiency syndrome; PWA = person with AIDS.

sources, self-help groups, and finances. Table 26–2 lists several psychosocial interventions for a person with AIDS.

Everyone—the general population, nurses, educators, and especially those who test HIV positive—needs to be continuously updated on the progression of AIDS and AIDS research. Nurses should review the *Morbidity and Mortality Weekly Report*, published by the Centers for Disease Control (CDC), to keep up to date on the rapid changes.

FAMILY AND FRIENDS. Because studies show that the immediate biological family and close friends are the social support that AIDS victims seek, families and friends also need to discuss their concerns, get current medical information, and receive help with the exhausting work of caring for their loved ones at home.

Stressors to family and friends are similar to those of the AIDS victim. Long periods of nonspecific illness during which there is uncertainty about the diagnosis and the prognosis, increasing physical and mental disability, lack of definitive treatment, and financial constraints, compounded by the constant stigma associated with the disease, tend to "burn out" family members and friends who comprise the support system of the AIDS client (Smith and Popp 1992).

Family members frequently need, and should receive, referrals for their own mental health (Baer et al. 1987). Self-help groups for families and friends are available in many areas.

Mr. Todd is a 27-year-old man who is initially seen in the outpatient clinic for nausea, vomiting, and fever. Initially he is treated with antibiotics. For the next six months he has periods of remission, but the symptoms continue to recur. As the months pass, Mr. Todd begins feeling depressed and fatigued and loses interest in his job and usual activities with his friends. Finally, he is admitted to the hospital on a medical unit, where he is found to be HIV positive. Two days later he is diagnosed with AIDS.

When he learns of his diagnosis, Mr. Todd withdraws from the staff and is observed sitting for long periods of time in his room with the lights off and the curtains drawn. He is immediately placed in a single room on reverse isolation and precautions for blood and body secretions. The staff who have frequently visited Mr. Todd begin avoiding his room. Many nursing staff and physicians are concerned and confused about proper gowning procedure when entering Mr. Todd's room. Several staff put on gowns, gloves, masks, and hairnets and cover their shoes before entering; however, some staff just wear masks. Ancillary health professionals refuse to enter his room to dis-

pose of waste or to deliver his meals or mail. Soon Mr. Todd refuses to see his family and will answer questions only in two-word phrases. A psychiatric liaison nurse consultation is initiated by the head nurse to assess and evaluate Mr. Todd for depression. The head nurse asks Mr. Todd, and he agrees to the consultation.

Initially, Mr. Todd is guarded and evasive when answering questions. After several visits, Mr. Todd tells the psychiatric liaison nurse that he does not know what to tell his friends, family, and lover about the reason for hospitalization. Many of his friends and co-workers do not know that he is homosexual. He thinks that his family is suspicious about his homosexuality, yet he has never confronted the issue with them. Because his father is a very conservative, traditional man, Mr. Todd is afraid of being rejected and "disowned" by his family. On the other hand, he believes that his lover will accept his diagnosis, but feels extremely guilty for probably transmitting the disease to someone he loves. He states that he is angry at the staff for treating him like a "leper" and wonders why some of the staff use the full isolation technique and some wear masks. Those staff that use gowns, gloves, and masks prior to entering his room are perceived by Mr. Todd as being afraid of and disgusted by him. On the whole, he is angry at the staff for rejecting him and not coming into his room as often as they once did.

Mr. Todd is encouraged to contact his lover and discuss his fears with him. The psychiatric liaison nurse calls the infection control nurse and schedules a case conference for the staff. During the conference, the psychiatric liaison nurse presents the client's perception and feelings of rejection. The infection control nurse also reiterates and describes hospital policy and procedure in working with people with AIDS.

After talking with his lover, Mr. Todd discovers that he is supported by him and feels encouraged to contact his family. His father is concerned about Mr. Todd's physical deterioration; however, he still had strong ambivalent feelings toward his son. The staff begin visiting more often and begin educating Mr. Todd about his disease and treatment. However, several staff members are still afraid of his disease and tend to avoid him. As Mr. Todd begins feeling more supported by his lover and staff, he begins talking more, and his room is no longer dark and desolate. Continuing infection control inservice conferences are held to allay newcomers' fears and answer questions. The major nursing interventions are establishing rapport with Mr. Todd by returning to visit, listening to his concerns, and accepting his views nonjudgmentally.

A PERSON WHO IS DYING

Concerns of the Dying Person

Nothing in life adequately prepares a person for his or her own death. The experience of terminal illness intensifies painful feelings of loss, including loss of personal existence and physical health, loss of loved ones and friends, and loss of financial resources.

After being told the diagnosis, a person may experience intense emotional reactions, ranging from feelings of emptiness and disbelief to feelings of rage and loss of control. Suddenly, a person is faced with fears unparalleled by any previous life experience. Fears of prolonged suffering, constant pain, imminent death, financial burdens left behind, alienation, and isolation are often mentioned by a dying person. The fear of abandonment may be a terrifying concern. Often, the dying client's care has been transferred from a family doctor to a team of specialists. Thus, the client loses his close relationship with his or her trusted physician to a team who are unfamiliar. If the person has had extensive hospitalization, friends and relatives who initially visited may no longer be available. Eventually, a person may fear that everyone may leave him or her to die alone.

The fear of pain and of financial ruin may be well founded. With some of the more lethal illnesses, the course of the disease is long, with only brief periods of remission. The nurse needs to be knowledgeable about the different types of terminal illnesses and the various prognoses. Armed with this knowledge and awareness of the client's understanding of his or her illness, the nurse is equipped to lend support and guidance for clients and their families.

Concerns of the Family

The family also experiences painful and conflicting emotions as they begin to deal with the diagnosis. Not only must they concern themselves with their individual emotional reactions to the diagnosis, they must also deal with the client's response. They may react with disbelief, with statements such as "Are you sure?" Fear of the future, anger, and guilt are all common responses. In addition, how to communicate the news to other family members and friends becomes an issue (Euster 1984).

Several helpful approaches have been identified for use when the medical staff discuss the terminality of a disease with a client and family (Guttenberg 1983; Sadovsky 1991):

● Discuss the prognosis with the family and client in private and allow for plenty of time to adjust.

● Encourage everyone to sit down.
● Expect that the client and family will have strength. "Expecting success fosters success; expecting failure fosters failure."
● Give the client and family reason to hope by being specific about the diagnosis and treatments, by describing staff role and efforts, by accentuating the positive, by displaying confidence, and by getting the client and family involved in daily activities and decision making.
● Discuss end-of-life treatments (e.g., life support, tube feeding, and intravenous medications) and options for family and client to make a decision prior to the later stages of dying.
● Keep visits brief but visit often.
● Express your caring verbally and nonverbally.
● Encourage the client to express ambivalent feelings associated with dying.
● Encourage the client to reminisce about life events.
● Allow the client to withdraw from his or her interests and friends (this usually occurs in the later stages of dying).
● Provide unconditional emotional support.
● Assist the client in using his or her individual coping pattern.

The approach, of course, needs to be individualized to meet the client's needs and coping styles.

As the client's hospitalization continues, the family must constantly deal with disequilibrium. Generally, the family are unfamiliar with the hospital system. Consulting physicians who come and go may only increase confusion for the family. Even though the family may have met the physicians, they are often unsure of what questions to ask. Even after learning some of the medical information, they are still unsure of its meaning. Eventually, the family is confronted with the physical realities of the disease, the weakness, the changes in skin coloring, the weight loss, and the surgical mutilation. They are worried about their response to their loved one and how he or she will perceive their response. All of these issues add to the family's frustration, fatigue, and feelings of helplessness as they attempt to deal with their own reactions.

Discharge of the client brings another set of problems for the client and family. "The continued stress of an ill family member creates feelings of anger in relatives" (Euster 1984). Sometimes, the illness necessitates role reversal, which may produce anger. Along with anger come feelings of guilt. Over time, the family members who experience no relief become depleted of emotional support, physical assistance, and financial support. As time progresses, their ability to cope may diminish along with social and financial support.

Concerns Among Staff Members

Staff also have strong reactions when faced with a terminally ill client. Nursing staff may withdraw because they do not know what to say to the person or they may not be aware of what the person has been told. Ideally, the nursing staff should accompany the doctor when the diagnosis is being explained to the client and family. Physicians and nurses may also withdraw when they overidentify with the client. Members of the health care team often experience loss through personal identification with the client.

Before planning interventions, staff must first examine their own reactions to a client who is terminally ill. The nurses' reactions are influenced by similar factors that influence the reactions of the dying person. Cultural, educational, and religious background affect the nurses' ability to deal with death. Past experiences with deaths of clients and deaths of family members also play a role in how the nurses will interact with the dying client and family. Besides these factors, Adams (1984) suggested six other variables that play a major role in how nurses respond to dying clients, as seen in Table 26–3.

All these factors and variables are reflected in the nurses' delivery of client care. If nurses find that they are not able to cope with the dying client, or that their response is negative, they should ask to be excused from the case.

Table 26–3 ■ FACTORS THAT INFLUENCE A NURSE'S REACTION TO A DYING PATIENT

FACTOR	REACTION
1. Length of hospitalization	The longer the hospitalization, the more time the nurse has to form a relationship with the client and family. Nurses may begin to experience their own sense of mortality and become uncomfortable and withdraw. Nurses who can accept personal feelings will develop more empathy and become more supportive.
2. Frequency of admissions	More frequent admissions to the hospital strengthen the relationship between the patient and staff. The closer the relationship, the more attached the nurse may become and the more grief will be experienced by the nurse when the patient dies. If the hospitalizations have been marked with prolonged pain and suffering, the nurse may experience a sense of relief when the client dies.
3. Role of the family	When the family is not available, the nurse may assume the role of the family. This tends to bond the nurse to the patient. If the family is present, the nurse may identify with the family, or avoid them if they react as his or her family would. If the family expresses their anguish openly, the nurse may feel like withdrawing, especially if the family is from a different culture.
4. Patient's condition	The nurse tends to withdraw or feel indifferent toward a person who is unconscious.
5. Patient's coping style	An angry or dependent coping style tends to promote withdrawal and avoidance in the nurse. Nurses accept better the person who uses intellectualization and rationalization as coping strategies.
6. Role of the subconscious	If the client's mannerisms stir a memory of someone else the nurse has known, then the nurse may react countertransferentially to the client as if the client were that other person.

Adapted from Adams F. Six very good reasons why we react differently to various dying patients. Nursing '84, 14:8, 1984. Adapted with permission from the June issue of Nursing '84, copyright 1984, Springhouse Corporation, 1111 Bethlehem Pike, Springhouse, PA 19477-0908. All rights reserved.

Stages in the Process of Dying

Dying is a difficult and often emotionally painful topic to discuss. Until Kübler-Ross (1969) published her classic work on how people deal with their own death, little attention was paid to this often-avoided subject. Even though Kübler-Ross named five distinct stages in the process of dying, her intent was not to "classify" the client into a stage but merely to understand the emotions of a dying individual so that health care providers could be more empathetic. Needless to say, dying clients may skip stages or return to the first stage after completing the fourth stage. The most important of these five stages is to understand the psychological dynamics that the dying person and family are experiencing so that the nurse can best facilitate adaptive coping and provide individualized client care.

STAGE ONE: DENIAL AND ISOLATION. The first stage usually begins after the person has just learned of his or her diagnosis. The initial reaction of *denial, shock, and disbelief* is experienced by almost all clients, not only during this first stage but also later on, from time to time. After being told about their terminal illness, people are in a temporary state of shock. Their affect may be blunted. The content of conversation is, "No, this can't be happening to me." Sometimes clients may even begin talking about death, only to change the topic and contradict themselves later in the conversation. This denial leads to feelings of loneliness and isolation as they attempt to protect themselves against the onslaught of emotions. "Denial is usually a temporary defense and will soon be replaced by partial acceptance." (Kübler-Ross 1969, p 40).

Mr. Dodds, a 50-year-old married man, is admitted to the hospital and diagnosed with adenocarcinoma of the pancreas. When told about his diagnosis, Mr. Dodds replies, "How can that be? I've never smoked. You must have the wrong client." His initial denial is replaced by anger after several unsuccessful operations to alleviate an obstructed pancreas.

STAGE TWO: ANGER. After the denial has dissipated, reality begins to take the form of *anger, rage, resentment,* and even *envy.* "Why me?" is the most frequently asked question and the most difficult one for family and staff to answer. There is never an answer to this question. Anger may be internalized or displaced onto staff and loved ones. Projected anger can take the form of demanding or intimidating behavior toward staff and family. It is important that the nurse not internalize the client's displaced anger but understand its source. Staff need to work on acceptance of the person during this stage and not withdraw and leave the dying person feeling abandoned (Kübler-Ross 1969).

Mr. Dodds exhibits his anger by constantly complaining about his room, the nursing care, and his pain medication schedule. When the nurses enter his room with his pain medication, he comments about their unprofessional appearance, or asks them to straighten the flowers in his vase. Finally, one of the nurses takes the time to sit down and talk with him. Her response to his demands is, "It must be really frustrating for you now. How can I best help you?" Her response takes Mr. Dodds by surprise because most people quickly leave the room in anger after completing a task. Mr. Dodds begins to discuss his fears and later asks the nurse to visit more often.

STAGE THREE: BARGAINING. Most of the *bargaining* is made with God in an effort to postpone the inevitable. Promises to be a better person may be associated with guilt, which may be the result of irrational fears. It is important that the nurse explore feelings of guilt and not brush these feelings aside. Usually this stage is marked by statements such as, "If I eat more, will you let me go?" and "If only I can live until my son graduates, I'll donate all my savings to the church" (Kübler-Ross 1969).

Sometimes bargaining helps the client muster the energy to accomplish a goal.

Mrs. Abrahams, a 65-year-old widow diagnosed with breast cancer with metastasis to the lung, has one wish. She has always talked about her only grandson graduating from high school. She wants to be there in the auditorium when he walks up the steps to receive his diploma. Even though her lung involvement is extensive and restricts her, she does attend her grandson's graduation in a wheelchair. Twenty-four hours after returning to the hospital, she dies.

STAGE FOUR: DEPRESSION. Soon the numbness of the denial and the rage of the anger are replaced by a great sense of loss. The dying client can no longer pretend that there is nothing wrong or that surgery can cure the disease. *Depression* becomes the emotional response as the client begins to cope with the actual losses or impending losses. Depression is also "the preparatory grief that the terminally ill client has to undergo in order to prepare himself for his final separation from this world" (Kübler-Ross 1969). During this phase, staff become more uncomfortable and may tend to avoid the client. Usually, psychiatric consultations are generated when the staff begin to feel hopeless and helpless to "cure" the client.

Mrs. Jewel, a 52-year-old married mother of two, is diagnosed with adenocarcinoma of the pancreas with metastasis to the liver. She has been ill for almost two years without a definitive diagnosis. On learning of her diagnosis, the woman replies, "Well, I'm glad to finally know what's been making me sick for all these months. I had a feeling it was cancer." Her major concern is how to tell her husband and two daughters. She feels hopeless and helpless to change her prognosis. Eventually, she stops interacting with the nursing staff. During the psychiatric liaison nursing consultation, the psychiatric liaison nurse learns of her concern about informing her family that she is dying. The nurse encourages Mrs. Jewel to "role-play" communicating her diagnosis to her family. Mrs. Jewel also wants to know if it is normal to be thinking of funeral arrangements. Mrs. Jewel discusses her wishes for her funeral and how to broach the subject with her husband. Two days after this interaction with the nurse, she shares her grief and last wishes with her family. Three weeks later, she dies.

STAGE FIVE: ACCEPTANCE. This last stage signifies that the client has had enough time and assistance to work through the previous stages of denial, anger, and depression. The person has mourned his or her losses and is left tired and weak. This is a difficult time for both the client and family. By this time, the person is void of feelings; the struggle is gone. The person withdraws and no longer desires to communicate. Many people like the quiet reassurance of someone sitting nearby just holding their hand (Kübler-Ross 1969). Those who see their illness as a challenge may fight this stage until, one day, they decide they are too weak and can no longer fight.

Mrs. Yolanda is a 68-year-old widow who is diagnosed with adenocarcinoma of the abdomen with extensive abdominal metastasis. She has previously been hospitalized several times in this particular unit and is well known to the staff. Prior to this admission, Mrs. Yolanda was known for her independent personality and her humorous jokes, which kept a constant stream of staff coming into her room. Her abdominal girth has extensively enlarged from her ascites, causing shortness of breath and dyspnea on exertion. She finds it difficult to sleep lying down and can rest only by lying her head on the bedside table while sitting. Even though fluid is drawn from her abdomen numerous times, Mrs. Yolanda's girth continues to expand. She becomes increasingly uncomfortable and listless. Gone are her entertaining jokes and witty remarks to the staff. She confides in the staff a week before she dies that she "prays to God to die. I'm no longer afraid . . . I'm ready to go; just let me go."

Interventions for a Dying Person

WHEN WORKING WITH A DYING PERSON. *During the first stage*, denial and isolation, the nurse needs to know what the physician told the client and family. Possible interventions include the following:

1. Stay with the client as the person expresses his or her anxieties.
2. Actively listen to the person and reflect emotions.
3. Give physical comfort if acceptable to the person, e.g., putting a hand on the client's arm.
4. Encourage the client to express thoughts and feelings and identify realistic problems.
5. Answer questions regarding the disease and treatments when asked.

Give essential information at this time and expect the client to repeatedly ask the same questions because he or she may be unable to concentrate (Ostchega and Jacob 1984; Wright 1985).

The client experiences anger and rage *during the second phase*. This phase may be difficult for staff. If the nurse internalizes the client's anger, the nurse may withdraw or become angry with the client. Suggested nursing interventions include the following:

1. Recognize client's anger as being displaced.
2. Reflect and acknowledge his or her right to be angry.
3. Assist family members in dealing with the client's anger.
4. If a client loses control, the nurse must take charge, talk with him or her in a quiet room, and give a sedative if necessary.
5. Involve the dying person in decision making, giving the person a sense of control over the situation.

During phase three, bargaining, the nurse continues to intervene by:

1. Encouraging the client to discuss fears that may be related to feelings of guilt
2. Suggesting that clergy assist in dispelling irrational religious beliefs
3. Focusing on client's strengths and abilities to cope with situations in the past
4. Giving the client some "time out" from staff intervention

During the fourth stage, the nurse can be helpful to the client by evaluating when to intervene. "Sometimes dying persons need to feel the pain of their losses, and not have attempts made to relieve their suffering" (Benoliel 1985). Besides continued supportive listening and communication, useful nursing interventions are as follows:

1. Assist the client to discover ways of normalizing his or her life in the face of discontinuity and change (Benoliel 1985).
2. Keep the client informed of treatments, procedures, medications, and adverse side effects.
3. Develop small, obtainable, measurable goals with the client's input (e.g., sitting up in the bed for 10 minutes twice a day).
4. Be careful of withdrawing from or avoiding the client at this stage.
5. Request psychiatric consultation if the client becomes suicidal.
6. Refer the client and family members to a support group, such as Cancer Care.
7. Be available to explore philosophical questions the client has about life, religious beliefs, or life hereafter.
8. Continue to provide needed relief for pain control.

In *the last stage*, acceptance, the major goal for the nurse is to keep the client as comfortable as possible. Nursing interventions focus on maintaining dignity, especially if the client is mentally alert yet control of bodily functioning has been lost. Because most clients are exhausted, shorter interactions are indicated in keeping the client informed of daily happenings and preserving strength. Table 26–4 summarizes nursing interventions during the five stages of dying for the client who is terminally ill.

WHEN WORKING WITH THE FAMILY. (Refer to Chapter 17 for guidelines for working with a grieving family.) Specifically, the nurse works with the family to deal with the physical realities of a terminal diagnosis. In order to assist the client, the nurse must also be aware of how the family is reacting to the crisis. Nursing interventions include the following:

1. Encourage the family to share their thoughts, fears, and feelings and help them identify problems.
2. Encourage the family to share their concerns with the dying member in order to facilitate open communication.
3. Orient the family to the hospital and unit, explaining visiting hours, parking, lodging, and other practical necessities.
4. Encourage the family to ask the doctor questions; writing down their questions on paper will help them to remember.
5. Give the family private time with the client to share feelings.
6. Involve the family, along with the client, in decision making regarding care, which helps foster a sense of control, and encourage the family members to give feedback to the staff about the client's likes and dislikes.

7. Encourage the family to prioritize problems and solve each problem one by one.
8. Discuss hospice care as a possible alternative in the terminal stages of the illness.
9. Encourage family members to attend a support group, such as Cancer Care, if available. This support can help the family feel less isolated and alone during this time.
10. If the client and family do not want to use life-sustaining support systems (ventilators), encourage them to talk with the physician to request an order. Be with the client and family when they talk to the physician about a do-not-resuscitate order.
11. Include the children in the grieving process.

Working with the terminally ill client can be difficult. However, communicating openly and honestly and offering a human presence during a period when most people withdraw can be a profound experience for both the nurse and the dying person. In assisting the client through the stages of dying, the nurse can gain a great deal from the client's experience and from the relationship with the dying person. An empathetic and caring relationship facilitates the person's progression through the dying process and can instill a sense of accomplishment and connectedness in the nurse. Although difficult and emotionally draining, working with a terminally ill client offers unique rewards.

A PERSON WITH A PSYCHOPHYSIOLOGICAL DISORDER

Unlike the patient populations that we have previously discussed, a patient with *psychophysiological disorder* has physical symptoms with psychological components, which play a significant role in the expression and manifestation of the physical symptoms. In other words, emotions act as precipitating or aggravating factors in physical illnesses, such as bronchial asthma, peptic ulcer disease, and ulcerative colitis (Kellner 1990).

In contrast, a person exhibiting a *somatization disorder* frequently complains of physical symptoms that either lack a physiological basis or are in excess of what one would expect from medical findings. In other words, the person's symptomatology cannot be explained by the results of medical tests, or the person presents an exaggerated scenario of symptoms (refer to Chapter 15). Therefore, *psychophysiological* or *psychogenic disorders* differ from *somatization disorders* in that they have a physiological basis for the disorder, and the symptoms are not "grossly in excess"; however, the physi-

Table 26–4 ■ NURSING INTERVENTIONS AND RATIONALES: WORKING WITH A PERSON WHO IS DYING

INTERVENTION	RATIONALE
Stage One: Denial and Isolation	
1. Examine own feelings about death.	1. Personal defenses and fears can be projected onto dying person if not identified and worked out.
2. Encourage the patient's expression of feelings, concerns and fears: ● Sit at bedside. ● Actively listen and reflect client's feelings. ● Hold hand or touch shoulder when appropriate.	2. ● Provides presence and decreases feelings of abandonment. ● Lessens feelings of isolation and keeps channels of communication open. ● For some, physical touch provides comfort and demonstrates concern.
3. Provide small amount of information at a time. Encourage questions when client is ready.	3. Having correct information can decrease anxiety and clarify information.
4. Encourage decisions regarding self-care.	4. Increases feelings of control and encourages functioning at optimum level.
Stage Two: Anger	
1. Acknowledge person's right to be angry.	1. Increases feelings of support and being understood.
2. Understand that anger directed at staff and family is not personal.	2. Feelings of helplessness and loss stimulate anger that is often projected onto staff and loved ones.
3. Work with client to rechannel anger into positive channels, e.g., making decisions, setting goals, and fighting disease.	3. Can help rechannel energy in ways that help increase self-esteem, feelings of control, and sense of being supported by staff and others.
Stage Three: Bargaining	
1. Offer to contact clergy or rabbi.	1. May assist in dispelling irrational religious beliefs.
2. Encourage discussion of feelings, especially guilt and loss.	2. Decreases feelings of guilt and possible thoughts of being punished for past actions.
3. Encourage client's positive coping strategies used in the past.	3. Positive reinforcement can strengthen positive behaviors.
4. Encourage periods of time to focus on more satisfying areas of life	4. Periods of time away from discussion of disease and death helps person put life in broader terms
Stage Four: Depression	
1. Focus on daily short term *obtainable* goals.	1. Emphasizes positive functioning and areas of independence.
2. Continue to spend time with client on regular basis.	2. Staff awareness of tendency to withdraw can help staff modify own behaviors.
3. Encourage client to participate in usual activities.	3. Can decrease time spent in brooding and offer broader focus of experience.
4. Encourage client to participate in support groups.	4. Discussion with others in similar circumstances can decrease feelings of isolation and increase feelings of being understood.
5. Maintain adequate pain control.	5. Physical comfort can increase ability to interact with others and may diminish tendency to withdraw.
Stage Five: Acceptance	
1. Sit with person—even when person does not want to talk.	1. Provides presence and support and decreases feelings of abandonment.
2. Allow appropriate privacy, e.g., during toileting and bathing.	2. Maintains sense of dignity.
3. Continue pain control.	3. Provides comfort during final stages of dying.

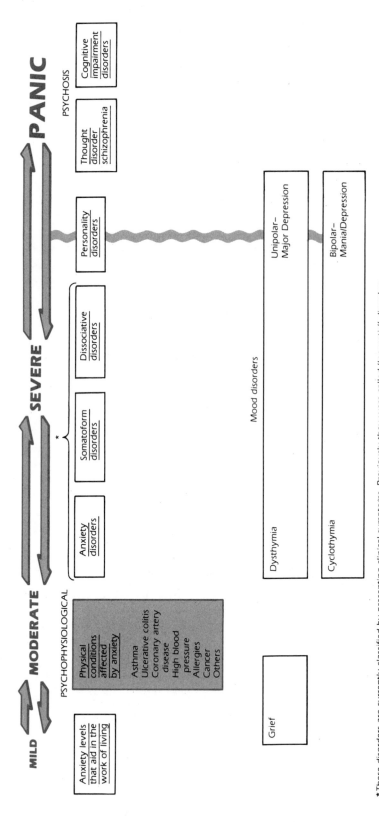

Figure 26–1. *Mental health continuum for the hospitalized person.*

*These disorders are currently classified by presenting clinical symptoms. Previously they were called "neurotic" disorders.

cal symptoms can be triggered by psychological factors. These disorders can be life threatening and often warrant hospitalization.

Essentially, a psychogenic disorder entails the following (Fig. 26–1):

1. The initiation or exacerbation of a specific physical condition or disorder can be related to specific stimuli that are psychologically meaningful to an individual (e.g., separation, death, or loss of job).
2. There is actual organ pathology (e.g., ulcers or asthma) or known pathophysiological process (e.g., migraine headache).
3. A somatization disorder is ruled out (APA 1987).

Physiological Correlates

In 1947, Flanders Dunbar suggested that specific personality profiles and behavioral patterns corresponded to specific organic disease. Likewise, Franz Alexander proposed that unconscious repressed conflicts, along with genetic predisposing factors, over time could result in specific organ diseases and named seven such diseases: ulcerative colitis, rheumatoid arthritis, hyperthyroidism, neurodermatitis, hypertension, peptic ulcer disease, and asthma.

Studies addressing psychophysiological disorders and their psychological determinants have yielded conflicting results. Some studies indicate that individuals with profound dependency needs and yearnings for affection are more likely to develop peptic ulcer disease. On the other hand, some studies have indicated that individuals with peptic ulcer disease have a genetic predisposition. Some studies indicate that people who have an exacerbation of their ulcers usually are experiencing a time of high anxiety and stress in their lives (Oken 1989). Currently, the trend is that peptic ulcer disease represents a group of disorders with different subgroups demonstrating different physiological and genetic characteristics. Table 26–5 gives

Table 26–5 ■ PSYCHOLOGICAL SUPPORTIVE MEASURES FOR SPECIFIC PERSONALITY PROFILES

CONFLICTS	POSSIBLE BEHAVIORS	CLINICAL EXAMPLES	PSYCHOLOGICAL SUPPORTIVE MEASURES
Gastrointestinal—Peptic Ulcers			
Intense dependency needs associated with underlying hostility May use reaction-formation as a defense	Very aggressive, overly independent or demanding Difficulty trusting or asking others for support Worry	Mr. Stubbs, 42, was a hard-driving man who was vice-president of a local insurance company. He prided himself on his self-sufficiency. When the work piled up, he was unable to admit to his boss he needed assistance. After three weeks of working until 11:00 P.M. and taking aspirin for stomach pain, he was admitted to the emergency room with a massive gastrointestinal bleed.	1. Meet needs but do not foster or reinforce dependency. 2. Foster activities for self-care. 3. Combine health teaching with psychological support. 4. Work with client to reduce environmental stress. 5. Encourage person to share thoughts and feelings directly.
Gastrointestinal—Ulcerative Colitis			
Issues of control Strong need for approval Difficulty with dependency issues and sensitivity to loss	Rumination, indecision, passive compliance, moral rigidity, perfectionism, conformity, orderliness (obsessive-compulsive trait), passive-aggressive tendencies	Ms. Lions, a 24-year-old computer operator, was prized by her boss for being efficient, attending to detail, and handing her work in on time. Although she did not seem to have a sense of humor, she complied with demands and never bothered anyone. Ms. Lions always thought her boss did not appreciate her enough. Three weeks after she broke up with her boyfriend, she noticed blood and mucus in her now frequent watery stools.	1. Encourage person's sense of control. 2. Simplify choices. 3. Work with the person to set realistic goals. 4. Encourage productive activities that will increase self-esteem and decrease self-rumination.

Table continued on following page

Table 26–5 ■ PSYCHOLOGICAL SUPPORTIVE MEASURES FOR SPECIFIC PERSONALITY PROFILES *Continued*

CONFLICTS	POSSIBLE BEHAVIORS	CLINICAL EXAMPLES	PSYCHOLOGICAL SUPPORTIVE MEASURES
Cardiovascular—High Blood Pressure			
Between dependent and aggressive drives	Outwardly pleasant and calm Use of reaction-formation to repress rage and suspicion	Tom Sharp, 52, lived most of his life with his invalid mother. Everyone said what a wonderful son he was to devote his life to his mother. He gave up a promotion involving moving to another state to stay with and care for his mother. The mother refused to let anyone but her son care for her and was sharply critical of any woman Tom wanted to date. Three months after his mother's death Tom complained of dizziness and was found to have a blood pressure of 210/140 on a routine examination.	1. Combine psychological support with health teaching. 2. Evaluate and assess unwanted side effects from antihypertensives, which could affect compliance (e.g., impotence, loss of sexual drive). 3. Teach relaxation techniques. 4. Evaluate situational, environmental, and interpersonal stressors.
Cardiovascular—Coronary Artery Disease			
Around dependency issues	Behaviors typical of type A personality Highly competitive, sense of time urgency, hard working, aggressive, unable to relax, hostile Doesn't adhere to medical regimen Use of denial	Max Bender, 46, started a construction company the year he finished high school. He prided himself on "being a man," that is, tough, lucky with women, and always on top of things. The fact that his business was the most successful in the area was not an accident. Max worked long hours, took charge of everything, and worked his men hard. He smoked, drank, and often overate. One year after his wife died from cancer and two months after an important client defaulted on his payments and went bankrupt, Max was admitted to the emergency room with a massive myocardial infarction.	1. Emotional support with health teaching. 2. Counseling directed toward reducing competitiveness and time urgency and creating lifestyle changes. 3. Teach relaxation training. 4. Sexual counseling, if indicated. 5. Marital counseling, if needed, to decrease family stress. 6. Referral and supervision for prescribed exercise regimen
Respiratory—Asthma			
High dependency needs Extreme vulnerability regarding issues of separation	Overly dependent Clinging behaviors (e.g., behaviors that indicate a strong need for protection and security) Use of reaction-formation, e.g., behavior that rejects need for protection or security such as acting independent or highly competitive	Telly Long's dad had left the family when Telly was 3 years old. Her mother was forced to go back to work as a nurse when Telly was 6 years old. When Telly's mom decided to go away for a week's vacation with a friend, Telly started having a serious asthma attack. Telly was brought to the emergency room and given epinephrine. Telly's mom canceled her vacation plans. As the years progressed, Telly continued to have attacks, especially when Telly's mom planned extended time away from home.	1. Explore events and situations that precede an attack. 2. Encourage verbalization of thoughts and feelings to lessen somatic expression of conflict. 3. Maintain a balance between overprotectiveness and denial of disorder. 4. Encourage outside supports (e.g., self-help groups). 5. Emphasize person's strengths, abilities, and accomplishments.

a clinical example of proposed behaviors seen in some psychophysiological disorders.

The most widely publicized personality type to correlate with psychophysiological disorders is the *type A personality*. Type A personality occurs in individuals who exhibit their anger in a hostile manner and who are extremely competitive and driven. In the last decade, several research studies have associated type A personality disorder to coronary artery disease. However, it is now believed that it is not the type A personality itself but rather the degree of *hostility* felt that may make some people more prone to coronary artery disease (Fischman 1987). Whatever part personality plays in disease, most agree that chronic, severe, and perceived stress plays some role in the development of many diseases (Kaplan and Sadock 1991).

Table 26–6 identifies genetic and biological correlates and stress-related findings of some common physical disorders with psychogenic components.

Table 26–6 ■ ETIOLOGIC CONSIDERATIONS FOR PSYCHOPHYSIOLOGICAL DISORDERS

HYPOTHESIZED PERSONALITY TRAITS	INCIDENCE	GENETIC AND BIOLOGICAL CORRELATES	COMMON PRECIPITATING FACTORS	USEFUL THERAPIES OTHER THAN MEDICAL MANAGEMENT
Migraine and Vascular Headaches				
Is obsessive, controlling, perfectionistic, suppresses anger. Excessive self-demands, highly competitive.	15–20% of all men, 20–30% of women between puberty and menopause Begins in mornings or on weekends Lasts a few hours to a few days	Two thirds have family history.	Can be brought on by foods (e.g., monosodium glutamate, tyramine, chocolate), fluctuating levels of estrogen. Often in unilateral, temporal, or frontal areas. May include prodromata (nausea, vomiting, and photophobia).	Prodromal stage treated most effectively with ergotamine or analgesics.
Tension Headaches and Muscular Contractions				
People with type A characteristics, e.g., tense, high-strung, and competitive.	Occurs in 80% of population when under stress Begins at the end of the workday or early evening		Associated with anxiety and depression. Begins suboccipitally; usually bilateral.	Psychotherapy usually prescribed for chronic tension headaches. Learning to cope or avoiding tension-creating situations or people. Relaxation techniques helpful for some.
Respiratory—Bronchial Asthma				
No one personality type identified. Some asthmatic children have poor impulse control, are babyish, overly polite, and emotionally explosive; boys—passively dependent, timid, and immature; girls—try to be self-sufficient, often chronically depressed.	Usually occurs in younger children Usually occurs in people 40 and over	**Extrinsic:** usually in 30–50% of younger children, immunoglobulin E–type antibody formation to specific antibodies as a predisposition. 1. Runs in families. 2. Occurrence is seasonal. 3. Allergens play a part. **Intrinsic:** often marked by sensitivity to drugs, intense emotions, exercise, or weather changes.		Children—removal from home can radically alter attacks in some children. Others—need for steroids is lessened when removed from home environment. Others—have attacks in home environment only, e.g., not in schools.

Table continued on following page

HYPOTHESIZED PERSONALITY TRAITS	INCIDENCE	GENETIC AND BIOLOGICAL CORRELATES	COMMON PRECIPITATING FACTORS	USEFUL THERAPIES OTHER THAN MEDICAL MANAGEMENT
Cardiovascular—Essential Hypertension				
Anecdotal accounts: longs for approval, superficially easygoing, suppresses rage and suspicion. Hard driving and conscientious.	Higher in males until age 60	Family history of cardiac disease and hypertension.	Life changes and traumatic life events. Stressful jobs, e.g., air traffic controller. Hypothesized to be found more in areas of social stress and conflict.	Behavioral: biofeedback, stress reduction techniques, meditation, yoga, hypnosis. However, *pharmacological treatment is considered primary.*
Cardiovascular—Coronary Heart Disease				
Type A personality traits. Time urgency—difficulty doing nothing, always harried. Excessive competitiveness and hostility—always plays to win, general distrust of others' motives (e.g., altruism), authoritarian.	Higher in males until age 60

Higher in white population than in black population | Family history of cardiac disease is a risk factor. Other risk factors include hypertension, increased serum lipid levels, obesity, sedentary lifestyle, and cigarette smoking. | Often myocardial infarction (MI) occurs after sudden stress preceded by a period of losses, frustration, and disappointments. | Progressive relaxation, autohypnosis, meditation, biofeedback; behavior modification; support groups for type A personalities; prescribed program of physical exercise (prophylaxis against post-MI depression). When indicated, anxiolytics (benzodiazepines) and antidepressants are prescribed. |
Gastrointestinal—Peptic Ulcer				
Ambitious, independent. Regressive, overly dependent, repressed.	Occurs in 12% of men, 6% of women (more prevalent in industrialized societies)	Elevated pepsinogen level identified as an autosomal recessive trait. Both peptic and duodenal ulcers cluster in families, but separately from each other.	Periods of social tension and increased life stress. After losses—often after menopause.	Biofeedback can alter gastric acidity; behavioral approaches are used to reduce stress.
Gastrointestinal—Ulcerative Colitis				
Compulsive personality traits; neatness, orderliness, cleanliness; punctuality; hyperintellectualism; obstinacy; humorlessness; timidity; inhibition of feelings (especially anger); extreme sensitivity to real or imagined hurts.	Occurs equally in men and women

Develops in second and third decades of life and around age 50

High in Jewish population

Higher in whites than in blacks | Possible autoimmune response. Runs in families; no genetic marker found. | Centered on losses, especially key relationships. Narcissistic loss—client thinks he or she has failed, feels hurt or humiliated, unable to please others he or she depends on. | Psychotherapy: treating issues of separation, loss, rejection, dependency. |
| **Cancer** | | | | |
| Suppression of emotions, e.g., anger; easy to please and unaggressive; stoic, self-sacrificing; inhibited; self-effacing; rigid; may appear strong, puts others' needs first, conscientious | Men—most common in lung, prostate, colon, and rectum

Women—most common in breast, uterus, colon, and rectum

Death rates higher in men (especially black men) than in women | Genetic evidence suggests dysfunction of cellular profusion. Familial patterns—breast cancer, colorectal cancer, stomach cancer, melanoma. | Prolonged and intensive stress. Stressful life events, e.g., separation from or loss of significant other two years before diagnosis. Feelings of helplessness, hopelessness, and despair (depression) may precede the diagnosis of cancer. | Relaxation, e.g., meditation, autogenic training, self-hypnosis. Visualization. Psychological counseling. |

Nursing Interventions

In order to intervene with a person with a psychophysiological disorder, the nurse initially may focus on the physical symptoms. In some cases, these symptoms can be a medical emergency (e.g., status asthmaticus or bleeding ulcer). The nurse wants to engage the patient in a therapeutic relationship, and denial of the physical symptoms would alienate the patient from the nurse. In other words, the patient would perceive that the nurse did not believe these symptoms exist.

Most people believe that a person with a psychophysiological disorder is unaware of the presence of distressing conflicts and disturbing feelings; instead, there is a tendency to express their feelings and anxiety in physical symptoms. Often, through talking with others about painful emotions, viable alternatives for stressful situations and feelings can be found.

Coping skills of those individuals with psychophysiological disorders are often limited. Somatization is the major defense used; therefore, whenever the person encounters a stressful situation, the distress is expressed in "organ language" or physical symptoms (i.e., an asthmatic will complain of shortness of breath during a stressful time or a person with ulcers will experience stomach pain).

The most effective means of intervening with this type of patient is to *include the patient in all planning goals*. Interventions should focus on the patient's ineffective coping, which may be in response to feelings of helplessness. The nurse can begin by:

1. Helping the patient to recognize when he or she becomes anxious by determining behavioral cues, such as nervously shaking a foot; drumming fingertips; showing increased distractibility, increased perspiration, increased pulse, increased respiration, and increased blood pressure; and being unable to concentrate and complete a task
2. Working with a client to identify one situation that precipitates an onset of physical symptoms
3. Encouraging the client to verbalize anger and frustration more readily and more appropriately
4. Assisting the client to name and demonstrate one new way of dealing with a stressful situation
5. Assisting the client in identifying potential support systems and working on developing these

In addition, when persons with psychophysiological disorders are unable to relax, the nurse can assist by:

1. Helping the client recognize one difficulty surrounding his or her inability to relax (e.g., fear of losing control, fear of what others may think, or fear of being viewed as weak)
2. Teaching the client methods of relaxing, such as progressive muscle relaxation, deep breathing, self-hypnosis, and meditation
3. Asking the physician to discuss the possibility of using biofeedback with the client if he or she is unable to relax

Table 26–7 ■ AUTOMATIC NURSE RESPONSES AND SUGGESTED ALTERNATIVES

PATIENT BEHAVIORS	NURSES' AUTOMATIC RESPONSES	NURSES' ALTERNATIVE RESPONSES	EXAMPLES
1. Patient elaborates in detail the discomforts that nurse has heard before.	Annoyed, bored, argumentative	Use the patient's focus as starting point for eliciting the circumstances that surround the client's experience.	"What was happening at home/ with your job when this first started?"
2. Patient asks for sympathy and help (overtly or covertly).	Annoyed, burdened, or possibly overprotective	Show compassion as for clients generally. Maintain clear boundaries of self vis-à-vis patient.	"I can see that you are feeling particularly vulnerable now. Let's look at what *you* can do to feel less upset."
3. Patient's somatization is resistant to change.	Impatient, having unrealistic expectations of change	Be consistently available (within professional strictures).	"I know these migraines can be painful. I have 5 minutes to talk about your thoughts or feelings of concern to you."
4. Patient manifests anger or hostility toward staff.	Fearful, having avoidance behavior	Help patient note the difference between effects and action. Accept person having feelings of anger.	"You seem so angry this morning. Let's try and figure out what's going on."

Nurses' Reactions

Nurses are accustomed to having patients exhibit and complain of physical disorders that have an organic basis. The patient with a psychogenic disorder, however, may present a different scenario. For instance, the client may experience an increase in anxiety, which may intensify physical symptoms and interfere with his or her ability to follow the recommended treatment. Nurses and physicians may become frustrated and experience a threat to their own feelings of competence. Health care professionals may become more annoyed if the client continues to complain, receive treatment, and exhibit no progress. Table 26–7 identifies four client behaviors that can become troublesome for nurses.

The following is a case study of a nurse working with a patient with a psychophysiological disorder.

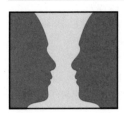

Case Study: Working with a Person Who Has a Psychophysiological Disorder

Mr. Hammond, 45, was brought to the emergency room after having a myocardial infarction. He had no history of coronary disease, although both his father and mother died of heart disease before the age of 65. Mr. Hammond is an executive in a large advertising firm, and according to his wife, he works many evenings and weekends to "beat the competition." Physical assessment reveals a blood pressure of 230/110 and a high serum cholesterol level of 290 mg/100 ml. He is considerably overweight and told the doctor that he has no time for exercise.

After five days in cardiac intensive care, Mr. Hammond was sent down to a medical unit. When Mr. Garcia, Mr. Hammond's primary nurse, went to visit, Mr. Hammond appeared restless, hostile, and demanding. Mrs. Hammond was in the room when the nurse arrived and seemed to be hovering over her husband's bed. Mrs. Hammond appeared greatly distressed, tired, and dejected. After Mrs. Hammond left, Mr. Garcia spent some time with Mr. Hammond. A sample of their interaction is provided subsequently.

Assessment

NURSE: Your wife seems concerned about you.

MR. HAMMOND: What does she know? She is treating me like a baby at a time I should be closing the Ford account. How much longer do I have to stay in this place?

NURSE: You have had a serious heart attack, and your body needs time to heal. You seem to have difficulty relaxing.

MR. HAMMOND: Relaxing . . . I never have time for relaxing. The minute you look away, someone gets in there ahead of you. Where is my phone? . . . I told them upstairs I needed a phone to make up for all this lost time.

NURSE: The doctor does not want you to have a phone at present. Your body needs the rest. Is there someone at the job who is taking over for you?

MR. HAMMOND: Are you kidding? Harry louses everything up. The only way to get anything done right is to do it yourself. If I could get out of here, I'd handle things myself. There is nothing wrong with me!

NURSE: It does sound like this has been very upsetting for you. We can talk about some of the things that are bothering you. Right now the doctor wants you to relax and has ordered a sedative for you.

MR. HAMMOND: I don't need anything to relax. I don't need anything or anybody. I am not a baby, and I don't need to be treated like one. Leave me alone. I've got a lot of good years ahead of me . . . I'm still the man I was . . . Get out of here!

NURSE: I can understand you are upset. I will be back in 15 minutes with your medication, and perhaps then we can talk about some of your concerns.

Mr. Garcia divided his data into objective and subjective components.

OBJECTIVE DATA

1. Serum cholesterol level of 290 mg/100 ml
2. Overweight
3. Restless and agitated
4. Male in his 40s
5. Both parents died of heart trouble in their early 60s
6. Blood pressure of 230/110

SUBJECTIVE DATA

1. Highly competitive
2. Has strong sense of time urgency
3. Has high performance standards
4. Appears angry and hostile
5. "I don't need anything or anybody."
6. "I'm not a baby and won't be treated like one."
7. "The only way to get things done is to do them yourself."
8. "There is nothing wrong with me."
9. "I never have time for relaxing."
10. "I'm still the man I was."

Nursing Diagnosis

Mr. Garcia realized that Mr. Hammond would need a lot of health teaching. At the same time, Mr. Garcia realized that Mr. Hammond had to accept the fact that he had a real medical problem and that certain changes in his diet and lifestyle could greatly increase the length and quality of his life. At the moment, Mr. Hammond did not appear receptive to health teaching. For a man who was accustomed to being in charge and productive, his heart attack appeared to be a great threat. Mr. Garcia thought that besides the threat to his role in business, Mr. Hammond might also be threatened in his role as a sexual partner.

Based on the initial data, Mr. Garcia made the following nursing diagnoses:

1. *Moderate to severe anxiety* related to threat to biological integrity, as evidenced by denial and irritability
   - "There is nothing wrong with me."
   - "I am still a man."
   - "I don't need anything or anyone."
   - "I am not a baby and won't be treated like one."

2. *Knowledge deficit* related to new diagnosis
   - "There is nothing wrong with me."
   - "I am still the man I was."
   - "I don't need anything to relax."
   - Overweight.
   - High cholesterol level.
   - Both parents died of coronary artery disease in their early 60s.
   - High blood pressure.

3. *Ineffective individual coping* related to inadequate relaxation
   - "I never have time for relaxing."
   - "The only way to get things done is to do them yourself."
   - "The minute you look away, someone gets in there ahead of you."
   - Strong sense of time urgency.
   - Highly competitive.

Planning

CONTENT LEVEL—PLANNING GOALS

Mr. Garcia thought that once Mr. Hammond felt less threatened and was better able to accept his illness, he would be more open to making positive change. Mr. Garcia realized that until a person recognizes that there is a problem and is motivated to make changes, medical compliance can be difficult. Only goals that a person thinks of as desirable will motivate him or her to take the time and energy needed for change. Therefore, Mr. Garcia planned to work closely with Mr. Hammond in planning nursing care.

Nursing Diagnosis	Long Term Goal	Short Term Goals
1. *Moderate to severe anxiety* related to threat to biologic integrity, as evidenced by denial and irritability	1. By (date), Mr. Hammond will be able to acknowledge that he has a cardiac problem.	1a. By (date), Mr. Hammond will discuss concerns of how his cardiac status might affect his work.

Continued on following page

Planning *(Continued)*	Nursing Diagnosis	Long Term Goal	Short Term Goals
			1b. By (date), Mr. Hammond will discuss concerns of how his cardiac status might affect his sexual activity.
	2. *Knowledge deficit* related to new diagnosis	2. Mr. Hammond will be able to discuss how diet, stress, and medication can influence the course of his disease.	2a. By (date), Mr. Hammond will be able to identify foods high in cholesterol and sodium and to name healthy foods he is willing to eat.
			2b. Mr. Hammond will lose two pounds per week for 20 weeks.
			2c. By (date), Mr. Hammond will state four changes in his work routine that can reduce stress.
			2d. By (date), Mr. Hammond will be able to name his medications, state their purpose, and discuss the side effects of each.
	3. *Ineffective individual coping* related to inadequate relaxation	3. By (date), Mr. Hammond will state that he feels less driven after following relaxation regime.	3a. By (date), Mr. Hammond will state that he understands benefits of relaxation both medically and emotionally.
			3b. Mr. Hammond will discuss with nurse various relaxation techniques by (date).
			3c. By (date), Mr. Hammond will choose one technique that he is willing to learn.

PROCESS LEVEL—NURSES' REACTIONS AND FEELINGS

Mr. Garcia had seen denial in men with coronary artery disease before. Initially, Mr. Garcia found this defense very annoying, because it diminished the effectiveness of his health teaching. When he began to appreciate denial as a defense against anxiety, fear, and helplessness, Mr. Garcia became more understanding. Mr. Garcia now attempts to explore some of the client's thoughts, feelings, and concerns about how the disease will affect his or her life. He finds that this often opens up avenues of discussion. Open communication channels pave the way for crucial and needed health teaching. Eventually, Mr. Garcia will discuss with Mr. Hammond acceptable changes in his lifestyle that can minimize stress and add to his quality of life.

Mr. Garcia is aware, however, that each person makes his or her own choices. The nurse can support, teach, and effect a variety of referrals in the least threatening manner possible. Clients will choose those measures or suggestions they are willing or able to follow.

Mr. Garcia no longer takes it personally or becomes angry with clients if they have difficulty accepting or following prescribed medical regimens. For some people, it takes a long time before defensive barriers break down, allowing major changes in health practices to take place.

Intervention

Initially, Mr. Garcia worked with Mr. Hammond to lower his anxiety and assist him in feeling more secure and in control. As Mr. Hammond's anxiety began to decrease, he was able to share some of his concerns. After a while, Mr. Hammond was more amenable to health teaching and more motivated to learn about how this heart attack would affect his life.

Mr. Garcia thought that a relaxation exercise might be useful for Mr. Hammond. Mr. Hammond's doctor agreed. After discussing some relaxation techniques, Mr. Hammond stated that he would be willing to try biofeedback: "That meditation mumbo-jumbo is not for me." Mr. Garcia agreed that Mr. Hammond would do better with a relaxation technique that had an external focus.

As Mr. Hammond became less tense and anxious, his wife appeared to relax. The nurse was concerned with the change that Mr. Hammond's coronary status would make on the whole family system. Mrs. Hammond seemed relieved when Mr. Garcia suggested that a visiting nurse come after discharge to check on medication, diet, and general progress. The nurse explained to Mrs. Hammond that illness could be a crisis for the whole family. Mr. Garcia explained to the couple that post-infarction despondency is an almost universal response to a heart attack (Kaplan 1985). Counseling during this time could be useful if the depression became severe. The nurse suggested that perhaps Mr. and Mrs. Hammond might speak with the social worker before discharge to acquaint themselves with the resources in their community.

Evaluation

By discharge, Mr. Hammond appeared to have a basic understanding of his illness and the risk factors. He seemed concerned about his cholesterol level and blood pressure, and he admitted that he was too heavy. He had worked out a diet with the dietitian, and his wife had been present at one of the meetings. He seemed pleased about the four pounds he had lost while in the hospital. He was well versed in his medications by discharge, and he shared the information with his wife two days before discharge.

Mr. Hammond still had some questions about the safety of future sexual activity. Both he and his wife decided to make a joint appointment with the doctor to discuss this further. Mr. Hammond was willing to make some changes in his work habits, although he knew that this would be hard for him to do.

An appointment was made for Mr. Hammond to start biofeedback training after discharge. He said that he would drop by and let Mr. Garcia know how everything was going.

Summary

Emotional reactions to physical illness are expected. Sometimes, emotional reactions to physical illness can impede recovery and block effective nursing care. This can leave both the client and the staff in conflict or crisis. In many institutions, the psychiatric liaison nurse is available to help staff assess the client's situation and plan care more effectively with the client. The psychiatric liaison nurse has a knowledge of physical illness and the clinical skills to help people deal more effectively with emotional problems.

All nurses need to be aware of the stresses a person encounters when hospitalized for the first time. The nurse also needs to assess the particular coping strategies a client is using. By supporting and encouraging adaptive coping strategies while minimizing and not reinforcing maladaptive coping strategies, the nurse can greatly affect the way a person copes with his or her illness. Nurses also need to be aware of the specific emotional issues involved with common though complex medical illnesses and conditions. Such awareness can increase the nurse's ability to better evaluate for health teaching, empathize with the person's experience, formulate more meaningful nursing diagnoses, and plan effective nursing care.

The emotional experiences a person may encounter during hospitalization were highlighted. Specific psychosocial approaches were discussed as they relate to a person (1) in chronic pain, (2) with AIDS, (3) who is dying, and (4) who has a psychophysiological disorder.

Research has repeatedly correlated mental and emotional processes with physical health and physical disease. In fact, there is probably no major health organ system or somatic defense that is not subject to the influence of interactions between the psychological and physiological. However, as yet, there is no one universally accepted model to explain the etiology of psychophysiological disease. It is believed that there are numerous contributing factors predisposing a person to a psychophysiological disorder. For example, personality profiles, genetic predisposition, environmental conditions, internal and external stressors, personal coping styles, and cultural background are all thought to play an important role. Table 26–6 lists some common psychophysiological disorders and outlines personality traits, biological and genetic correlates, environmental factors, and effective therapeutic approaches.

References

Adams F. Six very good reasons why we react differently to various dying patients. Nursing '84, 14:8, 1984.

AIDS Update. Know the early signs of HIV dementia complex. Nursing '88, 16(6):18, 1988.

American Nurses' Association. Standards of Psychiatric Consultation-Liaison Nursing Practice. Kansas City, MO: American Nurses' Association, 1990.

American Psychiatric Association. Diagnostic and Statistical Manual of Mental Disorders, 3rd ed, revised (DSM-III-R). Washington, DC: American Psychiatric Association, 1987.

Baer JW, Hall JM, Hulm K, et al. Challenges in developing an inpatient psychiatric program for people with AIDS and ARC. Hospital and Community Psychiatry, 38(12):1299, 1987.

Bell JP. AIDS and the hidden epidemic of grief: A personal experience. In Marcil WM, Tigges KN (eds). The Person with AIDS: A Personal and Professional Perspective. Thorofare, NJ: Charles B. Slack, 1992, pp 25–32.

Benoliel J. Loss and terminal illness. Nursing Clinics of North America, 20(2):439, 1985.

Breault J, Polifroni EC. Caring for people with AIDS: Nurses' attitudes and feelings. Journal of Advanced Nursing, 17(1): 21, 1992.

Centers for Disease Control. HIV/AIDS Surveillance Report. January: 1992:1–22.

Euster S. Adjusting to an adult family member's cancer. In Roback H (ed). Helping Patients and Their Families Cope with Medical Problems. San Francisco: Jossey-Bass Publishers, 1984, pp 428–452.

Faulstich ME. Psychiatric aspects of AIDS. American Journal of Psychiatry, 144(5):551, 1987.

Fife B. The challenge of the medical setting for the clinical nurse specialist in psychiatric nursing. Journal of Psychiatric Nursing and Mental Health Services, 21(1):8, 1983.

Fife B, Lemler S. The psychiatric nurse specialist: A valuable asset in the general hospital. Journal of Nursing Administration, 13(4):14, 1983.

Fischman J. Type A on trial. Psychology Today, 21(2):42, 1987.

Foley, K. The treatment of cancer pain. New England Journal of Medicine, 313(2):84, 1983.

Getty G, Stern P. Gay men's perceptions and responses to AIDS. Journal of Advanced Nursing, 15(8):895, 1990.

Gong V, Rudnick M. AIDS Facts and Issues. New Brunswick, NJ: Rutgers University Press, 1986.

Greenspan K. Biofeedback in the control of chronic pain. In Mark L (ed). Pain Control: Practical Aspects of Patient Care. New York: Masson Publishing, 1981, pp 89–94.

Guttenberg R. Softening the blow: How to break bad news to a patient's family. Nursing Life, July/August: 17, 1983.

Hackett T. The pain patient: Evaluation and treatment. In Hackett T, Cassem N (eds). Massachusetts General Hospital Handbook of General Hospital Psychiatry. St. Louis: CV Mosby, 1978.

Hendler N, Fernandez P. Alternative treatments for patients with chronic pain. Psychiatric Annals, 10(12):25, 1980.

Johnson B. Psychiatric nurse consultant in the general hospital. Nursing Outlook, 2:728, 1963.

Kaplan HI, Sadock BJ. Comprehensive Textbook of Psychiatry, vol 2, 5th ed. Baltimore: Williams & Wilkins, 1989.

Kellner R. Somatization: Theories and research. The Journal of Nervous and Mental Diseases, 178(3):150, 1990.

Kleinman A. Mental health and chronic pain. The Harvard Medical School Mental Health Letter, 8(2):4, 1989.

Kübler-Ross E. On Death and Dying. New York: Macmillan, 1969.

Lazarus R. Stress and coping as factors in health and illness. In Cohen J, Cullen J, Martin R (eds). Psychosocial Aspects of Cancer. New York: Raven, 1982, pp 163–190.

Leukefeld C, Fimbres M. Introduction. In Leukefeld C, Fimbres M (eds). Responding to AIDS: Psychosocial initiatives. Silver Spring, MD: National Association of Social Workers, 1987, as found in Leukefeld CG. Psychosocial initiatives in dealing with AIDS. Hospital and Community Psychiatry, 40(5):454, 1989.

Lewis A, Levy J. Psychiatric Liaison Nursing: The Theory and Clinical Practice. Reston, VA: Reston Publishing Company, 1982.

McGough RN. Assessing social supports of people with AIDS. Oncology Nursing Forum, 17(1):31, 1990.

McGuire L. Seven myths about pain relief. RN, 46(12):30, 1983.

Marcil WM, Tigges KN. The Person With AIDS: A Personal and Professional Perspective. Thorofare, NJ: Charles B. Slack, 1992.

Menenberg SR. Somatopsychology and AIDS victims. Journal of Psychosocial Nursing, 25(5):18, 1987.

Nyamathi A, Van Servellen G. Maladaptive coping in the critically ill population with acquired immune deficiency syndrome: Nursing assessment and treatment. Heart and Lung, 18(2):113, 1989.

Oken D. Gastrointestinal disorders. In Kaplan HI, Sadock BJ (eds). Comprehensive Textbook of Psychiatry, vol 2, 5th ed. Baltimore: Williams & Wilkins, 1989.

Ostchega Y, Jacob J. Providing "safe conduct": Helping your patient cope with cancer. Nursing '84: 42, 1984.

Perry SW, Markowitz JC. Psychiatric interventions for AIDS-spectrum disorders. Hospital and Community Psychiatry, 37(10):1001, 1986.

Robinson L. Liaison Nursing: Psychological Approach to Patient Care. Philadelphia: FA Davis, 1974.

Rogers A. 21 Problems in pain control—and ways to solve them. Your Patient and Cancer, 9(9):65, 1984.

Sadovsky R. Psychosocial issues in symptomatic HIV infection. American Family Physician, 44(6): 2065, 1991.

Schuman M. Biofeedback in the management of chronic pain. In Adrian C, Barker J (eds). Psychological Approaches to the Management of Pain. New York: Brunner-Mazel, 1982.

Smith MN, Popp SR. Family social support and AIDS. Virginia Nurse, 60(2):8, 1992.

Wain H. Pain control with hypnosis in consultation and liaison psychiatry. Psychiatric Annals, 16(2):106, 1986.

Weisman A. The Coping Capacity: On the Nature of Being Mortal. New York: Human Sciences Press, 1984.

Wright L. Life threatening illness. Journal of Psychosocial Nursing, 23(9):7, 1985.

Zahourek RP. Clinical and Therapeutic Suggestion in Nursing. Orlando, FL: Grune & Stratton, Inc., 1985.

Zborowski M. People in Pain. San Francisco: Jossey-Bass, 1969.

Further Reading

Bor R, Miller R, Johnson M. A testing time for doctors: Counseling patients before an HIV test. British Medical Journal, 303:905, 1991.

Cassem N, Hackett T. The setting of intensive care. In Hackett T, Cassem N (eds). Massachusetts General Hospital Handbook of General Hospital Psychiatry. St. Louis: CV Mosby, 1978.

Escobar P. Management of chronic pain. Nurse-Practitioner, 10:24, 1985.

Katzin L. HIV risk (still) low for health care workers. American Journal of Nursing, 88(7):950, 1988.

Lipowski Z. Physical illness, the individual, and the coping process. Psychiatry in Medicine, 1:91, 1970.

Lipowski Z. Somatization: The concept and its clinical application. American Journal of Psychiatry, 145(11):1358, 1988.

Nichols SE, Ostrow DG (eds). Psychiatric Implications of Acquired Immune Deficiency Syndrome. Washington, DC: American Psychiatric Press, 1984.

Ochitill H, Havassy B, Byrd R, et al. Leaving a cardiology service against medical advice. Journal of Chronic Disease, 38(1):78, 1985.

Schmitt M. The nature of pain with some personal notes. Nursing Clinics of North America, 12(4):621, 1977.

Sloand EM, Pitt E, Chiarello RJ, et al. HIV testing: State of the art. Journal of American Medical Association, 266(20):2861, 1991.

Swanson AR. Psychophysiological disorders. In Varcarolis EM (ed).

Foundations of Psychiatric-Mental Health Nursing. Philadelphia: WB Saunders, 1990.

Thornbury K. Coping: Implications for health practitioners. Patient Counseling and Health Education, 4(1):3, 1982.

Weisman A. Coping with illness. In Hackett T, Cassem N (eds). Massachusetts General Hospital Handbook of General Hospital Psychiatry. St. Louis: CV Mosby, 1978, pp 264–275.

Self-study Exercises

Place a T (true) or F (false) next to each statement.

1. _____ Most people have plenty of time to adjust to "the sick role."
2. _____ A person is forced to give up parts of his or her identity and independent functioning during the first few days of hospitalization.
3. _____ Financial worries and distance from support systems can be major concerns for the hospitalized person.
4. _____ Fear of death is often the ultimate concern for a surgical patient.

Put a + (plus) for positive coping strategies or a 0 for negative coping strategies used by a hospitalized patient.

5. _____ Seek information and get guidance for decision making.
6. _____ Deny as much as possible.
7. _____ Share and discuss concerns and find consolation.
8. _____ Blame or shame someone or something for what is happening.

Choose the letter that best answers the following questions:

9. Chronic pain is different from acute pain. Which statement is false regarding chronic pain?

   A. A person slowly adapts to the pain.
   B. The patient is the key for assessing the level of intensity.
   C. A placebo does not work for a person in chronic pain.
   D. There may be no increase in pulse or blood pressure in chronic pain as there is in acute pain.

10. All of the following can be useful for the management of chronic pain. Which of the following would be the *least* helpful in the management of chronic pain?

    A. Using relaxation techniques, hypnosis, and guided imagery.
    B. Giving a placebo without the person's knowledge helps separate physical from psychological pain.
    C. Encouraging the person to take an active role in his or her own pain management.
    D. Always assessing site, character, onset, and duration and suggesting that the patient keep a log.

Place T (true) or F (false) next to each statement.

11. _____ A person with AIDS should be in isolation that requires staff to gown and glove.
12. _____ AIDS is restricted to those in the homosexual community and those who use intravenous drugs.

13. _____ Staff inservice conferences and frequent discussion of fears and myths regarding working with a person with AIDS reduce staff anxiety and can increase a patient's emotional as well as physical comfort.

14. _____ Hugging, using the toilet, or eating off the dishes of an HIV-infected person can spread the disease.

15. _____ For two psychosocial nursing diagnoses applicable to a person with AIDS, identify at least two nursing interventions and explain their rationale. Refer to Table 26–2.

Place the behaviors next to the corresponding stage in Kübler-Ross's five stages in the process of dying.

16. _____ Denial and isolation
17. _____ Anger
18. _____ Bargaining
19. _____ Depression
20. _____ Acceptance

A. "If I take my medicine every day I will live."

B. "I feel so depressed. The staff seem to avoid coming into my room."

C. "I'm not afraid any longer, I'm ready to die now."

D. "I'm not dying . . . You have the wrong person."

E. "Why me? . . . How could God do this to me? It's not fair!"

21. For each of the above stages, name four nursing interventions and discuss the rationale for each.

Short Answer

22. For the following patient remarks (1) identify a negative reaction that a nurse might experience and (2) compose a useful response.

    A. "Oh I just don't know what to do . . . I can't seem to do anything without feeling pain . . . Do you have any idea how awful it is to be in pain when nobody seems to care?"

    B. "First it started in my left arm . . . then my right arm . . . now the rash has spread all over my body . . . (time goes on), and then I tried this new lotion . . . "

23. Name three therapeutic modalities that a nurse at the master's level might practice on a client with a psychophysiological disorder.

Infants, Children, and Adolescents

Beth Bonham

KEY TERMS AND CONCEPTS

The key terms and concepts listed here
also appear in bold where they are
defined or discussed in this chapter.

ART THERAPY

ATTENTION DEFICIT HYPERACTIVITY
DISORDER

BIBLIOTHERAPY

CLINICAL NURSE SPECIALIST

CONDUCT DISORDERS

GENOGRAM

INFANT PSYCHIATRY

MENTAL RETARDATION

MENTAL STATUS INTERVIEW

MILIEU THERAPY

PERVASIVE DEVELOPMENTAL
DISORDERS

PLAY THERAPY

REACTIVE ATTACHMENT DISORDER OF
INFANCY

SEPARATION ANXIETY DISORDER

OBJECTIVES ■

After studying this chapter, the student will be able to

1. Formulate a developmental framework for child and adolescent psychopathology.
2. Describe the roles of nurse generalist and clinical nurse specialist in child and adolescent psychiatric nursing.
3. Compare and contrast mental status interview, family history, and community relationships in assessing the infant, child, and adolescent.
4. Identify two assessment tools used with infants, children, and adolescents.
5. Discuss four intervention strategies that are shared by each age group.
6. Recognize psychopharmacological agents used in childhood disorders.
7. Explain why play therapy, art therapy, and bibliotherapy are useful interventions with children.
8. Describe the roles of psychodrama, music therapy, developmental games, and adventure-based programs in intervening with adolescents.
9. Describe the clinical features of the following DSM-III-R diagnostic categories and give a possible nursing diagnosis for each:
   A. Mental retardation
   B. Pervasive developmental disorders
   C. Attention deficit hyperactivity disorder
   D. Separation anxiety disorder
   E. Conduct disorders
   F. Depression

The specialty of child and adolescent psychiatric nursing evolved from a number of psychiatric and social reforms. Sigmund Freud, Melanie Klein, and Anna Freud were early pioneers in the analytical treatment of children (Clunn 1991). The first child guidance clinic, the Chicago Psychopathic Institute, was founded by William Healy in 1909. It was associated with the juvenile court. As the child guidance movement grew and nurses became involved because of new medications being used with children, the role of the nurse clearly needed to be defined. The visions of nursing leaders such as Claire Fagin, Patricia Pothier, Suzanne Goren, and Deane Critchley articulated the role and practice of the child psychiatric nurse (Fagin 1972, 1974; Pothier 1976).

The National Institute of Mental Health (NIMH) has estimated that at least 7.5 million children and adolescents in the United States suffer from some sort of mental disorder (NIMH 1991). Identification of this population is complicated by the long-held belief that childhood is a happy, stress-free time. Families seem to tolerate for a longer time behaviors in children and adolescents that have psychiatric implications (e.g., "It's just a stage.") Many behaviors are difficult to differentiate from normal growth and development, and many adults are unaware that abnormal behaviors have a psychiatric genesis. In addition, the stigma of mental illness unfortunately prevents people from seeking early intervention.

The beginning field of **infant psychiatry** is expanding as a result of stressors such as maternal deaths, domestic violence, and foster care. Child and adolescent care occurs in a variety of settings. The nurse who works with children and adolescents in settings such as pediatric well-child clinics, psychiatric units, and schools must possess a thorough knowledge of developmental theory. The nurse generalist must also possess assessment skills, interpersonal communication skills, and knowledge of psychotherapeutic interventions and community resources.

A psychiatric **clinical nurse specialist** (CNS) has a master's or doctoral degree and is usually certified by the American Nurses' Association in child and adolescent psychiatric–mental health nursing. The roles of the child and adolescent CNS include individual, group, and family psychotherapist; educator of nurses, other professionals, and community members; clinical supervisor of client care, staff, and students; consultant to professional and nonprofessional groups and organizations concerned with the health, education, and welfare of children; and researcher who contributes to theory development and the practice of child and adolescent psychiatric nursing (Grossman and Mayton 1988).

Research in child and adolescent mental health and psychiatric disorders has not occurred at the same rate as research in adult disorders. In response to a congressional request, the National Plan for Research on Child and Adolescent Mental Disorders has been developed. Some identified research needs focus on neurobiology, effective treatment techniques and intervention, and developmental factors of mental disorders of children (NIMH 1991). A historic event in child and adolescent psychiatric nursing occurred in 1991, when educators, clinicians, researchers, and consumers from across the United States met to debate and recommend *Collaboration for Improvement of Practice with Severely Mentally and Emotionally Disturbed Children and Adolescents* (Finke 1991).

Theory

A thorough grounding in various personality development theories is imperative for the nurse working with the child and adolescent psychiatric patient. Nursing education has traditionally used behavioral and social science theories. Normal child development has been studied for decades (Ilg and Ames 1955; Driekurs 1964; Erikson 1963; Fraiberg 1959; Freud 1967). There is not a single theoretical framework because a child develops along a life span continuum (Murray and Zentner 1985). The child's development is contingent on innate (genetic) personality characteristics and on social, cognitive, physical, and emotional factors. Moral development, children without consciences, separation and loss, and the effect of touch are promising new areas of developmental theory as it relates to children (Barnard and Brazelton 1990; Bloom-Feshbach and Bloom-Feshbach 1987; Kohlberg 1964; Magid and McKelvey 1987). Many of these studies, however, were done with male children. There is a need for research with female children, as well as for research emphasizing cultural differences and how they may influence growth and development.

ERIKSON AND PSYCHOSOCIAL DEVELOPMENT

Erik Erikson's theory of the eight stages of psychosocial development has provided a framework for understanding development across an individual's life span (Erikson 1963). Erikson expanded Freud's psychoanalytical theory to encompass the sociocultural aspects of development. Mastery of each task builds the foundation for the subsequent one (Table 27–1). If one task is unfinished or incomplete, difficulty in mastering the next task results.

Erikson's first stage is the development of *trust versus mistrust* (birth through one year of age). The first relationship a child has is with the parents. If consistent and compassionate care is provided, the infant develops a sense of security. With inconsistent nurturing, the infant does not feel that the world is a safe place and thus mistrusts the environment. Incomplete development of trust makes it difficult for the child to grow and to complete additional tasks (Barthel and Herrman 1991).

In Erikson's second stage, *autonomy versus shame and doubt* (1–3 years of age), the toddler seeks mastery with new-found independence. Acquiring a sense of competent self is facilitated by allowing the child to do what he or she can within a safe environment. The nurse can teach parents what normal developmental behaviors are and assist in constructing safe parameters.

Initiative versus guilt, the third stage, occurs between ages three and six. Family relationships not only give the child a sense of safety and security but also contribute to the child's sense of responsibility and conscience.

The fourth stage, *industry versus inferiority*, which occurs from six to 12 years of age, encompasses an active period of socialization for the child. An increasing level of competence is acquired.

The stage of *identity versus role confusion* spans the adolescent years and certainly continues into the second decade of life (12–21 years of age). The adolescent searches for self with much input from peers. Family individuation, sexual relationships, and career choices are but a few of the issues that confront the adolescent at this time. Refer to Chapter 1.

SEPARATION AND LOSS

John Bowlby provided original work on child attachment theory (1969, 1973, 1980). Bowlby maintained that the attachment between mother and child is so important that if it does not occur or is severed, the parent-child relationship will always be vulnerable. In-

Table 27-1 ■ OUTLINE OF TOOLS AND TASKS BY ERAS OF CHILD AND ADOLESCENT DEVELOPMENT

TASKS	TOOLS	IF TASKS NOT ACHIEVED
Infancy: Birth Through 1½ Years		
1. Learning to count on others to gratify needs; developing trust.	1. Crying and other prespeech vocalizations. 2. Mouth—used to express feelings (biting, spitting, pushing out) and satisfaction or dissatisfaction. 3. Empathetic observations: perceives feelings of other as his or her own. 4. Emergency reaction expressed by crying, increased motor activity, or apathy in the face of • Fear • Anxiety • Rage 5. Experimentation, exploration, and manipulation. 6. Autistic invention—allows for feelings of control, sees environment in highly personalized way.	If the child does not develop a strong sense of self, in later life problems of *mistrust, lack of self-confidence, dependency,* and *superficial relationships* may be experienced.
Early Childhood: 1½–3 Years		
1. Learning to accept interference with one's wishes in relation to comfort. 2. Developing a sense of autonomy, sense of self.	1. Language—uses meaningful sounds to communicate. 2. Anus—tool used to give or withhold, control significant people in the environment to express feelings of power. 3. Experimentation, exploration, and manipulation become more refined; behaviors seen include: • Exhibitionism • Imitation • Aggressive behavior • Increased locomotion • Masturbation	Autonomy does not develop. This lack may express itself as an excessive need for control or order; in overconforming behavior, and in irrational rituals. It is manifested in feelings of shame and doubt.
Late Childhood: 3–6 Years		
1. Learning to separate from parents and socialize outside the family: • Associates with age mates • Imitates roles and responses • Learns to stand alone • Develops sexual identity 2. Developing a sense of initiative; learning to • Select goals • Persevere • Recognize own worth • Feel worthy and competent	1. Self—functions as it develops in terms of ego strengths and superego structure. 2. Emergency reactions are • Shame • Anger • Guilt • Doubt • Anxiety	The child may lack initiative and belief in self-mastery. Problems can arise as to sexual or personal roles. Rigidity may be seen, and the child may experience guilt. The child will have a reluctance to explore new skills and to test abilities.
School Age: 6–9 Years		
1. Learning to form satisfactory relationships with peers. 2. Learning to win recognition by productivity. 3. Becoming intellectually able to encompass the abstract, objective, or general event, e.g., • Distinguishes fantasy from reality • Makes a rational connection between cause and effect	1. Competition—used to contest for affection and status. 2. Compromise—enables child to give and take in a reciprocal relationship to retain own position. 3. Cooperation—enables child to maintain own position by adjusting to the wishes of others.	The child may have difficulty relating to peers. The child feels inadequate and experiences low self-esteem and inferiority, which may persist into later life. The child may be unprepared for school. A reluctance to explore and form relationships and to explore the environment is also seen.

TASKS	TOOLS	IF TASKS NOT ACHIEVED
School Age: 6–9 Years		
4. Learning to see self in relation to others, e.g., • Accepts reasonable restraints • Begins to become self-reliant • Begins to accept responsibility and take consequences for behavior • Learns appropriate responses to situations	4. Experimentation, exploration, and manipulation are further refined: • Experiences learning as fun • Engages in cooperative play • Has recreational and sexual curiosity • Becomes more aware of self and the world around	
Preadolescence: 9–12 Years		
1. Moving to fully social state, e.g., • Identifying self with peers of same sex • Being more loyal to chum than to family members • Relating closely to chum of same sex • Expanding of interpersonal relationships	1. Capacity to love. 2. Consensual validation. 3. Collaboration. 4. Experimentation, exploration, and manipulation.	Sense of self in relationship to others is not well developed. The child has feelings of inferiority and isolation.
2. Seriously using learning to implement self for future life, e.g., • Developing own value system • Learning that recognition is won by directing activities toward constructive ends • Becoming familiar with the rational and irrational ideas, values, and mores of his or her culture		The child experiences uncertainty about self, abilities, and where he or she fits into life.
Early Adolescence: 12–15 Years		
1. Working through developmental crisis of physiological and psychological changes and moving toward independence, e.g., • Asserting self and challenging authority • Evaluating own limitations and powers • Examining and anticipating consequences of own decisions	1. Lust—awareness of sexual drive, which stimulates the integration of situations affecting the genital zones. 2. Greater recognition of powers. 3. Experimentation, exploration, and manipulation. 4. Anxiety.	Although a time of confusion and introspection for all at this age, the experience is especially pronounced and may persist into adulthood when the adolescent does not have the tools to negotiate this stage. The normal mood swings of adolescence may be intensified and prolonged.
2. Learning to establish satisfactory relations with members of the opposite sex, e.g., • Accepting self as sexual object • Finding suitable sexual objects • Experimenting socially • Learning healthy patterns for emotional release		Severe difficulty in heterosexual relationships is a result of identity confusion and low self-esteem.
Late Adolescence: 15 Years and Older		
1. Learning to become interdependent, e.g., • Tolerating anxiety and using it constructively • Establishing mature and reciprocal relationships with parents • Accepting other people as individuals of worth	1. Genital organs. 2. Experimentation, exploration, and manipulation. 3. Mature self-system.	Personal identity and role confusion result in • Deficits in assuming responsibility • Sense of inadequacy in controlling self • Inability to compete successfully • Dissatisfaction in personal relationships or isolation • Difficulties in sharing and experiencing intimate relationships
2. Learning to integrate conscious values in harmony with practical, realistic, scientific world, e.g., • Making decisions and choices of far-reaching importance for future		

Table continued on following page

Table 27–1 ■ OUTLINE OF TOOLS AND TASKS BY ERAS OF CHILD AND ADOLESCENT DEVELOPMENT *Continued*

TASKS	TOOLS	IF TASKS NOT ACHIEVED
Late Adolescence: 15 Years and Older		

- Selecting mate and preparing for productive family life
- Learning to become economically, intellectually, and emotionally self-sufficient
- Achieving socially responsible behavior as a citizen of the community, state, nation, and world

3. Forming durable sexual relationship with selected member of the opposite sex, e.g., wooing and winning mate with whom one develops the following:
   - Willingness to share mutual trust
   - Mutuality of sexual satisfaction
   - Willingness to share procreation
   - Willingness to regulate cycles of work and recreation
   - Willingness to assume responsibility for others

Adapted from Fagin C. Nursing in Child Psychiatry. St. Louis: CV Mosby, 1972; Haber J. Developmental processes. In Haber J, Hoskins PP, Leach AM, et al (eds). Comprehensive Psychiatric Nursing, 3rd ed. New York: McGraw-Hill Book Company, 1987.

fant or early childhood vulnerability not only leads to psychological sequelae but has implications for normal development and subsequent losses. Children's reactions to losses such as a chronic illness, moving to a new home, and death of a parent are further discussed in *The Psychology of Separation and Loss: Perspectives on Development, Life Transitions and Clinical Practice* (Bloom-Feshbach and Bloom-Feshbach 1987).

SYSTEMS THEORY

A thorough understanding of systems theory and family systems is helpful because the child or adolescent is affected by family dynamics, school, and peers. The family system contributes to child psychopathology, and because of the psychological and biological issues involved, work with family systems is helpful with psychosomatic illness (Minuchin et al. 1975).

A thorough discussion of theoretical foundations for child psychiatry can be found in *Child Psychiatric Nursing* (Clunn 1991), and one for adolescents can be found in *Adolescent Psychiatric Nursing* (Hogarth 1991).

PIAGET AND COGNITIVE DEVELOPMENT

Jean Piaget studied the biological, social, and physical worlds of the child to detail cognitive development (Piaget and Inhelder 1969). The child integrates past

and new experiences by assimilation. Possessed with his or her own cognitive structures or "schemas," the child uses accommodation to make the schemas fit or creates new ones. Piaget has described stages of development according to the child's physical prowess and chronological age (Table 27–2). Refer to Chapter 1.

The cognitive development theory is helpful to the nurse implementing intervention based on the child's age. The preoperational child is a concrete thinker who will not be able to abstractly "think through" all consequences of behavior. The stages of sensorimotor, preoperational, concrete operations, and formal operations are useful for understanding the child's readiness to learn new information. A more complete explanation of cognitive development and its relation to nursing assessment can be found in Clunn's *Child Psychiatric Nursing* (1991).

NEUROBIOLOGICAL THEORIES

The increasing complexity of care, and the agendas of consumer advocacy groups force the nurse to acknowledge biological research findings (McBride 1990). Brain research has identified more than 75 neurotransmitters. Genetics research has given new information to families and health professionals, so that counseling can prevent further tragedy. Cerebellar deficits have been identified in the brains of autistic children (Finke 1991). Brain glucose metabolism can

Table 27-2 ■ PERSONALITY DEVELOPMENT THEORIES

PSYCHOSOCIAL DEVELOPMENT (ERIKSON)	PSYCHOSEXUAL DEVELOPMENT (FREUD)	COGNITIVE DEVELOPMENT (PIAGET)
Birth to 1 Year: Infant		
Trust vs mistrust Oral needs are of primary importance. Adequate mothering is to meet the infant's needs. Acquisition of hope.	*Oral* Primary source of pleasure is the mouth. Uses mouth as a means of experiencing the world and meeting needs.	*Sensorimotor* World of here-and-now. Complete self-world. Experiences through senses and motor movements. Sucking • "Primary circular"—head moves in direction of visual and auditory stimuli • "Secondary circular"—grasps objects • "Tertiary circular"—looks for objects out of sight and identifies objects when requested to
1–3 Years: Toddler		
Autonomy vs shame Anal needs are of primary importance. Father emerges as an important figure. Acquisition of will.	*Anal* Primary sources of pleasure are through elimination and retention. First experience with discipline and authority. Development of object relationships..	
3–6 Years: Preschool		
Initiative vs guilt Genital needs are of primary importance. Family relationships contribute to an early sense of responsibility and conscience. Acquisition of purpose.	*Phallic* Primary source of pleasure is genital. Emergence of Oedipus and Electra complexes.	*Preoperational* Animistic thinking. (Inanimate objects have motives and intentions.) Phenomenalistic causality. Magical thinking. Egocentric thought. Language ability develops. Symbolic play.
6–12 Years: School Age		
Industry vs inferiority This is an active period of socialization for the child as the child moves from the family and into society. Acquisition of competence.	*Latency* Basically quiet stage of development marked by expanding peer relationships.	*Concrete operations* Concrete thinking still predominates. Begins to grasp concepts of reversibility, classification, and number. Is developing basic concepts of time, space, quantity, and causality.
12–21 Years: Adolescent		
Identity vs role confusion Peers play an important part in the search for self. A psychosocial moratorium is provided by society to aid the adolescent. Acquisition of fidelity.	*Genital* Sexual desires and urges become prominent, and the individual seeks to fulfill them.	*Formal operations* Abstract thought. Generality of thought. Propositional thinking. Hypothetical thinking. Strong idealism.

now be studied using positron emission tomography. Technological advances in brain imaging techniques such as positron emission tomography (PET), magnetic resonance imaging (MRI), single photon emission computerized tomography (SPECT), regional blood flow, and evoked potentials (EP) now allow the brain's structure, electrical activity, and metabolism to be studied in children and adolescents.

Assessment

Assessment of infants, children, and adolescents is based on the child's developmental stage; the presenting concern (usually behavior); and family, social, school, and peer relationships (Box 27–1). The nurse not only uses general communication and his-

---

Box 27–1. INFANT, CHILD, AND ADOLESCENT ASSESSMENT CRITERIA

Physical
- Neuromusculature
- Motor function
- General appearance

Developmental
- Speech
- Language
- Psychomotor

Behavioral, emotional, and social
- Conscience
- Interactions with family and peers

Cognitive and psychological
- Self-concept
- Coping mechanisms
- Defense mechanisms

Educational and intellectual
- Psychometric evaluation

Cultural
- National heritage
- Immigration status
- Role of religion in the family

---

tory-taking skills but also asks questions specific to the child, based on the child's developmental and chronological ages. Assessment or data collection directs the treatment planning and interventions.

INFANTS

At one time, it was thought that children were merely "little adults" and did not feel the same things that adults do. As social changes, clinical practice, and research have evolved, so have parental treatment and professional treatment of children (Clunn 1991). Failure to bond and failure to thrive are now known to have an emotional genesis in many cases. The infant who exhibits a feeding disorder may indeed need more than a physical investigation, with subsequent intervention. Prenatal care is a good example of primary intervention for the infant's mental health. A thorough prenatal history taking by the nurse may well uncover possible emotional problems (e.g., the mother who used substances during pregnancy). Parent-child interactions are assessed. The way in which

the caregiver holds and talks to the infant demonstrates interactional patterns that may need nursing intervention. A family assessment provides rich data concerning the infant, child, or adolescent (Box 27–2). Of particular importance is the assessment of trends now occurring in our society—incarcerated parents, children being born in prisons, and fathers and grandparents becoming legal guardians of children.

The Brazelton Neonatal Assessment Scale measures the newborn's integrative behavioral processes in response to various stimuli (Brazelton 1973). This assessment shows the nurse how the infant responds to stimuli and to other people, and how the infant calms him- or herself when distressed. Parent-child interaction is assessed, as is how parents respond to the baby's cues. These data provide indicators for nursing interventions regarding parental health teaching and anticipatory guidance.

Box 27–2. NURSING ASSESSMENT: FAMILY CHECKLIST

Presenting Problem

"What concerns you about your child?"
"What have you tried?"
"What would you like to have happen?"

Prenatal History

"Tell me about any prenatal problems that occurred."

Developmental History

"How old was your child when he or she walked, talked, and sat by him- or herself?"
"What significant injuries or illnesses has your child had?"

Social History

"Who lives in your house?"
"What does your family do for fun?"
"Where do you work?"

Family History

"Has there been anyone in your family with a history of psychiatric disease?"
"Tell me who your support systems are."
"Has there been a recent crisis in your family (divorce, death, or job loss)?"
"What are some of the family rules in your family?"

The Denver Developmental Screening Test is a common and easy instrument to use (Frankenburg et al. 1971). This test quickly assesses developmental delays in children; the children can then be referred for a more thorough assessment.

The Developmental Profile II is a skills inventory of children's development from birth to nine and a half years of age (Alpern et al. 1984). Physical, self-help, social, academic, and communication ages are the developmental areas assessed. For example, physical age can be used to measure sequential motor skills, whereas social age is a measure of interpersonal relationship abilities. This assessment tool is used, as are all others, in collaboration with the case history, family assessment, direct observation, and interviews with the child.

CHILDREN (1–12 YEARS OF AGE)

The nurse assesses the child's developmental, cognitive, and social behaviors, keeping normal developmental criteria in mind. The area or office where the assessment occurs may have various toys, including a dollhouse, stuffed toys, puppets, games, and age-appropriate toys such as soldiers. The nurse instructs the child to play with whatever he or she chooses,

and the nurse can then talk with the family and observe the play activity of the child. Asking the parent to leave the office is helpful to establish rapport with the child and to assess separation anxiety.

While conducting a **mental status interview,** the nurse can ask the child to draw pictures of him- or herself, a family, or a house, or can sit on the floor where the child is playing. Not only does this enhance the nurse-child relationship, but the drawings may be helpful in assessing developmental and cognitive strengths and family interactional patterns. The nurse observes verbal and nonverbal behaviors (Table 27–3). Other areas assessed are peer and family relationships; self-concept; thought processes; and fantasies, fears, and wishes. Sample questions are provided in Box 27–3. A child's answers to questions may be quite literal or may require further questioning from the nurse to assess reality orientation. For example, if the nurse asks, "What is your favorite thing to do outside?," and the child answers, "I sit in a circle of candles and drink red stuff that looks like blood," further questioning is certainly indicated. In this case, the child's sense of reality must be assessed, as well as the possibility of cult involvement. More than one interview may be indicated, especially if the child is nonverbal or extremely active.

Table 27–3 ■ VERBAL AND NONVERBAL AREAS TO BE OBSERVED

AREA TO BE OBSERVED	SOME OBSERVATIONS TO BE NOTED
Affects and anxiety	How does the child use the environment? What emotions are observed? When do emotions change? Are affects appropriate during play? Are affects appropriate to child's age?
Mood	What is the overall emotional tone of the child? Is the child sad, happy, or angry?
Capacity to relate	How does the child treat the nurse as a person? How much contact does the child initiate? Is the child affectionate, warm, or aloof?
Cognitive level	Is the child able to move from an activity to talking about what is on his or her mind? How does a child tell a story? How far does the story progress?
Physical and neurological development	Child's posture Skin condition Height and weight Gait and balance Fine motor coordination Gross motor coordination Speech—lisps or stutters Quality and tone of voice Sensorimotor coordination Sensory intactness

Box 27–3. NURSING ASSESSMENT: MENTAL STATUS INTERVIEW WITH CHILDREN AND ADOLESCENTS

Introduction

"Some kids would have some questions about why they were here, but they might be too nervous to ask."

Developmental

"How old are you?"
"What is your favorite thing to do outside?"

Cognitive/Insight

"What grade are you in?"
"Some kids have a favorite thing about school. What is yours?"
"Parents get worried about their kids sometimes. What do you think could worry your parents about you?"
"Kids get worried about parents too. What could worry you about them?"

Social Relationships

"What is your favorite television show (movie, book)?"
"Some kids save things. How about you?"
"Tell me about a friend you like very much."
"Some kids don't have friends. I wonder why."
"What do you and your friends do together?"

Family Relationships

"Tell me who is in your family. Let's make a chart."
"What happens at your house on the weekends?"

"What should good mothers be like? Good fathers?"
"How do good (bad) mothers (fathers) treat their kids?"

Emotional Development

"What would you like to be when you grow up?"
"Do you ever need help?"
"If trees could talk, what would they say to you?"
"What is neat about you?"
"What makes you mad?"

Thought Processes

"What would you miss the most if you could not touch or feel?"
"Are there ways you create beauty?"
"Do you have to be happy to learn?"

Fantasies, Fears, and Wishes

"If you could have three magic wishes, what would they be?"
"If you could be an animal, what would you be? How come?"
"Sometimes dreams are scary. Tell me about one you have had."

Adapted from Robinson M. Interviewing children as an assessment tool. *In* Babich KS (ed). A Workbook: Assessing the Mental Health of Children. Boulder, CO: Western Interstate Commission for Higher Education, 1982, pp 59–69.

ADOLESCENTS (13–19 YEARS OF AGE)

The adolescent is more able to think abstractly. Thus, the interview and assessment may be conducted with the nurse, the family, and the client facing each other. Drawing from developmental, social, and cognitive norms, the nurse will be able to differentiate abnormal patterns. Again, school, peer, and family relationships are assessed. A **genogram** displays family information over at least three generations and may

enable the nurse to formulate hypotheses about the connection between the family and the clinical problem (McGoldrick and Gerson 1985). A sample genogram is shown in Figure 27–1. The social life of an adolescent is more complex than that of a child, so the nurse will need to ask different questions. For example, when assessing peer relationships, questions pertaining to sexual activity and use of substances (e.g., nicotine, alcohol, and illegal drugs) are indicated.

Subject-specific projective story-telling cards can

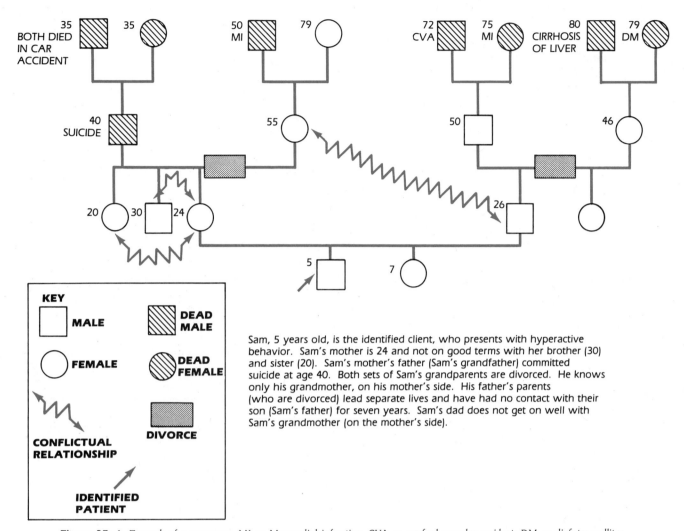

Figure 27–1. *Example of a genogram.* MI = *Myocardial infarction;* CVA = *cerebral vascular accident;* DM = *diabetes mellitus.*

elicit helpful assessment data. An assessment tool called the "Court Set" can be used with clients whose parents have divorced (Projective Story Telling Cards Court Set 1988). Sentence completion ("I feel to blame when . . . ") or word association ("Tell me the word you think of when I say 'hate'.") activities can also produce useful information about the child or adolescent.

Nursing Diagnosis

A nursing diagnosis for the infant, child, or adolescent client is extrapolated from the many sources of assessment—the clinical interview of the child and family, the mental status examination, and direct observations. The developmental stage of the child must also be considered. Some potential nursing diagnoses for each age group are as follows:

Infants
- Altered nutrition: less than body requirements
- Altered growth and development
- Feeding self-care deficit
- Pain
- Impaired social interaction
- Sleep-pattern disturbance

Children
- Impaired verbal communication
- Defensive coping
- Ineffective individual coping
- Ineffective family coping
- Denial
- Altered family processes

- Grieving
- Altered growth and development
- Altered thought processes
- Altered school performance

Adolescents

- Hopelessness
- Ineffective individual coping
- Altered family processes
- Self-esteem disturbance
- Self-care deficit
- Sensory perceptual alteration
- Social isolation
- Potential for violence directed at self or others
- Ineffective denial
- Altered sexuality patterns
- Personal identity disturbance

Planning

Planning involves both the content level—setting goals with the client and family—and the process level—nurses' reactions and feelings. With the child client, planning extends to the family, milieu, and community.

CONTENT LEVEL—PLANNING GOALS

Individual

1. Infant—*Altered nutrition*: less than body requirements related to poor sucking reflex, as evidenced by premature birth
   - Infant's emotional needs rather than physical needs will be stressed during feeding interventions by (date).
   - Infant will gain a specified amount of weight by (date).
   - Infant will demonstrate satiated behaviors (e.g., will sleep longer and show decreased agitation) by (date).
2. Child—*Grieving* related to mother's death, as evidenced by lack of spontaneity and poor school performance
   - Child will meet with the nurse once per day for 15 minutes to draw feelings.
   - Child will verbally demonstrate feelings by (date).
   - Child will initiate an activity with a peer by (date).

- Child will verbally demonstrate positive memories of mother by (date).
3. Adolescent—*Ineffective individual coping* related to school failure, as evidenced by suicidal ideation
   - Client will identify personal strengths and weaknesses by (date).
   - Client will identify feelings that occur before the client feels so bad that he or she wants to harm self by (date).
   - Client will sign a daily 24-hour no-suicide contract.
   - Client will meet with one teacher to discuss school progress by (date).

Family

1. *Altered family processes* related to adolescent's behavior, as evidenced by poor communication patterns
   - By (date), family members will identify normal adolescent behavior.
   - By (date), the family will discuss with the adolescent what behaviors are acceptable and what the consequences of unacceptable behaviors will be.
   - By (date), the family will effectively demonstrate two learned communication techniques.

Milieu and Community

If the child is hospitalized, the milieu must be managed to facilitate the goals for the client. Milieu therapy is further discussed in the next section. If the child is participating in outpatient therapy, the nurse must be aware of how other environments affect the client. A home visit, a classroom visit, or a visit to one of the child's extracurricular activities may be indicated.

It is extremely helpful to identify the child's or the adolescent's community. Does the client live in a public housing development where drugs and drive-by shootings are a daily occurrence? Does the child live in a shelter for the homeless because the parents have been evicted? What is the ethnic concentration of the child's neighborhood? The availability of community resources and support, such as bereavement groups for children or parent support groups, also needs to be considered during planning.

PROCESS LEVEL—NURSES' REACTIONS AND FEELINGS

Child and adolescent psychiatric nursing is demanding, and the child's or the adolescent's behavior may trigger reactions in the nurse. Transference and countertransference issues need to be identified and processed. The nurse's reaction to a child's or an adolescent's behavior may reflect unresolved or previously unknown feelings about the nurse's relationship with his or her parent. Clinical supervision, both individual and group, is of utmost importance for the nurse working with children and adolescents. Supervision with a clinical nurse specialist will provide personal and professional growth, prevent "burnout," and maintain the integrity of the treatment plan.

Intervention

Nursing interventions develop from ongoing assessment of the client. The nurse outlines a nursing care plan that includes short and long term goals and decides on the treatment modality and the particular techniques to be used (West and Evans 1992). Because of the age of the client, family interventions always need to be developed. Each age group has in common the interventions of milieu therapy, health teaching, activities of daily living programs, somatic treatments, and family and group therapy. These shared interventions are described, and then specific interventions for infants, children, and adolescents are presented.

MILIEU THERAPY

Whether the client is treated in an inpatient or outpatient setting, the concept of structure is integral to any plan. For example, the adolescent client may balk at rules, but children and adolescents need structured limitations to ensure both physical and emotional safety. **Milieu therapy** includes four common constructs:

1. Facilitation of open communication between the client and the environment.
2. Provision of an atmosphere in which the client can freely examine his or her feelings, thoughts, and behaviors.
3. Setting of limits on inappropriate behavior while supporting the client in his or her attempt to test new behavior patterns.
4. Provision of appropriate role models for behavior.

The individual treatment plan directs the therapeutic milieu. Interventions focus on self-governance through decision making; attaining progressive levels of responsibility; promoting meaningful activities; and establishing connections with the client's family and community.

Outpatient Programs

For the client who can safely function, intervention may be implemented in an outpatient setting such as a private office or a community mental health center. The therapy may be with just the client, with the entire family, or with the client and one parent. For example, individual therapy may reveal issues the adolescent has with his or her mother. Inviting the mother to participate in sessions with the daughter or son, the nurse can use family therapy techniques to change mother-child communication patterns.

Hospitalization

The client may need to be hospitalized if the situation is life-threatening, if the dysfunction severely impairs the child, if a thorough evaluation is needed, or if psychopharmacological therapies are initiated. The nursing care plan is part of the multidisciplinary team approach that includes psychiatrists, psychologists, social workers, and other mental health team members. A structured environment or milieu provides information and expectations. A sample milieu program for the adolescent client is presented in Table 27–4.

The one-to-one relationship the nurse generalist develops with the hospitalized child or adolescent is based on trust, knowledge of the developmental stage, and limit setting. Trust is an issue because the child or adolescent may never have had a trusting relationship with an adult. The client's developmental stage is significant because unlike adults, who enter into a therapeutic relationship willingly and ready to work, the child or adolescent may not be able to think abstractly or may not possess verbal skills. Further, limit setting is critical because the child or adolescent not only may perceive him- or herself as not having a problem but may see the nurse as all-knowing, all-powerful, and all-controlling. Common child and adolescent characteristics with corresponding positive nursing behaviors that direct therapeutic relationships and interventions are shown in Table 27–5.

Day Hospital Programs

Day hospital programs provide a less intensive structured environment. The client may attend his or her own school and then attend the day hospital for a specified time. Another option is for the client to both attend school at the day hospital and have specified therapeutic activities there and to return home in the evening. Therapeutic interventions may include individual and group therapies, participation in problem-solving groups, and work in skill-building groups. A

TIME	MONDAY	TUESDAY	WEDNESDAY	THURSDAY	FRIDAY	SATURDAY/SUNDAY
7–8 A.M.	Wake up/hygiene					
8–8:30	Breakfast					
8:30–9	Goal setting; patient government					Wake up/hygiene
9–11	School					9–9:30 Breakfast 9:30–11:30 OT/PT
11–11:30	Music therapy	Community exploration	Art therapy	Stress management	Music therapy	Activity
11:30–12	Lunch					Lunch
12–1 P.M.	Cooking class	Psychodrama	Survival group	ADL group	Social skills	Field trip
1–3	Social skills	Girls' group	Game therapy	Boys' group	Exercise	Game therapy
3–3:30	Quiet time					Quiet time
3:30–5	Group therapy	Crafts	Sex education	Community exploration	Semiactive games	Free time
5–5:30	Dinner					Dinner
5:30–6:30	Current events	Social skills	TV time	Current events	AA/NA/Alateen; movies	Movie
6:30–7:30	Study time				Alateen; movies	TV time
7:30–8:30	Family/TV	Parent support group	Family/TV	Parenting skills	Table games	
8:30–9	Prepare for bed					Prepare for bed
9:30	Bedtime					Bedtime

NA = Narcotics Anonymous; OT = occupational therapy; PT = play therapy.

problem-solving group, for example, may focus on activities to control anger.

Residential Treatment

Residential treatment programs are indicated for long term care in situations in which the client needs to be removed from the home environment or is homeless. Residential treatment settings range from a group home in a residential neighborhood to a large, campus-like environment. Again, the individualized treatment plan is used in a therapeutic milieu.

HEALTH TEACHING

The client's presenting concerns or behaviors indicate possible areas of knowledge deficit in the client's parents. The nurse generalist has an opportunity to practice primary prevention when he or she teaches a group of first-time parents how to distinguish a baby's

cries, models positive interactive behaviors (e.g., rocking, holding, and talking to the baby), and offers a list of community supports. If a client is to use medication, the nurse can teach the client and the family drug information. Normal growth and development is another area in which the nurse generalist can teach parents what to expect. The nurse uses teaching methods such as coaching, positive reinforcement, feedback, and modeling, as well as printed material or pictures (e.g., videos, brochures, and pamphlets). Role-playing is another example of a methodology for increasing client knowledge. Having information and verbally demonstrating knowledge increases compliance and facilitates family communication.

ACTIVITIES OF DAILY LIVING PROGRAMS

Self-care deficits, impaired communication skills, and *ineffective coping* are examples of problems that require intervention. For the child who is mentally retarded, a treatment program to teach dressing and toileting is

Table 27–5 ■ CHILD OR ADOLESCENT CHARACTERISTICS WITH POSITIVE NURSING INTERVENTIONS	
CHILD OR ADOLESCENT CHARACTERISTIC	**POSITIVE NURSING BEHAVIOR**
1. The cognitive and language abilities of the child or adolescent may require acting out feelings.	1a. Facilitate a creative approach to problem solving. 1b. Assist the child or adolescent in balancing verbal and nonverbal expressions. 1c. Use role-playing, games, drawings, books, TV and movie characters, computer games, and journals. 1d. Use language appropriate for the child's or adolescent's comprehension.
2. The child or adolescent does not see him- or herself as having a problem.	2a. Communicate the need to work together to facilitate problem-solving. 2b. Convey a sense of acceptance for negative feelings but emphasize limits in a caring, directive manner. 2c. Collaborate with the child or adolescent and the family in working together to problem-solve by avoiding taking sides. 2d. Communicate respect to the child or adolescent client by meeting the client at his or her own level. Avoid patronizing and "one up" behaviors.
3. The child or adolescent perceives the nurse as an all-knowing and powerful adult.	3a. Demonstrate positive role-modeling. 3b. Keep verbal and nonverbal behaviors congruent. 3c. Assess the reasons for the behavior. 3d. Provide positive feedback. 3e. Avoid reacting to the child's or the adolescent's verbal or nonverbal behavior with threats or a show of power. 3f. Give active direction and suggestions when necessary.

Adapted from Kunes-Connell M. Children and adolescents: Developmental issues and concerns. *In* McFarland GK, Thomas MD (eds). Psychiatric Mental Health Nursing: Application of the Nursing Process. Philadelphia: JB Lippincott, 1991, pp 609.

implemented. For the adolescent who cannot communicate effectively, interventions focus on training the client in assertiveness skills, such as maintaining eye contact (if culturally appropriate), making "I" statements, and requesting information. The client's developmental stage and the disease process must be considered in developing an activities of daily living plan. If a developmental task has been interrupted because the child became ill at that point in his or her development, nursing interventions are developed to assist in task completion. Not only does psychiatric illness impede developmental, cognitive, and social growth, but interventions may need to focus at chronological and emotional ages that are earlier than those at which the child presents with a problem.

SOMATIC THERAPIES

Psychopharmacological interventions are helpful, when indicated, for the child or adolescent client. The nurse generalist can administer medication and can teach the client and family about drug dosage, side effects, toxic effects, and expected responses. The clinical nurse specialist can monitor the progress of the patient through serum levels and symptom abatement. In some states, the clinical nurse specialist can write prescriptions. Nursing interventions include surveillance, teaching, collaboration, and advocacy (Hogarth 1991). The central nervous system stimulants methylphenidate (Ritalin), dextroamphetamine (Dexedrine), and pemoline (Cylert) are given to both children and adolescents with attention deficit hyperactivity disorder. Phenothiazines such as haloperidol (Haldol), fluphenazine (Prolixin), and chlorpromazine (Thorazine) are used to treat psychotic disorders in children and adolescents. Children and adolescents with an affective disorder may receive tricyclic antidepressants such as imipramine (Tofranil) and amitriptyline (Elavil, Endep). However, tricyclic antidepressants are not recommended for children younger than 12 years of age. Children with enuresis have been treated successfully with imipramine. Adolescents with bipolar disease may be treated with lithium. Measurement of baseline hormone levels and monthly serum levels is indicated. Currently, psychopharmacological intervention with children and adolescents is one of the most active areas of research.

FAMILY THERAPY

When the family is available, nursing interventions center on health teaching (e.g., about medicines and the disease process), communication techniques, and support. The nurse generalist teaches families drug information and observes family and client interaction. The clinical nurse specialist may use family therapy techniques. The family may be referred to a clinical nurse specialist certified in family or marital therapy, and one parent may consider individual psychotherapy for him- or herself. Work with families may extend from leading a large support group for parents of hospitalized children to family therapy.

GROUP THERAPY

Group therapy with children and adolescents is a powerful therapeutic modality because of the normalizing, social, and support behaviors that emerge. Children who have been identified as being undersocialized can benefit from learning age-appropriate behaviors in a group. Adolescents who have been sexually abused can hear similar stories from their peers that aid in the healing process. Support, peer, and therapy groups can be formed to focus on many issues facing children and adolescents. Examples of support groups are Alatot for children and Alateen for adolescents who have an alcoholic parent. Siepker and Kandaras (1985) fully describe the stages of group development with children and adolescents.

INFANTS

The ill infant may require hospitalization. Nursing interventions focus on relieving life-threatening symptoms. For example, the infant with a feeding disorder such as anorexia needs interventions such as scheduled and limited-time feedings and play activity after meals to seek and receive attention and affection.

Infant mental health intervention often occurs in the home, where nursing interventions include education, support, and developmental guidance. Dyadic, family, and group modalities help establish parent-child interactions and offer support (West and Evans 1992).

CHILDREN

Play Therapy

Play is the developmental continuum that children use to explore and communicate with their world.

Play therapy encourages exploring the self in relation to others, self-expansion, and self-expression. Children who cannot or do not talk can freely employ play as a therapeutic intervention. The role of the therapist may be either directive (guiding and interpreting the play) or nondirective (leaving the responsibility and direction to the child). Toys that encourage self-expression are dolls, puppets, crayons, paint, clay, soldiers, wooden blocks, toy animals, and cars.

Art Therapy

Drawings allow the child a safe, therapeutic avenue to express feelings of frustration, fear, aggression, or confusion (Oster and Gould 1987). In **art therapy** the client is encouraged to explore his or her own ability to resolve conflict and discover self-direction. The child's age and developmental level are important considerations in interpreting a child's drawings (DiLeo 1983). For example, when drawing a family, the three-year-old will use stick figures; if a 10-year-old uses stick figures, the interpretation will differ. The nurse can ask the child to explain the drawings, thereby enhancing communication. This artwork needs to be interpreted by nurses, art therapists, and other mental health professionals who have special training.

Bibliotherapy

Reading stories about children in a situation similar to the client's is a therapeutic intervention that is nonthreatening and also furthers the child's reading ability. In a supportive environment, **bibliotherapy** facilitates self-expression and resolution of the child's conflict (Cohen 1987). Using books as a therapeutic intervention helps children dealing with divorce, death, fears, and separation. *The Boys' and Girls' Book About Divorce* by Gardner (1970) is a book that is useful for children who are dealing with parental divorce. The reading, reciting, and performing of fairy tales is another therapeutic intervention that empowers the child to resolve conflicts and problem-solve (Franzke 1989).

ADOLESCENT

Psychodrama

Psychodrama was initially invented by Dr. J. L. Moreno, who recognized that spontaneity was crucial to creativity (Blatner 1988). Used as a therapeutic intervention, psychodrama facilitates interpersonal freedom and responsibility. The re-enactment of situations through role-playing, nonverbal communication, and imagination provides an intrapsychic modality for the adolescent, as well as for adults. Discovering alternative and constructive options, the adolescent is assisted in role definition, problem-solving, and conflict resolution.

Music Therapy

Music can evoke emotions that transcend words. For children or adolescents with poor verbal or social skills, music therapy provides a relaxed, creative intervention for self-expression and insight. Music can be used in a variety of ways. The adolescent can listen to music and then label the feelings experienced while listening. This assists in the identification of feelings and with verbal skills. In a group setting, adolescents can put their own words to music, which facilitates both social cooperation and verbal communication (Kunes-Connell 1991). Playing background music during play therapy has decreased anxiety and increased peer cooperation (Hinds 1980).

Developmental Games

Adolescents who have perceptual and learning disorders can be helped with the use of developmental games (Shapiro 1984). The adolescent plays a therapeutic game that has specific goals. One example of a goal is to attend to and complete a task. The therapeutic value consists of transferring what is learned from game playing to other situations.

Adventure-Based Programs

Adventure-based programs assist the adolescent in recognizing and developing internal skills of self-resiliency, survival, and problem-solving. A cooperative component is integral to this program. Adventures may range from scaling 10-foot wooden structures built in a hospital's play area to participating in a highly structured chaperoned trip to a wilderness area.

Issues That Affect the Mental Health of Children

Several psychiatric disorders develop in infancy, childhood, and adolescence. Prevalent disorders currently

seen are presented here with clinical vignettes to illuminate the disorder. Sample nursing diagnoses are suggested. Box 27–4 shows the DSM-III-R classification of childhood disorders.

INFANTS

Mental Retardation

Mental retardation is characterized by a significant subaverage intellectual function (IQ less than 70) that results in impaired adaptive behavior and is diagnosed before the age of 18. Retardation is chronic. Some kinds of mental retardation have a genetic cause (e.g., an extra chromosome) or result from an endocrine disorder (e.g., cretinism), but a large percentage can be prevented with prenatal care and education. Although an infant or a child may be mentally retarded, that does not mean he or she is mentally ill. However, a mentally retarded individual may also have a mental illness. Concomitant aggressive, irritable, tantrum, and stereotyped behaviors may be obvious. Vision and hearing deficits may occur, as may limited motor function and seizures. The intellectual functioning and characteristics listed in Table 27–6 assist the nurse in developing a care plan.

Rachel is a nine-year-old with an IQ of 42. She did not walk until she was three years old, and she now talks in two-word sentences. She gives hugs to any person next to her. She can put on a shirt, but her mother must put on Rachel's socks, pants, and shoes for her. She rarely smiles, and when she is tired or frustrated, she screams, which distracts her classmates in her special education classroom. She has just learned to print her first name.

Sample Nursing Diagnosis: *Altered grooming* related to neurological impairment, as evidenced by inability to dress self

Long Term Goal	Short Term Goals
1. Child will dress herself by the end of 12 months.	1. Child will select daily shirt, pants, socks, and shoes in three months.
	2. Child will differentiate right foot from left in five months.

Reactive Attachment Disorder of Infancy

Reactive attachment disorder of infancy is characterized by a lack of social responsiveness and by de-

---

Box 27-4. DISORDERS USUALLY SEEN IN INFANTS, CHILDREN, OR ADOLESCENTS

Disruptive behavior disorders
Attention deficit hyperactivity disorder
Conduct disorders
    Group type
    Solitary aggressive type
    Undifferentiated type
Oppositional defiant disorder

Anxiety disorders of childhood or adolescence
Separation anxiety disorder
Avoidant disorder of childhood or adolescence
Overanxious disorder

Eating disorders (see Chapter 25)
Anorexia nervosa
Bulimia nervosa
Pica
Rumination disorder of infancy
Eating disorder NOS

Gender identity disorders
Gender identity disorder of childhood
Transsexualism
    Specify sexual history: asexual, homosexual,
        heterosexual, unspecified
Gender identity disorder of adolescence or
    adulthood, nontranssexual type
    Specify sexual history: asexual, homosexual,
        heterosexual, unspecified
Gender identify disorder NOS

Tic disorders
Tourette's disorder
Chronic motor or vocal tic disorder
Transient tic disorder
    Specify: single episode or recurrent
Tic disorder NOS

Elimination disorders
Functional encopresis
    Specify: primary or secondary type
Functional enuresis
    Specify: primary or secondary type
    Specify: nocturnal only, diurnal only, nocturnal
        and diurnal

Other disorders of infancy, childhood, or adolescence
Elective mutism
Identity disorder
Reactive attachment disorder of infancy or early
    childhood
Stereotype/habit disorder
Undifferentiated attention deficit disorder

Mental retardation
Mild mental retardation
Moderate mental retardation
Severe mental retardation
Profound mental retardation
Unspecified mental retardation

Pervasive developmental disorders
Autistic disorder
    Specify: if childhood onset
Pervasive developmental disorder NOS

Specific developmental disorders
Academic skills disorders
    Developmental arithmetic disorder
    Developmental expressive writing disorder
    Developmental reading disorder
Language and speech disorders
    Developmental articulation disorder
    Developmental expressive language disorder
    Developmental receptive language disorder
Motor skills disorders
    Developmental coordination disorder
    Specific developmental disorder NOS

Other developmental disorders
Developmental disorder NOS

Speech disorders not elsewhere classified
Cluttering
Stuttering

Reprinted with permission from American Psychiatric Association: Diagnostic and Statistical Manual of Mental Disorders, Third Edition, Revised, Washington, DC, American Psychiatric Association, 1987.

Table 27–6 ■ CLASSIFICATION OF MENTAL RETARDATION	
IQ LEVEL	**CHARACTERISTICS**
Mild Mental Retardation (Educable)	
50–70	1. Social and communication skills 2. Minimal impairment in sensorimotor areas 3. Academic skills to sixth-grade level 4. Social and vocational skills, minimal self-support
Moderate Mental Retardation (Trainable)	
35–49	1. Poor awareness of social conventions 2. Can develop academic skills to about second-grade level 3. May contribute to own support under close supervision
Severe Mental Retardation	
20–34	1. Poor motor development 2. Little speech 3. May learn to talk in school and learn hygiene 4. May be able to learn simple work tasks
Profound Mental Retardation	
Below 20	1. Minimal capacity for sensorimotor functioning 2. Some motor development and minimal self-care in school 3. Very limited self-care

Data from American Psychiatric Association. Diagnostic and Statistical Manual of Mental Disorders, 3rd ed, revised (DSM-III-R). Washington, DC: American Psychiatric Association, 1987.

velopmental delays before the infant is eight months of age. The infant does not visually track or smile at two months, may not engage in games or vocalize at six months, and makes no attempt to crawl or reach out to be picked up by eight months.

Kara is a five-month-old infant seen at the health department's well-child clinic. She is listless, closes her eyes when the nurse takes her from her mother to weigh her, and has no vocalization. Her mother, a 14-year-old adolescent, states "everything's just fine."

Suggested Nursing Diagnosis: *Altered growth and development* related to adolescent parenting, as evidenced by listlessness and no vocalization

Long Term Goal	**Short Term Goals**
1. Infant will demonstrate normal vocal, behavioral, and interactive patterns in six months.	1. Infant will reach out arms when she wants to be picked up in one month. 2. Infant will imitate the mother's vocalizations in two months. 3. Infant will crawl in three months.

CHILDREN

Pervasive Developmental Disorders

Pervasive developmental disorders involve distortions in the development of social skills and language that include perception, motor movement, attention, and reality-testing distortions. Previous diagnoses in this category included childhood schizophrenia and symbiotic psychosis.

Autistic disorder is thought to be the most severe type of pervasive developmental disorder (APA 1987). The significant characteristic of autism is the child's failure to develop interpersonal skills. The disorder is chronic and can range from mild to severe. The infant fails to develop normal attachment behaviors such as cuddling, making eye contact, and using facial expressions. The child may exhibit asocial behavior and inappropriate clinging. Peer relationships are absent, which poses a special problem for the adolescent. As the child develops chronologically, behaviors that did not pose a threat when the child was younger may become more harmful. As adolescence is approached, pubertal and emotional changes may require environmental and medication adjustments. The child with a pervasive developmental disorder (autism) may demonstrate attachment to an object such as a top and spend countless hours repeatedly spinning the top. Any kind of change not only is difficult to adapt to but may exacerbate stereotypical behaviors such as arm flapping and spinning around. Practice and research in facilitated communication (e.g., the use of computers) show encouraging results in language development for the autistic child. Early identification, intervention, and family support are ways in which the nurse can provide primary prevention.

Scott is a 10-year-old enrolled in a public school's special education program. He rocks back and forth while listening to the teacher. When he walks down the hall, one hand is in constant contact with the wall. His only word is "mama," and when excited or rushed, he repeatedly screams, "Ai, ai, ai."

Sample Nursing Diagnosis: *Altered communication* related to language delay, as evidenced by use of one word

Long Term Goal	Short Term Goals
1. Child will verbally identify three objects accurately in six months.	1. Child will maintain eye contact in two months. 2. Child will use his arm to make a request in four months. 3. Child will match a word with a picture in five months.

ATTENTION DEFICIT HYPERACTIVITY DISORDER

Children with **attention deficit hyperactivity disorder** display difficulties with attention (Mash and Barkley 1989). A causative factor is not known, but theories regarding self-regulation, developmental delays, and inhibition to responding have been postulated. The disorder is manifest by incessant talking, constant movement, inability to attend to or finish a task, poor social relationships, and easy distractibility. Attention deficit hyperactivity disorder is the most common pediatric behavioral disorder. It has been studied in both the psychiatric and education disciplines. Many children respond to methylphenidate (Ritalin). This response has caused an increase in the number of medicated children, and the increased use of this drug has raised legal and ethical questions. A thorough multidisciplinary evaluation is indicated for the hyper-

active child. At one time, it was thought that children outgrew attention deficit hyperactivity disorder, but it is evident now that adolescents develop and use different coping mechanisms.

Monica is an eight-year-old second grader who, when not daydreaming in class, talks out loud and jumps up and down in her seat. She constantly moves her fingers, hands, and legs and stretches out on her desk. Other children inch away from her physically, and she is never picked as a team member for the recess games. At home, she does not complete tasks she starts and is a restless sleeper.

Possible Nursing Diagnosis: *Sensory alteration* related to neurological overload, as evidenced by restless and talking-out behaviors

Long Term Goal	Short Term Goals
1. Child will complete one written task without self-interruption in six months.	1. Child will be evaluated by a clinical nurse specialist, a child psychiatrist, the family doctor, and a school psychologist. 2. Child will select and complete one concrete task in two months. 3. Child will identify two thoughts or feelings that occur when she is distracted in three months.

SEPARATION ANXIETY DISORDER

In the school-age child, **separation anxiety disorder** is commonly seen as school phobia or school refusal. Whether this disorder is a recurrence of an earlier anxiety disorder or a precursor to an anxiety disorder such as obsessive-compulsive disorder is not known. The child displays behavioral symptoms of excessive fear, avoidance, and protest with regard to separation from an attachment figure. A panic level of anxiety may be seen. Onset is usually before age 18, and a duration of at least two weeks is needed to make a diagnosis. The anxious child worries unrealistically that a catastrophe will befall major attachment figures, is unable to sleep away from home, has nightmares with themes of separation, and displays somatic complaints of headache, stomach ache, or nausea when anticipating separation from the major attachment figure (Rapoport and Ismond 1990). Behavioral modification has been used as a treatment modality, as have family therapy and medication.

Kent, a six-year-old whose parents have been divorced for one year, has started first grade at a new school. When his mother drops him off at school, he begins screaming and wraps himself around her legs, beseeching her, "Don't leave me!"

Suggested Nursing Diagnosis: *Severe anxiety* related to maternal separation, as evidenced by screaming, crying, and clinging

Long Term Goal	Short Term Goals
1. Child will be able to stay in school in one month.	1. Child will say goodbye to his mother in the car daily.
	2. Child will be met by the principal at the door daily.
	3. Child will accompany the principal to the classroom daily.
	4. Child will be met by the classroom teacher daily.

ADOLESCENTS

Conduct Disorders

Conduct disorders are manifest by negativism, disobedience, and destructive acts. The adolescent with a conduct disorder infringes on the rights of others and when confronted states that other people are making unreasonable requests. The adolescent with a conduct disorder finds anything threatening, expects assault, and persists in oppositional behavior even when it is destructive to his or her well-being. For conduct disorder to be diagnosed, its duration must be at least six months. Behaviors include stealing, running away from home, destroying other people's property, and physical cruelty to animals and people. DSM-III-R categories include group type (conduct problems occur in group activity with peers), solitary aggressive type (conduct problems are initiated by the individual), and undifferentiated type (APA 1987).

Don is a 14-year-old boy who set his parent's garage on fire when he was 12, assaulted an elderly man "because my friends dared me to," and has run away from home three times in the past two months. He has a history of repeated truancy from school, and the school's truant officer visited his parents yesterday.

Possible Nursing Diagnosis: *High risk for violence* related to aggression, as evidenced by assaultive and fire-setting acts

Long Term Goal	Short Term Goals
1. Adolescent will comply with house rules set by parents within three months.	1. Adolescent will remain in school within one month's time.
	2. Adolescent will identify feelings of anger and helplessness in one month.
	3. Adolescent will define three constructive behaviors in two months.
	4. Adolescent will verbalize house rules in two months.
	5. Adolescent will state the consequences of noncompliance with house rules in two months.

Box 27–5. ADOLESCENTS AT RISK FOR SUICIDE

Characteristics of Suicidal Adolescents

1. Family history of suicide
2. Previous suicide attempt
3. Chronic illness
4. Suffering bereavement
5. Alcoholism
6. Chronic use of drugs
7. Domestic difficulties
8. Depression in teenagers marked by acting-out behaviors:
   - Delinquent behaviors, i.e., stealing, vandalism, academic failure, promiscuity, fights at school, and running away
   - Escape behaviors, i.e., drugs, sex, and withdrawal
9. Loss of girlfriend or boyfriend

Characteristics of a Family with a Suicidal Adolescent

1. Unproductive communications
2. Communications reveal much conflict between family members
3. Impaired problem-solving ability
4. Inconsistent positive reinforcements plus a greater number of negative reinforcements
5. Unstable home environment

Data from Hamlin WT. Adolescent suicide. Journal of the National Medical Association, 74(1):25, 1982; Hart NA, Keidel GC. The suicidal adolescent. American Journal of Nursing, 79(1):80, 1979.

Depression

Depression in children and adolescents is now recognized as a major mental health problem. Depression may be a factor in the increased rate of suicide and a sequela of sexual abuse. The depressed adolescent is sad, may overeat or undereat, experiences insomnia, and exhibits poor concentration that affects school performance. Learned helplessness, separation and loss, feelings of incompetence, and the role of shame are some of the etiologies postulated (Rutter et al. 1986). It may be difficult to diagnose adolescent depression because it may be masked by acting-out behaviors such as sexual promiscuity, conduct disorders, substance abuse, delinquency, and aggression. Children as well as adolescents have thoughts of suicide, so suicide ideation and lethality must always be assessed (Box 27–5). Hospitalization may be indicated for the adolescent at risk for self-injury. Other successful modalities include psychopharmacologic therapies and individual, group, and family therapies.

Jack is a 16-year-old high school junior who has played varsity football, is an honor roll student, and is well liked by his classmates. During the past month, he has secluded himself in his room, will not take phone calls, has lost weight, and no longer demonstrates his sense of humor or teases his little brother. His parents are quite concerned and can think of no recent loss or crisis that Jack or the family has had.

Possible Nursing Diagnosis: *Social isolation* related to unknown etiology, as evidenced by secluding self from family and friends

Long Term Goals	Short Term Goals
1. Adolescent will join in family activities within two months. 2. Adolescent will resume peer relationships in three months.	1. Adolescent will be evaluated by a psychiatrist by (date). 2. Adolescent will begin medication as necessary within one month. 3. Adolescent will verbalize feelings such as loneliness and helplessness in two months. 4. Adolescent will develop two alternative techniques for dealing with depression in three months. 5. Adolescent will identify two resources he can use by three months.

Other Disorders

Post-traumatic stress disorder in children and adolescents bears further investigation. The relationship between physical and sexual abuse in childhood and the later development of borderline and antisocial personality disorders is an area of current work. Bipolar disease and schizophrenia may begin in adolescence, but they are difficult to differentiate from other disorders.

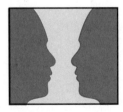

Case Study: Working with an Aggressive Child

Tim Perkins is a nine-year-old third grader who has a history of temper outbursts in the classroom. He was referred to the clinical nurse specialist (CNS) because he had become so enraged at a classmate during recess that he twisted the classmate's arm, causing a spiral fracture.

Assessment

When Tim was brought to the office, he was defiant, hostile, and guarded. Dressed in a plaid shirt and jeans, he refused to sit down and warily looked around the room. When invited to explore the toy shelves, his eyes widened with incredulity, but his expression then quickly became guarded. In response to questions, his speech was tense and stilted. Tim slowly inched his way to the toys, but an air of suspicion surrounded him. During the mental health assessment (see Box 27–3), when he was asked what his favorite thing about school was, he said, "Nothing" and denied having any friends. He related no hobbies and said that the TV was "broke." He became very guarded when questioned about his family. He said he had a mother, father, and baby sister, "but you don't want to know them." He did not respond to questions about what he wanted to be when he grew up or what he would miss if he could not touch. He exploded verbally with "NO-THING!" when asked what was neat about him or what made him mad. He did not answer to the three magic wishes question and shouted "stupid" when asked about being an animal or having scary dreams. By this time, he had discovered the crayons and hesitantly asked if he could draw. He then proceeded to draw an exquisite picture of a house using soft, pastel colors. When told that the interview was finished, he asked when he could return.

The CNS telephoned Tim's mother to discuss Tim's assessment and suggest Tim return the following week. Tim's mother brusquely replied that she didn't have a car. She said it would be "OK with me if Tim comes to your office once in a while." The CNS then reviewed the child's academic folder for results of standardized tests reflecting intellectual functioning. Test scores reported an above-average intelligence (IQ of 113).

Planning

Based on her assessment, the CNS formulated the following nursing diagnosis:

Nursing Diagnosis	Long Term Goal	Short Term Goals
1. *High risk for violence* related to aggressive behavior, as evidenced by rage and poor impulse control	1. Tim will refrain from angry outbursts that infringe on other people's rights.	1. Tim will identify three alternative behaviors to use when he is angry. 2. Tim will identify three thoughts or feelings he has before engaging in abusive behavior. 3. Tim will select a password to use in the classroom to let the teacher know that he is becoming angry.

Interventions

The CNS developed the following interventions:
1. Tim will meet with the CNS two times per week.
2. Play therapy will be initiated and directed by Tim.
3. Sessions will take place in the gym or outdoors to encourage the displacement of anger through more appropriate channels.
4. Art therapy will be used to begin the process of identifying feelings.

Evaluation

Tim's ability to control himself will be self-reported and teacher reported. Each time one week of controlled behavior has been accomplished, Tim will put a star on the chart he drew.

Summary

Assessment of infants, children, and adolescents requires a thorough investigation of the client, the family, and community relationships. Because the child or adolescent responds in a concrete, literal way, questions are couched in different ways to assess areas such as emotional development and thought processes. Infants can be assessed by observing their patterns of interaction with their parents. Children can be assessed through play, drawings, and interviews.

Genograms, sentence completion activities, and specific age-appropriate questions assist in assessing the adolescent.

Various intervention strategies were discussed because care of children may occur in many settings, among them the client's home, the hospital, and the community mental health care center. Play therapy, art therapy, and bibliotherapy are useful interventions for children; psychodrama and music therapy can tap into the adolescent's imagination and search for identity.

Common childhood psychopathological conditions were discussed, and potential nursing diagnoses to assist the student were suggested. Milieu, somatic, activities of daily living, and group and family interactions and interventions are used with clients of each age group—infants, children, and adolescents.

References

Alpern G, Boll T, Shearer M. Developmental Profile II. Los Angeles: Western Psychological Services, 1984.

American Psychiatric Association. Diagnostic and Statistical Manual of Mental Disorders, 3rd ed, revised (DSM-III-R). Washington, DC: American Psychiatric Association, 1987.

Barnard KE, Brazelton TB (eds). Touch: The Foundation of Experience. Madison, CT: International Universities Press, 1990.

Barthel R, Herrman C. Psychiatric mental health nursing with children. In Gary F, Kavanagh CK (eds). Psychiatric Mental Health Nursing. Philadelphia: JB Lippincott, 1991, pp 801–861.

Blatner A. Foundations of Psychodrama: History, Theory and Practice, 3rd ed. New York: Springer Publishing Company, 1988.

Bloom-Feshbach J, Bloom-Feshbach S. The Psychology of Separation and Loss: Perspectives on Development, Life Transitions and Clinical Practice. San Francisco: Jossey Bass Publishers, 1987.

Bowlby J. Attachment and Loss. Volume I: Attachment. New York: Basic Books, 1969.

Bowlby J. Attachment and Loss. Volume II: Separation. New York: Basic Books, 1973.

Bowlby J. Attachment and Loss. Volume III: Loss. New York: Basic Books, 1980.

Brazelton TB. Neonatal Behavioral Assessment. London: William Heinemann and Sons, 1973. National Spastics Society Monograph. Clinics in Developmental Medicine No. 50.

Clunn P. Child Psychiatric Nursing. St. Louis: Mosby–Year Book, 1991.

Cohen LJ. Bibliotherapy: Using literature to help children deal with difficult problems. Journal of Psychosocial Nursing and Mental Health Services, 22(10):20, 1987.

DiLeo JH. Interpreting Children's Drawings. New York: Brunner-Mazel, 1983.

Driekurs R. Children: The Challenge. New York: Hawthorn-Dutton, 1964.

Erikson EH. Childhood and Society, 2nd ed. New York: WW Norton, 1963.

Fagin C. Nursing in Child Psychiatry. St. Louis: CV Mosby, 1972.

Fagin C. Readings in Child and Adolescent Psychiatric Nursing. St. Louis: CV Mosby, 1974.

Finke LM (ed). Collaboration for Improvement of Practice with Severely Mentally and Emotionally Disturbed Children and Adolescents. Indianapolis, IN: Advocates for Child Psychiatric Nursing, Society for Education and Research in Psychiatric Mental Health Nursing, 1991. National Institute of Mental Health Contract No. 91MEF333156.

Fraiberg SH. The Magic Years: Understanding and Handling the Problems of Early Childhood. New York: Charles Scribner's Sons, 1959.

Frankenburg WK, Goldstein AD, Camp BW. The revised Denver Developmental Screening Test. Journal of Pediatrics, 70:988, 1971.

Franzke E. Fairy Tales in Psychotherapy: The Creative Use of Old and New Tales. Toronto: Hogrefe & Huber Publishers, 1989.

Freud A. Normality and Pathology in Childhood. New York: International Universities Press, 1967.

Gardner RA. The Boys' and Girls' Book About Divorce. Toronto: Bantam Books, 1970.

Grossman J, Mayton K. Applying the nursing process with children. In Wilson HS, Kneisl CR (eds). Psychiatric Nursing, 3rd ed. Reading, MA: Addison-Wesley, 1988.

Haber J. Developmental processes. In Haber J, Hoskins PP, Leach AM, et al (eds). Comprehensive Psychiatric Nursing, 3rd ed. New York: McGraw-Hill Book Company, 1987.

Hamlin WT. Adolescent suicide. Journal of the National Medical Association, 74(1):25, 1982.

Hart NA, Keidel GC. The suicidal adolescent. American Journal of Nursing, 79(1):80, 1979.

Hinds P. Music: A milieu factor with implications for the nurse therapist. Journal of Psychosocial Nursing and Mental Health Services, 18:28, 1980.

Hogarth C. Adolescent Psychiatric Nursing. St. Louis: Mosby–Year Book, 1991.

Ilg FL, Ames LB. The Gesell Institute's Child Behavior: From Birth to Ten. New York: Harper & Row, 1955.

Kohlberg L. Development of moral character and moral ideology. In Hoffman ML, Hoffman LW (eds). Review of Child Development Research. New York: Russell Sage Foundation, 1964.

Kunes-Connell M. Children and adolescents: Developmental issues and concerns. In McFarland GK, Thomas MD (eds). Psychiatric Mental Health Nursing: Application of the Nursing Process. Philadelphia: JB Lippincott, 1991, pp 597–613.

Magid K, McKelvey CA. High Risk: Children Without a Conscience. Golden, CO: M & M Publishing, 1987.

Mash EJ, Barkley RA. Treatment of Childhood Disorders. New York: Guilford Press, 1989.

McBride A. Psychiatric nursing in the 1990's. Archives of Psychiatric Nursing, 4(1):21, 1990.

McGoldrick M, Gerson R. Genograms in Family Assessment. New York: WW Norton, 1985.

Minuchin S, Baker L, Rosman B, et al. A conceptual model of psychosomatic illness. Archives of General Psychiatry, 32:1031, 1975.

Murray RB, Zentner JP. Nursing Assessment and Health Promotion Through the Life Span, 3rd ed. Englewood Cliffs, NJ: Prentice-Hall, 1985.

National Institute of Mental Health. Implementation of the National Plan for Research on Child and Adolescent Mental Disorders. Washington, DC: US Government Printing Office, 1991. Catalog of Federal Domestic Assistance 93.242, 93.281, and 93.282.

Oster GD, Gould P. Using Drawings in Assessment and Therapy: A Guide for Mental Health Professionals. New York: Brunner-Mazel, 1987.

Piaget J, Inhelder B. The Psychology of the Child. New York: Basic Books, 1969.

Pothier P. Mental Health Counseling with Children. Boston: Little, Brown & Company, 1976.

Projective Story Telling Cards Court Set. Redding, CA: Northwest Psychological Publishers, 1988.

Rapoport JC, Ismond DR. DSM-III-R Training Guide for Diagnosis of Childhood Disorders. New York: Brunner-Mazel, 1990.

Robinson M. Interviewing children as an assessment tool. In Babich KS (ed). A Workbook: Assessing the Mental Health of Children. Boulder, CO: Western Interstate Commission for Higher Education, 1982, pp 59–69.

Rutter M, Izard CE, Read PB. Depression in Young People: Developmental and Clinical Perspectives. New York: Guilford Press, 1986.

Shapiro LE. The New Short Term Therapies for Children: A Guide for the Helping Professions and Parents. Englewood Cliffs, NJ: Prentice-Hall, 1984.

Siepker BB, Kandaras CS (eds). Group Therapy with Children and Adolescents: A Treatment Manual. New York: Human Sciences Press, 1985.

West P, Evans CLS (eds). Psychiatric and Mental Health Nursing with Children and Adolescents. Gaithersburg, MD: Aspen Publishers, 1992.

Further Reading

Axline VM. Play Therapy. New York: Ballantine Books, 1947.

Barthel R, Herrman C. Psychiatric mental health nursing with children. In Gary F, Kavanagh CK (eds). Psychiatric Mental Health Nursing. Philadelphia: JB Lippincott, 1991, pp 801–861.

Self-study Exercises

Place an S (specialist) or a B (both specialist and generalist) next to each nursing role.

1. _____ Psychotherapeutic intervention.
2. _____ Psychotherapy (group, family, individual).
3. _____ Educator of nurses and other child care personnel in a variety of settings.
4. _____ Basic health teaching to families, groups, and clients.
5. _____ Researcher who contributes to theory and practice of child and adolescent psychiatric nursing.
6. _____ Administers and teaches medication.

Choose the letter that matches each of the following theories.

7. _____ A thorough knowledge is necessary because of family, school, and peer relationships.
8. _____ A psychosocial approach to life-span development.
9. _____ A sensorimotor explanation of child development.
10. _____ If severed, the parent-child relationship is always vulnerable.

A. Piaget's cognitive theory

B. Neurobiological

C. Erikson

D. Separation and loss

E. Systems

Match the assessment strategy with the correct age group or groups.

11. _____ Sentence completion
12. _____ Genogram
13. _____ Mental status interview
14. _____ Family
15. _____ Denver Developmental Screening Test
16. _____ Projective Story Telling Cards

A. Infant

B. Adolescent

C. Child

Short answer

17. Formulate one intervention for each of the following types of treatment.

    A. Outpatient program: _____
    B. Hospitalization: _____
    C. Residential care: _____
    D. Day hospital program: _____

Match the following:

18. _____ Used in enuresis
19. _____ IQ less than 70
20. _____ Assertiveness training

A. Mental retardation

21. _____ Methylphenidate
22. _____ Parent-child communication
23. _____ Amitriptyline
24. _____ Alatot
25. _____ Activity directed by child
26. _____ Re-enactment of situations by using imagination
27. _____ Intervention for adolescents with learning disorders

B. Attention deficit hyperactivity disorder

C. Depression

D. Play therapy

E. Imipramine

F. Activities of daily living

G. Family therapy

H. Support group

I. Lithium

J. Psychodrama

K. Developmental games

Short answer

28. Develop one intervention for each of the following disorders.

    A. Mental retardation: _____
    B. Separation anxiety: _____
    C. Pervasive developmental disorder: _____
    D. Attention deficit hyperactivity disorder: _____
    E. Depression: _____

CHAPTER 28

Adult Relationships and Sexuality

Mary Jane Herron
William G. Herron

KEY TERMS AND CONCEPTS · · · · · · · · · · · · · · · ·

The key terms and concepts listed here also appear in bold where they are defined or discussed in this chapter.

BLENDED FAMILY

EJACULATORY INCOMPETENCE

EJACULATORY OR POSTEJACULATORY
    PAIN

EXHIBITIONISM

FETISHISM

HOMOSEXUAL LIFESTYLE

INHIBITED DESIRE

OPEN MARRIAGE

ORGASMIC DYSFUNCTION

PARAPHILIAS

PEDOPHILIA

PREMARITAL RELATIONSHIPS

PREMATURE EJACULATION

SADISM AND MASOCHISM

TRANSSEXUAL

TRANSVESTISM

VAGINISMUS

VOYEURISM

OBJECTIVES ■

After studying this chapter, the student will be able to

1. Distinguish among levels of nursing education and appropriate assessment and intervention strategies.
2. Summarize the stages in the human sexual response.
3. Compare and contrast the major models of adult relationships discussed in this chapter.
4. Discuss the major sexual dysfunctions found among males and females.
5. Identify therapeutic interventions for the sexual dysfunctions.
6. Describe gender identity disorders and medical interventions for them.
7. Define various sexual behaviors.
8. Recognize the different sexually transmitted diseases by their symptoms.

The major mental disorders have been covered in preceding chapters. However, there are several issues that can affect the mental health of some adults. Contemporary men and women face numerous social issues that can cause conflict, anxiety, and stress in their daily lives and that may ultimately affect their mental health in various ways. The number of stressors has increased as the world population has expanded and the personal and political boundaries between people have shrunk.

Social mores affecting the more personal aspects of people's lives have also changed dramatically in recent years. In earlier times, religious leaders were often responsible for setting standards of behavior and establishing expectations for personal life and loving. By the 1990s, although religious affiliation has risen slightly from its low point of the 1980s, there is no commonly accepted authority to take the place religious leaders once held.

Standards for marriage, family life, and sexual practices have been particularly affected, and wide variations are now being reported. A second look was taken at the famed 1924 sociological study by Robert and Helen Lynd of the industrial city they called "Middletown, USA" in 1982. By that time, the most significant changes that had occurred in "Middletown" had been in the area of sexuality and adult relationships (Caplow et al. 1982). What had previously been unacceptable and even illegal had become commonplace, and freedom of choice had become a widely accepted concept.

Americans, especially, have experienced numerous variations in standards, possibly due to the many different cultural and ethnic groups that make up our population. One of the early sexuality researchers, Havelock Ellis (1938), proposed that sexual customs are relative to each individual society. Because we are a "melting pot" of cultures, our sexual practices are

widely different. Although these variations provide people with a wide range of possibilities, they also can create a sense of conflict about which choices are right for them.

Nurses are often the first to hear of concerns regarding sexuality that are affecting the mental health of clients. Concern about changing family situations, sexual development and desires, and physical diseases are all issues that many people have difficulty discussing, especially in a formal setting. Thus, nurses can often encourage discussion by being aware of the importance of these concerns and by being receptive when clients make seemingly casual references to issues that are really of vital concern to them. Nurses can face the taboo that dictates that sexual issues are not the focus of "polite" conversation by encouraging questions and giving factual information when needed. This chapter focuses on interpersonal issues that may affect the mental health of some adults. The role of the nurse at different educational levels is defined. Guidelines for psychosexual assessment at the generalist level as well as appropriate interventions are presented.

The Role of the Nurse

Although foundations for nursing practice hold a holistic view, a client's sexuality is often not addressed in the treatment process. See "Nurse Speaks" at the beginning of Chapter 26. The nurse's background reflects education in the physical, social, and behavioral sciences, as well as theory and practice in counseling techniques. Because of this training, the nurse is an ideal member of the health team to counsel clients in the sensitive and highly charged area of human sexuality (Zalar 1982).

Acute, chronic, or disabling conditions necessitate alterations in the ways in which individuals express their sexuality. Adolescents and the aged have special issues and concerns regarding their sexuality. A nurse who is knowledgeable, nonjudgmental, and has good communication skills can play an important role in identifying potential problem areas and providing effective sex counseling or referral (Zalar 1982).

An example of need is identified in a study by Krueger et al. (1979) of premenopausal women who had hysterectomies for nonmalignant conditions. When asked for suggestions about how nurses could have assisted them with their sexual adjustment after surgery, 45 of 51 respondents indicated they would have liked nurses to have provided more information about sexual adjustment after surgery (Zalar 1982). The crippling or disfigurement resulting from surgery, disease, or injury can negatively affect a person's sexual identity and sense of attractiveness. Because nurses spend more time with clients than perhaps any other member of the health team, they are in a prime position to assess, educate, and support clients in areas that threaten sexual identity or impair sexual function (Zalar 1982).

How does one define the nurse's role in helping selected clients meet their sexual needs? Masters and Johnson described nurses as intermediaries between physicians who are uncomfortable with the topic of sexuality and clients who lack the knowledge of, or who have misconceptions about, sexuality and sexual practices (Hogan 1980). The World Health Organization describes the role of the nurse in terms of having a supportive relationship with clients who have sexual problems and helping in such matters as feminine hygiene, family planning, parents' dealing with sexual behaviors and questions of their children, and assisting teachers with sex education (Hogan 1980). Many nurses have greatly expanded their roles and work as sex therapists with individuals who express unmet sexual needs and impaired functioning. Not all nurses will go on to become sex therapists, but all nurses should be knowledgeable about the bio-psycho-social aspects of sexuality throughout the life cycle, the effects of various illnesses on sexual functioning, and the effects of psychological and sociocultural deprivations on human sexual functioning (Hogan 1980).

Four levels of sexual counseling have been described (Annon 1978; Zalar 1982):

1. *Permission*: reassurance that the client's sexual practices are normal, and professional "permission" to continue his or her usual practice. Permission can prevent the escalation of a major problem.
2. *Limited information*: providing information directly related to the client's concerns. Limited information

directly relating to the client's problem can effect significant changes in attitudes and behaviors.
3. *Specific suggestions*: direct attempts to assist the client to change behavior in order to reach stated goals. At this level, the nurse offers specific suggestions related to the client's particular problem.
4. *Intensive therapy*: when brief therapy has not been effective. At this level, the client is often referred to a professional with specific knowledge, experience, skills, and time to devote to specialized treatment.

Nurses working in acute or chronic care settings, schools, or nursing homes, on the generalist level, "should be able to competently assist clients with needs involving (1) permission and (2) limited information. These aspects of sexual health care are usually preventive in nature" (Mims 1977). Interventions on these levels include limited sex education and limited information about sexual feelings, behaviors, and myths (Zalar 1982). The other two levels, (3) specific suggestions and (4) intensive therapy, can be carried out by nurses with more specific training and advanced knowledge in the area of human sexuality, for example, a nurse educated at the practitioner level or at the master's level prepared in the area of human sexuality and therapy. The important prerequisites for a nurse in counseling a client about human sexuality on any level are knowledge, skill, and ease in discussing sex as an activity of daily living (Schuster et al. 1982).

Many nursing leaders encourage more sex education for nursing students in the nursing curricula, and believe that without training in sexuality, students might not have the necessary skills for sensitive and effective counseling. For example, students might not have the cognitive knowledge, the ability to recognize personal feelings, or the sensitivity to respond in an effective manner to reduce anxiety and enhance positive change. It is also believed that when sexuality has been altered, affected, or denied during the acute or chronic phases of illness, nurses should become aware of special problems their clients might be experiencing (Magenity 1975; Jacobson 1974; Zalar 1982).

Unique Assessment Strategies

There may be times when a physical condition or the result of surgery will alter or impair a person's sexual desire, ability to function, or sexual self-concept.

During the process of people's lives, there are many situations that can increase sexual tension and alter sexual drive, for example (Felstein 1986):

- Moving to a new house or apartment
- Moving to a new town or country
- Increasing traveling in one's occupation
- Starting a new career
- Doing regular or heavy gambling
- Using drugs or alcohol

Nurses, as all health professionals, must always be aware that their own cultural, religious, and sexual experiences and backgrounds affect the way they react to client's patterns that may be different from their own. When working with clients who may be having difficulty in sex-related areas or with sexually transmitted diseases (STDs), the nurse must remain nonjudgmental and open to the uniqueness of each person. Organizations such as the Sex Education and Information Council of the United States (SEICUS) are very helpful in providing the most recent statistics and bibliographies in the field. Keeping current in terms of knowledge and understanding of changing behaviors is an important skill in an area where self-evaluation should be ongoing.

For a person struggling with a physical or emotional problem or entering adolescence or advanced age, difficulties and concerns with sexual functioning are valid and vital issues.

Numerous physical conditions as well as medical interventions can alter sexual functioning and require counseling and information for the client to find alternative and satisfying means to attain his or her sexual goals. The following are only a sample of common recurring health problems that can alter sexual function and greatly affect a person's sense of attractiveness and identification as a sexual being.

For example, clients who have experienced a myocardial infarction will have concerns about sexual function. The most common cause of sexual dysfunction is lack of knowledge, resulting in fear. A client often believes that sexual intercourse will cause another heart attack. Fatigue, pain, and shortness of breath related to cardiovascular disease may also cause sexual dysfunction (Stier 1986).

Clients who have had a leg amputated may be able to function sexually but may see themselves as less attractive and worry about their partner's reactions.

Clients with disorders of the musculoskeletal system may also experience sexual dysfunction and disturbance in self-concept related to prolonged hospitalization, traction, casts, deformity, and pain. Sexual dysfunction can also be related to depression and anxiety resulting from the musculoskeletal disorder. Often, problems occur when the partner's perception of the client as a sexual being is altered, affecting their usual sexual relationship (McCausland 1986).

Clients with nervous system dysfunction may complain of sexual dysfunction as a result of insult to parasympathetic fibers from spinal cord segments S-2, S-3, and S-4; sympathetic fibers from the lumbar spine; or peripheral nerves from these segments (Markarian 1986).

Surgical procedures, such as ostomies, mastectomies, hysterectomies, and prostatectomies, can profoundly affect a person's self-concept and require definite sexual counseling and encouragement of expression.

Often, other side effects of various medications can cause sexual dysfunctions. For example, drugs that may cause *impotence* or *delayed ejaculation* in men and *decreased responsiveness* in women are

- *Phenothiazines* (e.g., thioridazine [Mellaril], chlorpromazine [Thorazine], and fluphenazine [Prolixin].)
- *Sedatives-hypnotics-opiates* (e.g., morphine, barbiturates, diazepam, and lithium carbonate)
- *Tricyclic antidepressants* (e.g., imipramine and desipramine)

Drugs that may induce *depression* are

- Antihypertensive drugs (e.g., reserpine, methyldopa, and propranolol)
- Ethyl alcohol

The following suggestions have been outlined by Cole et al. (1979) to help the nurse obtain information regarding sexual concerns or dysfunctions the client may be experiencing:

- Do not force the person to talk about sex.
- Place sexuality in the context of other problems.
- Do not force your own moral standards on the client.
- Conduct discussions in a clear and frank manner.
- Do not assume that once the topic has been talked about it is resolved.

Hogan (1980) suggests that the nurse have an introductory statement prepared. For example, "As a nurse I am concerned about all aspects of your health. However, we often neglect helping clients in what may be a very important part of their lives—their sexual needs. I'm going to ask you some questions in this area."

Woods (1984) has suggested using a three-question form called "A Brief Sexual History" to obtain information about a person's sexual functioning and concerns. The first question asks about *sexual roles*, the second question identifies the person's *sexual image*, and the third, *sexual functioning*.

1. Has anything (e.g., illness, pregnancy, or health problems) interfered with your being a (wife, husband, mother, father)?
2. Has anything (e.g., heart attack or mastectomy)

changed the way you feel about yourself as a (man, woman)?

3. Has anything (e.g., surgery or disease) changed your ability to function sexually?

Table 28–1 suggests some statements the nurse can use to facilitate communication for identifying more specific areas and opening up channels for future teaching and clarifying.

It is important for the nurse to use correct terminology, even though the client may use slang words for parts of the body or sexual acts. Slang or street terms often have emotionalized connotations for the person using them. For the nurse to use such terms can cast doubts on the nurse's professionalism or competence. Always verify words the client may use to make sure that both the nurse and the client are talking about the same thing (Hogan 1980).

Unique Intervention Strategies

All health care professionals working in the area of emotional and sexual issues must be aware that the intensity of involvement that often arises between provider and patient can present difficulties. **Sexual involvement with patients during the course of treatment is unethical and is almost always harmful to the patient whose trust has been violated.** In addition, both the American Psychological and American Psychiatric Associations have taken strong positions in their ethical codes prohibiting sexual involvement with clients. Some (Lazarus 1992) feel that this prohibition should include the provision that sexual involvement is *never* acceptable, even with a former

Table 28–1 ■ STATEMENTS THAT FACILITATE COMMUNICATION

SITUATION BEING EXPLORED	FACILITATING STATEMENT
Giving rationale for question	As a nurse, I'm concerned about all aspects of your health. Many individuals have concerns about sexual matters, especially when they are sick or when they are having other health problems.
Giving statements of "generality" or "normality"	Most people are hesitant to discuss . . . Many people worry about feelings . . . Many people have concerns about . . .
Identifying sexual dysfunction	Most people have difficulties at some time during their sexual relationships. Have you had any problems?
Obtaining information from an unmarried individual	The degree to which unmarried persons have sexual outlets varies considerably. Some have sexual partners, others have none, some relieve sexual tension through masturbation, others need no outlet at all. What has been your pattern?
Identifying sexual myths	While growing up, most of us have heard some sexual myths or half-truths that continue to puzzle us. Are there any that come to mind?
Identifying feelings about masturbation	Many of us grown-ups have heard various stories about masturbation and what problems it supposedly causes. This can cause worry even into adulthood. What have you heard?
Determining if homosexuality is a source of conflict	What is your attitude toward your homosexual orientation?
Identifying older individuals' concern about sexual functioning	Many people, as they get older, believe or worry that this signals the end of their sex life. Much misinformation surrounds this myth. What is your understanding about sexuality during the later years? How has the passage of time affected your sexuality (sex life)?
Obtaining and giving information (miscellaneous areas)	Frequently, people have questions about . . . What questions do you have about . . . What would you like to know about . . . ?
Closing the history	Is there anything further in the area of sexuality that you would like to bring up now? I hope that if questions or concerns do come to mind in the future we'll be able to discuss them.

Adapted from Green R. Human Sexuality: A Health Practitioner's Text. Baltimore: Williams & Wilkins, 1975.

patient, no matter how long a time has passed since the professional relationship ended. Therapists from all disciplines need to be aware of the possibility of inappropriate transfer of feelings to clients and must know that any such involvement can lead to severe emotional harm to their client and even to themselves. Thirteen states have passed laws that forbid psychiatrists and mental health professionals to have sex with clients. Nine of these states opted for criminalization of offenders, and other states chose mandatory reporting by subsequent therapists (Debate 1993).

From the sample of possible situations a nurse may encounter in the hospital setting, numerous nursing diagnoses become apparent. First, the obvious *altered sexuality patterns* or *sexual dysfunctions* related to various pathophysiological conditions, treatment modalities, or situations are often present. Some problems may be due to a *knowledge deficit*. Problems identifying sexual identity should be assessed for and may take the form of *disturbance in self-esteem*. Not only may the individual experience *ineffective coping*, but a disruption of usual sexual patterns and methods of sexual expres-sion in one partner may lead to *altered family processes*. When a person is left with a deformity or altered body image (e.g., after mastectomy or ostomy), *grieving* is a natural reaction, one that can also alter a person's sexual desire or ability to function.

Nurses intervene in areas of sexuality on many levels. Watts (1979) has identified various levels of assessment and intervention appropriate for certain levels of training (Table 28–2). At the generalist level, the nurse screens for sexual function and dysfunction. Nurse generalists will intervene at level one, which entails giving education and limited information about sexual feelings, behaviors, and myths. Nursing knowl-edge includes a sound understanding of sexual devel-opment, reproduction, sexual expression, sexual dys-function, and disease.

Hogan (1980) stresses awareness of beliefs, atti-tudes, and values because these directly influence how a person interacts with others. Values clarifica-tion on such topics as masturbation, dating, petting leading to orgasm, abortion, and homosexuality is an important area for self-evaluation. As nurses, we are entitled to our own feelings, attitudes, beliefs, and

Table 28–2 ■ LEVELS OF ASSESSMENT AND INTERVENTION*

PROFESSIONAL COMPETENCE REQUIRED	LEVELS OF ASSESSMENT	LEVELS OF THERAPEUTIC INTERVENTION
Level 1		
Nurse generalist	Health history ● Screen for sexual function and dysfunc-tion	Limited education: ● Limited information about sexual feel-ings, behaviors, and myths ● Refer to levels 2 or 3, if necessary
Level 2		
Professional nurse with postgraduate train-ing in sex education and counseling	Sexual history	Sex education and counseling: ● Specific information about sex and sexu-ality ● Concise suggestions about sexual fears and adaptations to illness and anticipa-tory guidance ● Refer to level 3, if necessary
Level 3		
Professional nurse, physician, psychologist, or social worker, all qualified as trained sex therapists	Sexual problem history	Sex therapy: ● Individual or group therapy ● Couple therapy ● Refer to level 4, if necessary
Level 4		
Psychiatric nurse clinician with an MSN, physician, psychologist, or social worker, all with subordinate specialty in sex ther-apy	Psychiatric and psychosexual history	Eclectic approach: ● Intensive individual psychotherapy, sex therapy, and marital therapy

* There is linear relationship between the depth of a patient's sexual problems and the kind of professional competence that is needed to assess and treat them.
Watts DW. Dimensions of sexual health. American Journal of Nursing Company. Copyright 1979 The American Journal of Nursing Company. Reprinted from American Journal of Nursing, September, 1979, Volume 79, No. 9. Used with permission. All rights reserved.
MSN = Master of Science, Nursing.

standards regarding sexuality; however, clients under our care are equally entitled to theirs, without censure or criticism.

Specific sex education and counseling, sex therapy, and individual and marital therapy are appropriate for nurses with postgraduate training in sex education and above. Therefore, nurse generalists need to recognize when referrals are indicated and know whom to contact.

Hogan (1980) goes on to stress that skill and sensitivity in understanding the client's concerns and relating empathically to them are as important as specific knowledge to answer the client's concerns. Nurses are needed to promote sexual health in the home, schools, clinics, hospitals, nursing homes, and extended care facilities. Nurses at all levels are in prime positions to educate parents, community groups, school groups, and teachers on STDs, especially acquired immunodeficiency syndrome (AIDS) (refer to Chapter 26).

In the discussion to follow, dealing with psychosexual disorders, specific interventions are the province of the professional staff with specific training in sexuality and therapy—nurses, social workers, psychologists, or psychiatrists.

Issues That Affect the Mental Health of Some Adults

VARIETIES OF ADULT RELATIONSHIPS

People today are more unlikely than in the past to accept a static, unsatisfying marriage. Changing economic needs and societal norms are such that we are more open to various patterns. Concerns about the development of intimacy (close personal relationships) are widely discussed phenomena that affect the lifestyle choices of many adults (Herron and Rouslin 1984). By 1991, 45% of women aged 25–29 reported having cohabited with a man, and 35% of women aged 15–44 had done so. Some of the choices women make will be discussed in this chapter, with an emphasis on how they affect women's general mental health.

Premarital Relationships

Once believed to be the legal and moral right of only the married, sexual activity is now considered by some to be completely acceptable for any consenting adult. According to a report published by the National Center for Health Statistics (1985), more than 75% of American women are beginning sexual activity prior to

marriage, and almost all males are doing so. Marriage, formerly viewed by many as a necessity of adult life, is clearly no longer the only acceptable pattern. This is a sharp increase from a previous survey in the early 1960s, which showed 48% of women delaying intercourse until marriage. Indeed, the practice has become so commonplace that the Roman Catholic Council of Cardinals, meeting in 1985, felt it necessary to reiterate that premarital intercourse was not permitted according to that church's law.

For the young people involved, a new emotional difficulty has sometimes replaced the old one of "should we or shouldn't we?" It consists of a feeling reported especially by young women that they *must* have intercourse after a few dates. If one does not engage in sex, his or her maturity is suspect. The pressures of fear of pregnancy are largely dismissed (unrealistically, as one in every five babies born in the United States is out of wedlock and usually unplanned). The fear of the spread of disease does not appear to be sufficiently high to alter most heterosexual behavior, although the advent of AIDS has changed sexual practices for many. The change seems to be in the use of condoms and the practice of "safer sex," however, and not in abstinence. Most young people do marry, and thus the premarital sex issue is put to rest for them. There is, however, an increasingly large group of adults who have never married.

The Never-Married Adult

The ranks of the never-married adult are steadily increasing in the industrialized nations. Demographers predict that the number of never-married adults will double by the year 2000. This relatively new phenomenon has not been evident long enough to afford us much statistical information, but the impact of the group seems to be increasingly powerful. By 1980, nearly 18 million Americans were living alone, although some of these had been previously married (Wolfe 1982). However, this statistic does not reflect lesbians and gay men in relationships, just the "single" or the "unmarried." Typically, on completion of as much schooling as was thought desirable, young people would begin to actively look for marriage partners. Although this is still true in many cases, it has become much more acceptable for men and women to reach age 25 or older without having married. Indeed, in 1991, marriage rates were at the lowest level since 1967. Economic independence and opportunity have dramatically changed the lifestyles of many in this group, affording them the opportunity to live independent of their family of origin. Sexual activity is frequent and the stereotypical "old maid" image has all but disappeared. Numerous problems do exist for this group, as they begin to age and find fewer societal supports for themselves than do other groups. Potential partners often leave the group for marriage, making it increasingly hard to find suitable choices. As members of the family of origin die or move, single adults may find themselves lonely and lacking for companionship. Worries about who will care for them in their old age become significant, and financial support in times of trouble is more tenuous than for those with a more comprehensive family network. Nonetheless, more and more adults are making the choice to never marry and many report satisfaction with their independent and self-sufficient lives.

Traditional Marriage

Traditional marriage was, at one time, the goal of most of the American population. During most of this century it was considered inappropriate and even unlawful to have sex outside of marriage. Career choices outside of motherhood were very limited for women, and unmarried men beyond a certain age were often regarded with suspicion. Cross-racial and cross-religious unions were unusual, and divorce was considered quite scandalous and reserved for only the most serious of reasons.

A typical traditional marriage today contains many of these features, although there have been some significant changes. According to the National Center for Health Statistics (1985), the large numbers of people born after World War II (the "baby-boomers") have postponed marriage to further their education and careers. The marriage age for both men and women has been moving upward, with men having a first marriage at age 24 and women at 21. Once married, the age of women having their first baby has also risen, and the total number of children born to a married couple has declined. Although a 1991 survey of young women indicated that 66% would like to remain at home with children if possible, more than 80% of wives today work outside of the home. Sixty-seven percent of those with children under age 18 are in the work force. Thus a typical modern marriage might be like that of Ellen and Joe.

Ellen is a 24-year-old dental assistant. She has an associate's degree from a community college and is taking a night course working toward another degree. She works for a local dentist four days a week. She and Joe have been married for two years. They live in a condominium on which they have a large mortgage. Joe is a technician for a public utility. He has had two years of college. Because he is a union member, his job is secure, although his hours are long and he must work overtime during emergencies. Joe and Ellen met during high school. He was raised a Catholic and she a Protestant. They attend services at her parents' church on Easter and Christmas. They plan to have children in a few years when they can better afford a maternity leave for her.

Joe and Ellen had been seriously involved with other people during college. Although neither was a virgin at the time of their marriage, they expect that they will be sexually exclusive with one another. One area of conflict for them has been Joe's desire to continue to "hang out" with his buddies from work after hours. He often will stop for a beer or to watch a game with them. Ellen feels that this interferes with their relationship as a couple and reminds him that both their sets of parents had their spouses as their best friend.

Otherwise, they agree on most issues. Ellen does most of the housekeeping chores, although Joe does help her. Although their parents are pressuring them for grandchildren, they are very satisfied with their decision to wait a few more years. They have sex three or four times a week and have no fear of pregnancy because Ellen is taking birth control pills.

Open Marriage

Open marriage is the name given to a relatively new concept that accepts free sexual interaction with those other than one's spouse. First popularized in the 1960s (O'Neill and O'Neill 1974), it does not mean marital "cheating," in which one partner engages in extramarital sex without the knowledge or consent of the other. Instead, a couple agrees that together or separately, they will be involved in sexual activity with others. Although the phenomenon of open marriage has received a great deal of publicity, it does not appear to be prevalent in reality. In several surveys, only between 2% and 4% of married couples reported having engaged in this activity (Goldberg, 1985). Typical comments from couples who have attempted open sexual activities include, "We hardly have time for sex with each other let alone outsiders," and "It has taken so long to build an intimate and warm relationship with one partner. I wouldn't want to take the chance of destroying it," and the practical and true, "The risk of picking up a disease just isn't worth it."

Those few who do participate in open marriages over a period of time, however, seem very enthusiastic. Members of The Lifestyle Organization, based in Anaheim, California, actively promote open marriage and alternative lifestyles in human sexuality. They report enhancement of their marriages, relief from boredom, and openness and spontaneity, which they feel did not exist for them previously. They say, it is far better for a marriage to proceed on a foundation of honesty about sexual desire for others than to fall prey to the "cheating" type of extramarital behavior that prevails in so many traditional marriages. Both Kinsey and Hunt found that around 45% of men and 20% of women had at least one secret incident of extramarital sex. This kind of clandestine affair is much more devastating if discovered than an open sexual arrangement. Thus far, the social and legal codes of conduct of most cultures do not permit "open marriages," nor does this standard seem likely to change in the immediate future.

Divorce

Not many years ago, divorce was considered so unacceptable that it was grounds for expulsion from "polite society." Politicians who divorced were considered unelectable, and many legal statutes made it next to impossible to dissolve a marriage without grave cause. Yet divorce has become almost commonplace today, with approximately 45% (almost half) of all American marriages ending in divorce (McNeil 1992). Government studies show that 20% of first marriages end in divorce within five years (up from under 10%, 10 years ago) indicating that there is less interest than in earlier years in "sticking it out." Indeed, in 1991, marriage rates were at their lowest level since 1967. By 1991, 78.6% of every 1000 women and 109.7 of every 1000 men reported having been divorced.

Societal attitudes toward divorce have changed as the numbers of divorced people have increased. There is little if any taboo or social censure if children are not involved. Divorced persons almost always begin dating and resume sexual activity within a year of divorce, with 100% of the men and over 80% of the women reporting active sex lives.

Many divorced people express dissatisfaction with their lives, however. Society does not have a role for them, and many feel a sense of personal failure at not having made their marriage work. Financial pressures are often an additional burden in the form of alimony and child support issues. Loneliness can become a problem, and many divorced people begin to look for new partners as soon as possible. In fact, divorced people who do remarry tend to do so within five years of their breakup. Today, about 33% of all marriages involve at least one partner who has been married before (Glick 1980).

Remarried or Blended Family

As the divorce rate has risen, so has the rate of families in which one or both partners may have children from a former marriage. Given many names, such as "stepfamilies," **"blended families,"** and "remarried families," most of the participants seem to prefer to be thought of just as a "family." Because about 75% of divorced parents do remarry (Calderone and Johnson 1981), as do most widows and widowers with young children, many children become someone's stepchild for at least a portion of their lives.

These new family units becomes complicated as various new roles are created. There may be stepsiblings present in the home. New babies become a challenge for a half-sibling and create a bond between the adult partners that the older children may resent or fear. Some children end up with many sets of relatives, "old" and "new" grandparents, cousins, friends, and even homes.

Donna and Rory are examples of parents who have created a blended family. Donna was divorced three years ago from John. She receives child support payments from John, who has the children visit every other weekend and for one month in the summer. John has remarried a young woman, who is expecting a baby in several months. Rory is divorced from Cathy. He has joint custody of his son, who spends Monday through Thursday with his mother and Friday through Sunday with Rory. Cathy has remarried Jim, who has a 16-year-old daughter who lives in a distant state and who spends two weeks at Christmas and the entire summer with her father.

Donna and Rory would like to have a child together but fear the complication. At present, their combined three children have several sets of parents and siblings to deal with. It is virtually impossible to arrange family vacations, as Donna's children are with their father when Rory's son is with him, and the involvement of the new spouse's children makes it impossible to change plans.

The children in this "remarried" family must deal with various adults in different ways. Family rules and customs often vary from house to house. Religious convictions and financial status may differ, sometimes making the children feel as if they must fend for themselves in constantly changing situations. The parents involved have the problem of divided loyalty between new spouse, original child, new spouse's children by a previous marriage, and possibly new children produced in the new marriage. When former partners are hostile or are still involved in disputes concerning finances or child custody, the situation may become almost unworkable.

In intact families, family members can be expected to help one another in times of stress and difficulty. Each person's problem creates a network of responses that usually lead to emotional balance. The family becomes the mediator between its members and the world. This kind of response is altered in the blended family, but it does not have to disappear. Some extended family groups are able to continue to function in supportive ways even though traditional patterns have changed. Despite some times of confusion, the larger numbers of people involved can supply various resources and emotional experiences for those involved.

Single-Parent Family

Quite the opposite of the many adults usually found in a blended family is the ever-growing number of families led by one parent. Once almost exclusively the result of death or divorce, single parenthood has become an option of choice for more and more people.

As mentioned earlier, many adults are now choosing to never marry, but this situation may not mean a choice not to raise children. It is becoming more commonplace for women to have children although unmarried, and pregnancies are sometimes arranged via artificial insemination or unknowing partner with no thought that more than one parent will raise the child. Adoption by single people has become a possibility, especially in the case of the "hard-to-place" child. Despite media attention to the single father or deliberately pregnant single woman, the overwhelming majority of single parents are women who have reached that status accidentally, that is, via an unplanned pregnancy or divorce. About 45% of children today spend some of or all their early years with only one parent (McNeil 1992).

Often, the situation is one of stress and discomfort for both parent and child. In fact, income inequality and the lessening number of those in the middle class of the US economy are attributable to families headed by single mothers who are unable to work (McNeil 1992). Unless finances are no problem, a child may be left unattended or in an inadequate day care or babysitting arrangement while the parent works. Without a partner to confide in or share burdens with, a single parent can become overly confiding in the child and may give the child too many responsibilities too soon. In many two-parent families,

at least one parent is available, either part- or full-time during the day, and so is able to participate in school functions and activities. This is rarely the case for the single parent and can create added conflict.

The single parent who lives in close contact with an extended family or network of friends seems to have the best situation. If others are available to help with child-rearing and finances, the job is made easier.

Lesbian and Gay Men's Relationships

Sexual activity between members of the same sex has been evident throughout history and in every culture. In the last part of the twentieth century, old taboos and prejudices about homosexuality have begun to change, and legislative, religious, and social acceptance has become somewhat more widespread. Lesbians and gay men have become an increasingly visable part of society. Homophobic feelings still exist and are evident in the all-too-frequent incidents of physical violence against gays (gay bashing). Magazines such as *Out*, which targets the mature and openly gay market, are being published, and support groups such as "Parents and Friends of Gays and Lesbians" and "Gay Men's Health Crisis" count membership among heterosexual and homosexual people. Lesbians and gay men participate in all of the lifestyles already discussed, including marriage and single parenting. A change in recent years is that many lesbians and gay men no longer feel the need to hide their sexual orientation and in increasing numbers are openly stating their sexual orientation.

The process of "coming out," which is the recognition of one's homosexuality to oneself, family, or the greater community, is recognized as a pivotal experience for lesbians and gay men (Marcus 1992). This emotional and often political decision can be counted among life's stressors and as such may come to the attention of the nurse or counselor working with an individual or a family. Misinformation still abounds regarding the origins of this orientation, and fears concerning AIDS are reported to be foremost in families' minds when they learn that one of their members is homosexual.

In fact, the origin of homosexuality is an area of debate. Theories range from the concept that this sexual preference is genetically determined, to the idea that it is caused by early childhood experiences or is hormonally influenced. The majority of people with **homosexual lifestyles** are well adjusted and lead satisfying and productive lives.

The fear of AIDS is a valid one, with 58% of cases in 1992 resulting from male homosexual activity. Progress is being made in slowing the spread of this disease through the active participation of many gay men in safer-sex workshops. Lesbians are in the lowest AIDS risk group. The number of people involved in homosexual activity is difficult to estimate. Sometimes, the activity is only situational and exists because there are no other partners available, as might be the case with a person in prison. On the other hand, a person may be firmly convinced that he or she is homosexual and has sexual fantasies that involve only partners of the same sex. Due to religious or social pressure, the person may choose never to act on these fantasies, and yet could probably be called homosexual. We do know that about 37% of all men and 13% of all women have had at least one sexual same-sex experience (Kinsey et al. 1948, 1953). Among these, approximately 60% of both sexes have lived in a coupled relationship or a single one with numbers of partners, which they considered satisfactory (Bell and Weinberg 1978). In fact, over 50% of the men in Bell and Weinberg's lengthy study (1978) reported that they had had more than 500 sexual partners each. This percentage has decreased in recent years because the AIDS crisis has led to changes in the lifestyles of many gay men. Partners are fewer in number, and safer sex is being practiced on a more regular basis (Ecstrand and Coates 1990). One lifestyle of a gay man can be seen in the case of Bart.

Bart was born the third child and only son of middle-class Catholic parents. From early childhood on he had a strong interest in the games of his sisters, and in his earliest sexual fantasies, he almost exclusively chose other males as his partners. When Bart goes away to college, he is approached by an older boy, who initiates his first sexual experience. Thereafter, he is involved in a number of brief encounters with fellow male students and older men. He struggles with the issue of "coming out" for several years. Bart fears disapproval from his parents and fears for his chances at career advancement in the banking field. When Bart finally confides in his sister, she advises him to enter therapy to "cure" his homosexuality, but Bart has no desire to do this. He has not come out at work and in fact has felt the need to invent a broken engagement to protect himself from questions about his social life. He would like to have a permanent relationship, but that has not happened yet. Recent legislation protecting homosexuals from job discrimination has been encouraging, but he is not yet trusting of its usefulness in his competitive firm.

As attitudes and laws continue to change in a posi-

tive way, the chances for all people to live openly will increase.

Jamie was 20, married, and attending a local college when she met Rhoda. They quickly became friends and greatly enjoyed the political discussions begun in their history class. Jamie had been married to Ron at 18 at her parents' urging. Her parents believed a traditional role was best for women and were long-time friends of Ron's well-to-do parents. Jamie did not have much sexual experience when she was married and assumed that her lack of interest in sex with Ron was "just the way it is" for most women. Otherwise, her marriage was happy enough and she and Ron were good friends.

Rhoda had been involved with both men and women before she met Jamie. She was politically active in the campus women's movement and was becoming convinced of her own lesbianism. She was attracted to Jamie from the start and began to encourage her to join her friends in their activities. After a few months, Jamie and Rhoda became lovers. Jamie found sex with a woman an entirely different and better experience than with Ron. About one year after the women met, Ron and Jamie had their marriage annulled. Jamie immediately moved in with Rhoda and has been with her for 11 years. The women have been quite active in the lesbian liberation movement, and Rhoda, who became a teacher, successfully sued the city board of education for the right to be a classroom teacher even though openly gay. Jamie occasionally sees Ron, who has remarried, and neither bears any resentment.

Because of the somewhat dramatic nature of the marriage breakup, Jamie never had to worry about when to "come out" to her parents. They knew from the start. At first they were very upset and unaccepting, but as the years went by and their daughter seemed happy and in a stable relationship, their attitude softened. Rhoda and Jamie are quite content in their life together and have a large circle of friends both straight and gay.

The possibility of living in an open and accepted living relationship increases the quality of life for Rhoda and Jamie. As more people gain knowledge about homosexuality and as some of the homophobic bias of the past diminishes, it should be possible for more gay people to create a happy life for themselves. Deevey (1993) acknowledges the complications for gay men and lesbian women in sharing their lifestyles with others in a still-homophobic society. Table 28–3 offers suggestions to lesbian women for responding to the various reactions of people who are threatened by alternative sexual lifestyles.

Table 28–3 ■ HOMOPHOBIC REACTIONS TO LESBIAN SELF-DISCLOSURE

REACTION	PRIVATE RESPONSE	PUBLIC RESPONSE
"You're a sinner."	The God-Hates-You Attack	"I respect your religious beliefs, but I insist that you treat me with respect."
"You're fired."	The Financial-Ruin Attack	"This is a very emotional topic. Let's discuss it when we've both had a chance to think about this."
"Your mother/father was cold/sick/weak and caused you to be a lesbian."	The Child-of-Bad-Parents Attack	"We don't really know what causes either heterosexual or homosexual orientation. About 10% of all people are gay and lesbian, whatever their family background."
"You're an ugly woman who couldn't get a man."	The Body Image Attack	"Stereotypes about lesbians often include physical unattractiveness, man-hating, or lack of heterosexual experience, but none of these stereotypes are true."
"You should be ashamed—you bring danger/humiliation to this family/profession/neighborhood/nation."	The Guilt Trip Attack	"I am proud and happy to be a lesbian. I'd be glad to answer your questions about lesbian culture."
"I'll report you to the authorities. They'll take away your child."	The Unfit Mother Attack	"I am confident that I am a good parent to my child. She/he benefits from the courage and wisdom I have gained in dealing with my oppression as a lesbian."
"A patient complained to the head nurse that you asked him if he is gay. Why did you do that?"	The Professional Integrity Attack	"I believe each patient should be asked about sexual orientation to make clear that we offer good care to *all* patients."
"I'll tell your partner's parents/employer/grandmother."	The Attack on the Closeted Partner	"You can threaten me with scandal, but blackmail is illegal, and I will sue you."
"Are you the little boy or the little girl?"	The Lesbians-as-Pseudoheterosexuals Attack	(Some questions I don't dignify with an answer.)
"It's OK with me if you're a lesbian, so long as you keep your hands off my neck."	The Predatory Lesbian Attack	"We lesbians make pretty clear distinctions between courting and friendship with women. I think you'll continue to feel safe with me."
"You mean all this time you didn't tell me? Why don't you trust me?"	The Lesbians-Are-Liars Attack	"Try to imagine for the next 48 hours that you are a lesbian. It takes courage and compromise to survive in a hostile environment."
"You're so comfortable talking about lesbian issues, I can't believe you get angry or scared about homophobia."	The Looks-So-Easy Attack	"I do accept myself. But the world is still hostile and violent toward gay and lesbian people. I never can predict if I'll be safe in a new situation."
"There's no reason to do research on lesbian women, no need to provide special services. You have convinced me that lesbian women are no different from other women."	The Denial-of-Difference Attack	"It's true that lesbian women are not 'different' in the sense of being emotionally disturbed or sinful or criminal. But the prejudice against us causes minority stress and has generated a hidden lesbian culture that few straight people know about."
"When you get AIDS, I'll take care of you."	The So-Much-to-Learn Attack	"Lesbian women are actually the lowest-risk population for AIDS, but I appreciate your support."
"You're disgusting and sick."	The Blatant Attack	"I see you have a problem. I'd be glad to recommend a good therapist."
"I never met one before."	The Honest Truth Response—one I respect	"Well, you're in luck. If you want to know more about gay and lesbian culture, I love to answer questions. I've been asked all kinds of things, so don't be shy."

From Deevey S. Lesbian self-disclosure strategies for success. Journal of Psychosocial Nursing, 31(4):25, 1993.

SEXUALITY

Becoming a Sexual Being

We have come a long way since Freud first shocked his Victorian readers by arguing that sexual feelings and response did not just burst on the scene in adolescence. The sexual instinct, it turned out, was present from birth, and in a much more complex and encompassing way than had ever been previously imagined. *First,* human sexuality is an evolving concept that includes cognitive, affective, social, and instinctual-psychological responses. Second, this development takes place in stages that build on and can affect each other, both positively and negatively. Review Chapter 1 for psychosexual stages of development.

Sexuality is a part of human behavior throughout the life cycle. Now we know that infants, toddlers, and elementary school children are just as much sexual beings as adolescents and adults. We also know that the way parents and other adults respond to children affects subsequent psychosexual development. Still, many people remain reluctant to accept the facts of sexual development. Denial is too frequent, and ignorance about sexual behavior is found on all socioeconomic and educational levels. Nurses can help resolve a number of these problems with a straightforward presentation of facts that will help clients understand their children's needs. As Freud (1905) noted, children have sexual instincts that motivate a great deal of their lifelong behavior.

What Freud saw as a preadolescent latency period in regard to sex actually contains considerable private sexual activity. We are also learning a great deal about female sexuality, an area in which the early psychoanalysts had their confusions. In this regard, Masters and Johnson (1966) have shown the validity, and value, of the clitoral orgasm as opposed to the previously suggested superiority of the vaginal orgasm. Freud's greatest contribution was opening up the discussion of sexuality and sexual development. Previously, little was known or discussed, and as a result, parents had no idea how to view the sexual development of their children. We are now aware of the importance of our reactions as a child passes through the various stages. These early experiences in emotional relating have important consequences in later years. A positive and accepting attitude by parents provides a background for the child to have satisfactory adult relationships. An informed nurse is aware of developmental patterns and uses his or her knowledge to help parents adjust to the child in different ways at different times. For example, if a mother of a two-year-old expresses dismay at the child's unexpected resurgence of clinging behavior, it can be explained that this is a part of necessary reassurance and is to be expected, not feared. When working with adult clients, it is useful to relate their current state to earlier patterns. If the adult did not satisfactorily pass through each stage, he or she may become stuck or fixated at a given level. This fixation may occur because of parental errors, misfortunes, or pathologies and can range from severe to mild.

The Human Sexual Response

The importance of events in the early years of life on an adult's sexual patterns is indeed striking. For years, psychoanalytic theory has struggled with these issues in an attempt to assist adults in making fuller lives for themselves. Only recently, however, have we had adequate physiological knowledge of what occurs during a normal sexual response cycle.

In 1966, William Masters and Virginia Johnson published the results of their 12-year research project with almost 700 subjects (Masters and Johnson 1966). Using such devices as an electrocardiograph to measure changes in heart rate, a pH meter to measure acidity of the vagina, an electromyograph to measure muscular contractions, and an artificial penis, complete with a recording apparatus inside, they began to collect the first verifiable data on the sexual response cycle during intercourse and masturbation. Over 10,000 sexual cycles were observed in men and women under conditions including fatigue, drug use, pregnancy, and old age. The resulting information is of profound importance to the field of sexology and has provided a factual basis for the relatively new techniques of sex therapy. Basically, Masters and Johnson discovered that there is one sexual response pattern for males and three basic patterns for females (Figs. 28–1 and 28–2).

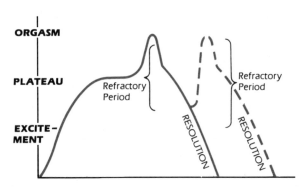

Figure 28–1. *Male sexual response cycle. (Redrawn from Masters WH, Johnson VE. Human Sexual Response. Boston: Little, Brown & Company, 1966.)*

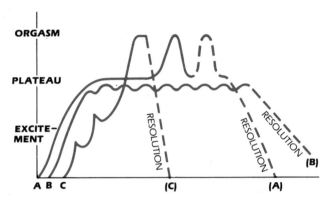

Figure 28-2. *Female sexual response cycle. (Redrawn from Masters WH, Johnson VE. Human Sexual Response. Boston: Little, Brown & Company, 1966.)*

In both males and females, the sexual response cycle begins with *stage one, the excitement phase.* During the onset of erotic feeling, males will experience erection of the penis, and females will begin vaginal lubrication and often have swelling of the breasts and labia and "tenting" of the cervix and uterus. Blood pressure and pulse increase, and some people experience a reddening of the skin called "sex flush." This leads to *stage two*, called *plateau*, if effective stimulation is continued. Here sexual tensions are intensified and will lead to the relatively brief *third stage* of orgasm. A sense of orgasmic inevitability is produced in which the person cannot stop the orgasm. During these 10 seconds or so males will usually expel semen and females will often experience uterine contraction.

After orgasm, both men and women will proceed to *stage four*, that of *resolution*. In males, this stage is usually rapid, with the penis returning to its unstimulated size. The female clitoris will also return to normal position, and the uterus begins to shrink. This phase generally takes 15-30 minutes in women.

During the resolution stage, males will enter the refractory period, during which they cannot be aroused again. Age, culture, and expectation seem to determine the length of this period, which varies from minutes to days and from male to male.

The information the sexology community obtained from this research has both educational and therapeutic value. Indeed, one of the primary motives for conducting these studies originally was to aid those experiencing some kind of sexual dysfunction. Masters and Johnson have estimated that over 30% of American couples suffer a dysfunction (Masters and Johnson 1970), and they and other sexologists have developed a number of very specific techniques to deal with various male and female sexual dysfunctions.

SEXUAL DISORDERS

Refer to Table 28-4 for an overview of the DSM-III-R classification of psychosexual disorders. Sexual dysfunctions are one group of sexual disorders. Paraphilias are another and will be discussed subsequently.

In both male and female charts, a disorder called **inhibited desire** is listed. Kaplan (1979) contends that this disorder is the most common among couples requesting sex therapy. The DSM-III-R refers to this disorder as *hypoactive sexual desire disorder.* Lack of desire is typified by deficient or absent sexual desire or fantasies, and a decline in sexual activity with no particular wish for this to improve. In cases where both partners, man and woman, suffer from this problem, there is usually no conflict. Only if there is a desire for a child, or if one of the partners becomes dissatisfied with the minimal or nonexistent sexuality, is a sex therapist consulted. This dysfunction is sometimes situational, for example, occurring during times of unusual stress at work or the birth of a child. Sometimes, the dysfunction can be accounted for when one of the partners becomes involved sexually elsewhere. Thus, a man having a secret love affair may not be suffering from the sexual disorder of inhibited desire but rather from the marital problem of no longer being interested in his wife. For married couples, sexual intercourse two to three times a week is considered average. Substantially less sex than this or failure of the male to have or maintain an erection 25% of the time or failure of the woman to lubricate much of the time are all symptoms of inhibited desire (Kaplan 1974).

Sexual Dysfunction

MALES. *Sexual aversion disorder* is a disorder characterized by persistent or recurrent extreme aversion to, and avoidance of, all, or almost all, genital sexual contact with a sexual partner.

Erective incapacity is a disorder of the excitement phase of the sexual response cycle, which is included in inhibited desire but which can be separate from it. Formally referred to as impotence, it is estimated that over half of the male population has this experience some of the time.

Premature ejaculation used to be the most commonly presented sexual difficulty of males, but the effective therapeutic techniques used with this difficulty have reduced it to second place, behind inhibited desire. There are many ways to define what is premature. Some have suggested that any ejaculation occurring before the partner is satisfied is premature.

Table 28-4 ■ PSYCHOSEXUAL DISORDERS*	
DISORDER (DEFINITION)	**EXAMPLE**
Paraphilias	
Arousal in response to sexual objects or situations that are not part of normal arousal activity patterns	Fetishism Transvestism Zoophilia Pedophilia Exhibitionism Voyeurism Sexual masochism Sexual sadism
Sexual Dysfunctions	
Inhibitions in the repetitive or psycho-physiological changes that character-ize the normal sexual response cycle	Inhibited sexual desire Inhibited sexual excitement Inhibited orgasm Premature ejaculation Functional dyspareunia Functional vaginismus
Ego-dystonic Homosexuality	
Persistent distress around unwanted homosexual arousal and absent or weak heterosexual arousal that inter-feres with wanted heterosexual rela-tionships	
Gender Identity Disorders	
Disorders first evidenced in childhood or adolescence	Transsexualism
Sense of discomfort and inappropriate-ness about one's anatomic sex and wish to be of the other sex	Gender identity disorder of childhood or adulthood

Adapted from American Psychiatric Association. Diagnostic and Statistical Manual of Mental Disorders, Third Edition, Revised (DSM-III-R). Washington, DC: American Psychiatric Association, 1987.
* Disorders related to sexuality in which psychological factors are assumed to be of major etiological significance.

Others suggest that ejaculation occurring before the man wishes it to more than 50% of the time is premature. However, this definition could include those who wish to engage in sex for hours before they ejaculate, so that hardly seems to be a fair description. The usual duration of coitus is between four and seven minutes, so anything less than a two-minute erection more than half the time could be considered premature. It is not uncommon for some males who suffer from this difficulty to come to orgasm even before they can proceed from foreplay to intercourse.

Ejaculatory incompetence, or retarded ejaculation, is a relatively rare phenomenon in which the male becomes repeatedly erect and wishes to ejaculate but cannot. This occurs in one in 700 men and is called *inhibited male orgasm* in the DSM-III-R. Pain in the testi-cles will often occur after a length of time of erection with no ejaculatory release.

Ejaculatory or postejaculatory pain can also lead to sexual dysfunction as the experience of intercourse becomes more and more unpleasant. While not very common, those afflicted can suffer for minutes or even hours. See Table 28–5 for an overview of male sexual dysfunctions.

FEMALES. In females, *inhibited desire* or *hypoactive sexual desire* is typified by lack of vaginal lubrication and a lack of interest in sex. Often referred to as *"frigidity,"* this disorder seems to affect many women at times of stress or physical illness, but only a small number of women all the time.

Orgasmic dysfunction, or inhibited female orgasm, is the most commonly presented female problem.

Table 28-5 ■ MALE SEXUAL DYSFUNCTIONS		
PROBLEM	**PHASE**	**MAJOR SYMPTOM**
Inhibited desire	Arousal-excitement	No erection, no sexual interest
Erective incapacity	Arousal-excitement	No or partial erection 50% of the time
Premature ejaculation	Orgasmic	Ejaculation before he wishes 50% of the time
Ejaculatory incompetence	Orgasmic	No or rare ejaculation
Ejaculatory pain	Orgasmic	Pain upon or just after ejaculation much of the time

Some of those women involved are not interested in orgasm in any case, but many are very interested in being able to fully enjoy sex. These women are taking an increasingly active role in assuring themselves of this experience.

Sexual Pain Disorders. Vaginismus is the disorder in which the vaginal muscles involuntarily go into spasms during intercourse. This can cause great pain and lead to inhibited desire as well.

Dyspareunia is persistent genital pain in either a male or female before, during, or after sex. Table 28-6 gives an overview of female sexual dysfunctions.

CAUSES. The difficulties people have in creating a satisfactory sexual life can often be treated through various behavioral and psychodynamic techniques by a professional with special training in this area. Many nurses have joined other health professionals in taking the additional training needed to become a certified sex educator/therapist through the American Association of Sex Educators, Counselors and Therapists (AASECT), based in Washington, DC.

It is believed that *biological causes* of sexual dysfunction occur in only 20% or fewer of presenting cases. Biological causes include general illness, e.g., the flu, colds, or fatigue, and certain diseases, in addition to those mentioned earlier, such as diabetes, hepatitis, and multiple sclerosis. Hormonal disorders in which medications cause a drop in androgen, such as hypopituitary problems and the feminization of testicular tumors, also may cause sexual dysfunction. Alcohol and hard drug use (cocaine and heroin) decrease sexual drive. As mentioned, hypertensive drugs and the phenothiazines can affect sexual performance in some clients. Other physical conditions that can cause pain are arthritis, back pain, obesity, vaginal infection, or late stages of pregnancy. Age can be a factor in sexual dysfunction in several ways. Postmenopausal women may need more lubrication, and older men may find they do not ejaculate as frequently as they did when they were younger. Also, if a partner is lost through death or divorce and the one remaining has no sexual activity for a period of years, he or she may find it hard to regain sexual function. Age in itself does not cause dysfunction, however, and many couples report active and satisfactory sex lives well into their eighties.

Psychological causes of sexual dysfunction can be attributed to the following:

- Ignorance as to what actions are stimulating for oneself or partner
- Anxiety due to fear of failure
- Demand for performance or an excessive need to please the partner
- Perceptual and intellectual defenses that get in the way of eroticism, such as "not feeling"
- Turning off with judgmental thoughts and becoming engrossed in self-observation instead of participation
- Poor relationship choices that can result in

Table 28-6 ■ FEMALE SEXUAL DYSFUNCTIONS		
PROBLEM	**PHASE**	**MAJOR SYMPTOM**
Inhibited desire	Arousal	No lubrication, little interest
Orgasmic dysfunction	Orgasmic	Inability to have orgasm most of the time
Vaginismus	Orgasmic	Involuntary, painful spasms during intercourse

partner rejection, lack of trust, power struggles, and other sexual sabotage that virtually guarantee that sex will not be rewarding

Various schools of psychology take different approaches to the causes of sexual problems. Adherents of psychoanalytic theory explore unconscious conflicts connected to critical childhood experiences, such as guilt regarding sexuality, incestuous wishes, and the inability to trust and love another person. Adherents of systems theory emphasize the pathological transactions between partners that can create a sexually destructive environment, and behavior theorists see specific conditioned reactions impairing sexual response as a result of aversive contingencies that have followed sexual behavior.

TREATMENT. Treatment of the various dysfunctions is based on much of the pioneering efforts of sexologists like Masters and Johnson and Helen Singer Kaplan. Specially trained nurses and other sex therapists seem to blend behavioral and psychodynamic techniques.

When a couple decides on sexual counseling, a sexual history will become part of the general history taken in the first session or two. Particular emphasis is on trying to ascertain specific details about what the couple actually does sexually. The therapist will want to rule out organic causes or require a medical consultation if in any doubt. Additionally, the therapist will want to determine what stage of the response cycle is impaired and if the problem is primary and one or both partners have never performed satisfactorily, or if it is secondary and not always in force. The couple's interaction, as in their communication patterns and expectations, will give the therapist clues as to the psychodynamic relationships. Sometimes, what is presented as a sexual difficulty may also be a greater problem in that the entire relationship is distressed. Also it is important to be alert for unconscious deceptions on the part of the couple. For example, many self-reported cases of female lack of orgasm can be more properly diagnosed as premature ejaculation. Also, often unconsciously, one or both partners may suffer from cultural attitudes that prohibit enjoyable sex. The idea that sex is for procreation not recreation still inhibits many people.

The therapeutic intervention required in all the possible cases of dysfunction will usually include anxiety reduction and a certain amount of "permission giving." The attitude that it is all right to enjoy sex is vital for successful treatment. Couples are urged to openly discuss their sexual needs and desires and to take turns, from time to time, in concentrating on giving pleasure to one or the other partner. The problem is treated as "theirs," not just his or hers. Information and education are considered crucial, as is the need for open communication, for changing destructive patterns.

Sex therapy cannot be very successful if the relationship is not a good one. Indeed, this is one of the reasons for discontinuing the use of surrogates, a procedure that was once thought more appropriate. The sexual area is but one in the complexity of a total relationship and, although important, is not exclusively the issue.

Gender Identity Disorders

Gender, the physical fact of maleness or femaleness, is usually the first significant item to be known about a person. Social groups immediately begin prescribing different role models for males and females. Boys and girls are treated differently from birth (Gorman 1992), from areas such as choice of toys and clothing to the amount of handling and cuddling each receives.

The child becomes aware early on of the psychological as well as physiological differences between the sexes and most are firmly committed to the societal expectations for their gender as early as 18 months of age. In rare cases in which gender was misassigned at birth due to physical abnormality or where accidental damage has been suffered, it is considered almost impossible to reassign a child to the opposite sex after age one and a half. By then, the sense of gender identity, of being male or female, is too firmly rooted to change (Money and Ehrhardt 1972).

For most people, the private sense they have of themselves as being male or female matches their physical makeup. As children grow into adolescence and become aware of sexual interactions, they are clearly aware that they are a man or a woman, and, regardless of heterosexual or homosexual preferences, they will be satisfied in their gender identity.

TRANSSEXUALISM. There are, however, other people who do not have this match between biological gender and psychological gender identity. These people, called **transsexuals,** have an early and persistent feeling that they are trapped in a body with the wrong genitals. In reality, they believe, they are and were always meant to be of the opposite sex. Experts at the Erickson Educational Foundation, which studies transsexualism, have estimated that there are approximately 10,000 such people in the United States. About 2000 of these have undergone sex reassignment surgery to correct what they believe to be their physically flawed bodies (Money 1986). Although both males and females are found in the greater group of transsexuals, men seem to outnumber women by about seven to one (Levine and Lothstein 1981).

Little is known of the origins of transsexualism, but childhood patterns seem to be fairly consistent. Typically, the child who becomes transsexual relates better to the other sex. Boys will prefer female friends and activities and will cross-dress whenever possible. Girls will develop masculine type behavior and refuse to be involved in activities usually assigned to females. Of course, not all children with such childhood behavior become transsexuals. At puberty, the true transsexual will be quite horrified at the physical changes taking place. This is not true for most homosexuals or transvestites. The opposite-sex behavioral style continues on into adulthood with transsexuals and often leads them to a desire for sexual reassignment as they find partners with whom they wish to live or marry. Transsexuals never consider themselves to be homosexual. The biological female who falls in love with a woman believes herself to really be a man who loves that woman. Thus a desire for congruity in gender identity and physiology becomes important for many.

Until 1964, Americans wishing such surgery were forced to go to other countries. In the last twenty years, however, such reassignment has been permitted at selected hospitals and clinics within the United States.

Treatment generally begins with psychotherapy for about two years. If the client is considered a potential candidate for surgery, he or she is urged to live in the cross-gender role for two years, e.g., dressing in the clothing of the opposite sex. After two years, if the client is still considered a good candidate for surgery, then hormone therapy is begun. Hormone therapy (males taking estrogen and females, androgen) helps develop the bodily characteristics desired, for example, hips and breasts in the biological male, and body hair and lack of menstruation in the biological female. The client continues cross-dressing and otherwise living as the "new" gender and continues psychotherapy. Legal and social arrangements are made, such as name change on various documents, and new employment if it is necessary to leave a former job owing to discrimination. Relationship issues are discussed in therapy, such as what to tell parents, children, and former spouses. Only after it appears that a successful outcome is likely is surgery performed.

Professionals debate the value of sex surgery, with conflicting studies making the issue rather unclear. Some transsexuals seem to live happy and productive lives without undergoing this expensive and painful surgery, whereas others seem unable to function without it. The number of people involved is so limited that each case must be treated individually, and until more information becomes available, few conclusive statements can be made about the desirability of sexual reassignment surgery.

Paraphilias

For some adults, the preferred expression of sexuality will include unusual behavior often found unpleasant or bizarre to the majority of people. Even when engaged in by consenting adults, these activities are usually criticized or even made illegal by the greater society.

The bias against these behaviors is such that there is an assumption by both the public and professional communities that the participants are disturbed and unable to relate well to others. These **paraphilias,** as they are often called, are described as unconventional activities that diminish the capacity of the person to have a close relationship with another (APA 1987).

Some people, of course, find that having a strong desire or need to engage in unconventional sexual behavior is a problem. They may suffer from guilt and fear of ridicule and may have difficulty finding partners. Others, however, do not experience these problems and are resentful of the mental health community's wish to "cure" them. The situation for many is similar to that of homosexuals not so many years ago. As long as a certain sexual activity is scorned and considered both illegal and disturbed, its adherents may suffer. As the general public, including those in the health care professions, becomes more educated and aware of its bias, more and more participants are free to be open and honest about the nature of their lives. As with all other groups, some people with a paraphilia may be unable to relate to others and are nongiving, whereas others may have few if any life difficulties.

Many people have no real wish to actually perform these behaviors but are sexually aroused by the fantasy. It is important to remember that this group of people also suffer and may be encumbered by guilt and shame.

The majority of people involved in the various paraphilias are male. There is no certainty as to why this is the case, although explanations include genetic, hormonal, and social influences. Perhaps as women become better educated sexually and more free to determine their own desires in terms of behavior, they will become involved in greater numbers.

Certainly, culture and experience play a role in what is considered a paraphilia. For someone who has never seen a male dressed in other than trousers or jeans, a flowing silk gown might be considered abnormal wear. Yet, in many countries and eras such a gown would be appropriate for a man. In some cultures, a casual kiss between acquaintances on the street is the norm. Elsewhere, such behavior could be considered lewd, immoral, and reason for arrest. We often see a conflict between the stated norms such as, "sex should be reserved for marriage," and the actual-ity, in which the majority of adults have been involved in sexual experiences outside of marriage. Standards regarding what is the norm and what is not are always changing, so it is difficult to predict what will be acceptable and what will not in future years. Currently the following are considered unusual enough to be called paraphilias: fetishism, pedophilia, exhibitionism, voyeurism, transvestism, sadism and masochism, and zoophilia.

FETISHISM. A person with a sexual fetish will find it necessary to have some external object present, either in fantasy or reality, in order to be sexually satisfied. The fetish may be mild and quite socially acceptable, such as black lace undergarments being worn by a woman as a necessary part of sex life with her husband. For many couples this would not present a problem but for some it might. If the fetish becomes more unusual and the partner needed his wife to wear a tightly fitting rubber corset, for example, she might well refuse. Some fetishists also develop problems when they do not have cooperative partners. They may assault women in public because they are wearing the fetish object, or they may commit robbery in an attempt to get a particular object.

Most fetishes develop during adolescence, and the object is often associated with the mother or other significant females. In some cases the fetish takes the form of objectification of a part of the body, such as the foot. This variation is known as partialism and often is undetected, especially if the object of excitement is also viewed as sexual by others (such as breasts and buttocks).

PEDOPHILIA. Pedophilia involves the desire or fantasy of an adult (16 years or older) to have sex with a prepubescent child, generally 13 years old or younger. The DMS-III-R states that there has to be at least five years' age difference. Almost universally prohibited, it is nonetheless an activity that has occurred both cross-culturally and over the centuries. In recent years, a great deal of attention has been paid to this sexual abuse of children, and it is now thought that approximately 80% of the victims know the adult as a family member, friend, or neighbor (Sanford 1980). The sexual activity often includes fondling and masturbation, with intercourse occurring more rarely. Because those involved often know one another, it is believed that large numbers of cases of pedophilia are unreported. Some of those involved maintain that the activity is not necessarily harmful to the child and that a responsible adult participant will become sexual only with a consenting young partner. The age at which a child can truly give consent is, of course, open to question. Most people would agree that a seven-year-old cannot, but the ability of a 15-year-old to understand and desire sex is more debatable. Both are legally children, however, and thus are not able to

engage in sexual activity with an adult according to the law.

Due to the secrecy about pedophilia, we do not have accurate information regarding its incidence or well-defined profiles of the pedophile. It is known, however, that the partners usually know one another and that the adult is often a married, somewhat conservative man. In cases of pedophilia among family members, which is called *incest*, the vast majority of cases include father or stepfather and daughter. Cases between mother and child are extremely unusual, with brother-sister incest believed to be more common.

EXHIBITIONISM. The intentional exhibition of one's genitals in a public place is deemed more harmless than many of the other paraphilias. Although **exhibitionism** is illegal, the exhibitionist is usually not interested in sexual assault or rape and prefers to startle his victims and then move on. This compulsive need to display the penis seems to often be triggered by stress in otherwise sedate, middle-class males. Females have been thought not to be involved as exhibitionists, although one might argue that the intent behind some strippers and porno models could be the same as that of the street flasher.

VOYEURISM. "Peeping" at others while they make love or watching a person undress is considered a paraphilia only when this activity becomes compulsive and preferable to other sexual activity. The voyeur is thought to be almost always a heterosexual male who wishes no contact with those on whom he is spying. Often the man is described as shy, socially unskilled, and without close friends. A man who enters a building where these activities are going on, however, can be dangerous, and he may commit crimes such as rape or robbery (Gebhard et al. 1965).

TRANSVESTIC FETISHISM. Transvestism involves obtaining sexual satisfaction via dressing in the clothing of the opposite sex. The desire to use such clothing is related to fetishism but often goes beyond the use of one particular object. Those involved usually develop their interest in the clothing of the opposite sex early, and, unlike transsexuals, they have no doubt as to their sexual orientation, nor do they have a wish to change their sex. Usually heterosexual, many transvestites cross-dress in only specific sexual situations and are often surprised to receive the cooperation and support of their partners in obtaining clothes and other articles.

SEXUAL SADISM AND MASOCHISM. Sexual sadism and masochism are two related paraphilias which include the giving **(sadism)** and receiving **(masochism)** of psychological or physical pain or domination. Although statistics show that actual involvement in sadomasochistic activity is not thought to be prevalent, the fantasy of such behavior is quite frequent among both homosexuals and heterosexuals (Masters and Johnson 1979). For some, roles are never switched, with the desire always the same—to be the dominant or to be the submissive one. More often, however, there is some mixing of roles, and pain is not necessarily a feature. Activities may range from mild restraint or biting to much more severe activity, including inflicting bodily harm (Herron and Herron 1982). Both homosexual and heterosexual people are involved in sadomasochistic lovemaking, and many do not follow the sex-role stereotypes that might be expected. Therefore, males who are thought to be more aggressive and dominant, in a psychological and social sense, are often interested in masochistic behavior. The same is true for females who wish to be sexually dominant (Herron et al. 1983).

OTHER PARAPHILIAS. There are numerous other nonstandard sexual behaviors that some people engage in as either a part of or as their major source of pleasure. As with the other paraphilias discussed, they may or may not cause a problem for the participant, depending on the availability of consenting partners and the societal norms at the time.

Some of these behaviors are zoophilia, or sexual contact with animals; coprophilia, klismaphilia, and urologia are all associated with feces, enemas, or urine; necrophilia, in which a corpse is desired; scatophilia, where obscene language is used; and frotteurism, where sexual gratification occurs in rubbing up against a stranger.

INTERVENTIONS. Many of the people involved in nonstandard sexual practices find no need for therapy. If their sexual activities are carried out with a consenting, adult partner and do not involve any illegality, or are not physically or emotionally harmful to either partner, they are in no more need of counseling than any other person might be.

If, however, the person is experiencing relationship difficulties, wishes to change sexual orientation, becomes involved in illegal activity, or is physically or emotionally harming others or is being harmed, then therapy is indicated.

The most usual treatment design used specifically with paraphilias is behavior therapy. An attempt will be made to help the person learn a new sexual response pattern that will eliminate the need for the activity that is causing the problem. Techniques range from positive reinforcement for appropriate object choices to aversion techniques, in which mild electric shocks may be used for inappropriate choices. The most successful treatments seem to be those that include psychodynamic techniques designed to help the patient understand the origin of the paraphilia. Substitution can be helpful, as in the case where a pedophile's wife agreed to play the role of a child in dress and manner during some sexual encounters. In this way, the man was able to achieve sexual satisfaction in a legal way, and his wife came to enjoy her role in helping him be involved with her instead of molesting children.

For many, however, therapy does not appear to alter criminal behavior. A relatively poor success rate has been shown for many sex offenders who have undergone treatment programs in prison.

Sexually Transmitted Diseases

Any disease that can be contracted by sexual contact can be classified as an STD. STDs are also called venereal diseases, and there are numerous types, which range from merely annoying to life threatening. The American Social Health Association estimates that more than 25 diseases are spread through sexual contact. STDs are among the most common contagious diseases in the United States, affecting more than 40 million Americans in 1989, with 12 million new cases expected each year.

AIDS. Recently an enormous amount of attention has been paid to the usually sexually transmitted disease of AIDS. Because the human immunodeficiency virus can incubate anywhere between six months to 10 or more years, there is grave concern among many people that they were exposed to AIDS years ago, and now they live with the dread of developing AIDS years after the fact.

AIDS involves a disruption of the body's immune system. The virus attacks certain white blood cells called T-4 lymphocytes, leaving the person open to many serious diseases. Weight loss, diarrhea, lesions that do not heal, cancers, infections, and severe motor dysfunction all may occur. However, people with the human immunodeficiency virus or AIDS can live for a long period of time in productive and satisfying lives. (Refer to Chapter 26 for further discussion of AIDS.)

The United States leads the world in reported cases of AIDS. In 1988, it was estimated that a million and a half persons in the United States were infected and that 100 new cases of AIDS per day were being reported (Jones 1988). By December 1990, the death toll from AIDS in the United States was over 100,000, according to the Centers for Disease Control. During sexual intercourse, infected semen enters the partner's bloodstream through abrasions in the mucous membranes. Intravenous drug users can be contaminated when the blood from one infected user is passed via a shared needle to another. Caretakers and relatives of AIDS victims are rarely at risk. The virus, which must enter a person's bloodstream to cause infection, is carried in the highest concentration in blood and semen and in low concentration in saliva and sweat. A caretaker is rarely in contact with the former and is thus not likely to contract the disease.

There is enormous public outcry and fear regarding the disease. Hospitals have refused to accept persons with AIDS as clients, and school systems throughout the country have rejected AIDS students in response to boycotts led by fearful and angry parents. Some nations, even our own, have considered requiring screening blood tests for any foreigners wishing to visit.

Although safer sex practices can be taught, and although early studies showed the gay community significantly changing its sexual habits (National Center for Health Education 1985), there is disturbing evidence that education is not controlling the problem to the extent formerly hoped for. Although dramatic behavior changes have occurred, especially in the gay community, infection of intravenous drug users and a smaller number of homosexuals continues. Seventy percent of AIDS victims are homosexual, and 17% are intravenous drug users. The number of cases among heterosexuals has risen in the last few years from 1% to 5% (Greenspan and Castro 1990) in the United States, although almost 80% of cases in Africa occur among heterosexuals (Eckholm 1990). In spite of massive health education programs aimed at high-risk groups, there are those who pay no more attention to these programs than many do to other health issues, such as cessation of smoking (Stall 1988). Meanwhile, research efforts are continuing in an effort to find a way to combat this dreaded disease. (Refer to Chapter 26).

HERPES. Another sexually transmitted disease that has received widespread attention in recent years is herpes simplex virus (*Herpesvirus hominis*) The United States Public Health Service (1982) reports that there is at least a 10-fold increase in cases in the last 10 years and that there is no cure for the viral infection as yet. Between 26 and 31 million people in the United States have contracted herpes. There is no permanent cure, although the drug acyclovir has been effective in reducing the frequency and duration of outbreaks. It is most often found in the 15–30 age group.

Herpes genitalis is an infection resulting in rupture of vesicles causing painful ulcers. Systemic symptoms include fever, malaise, and inguinal node enlargement. Symptoms occur approximately two to seven days after incubation.

The ulcers are usually present on the medial aspects of the labia minora, clitoris, vagina, urethra, and cervix. They can last from four to six weeks (Wardell 1986). The first attack tends to be the most severe, and about 66% of herpes victims do not have any more outbreaks, although the virus does remain in the system. One third of the victims do have recurring infections, which are contagious as long as the symptoms are present.

Other side effects of herpes can include keratitis, if the virus is transferred to the eyes. An association with cervical cancer and the infection of infants born vaginally to mothers with an outbreak of the disease is suspected. Psychological effects can also be quite profound, with some people losing all sexual desire because of fear of contracting or spreading the disease. Among some single adults, the question, "Are you healthy?" has become part of dating procedure, with the herpes client consequently left feeling most undesirable.

Health care professionals can do a great deal to educate the public about the prevention of herpes. Those having an outbreak can be taught to avoid sexual activity. Mothers can be encouraged to deliver their babies by cesarean section if an outbreak occurs. Washing of hands and towels and sheets can help prevent the spread of the virus.

CHLAMYDIA INFECTIONS. Chlamydial infections are contracted by an estimated 4 million Americans each year. They are twice as common as gonorrhea and 40 times more common than syphilis. About 80% of women have no observable symptoms and are diagnosed only when a partner is diagnosed. Symptoms can include genital discharge, burning during urination, and pain in the lower abdomen or testicles. Chlamydial infections are treated with antibiotics, and intercourse should be avoided until treatment is completed.

GENITAL WARTS. Genital warts, which are caused by a virus, affect almost 2 million Americans. Not always visible, they are often soft and flat and can grow and itch. If not treated medically, they can block openings of the vagina, anus, or throat and can lead to cancer of the cervix, vulva, or penis.

HEPATITIS B. Hepatitis B has been on the rise, with 26,000 new cases reported in 1986. When there are symptoms, they can include fatigue, headache, dark urine, light stools, and jaundice. This disease is very contagious and can be passed during intimate sexual encounters as well as during more casual contact. A vaccine is available to protect health care workers and those in intimate relationships with infected people. About 90% of adults recover completely from hepatitis B, but severe liver disease and even death can occur from lack of treatment.

GONORRHEA. Gonorrhea is one of the most common STDs. Gonorrhea is a bacterial infection (caused by *Neisseria gonorrhoeae*) that enters the body through warm, moist areas, such as the genitals or mouth. Approximately one million cases are reported each year, and three million are suspected. Males tend to experience pain when urinating and discharge; about 50–75% of females have less obvious early indications and may be asymptomatic, whereas others may experience painful urination and discharge. Sterility can be caused by untreated gonorrhea in both men and women.

Because the early stages are not obvious in women, it is likely that the disease will not be treated and secondary infections, such as pelvic inflammatory disease, can occur. A baby born to an infected mother will become blind if the bacteria enters his or her eyes. Therefore, all newborns' eyes are treated with tetracycline or silver nitrate to prevent possible blindness.

Early diagnosis of gonorrhea is important. Treatment is relatively simple with effective antibiotics. Gonorrhea is twice as prevalent as it was 15 years ago, and although rates dropped by 33% during the 1980s, there has been a new increase in strains that are resistant to the more commonly prescribed antibiotics.

Use of condoms, washing of the genitals, and visual inspection of a partner's genitals can help prevent the spread of this and other sexually transmitted diseases.

SYPHILIS. Syphilis, caused by the spirochete *Treponema pallidum*, remains a serious sexually transmitted disease, with over 25,000 cases reported each year between 1980 and 1986 (CDC 1986). An important factor contributing to the rise in the incidence of syphilis, according to the Centers for Disease Control, has been the exchange of sexual services for drugs, and by 1990, a 34% increase in the number of Americans being treated for syphilis was reported. Penicillin or other antibiotics are able to cure the disease at any stage, although damage that has already been caused by the disease cannot be reversed.

Syphilis appears to have existed for many centuries in all parts of the world. It is a chronic infection, which can be transmitted via the mouth, genitals, anus, or even a small lesion. It travels through the bloodstream to all parts of the body and can take many years to develop completely into a serious and life-threatening illness.

In its *primary stage*, syphilis can be detected by dark-field examination after the incubation period of 10–90 days. The only symptom is a painless sore called a chancre, which usually appears near the mouth, anus, or genitals within a week to several months after infection. The chancre grows for one to eight weeks and generally is open at the top, with a band of hard tissue around the base. Because it is quite painless or in females may be growing internally, this sore is often ignored or not seen. If it is not treated at this stage, the ulcers will heal in three to nine weeks, and the disease goes on to the second stage.

The *second stage* lasts between two and 10 weeks while the disease spreads, with sores or lesions appearing on the vulva, mouth and pharynx, axilla, and under the breasts. During this stage, systemic symptoms may occur, such as fever, sore throat, and headache. All these symptoms disappear even without treatment, and the disease can still be unknown to its victim.

The *third or latent stage* of syphilis can last for decades. No longer contagious, except to a child born of a carrier parent, the disease nonetheless may attack various parts of the body, including the circulatory and nervous systems.

Only in the *fourth or late stage* of syphilis does its presence become obvious. Serious illness, blindness, and mental and cardiovascular problems can all be present.

The treatment of syphilis in the primary and secondary stages is with penicillin G benzathine. Clients allergic to penicillin may be given erythromycin.

Fear of syphilis has waned some with the advent of more effective treatment procedures. Still, there are hundreds of thousands of cases reported in the United States each year and possibly many more that go undetected until it is too late to cure them.

Summary

Nurse generalists can take a health history and screen for sexual function and dysfunction and are in key positions to teach others (e.g., parents, community groups, and adolescents) about sexually transmitted diseases, bio-psycho-social aspects of sexuality throughout the life cycle, and the effects of certain illnesses on sexual functioning.

Many adults in our society experience stress surrounding changing social mores, relationship issues, and sexual behavior. In order to recognize these issues and to help clients come to terms with them, the nurse should become aware of the various kinds of difficulties and the developmental basis for them.

Personality patterns and sexual awareness and reactions begin to develop in the early years. Prevalent sexual dysfunctions among men and women have been discussed. Specific sexual disorders were mentioned, and an overview of prevalent STDs was presented. Knowledge and empathy are needed when working with people with these problems.

References

American Psychiatric Association. Diagnostic and Statistical Manual of Mental Disorders, 3rd ed, revised (DSM-III-R). Washington, DC: American Psychiatric Association, 1987.

Annon JS. The PLISSIT model: A proposed conceptual scheme for the behavioral treatment of sexual problems. Journal of Sex Education and Therapy, 2:1, 1978.

Bell AP, Weinberg MS. Homosexualities. New York: Simon & Schuster, 1978.

Campbell JW, Frisse M (eds). Manual of Medical Therapeutics. Boston: Little, Brown & Company, 1983, pp. 897–899.

Caplow T, et al. Middletown Families. Minneapolis: University of Minnesota Press, 1982.

Centers for Disease Control. Statistical data re syphilis. Morbidity and Mortality Weekly Report, 356, 1986.

Colderone MS, Johnson EW. The Family Book About Sexuality. New York: Morgan & Row, 1981.

Cole CM, Levin EM, Whitley JO, et al. Brief sexual counseling during cardiac rehabilitation. Heart and Lung, 8:124, 1979.

Debate on punishing patient-therapist sex: Not whether, but how. Psychiatric News, 28(13):5, 1993.

Deevey S. Lesbian self-disclosure strategies for success. Journal of Psychosocial Nursing, 31(4):25, 1993.

Eckholm E. An atlas of spreading tragedy. New York Times, September 16, 1990:15.

Ecstrand ML, Coates TJ. Maintenance of safer sexual behaviors and predictions of risky sex. American Journal of Public Health, 80:973, 1990.

Ellis H. Studies in the Psychology of Sex. New York: Basic Books, 1936.

Felstein I. Understanding Sexual Medicine. Lancaster, England: MTP Press, 1986.

Freud S. Three essays on the theory of sexuality. The Standard Edition of the Complete Psychological Works of Sigmund Freud, vol. 7. London: Hogarth Press, 1905, pp 125–145.

Gebhard P, Gagnon JH, Pomeroy WB, Christenson CV. Sex Offenders: An Analysis of Types. New York: Harper & Row, 1965.

Glick PC. Remarriage: Some recent changes and variations. Journal of Family Issues, 1:455, 1980.

Goldberg D (ed). Contemporary Marriage. Homewood, IL: Dorsey, 1985.

Gorman C. Sizing up the sexes. Time, 139(3)42, 1992.

Green R. Human Sexuality: A Health Practitioner's Text. Baltimore: Williams & Wilkins, 1975.

Greenspan A, Castro KG. Heterosexual transmission of HIV infection. SEICUS Report, 19:1, 1990.

Herron MJ, Herron WG. Meanings of sadism and masochism. Psychological Reports, 50:199, 1982.

Herron MJ, Herron WG, Schultz CL. Sexual dominance/submission, gender and sex-role identification. Perceptual and Motor Skills, 56:931, 1983.

Herron WG, Rouslin S. Issues in Psychotherapy, vol 1. Washington, DC: Oryn, 1984.

Hogan R. Human Sexuality, A Nursing Perspective. New York: Appleton-Century-Crofts, 1980.

Jacobson L. Illness and sexuality. Nursing Outlook, 22:50, 1974.

Jones JM. Section introduction: Psychology and AIDS. American Psychologist, 43(11):899, 1988.

Kaplan HS. The New Sex Therapy. New York: Brunner-Mazel, 1974.

Kaplan HS. Disorders of Sexual Desire. New York: Simon & Schuster, 1979.

Kinsey A, Pomeroy W, Martin C, et al. Sexual Behavior in the Human Male. Philadelphia: WB Saunders, 1948.

Kinsey A, Pomeroy W, Martin C, et al. Sexual Behavior in the Human Female. Philadelphia: WB Saunders, 1953.

Krueger JC, Hassell J, Goggin DB, et al. Relationship between nurse counseling and sexual adjustment after hysterectomy. Nursing Research, 28:145, 1979.

Lazarus J. Sex with former patients almost always unethical. American Journal of Psychiatry, 149(7):855, 1992.

Levine S, Lothstein LM. Transsexualism or the gender dysphoria syndromes. Journal of Sex and Marital Therapy, 7:85, 1981.

McCausland LH. Surgical approach to musculoskeletal system dysfunction. In Kneisl CR, Ames SW (eds). Adult Health Nursing. Reading, MA: Addison-Wesley Publishing Company, 1986.

McNeil J. Report. US Census Bureau, Washington, DC: US Census Bureau, February 21, 1992.

Magenity J. A plea for sex education in the nursing curriculum. American Journal of Nursing, 75:1171, 1975.

Marcus W. Making History: The Struggle for Gay and Lesbian Rights. New York: Harper, 1992.

Markarian MF. The nursing process for clients with nervous system disorders. In Kneisl CR, Ames SW (eds). Adult Health Nursing. Reading, MA: Addison-Wesley Publishing Company, 1986.

Masters WH, Johnson VE. Human Sexual Response. Boston: Little, Brown & Company, 1966.

Masters WH, Johnson VE. Human Sexual Inadequacy. Boston: Little, Brown & Company, 1970.

Masters WH, Johnson VE. Homosexuality in Perspective. Boston: Little, Brown & Company, 1979.

Mims FH. Sexuality in the nursing curriculum. Nursing Education, 11:23, 1977.

Money J. Lovemaps. Buffalo, NY: Prometheus Books, 1986.

Money J, Ehrhardt A. Man and Woman, Boy and Girl. Baltimore: Johns Hopkins Press, 1972.

National Center for Health Statistics. National Survey of Family Growth. Washington, DC: National Center for Health Statistics, 1985.

O'Neill GO, O'Neill N. Open Marriage. New York: M. Evans, 1974.

Sanford LT. The Silent Children. Garden City, NY: Dell, 1980.

Schuster EA, Unsain IG, Goodwin MH. Nursing practice in human sexuality. Nursing Clinics of North America, 17(3):345, 1982.

Stall R, Coates T, Hoff C. Behavioral risk reduction for HIV infection among gay and bisexual men. American Psychologist, 43(11):878, 1988.

Stier FL. The nursing process for clients with major blood vessel dysfunction. In Kneisl CR, Ames SW (eds). Adult Health Nursing. Reading, MA: Addison-Wesley Publishing Company, 1986.

US Public Health Service. Sexually transmitted diseases: Treatment guidelines. Morbidity and Mortality Weekly Report, 17:356, 1982.

Wardell DW. Specific disorders of the female reproductive system. In Kneisl CR, Ames SW (eds). Adult Health Nursing. Reading, MA: Addison-Wesley Publishing Company, 1986.

Watts RJ. Dimensions of sexual health. American Journal of Nursing, 79(9):1570, 1979.

Wolfe L. The good news. New York Magazine, 15(7):33, 1982.

Woods NF. Human Sexuality in Health and Illness, 3rd ed. St. Louis: CV Mosby, 1984.

Zalar MK. Role preparation for nurses in human sexual functioning. Nursing Clinics of North America, 17(3):351, 1982.

Further Reading

Bohannan P. Divorce and After. Garden City, NY: Doubleday, 1968.

Caldwell B, Landes A, Siegal M. Health: A Concern for Every American. Wylie, TX: Information Plus, 1991.

Chapple S, Talbot D. Burning Desires: Sex in America. New York: Doubleday, 1989.

Faderman L. Odd Girls and Twilight Lovers: A History of Lesbian Life in Twentieth Century America. New York: Columbia University Press, 1992.

Fairbairn WP. An object-relations theory of the personality. New York: Basic Books, 1952.

Ford C, Beach F. Patterns of Sexual Behavior. New York: Ace, 1951.

Hamilton R. The Herpes Book. Los Angeles, CA: JP Tarcher, 1980.

Kolodry RC, Masters WH, Johnson VE. Textbook of Human Sexuality for Nurses. Boston: Little, Brown & Company, 1979.

Ladas AK, Whipple B, Perry JD. The G Spot. New York: Dell, 1981.

Marriage rates drop. Contemporary Sexuality, 25(10):4, 1991.

National Center for Health Education. The emerging pandemic of AIDS. CENTER, 3:3, 1985.

Rubin J, Provanzano F, Luria Z. The eye of the beholder: Parents' view on sex of newborns. American Journal of Orthopsychiatry, 44:512, 1974.

Sexton RE, Sexton VS. Intimacy: A historical perspective. In Fischer M, Stricker G (eds). Intimacy. New York: Plenum Press, 1982.

Talese G. Thy Neighbor's Wife. Garden City, NY: Doubleday, 1980.

Tutliean L. Herpes update. New York, June 3, 1991.

Weinberg JS. Sexuality, human needs and nursing practice. Philadelphia: WB Saunders, 1982.

What you think. Time, 136(19):14, 1990.

Williams M (ed). Support of condoms in school. Contemporary Sexuality, 25(9):2, 1991.

Winslow R. Use of birth control. Wall Street Journal, August 20, 1991:B-9.

Women with children. Wall Street Journal, February 12, 1992:B-1.

Self-study Exercises

Using Watts levels, identify the following levels with either the assessment or the intervention level:

1. _____ Takes a psychiatric and psychosocial history.
2. _____ Is a professional nurse with postgraduate training in sex education and counseling.
3. _____ Sex therapy—individual or group.
4. _____ Imparts limited information about sexual feelings and behaviors.
5. _____ Screens for sexual function and dysfunction.

A. Level 1

B. Level 2

C. Level 3

D. Level 4

Match the stages in the human sexual response.

6. _____ Sex organs return to normal.
7. _____ Orgasm occurs.
8. _____ Sexual tension builds up.
9. _____ Onset of erotic feelings.

A. Stage 1— Excitement

B. Stage 2— Plateau

C. Stage 3— Orgasm

D. Stage 4— Resolution

Match the following paraphilias with their definition:

10. _____ Need for a specific object.
11. _____ Public display of genitals.
12. _____ Sexual arousal when cross-dressing.
13. _____ Pain or humiliation and sex.
14. _____ Sex with a child.

A. Sadomasochism

B. Pedophilia

C. Fetishism

D. Exhibitionism

E. Transvestic fetishism

Complete the statements by filling in the appropriate information.

15. Masters and Johnson discovered that males but not females have a _____ period in a typical sexual response cycle.
16. Approximately _____ % of American women begin sexual intercourse prior to marriage.
17. Approximately _____ % of all American marriages end in divorce.
18. The gender identity disorder resulting in a person believing he or she is really the other sex is called _____.
19. _____ is considered the most common sexual dysfunction.
20. Helen Singer Kaplan advocates a blending of _____ and _____ techniques in treating sexual dysfunction.

Brief essay

21. Write a paragraph comparing and contrasting a person who has a homosexual lifestyle with a person who is a transsexual living a cross-gender role.

The Elderly

Sally Kennedy Holzapfel

OUTLINE

KEY TERMS AND CONCEPTS

The key terms and concepts listed here also appear in bold where they are defined or discussed in this chapter.

AGEISM

CHEMICAL RESTRAINTS

DAY CARE PROGRAMS

DIRECTIVE TO PHYSICIAN

DURABLE POWER OF ATTORNEY FOR
    HEALTH CARE

GROUP PSYCHOTHERAPY

HIGH-RISK SUICIDE FACTORS IN THE
    ELDERLY

HOSPICE PHILOSOPHY

LIVING WILL

OMNIBUS BUDGET RECONCILIATION
    ACT

PATIENT SELF-DETERMINATION ACT

PHYSICAL RESTRAINTS

REMINISCING THERAPY

REMOTIVATION THERAPY

SOCIAL DYSFUNCTION RATING SCALE

ZUNG'S SELF-RATING DEPRESSION
    SCALE

OBJECTIVES ▪

After studying this chapter, the student will be able to

1. Discuss five myths on aging.
2. Compare the purpose, format, and desired outcomes among the following group treatments: remotivation, reminiscing, and psychotherapy.
3. List two characteristics of physical and chemical restraints.
4. List two institutional requirements of the Patient Self-determination Act.
5. List three differences between living wills, directives to physicians, and durable power of attorney for health care.
6. Recognize guidelines a nurse can employ in approaching issues of life and death with a client.
7. Discuss ways in which the nurse may assist families of a dying client.
8. Summarize the concept of the hospice program.
9. Identify the elderly group at highest risk for suicide.
10. Describe the characteristics of two types of elderly alcohol abusers.

The growing number and proportion of elderly in the United States have a significant impact on our economic, social, and health institutions, and mental health services. For example, at the turn of the century, 4% of the total population was over 65 (Schneider and Emr 1985). In 1989, 12.5% of the total population (about 31 million) was over 65, and by the year 2000, 13.2% of the population will be over 65. By the year 2030, this population is expected to number at 66 million, 2.5 times their number in 1980 (A Profile of Older Americans 1990).

The trend in the health of the elderly has shown that chronic illness and disability, as opposed to acute illnesses, are the major threats to the older person's health. At least 80% of individuals over 65 report at least one chronic condition; many elderly have multiple chronic conditions (Price and Feldman 1983). Thirty percent of older persons consider their health fair or poor, compared with only 10% of persons under 65 (A Profile of Older Americans 1990). The likelihood of developing one or more chronic illnesses increases significantly with age: individuals 75 years of age and older are the most prone to chronic illnesses and functional disabilities. Chronic illness is responsible for more than 70% of all deaths (Kayser-Jones 1986).

At birth, the life expectancy of the urban population, which comprises 74% of the US population, is 71 years for men and 79 years for women, with an average of 75 years for both sexes (Ebersole and Hess 1990). In 1989, there were 145 women for every 100 men in the over-65 category (A Profile of Older Americans 1990). The female-male sex ratio increases with age. Women's greater longevity has significant ramifications for society and for the health care professions in particular. More older women with more severe functional limitations are the people the health professions will be working with, both in the community and in nursing homes (Caserta 1983).

It is meaningful to separate the needs of persons in the older age groups, particularly the group 85 and older, from those of other aged persons; there are noticeable differences between individuals in their 60s (old) and people in their 80s (old-old). The younger group is relatively healthy; the older group is much more profoundly affected by the chronic diseases and disorders of aging. In fact, the fastest expanding age group is the group 85 years or older (Schneider and Emr 1985). This age group is expected to triple between 1980 and 2020 (Hogan 1990).

The following list identifies specific facts about mental health and the aged (Burnside 1988):

1. Mental illness is more prevalent among the elderly than among younger persons (18–25% of the elderly have mental problems).
2. Psychosis increases significantly after age 65.
3. Suicide occurs more frequently among the elderly than in any other age group.
4. Senile dementia is the fourth leading cause of death among the elderly.
5. Fifteen percent of the elderly have chronic physical problems that can result in negative psychological responses.

Dementia and depression are two major mental health concerns among the elderly.

Alzheimer's disease is the most common form of dementia in the elderly. Individuals in their 60s and early 70s have a 4% chance of developing Alzheimer's disease; there is a 10–15% risk of developing Alzheimer's when people reach their late 70s and early 80s; in the 85 and older age group, the risk is between 20 and 30%. Schneider and Emr (1985) predict Alzheimer's disease to be the leading cause of death in the next century. See Chapter 20 for a discussion of Alzheimer's disease.

The population of elderly persons has been increasing so steadily that questions of care for the elderly are highly apparent whenever issues about health care delivery are raised. Unfortunately, the elderly receive little attention in the positive areas of health education aimed at prevention and rehabilitation; they receive a great deal of notice in tertiary care, high-technology care, and, finally, institutional care (German 1981).

The increasing number and population of elderly persons are having a significant impact on the utilization and cost of health care services, and this has important implications for nursing (Kayser-Jones 1986), especially in hospitals and nursing homes.

The Role of the Nurse

Nurses have much to contribute to the care and promotion of health in the elderly. However, questions arise as to whether student nurses are given accurate information and sufficient exposure to the elderly. If not, sufficient theory and principles needed to provide safe and excellent care to the elderly are deficient (Burnside 1988). Lack of specific information necessary for a student nurse to make sound decisions in regard to elderly clients is in part a result of the following:

- Negative faculty attitudes toward the old
- Lack of exposure and lack of clinical emphasis on older persons
- Negative student attitudes toward the elderly because of information based on myths and stereotypes
- Unfamiliarity with gerontological information and resources

One of the factors that contribute to the negative view that nurses (generalists, educators, students) as well as the general population have toward the elderly are the myths that surround being old. These myths and stereotypes of the aged underlie the phenomenon of ageism.

AGEISM AND THE ELDERLY

Ageism has been defined as a bias against older people based solely on their age (Gambert 1983); it is a system of destructive, erroneous beliefs. In essence, ageism reflects a dislike by the young of the old (Preston 1986), depicting the disparaging effect of society's attitudes toward the elderly (Austin 1985). This age prejudice is based on the belief that aging makes people increasingly unattractive, unintelligent, asexual, unemployable, and senile (Atchley 1988).

Ageism is not limited to the way the young may look at the old; it also includes older people's views, which tend to be critical about themselves and their peers. The attitudes of the elderly toward the aged, particularly those with mental disabilities, are often more negative than the views held by the young. The threat of social contagion by association with the frail and infirm may simply be too strong to bear. Age proximity raises feelings of vulnerability (Ebersole and Hess 1990). This may explain why older persons often do not like to be referred to as "old." By seeing themselves as "young" rather than "old," they adjust better to their advancing years (Hogstel 1990).

Ageism differs from other forms of discrimination in that it cuts across gender, race, religion, and national origin (Neussel 1982). Old age does not award a desirable status or membership in a sought-after club; rather, it is a social category with negative connotations (Matthews 1979). Butler (1975) has written:

> Ageism is manifested in a wide range of phenomena, both on individual and institutional levels—stereotypes and myths, outright disdain and dislike, or simply subtle avoidance of contact; discriminatory practices in housing, employment, and services of all kinds; epithets, cartoons, and jokes.

Effects of ageism can be observed throughout different levels of society; even health care providers are not immune to its effects. Their attitudes reveal in many instances society's values as a whole, which are characterized by negativism and stereotyping (Benson 1982). Participating in the therapeutic milieu, they cannot easily dissociate themselves from the predetermined disapproval of society's attitudes toward the elderly. Negative values can surface in a myriad of ways in the health care system. Financial and political support for programs for the elderly are difficult to obtain; the needs of the elderly come second to those of smaller but younger population groups.

Studies have shown that almost all health professionals prefer to work with children or young adults, and that few choose to specialize in geriatrics (Green 1981). Student nurses and nurses are no exception: they prefer to work with clients of age groups other than the aged (Gomez et al. 1985). Younger caregivers may feel the prejudice of ageism and experience a fear of aging itself, that is, gerontophobia (Burnside 1988).

Medical care of aged clients has been characterized by pessimism, defeatism, and professional aversion. Such negative attitudes and stereotyped thinking have been found both among professionals and ancillary personnel in nursing homes and other institutional settings (Adelson et al. 1982).

Bower (1981) found that there is a relationship between nurses' attitudes, the characteristics of their elderly clients, the setting in which the nursing care takes place, and the educational background of the nursing personnel. It also appears that the longer nurses have worked with older clients, the more likely they are to hold stereotypical views of them. Gerontological nursing education and sensitization to the needs of the elderly can help change these attitudes and bring about a more positive approach.

According to Elliot and Hybertson (1982), the social conduct of older clients and their level of functional independence have a bearing on the feelings of, and approach taken by, nursing personnel. Nursing assistants expressed negative feelings about caring for extremely dependent elderly clients. Independence in self-care and pleasing client conduct elicited more positive feelings; socially unacceptable behaviors provoked unfavorable attitudes.

There is a need to foster more positive attitudes among nurses who provide direct service to their elderly clients (Benson 1982). Two interrelated reasons support this objective. First, the increase in the number of geriatric clients requiring nursing services has been accompanied by a decline in the number of nurses interested in working with elderly clients. Negative attitudes toward the elderly may be a contributing factor to this shortage (Penner et al. 1984). Second, it has been suggested that nurses who work with elderly clients and harbor such negative attitudes will engage in actions harmful to the best interests of their clients (Bower 1981).

Two types of inservice programs are recommended to improve negative attitudes: (1) *provide factual information about the aging process* and (2) *address and isolate the attitudes related to client care* (Elliot and Hybertson 1982). Educational programs need to discuss misconceptions about the elderly; this communication may increase the number of new nurses who are willing to work with elderly clients. These educational and training programs must address the dynamics of the nurse/staff-client interactions. Nursing personnel need to be made cognizant that their own actions may augment the very behaviors that they dislike in the elderly. Furthermore, consideration must be given to the effects that organizational policies and practices may have on the staff and their interaction with elderly clients (Penner et al. 1984).

Table 29–1A ■ QUIZ: FACTS AND MYTHS OF AGING

T F	1.	The majority of older adults past the age of 65 are demented.
T F	2.	The senses of vision, hearing, touch, taste, and smell all decline with age.
T F	3.	Muscular strength decreases with age.
T F	4.	Sexual interest declines with aging.
T F	5.	For the older adult, regular sexual expressions are important to maintain sexual capacity and effective sexual performance.
T F	6.	At least 50% of restorative sleep is lost as a result of the aging process.
T F	7.	As a group, the elderly are major consumers of prescription drugs.
T F	8.	Older adults are not able to learn new tasks.
T F	9.	The elderly have a high incidence of depression.
T F	10.	As individuals age, they become more rigid in their thinking and set in their ways.
T F	11.	The aged are well off and no longer impoverished.
T F	12.	Many individuals experience difficulty when they retire.
T F	13.	The elderly are prone to become victims of crime.
T F	14.	Most elderly are infirm and require help with daily activities.
T F	15.	Older individuals are more dependable and have fewer accidents than younger persons.
T F	16.	The majority of older adults are socially isolated and lonely.
T F	17.	Medicaid is a federally assisted program providing health care benefits to anyone over the age of 65.
T F	18.	The term "ageism" reflects society's positive views toward the elderly.
T F	19.	Widowers are more likely to remarry than widows.
T F	20.	Older widows appear to adjust better than younger ones.

Answers on page 853.

Even though advanced levels of education appear to be associated with decreased stereotyping of the aged, it does not seem to increase preference for working with the aged. Positive attitudes toward the elderly and to caring for them need to be instilled during basic nursing education and should be included in the curriculum (Gomez et al. 1985).

A better understanding of the aging process and the ability to differentiate between normal and abnormal, e.g., dementia versus normal aging, is necessary for a productive and positive interaction between nursing caregivers and their aging clients.

In defining one of the objectives of nursing care of the elderly, Preston (1986) comments:

> We must resist the ease of paternalism, which weakens our relationship with the elderly. We must endeavor to study them and their particular problems as vigorously as we study diseases. And we should love them, for that is the only way we can love ourselves when we take their places.

Refer to the Quiz: *Facts and Myths of Aging* in Table 29–1A. Answers at end of chapter.

GENERALIST VERSUS GERONTOLOGICAL NURSING PRACTICE

McConnell (1988) states that elements of nursing practice remain the same between generalist nursing practice and gerontological nursing practice. For example:

1. Goals of nursing
2. Generic nursing process and methods
3. Professional practice roles:
   Follow standard of practice
   Code of ethics
   Accountability to clients

Nurses in the levels of nursing practice shown in Table 29–1 have specific knowledge of aging and the interaction of health, aging, and illness, as well as knowledge and skill to modify and implement nursing methods. Box 29–1 outlines gerontological nursing skills.

Psychiatric nurse specialists who work with the elderly experiencing mental health problems also need to know about normal aging and interactions between aging and illness. Ronsman (1987) provides an overview of the nursing process in the care of the elderly client (Table 29–2).

Unique Assessment Strategies

Nurses who work with the elderly benefit from specific knowledge about normal aging, drug interactions, and chronic diseases. Those who work with elderly clients who have mental health problems also need to have special skills, e.g., interviewing, assessing, and knowing effective treatment modalities. Lekan-Rutledge (1988) outlines approaches to the elderly person dur-

Table 29–1 ■ NURSES PREPARED TO CARE FOR THE ELDERLY	
FUNCTION	**EDUCATION**
Nurse Practitioner	
Performs medical acts: • Prescribes medications • Diagnoses disease • Manages chronic disease	1. Certificate programs open to any registered nurse (RN) regardless of level of preparation 2. Master's level programs 3. RNs certified jointly by state boards of nursing and medicine
Clinical Specialist	
Advanced practitioner of nursing/clinical teacher	Master's degree (MSN, MN); also RNs
Nurse Scientist	
Nurse researcher or nurse educator	Doctor of Nursing Science (DNS) or Doctor of Philosophy (PhD) in Nursing or psychology, sociology, physiology, and anthropology

Adapted from McConnell ES. A conceptual framework for gerontological nursing practice. In Matteson MA, McConnell ES (eds). Gerontological Nursing: Concepts and Practice. Philadelphia: WB Saunders, 1988, p 35.

Box 29–1. SKILLS FOR GERONTOLOGICAL NURSING

Gerontological nurses should be skillful in applying generic nursing methods to care of the aged and be able to do the following:

- Use research findings from gerontology as well as from nursing and the biomedical and behavioral sciences to inform nursing practice.
- Interact with individuals who have sensory loss.
- Perform multidimensional assessment of the elderly person by using existing standardized tools and individualized approaches.
- Implement rehabilitative nursing techniques.
- Help clients integrate past life with present.
- Include the older person and family members in developing goals for nursing care, even if the individual has significant communication or cognitive impairments.
- Modify the environment to maximize the older person's ability to function independently.
- Provide excellent palliative, supportive, and spiritual care for those who are dying.
- Give counsel to the grieving.
- Consider ethical dilemmas encountered by old people, their kin, and their health care providers.
- Help families and communities overcome hostilities toward the elderly.
- Participate in professional activities designed to improve health care for the elderly.
- Supervise the efforts of paraprofessional and lay caregivers in providing nursing care to the aged.
- Teach paraprofessional and lay caregivers and old people about the impact of the aging process and the disease process on self-care abilities and requisites of older persons.
- Teach paraprofessional and lay caregivers and old people about techniques to achieve self-care objectives.
- Establish developmentally appropriate criteria for evaluation and nursing care.

Adapted from Matteson MA, McConnell ES (eds). Gerontological Nursing: Concepts and Practice. Philadelphia: WB Saunders, 1988, pp 37–38.

Table 29–2 ■ THE NURSING PROCESS AND THE CARE OF THE ELDERLY CLIENT

	ASSESSMENT	NURSING DIAGNOSIS	ESTABLISHING GOALS	INTERVENTION	EVALUATION
1. **Physiological needs:** Food/fluid Shelter/warmth Air Rest/sleep Avoidance of pain Sex	Usual and present nutritional, elimination, sleep, and sexuality patterns Physical activity exercise pattern Emotional pain and discomfort Suicide potential Physical health Medications	*Altered patterns of urinary elimination* *Altered nutrition* Dehydration *Constipation* *Sleep pattern disturbance* *Sexual dysfunction* *Knowledge deficits* Medications or physical illnesses that may cause depression *High risk for self-harm*	Establishing and maintaining adequate biological functioning in areas of sleep, nutrition, and elimination Relief from emotional pain and discomfort Elimination of drug- or disease-induced depression	Assist with ADLs Support of self-care abilities Encourage to start a physical activity regime Teach side effects of antidepressants Treat medical problems under poor control Change medications that may cause depression	Feelings of physical satiation Homeostasis Optimal physical health

Table continued on following page

Table 29–2 ■ THE NURSING PROCESS AND THE CARE OF THE ELDERLY CLIENT *Continued*

	ASSESSMENT	NURSING DIAGNOSIS	ESTABLISHING GOALS	INTERVENTION	EVALUATION
2. **Safety and security needs:** Feel free from danger Need for a predictable, lawful, orderly world Need to feel in control	Home environment assessment Mental status exam Assessment of visual acuity and hearing Knowledge of disease process Physical mobility	*Ineffective individual coping* *Powerlessness* *Fear* *Sensory/perceptual alterations* *Impaired physical mobility* *Self-care deficit*	Establish predictability and structure in environment Maintenance of a safe environment Realistic understanding of disease course and expected outcome Reversal of treatable confusion	ECT, hospitalization, antidepressive medications for the severely depressed Avoid relocations when possible Correct environmental hazards Encourage a structured daily routine Instruct about disease course and prognosis	Feeling in control of one's disease and optimistic about the future Confidence in the future Feelings of safety, peace, security, protection, lack of danger and threat
3. **Need for love, belonging, and affection:** Need for contact and intimacy Need for friends Need for feeling of having a place and "belonging" Need for interactions with others	Family relationships and members Friends that are supportive Recent losses Present and past social interactions	*Disruption in significant relationships* *Social isolation* *Lack of contact with, or absence of, significant others* *Impaired social interactions*	Maintenance of significant relationships with family and friends Establish community support system Resumption of previous level of social activity	Encourage social interactions that have been enjoyed in the past Encourage interactions with family members, friends, and health caregivers Provide reassuring, supportive atmosphere	Feelings of loving and being loved, of being one of a group, of acceptance
4. **Need for esteem and self-respect:** Need for achievement, mastery, and competence Need for reputation or prestige, appreciation, and dignity Need for love of self	Amount of pleasurable pursuits Emotional or mood assessment Role patterns Coping—stress-tolerance pattern Attitude about self, the world, the future	*Disturbance in self-esteem* *Loss of significant roles* *Unrealistic self-expectations* *Anxiety* *Lifestyle change* *Dependency on others*	Acceptance of realistic limitations Establish appropriate roles Achieve self-acceptance Accept ownership of consequences of one's own behavior	Teach problem-solving skills Cognitive therapy Promote self-care Counseling Behavior therapy Relaxation techniques	Feelings of self-confidence, worth, strength, capability and adequacy, of being useful and necessary in the world
5. **Need for self-actualization:** Need for beauty Need for self-expression Need for new situations and stimulation	Occupation, job history Value-belief patterns	Loss of zest for life *Spiritual distress* *Grieving*	Expression of self through meaningful recreational activities Exploring new interests	Encourage a non-restrictive environment Provide beauty in environment Read to the sick or hard of hearing Music	Autonomy Freshness of appreciation Creativeness Spontaneity Feelings of self-fulfillment

From Ronsman K. Therapy for depression. Journal of Gerontological Nursing, 13(12):21, 1987.
ADLs = activities of daily living; ECT = electroconvulsive therapy.

Table 29-3 ▪ GUIDELINES FOR THE FIRST INTERVIEW

APPROACH	PROCESS COMMENTS
1. Approach the client: note appearance, posture, spontaneous activity, grooming, hygiene, comfort, presence of others, facial expression, attentiveness, interest.	1. Cues gathered about musculoskeletal, neurological, genitourinary, gastrointestinal, cardiovascular, and pulmonary systems, cognitive and emotional function, senses, and social support.
2. Address the client by name. Introduce self: "My name is . . . I prefer to be called . . . What do you like to be called?"	2. Hearing. Ability to respond to social situation and to cues about cognitive and affective function.
3. Offer to shake hands or grasp client by the hand.	3. Neuromuscular function, strength, skin temperature, and texture.
4. Establish eye contact, ask about visual ability and use of glasses. Position self in full view of client. Adjust lighting for brightness, but avoid glare.	4. Assess vision.
5. Ask client about any hearing difficulties and if client can hear you clearly. Ask about the use of hearing aid, lip reading, better hearing in one ear than the other.	5. Cues about hearing and cognitive function.
"How are you feeling today?" If a clinic visit, "What brings you here today?" or "Is anything troubling you lately?" Probe specifically with open-ended questions, e.g., "Oh, you're hurting, tell me more about that."	Self-assessment of health, symptoms assessment, cognitive and verbal function, communication skills, optimism, and emotional response.
"What would you like help with today?" Note the issues identified and the order of concerns.	Cues about client's priorities, expectations, response to health, or social problems or concerns.
6. Summarize the interaction so far. "Mrs. J., we have approximately 45 minutes together to address your concerns. I think that will give us time to deal with the concerns you have voiced. I would like to proceed now by asking you a few more questions and then do the following exam procedures for these reasons."	6. Establish trust, contract for and set mutual expectations for the encounter, prioritize concerns, and validate inferences with the client.

From Matteson MA, McConnell ES (eds). Gerontological Nursing: Concepts and Practice. Philadelphia: WB Saunders, 1988, p 80.

Table 29-4 ▪ NURSING ASSESSMENT: SOCIAL DYSFUNCTION RATING SCALE

Directions: Score each of the items as follows:
1. Not present 2. Very Mild 3. Mild 4. Moderate 5. Severe 6. Very Severe

Self-esteem
1. _____ Low self-concept (feelings of inadequacy, not measuring up to self-ideal).
2. _____ Goallessness (lack of inner motivation and sense of future orientation).
3. _____ Lack of a satisfying philosophy or meaning of life (a conceptual framework for integrating past and present experiences).
4. _____ Self-health concern (preoccupation with physical health or somatic concerns).

Interpersonal System
5. _____ Emotional withdrawal (degree of deficiency in relating to others).
6. _____ Hostility (degree of aggression toward others).
7. _____ Manipulation (exploiting of environment or controlling at others' expense).
8. _____ Overdependency (degree of parasitic attachment to others).
9. _____ Anxiety (degree of feeling of uneasiness or impending doom).
10. _____ Suspiciousness (degree of distrust or paranoid ideation).

Performance System
11. _____ Lack of satisfying relationships with significant persons (spouse, children, kin, or significant persons serving in a family role).
12. _____ Lack of friends or social contacts.
13. _____ Expressed need for more friends or social contacts.

Table continued on following page

Table 29–4 ■ NURSING ASSESSMENT: SOCIAL DYSFUNCTION RATING SCALE *Continued*

Directions: Score each of the items as follows:
1. Not present   2. Very Mild   3. Mild   4. Moderate   5. Severe   6. Very Severe

14. _____ Lack of work (remunerative or nonremunerative, productive work activities that normally give a sense of useful-ness, status, or confidence).
15. _____ Lack of satisfaction from work.
16. _____ Lack of leisure time activities.
17. _____ Expressed need for more leisure, self-enhancing, and satisfying activities.
18. _____ Lack of participation in community activities.
19. _____ Lack of interest in community affairs and activities that influence others.
20. _____ Financial insecurity.
21. _____ Adaptive rigidity (lack of complex coping patterns to stress).

PATIENT: _____ RATER: _____ DATE: _____

From Linn MW, et al. A social dysfunction rating scale. Journal of Psychiatric Research, 6:299, 1969. Copyright 1969, with kind permission from Pergamon Press Ltd, Headington Hill Hall, Oxford OX3 0BW, UK.

ing the initial assessment. Because examination and interviews can produce anxiety in the elderly, and because the initial interview is often in unfamiliar surroundings, the guidelines in Table 29–3 are useful no matter what the setting or purpose of the interview.

Because effective coping, problem solving, and adaptive behaviors are necessary for healthy social functioning, the degree of social dysfunction needs to be assessed. The **Social Dysfunction Rating Scale** (Table 29–4) is widely used for this purpose.

Depression and substance abuse among the elderly are both major health problems. Because they both affect each other, a special scale for detecting the presence of depression among the elderly has been devised. **Zung's Self-rating Depression Scale** is one of the most widely used (Table 29–5). The client rates himself, unless he is illiterate or has vision problems.

Table 29–5 ■ NURSING ASSESSMENT: ZUNG'S SELF-RATING DEPRESSION SCALE*

	NONE OR LITTLE OF THE TIME	SOME OF THE TIME	A GOOD PART OF THE TIME	MOST OR ALL OF THE TIME
1. I feel down-hearted, blue, and sad.	1	2	3	4
2. Morning is when I feel the best.	4	3	2	1
3. I have crying spells or feel like it.	1	2	3	4
4. I have trouble sleeping through the night.	1	2	3	4
5. I eat as much as I used to.	4	3	2	1
6. I enjoy looking at, talking to, and being with attractive women/men.	4	3	2	1
7. I notice that I am losing weight.	1	2	3	4
8. I have trouble with constipation.	1	2	3	4
9. My heart beats faster than usual.	1	2	3	4
10. I get tired for no reason.	1	2	3	4
11. My mind is as clear as it used to be.	4	3	2	1
12. I find it easy to do the things I used to do.	4	3	2	1
13. I am restless and can't keep still.	1	2	3	4
14. I feel hopeful about the future.	4	3	2	1
15. I am more irritable than usual.	1	2	3	4
16. I find it easy to make decisions.	4	3	2	1
17. I feel that I am useful and needed.	4	3	2	1
18. My life is pretty full.	4	3	2	1
19. I feel that others would be better off if I were dead.	1	2	3	4
20. I still enjoy the things I used to do.	4	3	2	1

From Zung WK. A self-rating depression scale. Archives of General Psychiatry, 12:63, 1965. Copyright 1965, American Medical Association.
*A raw score of 50 or above is associated with depression requiring hospital treatment.

The score is derived by dividing the sum of the 20 items by 80 (the maximum score) (Lekan-Rutledge 1988). Scores above .38 or a raw score of 50 and over signify depression requiring hospital treatment (Zung 1965).

Unique Intervention Strategies

Pfeiffer (1978) emphasizes that the majority of older persons are well. Those that do present with mental problems are treatable and responsive. He stresses that psychotherapeutic approaches need to be simplified and modified for older clients. Certain psychotherapeutic techniques are useful for the elderly client:

1. Using crisis intervention techniques (see Chapter 11)
2. Understanding empathically
3. Encouraging ventilation of feelings
4. Re-establishing emotional equilibrium if the anxiety is out of hand
5. Explaining alternate solutions

Burnside (1988) offers specific guidelines for caring for an elderly client. She urges nurses to pace themselves, *not* to move quickly, rush, or joggle the client. She also urges nurses to "truly listen" and make the quality of their time important, not the quantity. Specific guidelines in the one-to-one relationships and interviews are listed subsequently (Burnside 1988):

1. Select a setting that provides privacy for the interview.
2. Make certain that the client is physically comfortable.
3. Ask the client what name he or she prefers to be called and then use it often.
4. Touch can be effective in getting the client's attention.
5. *Assess the client's mental status*, e.g., observe for any deficits in recent or remote memory and determine if any mental confusion exists. Be aware of *all* medications that the client is taking and their effects, any side effects, and possible drug interactions. A patient taking many medications can be confused.
6. *Ascertain the status of the client's sight and hearing faculties.* If the client has a hearing aid or glasses or both, make certain that they are being worn.
7. *Lighting in the interview setting is important*, as the older adult needs three times more light to see

than the teenager. Do not allow sunlight or bright lights to shine directly into the client's face, as the older adult's eyes are very sensitive to glare.

8. *Sit close to and speak directly to any clients who have hearing deficits.* Maintain direct eye contact with the client when sitting or standing not more than five feet away. When speaking, do *not* exaggerate lip movements; as this action distorts the mouth and what is being said. Talk in a moderate voice with a slower than normal rate of speech. Do *not* shout. This action accentuates the vowel sounds and obscures the consonants, which are already hard for the elderly person to hear.
9. *Observe the client for any signs of fatigue.* Gauge his or her attention span, and keep the interview short if necessary.
10. *Pace the interview*, slowing it, if necessary, to match the client's needs. At the same time, allow the client enough time to think and respond to any questions, instructions, or discussions.
11. Try to include the client in all decisions.
12. Explain clearly to the client all the possible options from which to choose when making a decision. (Remember that choices may be more limited for the aged.)
13. When possible, *use reminiscing strategies to keep obtaining information.* Stimulate memory chains by attempting to recall patterns of association that will improve the client's recollection.
14. If the client verbalizes low self-esteem or negative views of aging, pick up on his or her strengths and point them out.
15. *Give instructions to the client slowly and clearly; print them in letters large enough to be read later, when the client's anxiety level may be lower.* If you are using handouts, make sure that the type is large enough for the client to read.
16. *Make an appointment for the next meeting.* The client should understand what is expected both of the interviewer and of the client before the next meeting.
17. If possible, *include family members* in part of the interview for added input, clarification, support, and reinforcement.
18. Be an advocate for the elderly.

INPATIENT SETTINGS

When clients are institutionalized, group therapy is an economical way to provide therapeutic intervention. **Remotivation therapy, reminiscing therapy,** and **group psychotherapy** are three group modalities often led by nurses who have special training or education. Table 29–6 outlines the purpose, format, and

Table 29-6 ■ USEFUL GROUP MODALITIES FOR ELDERLY CLIENTS		
REMOTIVATION THERAPY	**REMINISCING THERAPY (LIFE REVIEW)**	**PSYCHOTHERAPY**
Purpose of Group		
• Resocialize *regressed* and *apathetic* clients.	• Share memories of the past. • Increase self-esteem. • Increase socialization. • Increase awareness of the uniqueness of each participant.	• Alleviation of psychiatric symptoms. • Increase ability to interact with others in a group. • Increase self-esteem. • Increase ability to make decisions and function more independently.
Format		

• Groups are made up of 10–15 clients.
• Meetings are held once or twice a week.
• Meetings are highly structured in a classroom-like setting.
• Group uses props.
• Each session discusses a particular topic.
• See Box 29–2 for the five basic steps used in each session.
	• Groups are made up of 6–8 people.
	• Meetings are held once or twice weekly for one hour.
	• Topics include holidays, major life events, birthdays, travel, and food.
		• Group size is 6–12 members.
		• Group members should share similar
		  a. Problems
		  b. Mental status
		  c. Needs
		  d. Sexual integration
		• Group meets at regularly scheduled times (number of times a week, duration of session) and place.

Desired Outcomes		

• Increases participant's sense of reality.
• Offers practice of health roles.
• Realizes more objective self-image.
	• Alleviates depression in institutionalized elderly.
	• Through the process of reorganization and reintegration provides avenue by which elderly can.
	  a. Achieve a new sense of identity.
	  b. Achieve a positive self-concept.
		• Decreases sense of isolation.
		• Facilitates development of new roles and re-establishes former roles.
		• Provides information for other group members.
		• Provides group support for effecting changes and increasing self-esteem.

Data from Matteson MA, McConnell ES (eds). Gerontological Nursing: Concepts and Practice. Philadelphia: WB Saunders, 1988.

desired outcomes for each type of group. Box 29–2 gives an example of a remotivation therapy session.

COMMUNITY-BASED PROGRAMS

The hazards of institutionalization are numerous and include increased mortality, decreased social opportunity, and "learned helplessness." The purpose of many community-based long term care services is to promote the elder's independent functioning and reduce stress on the family system (Henderson and McConnell 1988). One such program for the elderly is the **day care program.**

As a result of rising institutional costs and ever-longer waiting lists for in-home care, interest in alternatives to long term care is increasing. Much too often, individuals and their families can no longer afford the expense of a nursing home, and frequently

institutionalization is not the best answer. Therefore, help from federal, state, and local governments is required. The idea of establishing day care facilities should be seriously considered (Butrin 1985; Graham 1989).

The concept of day care is not new. It started in England in the early 1940s and came to the United States about a decade later. Essentially there are two types of day care programs: (1) supervised daytime recreation and social activities and (2) inclusive health care and rehabilitative programs (Koenen 1980). The boundaries of these programs do blend and overlap (O'Brien 1981).

The first program affords the participants the opportunity for recreation and social interaction; they usually do not receive rehabilitative care. This is the more common type and is less expensive to operate (Koenen 1980). The second program goes beyond meeting recreational and social needs; it provides re-

Box 29-2. EXAMPLE OF A REMOTIVATION SESSION
(BODIES OF WATER)

Step 1: Climate of Acceptance

The leaders personally welcomed each participant as he or she arrived at the group session. After the leaders introduced themselves, each group member made a self-introduction. The leader used a calendar to orient the members to the date and time of the current remotivation session. The theme for session 4 was introduced by the leader as "bodies of water—rivers, lakes, and oceans." All group members had some familiarity with bodies of water because of their residence in Seattle.

Step 2: Creating a Bridge to Reality

The world globe was used as a visual aid to stimulate discussion on bodies of water. The leader asked questions, such as "How are bodies of water formed from glaciers?" Pictures of glaciers, rivers, and lakes were shown.

The leader read poems about tide pools, sea shells, and fishing written by anonymous grade school children. Discussion was stimulated by the leader asking, "What can we do at the ocean?" Visual aids and props were provided for direct sensory stimulation. Some examples of these aids and props included (1) different types of sea shells, (2) fishing tackle and bait, (3) suntan lotion, (4) sun hat, and (5) sunglasses.

A poem by an anonymous author about fishing was read to the group. This was followed by recorded music with lyrics about fishing experiences.

Step 3: Sharing the World We Live In

Group discussion focused on jobs related to bodies of water. Topics the participants discussed in regard to self or others included crabbing, clamming, shrimping, and fishing. Visual aids were provided to stimulate further discussions of past-related experiences involving bodies of water. Pictures of river-rafting, canoeing, scuba diving, and sailing were shared.

Step 4: An Appreciation of the Work of the World

This time was used for the members to think about work in relation to others. More experiences in past-related work roles as well as hobbies and pastimes were discussed. The group then participated in singing a familiar old song, "Love Letters in the Sand," written in 1931 by J. Fred Coots and revived in 1957 when sung by Pat Boone.

Step 5: Climate of Appreciation

The group members were thanked individually by the leaders for coming to the group and sharing their experiences. The following remotivation session theme and meeting date were announced prior to terminating the session.

Group Response to Session 4

Most members of the group appeared to enjoy discussing their experiences in relation to bodies of water. Many members recalled fishing and boating experiences. Other members expressed interest in this topic by their nonverbal participation in touching and smelling some physical props and observation of visual aids. All but two participants touched the seashells and smelled the fish eggs. One lady in the group stood up and modeled the sun hat and glasses, while a man demonstrated how to reel in the line on a fishing pole. Several participants remarked on how beautiful the pictures of the glaciers were. All but a couple of group members sang to the recorded lyrics on fishing. One member stood up and danced to the music while many others clapped to her movements.

From Janssen JA, Giberson DL. Remotivation therapy. Journal of Gerontological Nursing, 14(6):31, 1988.

storative and posthospital care, health promotion, health maintenance and services for the high-risk elderly, and psychosocial services to the frail aged (O'Brien 1981). Nursing personnel, pharmacists, physicians, physiotherapists, occupational therapists, social workers, lay persons, and volunteers are available, forming a broad base of support necessary for such care. This program aims to prevent or slow down any mental, physical, or social deterioration in order to thus maximize the older adult's full potential regardless of disease or condition (Koenen 1980).

Payment for care depends on the facility and its funding source. Services may be paid for privately or by a federal or state governmental agency according to their eligibility requirements (Hogstel 1990). Most socially oriented centers derive their funding from clients, donations, and fundraising. Many of the medical models are funded through private insurance or Medicaid. Because of these sources, they are highly regulated and impose strict admission requirements.

For the disabled demented elderly, more units are currently being developed. They are meant to provide a safe and supportive environment that can give family members respite while providing a positive emotional atmosphere for the client. Emphasis is on maintaining competence in areas in which the individual is most capable. A high staffing ratio (ratio of staff members to clients), usually 1:3, is required. Although the inevitable cognitive decline cannot be prevented, the client's quality of life is enhanced, and psychosocial dysfunction is decreased. Restlessness, anxiety, and agitation that frequently occur in the demented client are kept to a minimum by providing a calm, nonthreatening environment (Ebersole and Hess 1990).

These programs are targeted to achieve the following: (1) furnish respite and support for caretakers, (2) provide socialization and stimulation appropriate for the demented client, and (3) assist family members to keep the individual in the community as long as is appropriate. To achieve these goals, the centers may emphasize therapeutic and recreational activities, mental and social stimulation, exercise and movement therapy, entertainment and music therapy, nursing and social work consultation, caregivers' support group, nutritional warm meals, and transportation (Simcox 1990).

Day care centers of one sort or another exist in nearly every state. Nationwide, there are more than 1,200 such centers, which is a great increase from the dozen that were present in 1970. With a combined annual budget of about $150 million, these centers care for an estimated 28,000 elderly. Approximately 75% are nonprofit institutions run by hospitals, centers for the elderly, or churches (Ansberry 1986).

Although the number of adult programs is growing, most limit themselves to recreation and social orientation. Even though many states are interested in developing health rather than social models, they look to the federal level for direction and participation in funding; consequently, the process has slowed down. Funding, or lack of it, continues to be a primary issue in the development of day care facilities.

Adult day care does provide a vital function for older adults and their families, thereby permitting them to continue their present living arrangements and to maintain their social ties to the community; this service relieves families of the burden of 24-hour daily care for their elderly dependents. If institutionalization becomes necessary, day care staff can work with their clients and their families to assess the present situation and make recommendations for placement.

Issues That Affect the Mental Health of Some Elderly

The issues chosen here for discussion are four of the most prevalent problems for many elderly: (1) *use of restraints* in the elderly comes into the forefront with changes in federal law; (2) *death and dying* of the elderly poses complex legal and ethical issues for the elderly client, the family, doctors, and nurses; (3) *suicide* is a growing phenomenon among the elderly; and (4) *alcoholism* is a "neglected disease" affecting both the physical and the mental health of some elderly. Elder abuse, another serious problem for many elderly, is covered in Chapter 12.

RESTRAINTS IN THE ELDERLY

The use of restraints in the elderly is an issue of ethical and legal interest. Restraints can be both physical and chemical. **Physical restraints** are any manual method or mechanical device, material, or equipment that inhibits free movement (Hogstel 1990; National Citizens' Coalition 1991). **Chemical restraints** are drugs given for the very specific purpose of inhibiting a specific behavior or movement (Hogstel 1990).

According to a recent Health Care Financing Administration report on state and federal licensure surveys of nursing facilities in the United States, 42% of all nursing home residents are tied at one time or another to their beds or chairs (Stilwell 1991). Furthermore, evidence suggests that once a resident is restrained, the individual will continue to be regularly restrained for an indefinite period of time (Blakeslee et al. 1991). Every day, more than 500,000 older people in hospitals and nursing homes are secured to their beds or chairs (Evans and Strumpf 1989).

Some of the questions about the practice of physical restraint include whether health care providers have the right to physically restrain another individual in such a manner and whether persons who are restrained are really safer (Masters and Marks 1990). Physical restraints are often used to prevent falls in the hospitalized or institutionalized confused elderly. Fear of litigation may often be the impetus for such action (Ebersole and Hess 1990).

In response to the use of restraints, the elderly have responded with anger, fear, humiliation, demoralization, discomfort, and resignation (Evans and Strumpf 1989). Even though physical restraints are used to prevent falls, *clients who were restrained were much more likely to be hurt than those who were not.* Residents in restraint-free facilities have experienced fewer injuries from falls than those in facilities using restraints. The risk of death through strangulation or asphyxiation when using physical restraints is of great concern (Blakeslee et al. 1991). In fact, several deaths have been reported as a result of restraints (Ebersole and Hess 1990).

In addition to these most severe consequences, immobilizing the elderly can result in many physical problems (Brower 1991; Blakeslee et al. 1991):

- Chronic constipation or impaction
- Disrupted vestibular function
- Reduced or impaired circulation
- Incontinence of urine and feces
- Abrasions and skin tears or pressure sores
- Loss of bone mass
- Reduced or impaired circulation
- Reduced metabolic rate
- Electrolyte losses
- Muscle atrophy, decreased tone and strength, and contractures

Any confused behavior exhibited by restrained residents may become intensified through immobilization. Restraints also have a dehumanizing effect on both the caregiver and the resident. Their use is in conflict with the concept of human dignity and individual independence (Blakeslee et al. 1991).

To correct these injustices, the **Omnibus Budget Reconciliation Act** (OBRA) came into law October 1, 1990. Nursing homes now are held accountable to a higher standard of care that focuses on the resident's "highest practicable, physical, mental, and psychosocial well-being" and are directed to support "individual needs and preferences" and to "promote mainte-

nance or enhancement of the quality of life" (National Citizens' Coalition 1991). OBRA mandates that each resident has the right to be free from unnecessary drugs and physical restraints and is provided treatment to reduce dependency on chemical and physical intervention (Hogstel 1990).

Restraints may be imposed only (1) to ensure *the physical safety of the resident or other residents*, and (2) upon the written order of a physician that *specifies the duration and the circumstances* under which the restraints are to be used (National Citizens' Coalition 1991).

The federal government has set standards of care for every nursing home receiving Medicare or Medicaid funds. The HCFA has been charged with enforcing these standards through inspections or "surveys." The guidelines direct HCFA surveyors to evaluate the use of physical restraint use and determine if (National Citizens' Coalition 1991):

- Less restraining measures were attempted
- Occupational or physical therapists were consulted
- The client and family received a complete explanation
- The device was used only for definite periods as an "enabler" to the resident or for brief periods to provide necessary life-saving treatment
- Use of restraints was detrimental to the resident's physical, mental, or psychosocial well-being

With respect to chemical restraints, HCFA will investigate to determine if:

- Residents are free from unnecessary drugs
- Residents are given antipsychotic drugs only to treat a specific condition
- Residents are given gradual dose reductions, drug holidays, and behavioral programming whenever possible, in lieu of medications

The guidelines on antipsychotic drugs list certain circumstances for which they can be prescribed, e.g., "organic mental syndromes" (including dementia) with associated psychotic or agitated features, specified by:

- Specific behaviors defined quantitatively and objectively that cause residents to present a danger to themselves or to others or actually hinder the staff in its ability to provide care
- Psychotic symptoms that cause the "resident frightful distress" (National Citizens' Coalition 1991)

Nurses can avoid liability by knowledge of the law, adherence to the policies and procedures of the institution, and by use of good nursing judgment. All nursing homes and hospitals should have written restraint procedures and policies to be made available to all health care providers. If restraints are used, the nurse is responsible for the safety of the client during that time. The client should be restrained only for a limited time and for a limited purpose (Hogstel 1990).

Restraints do not enhance resident care. Creative nursing skills and interventions are frequently more beneficial. The necessity of applying restraints "for the resident's safety" can often be avoided when effective communication and planning are used to decrease the client's anxiety and agitation. Nurses should be familiar with alternative methods of client control to produce desirable results. They should be aware of current research findings and support continued research in this sensitive area.

DEATH AND DYING AND THE ELDERLY

Life is bounded by two milestones: birth and death. To some, death is the completion of a life process; to others it is a passage to another life. For all, though, the thoughts and fears of death and its irreversibility have a particular significance.

As recently as 50 years ago, the elderly approaching death found themselves not in the hospital or nursing home but at home, with death usually taking place in familiar surroundings. The individual could thus progress through the dying process in the intimate environment of home (Olson 1981), with death to some extent being part of living.

As a youth-oriented society, Americans view death as not being of immediate concern but rather as a remote prospect. By turning their sick over to the medical experts, they expect the advanced technologies to answer all problems, including death. Thus, they insulate themselves from death (Ross 1981). Polls have been conducted on themes of death and prolonging life. When members in a retirement community were asked to assess the extent of intervention they would like should they be dying, the majority desired only comfort care; they were not interested in the life-extending processes. Many wanted to ensure that their wishes were followed by having a written document of such wishes accessible to their physicians (Snow and Atwood 1985). A Louis Harris poll of over 1000 adults found that 86% thought that terminally ill clients ought to be able to tell their physicians to let them die; almost an equal percentage favored withdrawal of feeding tubes, if this was the client's desire (Wallis 1986).

Another group was asked what they would desire if they had severe memory loss, were unable to care for themselves, or had no chance of recovery. A much greater percentage of older persons than younger ones said they would refuse intensive care or tube feeding.

Advances in Technology

Technological advances in medicine have brought about corresponding changes in life-sustaining machinery. Increasing efforts are made to keep alive elderly persons who otherwise would die. Physicians are having a difficult time making decisions affecting the care of their dying clients. The American College of Physicians Committee on Medical Ethics states that a physician has a responsibility to make certain that his or her hopelessly ill client dies with dignity and with as little suffering as possible (Jenike 1984).

These recommendations are not always easy to follow. As a rule, physicians feel compelled to apply treatment regardless of the client's prognosis—unless the client specifically objects or has a written living will (Kleiman 1985). Preserving life is what nurses and physicians have been educated and trained to do and what they have promised to do in their professional oaths. Their actions are geared toward sustaining and prolonging life (Wanzer et al. 1984). Withholding treatment from hopelessly ill clients may open physicians to malpractice charges (Kleiman 1985).

Medical technology has frequently outpaced our ability to apply it judiciously (Pinch and Parsons 1992). The lives of those who would have died sooner is often prolonged regardless of the client's mental capacity (Olson 1981). The percentage of elderly not dying at home but in a hospital or nursing home has been steadily increasing. Today, approximately 80% of all people die in hospitals or nursing homes, often surrounded by life-extending apparatuses (Wallis et al. 1986).

Although technology has resulted in decreased mortality in some areas, prevention of chronic illness has lagged behind. A definite aging population has evolved, which means that physicians, the elderly, and their families are facing more treatment decisions than ever before (Pinch and Parsons 1992). Society has never before faced the problem of so many people living for so long with such severe impairments. No specific cure exists for many of the chronic diseases afflicting the elderly, such as senile dementia, stroke, osteoporosis, advanced cancer, rheumatic disease, and arteriosclerosis (Nelson 1982).

Lower mortality rates and increased life expectancy have made death "less visible, less meaningful, and less controllable than it was in the past." For many persons, death has been "transposed, insulated, technologicalized, decontextualized" (Ross 1981). There is a growing concern that death in America is too often controlled by machines rather than by nature (Wallis 1986). Because of advances in medicine, the ability to extend life may carry "overwhelming emotional hardships, agonizing pain, and devastating financial costs" (Kaufman 1985). In the case of a terminally ill or demented client, a point may be reached in which the balance of what is to be "saved," when weighed against emotional and financial ruin, favors the latter. The question should be asked: "Should the quality of life become a weightier consideration than mere survival?" (Nelson 1982).

Technology has its price, and financing health care is a quickly escalating concern. Currently, 12.5% of the gross national product is allocated to health care. Cost should not determine ethical decisions, but financial considerations are important if technology is used when it is not desired or when the outcome does not warrant the risks involved (Pinch and Parsons 1992).

Since the 1960s, the public's desire to have a voice in making decisions about its care has been increasing. This interest in client advocacy has been recognized with the passage of the **Patient Self-Determination Act** (PSDA) of 1990.

Although the elderly are becoming better-educated consumers of health care, they are still reluctant to make health care decisions, such as the extent of medical interventions or a living will; instead, they prefer to rely informally on family members to make choices for them (Shawler et al. 1992). Before the passage of the PSDA, only about 10% of the population had some form of written advance directive, and less than 5% of acute care hospitals routinely inquired about the existence of such directives at the time of admission (Boyle 1992).

Patient Self-Determination Act (PSDA) of 1990

In June 1990, the US Supreme Court, in deciding the Nancy Cruzan "right-to-die" case, affirmed the right of a competent person to reject life-sustaining treatment (including hydration and nutrition). The court, however, held that states may ascertain the degree of proof required before a client's wishes set forth in an advance directive are honored. In response to the court's decision, Congress enacted the PSDA (Burke and Walsh 1992).

This act establishes guidelines regarding clients' requests before and during episodes of serious illness. It fosters clearer communication between them, their families, physicians, and health care workers (Smith 1992). Health care institutions that receive federal funds are now required to provide, at the time of admission, written information to each client regarding his or her right to execute "advance health care directives" and to inquire if such directives have been made by the client. The client's admission records should state whether such directives exist (Box 29-3).

Clients use such directives to indicate their preferences for the types of medical care they want or how much treatment they desire to have provided to them. The directives come into effect should physical or mental incapacitation prevent clients from making their health care decisions. These wishes can be communicated through one or more of the following instruments: (1) a living will, (2) a directive to physician, and (3) a durable power of attorney for health care. These documents must be in writing and witnessed; depending on state and institutional provisions, they may require notarization. Preprinted forms, varying from one to several pages, are available through various organizations (e.g., Concern for Dying/Society for Right to Die), hospitals, or stationery stores. These directives may be valid for up to seven years unless state law stipulates a shorter period. The individual must be of age and competent when signing the instrument (Table 29-7).

Living wills express clients' wishes about their future medical care. During times of crisis, living wills can influence the course of therapy. The idea originated in the late 1960s as a tool to allow individuals to restrict medical intervention when technology or treatment can no longer advance a reasonable quality of life or chance of recovery (MacKay 1992). Various sample forms are available if the individual does not want to have a lawyer draft his or her own living will.

The concept of a living will has been adopted nationwide. Corresponding living will statutes have been enacted in 44 states; other states should follow (MacKay 1992). These statutes, as a rule, allow terminally or irreversibly ill individuals to stipulate that life-sustaining procedures be limited, withheld, or withdrawn. Many states, however, do not recognize a request for the withdrawal of food, water, or both (Janofsky 1990).

A living will may not offer as much protection as the client might think—there are limitations. Only cases of terminal illnesses are covered. A living will does not extend to clients with chronic illnesses, such as Parkinson's disease, multiple sclerosis, or Alzheimer's disease. Living wills can be acted on only after a 14-day waiting period following verification by two physicians of the individual's terminal illness or irreversible condition (Rosenthal 1991).

Box 29–3. RESPONSIBILITIES OF HEALTH CARE PROVIDERS UNDER THE PATIENT SELF-DETERMINATION ACT OF 1990

Hospitals, skilled nursing facilities, home health agencies, hospice organizations, and health maintenance organizations servicing Medicare and Medicaid clients must

1. Maintain written policies and procedures for providing information to clients for whom they provide care.
2. Give written material to clients concerning their rights under state law to make decisions about medical care, including the right to accept or refuse surgical or medical care and to formulate advance directives and provide for written policies and procedures for the realization of these rights.
3. Document in clients' records whether they have advance directives.
4. Do not discriminate in care or other ways against clients who have or have not prepared advance directives.
5. Policies should be in place to ensure compliance with state laws governing advance directives.

The written information should be made available to clients as follows:

1. In hospitals, on admission as an inpatient
2. In skilled nursing facilities, on admission as a resident
3. By home health agencies, on coming under care of the agency
4. By hospice programs, on receiving care from the program
5. For health maintenance organizations, at the time of enrollment

From Schlossberg C, Hart MA. Legal perspectives. In Burke M, Walsh M (eds.): Gerontologic Nursing Care of the Frail Elderly. St. Louis: Mosby–Year Book, 1992, p 469.

The requirement that the living will be in writing ensures that there is no misunderstanding about the client's wishes at the time of the signing of the document. An oral declaration will not have the same effect. The living will can be revoked by the client orally (or by any other means) at any time, without regard to the individual's competency. The wish to rescind the living will can be made known to the health care provider directly or via a third person (e.g., a spouse) in front of the client (MacKay 1992). The health care provider must then follow the institution's protocol and act accordingly.

Executing a living will may not always guarantee its effectiveness. Notwithstanding the institution's legal obligation to inquire into the existence of any such directives, the client simply may not be in a state to respond to such questions at the time of admission. Almost half of all persons admitted to nursing homes may have serious cognitive defects (MacKay 1992). Thus, in many cases, the institution may not become aware of the existence of such a document, and the client's specified wishes may go unheeded. Consequently, it is advisable for anyone having such a document to keep it readily available and not hidden away. It would also be helpful if a family member, close friend, and the client's physician have copies or access to them.

The living will may designate a person to be contacted in the event that questions of interpretation arise. In the absence of such designation, the health care provider will follow an affirmative course under the maxim "when not certain, provide treatment."

A further shortcoming of the living will is the lack of specificity when it comes to naming the "heroic" measures the client chooses to relinquish (i.e., cardiopulmonary resuscitation, mechanical ventilation, or surgery). The use of vague terms, such as "hopeless" and "extraordinary" may also burden the usefulness of the living will (Rosenthal 1991).

With a **directive to physician,** a physician is appointed by the individual to serve as proxy. This directive must be completed on a prescribed form. Many of the features parallel those of a living will (i.e., presence of terminal illness, verification by the physician, and competency at time of signing).

The directive to physician can be particularly useful in cases in which a terminally ill individual with no family or close ties to others feels most comfortable with having his or her physician act as surrogate. The physician must agree in writing to be the client's

	Table 29–7 ■ ADVANCE DIRECTIVES		
FEATURES	**LW**	**DTP**	**DPAHC**
Client competent to initiate	Yes	Yes	Yes
Client competent to revoke	No	No	Yes
Special form needed	No	Yes	No
Lasts up to 5 years	Yes	Yes	Yes
Lasts at least 7 years	No	No	Yes
Client needs agent or surrogate decision maker	No	Yes	Yes
Physician required to be agent or surrogate decision maker.	No	Yes	No
Used only for terminal illness or when death is imminent	Yes	Yes	No
Can go into effect immediately	No	No	Yes
Need 14-day waiting period after terminal illness is determined	Yes	Yes	No
Two physicians needed to determine terminal illness	Yes	Yes	No

From MacKay S. Durable power of attorney for health care. Geriatric Nursing, 13(2):99, 1992.
DPAHC = durable power of attorney for health care; DTP = directives to physicians; LW = living will.

agent and he or she must also be one of the two physicians who made the original determination that the client is terminally ill (MacKay 1992). Like the living will, the directive to physician can be revoked orally at any time without regard to client competency.

The **durable power of attorney for health care** (DPAHC) differs from the two earlier instruments in that a person (other than a physician) is appointed to act as the client's agent, and there is no waiting period for implementation. Furthermore, with the DPAHC, the client must not only be competent and of age when making the appointment but must also be competent to revoke the power. Designating a health care proxy is generally a simple step (Rosenthal 1991). No waiting period is necessary for the DPAHC to go into effect. Furthermore, individuals do not have to be terminally ill or incompetent for the person appointed with the health care power of attorney to act on their behalf. No physician's certification is required.

Agents can make decisions for their clients whenever necessary. They need not be relatives but can be anyone in whom the clients trust and who are willing to accept the responsibilities. The scope of their au-

thority reaches beyond decisions on withholding interventions or treatment to more general aspects of medical care. The agent becomes the client's advocate in all medical matters and may even limit the institution from providing services to the client that he or she believes is not wanted.

Health care providers who have backed away from living wills because of frequent ambiguities may find the DPAHC more agreeable. Relying solely on a living will document to make a life-or-death decision can be uncomfortable for the provider. Under the DPAHC, a surrogate is named with whom the health care provider can consult and discuss treatment alternatives (Rosenthal 1991).

Because not all state laws authorize these instruments, they might not be binding in jurisdictions without explicit statutes. In such cases, the health care providers would decide whether to accept the advanced directives (Janofsky 1990).

In short, the DPAHC provides the best option for most clients (MacKay 1992). Still, some individuals may choose to supplement a DPAHC with a living will, keeping the latter "in reserve" in case of need for possible clarification of their wishes.

Hospice Care

One alternative to dying in hospitals or nursing homes is the hospice approach. The **hospice philosophy** is characterized by the acceptance of death as a natural conclusion to life; the clients have the right to live and die in a way decided by them, rather than a way set by the care providers (MacElveen-Hoehn and McIntosh 1981). One goal of hospice care is to establish a special bond between the individual who is dying and the family (Burggraf and Stanley 1989). Terminally ill clients thus receive supportive care in their homes or in a home-like setting. The focus is on keeping dying people comfortable, free of pain, as active as possible, and close to their families. They need not fear being subjected to prolonged medical care against their wishes. The hospice approach may constitute for many an acceptable equilibrium between the clients' needs and wishes and the emotional financial strain on their relatives.

Nurse's Role in the Decision-Making Process

If the client cannot decide for himself or herself, nurses may be in the best position to know whether "the remaining life is worth the suffering of the client." Not only do they spend more time with the client than the physician and often even family members, but they also have a broader understanding of the client because of their communication skills and concerns with the sociological and psychological basis of illness and health. The nurse is often involved in decisions of whether to treat the client aggressively or to allow the client to die without the use of life-support equipment (Olson 1981). Box 29–4 offers guidelines relating to issues of life and death (Alford 1986).

In working with the client's family, the nurse should orient family members and significant others about the ethicolegal policies of the institution and assist them to live with, and understand the concepts of, dying and death (Alford 1986). The nurse should explain that the family need not feel morally obligated to provide for all possible medical care, extending only the suffering of the client. This is especially true when such extraordinary measures do not represent the client's values and beliefs (Sherlock and Dingus 1984).

Maintaining an open and continuing dialogue among the client, family, nurse, and physician is of principal importance. The nurse should serve as an advocate for competent clients in their decision making and should be supportive of the client's surrogate when determinations need to be made (Alford 1986).

Any indication the clients might have given in the past about their views toward death and dying should have a bearing on their medical care. Existence of a living will is also an indication of their wishes. *Old age alone ought not to be a factor.* Age becomes significant only as expressed by the client, e.g., "I'm tired; I'm too old; I want to go" (Gadow 1979).

Each health care institution should have a written policy on "coding" to serve as a guideline for physicians and nurses. Affected clients should have orders in effect for implementation. **The nurse should never accept verbal "no-code" orders from physicians** (Alford 1986).

In addition, each health care facility receiving federal funds must have written policies and procedures and protocols in compliance with the PSDA. Such guidelines result in more, not less, involvement and responsibilities for nurses (Shawler et al. 1992). Nurses must prepare themselves for the legal, ethical, and moral issues involved when giving advance directive counseling (Moore 1992). The new law does not specify who must talk with clients about treatment

---

Box 29–4. GUIDELINES FOR RELATING TO ISSUES OF LIFE AND DEATH

1. Understand that it is the client's will, not health, that is all-important.
2. Assess the client for ethicolegal factors, e.g., living wills, guardianship, and competency.
3. Know the state's nursing practice act and understand the state laws and the institution's policies concerning death and the termination of life support systems.
4. Follow the American Nurses' Association (ANA) Code of Ethics and the ANA Standards of Gerontological Nursing.

Data from Alford D. Managing ethical and legal dilemmas in the care of the elderly. Presentation at Current Directions in Gerontological Nursing, Bethesda, MD, 1986.

decisions, but in many facilities nurses are being asked to do this.

When this is the case, policy and procedure manuals should outline the nurses' responsibility for discussing advanced directives with clients and for ensuring that such directives are included in the clients' charts.

Institutions are required to implement the mandates of the act. Although federal law, through the PSDA, requires institutions to develop corresponding policies and procedures, state law governs the specifics of such guidelines. **Nurses need to be cognizant of their state laws,** such as what advanced directives are permitted and what can be withheld. Nurses should be available to clients and their families to respond to questions on the ramifications of the act and to provide appropriate resources in answering their questions (Boyle 1992).

If the nurse becomes aware that the advance directive of a client is not being carried out, the nurse, as the client's advocate, should intervene on the client's behalf. If the problem is not resolved after the nurse talks with the individual's physician, the nurse should follow the facility's protocol by notifying the appropriate supervisor (Boyle 1992).

Making decisions regarding the treatment of an incapacitated client is never easy. The existence of an advance directive can guide the health care providers in this process. Clear-cut answers will not always be found. However, a conscientious and informed health care provider, together with clear and established written policies and procedures of the institution, will facilitate the process of following the client's wishes (Gobis 1992).

SUICIDE AND THE ELDERLY

Despite recent publicity about the growing number of suicides among the young, suicide rates of the elderly in the United States are 50% higher and continue to be the highest of any age group (McIntosh 1985; Osgood 1988). Comprising about 13% of the population, the elderly account for 25% of the total number of annual suicides (Eliopoulos 1987). The percentage of older persons taking their own lives is on the rise (Brant and Osgood 1990). Refer to Chapter 21 on suicide.

One study identifies despair as the major motive for suicide (Burnside 1988). Other significant factors are feelings of hopelessness and uselessness. For the older adult, suicide may be seen as a final gesture of control at a stage when independence is at risk or activities are limited. For this reason, a suicide attempt is more likely to succeed. Unlike with younger persons, there may be no history of previous suicidal gestures or attempts (Ebersole and Hess 1990).

Money can be a contributing factor to the high suicide rate. Federal reductions in programs like Medicare, Medicaid, and food stamps, along with state ordered medical-aid cuts, cause many elderly Americans to worry about their future. An inverse relationship between economic conditions and suicide rate has been identified (Marshall 1978).

Statistically, among the elderly, the white male consistently has the highest suicide rate, particularly if he is over 75 years of age (Burnside 1988; Eliopoulos 1987; Forbes and Fitzsimons 1981; Whall 1985). This rate seems to reflect the significant role that position and achievement play in the lives of the older white male. In old age, they may suffer more fundamental losses than women do. For example, an aging man may lose status, contact with fellow workers, and wage and station, whereas many older women retain many of the roles that they had during their earlier years (Ebersole and Hess 1981). Because men have been more likely to achieve and associate with high social standing more than women, a loss in status at retirement or otherwise can be more traumatic for them, although this is changing with the change in women's roles.

Assessing Suicide Risk in the Elderly

Other **high-risk suicide factors in the elderly** are (1) *widowhood*, (2) *illnesses and intractable pain*, (3) *status change*, and (4) *losses*. With respect to the latter, losses may be personal in nature (death of a family member or close friend), economic (loss of earnings or job), or social (loss of prestige or position) (McIntosh 1985; Boxwell 1988). The potential for suicide is intensified by these changes and losses.

Old age has been described as a "season of losses." Frequently, multiple losses accompany the aging process (Osgood 1988). These losses increase stress at a time when the older adult may be the most vulnerable and least resistant to stress, precipitating a depressive state. Nevertheless, the majority of older adults are able to function despite their losses. Those who give in may do so because of hopelessness (Boxwell 1988).

The technological advances that extend the lives of older adults sometimes bring a quality of life that is not acceptable to them. Some elderly people may decide that their lives are not worth living under such circumstances and opt for "rational" suicide. In these instances, they may have at least have the tacit support of their children, who may resent the cost and problems of keeping their parents alive (Tolchin 1989).

Vigilance with regard to suicide in later life should be maintained. The significant increase in the sheer number of elderly is expected to lead to a doubling in the number of suicides within the next 40 years. These rates are anticipated to swell as "baby boomers" grow older. Although life expectancy has increased, individuals continue to retire at about the same age. Fears about their livelihood, inflation, and possible collapse of pensions become critical factors. Any cutbacks in medical care will cause anxiety about continuing health care to increase. All these aspects are likely to contribute to an increase in the suicide rate (Blazer et al. 1986).

In assessing suicide risk, the health care provider must examine prior suicidal behavior and understand that the elderly make fewer suicidal gestures than the population at large. An inquiry into the client's idea of the future should also be examined (Boxwell 1988).

If suicide is contemplated, there is likely to be a strong determination to succeed, causing the elderly to choose a reliable method. Guns are the most common means of suicide (used by approximately 75% of men and 33% of women) (Suicide Rate Among Elderly Rises 1991). Jumping, hanging, and drowning are also relatively frequent methods. The ratio of attempts to completed suicides among all ages is about 10:1, whereas in those over 65, the ratio is 10:9 (Richardson et al. 1989).

Depression continues to be the most common factor in all suicide activities (Burnside 1988). As the most frequent functional psychiatric disorder of later life, causing between 50 and 70% of the late-life suicides (Richardson et al. 1989), it has also been the most underdiagnosed and undertreated disorder (St. Pierre et al. 1986).

Depression puts the client at an increased risk for suicide (Friedman 1976). It is the most frequent functional psychiatric disorder of later life, causing between 50 and 70% of the suicides among the elderly (Gurland and Cross 1983). It has also been the most underdiagnosed and undertreated disorder (St. Pierre et al. 1986).

Depression Versus Dementia

Depression is often confused with dementia. This is an important fact for nurses to keep in mind. Unlike dementia, depression is treatable with medication and other interventions. Depression is not always recognized as such. Assessment may be difficult because the depressed elderly may appear demented. They

may show profound memory and other intellectual impairments, become very unsociable, or agitated, and appear to be demented. A careful systematic assessment, therefore, is necessary to properly identify the illness (St. Pierre et al. 1986).

In making assessment, the health care provider needs to be familiar with the symptoms of later-life depression, which may include one or more of the following (Osgood 1988):

- Changes in sleep patterns and symptoms of insomnia
- Changes in eating patterns—particularly, loss of appetite
- Weight loss
- Excessive fatigue
- Increased concern with bodily functions
- Alterations in mood
- Expression of apprehension and anxiety without any reason
- Low self-esteem, feelings of insignificance, or pessimism

A careful evaluation of the etiology of any presenting depression is also necessary. Depression can be caused by drugs, such as reserpine, rauwolfia derivatives, steroids, and phenothiazines, as well as by metabolic and endocrine diseases, like hepatitis and adrenal and thyroid insufficiency. Generally, chronic health problems may also augment the suicide potential (Osgood 1988).

Antidepressants and the Elderly

In choosing a drug to treat depression in the elderly, primary emphasis should be placed on avoiding possible side effects rather than on efficacy. When starting therapy, low antidepressant dosages are generally recommended; they then can be slowly and gradually increased. Orthostatic hypotension is of particular concern in the elderly. *Nortriptyline* and *doxepin* are two drugs reported to have low orthostatic effects. The elderly male may have a pre-existing condition of prostatic hypertrophy. Desipramine and trazodone have the fewest anticholinergic effects on urinary retention. Drugs with a high degree of sedation, such as doxepin or trazodone, may be less desirable than desipramine or nortriptyline in the treatment of the elderly with coexisting symptoms of psychomotor retardation or hypersomnolence (Neshkes and Jarvik 1986).

Social networks to reduce suicide potential have not been as successful among older adults as they have been for younger persons (Ebersole and Hess 1990). The elderly with suicidal tendencies infrequently seek help; they have difficulty admitting that they have a weakness (Gottashalk 1986). They may be reluctant to turn to others because of the ethical and moral stigma of suicide and suicidal ideation or the social embarrassment of psychiatric illness. Instead of looking for assistance from the mental health professional, the suicidal geriatric client would rather go to his or her primary care provider and complain of depressive or somatic manifestations. Primary care providers, therefore, must have sensitive assessment skills for suicidal risk and be knowledgeable about methods of intervention (Boxwell 1988).

Right to Suicide

One concern of nursing is the question of whether an elderly individual has the right to commit suicide. Intensifying the ethical and moral dilemma of suicide is the distinction that must be made between suicide and voluntary active euthanasia (Boxwell 1988). Although society frowns on suicide in general, there seems to be a growing recognition that elderly persons with terminal illnesses should be able to take their own lives. If an elderly alert client is confronted with an intractable, lingering, and painful illness, with no hope of relief except for suicide, is the intervention of the health care provider to prevent suicide justifiable? If the determination is made to intervene, e.g., by hospitalization and physical restraint, it could be suggested that the health care provider has placed a higher value on the client's life than the client has (Boxwell 1988).

Although suicide is discussed in Chapter 21, there are specific factors that concern the elderly, such as retirement-related difficulties, physical illness, economic problems, loneliness, social isolation, and ageism. Innovative methods to deal with these factors need to be developed for the elderly. Education of the public in general and health care providers in particular is necessary to raise the level of awareness of this geriatric problem (McIntosh 1985).

ALCOHOLISM AND THE ELDERLY

Alcoholism, the country's most neglected disease, is a particular concern for the older adult (Lasker 1986). Although more than 10% of all older Americans are affected by it (Ostrander 1992), the vast majority (85%) receive no treatment for it (Parette et al. 1990). There are *two major types of alcohol abusers*: (1) the "*aging alcoholic*" and (2) the "*geriatric problem drinker*." The *aging alcoholic* has had alcohol problems intermittently throughout most of his early life, with regular alcohol-abusive pattern starting to evolve in late middle or older age. The *geriatric problem drinker*, on the other hand, has no history of alcohol-related problems but develops an alcohol-abusive pattern in response to the stresses of aging (Johnson 1989).

The stressful, or "reactive factors," that precipitate late-onset alcohol abuse are often caused by environmental conditions that may include retirement, widowhood, and loneliness. These stressors on the older adult, who may have retired, may not drive, and may be isolated from family and friends (Johnson 1989), are often greater than the problems faced by the middle-aged adult, who has to manage a job or career and care for a family and household. Work and family responsibilities may help keep a potential alcoholic from drinking too much. Once these demands are gone and the structure of daily life is disrupted, there is little impetus to remain sober. Older adults who lose a spouse through death, divorce, or legal separation are at highest risk of becoming late-in-life alcoholics (Brody 1988).

Alcohol abuse in the elderly may be difficult to identify. When a person is no longer in the familiar surroundings of work or relatives, family members, friends, and employers are not available to notice changes in behavior and personality attributable to abuse.

Alcohol and Aging

Excessive consumption of alcohol can create particular problems for the elderly. The older adult has an increased biological sensitivity to, or conversely, a decreased tolerance for, the effects of alcohol. This diminished resistance, combined with age-related changes, such as weakened manual dexterity, balance, and postural flexibility, can increase the likelihood of falls, burns, or other accidents (Valanis et al. 1987).

Some drinkers, as they get older, note changes in their response to alcohol, such as headaches, reduced mental abilities with memory losses or lapses, and a malaise rather than a feeling of well-being. These problems start to occur at lower levels of consumption than used to be the case in earlier years. Older persons are likely to drink more frequently but in lesser quantities than younger individuals, who tend to drink larger amounts less often (Gomberg 1980). Thus, the possibility of alcohol abuse in cases of only moderate ingestion by the elderly is not frequently recognized by the alcoholic's friends or family (Alcohol and the Elderly 1984).

With aging, the body becomes less resilient; healing from injury or infection is slower, and stress is more likely to cause a loss of physiological equilibrium. As the proportion of fatty tissues to lean body mass increases with age, the individual's metabolic rate usually slows down, increasing the amount of time it takes the body to eliminate drugs (Parette et al. 1990).

Alcohol and Medication

The interaction of drugs and alcohol in the elderly can have serious consequences. There is a decreased functioning of the liver enzymes that break down the alcohol, which on a short term basis has the effect of prolonging the action of many medications, potentiating their effect. On the other hand, chronic ingestion of alcohol enhances the metabolism of many drugs by causing faster turnover of medication.

Older individuals can expect higher blood alcohol levels than younger persons for an equivalent intake of alcohol (Schuckit 1982). Alcohol's effects on the brain may be one reason that alcohol abuse sometimes mimics or exacerbates normal changes of aging because even a moderate intake of alcohol can impair the cognition and coordination skills that are already decreased with age.

The effects of alcohol can be particularly harmful if an older person is taking antidepressants or tranquilizers (Hartford and Samorajski 1982). Extreme care is required in treating the older alcoholic with any medications. For example, the therapeutic use of disulfiram (Antabuse) to cause disagreeable psychological and physiological reactions when alcohol is drunk is not recommended because of possible cardiovascular side effects (Gulino and Kadin 1986).

Alcohol consumption produces a change in a person's sleep pattern, particularly affecting the older adult. Unlike younger persons, the elderly take longer to fall asleep and do not sleep as restfully. Although alcohol may decrease the time it takes to fall asleep, this benefit is offset by frequent awakenings caused by alcohol during the night (Hartford and Samorajski 1982).

Symptoms of Aging Versus Symptoms Seen in Alcohol Dependence

Health practitioners working with the elderly need to be concerned with, and sensitive to, possible alcohol abuse among their older clients. Careful assessment of the conditions is necessary to differentiate the normal physiological changes of the aging from those due to excessive drinking. Some of the symptoms of alcohol abuse are poor coordination, visual disturbances, slurred speech, and gastrointestinal complaints; they may often mimic the normal aging process (Gulino and Kadin 1986). Confusion and disorientation in an older client is not always caused by dementia or Alzheimer's disease but may be due to alcohol abuse (Hartford and Samorajski 1982).

Treatment for the Elderly Alcoholic

Because many elderly do not live in big families or have work-related contacts, they are less likely to be referred for treatment than are younger drinkers (Gulino and Kadin 1986). Too often, by the time the elderly alcoholic comes to the notice of any treatment agencies, the client's support systems and resources are severely decreased or depleted. Declining social, physical, and psychological performances are frequently found in the elderly alcoholic, thus exacerbating the difficulties of loneliness, depression, monotony, accidents, social conflict, loss, and physiological changes of aging (Burns 1988).

Ageism has deterred the development of treatment programs specially designed for the elderly. Beliefs about the elderly as being too isolated, too embedded in denial of their illness, and too old to function have been detrimental in encouraging health professionals to work with chemically dependent seniors (Lindblom et al. 1992).

Treatment plans for the elderly problem drinker should emphasize social therapies. Elderly alcoholics tend to be more passive than younger alcoholics and may benefit from interpersonal involvement with professional health care personnel (Burns 1988). The old respond easily to emotional and social support (Gulino and Kadin 1986). Family therapy should be encouraged. Group therapy made up of middle-aged and older alcoholics can be effective (Gomberg 1980).

The older alcoholic who does seek help may be confronted with serious gaps and inadequacies in the health care delivery system (Gulino and Kadin 1986). Substance abuse counselors, therefore, must be in contact with other agencies providing services to the elderly so that their help can be coordinated. They should be cognizant of the financial and transportation abilities of their elderly client (Gomberg 1980).

The aging alcoholic is difficult to treat. On the other hand, prognosis for the geriatric problem drinker—a person who had led his life up to this point without

Table 29–1A ■ ANSWERS TO QUIZ: FACTS AND MYTHS OF AGING

1. **False.** Ninety percent of older adults possess a healthy mental ability, 5% exhibit symptoms of chronic mental dysfunction, and another 5% display signs of acute mental impairment (Courtenay and Suharat 1980).

2. **True.** All the senses decrease with aging. Many of the changes begin slowly when the individual is in his or her mid-forties and increase with aging. (1) Vision: Particularly affected are peripheral vision, visual acuity, adaptation to dark, and accommodation (presbyopia). (2) Hearing: Decreased ability to hear high frequency sounds with later changes possibly involving middle and low frequency sounds (presbycusis); males tend to show hearing loss earlier than women. (3) Taste: The number of functioning taste buds is reduced, which particularly affects the ability to taste sweet and salty flavors. (4) Touch: Simultaneously occurring with age are the loss of receptors and an increased threshold for stimulation; pain and pressure are thus not as easily sensed. (5) Smell: A decline in the number of fibers in the olfactory nerve has been reported, leading to speculation that smell also undergoes age-related changes (Eliopoulos 1987).

3. **True.** As one ages, muscle fibers atrophy and decrease in number with fibrous tissue slowly displacing muscle tissue. Overall muscle mass, muscle strength, and muscle movements decrease. The arm and leg muscles, which become particularly flabby and weak, show these changes as well. Exercise is important to minimize the loss of muscle tone and strength (Eliopolous 1987).

4. **False.** Sexual interest and activity continue to play a pivotal role in providing life satisfaction (Atchley 1987).

5. **True.** Masters and Johnson in their work on human sexuality found that regular sexual expressions for the older adult are important for maintained sexual capacity and effective sexual performance (McCarthy 1979; Atchley 1987).

6. **True.** Changes in sleep patterns occur along the entire life span. Restorative sleep declines rapidly with aging and by age 50 is reduced by 50%. It not only takes the elderly more time to achieve restorative sleep than the younger adult, but with aging, sleep is less effective (Lerner 1982; Burke and Walsh 1992).

7. **True.** Comprising 11% of the population, the elderly accounted for 25% of all prescription drugs sold. This is not a surprising finding, since the incidence of chronic diseases among the elderly is high and prescription drugs are often used with chronic disease (Raffoul et al. 1981; Burggraf and Stanley 1989).

8. **False.** All age groups can learn. Limited, of course, by any physical limitations, older adults can usually master anything others can do if allowed a little more time. Jobs involving manipulation of objects or symbols or requiring discrete and clear responses are particularly well performed by older people (Atchley 1988; Burggraf and Stanley 1989).

9. **True.** Clinical depressive disorders increase in both prevalence and intensity with age. It may be called the "common cold" of the elderly and is expected to further increase in the years ahead (Steffl 1984; Ebersole and Hess 1990).

10. **False.** The ability to change and adapt has little to do with one's age but more with one's character (Judson 1985).

11. **False.** Although a small number of aged are very well off, and many are moderately comfortable, a large segment remains poor. According to government statistics, 12% of older adults live in poverty (Burke and Walsh 1992).

12. **True.** One out of three retirees encounters difficulty adjusting to retirement. Adapting to a diminished income and no longer being in a job-related environment were two of the most frequently listed causes of difficulty (Atchley 1988).

13. **True.** In May 1982, the House Select Committee on Aging conducted a study on crimes and fraud. Senior citizens make up 11% of the population but constitute about 30% of the victims of crime. Business and investment frauds rank high on the list of white-collar crimes perpetrated against the elderly (Chairman of the Select Committee on Aging 1982).

14. **False.** Eighty percent of older adults are healthy enough to carry on their normal lifestyles; 15% have chronic health conditions interfering with their lives; about 5% are institutionalized (Ebersole and Hess 1990).

15. **True.** Older persons are more reliable workers; their accuracy, performance, and stability are better and the number of accidents is lower except in situations requiring rapid reaction time (Palmore 1979).

16. **False.** Most elderly have relatives, friends, and organizations that are significant to them. About two-thirds do not consider loneliness a problem (Ebersole and Hess 1990).

17. **False.** Medicaid is a federally assisted state administered program that provides health care benefits to low income persons. Medicare, on the other hand, provides health insurance basically to individuals 65 and over (Atchley 1987).

18. **False.** The term "ageism" reflects the negative prejudicial views of older people that pervade our youth-oriented society (Hogsted 1990).

19. **True.** Nearly twice as many widowers wed annually as compared with widows in spite of the fact that older widows outnumber older widowers by four times. In addition, half of those widowers who do remarry choose wives under 65 years of age (Atchley 1988).

20. **True.** Sociologists have found that for the older widow, widowhood is viewed as ordinary with supports available from family, friends, and the community. The younger widow, however, is viewed differently: widowhood is not a normal occurrence. Young women are permitted to play the widow role for only a brief period of time, and they are considered to be single rather than widowed. Because they are in the minority, these women feel stigmatized by widowhood. The younger the widow, the more problems she encounters (Atchley 1988).

recourse to alcohol and whose drinking is caused by losses and stress—is excellent. It is important that health care providers recognize this recovery potential. Proper education and awareness of a positive out-

come for the geriatric problem drinker could increase the availability of resources: if the prognosis is good, providers and agencies should be more willing to spend resources on treatment. This knowledge is valuable to share with the older client because restorative outcome is so frequently a self-fulfilling prediction (Gomberg 1980).

Among health care providers, nurses in particular are in an excellent position to assess and recognize elderly clients with alcoholic problems—they can educate the problem drinkers and their families, physicians, and emergency room and other health personnel (Gomberg 1980). It is important for both older persons and practitioners in aging to realize that society's attitudes play a big role in determining how well older people recover. The myths that surround aging become entanglements for alcoholics: they are considered too old to change, or deemed to have earned the right to be left alone to do what they want (Ostrander 1992). The health care provider can overcome these myths by taking an affirmative position that the client, particularly in the case of the geriatric problem drinker, can still effectively function and become an active participant in society.

Considering the magnitude of the problems and the likelihood that numbers of older abusers will continue to increase, efforts need to be intensified to identify the causes and to develop appropriate interventions to treat alcohol dependence among the elderly. If not, such dependence can overwhelm those charged with meeting the health and social-service needs of the older adults (Parette et al. 1990).

Summary

There are a number of issues that older adults face as they age and many myths existing that foster negative attitudes. Ageism is found in all levels of society and even among health care providers, thereby affecting the way they render care to their elderly clients.

Nurses who care for the elderly in various settings may function at various levels, such as generalist, nurse practitioner, and a clinical specialist in gerontological nursing. Nurses working with the mentally ill elderly client should know about aging and about psychotherapeutic approaches to the elderly. Nurses with special training and education may lead remotivation, reminiscing, or psychotherapy groups geared toward the special needs of this population.

Older adults face increasing problems of alcohol and suicide. The OBRA sets guidelines and a philosophy of care for clients to be free from unnecessary drugs and physical restraints. When it comes to dying and death, older adults' wishes and those of their families are frequently ignored. The implementation of the PSDA of 1990 can afford some clients autonomy and dignity in death.

References

A Profile of Older Americans: 1990. Washington, DC: American Association of Retired Persons, 1990.

Adelson R, Nasti A, et al. Behavioral ratings of health professionals' interactions with the geriatric patient. Gerontologist, 22(3):227, 1982.

Alcohol and the elderly. Geriatrics 39(12):28, 1984.

Alford D. Managing ethical and legal dilemmas in the care of the elderly. Presentation at Current Directions in Gerontological Nursing. Bethesda, MD, 1986.

Ansberry C. Day care centers for the elderly spring up as alternatives to costly nursing homes. Wall Street Journal, December 8, 1986:29.

Atchley R. Social Forces and Aging. Belmont, CA: Wadsworth, 1988.

Austin D. Attitudes toward old age: A hierarchical study. Gerontologist, 25(4):431, 1985.

Benson E. Attitudes toward the elderly: A survey of recent nursing literature. Journal of Gerontological Nursing, 8(5):279, 1982.

Blakeslee JA, Goldman GD, et al. Making the transition to restraint-free care. Journal of Gerontological Nursing, 17(2):4, 1991.

Blazer D, Bachar J, Manton K. Suicide in late life: Review and commentary. Journal of the American Geriatrics Society, 34:519, 1986.

Bower HT. Social organization and nurses' attitudes toward older persons. Journal of Gerontological Nursing, 7(5):293, 1981.

Boxwell A. Geriatric suicide: The preventable death. Nurse Practitioner, 13(6):10, 1988.

Boyle L. Legal implications of the Patient Self-Determination Act. Nurse Practitioner Forum, 3(1):12, 1992.

Brant B, Osgood N. The suicidal patient in long-term care institutions. Journal of Gerontological Nursing, 16(2):17, 1990.

Brody J. Personal health—The reality of elderly alcoholics and acting to help them. New York Times, May 12, 1988:B6.

Brower HT. The alternatives to restraints. Journal of Gerontological Nursing, 17(2):18, 1991.

Burggraf V, Stanley M. Nursing the Elderly: A Care Plan Approach. Philadelphia: JB Lippincott, 1989.

Burke M, Walsh M. Gerontologic Nursing Care of the Frail Elderly. St. Louis: Mosby–Year Book, 1992.

Burns B. Treating recovering alcoholics. Journal of Gerontological Nursing, 14(4):18, 1988.

Burnside I. Nursing and the Aged. A Self Care Approach. New York: McGraw-Hill, 1988.

Butler R. Why Survive? Being Old in America. New York: Harper & Row, 1975.

Butrin J. Day Care. A new idea? Not really. Journal of Gerontological Nursing, 11(4):19, 1985.

Caserta J. Public policy for long term care. Geriatric Nursing, 4(4):244, 1983.

Ebersole P, Hess P (eds). Toward Healthy Aging Human Needs and Nursing Response. St. Louis: CV Mosby, 1990.

Eliopoulos C. Gerontological Nursing. Philadelphia: JB Lippincott, 1987.

Elliot B, Hybertson D. What is it about the elderly that elicits a negative response? Journal of Gerontological Nursing, 8(10):568, 1982.

Evans L, Strumpf N. Tying down the elderly: A review of the literature on physical restraints. Journal of the American Geriatrics Society, 37(1):65, 1989.

Forbes E, Fitzsimons V. The older adult: A process for wellness. St. Louis: CV Mosby, 1981.

Friedman J. Cry for help: Suicide in the aged. Journal of Gerontological Nursing, 2(3):28, 1976.

Gadow S. Advocacy nursing and new meanings of aging. Nursing Clinics of North America, 14:81, 1979.

Gambert S (ed). The geriatric patient: Effective management of behavioral and mental disorders. Spring House, PA: McNeil Pharmaceutical, 1983.

German P. Delivery of care to older people: Issues and outlooks. Topics in Clinical Nursing, 3(10):1, 1981.

Gobis L. Recent developments in health care law relevant to health care providers. Nurse Practitioner, 17(3):77, 1992.

Gomberg E. Drinking and problem drinking among the elderly. Publication #1 Alcohol, Drugs, and Aging: Usage and Problems. University of Michigan: Institute of Gerontology, 1980.

Gomez G, Otto D, et al. Beginning nursing students can change attitudes about the aged. Journal of Gerontological Nursing, 11(1):6, 1985.

Gottashalk E. Ending it all. Wall Street Journal, 1, 1986.

Graham R. Adult day care: How families of the dementia patient respond. Journal of Gerontological Nursing, 15(3):27, 1989.

Green C. Fostering positive attitudes toward the elderly: A teaching strategy for attitude change. Journal of Gerontological Nursing, 7(3):169, 1981.

Gulino C, Kadin M. Aging and reactive alcoholism. Geriatric Nursing, 7(3):148, 1986.

Gurland B, Cross P. Suicide among the elderly. In Aronson MK, et al (eds). The Acting Out Elderly. New York: Haworth Press, 1983, pp 456–465.

Hartford J, Samorajski T. Alcoholism in the geriatric population. Journal of the American Geriatrics Society, 30:18, 1982.

Henderson ML, McConnell ES. Gerontological care in community settings. In Matteson MA, McConnell ES (eds). Gerontological Nursing: Concepts and Practice. Philadelphia: WB Saunders, 1988.

Hogan S. Care for the caregiver: Social policies to ease their burden. Journal of Gerontological Nursing, 16(5):12, 1990.

Hogstel M. Geropsychiatric Nursing. St. Louis: CV Mosby, 1990.

Janssen JA, Giberson DL. Remotivation therapy. Journal of Gerontological Nursing, 14(6):31, 1988.

Janofsky J. Assessing competency in the elderly. Geriatrics, 45(10):45, 1990.

Jenike M (ed). Ethical considerations in the care of the hopelessly ill patient. Topics in Geriatrics, 3(4):13, 1984.

Johnson L. How to diagnose and treat chemical dependency in the elderly. Journal of Gerontological Nursing, 15(12):22, 1989.

Kaufman I. Life and death decisions. New York Times, October 6, 1985:21.

Kayser-Jones J. Doctoral preparation for gerontological nurses. Journal of Gerontological Nursing, 12(3):19, 1986.

Kleiman D. Uncertainty clouds of dying. New York Times, January 18, 1985:B1–2.

Koenen R. Adult day care: A northwest perspective. Journal of Gerontological Nursing, 6(4):218, 1980.

Lasker M. Aging alcoholics need nursing help. Journal of Gerontological Nursing, 12(1):16, 1986.

Lekan-Rutledge D. Functional assessment. In Matteson MA, McConnell ES (eds). Gerontological Nursing: Concepts and Practice. Philadelphia: WB Saunders, 1988.

Lindblom L, Kostyk D, et al. Chemical abuse: An intervention program for the elderly. Journal of Gerontological Nursing, 18(4):6, 1992.

Linn MW, et al. A social dysfunction rating scale. Journal of Psychiatric Research, 6:299, 1969.

MacElveen-Hoehn P, McIntosh E. The hospice movement: Growing pains and promises. Topics in Clinical Nursing, 3(3):29, 1981.

MacKay S. Durable power of attorney for health care. Geriatric Nursing, 13(2):99, 1992.

McConnell ES. A conceptual framework for gerontological nursing practice. In Matteson MA, McConnell ES (eds). Gerontological Nursing: Concepts and Practice. Philadelphia: WB Saunders, 1988.

McIntosh J. Suicide among the elderly: Levels and trends. American Journal of Orthopsychiatry, 55(2):287, 1985.

Marshall J. Changes in aged white male suicide: 1948–1972. Gerontologist, 33:763, 1978.

Masters R, Marks F. The use of restraints. Rehabilitation Nursing, 15(1):22, 1990.

Matteson MA, McConnell ES. Gerontological Nursing: Concepts and Practice. Philadelphia: WB Saunders, 1988.

Matthews S. The social world of old women: Management of self-identity. Sage Library of Social Research 78. Beverly Hills, CA: Sage Publications, 1979.

Moore CV. Self-determined advance directives: New issues in primary care. Nurse Practitioner Forum, 3(1):10, 1992.

National Citizens' Coalition for Nursing Home Reform. Nursing Home Reform Law: The Basics. Washington, DC: National Citizens' Coalition for Nursing Home Reform, 1991.

Nelson L. Questions of age. Doctors debate right to stop "heroic" effort to keep elderly alive. Wall Street Journal, September 7, 1982:20.

Neshkes R, Jarvik L. Depression in the elderly: Current management concepts. Geriatrics, 41(9):51, 1986.

Neussel F. The language of ageism. Gerontologist, 22(3):273, 1982.

O'Brien C. Adult day-care and the bottom line. Geriatric Nursing, 2(4):283, 1981.

Olson J. To treat or allow to die: An ethical dilemma in gerontological nursing. Journal of Gerontological Nursing, 7(3):141, 1981.

Osgood NN. Suicide in the elderly: Clues and prevention. Carrier Foundation Letter No. 133, April 1988.

Ostrander N. Alcoholism and aging—A rural community's response. Aging Today, February/March:19, 1992.

Parette H, Hourcade J, Parette P. Nursing attitudes toward geriatric alcoholism. Journal of Gerontological Nursing, 16(1):26, 1990.

Penner L, Ludenia K, et al. Staff attitudes: Image or reality. Journal of Gerontological Nursing, 10(3):110, 1984.

Pfeiffer E. Sexuality in the aging individual. In Solnick R (ed). Sexuality and Aging. CA: University of Southern California Press, 1978.

Pinch WJ, Parsons ME. The Patient Self-Determination Act. Nurse Practitioner Forum, 3(1):16, 1992.

Preston T. Ageism undermines relations with elderly. Medical World News, December 8, 1986:26.

Price D, Feldman J. Living longer in the United States: Demographic changes and health needs of the elderly. Milbank Memorial Fund Quarterly—Health and Society, 61:362, 1983.

Richardson R, Lowenstein S, Weissberg M. Coping with the suicidal elderly: A physician's guide. Geriatrics, 44(9):43, 1989.

Ronsman K. Therapy for depression. Journal of Gerontological Nursing, 13(12):18, 1987.

Rosenthal E. Filling the gap where a living will won't do. New York Times, January 17, 1991:B9.

Ross H. Society/cultural views regarding death and dying. Topics in Clinical Nursing, 3(3):3, 1981.

Schlossberg C, Hart MA. Legal perspectives. In Burke M, Walsh M (eds). Gerontologic Nursing Care of the Frail Elderly. St. Louis: Mosby–Year Book, 1992, p 469.

St. Pierre J, et al. Late life depression: A guide for assessment. Journal of Gerontological Nursing, 12(7):5, 1986.

Schneider E, Emr M. Alzheimer's disease. Geriatric Nursing, 6(3):136, 1985.

Schuckit M. A clinical review of alcohol, alcoholism, and the elderly patient. Journal of Clinical Psychiatry, 43(10):396, 1982.

Shawler C, Dallas M, et al. Clinical considerations: Surrogate decision making for hospitalized elders. Journal of Gerontological Nursing, 18(6):5, 1992.

Sherlock R, Dingus M. Families and the gravely ill: Roles, rules and rights. Journal of the American Geriatrics Society, 33:121, 1984.

Simcox. Day care for the Alzheimer's patient. In Ebersole P, Hess P (eds). Toward Healthy, Aging Human Needs and Nursing Response. St. Louis: CV Mosby, 1990.

Smith D. Advance directive editorial. Journal of Enterostomal Therapy, 19(4):109, 1992.

Snow R, Atwood K. Probable death: Perspectives of the elderly. Southern Medical Journal, 78:851, 1985.

Stilwell EM. Nurses' education related to the use of restraints. Journal of Gerontological Nursing, 17(2):23, 1991.

Suicide Rate Among Elderly Rises, Study Says. New York Times, September 19, 1991:A25.

Tolchin M. When long life is too much: Suicide rises among elderly. New York Times, July 19, 1989:A15.

Valanis D, Yeaworth R, et al. Alcohol use among bereaved and nonbereaved older persons. Journal of Gerontological Nursing, 13(5):26, 1987.

Wallis C. To feed or not to feed? Time, March 31, 1986:60.

Wanzer S, Adelstein S, et al. The physician's responsibility toward hopelessly ill patients. New England Journal of Medicine, 310(15):955, 1984.

Whall A. Suicide in older adults. Journal of Gerontological Nursing, 11(8):40, 1985.

Zung WK. A self-rating depression scale. Archives of General Psychiatry, 12:63, 1965.

Further Reading

Atchley R. Aging: Continuity and Change. Belmont, CA: Wadsworth Publishing Company, 1987.

Brown B. Professionals' perceptions and alcohol abuse among the elderly. Gerontologist, 22(6):519, 1982.

Boyle L. Legal implications of the Patient Self-Determination Act. Nurse Practitioner Forum, 3(1):12, 1992.

Chairman of the Select Committee on Aging. Business and Investment Frauds Perpetrated Against the Elderly: A Growing Scandal. Washington, DC: US Government Printing Office, 1982. Committee Publication no. 97-347.

Courtenay B, Suharat M. Myths and realities of aging. Athens, GA: University of Georgia, Georgia Center for Continuing Education, 1980.

Dupree L, Broskowski H, et al. The gerontology alcohol project: A behavioral treatment program for elderly alcohol abusers. Gerontologist, 24(5):51, 1984.

Heller B, Walsh E. Changing nursing students' attitudes toward the aged: An experimental study. Journal of Nursing Education, 15(5):9, 1976.

Judson D. Attitudes toward aging. Current Consumer and Life-studies, September 14, 1985.

Lerner R. Sleep loss in the aged: Implications for nursing practice. Journal of Gerontological Nursing, 8(6):323, 1982.

McCarthy P. Geriatric sexuality: Capacity, interest and opportunity. Journal of Gerontological Nursing, 5(1):20, 1979.

Miller M. Toward a profile of the older white male suicide. Gerontologist, 18(1):80, 1978.

Mion L, Frengley J, et al. A further exploration of the use of restraints in hospitalized patients. Journal of the American Geriatrics Society, 37:949, 1990.

Palmore E. Advantages of aging. Gerontologist, 17:220, 1970.

Patient Self-Determination Act. Nurse Practitioner Forum, 3(1):35, 1992.

Raffoul P, Cooper J, et al. Drug misuse in older people. Gerontologist, 21(2):146, 1981.

Salerno C. Alternatives to restraints. Geriatric Nursing, 13(2):63, 1992.

Sand B, Yeaworth R, Mccabe B. Alzheimer's disease: Special care units in long-term care facilities. Journal of Gerontological Nursing, 18(3):28, 1992.

Shook M. Health Decisions: Maintaining control of health care choices. Nurse Practitioner Forum, 3(1):30, 1992.

Spence D, Feigenbaum E, et al. Medical students' attitudes toward the geriatric patient. Journal of American Geriatrics Society, 16:976, 1968.

Steffl D. Handbook of Gerontological Nursing. New York: Van Nostrand Reinhold Company, 1984.

Self-study Exercises

Place T (true) or F (false) next to each statement.

1. _____ The elderly are prone to be crime victims.
2. _____ "Ageism" reflects society's positive view of the elderly.
3. _____ Older adults are able to learn new tasks.
4. _____ Most elderly are infirm and require help with daily activities.

Match the type of group—R (remotivational), REM (reminiscing), and P (psychotherapy)—with the following descriptions:

5. _____ Shares memories of past events and helps increase esteem and socialization.
6. _____ Can help resocialize regressed and apathetic clients. Structured setting with set agenda.
7. _____ Problems are discussed among people with similar problems; aim is to relieve psychiatric symptoms and solidify functioning.

Place T (true) or F (false) next to each statement.

8. _____ Alcohol provides a beneficial night's sleep.
9. _____ Alcohol can mimic the normal changes of aging.

10. _____ Alcohol exacerbates all chronic conditions.
11. _____ Residents in restraint-free facilities experience fewer injuries from falls than those in facilities using restraints.
12. _____ Chemical restraints are devices that inhibit free movement.
13. _____ If restraints are used, the written order of the physician need only specify the duration of their use.
14. _____ The Patient Self-Determination Act (PSDA) was passed to assist physicians in making health-care decisions about their patients.
15. _____ A Living Will, a Directive to Physician, and a Durable Power of Attorney for Health-Care are all forms of advance health-care directives.
16. _____ Among the elderly, the white male has the highest suicide rate.
17. _____ Guns are the most common means of suicide used by the elderly.
18. _____ Acute illnesses are the major threat to older persons' health.
19. _____ Ageism is a bias against older people based on their age.

CHAPTER 30

Chronic Mental Illness and the Mentally Ill Who Are Homeless

Peggy Miller
Anne Cowley Herzog

OUTLINE

KEY TERMS AND CONCEPTS

The key terms and concepts listed here also appear in bold where they are defined or discussed in this chapter.

CHRONIC DISAFFILIATION

CHRONIC HOMELESSNESS

OBJECTIVES

After studying this chapter, the student will be able to

1. Explain what is meant by the term *chronic mental illness.*
2. Compare and contrast chronic mental illness and chronic physical illness.
3. Discuss specific considerations needed for the chronically mentally ill population when these common intervention strategies are employed:
   A. Medication
   B. Psychosocial rehabilitation
   C. Psychotherapy
4. Define chronic homelessness.
5. Explain the process of homelessness.

6. Discuss the physiological, behavioral, affective, cognitive, and sociocultural characteristics common among the homeless population.
7. Describe the nurse's roles in the interdisciplinary treatment team process.
8. Develop a plan of care for a chronically mentally ill homeless person using the case study of Evelyn.

The Chronically Mentally Ill Population

DEFINITION

The term *chronic mental illness* refers to a phenomenon whereby mental illness extends in time beyond the acute stage into a long term stage that is marked by persistent impairment of functioning. This decrease in functioning pervades the person's abilities to perform in all, or nearly all, aspects of daily living. Skill deficits range from an inability to prepare meals to an inability to cope with everyday stressors. Chafetz (1988) stated that "chronicity tends to go hand in hand with social and economic disadvantage." The chronically mentally ill population is at risk for multiple physical, emotional, and social problems, and homelessness is all too often the final result.

DEMOGRAPHICS

Precise calculation of the extent of chronic mental illness in the United States is difficult. Before deinstitutionalization, the mentally disabled population was easier to count. People with chronic mental illness were hospitalized, sometimes for the remainder of their lives. With the move to community-based mental health centers, and with changes within the population itself, there is no way to accurately tabulate this population. However, it is estimated that two thirds of those with major mental illness will have persistent physical and emotional problems (Worley 1990).

Chronicity can occur with persons of any gender, age, culture, or geographic location. However, this population includes two subgroups with unique characteristics: (1) persons old enough to have experienced institutionalization (before approximately 1975) and (2) persons young enough to have been hospitalized only during acute exacerbations of their disorders.

OLDER POPULATIONS. Before the move to deinstitutionalize the chronically mentally ill in 1975, psychiatric hospitals were the long term residences for

many people. A pervasive philosophical stance at that time was medicinal paternalism. The hospital's approach to the chronically mentally ill disabled person was that of making all decisions for the client. The daily institutional routine left little room for the client to exercise what social and problem-solving skills remained. Much of the client's behavior was a combination of the disease process and the decreased sense of self that resulted from the lack of autonomy.

Vignette

Marian was a resident at a facility for the chronically impaired during her adolescence and young adulthood. On discharge, she moved to a community home, where she spends long periods sitting in front of the living room window. Marian does not ask to go out into the garden she watches for so many hours. Indeed, she rarely asks for anything, including snacks or recreational activities. The caregivers must work with Marian for several months to get her to recognize her need of the moment and then to articulate or act on it. There is a major celebration the day that she walks into the kitchen and makes a peanut butter sandwich of her own volition. Some of the institutionalization-caused dependency is gone.

YOUNGER POPULATIONS. People young enough never to have been institutionalized may not have the problems of passivity and lack of autonomy that long term hospitalization may cause. However, this very lack of experience within the system may contribute to their denying that they even have a difficulty (Chafetz 1988). This denial, often coupled with the use of recreational drugs that further impair already faulty judgment and impulse control, makes chronically ill young adults at particular risk for many additional problems, including brushes with the law and frequent loss of employment after short periods of time.

Vignette

Joshua has had several short hospitalizations for treatment of his schizophrenia. Between admissions, he lives in unstable short term places varying from rooming houses to his car. He has been jailed several times for misdemeanors such as shoplifting and creating a public nuisance (e.g., loud arguments in public *places).* He has difficulty finding and keeping jobs as a laborer.

DEVELOPMENT OF CHRONICITY

Chronic psychosocial illness has much in common with chronic physical illness. The original problem sets in motion an erosion of basic mechanisms and compensatory processes. As the disorder extends beyond the acute stage, more and more of the neighboring systems are involved. For example, with chronic congestive heart failure, the lungs and kidneys begin to deteriorate. In the case of a chronic mental illness such as schizophrenia, the person's thought processes, ability to maintain contact with others, ability to stay employed, and so on frequently deteriorate.

Another similarity between physical illness and mental illness is the unpredictability of the disease course. Not knowing when the problem will exacerbate contributes additional stress. Adequate coping mechanisms for stress are a major deficit for those with chronic mental disorders. The fear of exacerbation and avoidance of stress can cause a withdrawal from life that eventually heightens the person's social isolation and apathy (Chafetz 1988).

INTERVENTION STRATEGIES

Many of the strategies used for chronic mental illness are the same as those used for acute problems. However, with chronic illness there are often special considerations to the otherwise basic intervention strategies.

MEDICATION. Neuroleptics have significantly improved the overall treatment of many major mental illnesses. Despite serious side effects, they are very effective in reducing or removing delusions and hallucinations for the majority of clients. However, they are not effective in treating many of the negative signs and symptoms of the disorders, such as withdrawal and apathy (see Chapter 19). The use of neuroleptics is only one step in providing a basis for treatment.

Numerous problems are inherent in the use of medications in a community setting; these problems include compliance and the occurrence of side effects and other adverse reactions. The cognitive impairment caused by the chronic mental illness makes it difficult for the client to take the medication as prescribed. Side effects that make the use of the medications unpalatable to the client further decrease compliance. Adverse reactions may go unnoticed and become dangerous or may even go on to cause permanent dam-

age. Adequate monitoring of efficacy by a community-based health care provider is difficult, if not often impossible.

PSYCHOSOCIAL REHABILITATION. During rehabilitation, it is important to view the person as capable of positive change. With this approach, skills training and the building of self-esteem can begin. Teaching emphasizes the skills necessary for basic everyday life, such as social, problem-solving, communication, and vocational skills. When clients are able to master certain basic skills, get their needs met more effectively through communication, increase their social support system, and learn important job skills, a sense of hopefulness and empowerment often follows. These important skills can aid many people with chronic mental problems to lead more satisfying and productive lives. These skills can also help clients become more involved with the people and opportunities around them and can help prevent the downward shift to the least desirable of all sequelae, homelessness.

CASE MANAGEMENT. Whether as a broker of services or as a therapist, the case manager can provide entrance into the system of care. Loosely made multiple referrals can be beyond the coping capabilities of the chronically ill. With one person coordinating services, help can be more efficiently used. In addition, the basic needs of the person (i.e., food, shelter, and clothing) are more likely to be addressed.

PSYCHOTHERAPY. Psychotherapy has a more restricted part in the total constellation of strategies. It is currently thought that attention must first be given to meeting very basic physical needs through the use of medication and skills training.

Homelessness

The homelessness issue has commanded public attention and discussion for many years. An adequate definition of homelessness has yet to be found, but the consensus is that there is no single explanation for this complex problem. Homelessness does not confine itself to a particular race, age, or sex, and it is more than a lack of a place to live. The homeless also suffer from a lack of food, appropriate clothing, access to health care and social services, and educational opportunities (Riesdorf-Ostrow 1989).

This chapter considers those people with chronic mental illness who reside long term in public shelters, on the street, or in other temporary living quarters. To be chronically homeless is to have a lifestyle completely ravaged by **chronic disaffiliation:** that is, to be cut off and estranged from family, community, and peer support and involvement. For many, then, homelessness is a lifestyle problem. It is a process that exists on a continuum and leads to long term residency in a mental hospital or public shelter. Many of the people who currently suffer from this lifestyle problem once had residences of their own or shared dwellings with family members or friends.

CAUSES OF HOMELESSNESS

The reasons for homelessness are many. The high rates of unemployment and underemployment and the reductions in public support programs and in low-cost housing are a few sources of the homeless problem today. Deinstitutionalization of the mentally ill from mental institutions into the community is another undisputed cause. Deinstitutionalization was based on the principle that patients can receive more humane and therapeutic care in the community than in institutions (Lamb 1984). However, multiple factors contributed to deinstitutionalization's side effect of homelessness. New drugs and treatments that control symptoms have made it possible for the mentally ill to live in the community. On the other hand, being homeless and living in a shelter could result in an emotional crisis that could in itself produce a mental disorder (Johnson 1990). There is a strong relationship between life without a home and mental disorder. Life on the street or in a shelter, whether temporary or not, can have a very negative influence on a person's self-esteem. Homelessness on top of a fragile mental status could be all that is necessary to provoke a crisis or exacerbate an existing mental disorder. People found wandering the streets in a daze and talking to themselves have often been taken to hospitals and labeled with an unwarranted psychiatric diagnosis. Their response in this way to a life of hardship and the loss of one's home is not unexpected. In any case, the homeless population presents a growing social problem with no simple solution. In describing the problem, it is necessary to discuss some of the subgroups that compose the homeless population.

SUBGROUPS OF HOMELESS PEOPLE

Subgroups of the homeless addressed in this section are (1) the chronically mentally ill, (2) chronic substance abusers, and (3) age-related populations, including families with children, adolescents, and the elderly.

THE CHRONICALLY MENTALLY ILL. The chronically mentally ill are well represented in each of these subgroups. Deinstitutionalization left many chronically mentally ill persons without shelter, as previously mentioned. State mental institutions drastically reduced their populations by returning patients to the community. Community mental health centers were supposed to provide inpatient and outpatient care, day care, outreach services, emergency treatment, consultation, and educational services, as well as specific services for children, adolescents, and the elderly. However, the community was usually unprepared to support the chronically mentally ill because of the lack of funding for these centers. As a result, many of the chronically mentally ill receive no social or medical support. Mental health authorities are reluctant to make homelessness a "mental health problem" because this might result in the reinstitutionalization of people in this population (Riesdorf-Ostrow 1989).

The chronically mentally ill homeless population consists of men and women who may have primary DSM-III-R diagnoses, including psychotic disorders (schizophrenia, bipolar, and depression disorders), personality disorders (borderline, dependent, and antisocial disorders), organic mental dysfunctions, and numerous other disorders. Characteristics common to this population include fragile ego development, extreme suspiciousness, vulnerability to stress, and impairments in thinking, perception, attention span, and concentration. Pathological defenses against anxiety are evidenced by frequent incidences of suicide, violence, substance dependence, retreat to psychosis, or complete denial of needing help. Mentally ill young adults also demonstrate tremendous deficits in their ability to form satisfactory interpersonal relationships, their social skills, and their competence in performing activities of daily living (Brunger 1986). As previously mentioned, the chronically mentally ill experience major problems with money management, transportation, compliance with medication instruction, meal preparation, and articulating their needs for other basic services. As a result, the chronically mentally ill in the community frequently live impoverished lives void of basic services that were available in state hospitals and other institutions (Lamb 1984).

CHRONIC SUBSTANCE ABUSERS. Chronic substance abusers may become homeless as a result of their addictions, which interfere with getting and keeping a job. Disaffiliation from family and friends may bring the abuser to a life on the streets. A study by Drake and Wallach (1989) showed that substance abuse added to the problems of disruptive, disinhibited, and noncompliant behaviors in patients dually diagnosed with substance abuse and chronic mental illness. These patients are younger, more often male, and less able to manage their lives in the community by maintaining regular meals, adequate finances, and stable housing. They are also less able to comply with the rules in available living situations, such as boarding homes, and are often evicted or choose to leave.

AGE-RELATED POPULATIONS. Homelessness can occur during any of the developmental stages of life. Therefore, age-related populations to be considered include families with children, adolescents, and the elderly. *Families with children* are the fastest-growing group of homeless in the United States. This is a consequence of cuts in welfare programs, specifically Aid to Families with Dependent Children (AFDC), and reductions in food stamp and affordable housing programs (Tower and White 1989). The problem becomes much more complex if a parent is diagnosed with a chronic mental illness. *Adolescents* find themselves homeless as a result of running away from home or being thrown out by their families. One study (Bassuk 1987) found that more than half of these youths had left home by age 13 and since that time had averaged nine moves a year. These adolescents come from chaotic families: The majority have a parent with a criminal history or a substance abuse problem, and one half have been physically abused (Bassuk 1987). An increasing number of *elderly* are finding themselves at risk for homelessness at a time when the demand for low-income housing is larger than the supply and the federal allocations for public housing have been severely cut. It is predicted that persons over 60 years of age will be the next group hit hard by homelessness. A single medical emergency or tragic incident could place many older persons living near the poverty level at risk for homelessness.

INCIDENCE OF HOMELESSNESS

Although attempts have been made to estimate the dimensions of the homeless population, it is difficult to count this population accurately. Until an accepted definition of homelessness is determined and greater accessibility of the homeless population can be achieved, no accurate count is possible. Many of the homeless, in fact, do not consider themselves to be homeless. This is true especially if their situation is the same as or better than that during childhood. Estimates of the homeless in the United States range from 1–4 million, one third to one half of whom may be suffering from a chronic mental disorder. Figure 30–1 depicts the homeless and severely mentally ill populations.

About 40–50% of the homeless abuse alcohol, and 10–15% abuse drugs. The average age of the homeless population has dropped from middle age to the early thirties. Homeless families account for more than 40% of the homeless population, and it is esti-

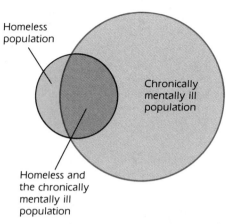

Figure 30–1. *The homeless and chronically mentally ill populations. (From Federal Task Force on Homelessness and Severe Mental Illness. Outcasts on Main Street, 1992.)*

mated that there are 750,000 to 1 million children in homeless families. The number of adolescents living on their own ranges between 100,000 and 400,000, and people over 60 years of age account for approximately 10% of the homeless population (Damrosch and Strasser 1988; Ryan 1989).

THE PROCESS OF HOMELESSNESS

Some people have a brief episode of homelessness as the result of a sudden crisis such as unemployment, eviction, or domestic upheaval. Many, however, experience homelessness as a situation that exists for a significant length of time. Disaffiliation, arrested social development, dealings with clinics, conflicts with employers, being on welfare, psychosexual difficulty, limited insight, and self-mutilation are life experiences that thousands of homeless men and women share across the country. Bassuk (1984) found that 74% of shelter residents had no family relations and that 73% had no friends. The figure jumps to 90% for homeless persons who also had psychiatric histories. The study concluded that **chronic homelessness** is often the final stage in a lifelong series of crises and missed opportunities, the culmination of a gradual disengagement from supportive relationships and institutions.

Many chronically homeless people are treated by a number of hospitals and clinics, and over time a homeless person may be given various psychiatric diagnoses. This does not so much point to psychiatric confusion or to a lack of communication among treatment facilities as make a case for the complexity of the chronically homeless person. A look at the hospital records indicates that although a person presents with an array of symptoms appropriate to warrant a specific diagnosis, the person does not stay in one place long enough to allow any sort of diagnostic fine-tuning to take place. Before a more accurate diagnosis can be developed, great and more prolonged care must be used to establish a therapeutic alliance. Because persons who suffer from homelessness as a lifestyle problem are severely and actively disaffiliated and estranged from themselves, others, and their environment, one or two hours, or even one or two sessions, are not enough to develop the necessary therapeutic alliance. It may take several months or more than a year before substantial treatment or accurate diagnoses can be established. This fact should warn the practitioner against rigidity when approaching the treatment of the homeless person (Grunberg 1990).

Complicating this already complex picture is the unfortunate occurrence of caseload transfers or the introduction of new or replacement staff. Inconsistent staffing and use of registry personnel also compound the issue, making it difficult to coordinate the multiple problems presented by the homeless person. Even though a homeless person may be involved in effective treatment, if a new staff person takes over all or part of the client's treatment, a new therapeutic alliance must be established, which prolongs treatment.

FUTURE DIRECTIONS

For a while, everyone seemed to be getting involved in helping the many thousands of homeless men and women throughout the United States: politicians, advocates, architects, welfare workers, psychiatrists, religious leaders, and others took part. The more they participate, the more city, state, and federal funding will follow. Chronically mentally ill homeless persons will crowd more and more shelters. As more programs open up, there will be a growing job market for those who wish to work with this population. There will be a need for experienced professionals to "change gears" and accept specialized training with this "new" population. Colleges are already beginning to teach subjects both directly and indirectly related to the problem, and some offer specialty degrees in the field of homelessness.

If the problem is clearly defined, there may be a solution. That is, if deinstitutionalization is considered the primary cause, reinstitutionalization will be seen as the solution. If the lack of low-cost housing is considered the main cause, a housing solution will be sought. Unfortunately, such a complex problem cannot be corrected by any single solution. If, however, this problem is viewed and defined as an encompassing lifestyle problem that results in severe and chronic

disaffiliation, possible solutions become clearer (Grunberg 1990).

Carol Johnson, director of the homeless services for the Massachusetts Department of Mental Health, has stated, "Mental health issues are an integral part of the experience of homelessness. . . . You can't separate homelessness, mental illness and bureaucratic structures. . . . The opposite of homelessness is community, not shelter" (JOC 1988).

There are great opportunities for nursing within the wide range of services for the mentally ill who are homeless. Aiken (1987) suggests the following strategies for nurses in assisting the mentally ill: (1) consolidating authority and the accountability in the fiscal management of clinical programs; (2) rooting authority in local government, where local officials can manage broad-based programs; (3) developing new service settings to include group homes, foster homes, mobile clinics, and the streets; (4) creating outreach programs much like the public health nursing model, in which nurses meet patients in the home, on the streets, and on the job; (5) reforming financial methods of reimbursement; (6) attracting professionals to public sector careers; and (7) joining the national public debate about homelessness and the chronically mentally ill. In these ways, nursing can assume a key role in delivering services and providing care to the chronically mentally ill who are homeless.

The Role of the Nurse

The nurse's delivery of care to the chronically mentally ill homeless person can be viewed in terms of the nine roles of the professional nurse, as defined by Kozier and Erb (1983): healing, caring, communicating, teaching, planning, coordinating, protecting, rehabilitating, and socializing (Table 30–1). All of these functions are applicable to both psychosocial and physical concerns and are accomplished through the nursing process.

PSYCHOSOCIAL CONCERNS

Basic psychosocial needs do not change simply because a person is homeless. However, ways in which health care workers meet these needs need to be adapted in order to reach those in need. The homeless person's problem of chronic disaffiliation makes the first step in caring for this client's health care needs (i.e., establishing a rapport) more problematic.

Table 30–1 ■ ROLES OF THE PROFESSIONAL NURSE

1.	**Healing**	Facilitating normal health and healing processes
2.	**Caring**	Providing comfort and support
3.	**Communicating**	Developing the patient's data base and disseminating information to other members of the health care team
4.	**Teaching**	Instructing on health problems and ways to change behavior
5.	**Planning**	Participating with other members of the health care team in developing approaches to care
6.	**Coordinating**	Organizing various aspects of care to maximize the use of resources (including time and patient energy)
7.	**Protecting**	Safeguarding against injury and complications
8.	**Rehabilitating**	Facilitating maximal return to function with minimal limitations
9.	**Socializing**	Providing activities that address the unique human side of each patient

From Kozier B, Erb G. Fundamentals of Nursing. Menlo Park, CA: Addison-Wesley Publishing Company, 1983.

HEALING, CARING, AND PROTECTING. Fear, anxiety, and distrust are pervasive in the lives of chronically mentally ill persons, especially those who are homeless. These people have a decreased ability to deal successfully with stress. Further, living on the street produces additional problems such as exposure to violence and the lack of physical necessities. These people are vulnerable to muggers, street gangs, starvation, and exposure to the physical elements.

Vignette

Susie is brought to a community psychiatric hospital by the police when local shopkeepers complain about her frequent bizarre behavior. She screams that the red traffic light at the corner is making the worms in her head angry. At first, the nurse can only attempt to make Susie feel less threatened in this new environment by providing plenty of physical distance and making no demands. The room is cleared of any objects that Susie could use to hurt herself or others.

Later, as Susie begins to trust a little more, the nurse coaxes her into eating a hot meal. Still later, Susie agrees to take her first dose of medications. Before she falls asleep that night, Susie takes the blankets off the bed and curls up in the corner of her room to sleep for a few hours. In the morning, Susie will not shower, but the nurse is able to persuade her to wash from the basin. Later that morning, after another dose of medications, Susie is calm enough to consider attending a group therapy session. There, the nurse is able both to begin connecting Susie to her peers and to help her discuss her altered thoughts.

TEACHING, REHABILITATING, AND SOCIALIZING. The nurses leading various groups and activities addressed some of Susie's problems. One of these was that Susie needed to continue her medications after discharge. Susie also needed help in improving her independence in activities of daily living. The staff wanted to help Susie deal with people in a more productive and satisfying manner. Throughout her stay, Susie saw how the nurses behaved toward her, toward her peers, and toward other health care workers. These interactions gave her a model of alternative methods of relating to others.

COMMUNICATING, PLANNING, AND COORDINATING. The health care team (social workers, activity therapists, psychiatrists, and others) relied on the nurses' assessment data. Only nurses observed Susie's functioning and were available for interventions 24 hours a day. The admitting nurse suggested getting Susie involved in the art therapy group. An evening nurse continued the health care teaching started during a day session. All staff members addressed discharge planning from the first day of Susie's admission. At their suggestion, before discharge, the psychiatrist changed the oral fluphenazine (Prolixin) to fluphenazine decanoate (Prolixin D). The long term decanoate preparation facilitated Susie's maintenance of an adequate serum level of antipsychotic drug. This was important because Susie's compliance with her drug regimen was doubtful once she was discharged. Susie was also referred to a shelter that had provision for mental health therapies. Action was then taken to ease some of Susie's financial problems.

Physical Concerns

The nurse must be involved with two areas of physical need: environment and health. Environmental needs include areas of concern such as safe shelter, clothing appropriate to the weather, accessibility of sanitary facilities, food, and money. Absence of these basic necessities increases the risk of decompensation in a person whose mental and physical health is already fragile.

HEALING AND PROTECTING. Once the person has obtained refuge at a shelter or multiservice center, he or she is relatively protected from the elements and the pervasive violence of the streets. With these basic needs attended to, the nurse can concentrate on providing other essentials of health and well-being, such as adequate nutrition, appropriate clothing, and hygiene. Without these, acute health problems will develop, and acute dysfunction will quickly become chronic. Consider the case of Jack.

Vignette

Jack suffers from chronic depression and the simple need for shoes. He finds a pair of shoes in a trash can, but they don't fit him very well. The rain and snow made the shoes wet, and there is no place he can dry them. While Jack is living on the street, he cannot take off the shoes, even in sleep, for fear that they will be stolen. Jack has no place to bathe, and he develops foot wounds that quickly become infected. Long term stress and the lack of proper nutrition deplete his immunological reserves. The result is cellulitis that extends nearly to his knee, as well as necrotic areas on three toes.

Jack presents to the emergency department of a local hospital for care. The emergency department nurse obtains information about a nearby shelter that has a program for intermittent nursing care. Once Jack is hooked into the system, he has a clean, safe place to sleep, sanitary facilities, and meals. His shelter nurse can perform the foot soaks, change the dressings, and administer the medications with some hope of their effectiveness. Jack has a chance to get well and not lose his foot.

TEACHING AND REHABILITATING. As Jack's infection resolved, the nurse taught him how to care for the problem and prevent its recurrence. The nurse discussed foot care and the signs that signal the beginning of a problem. The nurse's knowledge of available resources enabled the nurse to eventually find Jack a pair of shoes that fit.

COMMUNICATING, PLANNING, AND COORDINATING. At staff meetings, the nurse was an important source of information about Jack and his needs. The nurse helped identify both short and long term goals and discussed with the team how they could help Jack achieve these goals. Because of the nurse's referral, the social worker arranged Jack's placement in a work program in which he could sit while receiving job training. The social worker also arranged the schedule so that Jack was able to attend all his therapy group activities.

CARING AND SOCIALIZING. Through all her dealings with Jack, the nurse conveyed a sense of Jack's personal worth. In all contacts with him, the nurse treated him with dignity and warmth. The nurse's behavior toward people was a model for him to emulate.

THE NURSING PROCESS

The systematic approach to the nursing process is the backbone of the art and science of nursing. The careful use of each step provides the nurse with an organized system for addressing patient health problems.

Assessment

During the initial data gathering, information regarding the "where" and "what" of home is important information for both current and discharge planning. People rarely start a conversation with a statement of their homelessness. However, the nurse can get important clues from their hygiene status, signs of previous violence (e.g., scars, bruises, or abrasions), and their wearing of all their clothes and carrying of all their possessions. These cues, coupled with patterns such as poor nutrition, untended infections (including tuberculosis), infestations (e.g., lice and scabies), and climatic trauma (e.g., frostbite and heatstroke), raise the nurse's index of suspicion about homelessness. Frequently, during the taking of the nursing history, the person may be vague about sleeping, eating, and activities of daily living routines. When in doubt, the nurse should ask directly about living arrangements.

It is important to remember that from a health care provider's point of view, homelessness is not a reason for admission to a health care facility, however strong a contributor it is to health and other problems. It is not uncommon for a person who feels the need for respite from the street to seek admission on the basis of what are actually unchanged physical or mental problems. Initially, the nurse may wonder why anyone would want to be in a hospital. However, when the warm, dry, relatively safe hospital with plenty of food ("three hots and a cot") is weighed against living on the street, with minimal or no resources, it is easier to understand. Indeed, such behavior could be interpreted as quite reasonable and adaptive.

Planning

The assessment data often show patterns or cues that revolve around basic issues: independence in self-care (i.e., hygiene, nutrition, health care) and difficulties in relationships with others. Other problems, such as infection, hallucination, or injury, may widen the constellation of concerns.

Nursing diagnoses are the matrix on which the plan of care rests. Great care must be taken to ensure that the definitions and defining characteristics of the nursing diagnoses are actually drawn from the nurse's data and that colloquial meanings are not allowed to take over. For example, *noncompliance* is not defined as the patient's refusal to follow medical advice but as "the state in which an individual . . . *desires* to comply but is prevented from doing so by factors that deter adherence to health-related advice given by health professionals" (Carpenito 1992). Table 30–2 lists possible nursing diagnoses applicable to a chronically mentally ill homeless person.

Intervention

The duality of severe psychosocial and physical needs may strain the health care provider's available resources, especially time and talent. Complicated physical interventions can be an additional burden on the nurse already busy with groups and activities, and a patient with significant psychosocial dysfunction may compound the problems of the nurse attempting to care for several people with physical needs. Many mental health nurses find ample opportunity to perfect their psychosocial communication skills but may have far less need for "medical-type" skills. Conversely, the nurse in the medical-surgical setting may be proficient at applying complicated dressings and energy conservation techniques but less adept at using common psychotherapy strategies. A nurse equally expert in both these areas is ideally suited to working with this population.

However, the team approach to patient care enables the nurse to connect "the person with the skills" with "the person with the needs"; thus, the nurse is in a position to individualize client care. Current care-planning references should be readily available to the staff to jog a memory or to suggest something novel. If a new or infrequently used intervention is to be implemented, information on it should be available in the nurses' station or lounge as well. However, not only chronically mentally ill homeless persons may have dual problems. People with psychosocial problems frequently have acute and chronic physical health needs, whether they are cared for at home, in a psychiatric facility, or in a medical-surgical hospital. The professional nurse must be prepared.

Evaluation

The goals of intervention are patient centered; therefore, the final evaluation is based on (1) patient satisfaction with the new health status and (2) the health care team's estimation of improvement. Achieving these goals may take much longer than current funding allows. Therefore, referrals and plans for continued care are often essential to success. Although resources are available for the homeless population, local community programs vary widely.

The problem of homelessness is becoming even more widespread and the issues are becoming more complex. Nurses, in conjunction both with their health care facilities and with other supportive groups who care, could be instrumental in developing more help for the mentally and physically ill who are homeless. Patient advocacy is a primary function of the professional nurse.

Table 30–2 ■ NURSING DIAGNOSES: THE HOMELESS MENTALLY ILL

Impaired adjustment	High risk for infection
Anxiety	Alteration in nutrition: less than body requirements
Alteration in comfort	Powerlessness
Ineffective individual coping	Post-trauma response
Ineffective denial	Self-care deficit
Ineffective family coping	Sleep-pattern disturbance
Fluid volume deficit	Alteration in thought processes
Alteration in health maintenance	Impaired skin/tissue integrity
Hopelessness	Social isolation
High risk for injury	

Resources for the Mentally Ill Who Are Homeless

With the advent of deinstitutionalization, an emphasis was placed on discharging patients with chronic mental disorders from large state institutions into community-based care. Many of the outpatient services sounded good but in reality fell short in meeting the complex needs of the population they served. The concept of a national network of strong, community-based mental health centers that work to maintain a patient's ability to function independently out of the hospital setting has yet to be realized. Today, both large state hospitals and small private institutions house and care for the chronically mentally ill who are unable to live on their own, either temporarily or for an extended period. Most often, improvements seen in a patient's behavior in the hospital setting do not last long after the patient has been discharged. One of the main reasons for this inability to maintain more effective behaviors is the inability to take the prescribed medications and the "revolving door syndrome." Chronically mentally ill persons need appropriate resources as well as medication to be able to function in the community. A well-coordinated, comprehensive, and cost-effective system of care that is individualized and available to all in need is the ideal situation.

Community mental health services are designed to provide outreach and case management for the persistently and seriously mentally disabled who are also homeless. Patient participation in the program is voluntary. State and county monies fund these programs, which operate through three components: outreach programs, short term housing, and multiservice centers. Shelter beds and multiservice center services are contracted out to private service providers. Liaison is maintained with law enforcement and with governmental and nonprofit agencies that provide services to the homeless. Services are delivered in an individualized, self-enabling manner based on a philosophy that respects each individual's dignity, privacy, and right to refuse treatment. This service approach allows the patient to achieve the highest level of independence and self-sufficiency possible.

Community outreach programs, send professional and nonprofessional workers into streets, parks, temporary shelters, bus stations, beaches, and anywhere else the mentally ill may be. A team approach is used to gain access to patients and to connect them with the various services available to meet their needs. A trusting relationship must be established and maintained between the outreach worker and the patient

before communication can be developed. In this way, the patient's needs can best be considered and met. Outreach services provide liaison with community services and case management to include assistance in obtaining benefits (e.g., general relief, food stamps, and Social Security Income [SSI]), mental health services, medical treatment, and transportation. The role of the outreach worker is to be an advocate in all areas of patient need and to foster patient independence and terminate outreach services when appropriate.

Temporary shelters do not provide the ideal living situation but are a safe and supportive environment for individuals who have no other option. The mentally ill do need a place to live, even if it is a temporary location. A life can go either way in a public shelter. A person can become more chronically entrenched or can take steps toward improving his or her quality of life. Often, the longer a person stays in a shelter setting, the less likely the person is to emerge from it.

Multiservice centers collaborate with the outreach unit in implementing individualized service plans for the chronically mentally ill. They supply hot meals, laundry and shower facilities, clothing, social activities, transportation to and from shelters, access to a telephone, and a mailing address for the individual.

For example, at the Weingart Center in Los Angeles, the various programs and services that are available to the mentally ill who are homeless include Screening and Referral/High Risk Homeless, Short-Term Action Integration Referral Service (STAIRS), Testing Living Center (TLC), Recuperative Care, and the Specialized Shelter Program for severely and chronically mentally ill homeless individuals. This special program for the mentally ill is funded through the County of Los Angeles Department of Mental Health. The Weingart Center provides basic living support in the form of short term transitional housing, food, clothing, hygiene supplies, and limited supervision for homeless adults who are also chronically mentally ill and considered to be vulnerable on the streets. This temporary housing program provides the staff with an opportunity to stabilize clients' conditions by using medications, resolve benefit problems, and provide placement in more permanent housing.

Vignette

Carl, a 36-year-old black man, is admitted to the Specialized Shelter Program in March. He has recently moved from Salt Lake City, Utah, where he resided with his sister. Carl is diagnosed as a paranoid schizophrenic and is also mildly developmentally disabled. He is a pleasant gentleman who wants to stay in Los Angeles because of the mild climate. He has never been homeless before but finds himself without funds to rent an apartment. Because Carl is an affable person who is eager to please, he is very easy to manipulate, making him very vulnerable on the streets. His mental health case manager requests close monitoring via shelter placement. With the support of his case manager and the Specialized Shelter Program, Carl realizes his goals to move into a hotel where he can be taught additional independent living skills and to obtain his own apartment eventually.

Johnson (1990) cites housing as the first need of the mentally ill once they are discharged from a hospital setting. They have no hope of recovering from any illness on the streets. These people also need a place where they can belong—a refuge or haven. The mentally ill also require aggressive outreach programs and a mental health program that creates and adjusts its services to the limited abilities of its chronically ill patients. They need ready access to hospitals and permission to regress. Also needed is training in living skills, including personal hygiene and grooming, shopping, budgeting, traveling, and social skills. Next, the mentally ill need work to occupy their time and give them an idea of what it is like to live in the real world. Johnson addressed the need of this population for cigarettes and coffee and suggests setting up clinics to thus attract patients with chronic conditions. She concludes that the chronically mentally ill deserve treatment free of condescension for as long as they need it. A lifetime disability requires long term access (Johnson 1990).

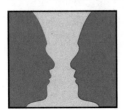

Case Study: Working with a Person Who Is Mentally Ill and Homeless

Evelyn Sun is a 42-year-old woman who was originally diagnosed with schizophrenia approximately 20 years ago. During the last two decades, she has been hospitalized several times in acute care psychiatric facilities. Her last admitting diagnosis was borderline personality disorder. Evelyn married for the first time at age 20 and was divorced a few years later. She has been married and has had more informal relationships several times since then. She has a 10-year-old daughter, Marie. Evelyn states that she doesn't have any friends: "There just aren't any people who want to be friendly."

During her last separation and divorce, which took place two years ago, her clinical presentation became more exaggerated. Evelyn had worked intermittently up to that time as a temporary clerical worker through a local personnel agency. However, her overreactions to office stress and her manipulating behaviors became so pronounced that she was fired.

Jobless, she and Marie were evicted from their tiny apartment for nonpayment of rent. For a time, they stayed with a former coworker named Gladys, but Evelyn began to say that Gladys didn't really care. So they lived in Evelyn's car, until it was stolen.

When Evelyn is not an inpatient at a mental health facility, they live at various shelters or in nearby parks with tents made of garbage bags and boxes. Marie is in and out of foster care homes. She attends school occasionally but is rarely at the same school more than a few weeks in a row. She can read on a first-grade level.

Evelyn is seeking admission because "there's a man down the street that says he's going to hurt me. You've got to let me in!" Although the weather is cold and rainy, she wears no coat, only layers of dirty blouses and sweaters with at least two pairs of torn slacks, sneakers without laces, and no socks. Her face, hands, and hair are dirty as well. She is carrying a bundle encased in many torn plastic bags.

In addition to her psychiatric difficulties, she has medical problems: a large weeping ulcer (5 cm, stage 3) on a swollen left ankle (4+/4+ to midcalf) and high blood pressure in both arms (right, 154/96; left, 160/98). Although the nurse is unable to completely undress Evelyn initially owing to her agitation, the nurse does feel protruding bones under her clothes. Evelyn's skin is dry and flaky, with multiple scars, abrasions, and bruises. Her feet are callused and cracked. Her heart rate is 98, her respiration rate is 22, and she refuses to have her temperature taken.

Assessment

The nurses assessed the following:

OBJECTIVE DATA

1. Several psychiatric admissions over 20 years
2. Multiple short term relationships with men
3. Difficulty maintaining relationships with friends and co-workers
4. Has a 10-year-old daughter
5. Homeless and jobless for two years

6. Poor hygiene
7. Clothes inappropriate for weather
8. Large leg ulcer and high blood pressure
9. Undernourished
10. Multiple signs of past injuries
11. Difficulty keeping focused during intake

SUBJECTIVE DATA

1. "A man . . . says he's going to hurt me."
2. "I'm tired and hungry."

3. "Marie is in school today. I got scared and couldn't wait for her."
4. "My leg gets real tired sometimes."
5. "There are a lot of nasty, mean people out there. You just can't get away from them."
6. "I don't remember when my leg got sore."

Nursing Diagnosis

The following nursing diagnoses were formulated:

1. *Altered thought processes* related to psychiatric dysfunction, as evidenced by distractibility and cognitive defects
   - "A man says he's going to hurt me."
   - Difficulty staying focused.
   - "I don't remember when my leg got sore."
   - Inability to obtain and retain a job.

2. *Ineffective family coping: disabling* related to psychiatric dysfunction and homelessness, as evidenced by neglect of 10-year-old daughter
   - Homeless and jobless for two years.
   - Marie's infrequent school attendance and poor academic function.
   - Not being where Marie expects to find her after school.

3. *Impaired tissue integrity* related to venous stasis, as evidenced by large ulcer on left ankle
   - 5-cm, stage 3 ulcer.
   - 4+/4+ edema to midcalf on left leg.
   - "My leg gets real tired sometimes."

Other nursing diagnoses that deserve attention are

1. *Hygiene self-care deficit* related to homelessness and decreased cognitive function, as evidenced by dirty, torn clothing and dirty hair and skin
2. *Altered nutrition: less than body requirements* related to poverty, as evidenced by emaciation
3. *High risk for injury* related to disease process and homelessness, as evidenced by scars, bruises, and abrasions

---

Planning

CONTENT LEVEL—PLANNING GOALS

Diagnosis	Long Term Goals	Short Term Goals
1. *Altered thought processes* related to psychiatric dysfunction, as evidenced by distractibility and cognitive defects	1. Evelyn will demonstrate improved thought processes during this admission.	1a. Evelyn will be able to concentrate on learning or therapy activities for at least 10 minutes. 1b. Evelyn will identify three appropriate actions that can be taken to decrease anxiety in the event of stress by discharge.
2. *Ineffective family coping: disabling* related to psychiatric dysfunction and homelessness, as evidenced by neglect of 10-year-old daughter	2. Evelyn will demonstrate improved nurturing behavior toward daughter by discharge.	2a. Evelyn will verbalize an appropriate plan for the care of Marie during Evelyn's hospitalizations. 2b. Evelyn will discuss with the social worker how to access benefits and programs for Marie's support and education by discharge. 2c. Evelyn will demonstrate nurturing behaviors toward Marie during visits throughout this hospitalization.

PROCESS LEVEL—NURSES' REACTIONS AND FEELINGS

Most nurses become skilled in dealing with both the medical and the psychosocial needs of the hospital's population. Through close work with social workers, often much help is available to the homeless. However, dealing with child neglect and abuse is often difficult for nursing staff. Neglected and abused children do not learn or experience healthy bonding, and they do not develop effec-

tive social skills, problem-solving techniques, competencies necessary for employment, and many other skills needed to succeed in life. To adequately care for Evelyn, and indirectly for Marie, the staff realized that the social worker would be an important resource person providing access and referrals to meet some of this family's needs.

Intervention

Initially, during the first few hours, the focus was on lowering Evelyn's anxiety so that she would accept care. Meeting some of her physiological needs (e.g., food and rest) gave the staff the opportunity to make contact with Evelyn. The social worker was contacted and informed that Marie would come back from school and not be able to find her

mother. The social worker, Mr. Todd, located Marie at school and explained the problem. He then brought her to the hospital to see Evelyn before taking her to an emergency foster home. This activity was necessary not only to protect Marie but to emphasize to Evelyn how important such interventions were to Marie's well-being.

Evaluation

Evelyn's psychosocial and medical health improved slowly during the short admission. Her ability to think increased modestly. Her leg ulcer began to show signs of granulation. The edema decreased to 1+/4+ and remained at ankle level. Evelyn articulated plans for job training and living at a halfway house during the training period. She also talked about keeping Marie in a stable foster

care home until she was working and had a home for the two of them. Evelyn agreed to continuing parenting classes through the child welfare agency. However, Marie was demonstrating various acting-out behaviors both in the foster home and at school. She stated, "My mother loves me and I want to be with her now. The way we lived was just fine."

Summary

Homelessness is a complex problem that affects a growing number of Americans today. The number of persons who are both chronically mentally ill and homeless is also escalating. Homelessness reflects a lifestyle problem characterized by chronic disaffiliation from society and personal supports. The causes of homelessness are many, including high unemployment rates, reduction in public support programs and low-cost housing, and deinstitutionalization of the mentally ill from institutions into the community. Homelessness may be a cause as well as a consequence of mental illness.

Various subgroups of the homeless population include the chronically mentally ill, chronic substance abusers, and age-related groups such as families with children, adolescents, and the elderly. The problem of homelessness affects persons regardless of race, sex, and age. Common DSM diagnoses in the chronically

mentally ill subgroup include psychotic disorders, personality disorders, organic mental dysfunctions, and others. Characteristics of this population were also discussed.

Difficulty in accurately counting the number of homeless persons is due to varying definitions of homelessness and inadequate access to this population. Homelessness may be acute, the result of a sudden crisis, or more chronic, the result of gradual disengagement from supportive relationships. Developing a therapeutic relationship with the homeless individual is very important if effective treatment is to occur.

Nurses should take advantage of the many opportunities for assisting the mentally ill who are homeless and should play a key role in providing care and services. The nine roles of the nurse were illustrated and applied to a case study. These roles are healing, caring, communicating, teaching, planning, and coordinating, protecting, rehabilitating, and socializing. Some selected nursing diagnoses to be aware of in caring for the chronically mentally ill who are homeless were also presented. Each step of the nursing process was used to provide a systematic method of addressing the psychosocial and physical needs of an individual patient. Evelyn's story provides an example of the complex needs of a homeless person with a long history of mental illness.

Resources for the mentally ill who are homeless do not meet all the needs of this population. Community mental health services provide much support in the form of community outreach programs, temporary shelters, and multiservice centers. Housing is the first of many needs that chronically mentally ill homeless persons have when they are discharged from the hospital. Resources must be available on an ongoing basis to meet these complex needs. Services may also need to be adjusted to the specific needs of the individual. There is no simple solution to this perplexing problem.

References

Aiken L. Unmet needs of the chronically mentally ill: Will nursing respond? Image: Journal of Nursing Scholarship, 19(3):121, 1987.
Bassuk EL. The homeless problem. Scientific American, 251(1):40, 1984.
Bassuk EL. Homelessness. The Harvard Medical School Mental Health Letter, 3(7):4, 1987.
Brunger JB. The young chronic client in mental health today. Nursing Clinics of North America, 21(3):451, 1986.
Carpenito LJ. Nursing Diagnosis: Application to Clinical Practice, 4th ed. Menlo Park, CA: JB Lippincott, 1992.
Chafetz L. The chronically mentally ill. In Wilson HS, Kneisl CR (eds). Psychiatric Nursing, 3rd ed. Menlo Park, CA: Addison-Wesley Publishing Company, 1988.
Cook JS, Smith JE. Issues facing mental health nursing. In Cook JS, Fontaine KL (eds). Essentials of Mental Health Nursing. Redwood City, CA: Addison-Wesley Nursing, 1991.
Damrosch S, Strasser JA. The homeless elderly in America. Gerontological Nursing, 14(10):26, 1988.
Drake RE, Wallach MA. Substance abuse among the chronic mentally ill. Hospital and Community Psychiatry, 40(10):1041, 1989.
Federal Task Force on Homelessness and Severe Mental Illness. Outcasts on Main Street, 1992.
Grunberg JS. The mentally ill who are chronically homeless. In Varcarolis EM (ed). Foundations of Psychiatric-Mental Health Nursing, 1st ed. Philadelphia: WB Saunders, 1990.
JOC. Building a sense of community cooperation among agencies key to helping the homeless. Psychiatric News, 23(8):29, 48, 1988.
Johnson AB. Out of Bedlam: The Truth About Deinstitutionalization. New York City: Basic Books, 1990.
Kozier B, Erb G. Fundamentals of Nursing. Menlo Park, CA: Addison-Wesley Publishing Company, 1983.
Lamb HR. Deinstitutionalization and the homeless mentally ill. In Lamb HR (ed). The Homeless Mentally Ill: A Task Force Report of the American Psychiatric Association. Washington, DC: American Psychiatric Association, 1984.
Riesdorf-Ostrow W. The homeless chronically mentally ill: Deinstitutionalization: A public policy perspective. Journal of Psychosocial Nursing, 27(6):4, 1989.
Ryan MT. Providing shelter. Journal of Psychosocial Nursing, 27(6):15, 1989.
Tower CC, White DJ. Homeless Students. National Educational Association, 1989.
Worley N. The chronically mentally disabled. In Burgess AW (ed). Psychiatric Nursing in the Hospital and the Community, 5th ed. Norwalk, CT: Appleton & Lange, 1990.

Self-study Exercises

1. List some diagnoses of chronic psychiatric disorders and personality disorders common among the homeless population.

2. Describe what it means to be homeless in terms of chronic disaffiliation from family, friends, and community.

3. Explain the process of homelessness with regard to the complexity of the problem, as well as the difficulties in diagnosis and treatment.

4. Discuss the importance of establishing a trusting, therapeutic relationship with the mentally ill person who is chronically homeless.

5. List at least three characteristics of the chronically mentally ill homeless population for each of the following:
   Behavioral: _____
   Cognitive: _____
   Physiological:_____

6. Define the term *chronic mental illness*.

7. Prepare a preliminary plan of care for the following homeless patient. Remember to include the top two to three nursing diagnoses, patient outcomes, and key interventions.

TC is 39 years old and was first diagnosed with schizophrenia 15 years ago. He has had several acute psychiatric hospitalizations since then. Over the years, he has been intermittently employed as a day laborer, but he has not worked at all for nearly two years. TC was admitted a few hours ago. He is agitated, suspicious, dirty, and emaciated and is wearing torn, smelly, and ill-fitting clothing. He paces the halls, occasionally leaning against the wall and closing his eyes for a moment.

Appendices

Drug Information

CHLORPROMAZINE
(Thorazine, Chlorazine)

USES:
1. Management of acute psychotic disorders (schizophrenia, manic phase of a bipolar disorder) and to maintain remission of these psychotic disorders.
2. Management of severe behavioral disturbances in (a) children or (b) clients with organic mental disorders.
3. Other: Intractable hiccups, acute intermittent porphyria, tetanus, preoperatively, or to control nausea and vomiting.

ACTION: Blocks postsynaptic dopamine receptors in the cerebral cortex basal ganglia, hypothalamus, limbic system, brain stem, and medulla. Therefore, there is inhibition or alteration of dopamine release, which is thought to be related to the suppression of the clinical manifestations of schizophrenia.

DOSAGES & ROUTES

Hospitalized: Acute Psychotic Disorders

	PO	IM
Adult	Gradually increase over several days to maximum of 400 mg every 4–6 hours	25 mg—may give an additional 25–50 mg in 1 hour if needed

Outpatient: Maintenance Dose

	PO	IM	RECTAL SUPPOSITORY
Adult	10–50 mg twice daily to every 4 hours	25–50 mg 1–4 times daily	50–100 mg 3–4 times daily
Child	0.55 mg/kg every 4–6 hours	None	1.1 mg/kg every 6–8 hours
Elderly	(Debilitated) 25 mg 3 times daily		

CONTRAINDICATIONS: Comatose states, alcohol or barbiturate withdrawal states, bone marrow depression, pregnancy, lactation.

CAUTIONS: Seizure disorders, diabetes, hepatic disease, cardiac disease, glaucoma, prostatic hypertrophy, asthma.

REMARKS: A "low potency" neuroleptic (low neurological symptoms (extrapyramidal symptoms [EPS])), but with high sedation and autonomic side effects (e.g., hypotension, cardiac, allergic). Food or antacids decrease absorption. Liquid preparation is more rapidly absorbed.

SIDE EFFECTS **AUTONOMIC:** Dry mouth, nasal congestion, constipation or diarrhea, urinary retention or urinary frequency, inhibition of ejaculation and impotence in men.

CNS: *Extrapyramidal symptoms* (pseudoparkinsonism, akathisia, dystonia). Possible vertigo or insomnia.

CARDIOVASCULAR: Orthostatic hypotension, hypertension, vertigo, EEG changes.

ENDOCRINE: Changes in libido, galactorrhea in women, gynecomastia in men.

OCULAR: Photophobia, blurred vision, aggravation of glaucoma.

OTHER: Weight gain, allergic reactions such as eczema and skin rashes.

ADVERSE REACTIONS **CNS:** *Acute dystonias* (e.g., painful neck spasms, torticollis, oculogyric crisis, convulsions). *Tardive dyskinesia* (choreiform movements of the tongue, face, mouth, jaw, and possibly extremities). The elderly and those on the drug for extended periods of time are more susceptible; often the condition is irreversible.

HEMATOLOGIC: Agranulocytosis—drug immediately stopped.

HEPATIC: Jaundice; clinical picture resembles hepatitis.

NEUROLEPTIC MALIGNANT SYNDROME (NMS): Rare life-threatening syndrome. Includes severe rigidity, fever, increased white blood cell count, unstable BP, renal failure, tachycardia, tachypnea. Hold all drugs. Immediate administration of dantrolene sodium and bromocriptine is the most successful somatic prescription.

NURSING MEASURES:
1. Take BP lying and standing (withhold if systolic is 90 or below) and notify physician.
2. Hold dose if EPS or jaundice.
3. Check frequently for urinary retention.
4. Check for constipation (avoid impaction).
5. Observe for fever, sore throat, and malaise, and monitor complete blood count, indicating a blood dyscrasia.

INFORM CLIENT:
1. Rise slowly to a sitting position and dangle the legs five minutes before standing to minimize orthostatic hypotension.
2. Avoid sun. Use sunscreen when in direct light to avoid skin blotching. Wear long sleeves and hats.
3. Avoid sun. Client may experience severe photosensitivity. Advise wearing sunglasses to minimize photophobia.
4. Avoid use of alcoholic beverages because they enhance CNS depression.
5. Do not operate machinery if drowsiness occurs.

ANTIPSYCHOTIC/NEUROLEPTIC

HALOPERIDOL
(Haldol)

BUTYROPHENONE

USES:
1. Management of psychotic disorders.
2. Helps control remissions in schizophrenia.
3. Controversial use for children with combative, explosive hyperexcitability.
4. Control of tic and vocal utterances of Gilles de la Tourette's disorder.
5. Useful in acute mania and acute and chronic organic psychosis.
6. Management of drug-induced psychosis (LSD).

ACTION: Blocks the binding of dopamine to the postsynaptic dopamine receptors in the brain.

DOSAGES & ROUTES

	PO	IM
Adult	0.5–2.0 mg 2–3 times daily	(Severe) 3–5 mg every 1–8 hours to control symptoms, then give PO
Child	Not for children under 3 years; for children 3–12 years, 0.05–0.15 mg/kg/day in 2–3 divided doses	
Elderly	Elderly or debilitated clients may require smaller doses than adults	

CONTRAINDICATIONS: Hypersensitivity, Parkinson's disease, depression, seizures, coma, alcoholism, during lithium therapy.

CAUTIONS: The elderly; clients on anticoagulant therapy; clients with glaucoma, prostatic hypertrophy, urinary retention, asthma, or pregnancy/lactation.

REMARKS: A "high potency" neuroleptic; higher incidence of EPS but lower incidence of sedation and orthostatic hypotension. Haldol Decanoate E or D given intramuscularly can have lasting effects from one to three weeks.

SIDE EFFECTS   **AUTONOMIC:** Dry mouth, nasal congestion, constipation or diarrhea, urinary retention or urinary frequency, inhibition of ejaculation and impotence in men.

CNS: *Extrapyramidal symptoms* (pseudoparkinsonism, akathisia, dystonia), vertigo, insomnia, headache.

CARDIOVASCULAR: Orthostatic hypotension, hypertension, dizziness, EEG changes.

ENDOCRINE: Changes in libido, galactorrhea in women, gynecomastia in men.

OCULAR: Photophobia, blurred vision, aggravation of glaucoma.

OTHER: Weight gain, allergic reactions such as eczema and skin rashes.

ADVERSE REACTIONS   **CNS:** *Acute dystonias* (e.g., painful neck spasms, torticollis, oculogyric crisis, convulsions). *Tardive dyskinesia* (choreiform movements of the tongue, face, mouth, jaw, and possibly extremities). The elderly and those on the drug for extended periods are more susceptible; often irreversible.

HEMATOLOGIC: Agranulocytosis—drug immediately stopped.

HEPATIC: Jaundice; clinical picture resembles hepatitis.

NEUROLEPTIC MALIGNANT SYNDROME (NMS): Occurs within 24–72 hours. Fever, rigidity, renal failure, arrhythmias, and more. Hold drug and give dantrolene sodium or bromocriptine immediately.

NURSING MEASURES: 1. Check for signs of tardive dyskinesia (protrusion of tongue, puffing of cheeks, chewing or puckering of the mouth) and report them to physician immediately.
2. Observe for other signs of EPS and jaundice.
3. Check for orthostatic hypotension (take BP lying and standing). Withhold if systolic is 80 or below.
4. Check frequently for urinary retention.
5. Check for constipation (avoid impaction).

6. Observe for fever, sore throat, and malaise, and monitor complete blood count, indicating a blood dyscrasia.
7. Monitor renal function during long term therapy.
8. Monitor blood levels every week.

INFORM CLIENT:
1. Rise slowly to a sitting position and dangle the legs five minutes before standing to minimize orthostatic hypotension.
2. Use sunscreen when in direct light to avoid skin blotching, and wear sunglasses to prevent photophobia.
3. Avoid the use of alcoholic beverages because they enhance CNS depression.
4. Refrain from operating machinery if drowsiness occurs.

BENZTROPINE MESYLATE
(Cogentin)

ANTIPARKINSONIAN

USES:
1. Treating Parkinson's disease.
2. Treatment of extrapyramidal symptoms (except tardive dyskinesia) due to use of neuroleptic/antipsychotic medications.

ACTION: Cogentin is an anticholinergic agent. This drug increases and prolongs the action of dopamine activity in the CNS, thereby correcting neurotransmitter imbalances and minimizing involuntary movements.

DOSAGES & ROUTES

	PO	IM/IV
Adult	0.5–2 mg every day initially; gradually increase to 4–6 mg/day. For drug-induced extrapyramidal symptoms, 1–4 mg once or twice a day IM or PO	For acute dystonic reactions, 0.5–2 mg Im or IV
Elderly	Use lower doses	

CONTRAINDICATIONS: Narrow-angle glaucoma, pyloric or duodenal obstruction, peptic ulcers, prostatic hypertrophy, obstructions of the bladder neck, myasthenia gravis, and in children under three years of age. Rarely indicated for children.

CAUTIONS: The elderly and clients with cardiac, liver, or kidney disease or hypertension. Also used with caution in clients taking barbiturates or alcohol.

REMARKS: The effects of benztropine are cumulative and may not be evident for two or three days. After four to six months of long term maintenance antipsychotic therapy, antiparkinsonian drugs can be used on an as-necessary basis or withdrawn. Some clients respond best to the medication given every day. Others do better with divided doses. Long term use of benztropine with a neuroleptic can predispose a patient to tardive dyskinesia.

SIDE EFFECTS **AUTONOMIC:** Dry mouth, blurred vision, nausea, restlessness.

CNS: Sedation, vertigo, paresthesias.

CARDIOVASCULAR: Palpitations, tachycardia.

GASTROINTESTINAL: Nausea, vomiting, constipation, paralytic ileus.

GENITOURINARY: Dysuria, urinary retention.

OCULAR: Blurred vision, mydriasis, photophobia.

OTHER: Anhidrosis (abnormal deficiency of sweat).

ADVERSE REACTIONS **CNS:** CNS depression, mild agitation, hallucinations, delirium, toxic psychosis, muscle weakness, ataxia, numbness of the fingers.

NURSING MEASURES:
1. Monitor intake and output. Observe for urinary retention.
2. Give medication after patient voids to reduce possibility of urinary retention.
3. Monitor for constipation; abdominal pain or distention may indicate potential for paralytic ileus.
4. Indications of CNS toxicity (depression or excitement, hallucinations, psychosis, or other) warrant withholding the drug and informing the physician immediately.

INFORM CLIENT:
1. Avoid driving or operating hazardous equipment if drowsiness or dizziness occurs.
2. Tolerance to heat may be reduced owing to diminished ability to sweat. Plan periods of rest in cool places during the day.
3. Stop taking the medication if CNS toxic effects, or difficulty swallowing or speaking, or vomiting occurs. Inform physician immediately.
4. Monitor urinary output and watch for signs of constipation.
5. Consult with physician before using any medication, prescribed or over the counter, once started on benztropine.

DIAZEPAM
(Valium)

ANXIOLYTIC (ANTIANXIETY AGENTS)

BENZODIAZEPINE

USES:
1. Management of anxiety disorders, for short term relief of anxiety symptoms.
2. Presurgical sedation to allay anxiety and tension.
3. Alcohol withdrawal.
4. Seizure disorders.
5. Anticonvulsant.
6. Relief of skeletal muscle spasticity.

ACTION: One action of the benzodiazepines is to increase the action of gamma-aminobutyric acid (GABA). The benzodiazepines help GABA open a chloride channel in the postsynaptic membrane of many neurons, thereby reducing the neuron's excitability.

DOSAGES & ROUTES

	PO	IM/IV
Adult	Anxiety: 2–10 mg 2–4 times daily	2–10 mg 2–4 times daily
	Muscle relaxant: 2–10 mg 2–4 times daily	5–10 mg every 3–4 hours
	Convulsions: 2–10 mg 2–4 times daily	5–10 mg at 10-minute intervals
	Alcohol withdrawal: 10 mg 3–4 times daily	10 mg initially, followed by 5–10 mg every 3–4 hours
Elderly	2.5 mg twice daily	Convulsions: 2–5 mg (increase gradually as needed)

CONTRAINDICATIONS: Acute narrow-angle glaucoma, untreated open-angle glaucoma, during or within 14 days of monoamine oxidase inhibitor therapy, depressed or psychotic patients in the absence of anxiety, first-trimester pregnancy, breast-feeding, shock, coma, acute alcohol intoxication.

CAUTIONS: Epilepsy, myasthenia gravis, impaired hepatic or renal function, drug abuse, addiction-prone individuals. Injectable diazepam is used with extreme caution in the elderly, the very ill, and people with chronic obstructive pulmonary disease. May elicit rage reactions in some clients.

REMARKS: The benzodiazepines can produce psychological and physical habituation, dependence, and withdrawal. Therefore, they are recommended for short term therapy (2–4 weeks). These drugs need to be used with caution in individuals who have histories of addiction. Withdrawal from these drugs should be gradual in order to minimize withdrawal symptoms.

SIDE EFFECTS **CNS:** Sedation, vertigo, weakness, ataxia, decreased motor performance, confusion.

OCULAR: Double or blurred vision.

SKIN: Urticaria, rash, photosensitivity.

GASTROINTESTINAL: Change in weight, dry mouth, constipation.

ADVERSE EFFECTS **CNS:** Benzodiazepines are CNS depressants. They are fairly safe when used on their own, but when used in combination with other CNS depressants, they can cause death.

CARDIOVASCULAR: Tachycardia to cardiovascular collapse.

METABOLIC: Changes in liver or renal function test results.

INJECTION SITES: Can cause venous thrombosis or phlebitis at injection sites.

NURSING MEASURES:
1. Obtain drug history of prescribed and over-the-counter medications.
2. Periodically monitor blood cell count and liver function test results during prolonged therapy.
3. Assess for unexplained bleeding, petechiae, fever, and so forth.
4. Intramuscular therapy: Aspirate back, administer deeply into large muscle mass; inject slowly; rotate injection sites.

INFORM CLIENT:
1. Avoid alcohol or any other central nervous system depressants (anticonvulsants, antidepressants) while taking a benzodiazepine—can lead to respiratory depression. Check with physician before taking.
2. Avoid driving or operating hazardous machinery if drowsiness or confusion occurs.
3. Avoid abrupt withdrawal of benzodiazepine.

ANTIDEPRESSANT

IMIPRAMINE HYDROCHLORIDE

(Tofranil)

TRICYCLIC

USES:
1. The principal indication for tricyclic antidepressants (TCAs) is the treatment of depression (major, bipolar, or dysthymia).
2. Imipramine is effective in some organic affective disorders and obsessive-compulsive disorders.
3. Imipramine is used as adjunctive treatment in childhood enuresis and in bulimia.
4. Found useful in the treatment of agoraphobia with panic attacks and generalized anxiety disorder.

ACTION: TCAs block the reuptake of norepinephrine and serotonin into their presynaptic neurons.

DOSAGES & ROUTES		
	PO	**IM**
Adult	50 mg/day to start, given in 1–4 divided doses up to 200 mg daily for outpatients. Maintenance level 50–150 mg/day.	Do not exceed 100 mg/day in divided doses
Child	For childhood enuresis, 25 mg before bedtime; for depression in children *over* 12 years, 30–40 mg daily initially	
Elderly	Used with caution—usually start at lower dose. Geriatric clients start on 30–40 mg daily initially	

CONTRAINDICATIONS: Recent myocardial infarction or cardiac disease, severe renal or hepatic impairment. Death may occur if used with a monoamine oxidase inhibitor. However, the two may be cautiously used together in cases of refractory depression. TCAs may also cause fatal cardiac arrhythmias in clients with hyperthyroidism. Use with caution in children and adolescents. Special cautions for the elderly, especially those with cardiac, respiratory, cardiovascular, hepatic, or gastrointestinal diseases.

CAUTIONS: Other cautions include people with renal or hepatic disease, and narrow-angle glaucoma. The potential for suicide must be assessed. TCAs lower the seizure threshold: any client with a seizure disorder needs careful monitoring.

REMARKS: 1. Before receiving TCAs, clients need a thorough physical and cardiac work-up.
2. Patients need to know that mood elevation may not occur for two to four weeks.

SIDE EFFECTS **ANTICHOLINERGIC:** Dry mouth and nasal passages, constipation, urinary hesitancy, esophageal reflux, blurred vision.

CARDIOVASCULAR: Orthostatic hypotension, hypertension, palpitations.

CNS: Tachycardia, vertigo, tinnitus, numbness and tingling of extremities, stimulation.

ENDOCRINE: Galactorrhea, increased or decreased libido, ejaculatory and erectile disturbances, delayed orgasm.

OTHER: Weight gain and impotence, cholestatic jaundice, fatigue.

ADVERSE REACTIONS **AUTONOMIC:** Intracardiac conduction slowing.

CARDIOVASCULAR: Myocardial infarction, congestive heart failure, arrhythmias, heart block, cardiotoxicity, cerebrovascular accident, shock.

CNS: Ataxia, neuropathy, EPS, lowered seizure threshold, delirium.

HEMATOLOGIC: Bone marrow depression, agranulocytosis.

PSYCHIATRIC: Hallucinations, shift to hypomania, mania, exacerbation of psychosis.

NURSING MEASURES: 1. Monitor BP (both lying and standing) every two to six hours when initiating therapy.
2. Observe suicidal clients closely during initial therapy.

3. Supervise drug ingestion to prevent hoarding of drug.
4. Assess for urinary retention.
5. Monitor liver function test results and complete blood count (assess for signs of cholestatic jaundice and agranulocytosis).
6. Small amount of drugs should be dispensed if client is to be discharged.
7. Diabetic clients should be closely monitored especially during early therapy, since hypo- or hyperglycemia may occur in some clients.
8. All clients on TCAs need to be observed for the occurrence of hypomania or manic episodes, urinary retention, orthostatic hypotension, and seizure activity.

INFORM CLIENT:
1. Rise slowly to prevent hypotensive effects.
2. Do not drive or use hazardous machinery if drowsiness or vertigo occurs.
3. Do not use over-the-counter drugs in conjunction with a TCA without a physician's approval.
4. The effects of alcohol and imipramine are potentiated when used together, and alcohol use should be discussed with a physician before taking the drug.
5. One to four weeks may pass before the therapeutic effects are experienced.

ANTIDEPRESSANT

PHENELZINE SULFATE
(Nardil)

MONOAMINE OXIDASE INHIBITOR (MAOI)

USES:
1. MAOIs are used primarily for depression that is refractory to tricyclic antidepressant therapy.
2. MAOIs are particularly effective in atypical depression, agoraphobia, or hypochondriasis.
3. Panic disorders.

ACTION: Antidepressant effect thought to be due to irreversible inhibition of MAO, thereby increasing the concentration of epinephrine, norepinephrine, serotonin, and dopamine within the pre-synaptic neurons and at the receptor site.

DOSAGES & ROUTES

	PO
Adult	15 mg 3 times daily; increase rapidly to 60 mg daily until therapeutic level is noted
Elderly	Are prone to side effects and if > 60 may be contraindicated
Child	Not used with children

CONTRAINDICATIONS: MAOIs can cause untoward interactions with certain foodstuffs or cold remedies, which may produce hypertensive crises, CVA, or hyperpyrexia states that can lead to coma or death. Therefore, a confused or noncompliant client is at risk with an MAOI.

Other contraindications include people with congestive heart failure, cardiovascular or cerebrovascular disease, impaired renal function, glaucoma, history of severe headaches, or liver disease; elderly or debilitated patients; and people who are pregnant or who have paranoid schizophrenia.

CAUTIONS: Depression accompanying alcoholism or drug addiction, manic-depressive states, suicidal tendencies, agitated clients, and people with chronic brain syndromes or a history of angina pectoris.

REMARKS: Because of the severe interactions of some foodstuffs and medication, clients need comprehensive teaching, teaching aids, and supervision.

High-tyramine foods include beer, red wine, aged cheese, dry sausage, fava beans (Italian green beans), brewer's yeast, smoked fish, any kind of liver, avocados, and bologna. Chocolate and coffee should be used in moderation.

Drugs causing severe medication interactions include meperidine (Demerol), epinephrine, local anesthetics, decongestants, cough medications, diet pills, and most over-the-counter medications.

SIDE EFFECTS **GENERAL:** Constipation, dry mouth, vertigo, orthostatic hypotension, drowsiness or insomnia, weakness, fatigue, weight gain, hypomania, mania, blurred vision, skin rash. Muscle twitching is common.

ADVERSE REACTIONS **HYPERTENSIVE CRISIS:** Intense occipital headache, palpitation, stiff neck, fever, chest pain, bradycardia or tachycardia, intracranial bleeding.

HEPATIC: Jaundice, malaise, right upper quadrant pain, change in color or consistency of stools.

NURSING MEASURES:
1. Monitor BP for orthostatic hypotension every two to four hours during initial therapy.
2. Assess for other potential signs of hypertensive crises.
3. Observe for marked changes in mood (e.g., hypomania, mania).
4. Monitor intake and output and frequency of stools.
5. Have client dangle legs five minutes before standing.
6. Depressed persons are at risk for suicide; continue to monitor and observe for potential suicidal behaviors.

INFORM CLIENT:
1. Inform clients and their families clearly and carefully about foodstuffs and medications to avoid. REVIEW IN DETAIL.
2. Instruct clients taking MAOIs to wear a medical identification tag or bracelet.
3. Caution clients to avoid all over-the-counter drugs unless a physician's approval has been obtained.
4. Caution clients to avoid all alcohol.
5. Encourage clients and their families to go to the emergency room immediately if signs and symptoms of hypertensive crises are suspected. Phentolamine (Regitine) can be given for hypertensive crises.

FLUOXETINE HYDROCHLORIDE
(Prozac)   ANTIDEPRESSANT

USES:
1. Prozac is an atypical antidepressant medication that is chemically unrelated to tricyclic antidepressants or monoamine oxidase inhibitors.
2. Has been found effective in clients with bulimia and obsessive-compulsive disorders.

ACTION: Is a potent serotonin reuptake blocker whose use results in an increase in the amount of active serotonin within the synaptic cleft and at the serotonin receptor site. Increased serotonin in these areas appears to modify affective and behavioral disorders.

DOSAGES & ROUTES	
Adult	20 mg per day; may reach 40–60 mg in divided doses; do not exceed 80 mg daily
Elderly	Same as for adults
Child	No dosage for children as yet established

CONTRAINDICATIONS: Not to be taken within 14 days of an MAO inhibitor. Also, client must wait 5 weeks when going from fluoxetine to an MAO inhibitor.

CAUTIONS: Use with clients with concomitant systemic illness has not been studied extensively. Caution should be used with pregnant women or women who are breast-feeding, children, and the elderly. Caution should also be used with clients with liver disease or renal impairment or in a client who has had a recent myocardial infarction.

REMARKS: Fluoxetine, like the tricyclic antidepressants and monoamine oxidase inhibitors, takes from two to five weeks to produce an elevation of mood. Advantages of this drug are that there are fewer anticholinergic side effects and that there is a low incidence of cardiovascular effects. However, fluoxetine may impair judgment, thinking, and motor skills.

SIDE EFFECTS **GENERAL:** The most common side effects reported with fluoxetine hydrochloride are nausea, nervousness and anxiety, insomnia, and vertigo. When these side effects are severe, the drug is discontinued. If a rash or urticaria or both develop, the drug should be discontinued. Anorexia may appear in some people.

ADVERSE REACTIONS See side effects.

NURSING MEASURES:
1. Fluoxetine hydrochloride is given in the early morning without consideration to meals.
2. Clients who are potentially suicidal are assessed for suicidal thoughts or actions. Carefully observe taking of medication.
3. If client is underweight and experiences anorexia, the physician should be alerted to re-evaluate continuation of medication.

INFORM CLIENT:
1. If rash or urticaria appears, notify physician immediately.
2. Do not drive or operate machinery if drowsiness occurs.
3. Avoid alcoholic beverages.

LITHIUM CARBONATE/CITRATE

ANTIMANIC
___

(Carbolith, Eskalith, Lithane, Lithizine, Lithonate, Lithobid)

LITHIUM

USES:
1. Primarily used to control, prevent, or diminish manic episodes in people with bipolar depression (manic-depressive psychosis).
2. Used *experimentally* in alcoholism, premenstrual syndrome, drug abuse, phobias, eating disorders, and rage reactions.

ACTION: Lithium is an alkali metal salt that behaves in the body much like a sodium ion. Lithium acts to lower concentrations of norepinephrine and serotonin by inhibiting their release and enhancing their reuptake by neurons. The therapeutic effects, as well as the side effects and toxic effects, of lithium are thought to be related to the partial replacement of sodium by lithium in membrane action.

DOSAGES & ROUTES	
	PO
Adult	Acute mania, 600 mg 3 times daily; maintenance dose, 300 mg 3 times daily or 4 times daily
Child	Not labeled for pediatric use
Elderly	Reduce to 600–900 daily to produce low serum concentration of about 0.5 mEq/l

CONTRAINDICATIONS: Pregnancy, nursing mothers, significant cardiovascular or renal disease, schizophrenia, severe debilitation, dehydration, sodium depletion.

CAUTIONS: The elderly, thyroid disease, epilepsy, concomitant use with haloperidol or other antipsychotics, parkinsonism, severe infections, urinary retention, diabetes.

REMARKS: Serum lithium levels must be monitored during drug therapy. The therapeutic range is very narrow, and the potential for toxic effects is high if blood levels are not monitored. During the acute stage, blood levels are raised to 1.0–1.4 mEq/l. Maintenance therapy blood levels run from 0.8–1.2 mEq/l. Side effects and toxic effects are common at higher doses (1.5 mEq/l or more). Before a patient is started on lithium, BUN, T4, T3, and TSH levels should be measured, and an ECG should be done.

SIDE EFFECTS: The major long-term risks of lithium therapy are hypothyroidism and impairment of the kidney's ability to concentrate urine.
  Below 1.5 mEq/l: Polyuria, polydipsia, lethargy, fatigue, muscle weakness, headache, mild nausea, fine hand tremor, and inability to concentrate. May experience ankle edema. Symptoms disappear during continued therapy.

ADVERSE AND TOXIC EFFECTS **1.5–2.0 mEq/l:** Vomiting, diarrhea, muscle weakness, ataxia, dizziness, slurred speech, confusion.
  2.0–2.5 mEq/l: Blurred vision, muscle twitching, severe hypotension, persistent nausea and vomiting. Thyroid toxicity is common.
  2.5–3.0 mEq/l or more: Urinary and fecal incontinence, seizures, cardiac arrhythmias, peripheral vascular collapse, death.

NURSING MEASURES:
1. If serum lithium levels are above 1.5 mEq/l or if client has persistent diarrhea, vomiting, excessive sweating in hot weather, infection, or fever, check with physician before giving dose.
2. Check urine specific gravity periodically and teach patient to do so at home (normal: 1.005–1.025).
3. Administer lithium with meals.
4. Ensure that client is well hydrated.

INFORM CLIENT:
1. Drink plenty of liquids (2–3 liters/day) during initial therapy and 1–1.5 liters/day during remainder of therapy.
2. Know the side effects and toxic effects of lithium therapy and seek out physician immediately if problems arise.
3. Have blood lithium levels measured at regular intervals as directed in order to regulate dosage and prevent toxicity.
4. Maintain a regular diet, thus maintaining average salt intake (6–8 g) required to keep the serum lithium level in the therapeutic range.
5. Avoid alcohol.
6. Be aware that antibiotics (metronidazole and tetracycline) and nonsteroidal anti-inflammatory agents (indomethacin) can increase lithium levels.
7. Know that caffeine can lower lithium levels.

ALCOHOL DETERRENT

DISULFIRAM
(Antabuse)

ALDEHYDE DEHYDROGENASE INHIBITOR

USES: Adjunct treatment for selected clients with chronic alcoholism who want to remain in a state of enforced sobriety. A form of aversion therapy.

ACTION: Inhibits hepatic enzymes from normal metabolic breakdown of alcohol, resulting in high levels of acetaldehyde. It is this substance that causes the distressing symptoms of disulfiram-alcohol reaction.

DOSAGES & ROUTES	
	PO only
Adult	Initially, a maximum of 500 mg daily given as a single dose for 1–2 weeks; maintenance, 250 mg daily; not to exceed 500 mg daily.

CONTRAINDICATIONS: Severe heart disease, psychosis, and hypersensitivity to disulfiram.

CAUTIONS: Diabetes, hypothyroidism, epilepsy, cerebral damage, nephritis, hepatic disease, pregnancy.

REMARKS: Clients must abstain from alcohol intake for at least 12 hours before the initial dose of drug is administered.

SIDE EFFECTS: Common side effects experienced during the first two weeks of therapy include mild drowsiness, fatigue, headache, metallic or garlic aftertaste, allergic dermatitis, and acne eruptions. Symptoms disappear spontaneously with continued therapy or reduced dosage.

ADVERSE REACTIONS DISULFIRAM-ALCOHOL REACTION Flushing or throbbing in head and neck, throbbing headache, nausea, copious vomiting, diaphoresis, dyspnea, hyperventilation, tachycardia, hypotension, marked uneasiness, vertigo, blurred vision, confusion. Can cause death.

NURSING MEASURES:
1. Client must be able to demonstrate sobriety.
2. Client must be fully aware of drug's action when taken along with alcohol before treatment commences.
3. In severe disulfiram-alcohol reactions, supportive measures to restore BP and treat for shock in a medical facility are vital.

INFORM CLIENT AND FAMILY:
1. Avoid any substances that contain alcohol
   a. *Ingestion:* Elixirs, cough syrups, vinegars, vitamin/mineral tonics; be aware that some sauces, soups, ciders, flavor extracts (vanilla, cherry) and some desserts (flaming, and some cakes and pies) are made with alcohol.
   b. *Topical:* Mouth wash, body lotions, liniments, shaving lotion.
   c. *Inhalation:* Avoid inhaling fumes from substances that may contain alcohol, such as paints, wood stains, varnishes, and "stripping" compounds.
2. Carry a card stating that if they are found disoriented or unconscious, they may be having a disulfiram-alcohol reaction and telling the finder who to contact for medical care.
3. A disulfiram-alcohol reaction can occur within five to 10 minutes after ingestion of alcohol and can last 30–60 minutes or longer.
4. Reaction may occur with alcohol up to 14 days after ingesting disulfiram.

CARBAMAZEPINE
(Tegretol, Epitol, Mazepine)   ANTICONVULSANT, ANTINEURALGIC

USES:
1. Management of generalized tonic-clonic seizures (grand mal) and psychomotor seizures.
2. Trigeminal neuralgia.
3. Potential mood stabilizer, particularly in acute mania. Used clinically, but not FDA approved at present for this use.

ACTION: Reduces post-tetanic potentiation at the synapse, preventing repetitive discharge.

DOSAGES & ROUTES
(Seizures)

Adult	**PO only** (tablets, suspension, and chewable tablets) 200 mg twice daily, gradually increase until response is attained; maintenance, 800–1200 mg/day
Child **(6–12)**	100 mg twice daily, gradually increase until response is attained; maintenance, 400–800 mg/day in 3–4 equally divided doses. **Note:** Oral suspensions produce higher peak concentrations. Going from tablets to suspension, give in smaller and more frequent doses.

CONTRAINDICATIONS: History of bone marrow depression, history of hypersensitivity to tricyclic antidepressants.

CAUTIONS: Impaired cardiac, hepatic, and renal function; pregnancy or lactation (crosses placenta, distributed in breast milk, accumulates in fetal tissues).

REMARKS: Monitoring drug levels has increased the safety of anticonvulsant therapy.

SIDE EFFECTS **FREQUENT:** Drowsiness, dizziness, nausea and vomiting.

INFREQUENT: Lethargy, visual abnormalities (spots before the eyes, difficulty focusing), dry mouth, headache, urinary frequency or retention, rash.

ADVERSE REACTIONS **HEMATOLOGIC:** Blood dyscrasias (e.g., aplastic anemia, agranulocytosis, thrombocytopenia, leukopenia, bone marrow depression).

HEPATIC: Abnormal hepatic function test results; jaundice may be noticed; hepatitis.

CARDIOVASCULAR: Congestive heart failure, edema, aggravation of coronary artery disease, arrhythmias and atrioventricular block, primary thrombophlebitis. Some complications have resulted in fatalities.

CNS: Abrupt withdrawal may precipitate status epilepticus.

NURSING MEASURES:
1. Monitor for therapeutic serum level (3–12 μg/ml).
2. Assess for clinical evidence of early toxic signs (fever, sore throat, mouth ulcerations, easy bruising, unusual bleeding, joint pain).
3. Observe frequently for recurrence of seizure activity.

INFORM CLIENT AND FAMILY:
1. Blood tests should be repeated frequently during the first three months of therapy and at monthly intervals thereafter for two to three years.
2. Do *not* abruptly withdraw medications following long term use (may precipitate seizures).
3. Avoid tasks that require alertness until response to drug is established.
4. Report visual abnormalities.

BUSPIRONE HYDROCHLORIDE
(BuSpar)

ANTIANXIETY AGENT

USES: Management of anxiety disorders.

ACTION: The exact action of buspirone is not clear. It may exert a potent presynaptic dopamine antagonist effect in the CNS, resulting in increased dopamine at the synapses. It may also have an effect on serotonin receptors.

DOSAGES & ROUTES	
	PO only
Adult and Elderly	5 mg 2–3 times daily; may increase 5 mg every 3–4 days; maintenance, 15–30 mg/day in 2–3 divided doses; not to exceed 60 mg/day

CONTRAINDICATIONS: In clients with severe renal or hepatic impairment and clients on monoamine oxidase inhibitors (MAOIs).

CAUTIONS: Renal or hepatic impairment, pregnant or lactating women, elderly or debilitated clients.

REMARKS: The advantages of buspirone (BuSpar) are that it is not sedating, does not develop a tolerance, and is not addicting. The drug has a more favorable side effect profile than do the benzodiazepines.

SIDE EFFECTS: Dizziness, nausea, headache, nervousness, lightheadedness, and excitement, which generally are not major problems. Other less common problems may occur (e.g., blurred vision, tachycardia, palpitations, paresthesia, abdominal distention).

ADVERSE REACTIONS: Overdose may produce severe nausea, vomiting, dizziness, drowsiness, abdominal distention, excessive pupil constriction.

NURSING MEASURES:
1. Offer emotional support to anxious clients.
2. Liver and renal function tests and blood counts should be done regularly for clients on long term therapy.
3. Assist with ambulation and put in place other safety features if dizziness and lightheadedness occur.

INFORM CLIENT AND FAMILY:
1. Teach clients to inform their physicians:
   a. About any medications (prescription or nonprescription), alcohol, or drugs that they are taking.
   b. If they are now or plan to get pregnant.
   c. If they are breast-feeding an infant.
2. Do not drive a car or operate potentially dangerous machinery until they experience how this medication will affect them.
3. Notify physician of difficulty breathing, change in vision, sweating, flushing, or cardiac problems.
4. Improvement may be noted in seven to 10 days, but it may take three to four weeks or longer to note therapeutic effects.

CLOZAPINE
(Clozaril)

ANTIPSYCHOTIC/NEUROLEPTIC

TRICYCLIC DIBENZODIAZEPINE DERIVATIVE

USES: Management of severely ill schizophrenic patients who fail to respond to other antipsychotic therapy.

ACTION: May involve antagonism of dopaminergic, serotonergic, adrenergic, cholinergic neurotransmitter systems. Exact action unknown.

DOSAGES & ROUTES

	PO only
Adult	Initially, 25 mg 1–2 times daily; may increase by 25–50 mg/day over 2 weeks until 300–450 mg/day achieved; range, 200–600 mg/day; not to exceed 900 mg/day

CONTRAINDICATIONS: Clients who are hypersensitive to tricyclics, have a history of severe granulocytopenia; concurrent administration with other drugs having potential to suppress bone marrow function; clients who are CNS depressed or comatose or have myeloproliferative disorders.

CAUTIONS: Clients with a history of seizures; cardiovascular disease; impaired respiratory, hepatic, or renal function; alcohol withdrawal; urinary retention. Drug has potent anticholinergic effects, and extreme caution is advised for clients with prostatic enlargement or narrow-angle glaucoma. Also use with caution in pregnant or lactating women.

REMARKS: May take two to four weeks for therapeutic effects or as long as three to six months. Since 1–2% of people on clozapine develop agranulocytosis, weekly white blood cell (WBC) counts must be done.

SIDE EFFECTS **FREQUENT:** Sedation, salivation, tachycardia, dizziness, constipation (in order of frequency).

OCCASIONAL: Hypotension or hypertension, gastrointestinal upset, nausea and vomiting, sweating, dry mouth, weight gain.

RARE: Visual disturbances, diarrhea, rash, urinary abnormalities.

ADVERSE REACTIONS **HEMATOLOGIC:** 1–2% of clients develop agranulocytosis; mild leukopenia may develop.

CNS: *Seizures* develop in about 5% of patients on clozaril and up to 15% of patients on dosages over 550 mg/day.
Neuroleptic malignant syndrome (NMS) has been reported when clozapine is used concurrently with lithium or other CNS-active agents.
Other: Dizziness or vertigo, drowsiness, restlessness, akinesia, agitation.

CARDIOVASCULAR: Severe orthostatic hypotension (with or without syncope); marked tachycardia may occur in 25% of clients.

NURSING MEASURES:
1. Check baseline WBC count before initiating treatment.
2. Check weekly WBC count; hold drug if the count falls below 3000 mm^3 and notify physician.
3. Check BP lying and standing to assess for potential orthostatic hypotension.
4. Observe for signs of agranulocytosis (e.g., sore throat, fever, malaise).
5. Make baseline assessment of behavior, appearance, emotional status, response to environment, speech pattern, and thought content.

INFORM CLIENT AND FAMILY:
1. Teach about the side effects and toxic effects of the drug and the need for a weekly WBC count.
2. Avoid the use of over-the-counter medications, alcohol, or CNS medication because of potential and severe drug interactions.
3. Report immediately the appearance of lethargy, weakness, fever, sore throat, malaise, mucous membrane ulceration, or other possible signs of infection.
4. Refrain from operating machinery, driving, and other tasks that require alertness until response to the drug is established.
5. Inform the physician if pregnancy occurs.
6. Do not breast-feed an infant if clozaril is being taken.

APPENDIX B

Self-help Clearinghouses

UNITED STATES

ARIZONA The Rainy Day People Clearinghouse in Scottsdale (closed July, 1991).

CALIFORNIA CALIFORNIA SELF-HELP CENTER UCLA Psychology Department, 405 Hilgard Avenue, Los Angeles, CA 90024.
(800) 222-LINK (in CA only); (213) 825-1799; fax 206-4422 Fran Jemmott Dory, Executive Director.

> **NORTHERN REGION SELF-HELP CENTER— EASTERN DIVISION** Mental Health Association, 8912 Volunteer Lane, Suite 210, Sacramento, CA 95826.
> (916) 368-3100, Ms. Pat Camper, Coordinator.

> **NORTHERN SELF-HELP CENTER—WESTERN DIVISION** Mental Health Association, PO Box 447, Davis, CA 95617.
> (916) 756-8181, Elaine Talley, Coordinator.

> **SOUTHERN REGION SELF-HELP CENTER** Mental Health Association of San Diego, 3958 Third Avenue, San Diego, CA 92103.
> (619) 298-3152, Joe Horton, Coordinator.

> **SHRINE OF THE INLAND EMPIRE** Riverside Mental Health Association, 3763 Arlington Avenue, Suite 103, Riverside, CA 92506.
> (714) 684-6051, Karen Banker, Secretary.

> **CENTRAL REGION SELF-HELF CENTER** Merced County Department of Mental Health, 650 West 19th Street, Merced, CA 95340.
> (209) 725-3752, Mary Jo Burns, Coordinator.

> **SOUTHERN TRI-CITY REGIONAL SELF-HELP CTR** 5839 Green Valley Circle, Suite 100, Culver City, CA 90230.
> (213) 645-9890, Al Jenkins, Coordinator.

> **BAY AREA SELF-HELP CENTER** Mental Health Association, 2398 Pine Street, San Francisco, CA 94115.

(415) 921-4044; fax 921-1911, Duff Axsom, Coordinator.

CONNECTICUT CONNECTICUT SELF-HELP/MUTUAL SUPPORT NETWORK 389 Whitney Avenue, New Haven, CT 06511.
(203) 789-7645, Vicki Spiro Smith, Coordinator; Carol Shaff, Associate Director.

ILLINOIS ILLINOIS SELF-HELP CENTER 1600 Dodge Avenue, Suite S-122, Evanston, IL 60201.
Information and referrals (708) 328-0470; administrative (708) 328-0471, Pat Broughton Marketing Director, Daryl Isenberg, Executive Director.

> **SELF-HELP CENTER** Family Service of Champaign County, 405 South State Street, Champaign, IL 61820.
> (217) 352-0099, Mellen Kennedy, Coordinator.

IOWA IOWA SELF-HELP CLEARINGHOUSE Iowa Piot Parents, Inc., 33 North 12th Street, Fort Dodge, IA 50501.
(515) 576-5870; (800) 383-4777 (from within Iowa only), Carol Reed, Coordinator; Carla Lawson, Director.

KANSAS SELF-HELP NETWORK Campus Box 34, Wichita State University, Wichita, KS 67208-1595.
(800) 445-0116 (in KS only); (316) 689-3843, Greg Meissen, Director; Sherry Greenwood, Assistant.

MASSACHUSETTS MASSACHUSETTS CLEARING-HOUSE OF MUTUAL HELP GROUPS Massachusetts Cooperative Extension, 113 Skinner Hall, University of Massachusetts, Amherst, MA 01003.
(413) 545-2313, Warren Schumacher, Director.

MICHIGAN MICHIGAN SELF-HELP CLEARING-HOUSE Michigan Protection and Advocacy Service, 109 West Michigan Avenue, Suite 900, Lansing, MI 48933.
(517) 484-7373; (800) 752-5858 (in MI only); fax (517) 487-0827 (specify for the Self-help clearinghouse), Ms. Toni Young, Coordinator.

CENTER FOR SELF-HELP (Berrien County area), Riverwood Center, PO Box 547, Benton Harbor, MI 49022.
(616) 925-0594; (800) 336-0341 (in MI only), Pat Friend, Coordinator.

MINNESOTA FIRST CALL FOR HELP (only provides information on existing self-help groups statewide), 166 East 4th Street, Suite 310, St. Paul, MN 55101.
(612) 224-1133; administrative (612) 291-8427, Diane Faulds, Coordinator.

MISSOURI SUPPORT GROUP CLEARINGHOUSE (Kansas City area only), Kansas City Association for Mental Health, 1009 Baltimore, 5th Floor, Kansas City, MO 64105.
(816) 472-HELP, Julie Broyle, Coordinator.

   SELF-HELP CLEARINGHOUSE Greater St. Louis Mental Health Association, 1905 South Grand, St. Louis, MO 63104.
   (314) 773-1399, Peggy Corski, Coordinator.

NEBRASKA SELF-HELP INFORMATION SERVICES 1601 Euclid Avenue, Lincoln, NE 68502.
(402) 476-9668, Barbara Fox, Director.

NEW JERSEY NEW JERSEY SELF-HELP CLEARINGHOUSE St. Clares–Riverside Medical Center, Denville, NJ 07834.
(800) FOR MASH (Mutual Aid Self-help) (in NJ); (201) 625-9565; TDD 625-9053; fax 625-8848, Dennis Jarry, State Program Coordinator; Barbara White, I&R Service Coordinator; Ed Madara, Director.

NEW YORK BROOKLYN SELF-HELP CLEARINGHOUSE 30 Third Avenue, Brooklyn, NY 11217.
(718) 875-1420, Rose Langfelder, Director.

   LONG ISLAND SELF-HELP CLEARINGHOUSE New York Institute of Technology, Central Islip Campus, Central Islip, NY 11722.
   (516) 348-3030, Ms. Pat Verdino, Director.

   NEW YORK CITY SELF-HELP CLEARINGHOUSE, INC. (closed in 1990).

   NEW YORK STATE SELF-HELP CLEARINGHOUSE (closed May 1991), Richardson Hall, SUNY School of Social Welfare, 135 Western Avenue, Albany, NY 12222.
   (518) 442-5845 administrative.

   WESTCHESTER SELF-HELP CLEARINGHOUSE 456 North Street, White Plains, NY 10605.
   (914) 949-6301, Leslie Borck Jameson, Director; Lenore Rosenbaum, Coordinator.

   Note: Maintains a listing of additional local county self-help clearinghouses in upstate New York area.

NORTH CAROLINA SUPPORTWORKS (serving greater Mecklenberg area), 1012 Kings Drive, Suite 923, Charlotte NC 28283.
(704) 331-9500, Joal Fischer, Director.

OHIO GREATER DAYTON SELF-HELP CLEARINGHOUSE (Dayton area only), Family Services Association, 184 Salem Avenue, Dayton, OH 45406.
(513) 225-3004, Shari Peace, Coordinator.

OREGON NORTHWEST REGIONAL SELF-HELP CLEARINGHOUSE (includes Seattle, WA area), 718 West Burnside Street, Portland, OR 97209.
(503) 222-5555 I&R (503) 226-9360 administrative, Judy Hadley, Coordinator.

PENNSYLVANIA SELF-HELP GROUP NETWORK OF THE PITTSBURGH AREA 1323 Forbes Avenue, Suite 200, Pittsburgh, PA 15219.
(412) 261-5363, Betty Hepner, Coordinator.

   SHINE (SELF-HELP INFORMATION NETWORK EXCHANGE) c/o Voluntary Action Center, 225 North Washington Avenue, Park Plaza, Lower Level, Scranton, PA 18503.
   (717) 961-1234, Gail Bauer, Director.

   SELF-HELP INSTITUTE (clearinghouse services being developed), 462 Monastery Avenue, Philadelphia, PA 19128.
   (215) 482-4316, Gwen Olitsky, Contact Person.

RHODE ISLAND (The Support Group Helpline at the RI State Department of Health closed January 1992.)

SOUTH CAROLINA MIDLAND AREA SUPPORT GROUP NETWORK Lexington Medical Center, 2720 Sunset Boulevard, West Columbia, SC 29169.
(803) 791-9227 I&R; 791-2049 administrative, Nancy T. Farrar, Director.

TENNESSEE SUPPORT GROUP CLEARINGHOUSE Mental Health Association of Knox County, 6712 Kingston Pike, No. 203, Knoxville, TN 37919.
(615) 584-6736, Judy Balloff, Program Coordinator.

   SELF-HELP CLEARINGHOUSE Mental Health Association of Memphis, 2400 Poplar, Suite 410, Memphis, TN 38112.
   (901) 323-0633, Carol Barnett, Coordinator.

TEXAS TEXAS SELF-HELP CLEARINGHOUSE Mental Health Association in Texas, 8401 Shoal Creek Boulevard, Austin, TX 78758-7544.
(512) 454-3706, Christine Devall, Coordinator.

   SELF-HELP CLEARINGHOUSE Mental Health Association in Houston and Harris County, 2211 Norfolk, Suite 810, Houston, TX 77098.
   (713) 523-8963, Dianne Long, Coordinator.

TARRANT COUNTY SELF-HELP CLEARING-HOUSE Mental Health Association of Tarrant County, 3136 West 4th Street, Fort Worth, TX 76107-2113.
(817) 335-5405, Joyce Bishop, Coordinator.

DALLAS SELF-HELP CLEARINGHOUSE Mental Health Association of Dallas County, 2929 Carlisle, Suite 350, Dallas, TX 75204.
(214) 871-2420, Carol Madison, Director.

GREATER SAN ANTONIO SELF-HELP CLEAR-INGHOUSE Mental Health in Greater San Antonio, 901 NE Loop 410, Suite 500, San Antonio, TX 78209.
(512) 826-2288.

WASHINGTON, DC SELF-HELP CLEARINGHOUSE OF GREATER WASHINGTON (Washington, DC, northern Virginia, and southern Maryland), Mental Health Association of Northern Virginia, 7630 Little River Turnpike, Suite 206, Annandale, VA 22003.
(703) 941-LINK, Lisa Saisselin, Coordinator.

NATIONAL INFORMATION AND DIRECTORIES—UNITED STATES

AMERICAN SELF-HELP CLEARINGHOUSE Saint Clares–Riverside Medical Center, Denville, NJ 07834.
(201) 625-7101; TDD (201) 625-9053; fax (201) 625-8848, Edward J. Madara, Director.

NATIONAL SELF-HELP CLEARINGHOUSE Graduate School and University Center, CUNY, Room 620, 25 West 43rd Street, New York, NY 10036.
(212) 642-2944, Frank Riessman, Director.

CANADA

CANADIAN COUNCIL ON SOCIAL DEVELOPMENT Conseil Canadien de Developpment Social, PO Box 3505, Station C, Ottawa, Ontario, Canada K1Y 4G1.
(613) 728-1865; fax 728-9387, Hector Balthazar.

FAMILY LIFE EDUCATION COUNCIL 233 12th Avenue SW, Calgary, Alberta, Canada T2R OG9.
(403) 262-1117, Sonia Eisler, Executive Director.

CAMAC—CENTRE D'AIDE MUTUELLE, INC. (inactive at this time), Montreal, Quebec.

THE SELF-HELP CONNECTION Mental Health Association, 1496 Lower Water Street, Halifax, Nova Scotia, Canada B3J 2R7.
(902) 422-5831, Linda Bayers, Director.

SELF-HELP DEVELOPMENT UNIT (temporarily closed), for now direct mail
c/o Sharon Miller
10 Porteouf Crescent, Saskatoon, Saskatchewan, Canada S7J 2S8.
(306) 966-5580 administrative only, ask for Sharon.

SELF-HELP CLEARINGHOUSE OF METROPOLITAN TORONTO 40 Orchard View Boulevard, Suite 215, Toronto, Ontario, Canada M4R 1B9.
(416) 487-4355, Randi Fine, Director.

SELF-HELP COLLABORATION PROJECT United Way of the Lower Mainland, 1625 West 8th Avenue, Vancouver, British Columbia, Canada V6J 1T9.
(604) 731-7781, Rae Folster, Contact Person.

WINNIPEG SELF-HELP RESOURCE CLEARING-HOUSE NorWest Coop and Health Center, 103–61 Tyndall Avenue, Winnipeg, Manitoba, Canada R2X 2T4.
(204) 589-5500 or 633-5955, Bernice Marmel, Director.

INTERNATIONAL INFORMATION CENTRE ON SELF-HELP AND HEALTH

E. Van Evenstraat 2C, B-3000 Leuven, Belgium.
Telephone 30-891-4019, Peter Gielen, Coordinator.

AUSTRALIA WESTERN INSTITUTE OF SELF-HELP 80 Railway Street, Cottesloe, 6011, Western Australia.
Telephone (09) 383-3188, Cheryl A. Dimmack, Contact Person.

THE COLLECTIVE OF SELF-HELP GROUPS PO Box 159, East Brunswick 3057, 155 Lygon Street, Brunswick, Australia.
Telephone (03) 388-1777.

AUSTRIA SERVICESTELLE FÜR SELBSTHILFE-GRUPPEN Schottenring—24/3/31, 1010 Vienna, Austria.
Telephone 222-66-14405, Ilse Forster, Director.

BELGIUM TREFPUNT ZELF HULP E. Van Evenstraat 2C, B:3000 Leuven, Belgium, Linda Verwimp, Director.

DENMARK LAIKOS—National, Tordenjkjoldsvei 20, 3000 Helsinor, Denmark, Ulla-Britta Buch, Coordinator.

SR—BISTAND Social Radgivning og Bistand, Sortedam Dosseringen 3, st. th., 2200 Kobenhavn N, Denmark.
Telephone 31-31-71-97, Birthe Gamst, Director; Ann Gamst, Coordinator.

SELVJHAELPS-GRUPPER CENTRE IN KOLDING Vesterskovog 19, 6091 Bjest, Denmark, Lisbeth Bonde Petersen, Director.

ENGLAND NATIONAL SELF-HELP SUPPORT CENTRE National Council for Voluntary Organizations, 26 Bedford Square, London WC1B 3HU, England.
Telephone 01-636-4066, Ms. Katrina McCormick, Director.

THE SELF-HELP TEAM 20 Pelham Road, Nottingham NG5 1AP, England.
Telephone 44-0602-691212, Judy Wilson, Team Leader.

THE SELF-HELP ALLIANCE Lower King's Road 29, Berkhamsted, Herbs HP 4 2AB, England.

THE SELF-HELP GROUP PROJECT Leicester Council for Voluntary Services, De Montfort Street 32, Leicester LEI 7GD, England.
Telephone 0533-55-56.

HELP FOR HEALTH PROJECT Wessex Regional Library Unit, South Academic Bloc, Southampton General Hospital, Southampton SO9 4XY, England.
Telephone 703-77-90-91.

GERMANY (has over 100 clearinghouses; a few are given after the national clearinghouse).

NATIONALE KONTAKT UND INFORMATIONSSTELLE ZUR ANREGUNG UND UNTERSTUTZUNG VON SELBSTHILFEGRUPPEN (NAKOS) Albrecht-Achilles-Strasse 65, 1000 Berlin 31, Germany.
Telephone 30-891-4019, Klaus Balke, Director.

DEUTSCHE ARBEITSGEMEINSCHAFT SELBST-HILFEGRUPPEN e.V. (DAG SHG) c/o Friedrichstrasse 28, 6300 Giessen, Germany.
Telephone 641-702-2478, Jurgen Matzat, Contact Person.

KONTAKT UND INFORMATIONSSTELLE FÜR SELBSTHILFEGRUPPEN (KISS) Gaubstrasse 21, 2000 Hamburg 50, Germany.
Telephone 40-390-57-67 or 40-390-99-98.

LÄNDESARBEITSGEMEINSCHAFT Regierungsprasidium Chemnitz, PF 848, Zwickaub Strasse 38, 9001 Chemnitz, Germany, Jurgen Dudeck.

MUNICH SELF-HELP RESOURCE CENTER Bayerstrasse 77A, 8000 München 2, Germany, Wolfgang Stark, Director.

HUNGARY NATIONAL COMMITTEE OF MENTAL HEALTH PROMOTION PO Box 39, 1525 Budapest, Hungary, Bela Buda, Coordinator.

ISRAEL NATIONAL SELF-HELP CLEARINGHOUSE 37 King George Street, PO Box 23223, Tel-Aviv 61231, Israel.
Telephone 03-299389, Martha Ramon, Director.

JAPAN SOCIETY FOR THE STUDY OF SELF-HELP GROUPS Department of Social Welfare, Faculty of Humanities, Sophia University, 7-1, Kioicho, Chiyoda-ku, Tokyo 102, Japan, Office 011-81-03-3238-3645; fax/voice line 011-81-297-72-3118, Tomofumi Oka, Director.

POLAND NATIONAL CENTRE FOR HEALTH SYSTEM MANAGEMENT Dluga 38/40, 00-238 Warszawa, Poland, Elzbieta Bobiatynska, Coordinator.

SPAIN INSTITUT MUNICIPAL DE LA SALUT Pa. Lesseps, 1, 08023 Barcelona, Spain, Francina Roca, Coordinator.

PROGRAMME 'CRONICAT' Facultad de Medicina (Despacho 15), Hospital de San Pablo, Padre Claret 167, Barcelona 08026, Spain.
Telephone 93-256-3612, Elvira Mendez, Director.

SWEDEN DISTRIKTLAKARE Villavagan 14, 9390 Arjeplog, Sweden.
Telephone 961-11230, Bo Henricson, M.D., Contact Person.

SWITZERLAND SELBSTHILFEZENTRUM HINDER-HUUS Feldbergstrasse 55, 4057 Basel, Switzerland, Verena Vogelsanger.

TEAM SELBSTHILLFE ZURICH Wilfiedstrasse 7, 8032 Zurich, Switzerland.
Telephone 01-252-3036, Midi Muheim, Contact Person.

YUGOSLAVIA COLLEGE OF NURSING University of Zagreb, Mlinarska 38, 41000 Zagreb, Yugoslavia.
Telephone (050) 28-666, Arpad Barath, Contact Person.

OTHER RESOURCES

RESOURCES FOR RARE DISORDERS The most important organization that can be counted on to be the most helpful in providing you with information on what agencies, networks, and resources already exist for rare disorders is **NORD—National Organization for Rare Disorders, Inc.** Call them toll-free at (800) 999-NORD or (203) 746-6518, or write to PO Box 8923, New Fairfield, CT 06812. Begun as an informal coalition of national voluntary health agencies, NORD now provides information (to include a computer-accessible database through CompuServe), referral, and advocacy for orphan illness research. Most importantly, NORD provides a "networking program" service, linking together persons or families with the same disorder.

National Information Center for Orphan Drugs and Rare Diseases of the National Health Information Clearinghouse is another resource that responds to questions on rare disorders using the NHIC's computer database and library. Call them at (800) 456-3505 (toll-free in US) or (301) 565-4167, or write to NICODARD, PO Box 1133, Washington, DC 20013-1133.

RESOURCES FOR GENETIC DISORDERS The Alliance of Genetic Support Groups, Suite 800, 1001 22nd Street, NW, Washington, DC 20037, phone (800) 336-GENE or (202) 331-0942. The alliance is a partnership of self-help groups and professionals addressing communication, service delivery, and advocacy issues for member support groups that are composed of individuals and families affected by genetic disorders. The alliance seeks to sponsor special projects and publishes a newsletter.

The National Center for Education in Maternal and Child Health, 38th & R streets, NW, Washington, DC 20057, phone (202) 625-8400, was formerly the National Clearinghouse for Human Genetic Diseases. They continue to provide information on genetic disorders and resources, and among the publications available from them is one focused on how to start a self-help group for a genetic illness, *Learning Together: A Guide for Families with Genetic Disorders.*

The March of Dimes Birth Defects Foundation, 1275 Mamaroneck Avenue, White Plains, NY 10605, phone (914) 428-7100, provides information and publications that deal with all types of birth defects, including many genetic disorders. One of their publications is the *Guide for Organizing Parent Support Groups.*

The National Easter Seal Society, 2023 West Ogden Avenue, Chicago, IL 60612, phone (312) 243-8400, publishes information on all types of physical disabilities, including genetic disorders. Consider contacting them for a copy of their publication list.

RESOURCES FOR MENTAL HEALTH CONSUMERS

In addition to the national self-help groups previously cited, there is a national technical assistance center:

The National Mental Health Consumer Self-help Clearinghouse
311 South Juniper Street, Room 902, Philadelphia, PA 19107 (215) 735-2481

Funded by the National Institute of Mental Health's Community Support Program, the purpose of the clearinghouse is to encourage the development of consumer self-help groups. This is done by providing individuals and groups with information, materials, help, and referrals for a wide range of technical assistance issues, from fundraising to the development of consumer-run drop-in centers.

OTHER SELF-HELP RESOURCES

National Council on Self-Help and Public Health
310 Maple Avenue West, Suite 182, Vienna, VA 22180. Howard E. Stone, Chairperson.
The council works to implement recommendations from the Surgeon General's Workshop on Self-help and Public Health, which was held in 1987. The project has developed a national network of researchers examining and working with self-help groups.

Interest Group on Self-Help and Mutual Support
This organization is part of the Society for Community Research and Action (Division 27), American Psychological Association. It is a network of different professionals who share information on research work and interests and action projects. For more information, write to Greg Meissen, Department of Psychology, Wichita State University, Wichita, KS 67208.

SHALL—The Self-Help ALLiance
The Self-help Alliance is a developing national coalition of self-help groups with purposes of mutual support, education, and empowerment for self-help groups. For example, in coordination with the National Network for Mutual Help Centers, the Alliance is initially planning to use a portion of the Network's newsletter for self-help groups to share news, ideas, problems, and insights. To aid in alliance efforts, or for information, write to Ms. Lee Miller, Apartment C-41, 68-37 Yellowstone Boulevard, Forest Hills, NY 11375.

National Network for Mutual Help Centers
(an association of self-help clearinghouses in the US) Contact **Toni Young**, President, at Michigan Self-help Clearinghouse, listed earlier.

International Network for Mutual Help Centers
(an association of self-help clearinghouses in the US and Canada) Contact Lori Dessau, Chairperson, 2 Mount Royal Avenue, Hamilton, Ontario, Canada L8P 4H6, (416) 529-3480.

From Madara EJ: How to ideas. In Madara EJ, Meese A (eds). The Self-help Sourcebook: Finding and Forming Mutual Aid, 2nd ed. Denville, NJ: Self-help Clearinghouse, 1992. Reprinted with permission from the author, the NJ Self-help Clearinghouse, St. Clares–Riverside Medical Center, Denville, NJ.

Please note: This directory listing is an update of one we first started distributing in 1981. It includes all the general clearinghouse operations and associations that we know of at this time. Please advise us of any new clearinghouses that come to your attention.

APPENDIX C

Reporting Procedures for State Child Protection Agencies*

Because the responsibility for investigating reports of suspected child abuse and neglect rests at the state level, each state has established a child protective services (CPS) reporting system. Listed below are the name and address of the CPS agency in each state, followed by the procedures for reporting suspected child maltreatment. A number of states have toll-free (800) telephone numbers that can be used for reporting. Some states have two numbers, one for individuals calling within the state and the other for those calling outside of the state. Normal business hours vary from agency to agency but are typically from 8 or 9 A.M. to 4:30 or 5 P.M.

Alabama ALABAMA DEPARTMENT OF HUMAN RESOURCES Division of Family and Children's Services, Office of Protective Services, 50 Ripley Street, Montgomery, AL 36130-1801.
During business hours, make reports to the County Department of Human Resources, Child Protective Services Unit. After business hours, make reports to local police.

Alaska DEPARTMENT OF HEALTH AND SOCIAL SERVICES Division of Family and Youth Services, Box H-05, Juneau, AK 99811.
Make reports in state to (800) 478-4444. Out of state, use area code 907. This telephone number is toll-free.

American Samoa DEPARTMENT OF HUMAN RESOURCES Director of Human Resources, American Samoa Government, Pago Pago, AS 96799.

Arizona DEPARTMENT OF ECONOMIC SECURITY Administration for Children, Youth and Families, PO Box 6123, Site COE 940A, Phoenix, AZ 85005.
Make reports to Department of Economic Security local offices.

Arkansas ARKANSAS DEPARTMENT OF HUMAN SERVICES Division of Children and Family Services, PO Box 1437, Little Rock, AR 72203.
Make reports in state to (800) 482-5964.

California
Make reports to county departments of welfare or law enforcement agency.

Colorado DEPARTMENT OF SOCIAL SERVICES AND CHILD WELFARE SERVICES 225 East 16th Street, Denver, CO 80203-1702
Make reports to county departments of social services.

Connecticut CONNECTICUT DEPARTMENT OF CHILDREN AND YOUTH SERVICES Division of Children and Protective Services, 170 Sigourney Street, Hartford, CT 06105.
Make reports in state to (800) 842-2288 or out of state to (203) 344-2599.

Delaware DELAWARE DEPARTMENT OF SERVICES FOR CHILDREN, YOUTH AND THEIR FAMILIES Division of Child Protective Services, 1825 Faulkland Road, Wilmington, DE 19802.
Make reports in state to (800) 292-9582.

District of Columbia DISTRICT OF COLUMBIA DEPARTMENT OF HUMAN SERVICES Commission on Social Services, Family Services Administration, Child and Family Services Division, 609 H Street, NE, Washington, DC 20001.
Make reports to (202) 727-0995.

Florida FLORIDA PROTECTIVE SERVICE SYSTEM 2729 Fort Knox Boulevard, Tallahassee, FL 32308.
Make reports in state to (800) 342-9152 or out of state to (904) 487-2625.

* From Public Health Service. Child Abuse and Neglect: A Shared Community Concern. Washington, DC: Department of Health and Human Services, 1992.

Georgia **GEORGIA DEPARTMENT OF HUMAN RESOURCES** Division of Family and Children Services, 878 Peachtree Street, NW, Room 502, Atlanta, GA 30309.
Make reports to county departments of family and children services.

Guam **DEPARTMENT OF PUBLIC HEALTH AND SOCIAL SERVICES** Child Welfare Services, Child Protective Services, PO Box 2816, Agana, GU 96910.
Make reports to the State Child Protective Services Agency at (671) 646-8417.

Hawaii **DEPARTMENT OF HUMAN SERVICES** Public Welfare Division, Family and Adult Services, PO Box 339, Honolulu, HI 96809
Make reports to each island's Department of Human Services CPS reporting hotline.

Idaho **DEPARTMENT OF HEALTH AND WELFARE** Field Operations Bureau of Social Services and Child Protection, 450 West State Street, Boise, ID 83720.
Make reports to Department of Health and Welfare regional offices.

Illinois **ILLINOIS DEPARTMENT OF CHILDREN AND FAMILY SERVICES** Station 75, State Administrative Offices, 406 East Monroe Street, Springfield, IL 62701.
Make reports in state to (800) 25-ABUSE or out of state to (217) 785-4010.

Indiana **INDIANA DEPARTMENT OF PUBLIC WELFARE—CHILD ABUSE AND NEGLECT** Children and Families Division, 402 West Washington Street, Room W-364, Indianapolis, IN 46204.
Make reports to county departments of public welfare.

Iowa **IOWA DEPARTMENT OF HUMAN SERVICES** Bureau of Adult, Children and Family Services, Central Child Abuse Registry, Hoover State Office Building, Fifth Floor, Des Moines, IA 50319.
Make reports in state to (800) 362-2178. Make reports out of state to (515) 281-5581 during business hours and to (515) 281-3240 after business hours.

Kansas **KANSAS DEPARTMENT OF SOCIAL AND REHABILITATION SERVICES** Division of Social Services, Child Protection and Family Services Section, Smith-Wilson Building, 300 SW Oakley Street, Topeka, KS 66606.
Make reports to Department of Social and Rehabilitation services area offices and in state to (800) 922-5330.

Kentucky **KENTUCKY CABINET OF HUMAN RESOURCES** Division of Family Services, Children and Youth Services Branch, 275 East Main Street, Frankfort, KY 40621.
Make reports to county offices in 14 state districts.

Louisiana **LOUISIANA DEPARTMENT OF SOCIAL SERVICES** Office of Community Services, PO Box 3318, Baton Rouge, LA 70821.
Make reports to parish protective service units.

Maine **MAINE DEPARTMENT OF HUMAN SERVICES** Child Protective Services, State House, Station 11, Augusta, ME 04333.
Make reports to Regional Office of Human Services; in state to (800) 452-1999 or out of state to (207) 289-2983. Both lines operate 24 hours a day.

Maryland **MARYLAND DEPARTMENT OF HUMAN RESOURCES** Social Services Administration, Saratoga State Center, 311 West Saratoga Street, Baltimore, MD 21201.
Make reports to county departments of social services or to local law enforcement agencies.

Massachusetts **MASSACHUSETTS DEPARTMENT OF SOCIAL SERVICES** Protective Services, 24 Farnsworth Street, Boston, MA 02210.
Make reports to area offices or Protective Screening Unit or interstate to (800) 792-5200.

Michigan **MICHIGAN DEPARTMENT OF SOCIAL SERVICES** PO Box 30037, 235 South Grand Avenue, Suite 412, Lansing, MI 48909.
Make reports to county departments of social services.

Minnesota **MINNESOTA DEPARTMENT OF HUMAN SERVICES** Children's Services Division, Human Services Building, St. Paul, MN 55155.
Make reports to county departments of human services.

Mississippi **MISSISSIPPI DEPARTMENT OF HUMAN SERVICES** Office of Social Services Protection Department, PO Box 352, Jackson, MS 39205.
Make reports in state to (800) 222-8000 or out of state (during business hours) to (601) 354-0341.

Missouri **MISSOURI CHILD ABUSE AND NEGLECT HOTLINE** Department of Social Service, Division of Family Services, PO Box 88, Broadway Building, Jefferson City, MO 65103.
Make reports in state to (800) 392-3738 or out of state to (314) 751-3448. Both lines operate 24 hours a day.

Montana **DEPARTMENT OF FAMILY SERVICES** Child Protective Services, PO Box 8005, Helena, MT 59604.
Make reports to county departments of family services.

Nebraska **NEBRASKA DEPARTMENT OF SOCIAL SERVICES** Human Services Division, 301 Centennial Mall South, PO Box 95026, Lincoln, NE 68509.
Make reports to local law enforcement agencies or to

local social services offices, or in state to (800) 652-1999.

Nevada DEPARTMENT OF HUMAN RESOURCES WELFARE DIVISION 2527 North Carson Street, Carson City, NV 89710.
Make reports to Welfare Division local offices.

New Hampshire NEW HAMPSHIRE DIVISION FOR CHILDREN AND YOUTH SERVICES 6 Hazen Drive, Concord, NH 03301-6522.
Make reports to Division for Children and Youth Services district offices or in state to (800) 852-3345 (extension 4455).

New Jersey NEW JERSEY DIVISION OF YOUTH AND FAMILY SERVICES Department of Human Services (CN717), 50 East State Street, Sixth Floor, Trenton, NJ 08625.
Make reports in state to (800) 792-8610. District offices also provide 24-hour telephone services.

New Mexico NEW MEXICO HUMAN SERVICES DEPARTMENT Children's Bureau, Pollon Plaza, PO Box 2348, Santa Fe, NM 87503-2348.
Make reports to county social services offices or in state to (800) 432-6217.

New York NEW YORK STATE DEPARTMENT OF SOCIAL SERVICES Division of Family and Children Services, State Central Register of Child Abuse and Maltreatment, 40 North Pearl Street, Albany, NY 12243.
Make reports in state to (800) 342-3720 or out of state to (518) 474-9448.

North Carolina NORTH CAROLINA DEPARTMENT OF HUMAN RESOURCES Division of Social Services, Child Protective Services, 325 North Salisbury Street, Raleigh, NC 27603.
Make reports in state to (800) 662-7030.

North Dakota NORTH DAKOTA DEPARTMENT OF HUMAN SERVICES Division of Children and Family Services, Child Abuse and Neglect Program, 600 East Boulevard, Bismarck, ND 58505.
Make reports to county social services offices.

Ohio OHIO DEPARTMENT OF HUMAN SERVICES Bureau of Children's Protective Services, 30 East Broad Street, Columbus, OH 43266-0423.
Make reports to county departments of human services.

Oklahoma OKLAHOMA DEPARTMENT OF HUMAN SERVICES Division of Children and Youth Services, Child Abuse/Neglect Section, PO Box 25352, Oklahoma City, OK 73125.
Make reports in state to (800) 522-3511.

Oregon DEPARTMENT OF HUMAN RESOURCES Children's Services Division, Child Protective Services, 198 Commercial Street, SE, Salem, OR 97310.
Make reports to local Children's Services Division offices and to (503) 378-4722.

Pennsylvania PENNSYLVANIA DEPARTMENT OF PUBLIC WELFARE Office of Children, Youth and Families, Child Line and Abuse Registry, Lanco Lodge, PO Box 2675, Harrisburg, PA 17105.
Make reports in state to CHILDLINE (800) 932-0313 or out of state to (713) 783-8744.

Puerto Rico PUERTO RICO DEPARTMENT OF SOCIAL SERVICES Services to Family With Children, PO Box 11398, Santurci, PR 00910.
Make reports to (809) 724-1333.

Rhode Island RHODE ISLAND DEPARTMENT FOR CHILDREN AND THEIR FAMILIES Division of Child Protective Services, 610 Mt. Pleasant Avenue, Building no. 9, Providence, RI 02908.
Make reports in state to (800) RI-CHILD or 742-4453, or out of state to (401) 457-4996.

South Carolina SOUTH CAROLINA DEPARTMENT OF SOCIAL SERVICES 1535 Confederate Avenue, PO Box 1520, Columbia, SC 29202-1520.
Make reports to county departments of social services.

South Dakota DEPARTMENT OF SOCIAL SERVICES CHILD PROTECTION SERVICES Kneip Building, 700 Governors Drive, Pierre, SD 57501.
Make reports to local social services offices.

Tennessee TENNESSEE DEPARTMENT OF HUMAN SERVICES Child Protective Services, Citizen Bank Plaza, 400 Deadrick Street, Nashville, TN 37248.
Make reports to county departments of human services.

Texas TEXAS DEPARTMENT OF HUMAN SERVICES Protective Services for Families and Children Branch, PO Box 149030, MC-E-206, Austin, TX 78714-9030.
Make reports in state to (800) 252-5400 or out of state to (512) 450-3360.

Utah DEPARTMENT OF SOCIAL SERVICES Division of Family Services, 120 North 200 West, Salt Lake City, UT 84145-0500.
Make reports to Division of Family Services district offices.

Vermont VERMONT DEPARTMENT OF SOCIAL AND REHABILITATIVE SERVICES Division of Social Services, 103 South Main Street, Waterbury, VT 05676.
Make reports to district offices or to (802) 241-2131.

Virgin Islands DIVISION OF CHILDREN, YOUTH AND FAMILIES DEPARTMENT OF HUMAN SER-

VICES Government of the Virgin Islands, Barbel Plaza South, Charlotte Amalie, St. Thomas, VI 00802.

Make reports to Division of Social Services at (809) 773-2323.

Virginia COMMONWEALTH OF VIRGINIA DEPARTMENT OF SOCIAL SERVICES Bureau of Child Protective Services, Blair Building, 8007 Discovery Drive, Richmond, VA 23229-8699.

Make reports in state to (800) 552-7096 or out of state to (804) 662-9084.

Washington DEPARTMENT OF SOCIAL AND HEALTH SERVICES Division of Children and Family Services, Child Protective Services, Mail Stop OB 41-D, Olympia, WA 98504.

Make reports in state to (800) 562-5624 or to local social and health services offices.

West Virginia WEST VIRGINIA DEPARTMENT OF HUMAN SERVICES Office of Social Services, Building 6, Room 850, State Capitol Complex, Charleston, WV 25305.

Make reports in state to (800) 352-6513.

Wisconsin WISCONSIN DEPARTMENT OF HEALTH AND SOCIAL SERVICES Department of Health and Social Services, Bureau for Children, Youth, and Families, 1 West Wilson Street, PO Box 7851, Madison, WI 53707.

Make reports to county social services offices.

Wyoming DEPARTMENT OF FAMILY SERVICES Hathaway Building, No. 322, Cheyenne, WY 82002.

Make reports to county departments of public assistance and social services.

G*lossary*

Abstract thinking The ability to conceptualize ideas (e.g., finding meaning in proverbs).

Abuse An act of misuse, deceit, or exploitation; wrong or improper use or action toward another, resulting in injury, damage, maltreatment, or corruption.

Accommodation The ability to change one's way of thinking in order to introduce new ideas, objects, or experiences.

Acrophobia Fear of high places.

Acting-out behaviors Behaviors that originate on an unconscious level to reduce anxiety and tension. Anxiety is displaced from one situation to another in the form of observable behavioral responses (e.g., anger, crying, or violence).

Activities of daily living For a person with a chronic mental illness, this term refers to the skills necessary to live independently as an adult.

Acute anxiety Anxiety that is precipitated by an imminent loss or a change that threatens an individual's sense of security.

Addiction Addiction incorporates the concepts of loss of control with respect to use of a drug (e.g., alcohol), taking the drug despite related problems, and a tendency to relapse. *Addiction* is an older term that has been replaced by the term *drug dependence.*

Adult Children of Alcoholics (ACOA) A support group for adult children of alcoholics, who often experience similar difficulties and problems in their adult lives as a result of having an alcoholic parent or parents.

Adventitious crises Crises that are not part of everyday life; they are unplanned and accidental. They include natural disasters, national disasters, and crimes of violence such as rapes or muggings.

Affect An objective manifestation of an experience of emotion accompanying an idea or feeling. The observations one would make on assessment. For example, a client may be said to have a flat affect, meaning that there is an absence or a near absence of facial expression. Some people, however, use the term loosely to mean a feeling, emotion, or mood.

Ageism A system of destructive, erroneous beliefs about the elderly; defined as a bias against older people based solely on their age.

Aggression Any verbal or nonverbal, actual or attempted, forceful abuse of the self on another person or object.

Agnosia Loss of the ability to recognize familiar objects. For example, a person may be unable to identify familiar sounds, such as the ringing of a doorbell (auditory agnosia), or familiar objects, such as a toothbrush or keys (visual agnosia).

Agoraphobia The most serious and the most common phobia for which people seek treatment. It is fear and avoidance of being alone or being in open spaces from which escape might be difficult. At its most severe, a person with agoraphobia may not be able to leave his or her own home.

Agraphia Loss of a previous ability to write, resulting from brain injury or brain disease.

Akathisia Regular rhythmic movements, usually of the lower limbs; constant pacing may also be seen; often noticed in people taking antipsychotic medication.

Akinesia Absence or diminution of voluntary motion. Akinesia is usually accompanied by a parallel reduction in mental activity.

Al-a-Teen A nationwide network for children over 10 years of age who have alcoholic parents.

Al-Anon A support group for spouses and friends of alcoholics.

Alcohol withdrawal delirium An organic mental disorder that occurs 40–48 hours after cessation or reduction of long term heavy alcohol intake and that is considered a medical emergency; often referred to by the older term *delirium tremens* (DTs).

901

Alcoholic hallucinations Auditory hallucinations reported to occur approximately 48 hours after heavy drinking by alcohol-dependent clients.

Alcoholics Anonymous (AA) A self-help group of recovering alcoholics that provides support and encouragement to those involved in continuing recovery.

Alcoholism The end stage of the continuum that includes addiction to and dependence on the drug alcohol.

Alliance for the Mentally Ill A national support group for families of the mentally ill, with many local and state affiliates; provides educational programs and political action.

Alzheimer's disease A primary cognitive impairment disorder characterized by progressive deterioration of cognitive functioning, with the end result that a person may not recognize once-familiar people, places, and things. The ability to walk and talk is absent in the final stages.

Ambivalence The holding, at the same time, of two opposing emotions, attitudes, ideas, or wishes toward the same person, situation, or object.

Amnesia Loss of memory for events within a specific period of time; may be temporary or permanent.

Anergia Lack of energy; passivity.

Anhedonia The inability to experience pleasure.

Anorexia A medical term that signifies a loss of appetite. A person with *anorexia nervosa*, however, may not have any loss of appetite and often is preoccupied with food and eating. A person with this condition may suppress the desire for food in order to control his or her eating.

Antabuse (disulfiram) A drug given to alcoholics that produces nausea, vomiting, dizziness, flushing, and tachycardia if alcohol is consumed.

Anticholinergic side effects Side effects caused by the use of some medications, e.g., neuroleptics, tricyclics. Symptoms include dry mouth, constipation, urinary retention, blurred vision, and dry mucous membranes.

Anticipatory grief Grief that occurs before an actual loss. During this time, painful feelings may be partially resolved.

Antidepressants Drugs predominantly used to elevate mood in people who are depressed.

Antimanic drugs Drugs used in the treatment of a manic state to lower an elevated and unstable mood and to reduce irritability and aggressiveness.

Antipsychotic drugs (neuroleptics, major tranquilizers) Drugs that have the ability to decrease psychotic, paranoid, and disorganized thinking and positively alter bizarre behaviors; thought to reduce the effects of the neurotransmitter dopamine by blocking the dopamine receptors.

Antisocial (sociopath, psychopath) These terms are often used interchangeably to refer to a syndrome in which a person lacks the capacity to relate to others. These people do not experience discomfort in inflicting or observing pain in others, and they constantly manipulate others for personal gain. Common behaviors seen in people with this disorder include crimes against society, aggressiveness, inability to feel remorse, untruthfulness and insincerity, unreliability, failure to follow any life plan, and others.

Anxiety A state of feeling apprehension, uneasiness, uncertainty, or dread resulting from a real or perceived threat whose actual source is unknown or unrecognized.

Anxiolytics (antianxiety drugs, minor tranquilizers) Drugs prescribed usually on a short term basis to reduce anxiety.

Apathy A state of indifference.

Aphasia Difficulty in the formulation of words; loss of language ability. In extreme cases, a person may be limited to a few words, may babble, or may become mute.

Apraxia Loss of purposeful motor movements. For example, a person may be unable to shave, to dress, or to do other once-familiar and purposeful tasks.

Aristotle (384–322 B.C.) A philosopher and physician who made significant contributions in the area of clinical observation; observed a continuum in psychological reactions from normal to pathological behaviors.

Asclepiades (around 100 B.C.) Known as the Father of Psychiatry, he was a pioneer in humane treatment methods. He prescribed occupational therapy and introduced music therapy for mentally ill patients.

Assault An intentional act that is designed to make the victim fearful and that produces reasonable apprehension of harm.

Assertiveness Asking for what one wants or acting to get what one wants in a way that respects the rights and feelings of other people.

Assimilation The ability to incorporate new ideas, objects, and experiences into the framework of one's thoughts.

Associative looseness Disturbance of thinking in which ideas shift from one subject to another in an oblique or unrelated manner. When this condition is severe, speech may be incoherent.

Attention deficit disorder A behavioral disorder usually manifested before the age of seven that includes overactivity, chronic inattention, and difficulty dealing with multiple stimuli.

Autistic thinking Thoughts, ideas, or desires derived from internal, private stimuli or perceptions that often are incongruent with reality.

Automatic obedience The performance of all simple commands in a robot-like fashion; may be present in catatonia.

Battery The harmful or offensive touching of another's person.

Behavioral modification A treatment modality that focuses on modifying and changing specific observable dysfunctional patterns of behavior by means of stimulus-and-response conditioning. Examples of behavioral therapy techniques include operant conditioning, token economy, systematic desensitization, aversion therapy, and flooding.

Benjamin Rush The Father of American Psychiatry; wrote the first American textbook of psychiatry in 1812.

Binge-purge cycle An episodic, uncontrolled, rapid ingestion of large quantities of food over a short period of time, often followed by "purging" (vomiting); a characteristic seen in people with bulimia nervosa.

Biofeedback A technique for gaining conscious control over unconscious body functions, such as blood pressure and heartbeat, to achieve relaxation or the relief of stress-related physical symptoms; involves the use of self-monitoring equipment.

Bipolar disorders Mood disorders that include one or more manic episodes and usually one or more depressive episodes.

Bisexuality Sexual attraction toward both males and females, which may be acted on by engaging in both heterosexual and homosexual activities.

Blocking A sudden obstruction or interruption in the spontaneous flow of thinking or speaking that is perceived as an absence or deprivation of thought.

Body image One's internalized sense of self.

Borderline personality disorder Disorder characterized by impulsive and unpredictable behavior and marked shifts in mood. Instability is seen predominantly in the areas of behavior, mood, relationships to others, and images of self.

Bulimia An eating disorder characterized by the excessive and uncontrollable intake of large amounts of food (binges), alternating with purging activities such as self-induced vomiting; use of cathartics, diuretics, or both; and self-starvation. These alternating behaviors characterize the eating disorder *bulimia nervosa*.

Catatonia A state of psychologically induced immobilization at times interrupted by episodes of extreme agitation.

Catecholamines A group of biogenic amines derived from phenylalanine and containing the catechol nucleus. Certain of these amines, such as *epinephrine*, *norepinephrine*, and *dopamine*, are neurotransmitters and exert an important influence on peripheral and central nervous system activity.

Cathexis A psychoanalytical term used to describe the emotional attachment or bond to an idea, an object, or most commonly, a person.

Character The sum of a person's relatively fixed personality traits and habitual modes of response.

Child abuse—neglect This abuse can be *physical* (e.g., failure to provide medical care), *developmental* (e.g., failure to provide emotional nurturing and cognitive stimulation), *educational* (failure to provide educational opportunities to the child according to the state's education laws), or a combination.

Child abuse—physical battering Physical assaults such as hitting, kicking, biting, throwing, and burning.

Child abuse—physical endangerment The reckless behaviors toward a child that could lead to the child's serious physical injury, such as leaving a young child alone or placing a child in a hazardous environment.

Child abuse—sexual Sexual abuse of children can take many forms. Essentially it is those acts designated to stimulate the child sexually, or use a child for sexual stimulation, either of the perpetrator or of another person.

Chronic anxiety Anxiety that a person has lived with for a long period of time. Chronic anxiety may take the form of chronic fatigue, insomnia, discomfort in daily activities, or discomfort in personal relationships.

Chronic illness The process of progressive deterioration, with a resulting increase in (1) functional impairment, (2) symptoms, and (3) disability over time.

Chronic pain Pain is classified as chronic when a client has had it for more than six months.

Circumstantial speech A pattern of speech that is indirect and delayed: before getting to the point or answering a question, the person gets caught up in countless details and explanations.

Clang association The meaningless rhyming of words, often in a forceful manner.

Codependent Maladaptive coping behaviors that prevent individuals from taking care of their own needs and have as their core a preoccupation with the thoughts and feelings of another or others. It usually refers to the dependence of one person on another person who is addicted.

Cognition The act, process, or result of knowing, learning, or understanding.

Cognitive therapy A treatment method (particularly useful for depressive disorders) that emphasizes the rearrangement of a person's maladaptive processes of thinking, perceptions, and attitudes.

Compensation Making up for deficits in one area by excelling in another area in order to raise or maintain self-esteem.

Compulsions Repetitive, purposeless-seeming behaviors performed according to certain rules known to the client in order to temporarily reduce escalating anxiety.

Concrete thinking Thinking characterized by immediate experience rather than abstraction. There is an overemphasis on specific detail as opposed to general and abstract thinking.

Confabulation Filling in a memory gap with a detailed fantasy believed by the teller. The purpose is to maintain self-esteem. This is seen in organic conditions, such as Korsakoff's psychosis.

Confidentiality The ethical responsibility of a health care professional that prohibits the disclosure of privileged information without the patient's informed consent.

Conscious All experiences that are within a person's awareness.

Consensual validation The reality checking of thoughts, feelings, and actions with others. If a child grows up in an environment in which the chance to validate thoughts, feelings, and behaviors is decreased, the child's ability to perceive reality is greatly impaired.

Conversion The unconscious transfer of anxiety to a physical symptom that has no organic cause.

Coping mechanisms Ways of adjusting to environmental stress without altering one's goals or purposes; include both conscious and unconscious mechanisms.

Cotherapy The sharing of responsibility for therapeutic work, usually in groups or with families.

Countertransference The tendency of the nurse-counselor to displace feelings that are a response to people in the counselor's past onto the client. Strong positive or strong negative reactions to a client may indicate possible countertransferential reactions.

Crisis A temporary state of disequilibrium (high anxiety) in which a person's usual coping mechanisms or problem-solving methods fail. Crisis can result in personality growth or personality disorganization.

Crisis intervention A brief, active, and collaborative therapy that uses an individual's personal coping abilities and resources within the family, health care setting, or community.

Culture The total lifestyle of a people, the social legacy the individual acquires from his or her group, or the environment that is the creation of humankind.

Cunnilingus Oral stimulation of the female genitalia.

Cyclothymia A chronic mood disturbance (of at least two years' duration) involving both hypomanic and dysthymic mood swings. Delusions are never present, and these mood swings usually do not warrant hospitalization or grossly impair a person's social, occupational, or interpersonal functioning.

Decode Interpreting the meaning of autistic communications, such as in looseness of associations.

Defense mechanisms (DMs) Unconscious intrapsychic processes used to ward off anxiety by preventing conscious awareness of threatening feelings. They can be used in a healthy and a not-so-healthy manner. Examples of defense mechanisms include repression, projection, sublimation, denial, and regression.

Delayed grief A dysfunctional reaction to grief in which a person may not experience the pain of loss; however, that pain is modified by chronic depression, intense preoccupation with body functioning (hypochondriasis), phobic reactions, or acute insomnia.

Delirium An acute, usually reversible brain syndrome with multiple causes (APA 1987).

Delirium tremens (DTs) An older term now replaced by *alcohol withdrawal delirium*.

Delusions A false belief held to be true even with evidence to the contrary (e.g., the false belief that one is being singled out for harm by others).

Dementia An insidious, chronic, often irreversible brain syndrome (APA 1987).

Denial Escaping unpleasant realities by ignoring their existence.

Depersonalization A phenomenon whereby a person experiences a sense of unreality or self-estrangement. For example, one may feel that one's extremities have changed, that one is seeing oneself from a distance, or that one is in a dream.

Depressive mood syndrome This term can be defined as "a depressed mood or loss of interest, of at least two weeks' duration, accompanied by several associated symptoms, such as weight loss and difficulty concentrating" (APA 1987).

Derealization The false perception by a person that his or her environment has changed. For example, everything seems bigger or smaller, or familiar objects have become strange and unfamiliar.

Desensitization The reduction of intense reactions to a stimulus (e.g., phobia) by repeated exposure to the stimulus in a weaker or milder form.

Detachment An interpersonal and intrapersonal dissociation from affective expression. Therefore, individuals appear cold, aloof, and distant. This behavior is thought to be learned and is viewed as defensive.

***Diagnostic and Statistical Manual of Mental Disorders, 3rd edition, revised* (DSM-III-R 1987) *and* DSM IV** Classification of mental disorders that includes descriptions of diagnostic categories. The DSM IV is the most widely accepted system of classifying abnormal behaviors used in the United States today.

Disorientation Confusion and impaired ability to identify time, place, and person.

Displacement Transfer of emotions associated with a particular person, object, or situation to another person, object, or situation that is nonthreatening.

Dissociation Threatening thoughts or feelings are put out of conscious awareness before they are able to trigger overwhelming and intolerable anxiety; similar to Freud's defense mechanisms of repression.

Dissociative disorders Disorders that involve sudden temporary disturbances or loss of one's normal ability to integrate identity or motor behavior. Psychogenic amnesia and fugue are two examples.

Distractibility Inability to maintain attention; shifting from one area or topic to another with minimal provocation.

Double-bind message A message that contains two contradictory messages given by the same person at the same time, to which the receiver is expected to respond. Constant double-bind situations result in feelings of helplessness, fear, and anxiety in the receiver of the message.

Drug abuse The maladaptive and consistent use of a drug despite (1) social, occupational, psychological, or physical problems exacerbated by the drug, (2) recurrent use in situations that are physically hazardous, such as driving while intoxicated (APA 1987).

Drug dependence Impaired control of drug use despite adverse consequences, the development of a tolerance to the drug, and the occurrence of withdrawal symptoms when drug intake is reduced or stopped.

Drug interaction The effects of two or more drugs taken simultaneously, producing an alteration in the usual effects of either drug taken alone. The interacting drugs may have a potentiating or an additive effect, and serious side effects may result.

Dual diagnosis Studies support the impression that identified addicts have a high prevalence for other psychiatric disorders (Talbott et al. 1988). A person with a dual diagnosis is chronically dependent on a drug or alcohol and also has another psychiatric disorder such as a depressive or personality disorder.

Dyskinesia Involuntary muscular activity, such as tic, spasm, or myoclonus.

Dyspareunia Persistent genital pain in either a male or female before, during, or after sex.

Dysthymia A depression that is mild to moderate in degree and is characterized by a chronic depressive syndrome that is usually present for many years. The depressive mood disturbance is hard to distinguish from the person's usual pattern of functioning, and the person has minimal social or occupational impairment.

Dystonia Muscle spasms of the face, head, neck, and back; usually an acute side effect of neuroleptic (antipsychotic) medication.

Echolalia Mimicking or imitating the speech of another person.

Echopraxia Mimicking or imitating the movements of another person.

Ego One of three psychological processes that make up the Freudian system of personality (id, ego, and superego). The ego is one's "sense of self" and provides such functions as problem-solving, mobilization of defense mechanisms, reality testing, and the capacity for one to function independently. The ego is said to be the mediator between one's primitive drives (the id) and internalized parental and social prohibitions (the superego).

Ego boundaries A person's perception of the boundaries between him- or herself and the external environment.

Ego-alien/Ego-dystonic Synonymous terms used to describe symptoms that are unacceptable to the person who has them and not compatible with the person's view of him- or herself (e.g., fear of cats).

Ego-syntonic Symptoms that include behaviors or beliefs that do not seem to bother the owner or "seem right" to the owner. For example, a very paranoid person who wrongly believes that the government is out to get him or her truly believes this thought, and it is consistent with the way this person experiences life.

Egocentric Self-centered.

Ethics The discipline concerned with standards of values, behaviors, or beliefs adhered to by individuals or groups.

Electroconvulsive therapy (ECT) An effective treatment for depression that consists of inducing a grand mal seizure by passing an electrical current through electrodes that are applied to the temples. The administration of a muscle relaxant minimizes seizure activity, preventing damage to long bones and cervical vertebrae.

Emotional abuse This takes many forms (e.g., terrorizing, demeaning, consistently belittling, withholding warmth). Essentially, emotional abuse is depriving a child of a nurturing atmosphere in which the child can thrive, learn, and develop.

Empathy The ability of one person to get inside another's world and see things from the other person's perspective and to communicate this understanding to the other person.

Enabling Helping a chemically dependent individual avoid experiencing the consequences of his or her drinking or drug use. It is one component of a person in a codependency role.

Endorphins A naturally produced chemical (peptide) with morphine-like action; usually found in the brain and associated with the reduction of pain and feelings of well-being.

Enuresis Nocturnal and daytime involuntary discharge of urine.

Epinephrine (adrenalin) A catecholamine secreted by the adrenal gland and by fibers of the sympathetic nervous system. It is responsible for many of the physical manifestations of fear and anxiety.

Extrapyramidal side effects A variety of signs and symptoms that are often side effects of the use of certain psychotropic drugs, particularly the phenothiazines. Three reversible side effects include acute dystonia, akathisia, and pseudoparkinsonism. A fourth, tardive dyskinesia, is most serious and is *not* reversible.

Family system Those individuals who make up the family unit and contribute to the functional state of the family as a unit.

Family therapy A treatment modality that focuses on the relationships within the family system.

Fantasy A retreat from reality and an attempt to solve problems in a private world. The difference between a healthy person and a schizophrenic, for example, is that a schizophrenic may not know where fantasy leaves off and reality begins.

Fear A reaction to a specific danger.

Fellatio Oral sexual contact with the penis.

Fetish An object or part of the body to which sexual significance or meaning is attached.

Flight of ideas A continuous flow of speech in which the person jumps rapidly from one topic to another. Sometimes the listener can keep up with the changes; at other times, it is necessary to listen for themes in the incessant talking. Themes often include grandiose and fantasied estimation of personal sexual prowess, business ability, artistic talents, and so on.

Fight-or-flight response (sympathetic response) The body's physiological response to fear or rage that triggers the sympathetic branch of the autonomic nervous system as well as the endocrine system. This response is useful in emergencies; however, a sustained response can result in pathophysiological changes such as high blood pressure, ulcers, cardiac problems, and more.

Formication Tactile hallucination or illusion involving insects crawling on the body or under the skin.

Frustration Curtailment of personal goals, satisfaction, or security by conditions of external reality or by internal controls.

Fugue Fugue involves memory loss, as does psychogenic amnesia, but it also includes traveling away from home or from one's usual work locale. Therefore, fugue involves flight as well as forgetfulness.

General adaptation syndrome (GAS) Hans Selye demonstrated the body's organized response to stress. The focus was more on the adrenocorticotropic hormone (ACTH). The general adaptation syndrome progresses through three stages: (1) the stage of alarm, (2) the stage of resistance, and (3) the stage of exhaustion.

Genogram A systematic diagram of the three-generational relationships within a family system.

Grandiosity Exaggerated belief in or claims about one's importance or identity.

Grief The subjective feelings and affect that are precipitated by a loss.

Group Two or more individuals who have a relationship with one another, are interdependent, and may share some norms.

Group dynamics The interactions and interrelations among members of a therapy group and between members and the therapist. The effective use of group dynamics is essential in group treatment.

Group process Interaction continually taking place between members of a group.

Group therapy Psychotherapy based on the examination of group interaction with a view toward understanding and eventually changing the ways in which clients interact with others.

Hallucination A sense perception (seeing, hearing, tasting, smelling, or touching) for which no external stimulus exists (e.g., hearing voices when none are present).

Hippocrates (460–377 B.C.) The Father of Medicine. He devised a code of ethical behavior that continues to guide physicians. He advocated the belief that mental illness was the result of natural causes rather than supernatural causes.

Homelessness—chronic The final stage in a lifelong series of crises and missed opportunities. It is the culmination of a gradual disengagement from supportive relationships and institutions.

Homosexual panic An acute and severe attack of anxiety based on unconscious conflicts involving gender identity.

Homosexuality Sexual attraction to or preference for persons of the same sex.

Hopelessness The belief by a person that no one can help him or her; extreme pessimism about the future.

Hostility Anger that is destructive in nature and purpose.

Hotline A telephone crisis counseling service often used in crisis intervention centers to provide immediate contact between a person in crisis and a counselor.

Hypermetamorphosis The need to touch everything in sight.

Hyperorality The need to taste, chew, and put everything in one's mouth.

Hypersomnia The increased time spent in sleep, possibly to escape from painful feelings; however, the increased sleep is not experienced as restful or refreshing.

Hypochondriasis Excessive preoccupation with one's physical health, without any organic pathology being present.

Hypomania An elevated mood with symptoms less severe than those of mania. A person in hypomania does *not* experience impairment in reality testing, nor do the symptoms markedly impair the person's social, occupational, or interpersonal functioning.

Hysterical personality disorder A disorder characterized by dramatic, emotionally intense, unstable behavior.

Id One of three psychological processes that make up the Freudian system of personality (id, ego, and superego). The id is the source of all primitive drives and instincts and is thought of as the reservoir of all psychic energy.

Ideas of reference False impressions that outside events have special meaning for oneself.

Identification Unconsciously taking on the thoughts, mannerisms, or behaviors of a person or group, in order to decrease anxiety.

Identity The sense of one's self based on experience, memories, perceptions, and emotions.

Illusion An error in the perception of a sensory stimulus. For example, a person may mistake polka dots on a pillow for hairy spiders.

Impotence The inability to achieve or maintain a penile erection of sufficient quality to engage in successful sexual intercourse.

Impulsiveness Impulsiveness is an action that is abrupt, unplanned, and directed toward immediate gratification.

Incest A sexual relationship between persons related biologically.

Insomnia Inability to fall asleep or to stay asleep, early morning awakening, or both.

Intellectualization The use of thinking and talking to avoid emotions and closeness.

Intimacy Emotional closeness.

Intoxication Excessive use of a drug or alcohol that leads to maladaptive behavior.

Intrapsychic Within the self.

Introjection Process by which a person incorporates or takes into his or her own personality qualities or values of another person or group with whom or with which intense emotional ties exist.

Intuition Emotional knowing without thinking or talking.

Isolation Separation of thoughts, ideas, or actions from their emotional aspects.

Johann Weyer (1515–1588) Weyer made the greatest contributions to psychiatry during the Renaissance. He is identified with the humane treatment of the mentally ill and known as the Father of Modern Psychiatry.

Judgment The ability to make logical, rational decisions.

La belle indifférence The affect or attitude of unconcern about a symptom that is used when the symptom is unconsciously used to lower anxiety. The lack of concern is thought to be a sign that the primary gain has been achieved.

Labile Having rapidly shifting emotions; unstable.

Lesbian A female homosexual.

Libido Sexual drive.

Limit setting The reasonable and rational setting of parameters for client behavior that provide control and safety.

Lithium carbonate This agent is known as an antimanic drug because it can stabilize the manic phase of a bipolar disorder. When effective, it can modify future manic episodes and protect against future depressive episodes.

Living will An expression by a person, while competent, that states the individual's preference that life-sustaining treatment be withheld or withdrawn if he or she becomes terminally ill and no longer able to make health care decisions (Weiler and Buckwalter 1988).

Looseness of association Thinking is haphazard, illogical, and confused; connections in thought are interrupted; seen mostly in schizophrenic disorders.

Magical thinking The belief that thinking something can make it happen; seen in children and psychotic clients.

Malingering A conscious effort to deceive others, often for financial gain, by pretending physical symptoms.

Mania An unstable elevated mood in which delusions, poor judgment, and other signs of impaired reality testing are evident. During a manic episode, clients have marked impairment in their social, occupational, and interpersonal functioning.

Manipulation Purposeful behavior directed at getting needs met. According to Chitty and Maynard (1986), manipulation is maladaptive when (1) it is the primary method used for getting needs met, (2) the needs, goals, and feelings of others are disregarded, and (3) others are treated as objects in order to fulfill the needs of the manipulator.

Masochism Unconscious or conscious gratification is obtained when a person experiences mental or physical pain; often used to refer to deviant sexual behaviors.

Maturational crisis Normal state in growth and development in which specific maturational tasks must be learned while old coping mechanisms are no longer acceptable.

Mental status exam A formal assessment of cognitive functions such as intelligence, thought processes, capacity for insight, and others.

Milieu The physical and social environment in which an individual lives.

Milieu therapy Therapy focused on positive environmental manipulation (both physical and social) in order to effect positive change.

Mnemonic disturbance Loss of memory.

Modeling A technique in which desired behaviors are demonstrated. The client learns to imitate these behaviors in appropriate situations.

Mood A "pervasive and sustained emotion that, in the

extreme, markedly colors the person's perception of the world" (APA 1987).

Mood syndrome An alteration in mood along with associated symptoms that occur for a minimal period.

Mourning The processes (grief work) by which grief is resolved.

Multiple personality disorder A severe dissociative disorder in which one or more distinct subpersonalities exist within an individual, each of which may be dominant at different times. Each subpersonality is a complex unit with its own memories, behavioral patterns, and social relationships, which may be very different from those of the primary personality.

Narcissism (narcism) Self-love or self-involvement; normal in children but pathological when experienced in adults to the same degree.

Narcissistic personality disorder A disorder characterized by an exaggerated sense of self-importance.

Negativism Opposition or resistance, either covert or overt, to outside suggestions or advice.

Negligence The act, or failure to act, that breaches the duty of due care and results in or is responsible for a person's injuries.

Neologisms Words a person makes up that have meaning only for that person; often part of a delusional system.

Neuroleptic malignant syndrome A rare and sometimes fatal reaction to high-potency neuroleptic drugs. Symptoms include muscle rigidity, fever, and elevated white blood cell count. It is thought to result from dopamine blockage on the basal ganglia and hypothalamus.

Nihilism A delusion that the self or part of the self does not exist.

No-suicide contract A contract made between a counselor-nurse and client, outlined in clear and simple language, in which the client states that he or she will *not* attempt self-harm and in which specific alternatives are given for the person to do instead.

Nonverbal communication Communication without words, such as body language, facial expressions, or gestures.

Nursing The diagnosis and treatment of human responses to actual or potential health problems.

Obesity A weight gain of at least 20% over the acceptable standard or ideal weight.

Obsession An idea, impulse, or emotion that a person cannot put out of his or her consciousness; can be mild or severe.

Organic mental disorders Specific brain syndromes in which an etiology is known. For example, alcohol withdrawal delirium and Alzheimer's disease are specific organic mental disorders (APA 1987).

Organic mental syndrome A general term used to refer to disturbances in orientation, memory, intellect, judgment, and affect due to physiological changes in the brain. Delirium and dementia are examples of two organic mental syndromes. A newer term is cognitive impairment syndromes or disorders.

Orientation The ability to relate the self correctly to time, place, and person.

Overt anxiety Anxiety in which the attendant physical, physiological, and cognitive symptoms are evident and may be assessed.

Panic Sudden, overwhelming anxiety of such intensity that it produces disorganization of the personality, loss of rational thought, and inability to communicate, along with specific physiological changes.

Paranoia Any intense and strongly defended irrational suspicion. These ideas cannot be corrected by experiences and cannot be modified by facts or reality.

Passive-aggressive behavior Indirect expression of anger. Behavior may seem passive but is motivated by unconscious anger, often triggering anger and frustration in others. Examples of passive-aggressive behavior include lateness, forgetting, "mistakes," and obtuseness.

Peer review Review of clinical practice with peers, supervisors, or consultants.

Perception Mental processes by which intellectual, sensory, and emotional data are organized logically or meaningfully.

Perseveration The involuntary repetition of the same thought, phrase, or motor response (e.g., brushing teeth, walking); associated with brain damage.

Personality Deeply ingrained personal patterns of behavior, traits, and thoughts that evolve, both consciously and unconsciously, as a person's style and way of adapting to the environment.

Philippe Pinel (1745–1826) A reformer and humanitarian who introduced psychotherapeutic methods in the treatment of the mentally ill.

Phobia An intense irrational fear of an object, situation, or place. The fear persists even though the object of the fear is perfectly harmless and the person is aware of the irrationality.

Pierre Janet (1859–1947) Janet advanced the knowledge of the functioning of the mind. By the use of hypnosis, he was the first to demonstrate that many symptoms of "neurosis" lay in the subconscious mind.

Pleasure principle Seeking immediate gratification of impulses and tension reduction. The id operates according to the pleasure principle.

Polydrug abuse The pathologic use of more than one drug.

Polypharmacy The taking of more than one drug at any given time.

Postvention Therapeutic interventions with the significant others of an individual who has committed suicide.

Poverty of speech Speech that is brief and uncommunative.

Pressure of speech Forceful energy heard in a manic individual's frantic, jumbled speech as he or she struggles to keep pace with racing thoughts.

Primary anxiety Anxiety that is due to intrapersonal or intrapsychic causes, such as a phobia.

Primary depression A depressive mood episode that is *not* due to a known organic factor and is *not* part of another psychotic disorder, such as schizophrenia (APA 1987).

Primary gain The anxiety relief resulting from the use of defense mechanisms or symptom formation, such as somatizing (e.g., getting a headache instead of feeling angry).

Primary process A primitive and unconscious psychological activity in which the id attempts to reduce tension through formation of an image or by hallucinating the object that would satisfy its need.

Projection The unconscious attributing of one's own intolerable wishes, emotional feelings, or motivation to another person.

Projective identification A "primitive form of projection used to externalize aggressive feelings. Once projection has occurred, fear of the person is coupled with a desire to control the person" (Smith and Lego 1984).

Prolonged grief A dysfunctional reaction to grief in which the bereaved remains intensely preoccupied with the memories of the deceased many years after the person has died.

Psychiatry The science of treating disorders of the psyche. It is the medical specialty that is derived from the study, diagnosis, treatment, and prevention of mental disorders.

Psychogenic Physical conditions affected by psychological factors.

Psychogenic amnesia The loss of memory for an event or period of time that contains overwhelming anxiety and pain. The loss of memory is related to psychological stress.

Psychomotor agitation The constant involvement in some tension-relieving activity, such as constantly pacing, biting one's nails, smoking, tapping one's fingers on a table top, and so on.

Psychomotor retardation Extremely slow and difficult movements that in the extreme can entail complete inactivity and incontinence.

Psychophysiological A newer term that refers to all physical symptoms in which psychic elements play a significant role in initiating or maintaining chemical, physiological, or structural alterations responsible for the client's complaint. Referred to in the DSM-II.

Psychosexual development Emotional and sexual growth from birth to adulthood.

Psychosis An extreme response to psychological or physical stressors that affects a person's affective, psychomotor, and physical behavior. Evidence of impairment in reality testing is evident by hallucinations or delusions.

Psychosocial rehabilitation The development of the skills necessary for people with chronic mental illness to live independently.

Psychosomatic An older term describing the interaction of the mind (psyche) and the body (soma). The term was used in reference to certain diseases thought to be caused by psychological factors. Referred to in the DSM-I.

Psychotherapy A treatment modality based on the development of a trusting relationship between client and therapist for the purpose of exploring and modifying the client's behavior in a satisfying direction.

Psychotropic Affecting the mind.

Psychotropic drugs Drugs that have an effect on psychic function, behavior, or experience.

Rape See *sexual assault.*

Rape-trauma syndrome This syndrome comprises (1) the acute phase and (2) the long term reorganization process that occur after an actual or attempted sexual assault. Each phase has separate symptoms.

Rationalization Justifying illogical or unreasonable ideas, actions, or feelings by developing acceptable explanations that satisfy the teller as well as the listener.

Reaction-formation (overcompensation) The process of keeping unacceptable feelings or behaviors out of awareness by developing the opposite emotion or behavior.

Reality principle The gradual development of the ability to delay immediate gratification and modify desires in accordance with the demands of society and external reality.

Regression In the face of overwhelming anxiety, the ego returns to an earlier, more comforting (although less mature) way of behaving.

Relaxation response The opposite of the fight-or-flight response. This response is synonymous with the functioning of the parasympathetic branch of the nervous system. The relaxation response has a stabilizing effect on the nervous system.

Repression The exclusion of unpleasant or unwanted experiences, emotions, or ideas from conscious awareness. Thought of as the first line of psychological defense.

Respite care Temporary supervision and care of a client who lives with his or her family. The purpose of respite care is to provide the family with some relief from the demands of the client's needs for continuous care.

Rituals Repetitive actions that people must do over and over until they are exhausted or anxiety is decreased; often done to lessen the anxiety triggered by an obsession.

Role-playing A technique used in group or family therapy in which a member acts out the behavior of another member in order to increase the other member's ability to see a situation from another point of view.

Sadism Sexual pleasure and erotic gratification obtained by inflicting pain, abuse, or humiliation on another.

Scapegoat A member of a group or family who becomes the target of aggression from others but who may not be the actual cause of hostility or frustration in them.

Schizoaffective disorder A disorder that includes a mixture of schizophrenic and affective symptoms (i.e., alterations in mood as well as disturbances in thought); thought by some to be a severe form of bipolar disorder.

Schizoid personality disorder A personality disorder in which there is a serious defect in interpersonal relationships. Other characteristics include lack of warmth, aloofness, and indifference to the feelings of others.

Schizophrenia A severe disturbance of thought or association, characterized by impaired reality testing, hallucinations, delusions, and limited socialization.

Seasonal affective disorder (SAD) A recently studied syndrome that appears to affect mostly women. It is characterized by hypersomnia, fatigue, weight gain, irritability, and interpersonal difficulties during the winter months. It has been successfully managed with daily treatments of two to three hours of bright light.

Secondary anxiety Anxiety that is due to physiological abnormalities such as certain medical disorders (e.g., neurological, endocrine, or circulatory) or is secondary to a pervasive psychiatric disorder such as depression.

Secondary dementia A result of some other pathological process, such as a metabolic, nutritional, or neurological one. AIDS-related dementia is an example.

Secondary depression A depressive mood syndrome that is caused by a physical illness or another psychiatric disorder or is part of an organic mental disorder; essentially, depression secondary to other causes.

Secondary gain Those advantages a person realizes from whatever symptoms or relief behaviors he or she employs. These advantages include increased attention from others, getting out of expected responsibilities, financial gain, and the ability to manipulate others in the environment.

Secondary process Consistent with the ego functioning by way of the reality principle: that is, realistic thinking.

Selective inattention Sullivan defines a person with selective inattention as "an individual who doesn't happen to notice an almost infinite series of more-or-less meaningful details of one's own living" that might cause anxiety.

Self-concept A person's image of the self.

Self-esteem Feelings individuals have about their own worth and value.

Self-help group An organization of people who share similar problems and meet to receive peer support and encouragement.

Sexual assault/rape Rape is the forced and violent (without consent) vaginal or anal penetration against the victim's will and without the victim's consent. Legal definitions vary from state to state.

Simple (specific) phobias Very common in the general population; essentially, fear and avoidance of a single object, situation, or activity.

Situational crises Crises arising from external sources, as opposed to internal sources; most people have them to some extent during the course of their lives (e.g., with the death of loved one, marriage, divorce, or a change in health status).

Social phobias These include phobias of an interpersonal nature, such as fear of public speaking, fear of eating in front of others, or fear of writing or performing in public.

Social skills training Training that focuses on such skills as introducing oneself, starting and ending a conversation, asking for assistance, and other simple yet essential social interactions; often helpful in combatting the negative symptoms of schizophrenia.

Somatic therapy Treatment that involves manipulations of the body, such as the use of medications or electroconvulsive therapy.

Somatization The expression of psychological stress through physical symptoms.

Somatizing Experiencing an emotional conflict as a physical symptom.

Splitting A primitive defense in which persons see themselves or others as all good or all bad, failing to integrate the positive and negative qualities of the self and others into a cohesive whole.

Spouse abuse The intentional act or perceived intention of physically injuring one's spouse. It is an act of mental cruelty.

Stereotyped behaviors Motor patterns that originally had meaning to the person (e.g., sweeping the floor or washing windows) but have become mechanical and lack purpose.

Stress The body's arousal response to any demand, change, or perceived threat.

Stupor A state in which a person is dazed and awareness of reality in his or her environment appears deadened. For example, a person may sit motionless for long periods of time and in extreme cases may appear to be in a coma.

Subconscious Often called the preconscious; includes experiences, thoughts, feelings, and desires that might not be in immediate awareness but can be recalled to consciousness. The subconscious mind helps repress unpleasant thoughts or feelings.

Subintentioned suicide Schneidman's (1963) term used to describe self-destructive behaviors people employ that could hasten their own death, such as compulsive use of drugs, hyperobesity, and medical noncompliance.

Sublimation The unconscious process of substituting constructive and socially acceptable activities for strong impulses that are not acceptable in their original form, such as strong aggressive or sexual drives.

Suicidal ideation Thoughts a person has regarding killing him- or herself.

Suicide The ultimate act of self-destruction in which a person purposefully ends his or her own life.

Suicide attempt All willful, self-inflicted, life-threatening attempts that have not led to death.

Suicide gesture A suicide attempt that is planned to be discovered and is made for the purpose of influencing or manipulating.

Superego One of three psychological processes that make up the Freudian system of personality (id, ego, and superego). The superego is the internal representative of the values, ideals, and moral standards of society. The superego is the moral arm of the personality.

Suppression The conscious putting off of awareness of disturbing situations or feelings. The only defense mechanism that operates on a conscious level.

Symbolization The process by which one object or idea comes to represent another. For example, the nurse's keys on a locked unit may represent power and autonomy, or a fancy house may represent prestige and power.

Synesthesia A phenomenon experienced by people on hallucinogenic drugs; described as hearing colors or seeing sounds.

Tangentiality An association disturbance in which the speaker goes off the topic. When it happens frequently and the speaker does not return to the topic, interpersonal communication is destroyed.

T*arasoff* decision A California court decision that imposes a duty on the therapist to warn the appropriate person or persons when the therapist becomes aware that a client may present a risk of harm to a specific person or persons.

Tardive dyskinesia A serious and irreversible result of the use of phenothiazine-like drugs. It consists of involuntary tonic muscular spasms typically involving the tongue, fingers, toes, neck, trunk, or pelvis.

Therapeutic encounter A brief, informal meeting between nurse and client in which the relationship is useful and important for the client.

Therapeutic nurse-patient relationship A therapeutic relationship requires that the nurse maximize his or her communication skills, understanding of human behaviors, and personal strengths in order to enhance personal growth in the client. This relationship applies to *all* clinical settings, not just those on a psychiatric unit.

Token economy A behavioral approach to eliciting desired behaviors involving the application of the principles and procedures of operant conditioning; usually used in the management of a social setting such as a ward, classroom, or halfway house. Targeted behaviors are awarded "tokens" that can be exchanged for desired goods or privileges.

Tolerance A need for higher and higher doses of a drug in order to achieve intoxication or the desired effect.

Torts Civil wrongs for which money damages are collected by the injured party (plaintiff) from the wrongdoer (defendant).

Transference The experiencing of thoughts and feelings toward a person (often the therapist) that belong to a significant person in one's past. Transference is a valuable tool used by therapists in psychoanalytical psychotherapy.

Transsexuals People who have an early and persistent feeling that they are trapped in a body with the wrong genitals. They believe they are, and were always meant to be, of the opposite sex.

Type A personality Personality characteristics such as excessive competitiveness, strong sense of time urgency, irritation, authoritarian, distrustful of others' motives. Type A people were once thought to be at high risk for coronary artery disease. However, a type A personality alone is no longer thought to be a risk factor in and of itself. The trait thought to have a high correlation to coronary artery disease, however, is hostility.

Unconscious Repressed memories, feelings, thoughts, or wishes that are not available to the conscious mind. Usually, unconscious material harbors intense anxiety and can greatly affect an individual's behavior.

Undoing An act or behavior unconsciously motivated to make up for or negate a previous act or behavior (e.g., bringing the boss a present after talking about him unfavorably to other coworkers).

Vegetative signs of depression A significant change from normal functioning during a depressive episode of those activities necessary to support physical life and growth, such as eating, sleeping, elimination, and sex.

Waxy flexibility Having one's arms or legs placed in a certain position and holding that same position for hours.

Withdrawal symptoms The negative physiological and psychological reactions that occur when a drug taken for a long period of time is reduced or no longer taken.

Word salad A mixture of phrases meaningless to the listener and to the speaker as well.

APPENDIX E

DSM-IV *Classification*

Multiaxial System

Axis I Clinical disorders
Other conditions that may be a focus of clinical attention
Axis II Personality disorders
Mental retardation
Axis III General medical conditions
Axis IV Psychosocial and environmental problems
Axis V Global assessment of functioning

NOS = Not Otherwise Specified.

An *x* appearing in a diagnostic code indicates that a specific code number is required.

Disorders Usually First Diagnosed in Infancy, Childhood, or Adolescence

Mental Retardation

Note: *These are coded on Axis II.*

317	Mild mental retardation
318.0	Moderate mental retardation
318.1	Severe mental retardation
318.2	Profound mental retardation
319	Mental retardation, severity unspecified

Learning Disorders

315.00	Reading disorder
315.1	Mathematics disorder
315.2	Disorder of written expression
315.9	Learning disorder NOS

Motor Skills Disorder

315.4	Developmental coordination disorder

Communication Disorders

315.31	Expressive language disorder
315.31	Mixed receptive-expressive language disorder
315.39	Phonological disorder
307.0	Stuttering
307.9	Communication disorder NOS

Pervasive Developmental Disorders

299.00	Autistic disorder
299.80	Rett's disorder
299.10	Childhood disintegrative disorder
299.80	Asperger's disorder
299.80	Pervasive developmental disorder NOS

From Diagnostic and Statistical Manual of Mental Disorders, 4th ed. (DSM-IV). Washington, DC: American Psychiatric Association, 1994.

Attention-deficit and disruptive behavior disorders

314.xx	Attention-deficit/hyperactivity disorder
.01	Combined type
.00	Predominantly inattentive type
.01	Predominantly hyperactive-impulsive type
314.9	Attention-deficit/hyperactivity disorder NOS
312.8	Conduct disorder
313.81	Oppositional defiant disorder
312.9	Disruptive behavior disorder NOS

Feeding and Eating Disorders of Infancy or Early Childhood

307.52	Pica
307.53	Rumination disorder
307.59	Feeding disorder of infancy or early childhood

Tic Disorders

307.23	Tourette's disorder
307.22	Chronic motor or vocal tic disorder
307.21	Transient tic disorder
	Specify if: single episode/recurrent
307.20	Tic disorder NOS

Elimination Disorders

—.—	Encopresis
787.6	With constipation and overflow incontinence
307.7	Without constipation and overflow incontinence
307.6	Enuresis (not due to a general medical condition)

Other Disorders of Infancy, Childhood, or Adolescence

309.21	Separation anxiety disorder
313.23	Selective mutism
313.89	Reactive attachment disorder of infancy or early childhood
307.3	Stereotypic movement disorder
313.9	Disorder of infancy, childhood, or adolescence NOS

Delirium, Dementia, and Amnestic and Other Cognitive Disorders

Delirium

293.0	Delirium due to . . . [*indicate the general medical condition*]
—.—	Substance intoxication delirium (*refer to Substance-Related Disorders for substance-specific codes*)
—.—	Substance withdrawal delirium (*refer to Substance-Related Disorders for substance-specific codes*)
—.—	Delirium due to multiple etiologies (*code each of the specific etiologies*)
780.09	Delirium NOS

Dementia

290.xx   Dementia of the Alzheimer's type, with early onset (*also code on Axis III*)

    .10   Uncomplicated
    .11   With delirium
    .12   With delusions
    .13   With depressed mood

290.xx   Dementia of the Alzheimer's type, with late onset (*also code on Axis III*)

    .0   Uncomplicated
    .3   With delirium
    .20   With delusions
    .21   With depressed mood

290.xx   Vascular dementia

    .40   Uncomplicated
    .41   With delirium
    .42   With delusions
    .43   With depressed mood

294.9   Dementia due to HIV disease (*also code HIV affecting central nervous system on Axis III*)

294.1   Dementia due to head trauma (*also code on Axis III*)

294.1   Dementia due to Parkinson's disease (*also code on Axis III*)

294.1   Dementia due to Huntington's disease (*also code on Axis III*)

290.10   Dementia due to Pick's disease (*also code on Axis III*)

290.10   Dementia due to Creutzfeldt-Jakob disease (*also code 046.1 Creutzfeldt-Jakob disease on Axis III*)

294.1   Dementia due to . . . [*indicate the general medical condition not listed above*] (*also code the general medical condition on Axis III*)

——.–   Substance-induced persisting dementia

——.–   Dementia due to multiple etiologies

294.8   Dementia NOS

Amnestic Disorders

294.0   Amnestic disorder due to . . . [*indicate the general medical condition*]
     Specify if: transient-chronic

——.–   Substance-induced persisting amnestic disorder

294.8   Amnestic disorder NOS

Other Cognitive Disorders

294.9   Cognitive disorder NOS

Mental Disorders Due to a General Medical Condition Not Elsewhere Classified

293.89   Catatonic disorder due to . . . [*indicate the general medical condition*]

310.1   Personality change due to . . . [*indicate the general medical condition*]

293.9   Mental disorder NOS due to . . . [*indicate the general medical condition*]

Substance-Related Disorders

ª *The following specifiers may be applied to Substance Dependence:*
    With physiological dependence/without physiological dependence

Early full remission/early partial remission
Sustained full remission/sustained partial remission
On agonist therapy/in a controlled environment

The following specifiers apply to Substance-Induced Disorders as noted:
ᴵWith onset during intoxication/ᵂwith onset during withdrawal

Alcohol-Related Disorders

Alcohol Use Disorders

303.90   Alcohol dependenceª
305.00   Alcohol abuse

Alcohol-Induced Disorders

303.00   Alcohol intoxication
291.8   Alcohol withdrawal
291.0   Alcohol intoxication delirium
291.0   Alcohol withdrawal delirium
291.2   Alcohol-induced persisting dementia
291.1   Alcohol-induced persisting amnestic disorder
291.x   Alcohol-induced psychotic disorder
    .5   With delusions
    .3   With hallucinations
291.8   Alcohol-induced mood disorder
291.8   Alcohol-induced anxiety disorder
291.8   Alcohol-induced sexual dysfunction
291.8   Alcohol-induced sleep disorder
291.9   Alcohol-related disorder NOS

Amphetamine (or Amphetamine-Like)–Related Disorders

Amphetamine Use Disorders

304.40   Amphetamine dependenceª
305.70   Amphetamine abuse

Amphetamine-Induced Disorders

292.89   Amphetamine intoxication
292.0   Amphetamine withdrawal
292.81   Amphetamine intoxication delirium
292.xx   Amphetamine-induced psychotic disorder
    .11   With delusionsᴵ
    .12   With hallucinationsᴵ
292.84   Amphetamine-induced mood disorder
292.89   Amphetamine-induced anxiety disorder
292.89   Amphetamine-induced sexual dysfunction
292.89   Amphetamine-induced sleep disorder
292.9   Amphetamine-related disorder NOS

Caffeine-Related Disorders

Caffeine-Induced Disorders

305.90   Caffeine intoxication
292.89   Caffeine-induced anxiety disorderᴵ
292.89   Caffeine-induced sleep disorderᴵ
292.9   Caffeine-related disorder NOS

Cannabis-Related Disorders

Cannabis Use Disorders

304.30   Cannabis dependence
305.20   Cannabis abuse

Cannabis-Induced Disorders

292.89   Cannabis intoxication
292.81   Cannabis intoxication delirium

292.xx   Cannabis-induced psychotic disorder
  .11   With delusions[I]
  .12   With hallucinations[I]
292.89   Cannabis-induced anxiety disorder[I]
292.9   Cannabis-related disorder NOS

Cocaine-Related Disorders

Cocaine Use Disorders

304.20   Cocaine dependence[a]
305.60   Cocaine abuse

Cocaine-Induced Disorders

292.89   Cocaine intoxication
        Specify if: with perceptual disturbances
292.0   Cocaine withdrawal
292.81   Cocaine intoxication delirium
292.xx   Cocaine-induced psychotic disorder
  .11   With delusions[I]
  .12   With hallucinations[I]
292.84   Cocaine-induced mood disorder
292.89   Cocaine-induced anxiety disorder
292.89   Cocaine-induced sexual dysfunction[I]
292.89   Cocaine-induced sleep disorder
292.9   Cocaine-related disorder NOS

Hallucinogen-Related Disorders

Hallucinogen Use Disorders

304.50   Hallucinogen dependence[a]
305.30   Hallucinogen abuse

Hallucinogen-Induced Disorders

292.89   Hallucinogen intoxication
292.89   Hallucinogen persisting perception disorder (flashbacks)
292.81   Hallucinogen intoxication delirium
292.xx   Hallucinogen-induced psychotic disorder
  .11   With delusions[I]
  .12   With hallucinations[I]
292.84   Hallucinogen-induced mood disorder[I]
292.89   Hallucinogen-induced anxiety disorder[I]
292.9   Hallucinogen-related disorder NOS

Inhalant-Related Disorders

Inhalant Use Disorders

304.60   Inhalant dependence[a]
305.90   Inhalant abuse

Inhalant-Induced Disorders

292.89   Inhalant intoxication
292.81   Inhalant intoxication delirium
292.82   Inhalant-induced persisting dementia
292.xx   Inhalant-induced psychotic disorder
  .11   With delusions[I]
  .12   With hallucinations[I]
292.84   Inhalant-induced mood disorder[I]
292.89   Inhalant-induced anxiety disorder[I]
292.9   Inhalant-related disorder NOS

Nicotine-Related Disorders

Nicotine Use Disorder

305.10   Nicotine dependence[a]

Nicotine-Induced Disorder

292.0   Nicotine withdrawal
292.9   Nicotine-related disorder NOS

Opioid-Related Disorders

Opioid Use Disorders

304.00   Opioid dependence[a]
305.50   Opioid abuse

Opioid-Induced Disorders

292.89   Opioid intoxication
292.0   Opioid withdrawal
292.81   Opioid intoxication delirium
292.xx   Opioid-induced psychotic disorder
  .11   With delusions[I]
  .12   With hallucinations[I]
292.84   Opioid-induced mood disorder[I]
292.89   Opioid-induced sexual dysfunction[I]
292.89   Opioid-induced sleep disorder
292.9   Opioid-related disorder NOS

Phencyclidine (or Phencyclidine-Like)–Related Disorders

Phencyclidine Use Disorders

304.90   Phencyclidine dependence[a]
305.90   Phencyclidine abuse

Phencyclidine-Induced Disorders

292.89   Phencyclidine intoxication
292.81   Phencyclidine intoxication delirium
292.xx   Phencyclidine-induced psychotic disorder
  .11   With delusions[I]
  .12   With hallucinations[I]
292.84   Phencyclidine-induced mood disorder[I]
292.89   Phencyclidine-induced anxiety disorder[I]
292.9   Phencyclidine-related disorder NOS

Sedative-, Hypnotic-, or Anxiolytic-Related Disorders

Sedative, Hypnotic, or Anxiolytic Use Disorders

304.10   Sedative, hypnotic, or anxiolytic dependence[a]
305.40   Sedative, hypnotic, or anxiolytic abuse

Sedative-, Hypnotic-, or Anxiolytic-Induced Disorders

292.89   Sedative, hypnotic, or anxiolytic intoxication
292.0   Sedative, hypnotic, or anxiolytic withdrawal
        Specify if: with perceptual disturbances
292.81   Sedative, hypnotic, or anxiolytic intoxication delirium
292.81   Sedative, hypnotic, or anxiolytic withdrawal delirium
292.82   Sedative-, hypnotic-, or anxiolytic-induced persisting dementia
292.83   Sedative-, hypnotic-, or anxiolytic-induced persisting amnestic disorder
292.xx   Sedative-, hypnotic-, or anxiolytic-induced psychotic disorder
  .11   With delusions
  .12   With hallucinations
292.84   Sedative-, hypnotic-, or anxiolytic-induced mood disorder[I,W]

292.89 Sedative-, hypnotic-, or anxiolytic-induced anxiety disorder[W]

292.89 Sedative-, hypnotic-, or anxiolytic-induced sexual dysfunction[I]

292.89 Sedative-, hypnotic-, or anxiolytic-induced sleep disorder[I,W]

292.9 Sedative-, hypnotic-, or anxiolytic-related disorder NOS

Polysubstance-Related Disorder

304.80 Polysubstance dependence[a]

Other (or Unknown) Substance-Related Disorders

Other (or Unknown) Substance Use Disorders

304.90 Other (or unknown) substance dependence[a]

305.90 Other (or unknown) substance abuse

Other (or Unknown) Substance-Induced Disorders

292.89 Other (or unknown) substance intoxication

292.0 Other (or unknown) substance withdrawal

292.81 Other (or unknown) substance-induced delirium

292.82 Other (or unknown) substance-induced persisting dementia

292.83 Other (or unknown) substance-induced persisting amnestic disorder

292.xx Other (or unknown) substance-induced psychotic disorder

   .11 With delusions[I,W]

   .12 With hallucinations[I,W]

292.84 Other (or unknown) substance-induced mood disorder[I,W]

292.89 Other (or unknown) substance-induced anxiety disorder[I,W]

292.89 Other (or unknown) substance-induced sexual dysfunction[I]

292.89 Other (or unknown) substance-induced sleep disorder[I,W]

292.9 Other (or unknown) substance-related disorder NOS

Schizophrenia and Other Psychotic Disorders

295.xx Schizophrenia

The following Classification of Longitudinal Course applies to all subtypes of Schizophrenia:

Episodic with interepisode residual symptoms (*specify if:* with prominent negative symptoms)/episodic with no interepisode residual symptoms/continuous (*specify if:* with prominent negative symptoms)

Single episode in partial remission (*specify if:* with prominent negative symptoms)/single episode in full remission

Other or unspecified pattern

   .30 Paranoid type

   .10 Disorganized type

   .20 Catatonic type

   .90 Undifferentiated type

   .60 Residual type

295.40 Schizophreniform disorder

   Specify if: without good prognostic features/with good prognostic features

295.70 Schizoaffective disorder

   Specify type: bipolar type/depressive type

297.1 Delusional disorder

   Specify type: erotomanic type/grandiose type/jealous type/persecutory type/somatic type/mixed type/unspecified type

298.8 Brief psychotic disorder

   Specify if: with marked stressor(s)/without marked stressor(s)/with postpartum onset

297.3 Shared psychotic disorder

293.xx Psychotic disorder due to . . . [*indicate the general medical condition*]

   .81 With delusions

   .82 With hallucinations

———.— Substance-induced psychotic disorder

   Specify if: with onset during intoxication/with onset during withdrawal

298.9 Psychotic disorder NOS

Mood Disorders

Code current state of major depressive disorder or bipolar I disorder in fifth digit:

   1 = Mild

   2 = Moderate

   3 = Severe without psychotic features

   4 = Severe with psychotic features

      Specify: Mood-congruent psychotic features/mood-incongruent psychotic features

   5 = In partial remission

   6 = In full remission

   0 = Unspecified

The following specifiers apply (for current or most recent episode) to mood disorders as noted:

   [a]Severity/psychotic/remission specifiers/[b]chronic/[c]with catatonic features/[d]with melancholic features/[e]with atypical features/[f]with postpartum onset

The following specifiers apply to mood disorders as noted:

   [g]With or without full interepisode recovery/[h]with seasonal pattern/[i]with rapid cycling

Depressive Disorders

296.xx Major depressive disorder

   .2x Single episode

   .3x Recurrent

300.4 Dysthymic disorder

   Specify if: early onset/late onset

   Specify: with atypical features

311 Depressive disorder NOS

Bipolar Disorders

296.xx Bipolar I disorder

   .0x Single manic episode

   .40 Most recent episode hypomanic

   .4x Most recent episode manic

   .6x Most recent episode mixed

   .5x Most recent episode depressed

   .7 Most recent episode unspecified

296.89   Bipolar II disorder
         Specify (current or most recent episode): hypomanic/
         depressed
301.13   Cyclothymic disorder
296.80   Bipolar disorder NOS
293.83   Mood disorder due to . . . *[indicate the general
         medical condition]*
         Specify type: with depressive features/with major
         depressive-like episode/with manic features/with
         mixed features
——.—   Substance-induced mood disorder
         Specify type: with depressive features/with manic
         features/with mixed features
         Specify if: with onset during intoxication/with onset
         during withdrawal
296.90   Mood disorder NOS

Anxiety Disorders

300.01   Panic disorder without agoraphobia
300.21   Panic disorder with agoraphobia
300.22   Agoraphobia without history of panic disorder
300.29   Specific phobia
         Specify type: animal type/natural environment type/
         blood-injection-injury type/situational type/other type
300.23   Social phobia
         Specify if: generalized
300.3   Obsessive-compulsive disorder
         Specify if: with poor insight
309.81   Posttraumatic stress disorder
         Specify if: acute/chronic
         Specify if: with delayed onset
308.3   Acute stress disorder
300.02   Generalized anxiety disorder
293.89   Anxiety disorder due to . . . *[indicate the general
         medical condition]*
         Specify if: with generalized anxiety/with panic attacks/
         with obsessive-compulsive symptoms
——.—   Substance-induced anxiety disorder
         Specify if: with generalized anxiety/with panic attacks/
         with obsessive-compulsive symptoms/with phobic
         symptoms
         Specify if: with onset during intoxication/with onset
         during withdrawal
300.00   Anxiety disorder NOS

Somatoform Disorders

300.81   Somatization disorder
300.81   Undifferentiated somatoform disorder
300.11   Conversion disorder
         Specify type: with motor symptom or deficit/with
         sensory symptom or deficit/with seizures or
         convulsions/with mixed presentation
307.xx   Pain disorder
   .80   associated with psychological factors
   .89   Associated with both psychological factors and
         a general medical condition
         Specify if: acute/chronic
300.7   Hypochondriasis
         Specify if: with poor insight

300.7   Body dysmorphic disorder
300.81   Somatoform disorder NOS

Factitious Disorders

300.xx   Facititious disorder
   .16   With predominantly psychological signs and
         symptoms
   .19   With predominantly physical signs and
         symptoms
   .19   With combined psychological and physical
         signs and symptoms
300.19   Facititious disorder NOS

Dissociative Disorders

300.12   Dissociative amnesia
300.13   Dissociative fugue
300.14   Dissociative identity disorder
300.6   Depersonalization disorder
300.15   Dissociative disorder NOS

Sexual and Gender Identity Disorders

Sexual Dysfunctions
*The following specifiers apply to all primary Sexual
Dysfunctions:*

         Lifelong type/acquired type/generalized type/
         situational type due to psychological factors/due to
         combined factors

Sexual Desire Disorders
302.71   Hypoactive sexual desire disorder
302.79   Sexual aversion disorder

Sexual Arousal Disorders
302.72   Female sexual arousal disorder
302.72   Male erectile disorder

Orgasmic Disorders
302.73   Female orgasmic disorder
302.74   Male orgasmic disorder
302.75   Premature ejaculation

Sexual Pain Disorders
302.76   Dyspareunia (not due to a general medical
         condition)
306.51   Vaginismus (not due to a general medical
         condition)

Sexual Dysfunction Due to a General Medical Condition
625.8   Female hypoactive sexual desire disorder due
         to . . . *[indicate the general medical condition]*
608.89   Male hypoactive sexual desire disorder due
         to . . . *[indicate the general medical condition]*
607.84   Male erectile disorder due to . . . *[indicate the
         general medical condition]*
625.0   Female dyspareunia due to . . . *[indicate the
         general medical condition]*
608.89   Male dyspareunia due to . . . *[indicate the
         general medical condition]*
625.8   Other female sexual dysfunction due
         to . . . *[indicate the general medical condition]*

608.89 Other male sexual dysfunction due
to . . . [*indicate the general medical condition*]
——.– Substance-induced sexual dysfunction
302.70 Sexual dysfunction NOS

Paraphilias

302.4 Exhibitionism
302.81 Fetishism
302.89 Frotteurism
302.2 Pedophilia
302.83 Sexual masochism
302.84 Sexual sadism
302.3 Transvestic fetishism
302.82 Voyeurism
302.9 Paraphilia NOS

Gender Identity Disorders

302.xx Gender identity disorder
.6 in children
.85 in adolescents or adults
Specify if: sexually attracted to males/sexually
attracted to females/sexually attracted to both/
sexually attracted to neither
302.6 Gender identity disorder NOS
302.9 Sexual disorder NOS

Eating Disorders

307.1 Anorexia nervosa
Specify type: restricting type; binge-eating/purging type
307.51 Bulimia nervosa
Specify type: purging type/nonpurging type
307.50 Eating disorder NOS

Sleep Disorders

Primary Sleep Disorders

Dyssomnias
307.42 Primary insomnia
307.44 Primary hypersomnia
Specify if: recurrent
347 Narcolepsy
780.59 Breathing-related sleep disorder
307.45 Circadian rhythm sleep disorder
307.47 Dyssomnia NOS

Parasomnias
307.47 Nightmare disorder
307.46 Sleep terror disorder
307.46 Sleepwalking disorder
307.47 Parasomnia NOS

Sleep Disorders Related to Another Mental Disorder

307.42 Insomnia related to . . . [*indicate the disorder*]
307.44 Hypersomnia related to . . . [*indicate the disorder*]

Other Sleep Disorders

780.xx Sleep disorder due to . . . [*indicate the general medical condition*]
.52 Insomnia type

.54 Hypersomnia type
.59 Parasomnia type
.59 Mixed type
——.– Substance-induced sleep disorder
Specify type: insomnia type/hypersomnia type/
parasomnia type/mixed type
Specify if: with onset during intoxication/with onset
during withdrawal

Impulse-Control Disorders Not Elsewhere Classified

312.34 Intermittent explosive disorder
312.32 Kleptomania
312.33 Pyromania
312.31 Pathological gambling
312.39 Trichotillomania
312.30 Impulse-control disorder NOS

Adjustment Disorders

309.xx Adjustment disorder
.0 With depressed mood
.24 With anxiety
.28 With mixed anxiety and depressed mood
.3 With disturbance of conduct
.4 With mixed disturbance of emotions and
conduct
.9 Unspecified
Specify if: acute/chronic

Personality Disorders

Note: *These are coded on Axis II.*
301.0 Paranoid personality disorder
301.20 Schizoid personality disorder
301.22 Schizotypal personality disorder
301.7 Antisocial personality disorder
301.83 Borderline personality disorder
301.50 Histrionic personality disorder
301.81 Narcissistic personality disorder
301.82 Avoidant personality disorder
301.6 Dependent personality disorder
301.4 Obsessive-compulsive personality disorder
301.9 Personality disorder NOS

Other Conditions That May Be a Focus of Clinical Attention

Psychological Factors Affecting Medical Condition

316 . . . [*Specified psychological factor*]
affecting . . . [*indicate the general medical condition*]
Choose name based on nature of factors:
Mental disorder affecting medical condition
Psychological symptoms affecting medical
condition
Personality traits or coping style affecting
medical condition
Maladaptive health behaviors affecting medical
condition
Stress-related physiological response affecting
medical condition

Other or unspecified psychological factors
affecting medical condition

Medication-Induced Movement Disorders

332.1   Neuroleptic-induced parkinsonism
333.92 Neuroleptic malignant syndrome
333.7   Neuroleptic-induced acute dystonia
333.99 Neuroleptic-induced acute akathisia
333.82 Neuroleptic-induced tardive dyskinesia
333.1   Medication-induced postural tremor
333.90 Medication-induced movement disorder NOS

Other Medication-Induced Disorder

995.2   Adverse effects of medication NOS

Relational Problems

V61.9   Relational problem related to a mental
        disorder or general medical condition
V61.20 Parent-child relational problem
V61.1   Partner relational problem
V61.8   Sibling relational problem
V62.81 Relational problem NOS

Problems Related to Abuse or Neglect

V61.21 Physical abuse of child
V61.21 Sexual abuse of child
V61.21 Neglect of child
V61.1   Physical abuse of adult
V61.1   Sexual abuse of adult

Additional Conditions That May Be a Focus of Clinical Attention

V15.81 Noncompliance with treatment
V65.2   Malingering
V71.01 Adult antisocial behavior
V71.02 Child or adolescent antisocial behavior
V62.89 Borderline intellectual functioning
        Note: *This is coded on Axis II.*
780.9   Age-related cognitive decline
V62.82 Bereavement
V62.3   Academic problem
V62.2   Occupational problem
313.82 Identity problem
V62.89 Religious or spiritual problem
V62.4   Acculturation problem
V62.89 Phase of life problem

Key to Self-Study Exercises

Chapter 1

1. True (p. 7)
2. True (p. 6)
3. True (p. 7)
4. True (p. 21)
5. False (pp. 22–23)
6. C (p. 9)
7. A (p. 9)
8. E (p. 9)
9. H (p. 10)
10. B (p. 10)
11. F (p. 11)
12. D (p. 10)
13. G (p. 10)
14. D
15. A
16. C
17. C
18. D
19. A
20. C
21. C
22. E
23. G
24. H
25. B
26. F
27. A
28. D
29. D (refer to Table 1–7)
30. A
31. C
32. B
33. D

Chapter 2

1. C (p. 31)
2. A (p. 32)
3. D (p. 31)
4. B (p. 31)
5. behavior therapy (operant conditioning, p. 34)
6. Gestalt (p. 35)
7. psychoanalysis (p. 32)
8. transactional analysis (p. 33)
9. short term dynamic psychotherapy (p. 32)
10. psychoanalytic psychotherapy (p. 33)
11. A. See p. 35
11. B. See pp. 35–36
11. C. See p. 35
12. A. See p. 36

12. B. See p. 36
12. C. See p. 36
12. D. See pp. 36–37

Chapter 3

1. D
2. C
3. A
4. G
5. F
6. True
7. True
8. See pp. 51–56
9. See p. 50
10. See pp. 58–59
11. See p. 59
12. See pp. 64–66

Answers to Questions for Discussion
Page 59
1. Yes
2. Yes
3. Yes. If unfamiliar with current practice, the RN should seek continuing education prior to working with patients in a specialty area. To avoid insubordination charges, the nurse must clarify the expectations and areas of care he or she will be assigned to when being hired.
4. Misrepresentation, negligence, liability if injured patient.
5. Insubordination; charges of abandonment.
6. Clarify expectations with employer when being hired (in writing).
7. Require the assistance of another professional during nurse B's absence— such as a unit supervisor or doctor.
8. Both the hospital and nurse A will likely be named as defendants. The hospital breached its duty to provide competent care providers, especially if they knew of nurse A's limited scope of practice abilities.

Page 60
1. Yes, but the nasal packs in this case call for a higher standard of care, i.e., more frequent checks. The question will revolve around what behavior was/is reasonable and prudent to protect the patient (Negligence Standard).
2. Not totally, see comment earlier.
3. No. The doctor does not avoid some responsibility, but nurses are licensed professionals who much exercise their

own sound judgment when patient safety is jeopardized.
4. No.
5. Nasal packs; private room (isolated and less opportunity to observe patient); no restraints for "possible delirium tremens."
6. No
7. No, the statute identified a standard found acceptable by the state, but more frequent checks (every 15 to 30 minutes) are generally recommended. Federal regulations would overrule less restrictive state regulations.
8. No restraints. Check on patient more frequently. Don't place in isolated private room. Question the doctor on the order to restrain and refuse to place patient in this unsafe position. (Don't confront the doctor, but rather share your concerns in a professional manner.)

Page 61
1. On a protected incident report until the allegations can be investigated.
2. Follow agency protocols for incident reporting. Perhaps the charges are premature and could defame the psychiatrist.
3. Yes
4. With the supervisor, if agency policies suggest this chain of communication. Patients rights must also be considered.
5. Follow agency policy for channels of communication.
6. Follow agency policy for channels of communication.
7. If the allegations have foundation, the agency should report the incident, especially if the State Medical Practice Act directs reporting.
8. If the allegations have foundation, the agency should report the incident, especially if the State Medical Practice Act directs reporting.
9. The nurse should allow the agency administrators to follow necessary procedures for reporting.
10. Yes, even if Beth denies taking the medications, he should discuss the problem with the supervisor.
11. The supervisor and agency will report after investigating.
12. If Beth has admitted, Joe should identify Beth.
13. Yes, but the agency will usually accept this responsibility (not suspicions, but admitted facts).
14. No, this is a legal duty to intervene.

Page 63
1. Not keeping a safe environment (i.e., bed frame). Locking the room with knowledge that patient will foreseeably harm herself (because she hears voices).
2. Bed frame removed; frequent checks on patient; notify doctor of patient's statement; provide nursing interventions and support by staying with the patient.
3. Never falsify records. Fraudulent change to records could result in criminal as well as civil charges. Unethical and illegal.

Page 66
1. No, she has a legal duty to notify the boy's therapist, who, in turn, should warn the boy's mother.
2. Ethical principles cannot be valued over a human life that is threatened. The patient will be in greater trouble if the nurse does not intervene and allows the patient to harm his mother. Preventing this legal and human dilemma is more ethical toward the patient than maintaining confidentiality. Preventing a crime is in the patient's best interest (beneficence); justice could not allow harm to an innocent victim; our society cannot allow total autonomy or we'd have no law and order.
3. The "special relationship" recognized by the law is with the therapist, whom the nurse must notify, who, in turn, should warn the mother.
4. No, not the duty to warn.
5. No difference when discussing legal duty to warn and ethics.
6. If the jurisdiction where you are practicing does not recognize a duty to warn, then you might have more of an ethical dilemma than a legal duty.
7. Notify the treatment therapist as soon as possible—don't wait until the patient is discharged!
8. Statutes require child abuse to be reported. However, to avoid violating federal confidentiality laws, do not share the information that the abuser is in an alcoholic treatment program. It was not the patient who shared the information, but still the nurse must avoid disclosing that the abuser is in treatment.

Chapter 4

1. A. Refer to p. 72
1. B. Refer to p. 72
1. C. Refer to p. 71
1. D. Refer to p. 73
2. Discuss from your reading of Chapter 4.
3. Discuss from your reading of Chapter 4.
4. Discuss with classmate or neighbor of a different culture.
5. From your reading of Chapter 4.
6. Discussion
7. Discussion
8. Discussion
9. Writing these thoughts in a personal journal could be helpful.

Chapter 5

1. See p. 90 and Table 5–1, p. 91
2. See p. 94
3. See pp. 92–93
4. See pp. 94–95
5. See p. 95
6. Discussion—see p. 97
7. Write a brief paragraph.
8. See pp. 97–98
9. See p. 98
10. See p. 97
11. See p. 101

Chapter 6

1. False
2. True
3. True
4. False. (Review the part these factors play on p. 115)
5. True
6. True
7. N
8. V
9. N
10. V
11. N Belittling feelings
12. T Seeking clarification
13. T Making observation
14. N Advising
15. T Exploring
16. T Reflection
17. T Summarizing if people know each other; also is making observations.
18. S
19. I
20. I
21. T
22. S
23. T
24. I
25. S/I
26. True (p. 133)
27. True
28. True (p. 133)
29. Discussion
30. Discussion
31. T
32. O
33. W
34. T

Chapter 7

1. H
2. F
3. E
4. D
5. A
6. B
7. C
8. G
9. D
10. B
11. True
12. True
13. True
14. True

15. E
16. D
17. C
18. A
19. B
20. F
21. A
22. D
23. D
24. False
25. False
26. True
27. True
28. D (p. 155 and Table 7–10)
29. D (p. 155 and Table 7–11)
30. D

Chapter 8

1. A. Gathering data
1. B. Verifying data
2. A. Problem
2. B. Etiology
2. C. Supporting data
3. A. Determining desired outcomes
3. B. Identifying appropriate nursing interventions
4. A. Validating the care plan
4. B. Giving nursing care
4. C. Continued data collection
5. A. Evaluation of good achievement
5. B. Review of the nursing care plan
6. P
7. C-H
8. C-M/E
9. C-H
10. C-M/E
11. C-H
12. C-H
13. C-M/E
14. A. See Table 8–4
14. B. Use data given, review p. 178
14. C. Use data given, review p. 178
15. A. Review pp. 180–181
15. B. Review pp. 180–181
15. C. Review pp. 180–181
16. A. See p. 181
16. B. See p. 181
16. C. See p. 181
16. D. See p. 181
17. A. Review p. 186
17. B. Review p. 186
17. C. Review p. 186

Chapter 9

1. True
2. False (p. 198)
3. False (p. 198)
4. F
5. H
6. C
7. G
8. D
9. B
10. E
11. A
12. C
13. D

14. D
15. E
16. B
17. A
18. C
19. Reaction formation
20. Table 9–2, p. 200
21. Table 9–2, p. 200
22. Table 9–2, p. 200
23. Table 9–2, p. 200
24. Moderate
24. A. Table 9–4
24. B. Table 9–4
24. C. Table 9–4
25. Severe
25. A. Table 9–5
25. B. Table 9–5
25. C. Table 9–5

Chapter 10 *p. 228*

1. C
2. F
3. A
4. D
5. B
6. H
7. E
8. I
9. G
10. A, B, C, and D
11. C
12. A
13. B
14. A
15. A

Chapter 11

1. B
2. C
3. A
4. C
5. C
6. A
7. False
8. False
9. True
10. False
11. True
12. False
13. True
14. False
15. Refer to pp. 239–240
16. A. See pp. 242–243
16. B. See pp. 242–243
16. C. See pp. 242–243
17. A. See p. 243
17. B. See p. 243
17. C. See p. 243
18. See Table 11–2
19. A
20. C
21. B
22. A
23. Review p. 250
24. From reading chapter

Chapter 12

1. False (p. 258 and Tables 12–2 and 12–3)
2. False
3. False
4. False
5. True
6. True
7. False
8. True
9. True
10. True (Table 12–8)
11. True (Box 12–3)
12. False
13. E
14. F
15. G
16. A
17. F
18. C
19. D
20. B
21. B/G
22. G/E
23. A
24. B
25. A
26. C
27. B
28. C
29. A
30. A
31. A
32. A, B, and C
33. A, B, and C
34. A, B, and C
35. B
36. A
37. Review p. 271
38. See text and Table 12–8
39.1. The abuser will recognize inner indications of anger and identify alternative ways to deal with his or her anger.
39.2. The family will develop and describe support systems.
39.3. The incidence of abuse will decrease.
39.4. The presence of healthier defense mechanisms and increased family communication.
40. C
41. C
42. C
43. I
44. I
45. C
46. I

Chapter 13

1. True
2. True
3. False
4. False
5. False (Table 13–2)
6. False
7. False
8. False
9. A
10. LT

11. A
12. LT
13. A
14. LT
15. A
16. D
17. B
18. D
19. D
20. D
21. D
22. A. Verbatim statements (p. 294)
22. B. Detailed observation of emotional status
22. C. Detailed observation of physical status
22. D. Results of physical examination
23. A. Takes a brief medical history (p. 294)
23. B. Careful documentation for legal evidence
23. C. Explains the procedures before the examination
23. D. Stays with the client during the examination

Chapter 14 *p 339*

1. C
2. A
3. A
4. C
5. D
6. D
7. N (pp. 319–320 and Table 14–7, p. 322)
8. Y
9. Y
10. Y
11. Y
12. N
13. N
14. B (Table 14–1, p. 313)
15. A
16. C
17. N
18. N
19. Y
20. Y
21. N
22. Y

Chapter 15 *p. 367*

1. C
2. B
3. Y
4. Y
5. Y
6. Y
7. Y
8. Y
9. Y
10. Y
11. Y
12. Y
13. N
14. A
15. C
16. N
17. N
18. H

19. N
20. N
21. N
22. Y
23. Y
24. C
25. C

Chapter 16

1. True
2. False
3. True
4. False
5. Refer to p. 379
6. Refer to Box 16–1, p. 377 and Box 16–2, p. 378
7. See text
8. D
9. E
10. C
11. D
12. C
13. D
14. B
15. True (Refer to p. 395)
16. True
17. False
18. True
19. False
20. True
21. False (Refer to p. 396)
22. True
23. False
24. True
25. True
26. True (Refer to Box 16–6, p. 399)
27. False
28. True
29. False
30. True
31. False
32. True
33. True
34. False
35. True
36. D
37. Refer to p. 402 under Evaluation
38. Refer to p. 400
39. See Table 16–8, p. 402
40. A, B, D, F

Chapter 17

1. Developing awareness
2. Restitution
3. Shock
4. False (See p. 418)
5. True
6. False (See pp. 418, 420)
7. D
8. C
9. A
10. E
11. B
12. F
13. U
14. S
15. U

16. S
17. C
18. C
19. Refer to Table 17–2, p. 420
20. Refer to Table 17–2, p. 420
21. Refer to Table 17–2, p. 420
22. MD
23. D
24. MD
25. D
26. B
27. C
28. P
29. C or L
30. Refer to Table 17–3, p. 428
31. Refer to p. 428
32. Refer to pp. 428–429
33. Refer to p. 429
34. Refer to p. 429
35. Refer to pp. 429 and 431
36. Refer to pp. 431, 432
37. Refer to pp. 431, 432
38. Refer to pp. 431, 432
39. NP
40. P
41. P
42. NH
43. NH
44. NH
45. H
46. NH
47. NH
48. See Table 17–6
49. See Table 17–6
50. See Table 17–6
51. See Table 17–6
52. C
53. A (Box 17–3)
54. C
55. C
56. B

Chapter 18

1. D
2. C
3. Refer to p. 473
4. Refer to p. 473
5. Refer to p. 473
6. Refer to p. 473
7. Refer to p. 473
8. Refer to p. 473
9. Refer to p. 474
10. Refer to p. 474
11. Refer to p. 474
12. Refer to p. 474
13. See Table 18–4, p. 477
14. See Table 18–4, p. 477
15. See Table 18–4, p. 477
16. See Table 18–4, p. 477
17. See p. 478
18. See p. 478
19. See p. 478
20. Refer to p. 480
21. Refer to p. 480
22. Refer to p. 480
23. H
24. H
25. NH
26. NH
27. NH
28. H

Chapter 19

1. D
2. C
3. E
4. B
5. E
6. C
7. A
8. False
9. True
10. False
11. True
12. Review Delusions, p. 500; Hallucinations, pp. 502–503
13. Loss of Ego Boundaries
14. A. (p. 502)
14. B. (p. 501)
14. C. (p. 502)
15. Refer to pp. 506–507
16. A, B, D
17. A, B, C, D, E
18. A, B, D
19. D
20. H
21. HD
22. H
23. D
24. HD
25. HD
26. D
27. D
28. False
29. True
30. False
31. True
32. True
33. False
34. True
35. True
36. True
37. True
38. True
39. True
40. False
41. True
42. C
43. C
44. C
45. C
46. D
47. B

Chapter 20

1. DEL
2. DEM
3. DEM
4. DEL
5. DEM
6. DEL
7. DEM
8. DEL
9. F
10. G
11. D
12. C
13. B
14. Review pp. 550–551
15. A. See p. 560

15. B. See p. 561
15. C. See p. 561
15. D. See p. 562
16. See pp. 562–563
17. Review Tables 20–5, 20–6, and 20–7
18. Review Tables 20–5, 20–6, and 20–7
19. See Health Teaching, pp. 565–566

Chapter 21

1. True
2. True
3. False
4. False
5. False
6. True
7. True
8. C
9. D
10. D
11. C
12. C
13. T
14. S
15. S
16. P
17. P
18. S
19. Review pp. 593–594
20. Review pp. 593–594
21. Review p. 593

Chapter 22

1. See p. 609
2. See p. 609
3. See p. 610
4. See p. 610
5. See p. 610
6. See p. 610
7. See p. 610
8. B (Refer to Table 22–1, p. 612)
9. D
10. D
11. C
12. A
13. B
14. C
15. D
16. C
17. A
18. D
19. Refer to Box 22–1, p. 613
20. Refer to Box 22–1, p. 613
21. Refer to Box 22–1, p. 613
22. Refer to Box 22–1, p. 613
23. Refer to Box 22–1, p. 613
24. Refer to Box 22–1, p. 613
25. Refer to Box 22–1, p. 613
26. Refer to Box 22–1, p. 613
27. Refer to Box 22–1, p. 613
28. Refer to Box 22–1, p. 613
29. Refer to Table 22–2, p. 613
30. Refer to Table 22–2, p. 613
31. Refer to Table 22–2, p. 613
32. Refer to Table 22–2, p. 613
33. Refer to Table 22–2, p. 613
34. Review pp. 614–615
35. Refer to p. 614

36. Review pp. 614–615
37. Refer to p. 615
38. Refer to p. 615
39. Refer to Table 22–3, p. 616
40. Refer to Table 22–3, p. 616

Chapter 23

1. F
2. J
3. K
4. H
5. A
6. D
7. Review pp. 640–643
8. Review pp. 640–643
9. A
10. Review p. 644
11. Review p. 649
12. Review pp. 649–653
13. Review p. 653
14. E
15. B
16. A
17. F
18. G
19. F
20. E
21. C
22. A
23. D
24. Refer to p. 649

Chapter 24

1. G
2. D
3. C
4. B
5. I
6. A
7. P
8. S
9. P
10. True
11. True
12. Psychotherapeutic
13. A. Attend educational sessions on effects of substance abuse.
13. B. Plan for use of leisure time.
13. C. Learn to cope with painful feelings.
13. D. Make a commitment to ongoing treatment (recovery process).
14. I
15. W
16. O
17. I
18. Discussion
19. A. Document the problem
19. B. Be patient
19. C. Do not enable by covering up
19. D. Confront individual about false statements
19. E. Do not lecture, blame, scold
19. F. Follow through with objective documentation
20. C
21. D
22. B

23. A
24. B
25. C
26. C
27. B
28. B
29. D
30. B
31. D
32. C
33. D
34. B
35. A
36. True
37. True
38. True
39. C
40. A
41. B
42. B
43. D
44. B
45. C
46. True
47. True
48. A. Memory impairment
48. B. Difficulty concentrating
48. C. Lethargy and anhedonia

Chapter 25

1. C
2. E
3. C
4. B
5. C
6. E
7. C
8. E
9. A
10. D
11. B
12. B
13. C
14. B
15. B
16. C
17. C
18. D
19. B
20. D

Chapter 26

1. False
2. True
3. True
4. True
5. + Plus (Review Box 26–1, p. 751)
6. 0 Negative
7. + Plus
8. 0 Negative
9. C
10. B
11. False
12. False
13. True
14. False
15. Refer to Table 26–2, p. 758

16. D
17. E
18. A
19. B
20. C
21. See Table 26-4, p. 765
22. Review Table 26-7, p. 771
23. Review Table 26-7, p. 771

Chapter 27

1. B
2. S
3. S
4. B
5. S
6. B
7. E
8. C
9. A
10. D
11. B
12. B
13. C
14. A
15. A
16. B
17. A. (p. 791)
17. B. (p. 791)
17. C. (p. 792)
17. D. (p. 791)
18. E
19. A
20. F
21. B
22. G
23. C
24. H
25. D
26. J
27. K
28. A. (p. 795)
28. B. (p. 798)
28. C. (p. 797)
28. D. (p. 798)
28. E. (p. 800)

Chapter 28

1. D
2. B
3. C
4. A
5. A
6. D
7. C
8. B
9. A
10. C
11. D
12. E
13. A
14. B
15. Refractory (see p. 818)
16. 75% (see p. 811)

17. 45% (see p. 813)
18. Transsexual (p. 821)
19. Inhibited desire (p. 818)
20. Behavioral and psychodynamic (p. 821)
21. Review pp. 814, 815; 821, 822

Chapter 29

1. True (p. 853)
2. False (p. 832)
3. True (p. 853)
4. False (p. 853)
5. REM (See Table 29-6, p. 840)
6. R (See Table 29-6, p. 840)
7. P (See Table 29-6, p. 840)
8. False (p. 852)
9. True (p. 852)
10. True (p. 852)
11. True (p. 843)
12. True (p. 842)
13. False (p. 844)
14. True (p. 845)
15. True (p. 845)
16. True (p. 849)
17. True (p. 850)
18. False (p. 831)
19. True (p. 832)

Chapter 30

1. Some chronic psychiatric disorders and personality disorders common among the homeless population include schizophrenia, bipolar disorder, depression, borderline personality, dependent, antisocial, and organic mental dysfunctions (see pp. 859–860).
2. To be chronically disaffiliated is a lifestyle problem that means to be cut off and estranged from family, community, peer support, and involvement. This results in a gradual disengagement from supportive relationships and institutions (see pp. 860–861).
3. The process of homelessness involves a lifelong series of crises and missed opportunities that multiply and intensify with time. Every aspect of a person's life becomes affected. Many treatment facilities become involved, making continuity of care, accuracy of diagnosis, and efficacy of treatment very difficult. The homeless person also often is not in a position or able to adhere to treatment or recommended follow-up care (see p. 862).
4. Because the problems of the mentally ill who are homeless are so complex, it is very important to have consistent care by professional that a person can trust. Trust is the basis of the therapeutic relationship without which treatment will be ineffective and unnecessarily prolonged (see p. 864).
5. Behavioral: difficulty reestablishing

meaningful relationships, difficulty maintaining relationships, problems achieving and maintaining demeanor appropriate to the culture and situation, and poor hygiene and grooming.
Cognitive: impaired ability to follow directions, difficulty with independent action, problems with logical thought, ineffective at controlling thought processes.
Physiological: poor nutrition, clinical and subclinical infections, trauma, cardiopulmonary difficulties, digestive disorders, anemia.
6. Chronic mental illness refers to a phenomenon whereby mental illness extends in time beyond the acute stage into a long term stage that is marked by persistent impairment of functioning (see p. 859).
7. A. Nursing Diagnosis: Alteration in Thought Processes
Patient Outcome: TC will demonstrate improved thought processes via increased ability to (1) differentiate between delusional thinking and reality, (2) communicate clearly, (3) participate in self-sustaining behaviors (i.e., unit activities, nutrition, hygiene, job counseling, etc.) by date of discharge.
Key Nursing Interventions:
1. Establish an open rapport.
2. Consistent reality orientation.
3. Maintain TC's personal space.
4. Encourage verbalization of experiences, including "triggers" of anxiety.
5. Facilitate TC's learning improved communication techniques.
6. Teach productive methods of short-circuit escalating anxiety.
7. Support TC's efforts to improve participation in self-sustaining behaviors via role modeling, verbalization of logical decision making, communication with others, etc.
8. Problem-solve with TC and case manager about how to continue post-discharge care.
7. B. Nursing Diagnosis: Hygiene Self-Care Deficit
Patient Outcome: TC will demonstrate consistent and adequate hygiene/grooming by discharge.
Nursing Interventions:
1. Provide TC with personal care articles and clothing, and a storage area for them.
2. Demonstrate use of shower, razor, washing machine and dryer.
3. Facilitate development of habits via schedule times, consistency of expectation, and support as needed.
4. Praise efforts and successes appropriately.
5. Initiate health teaching about hygiene and grooming.
6. Problem-solve with TC and case manager about how to continue post-discharge care.
7. C. Nursing Diagnosis: Alteration in Nutrition: Less Than Body Requirements

Patient Outcome: TC will improve nutritional state, as evidenced by (1) increase in weight, (2) oral intake of essential nutrients and calories to achieve/maintain recommended levels, (3) sharing a plan with the case manager about continued good nutritional post-discharge, by the data of discharge.

Nursing Interventions:

1. Consult dietitian for full evaluation, including preferred foods.

2. Monitor effectiveness of GI functioning. Provide support as indicated.

3. Provide a calm, nonthreatening environment for eating. Stay with TC, as indicated, to support his efforts.

4. Encourage TC's use of high-protein, high-calorie foods and supplements.

5. Provide food in portable, finger-ready forms when agitation makes sitting down for a meal impossible.

6. Encourage frequent, small meals.

7. Obtain prescription for multivitamin with minerals.

8. Maintain careful I&O and calorie counts. Weigh daily, prior to breakfast.

9. Initiate health teaching about proper nutrition.

10. Problem-solve with TC and case manager about how to continue post-discharge care.

7. D. Other Nursing Diagnoses to be considered:

1. Anxiety

2. Impaired Individual Coping

3. Alteration in Health Maintenance

4. High Risk for Injury

5. High Risk for Infection

6. Sleep Pattern Disturbance

7. Social Isolation

Index

Note: Page numbers in *italics* refer to illustrations. Page numbers followed by b refer to boxed material; those followed by t refer to tables.

933